INTERNATIONAL ENCYCLOPEDIA OF
PHARMACOLOGY AND THERAPEUTICS

Executive Editor: A. C. SARTORELLI, *Yale University*

Section 111

VIRAL CHEMOTHERAPY
Volume 1

EDITORIAL BOARD

NOTICE TO READERS
Dear Reader
If your library is not already a standing order customer or subscriber to this series, may we recommend that you place a standing or subscription order to receive immediately upon publication all new issues and volumes published in this valuable series. Should you find that these volumes no longer serve your needs your order can be cancelled at any time without notice.

The Editors and the Publisher will be glad to receive suggestions or outlines of suitable titles, reviews or symposia for consideration for rapid publication in this series.

Robert Maxwell
Publisher at Pergamon Press

INTERNATIONAL ENCYCLOPEDIA OF
PHARMACOLOGY AND THERAPEUTICS

Section 111

VIRAL CHEMOTHERAPY
Volume 1

SECTION EDITOR

D. SHUGAR

Polish Academy of Sciences
Warsaw, Poland

PERGAMON PRESS

OXFORD · NEW YORK · TORONTO · SYDNEY · PARIS · FRANKFURT

U.K.	Pergamon Press Ltd., Headington Hill Hall, Oxford OX3 0BW, England
U.S.A.	Pergamon Press Inc., Maxwell House, Fairview Park, Elmsford, New York 10523, U.S.A.
CANADA	Pergamon Press Canada Ltd., Suite 104, 150 Consumers Road, Willowdale, Ontario M2J 1P9, Canada
AUSTRALIA	Pergamon Press (Aust.) Pty. Ltd., P.O. Box 544, Potts Point, N.S.W. 2011, Australia
FRANCE	Pergamon Press SARL, 24 rue des Ecoles, 75240 Paris, Cedex 05, France
FEDERAL REPUBLIC OF GERMANY	Pergamon Press GmbH, Hammerweg 6, D-6242 Kronberg-Taunus, Federal Republic of Germany

First edition 1984

Library of Congress Cataloging in Publication Data

Main entry under title:
Viral chemotherapy.
(International encyclopedia of pharmacology and therapeutics; section 3)
"Published as Supplement no. 11 1983, to the review journal Pharmacology & therapeutics"—
Verso t.p., v. 1.
1. Antiviral agents. 2. Virus diseases—
Chemotherapy. I. Shugar, D. II. Series. [DNLM:
1. Antiviral agents—Pharmacodynamics. 2. Antiviral agents—Therapeutic use. 3. Viruses. 4. Virus diseases—Drug therapy. WV 4 I58 section 111]
RM411.V57 1983   616.9'25061   82-24530

British Library Cataloguing in Publication Data

Viral chemotherapy.—(International encyclopedia of pharmacology and therapeutics; section 111)
Vol. 1
1. Viral chemotherapy
I. Shugar, D.   II. Series
615.5'8   RM411
ISBN 0-08-029821-4

Published as Supplement No. 11 (1983) to the review journal *Pharmacology & Therapeutics*

Photo typeset by Macmillan India Ltd., Bangalore

Printed in Great Britain by A. Wheaton & Co. Ltd., Exeter

PREFACE

SINCE viruses are obligate intracellular parasites, fully dependent on the host cells, which furnish the necessary apparatus required for the transformation of the genetic information of the viral nucleic acid into progeny viral particles, considerable scepticism existed up to only a few years ago as to the feasibility of developing antiviral agents sufficiently specific to readily traverse the host cell membrane and to inhibit such processes as viral uncoating, replication and assembly without adversely affecting the normal metabolic functions of the cell.

The early, frequently vociferous and even vituperative, opposition to viral chemotherapy came largely from some of the proponents of immunization. The successes achieved by vaccination are indisputable, and include virtual eradication of smallpox, and effective control of such diseases as poliomyelitis. However, both the development and subsequent production of vaccines are by no means free of problems, some of them rather formidable. The recent FDA approval of a vaccine for hepatitis B, prepared by isolation of hepatitis B surface antigen (HBsAg) from viral particles collected from the blood of human carriers, represents a significant new achievement in this field. But it should not be overlooked that it is "the first completely new viral vaccine in 10 years", while its use is to be limited only to those considered at high risk of developing the disease. Furthermore, development of vaccines against, for example, herpes, influenza and rhino viruses poses even more formidable theoretical and practical problems. One of the new approaches, involving the use of chemically synthesized peptides, and exemplified by the recent report of an effective vaccine against foot-and-mouth disease in guinea pigs and rabbits, holds out considerable promise for further advances, particularly when considered with the possible applications of recombination techniques. Meanwhile, it would appear obvious that chemotherapy offers the only alternative, in those instances where a fully effective vaccine is not already available, and, in those instances where it is by itself sufficiently effective, may be preferable to immunization.

During the past 10 years, scepticism regarding the possibilities of viral chemotherapy have been largely dispelled, in large part by practical demonstrations which have already resulted in official approval, in a number of countries, of several compounds for clinical use. As in the case of many other drugs, initial potential candidates for viral chemotherapy were uncovered during the course of *in vitro* random screening programs, with attempts at subsequent improvements based on structure-activity studies, i.e. evaluations of relative activities and cytotoxicities of various synthetically modified analogues of the parent compound with proven activity. The number of promising new agents is presently increasing at an impressive rate, and an appreciable number of these have attained the stage of being subjected to preclinical trials. One of the impressive recent achievements is the FDA approval for use of Acyclovir (or Acycloguanosine) in treatment of primary genital herpes less than 5 years following the initial report on the discovery of this compound and its *in vitro* activity against herpes viruses types 1 and 2.

Concurrently with the foregoing, remarkable progress has been achieved during the 1970s in the elucidation of the molecular biology of viral replication. This has led to the pin-pointing of a variety of 'targets', especially viral-encoded enzymes and proteins, with specificities frequently sufficiently different from the corresponding constituents of the host cells to provide a reasonably solid basis for further, and more fundamental, research in this field. As a result of this, one of the interesting features of a number of new antiviral agents, currently in course of development, has been the success achieved in delineating their

v

mode(s) of action. It is to be anticipated that this will significantly contribute to the design of more effective compounds. An important result of the foregoing is the gradual introduction of so-called more 'rational' approaches in the search for new, and more effective, agents, which is esthetically more satisfying and stimulating to the organic chemists who participate in the necessary synthetic programs and to the virologists, biochemists, enzymologists, pharmacologists, clinicians (and physical chemists and theoretical chemists involved in structure-activity relationships), all of whose collaborative efforts contribute to the eventual introduction of a useful compound into the clinic. Current progress is now such as to envisage the use of combination therapy, based on employment of two or more agents, each of which may affect a different step in viral replication, a field as yet relatively little explored.

With the foregoing in mind, contributors to this volume and to succeeding ones have been asked to concentrate as much as possible on fundamental aspects of their respective fields, so that these will prove useful in further research, and, wherever possible, to present as much detail as possible regarding the mechanism(s) of action of the agents described. I am indebted to most of the contributors for their assistance in attempts to attain this objective. I am also grateful to friends and colleagues who have been kind enough to offer suggestions and advice as to the nature and scope of the contributions required in such a volume and, particularly, to Dr. Ernest C. Herrmann, Jr., and Dr. William H. Prusoff, both well-known pioneers in the development and application of antiviral agents, and to Dr. Alan Sartorelli and Dr. Barbara Z. Renkin, whose assistance in dealing and processing of contributions has been invaluable.

DAVID SHUGAR
Institute of Biochemistry and Biophysics,
Academy of Sciences; and Department of Biophysics,
University of Warsaw, Warsaw

CONTENTS

LIST OF CONTRIBUTORS

BLACK, Francis L.
Yale University School of Medicine
Department of Epidemiology and Public Health
New Haven, Connecticut 06510
USA

BOCKSTAHLER, Larry E.
Bureau of Radiological Health
Food and Drug Administration
Rockville, Maryland 20857
USA

CARRASCO, Luis
Departamento de Microbiología de la UAM
Centro de Biología Molecular
Canto Blanco, Madrid-34
Spain

CHEN, Ming S.
Applebrook Research Center
Smith Kline Animal Health Products
1600 Paoli Pike
Westchester, Pennsylvania 19380
USA

COHEN, Seymour S.
Department of Pharmacological Sciences
State University of New York at Stony Brook
Stony Brook, New York 11794
USA

COOHILL, Thomas P.
Biophysics Program
Western Kentucky University
Bowling Green, Kentucky 42101
USA

DOSKOČIL, Jiří
Institute of Molecular Genetics
Czechoslovak Academy of Sciences
160000 Prague
Czechoslovakia

FENNER, Frank
John Curtin School of Medical Research
The Australian National University
Canberra, Australia

FISCHER, Paul H.
Department of Human Oncology
University of Wisconsin
Madison, Wisconsin 53706
USA

GALBRAITH, Alan
Pharmaceuticals Division
Ciba-Geigy (UK)
Horsham, Sussex
England

HELLMAN, Kiki B.
Bureau of Radiological Health
Food and Drug Administration
Rockville, Maryland 20857
USA

HERRMANN, Ernest C., Jr.
Department of Basic Sciences
Peoria School of Medicine
University of Illinois College of Medicine
Peoria, Illinois 60656
USA

HERRMANN, Judith A.
Department of Basic Sciences
Peoria School of Medicine
University of Illinois College of Medicine
Peoria, Illinois 60656
USA

LIN, Tai-Shun
Department of Pharmacology
Yale University School of Medicine
333 Cedar Street
New Haven, Connecticut 06510
USA

LYTLE, C. David
Bureau of Radiological Health
Food and Drug Administration
Rockville, Maryland 20857
USA

MANCINI, William R.
Department of Pharmacology
Yale University School of Medicine
333 Cedar Street
New Haven, Connecticut 06510
USA

NORTH, Thomas W.
Department of Biochemistry and Pharmacology
Tufts University Schools of Medicine
136 Harrison Avenue
Boston, Massachusetts 02111
USA

OTTO, Michael J.
Department of Pharmacology
Yale University School of Medicine
333 Cedar Street
New Haven, Connecticut 06510
USA

OXFORD, John S.
Division of Virology
National Institute for Biological Standards and
  Control
Holly Hill, London NW3, England

PERRIN, D. D.
Medical Chemistry Group
John Curtin School of Medical Research
Australian National University
Canberra City, ACT 2600, Australia

PRUSOFF, William H.
Department of Pharmacology
Yale University School of Medicine
333 Cedar Street
New Haven, Connecticut 06510
USA

RADA, Brětislav
Institute of Virology
Slovak Academy of Sciences
817 03 Bratislava
Czechoslovakia

ROBERTS, Joan E.
Fordham University
Lincoln Center Campus
New York, New York 10023
USA

SCHINAZI, Raymond F.
  Department of Pediatrics
  Emory University School of Medicine
  Atlanta, Georgia
  USA
SHIAU, George T.
  Department of Chemistry
  National Taiwan Normal University
  Taipei, Taiwan
SHUGAR, David
  University of Warsaw
  Institute of Experimental Physics
  Department of Biophysics
  93 Zwirki & Wigury
  02-089 Warszawa
  Poland
SMITH, Alan E.
  National Institute for Medical Research
  Medical Research Council
  The Ridgeway Mill Hill
  London NW7 1AA
  England

STEBBING, N.
  AMGen, Inc.
  1900 Oak Terrace Lane
  Newbury Park, California 91320
  USA
STÜNZI, H.
  Institut de Chimie
  Université de Neuchâtel
  Avenue de Bellevaux 51
  CH-2000 Neuchâtel, Switzerland
WALKER, Jamieson
  Department of Pharmacology
  University of Edinburgh
  Edinburgh, Scotland
WERNER, Georges H.
  Centre de Recherches de Vitry
  13, quai Jules Guesde
  B.P. 14 F-94400 Vitry-sur-Seine, France
ZERIAL, Aurelio
  Centre de Recherches de Vitry
  13, quai Jules Guesde
  B.P. 14 F-94400 Vitry-sur-Seine, France

CHAPTER 1

THE NATURE AND CLASSIFICATION OF VIRUSES OF MAN

Frank Fenner

John Curtin School of Medical Research, The Australian National University, Canberra, Australia

CONTENTS

1.1. INTRODUCTORY REMARKS

Studies on viral chemotherapy begin with experiments on virus-infected cultured cells, then move to viral infections in intact experimental animals, and finally, in the few cases where the earlier experiments are sufficiently promising, to clinical trials in man. The initial investigations are usually carried out with particular 'model' viruses that lend themselves to experimental manipulation. In order to appreciate the significance of discoveries made with such model systems it is necessary to understand how generally any discovered effect may extend among viruses pathogenic for man. This involves a knowledge of viral classification; if a chemotherapeutic effect is discovered which operates through its effect on a particular viral enzyme, for example, it can be expected to behave similarly in other viruses that possess that enzyme, but not in viruses of other families that do not.

This review begins with a description of the chemical composition and physical structure of the virions of the viruses that affect vertebrate animals. There follows a brief account of each of the twenty families of viruses that encompass almost all the viruses that affect man and other vertebrates.

1.2. INTRODUCTION

Virology began as a branch of pathology. At the end of the nineteenth century, when the microbial etiology of many infectious diseases had been established, pathologists recognized that there were a number of common infectious diseases of man and his domesticated animals for which neither a bacterium nor a protozoan could be incriminated as the causal agent. In 1898 Loeffler and Frosch demonstrated that foot-and-mouth disease could be transferred from one animal to another by material which could pass through a filter that retained the smallest bacteria. Following this discovery such diseases were tentatively ascribed to what were first called 'ultramicroscopic filterable viruses', then 'ultrafilterable viruses', and, ultimately, just 'viruses'. The word 'virus' itself, originally meaning a disease-producing poison, was appropriated to this particular class of agents because of the currency that Jenner had given to the term in describing cowpox and smallpox viruses a hundred years earlier.

1.3. THE NATURE OF VIRUSES

Unicellular microorganisms can be arranged in order of decreasing size and complexity: protozoa, yeasts and certain fungi, bacteria, mycoplasmas, rickettsiae and chlamydiae. Then there is a major discontinuity, for in one sense the viruses cannot be regarded as microorganisms at all. True microorganisms, however small and simple, are cells. They always contain DNA as the repository of their genetic information, and they also have their own machinery for producing energy and macromolecules. Microorganisms grow by synthesizing their own macromolecular constituents (nucleic acid, protein, carbohydrate and lipid), and they multiply by binary fission.

Viruses, on the other hand, contain only one type of nucleic acid, which may be either DNA or RNA, double-stranded or single-stranded. Furthermore, since viruses have no ribosomes or other organelles, they are completely dependent upon their cellular hosts for the machinery of protein synthesis, energy production, and so on. Unlike any of the microorganisms, many viruses can, in suitable cells, reproduce themselves from a single nucleic acid molecule. The key differences between viruses and microorganisms are listed in Table 1.

TABLE 1. *Properties of Microorganisms and Viruses**

	Growth on nonliving media	Binary fission	DNA and RNA	Ribosomes	Sensitivity to antibiotics	Sensitivity to interferon
Bacteria	+	+	+	+	+	−
Mycoplasmas	+	+	+	+	+	−
Rickettsiae	−	+	+	+	+	−
Chlamydiae	−	+	+	+	+	+
Viruses	−	−	−	−	−	+

*From Fenner and White (1976).

Viruses differ from cellular microorganisms in that they exist in two or sometimes three physically and functionally different states. Firstly, they exist as viral particles, or virions, which are the inert form that carries the viral genome from one host cell and/or one host organism to another one. Commonly, but incorrectly, the word 'virus' is often used as a synonym for 'virion'. The second functional state is 'vegetative virus', in which the viral genome undergoes replication, directs the formation of polypeptides and controls the assembly and often the release of progeny virions. In this state the 'virus' is part of the host cell that it infects; the unit is the virus-infected cell. Finally, with a few families of viruses, including lysogenic bacteriophages, papovaviruses and retroviruses, the viral genome, in whole or in part, is at times integrated into the host cell DNA as a 'provirus'. In the case of retroviruses, the provirus is a DNA copy of the RNA genome of the virion.

Virions consist of a genome of either DNA or RNA enclosed within a protective coat of virus-specified protein molecules, some of which may be associated with carbohydrates or lipids specified by the viral or more commonly the host cell genome. In the vegetative state and as 'provirus', viruses are reduced to their constituent genomes. The simplest 'viruses' (viroids) (Diener, 1979) may be transmitted from one host to another and exist only as naked molecules of nucleic acid, possibly associated with certain cellular components. At the other extreme, the virions of the larger animal viruses, e.g. the poxviruses and the retroviruses, have a relatively complex structure.

Viruses parasitize every kind of organism; possibly, indeed, every individual organism, prokaryote and eukaryote, is infected with one or more viruses. For our purposes we need consider only the viruses of vertebrate animals—mainly those of man, but also some viruses that infect domestic or experimental animals and are important in experimental virology, including viral chemotherapy.

1.4. THE CHEMICAL COMPOSITION OF ANIMAL VIRUSES

The virions of the simpler viruses consist solely of nucleic acid and a few virus-specified polypeptides. More complex viruses usually also contain lipids and carbohydrates; in the great majority of viral families these chemical components are not specified by the viral genome but are derived from the cells in which the viruses multiply. In exceptional situations, cellular nucleic acids or polypeptides may be incorporated in viral particles.

1.4.1. NUCLEIC ACIDS

Viruses, unlike microorganisms, contain only a single species of nucleic acid, which may be DNA or RNA. In different families of viruses the nucleic acid is single- or double-stranded, a single molecule or several, and if a single molecule either linear or cyclic. About 20 per cent of the cytosine residues in the ranavirus FV3 are methylated, but neither 5-methyl cytosine nor novel bases of the type encountered in some bacterial viruses have been found in other vertebrate viral nucleic acids. However, the nucleic acids of some viruses contain oligonucleotides rich in adenylate, of unknown function. The base composition of DNA from animal viruses covers a far wider range than that of the vertebrates, for the guanine plus cytosine $(G+C)$ content of different viruses varies from 35 to 74 per cent, compared with 40 to 44 per cent for all chordates. Indeed, the $G+C$ content of the DNA of viruses of one family (Herpesviridae) ranges from 46 to 74 per cent.

The molecular weights of the DNAs of different animal viruses vary from 1.5 to 185 million; the range of molecular weights of viral RNAs is much less, from just over about 2.5 to 15 million. The nucleic acid can be extracted from viral particles with detergents or phenol. The released molecules are often easily degraded but if kept intact the isolated nucleic acid of viruses belonging to certain families is infectious. In other cases, the isolated nucleic acid is not infectious even though it contains all the necessary genetic information, for its transcription depends upon a virion-associated transcriptase without which multiplication cannot proceed.

The genomes of all DNA viruses consist of a single molecule of nucleic acid, but the genomes of many RNA viruses consist of several different molecules, which are probably loosely linked together in the virion. In viruses whose genome consists of single-stranded nucleic acid, the viral nucleic acid is either the 'positive' strand (in RNA viruses, equivalent to messenger RNA) or the 'negative' (complementary) strand. Preparations of some Parvoviridae, which have genomes of single-stranded DNA, consist of particles that contain either the positive or the complementary strand.

Viral preparations often contain some particles with an atypical content of nucleic acid. Host-cell DNA is found in some papovaviruses, and what appear to be cellular ribosomes in some arenaviruses. Several copies of the complete viral genome may be enclosed within a single particle (as in paramyxoviruses) or viral particles may be formed that contain no nucleic acid ('empty' particles) or that have an incomplete genome ('defective interfering' particles), lacking part of the nucleic acid that is needed for infectivity.

Terminal repetition occurs in the DNA of some vertebrate viruses and the genome of retroviruses consists of two or three identical single-stranded RNA molecules linked end to end, but most sequences are unique. The largest viral genomes contain several hundred genes, while the smallest carry only sufficient information to code for about three proteins.

1.4.2. PROTEINS

The major constituent of the virion is protein, whose primary role is to provide the viral nucleic acid with a protective coat. The protein shells of the simpler viruses consist of repeating protein subunits. Sometimes the capsid protein consists of only one sort of polypeptide; more commonly there are two or three different polypeptides in the protein shell. Often certain of these surface polypeptides have a special affinity for complementary 'receptors' present on the surface of susceptible cells. They also contain the antigenic determinants that are responsible for the production of protective antibodies by the infected animal. Viral polypeptides are quite large, with molecular weights in the range

10,000–150,000 daltons. The smaller polypeptides are often, but not always, internal; the larger ones often, but not always, external. There are no distinctive features about the amino acid composition of the structural polypeptides of the virion, except that those intimately associated with viral nucleic acid in the 'core' of some icosahedral viruses are often relatively rich in arginine.

Viral envelopes usually originate from the cellular plasma membrane from which the original cellular proteins have been totally displaced by viral peplomers and a viral "membrane protein" (see Fig. 1). The peplomers consist of repeating units of one or two glycoproteins, the polypeptide moiety of which is virus-specified while the carbohydrate is added by cellular transferases. In many but not all enveloped viruses, the inside of the viral envelope is lined by a viral protein called the membrane or matrix protein.

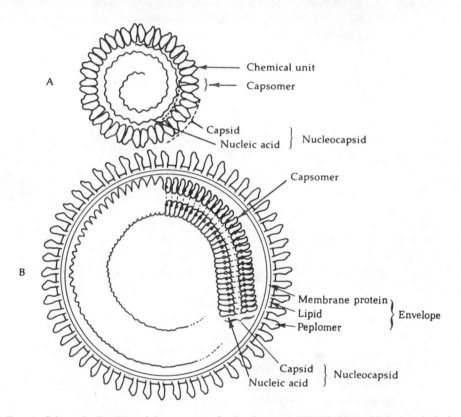

Fig. 1. Schematic diagrams of the structure of a simple non-enveloped virion with an icosahedral capsid (A) and an enveloped virion with a tubular nucleocapsid with helical symmetry (B). The capsids consist of morphological subunits called capsomers, which are in turn composed of structural subunits that consist of one or more chemical subunits (polypeptide chains). Many icosahedral viruses have a 'core' (not illustrated), which consists of protein(s) directly associated with the nucleic acid, inside the icosahedral capsid. In viruses of type B the envelope is a complex structure consisting of an inner virus-specified protein shell (membrane protein, made up of structural subunits), a lipid layer derived from cellular lipids, and one or more types of morphological subunits (peplomers), each of which consists of one or more virus-specified glycoproteins (from Fenner and White, 1976).

Not all structural viral proteins are primary gene products, since in viruses of several families the viral mRNA is translated into a large polypeptide that is enzymatically cleaved to yield two or more smaller virion proteins. Cleavage is often one of the terminal events in the assembly of the virion and it can occur on the virion after most of the proteins are already in place.

Although most virion polypeptides have a structural role, some have enzymatic activity. Many viruses contain a few molecules of an internal protein that functions as a transcriptase, one of the two kinds of peplomers in the envelope of orthomyxoviruses has neuraminidase activity, and several other enzymes are found in the virions of the larger, more complex viruses.

In addition to polypeptides that occur as part of the virion, part of the viral genome codes for polypeptides that have a functional role during viral multiplication but are not incorporated into viral particles. Few of these 'nonstructural viral proteins' have been characterized.

1.4.3. LIPID AND CARBOHYDRATE

Lipids and to a large extent carbohydrates are usually found only in viral envelopes except in the virions of poxviruses and some iridoviruses, where they occur in the outer membrane as well as the envelope. The lipids of viral envelopes are characteristic of the cell of origin, though minor differences may be demonstrable. About 50–60 per cent of the lipid is phospholipid and most of the remainder (20–30 per cent) is cholesterol. Some of the viral carbohydrate occurs in the envelope as glycolipid characteristic of the cell of origin, but most of it is part of the glycoprotein peplomers that project from the viral envelope.

1.5. THE STRUCTURE OF ANIMAL VIRUSES

Three structural classes of viruses of vertebrates can be distinguished: isometric particles, which are usually 'naked' but in some families are enclosed within a lipoprotein envelope; long tubular nucleoprotein structures, always surrounded by a lipoprotein envelope; and in a few groups, a more complex structure.

1.5.1. TERMINOLOGY

Virion (plural, virions) is used as a synonym for 'virus particle'. The protein coat of an isometric particle, or the elongated protein tube of viruses with helical symmetry, is called the *capsid* (Fig. 1). It may be 'naked', or it may be enclosed within a lipoprotein *envelope* (peplos) which is derived from cellular membranes as the virus matures by budding. Where the capsids directly enclose the viral nucleic acid, as is usual with tubular capsids but less common with isometric capsids, the complex is called the *nucleocapsid*. With most isometric particles, and in all complex virions, the capsid encloses another protein structure containing the viral genome, called the *core*.

Capsids consist of repeating units of one or a small number of protein molecules. Three levels of complexity can be distinguished. *Chemical units*, the ultimate gene products, are single polypeptides that may themselves constitute the *structural units*, or several poly-peptides may form homo- or heteropolymers which constitute structural units. The structural units, or groups of them, may be visualized in the electron micrographs as *morphological units*. Morphological units that form part of a capsid are called *capsomers*; those projecting from the envelope are the *peplomers* (sometimes called 'spikes', an unsatisfactory term since they are never pointed and may, indeed, have knob-shaped ends).

The chemical units are sometimes held together by disulfide bonds to form the structural units, hence the practice of using reducing agents in polyacrylamide gel electrophoresis when analyzing viral proteins to determine their constituent polypeptides. The structural units are held together to form the capsid by noncovalent bonds, which may be polar (salt and hydrogen bonds) or nonpolar (van der Waals and hydrophobic bonds). The capsids of some viruses are readily disrupted in molar calcium or sodium chloride, suggesting electrovalent bonds between the structural units; others are unaffected by salt and can only be disrupted by detergents, suggesting that they are hydrophobically bonded.

1.5.2. ISOMETRIC VIRUSES

The capsomers of isometric viruses are arranged with icosahedral symmetry, because the icosahedron is that polyhedron with cubic symmetry which, if constructed of identical subunits, would least distort the subunits or the bonds between them.

An icosahedron (Fig. 2) has twenty equilateral triangular faces, twelve vertices, where the corners of five triangles meet, and thirty edges, where the sides of adjacent pairs of triangles meet. It shows two-fold symmetry about an axis through the center of each edge (Fig. 2A), three-fold symmetry when rotated around an axis through the center of each triangular face (Fig. 2B), and five-fold symmetry about an axis through each vertex (Fig. 2C). Each triangular face may be thought of as containing, and being defined by, three asymmetric units (i.e. units that have no regular symmetry axes themselves) so that a minimum of sixty asymmetric units are required to construct an icosahedron.

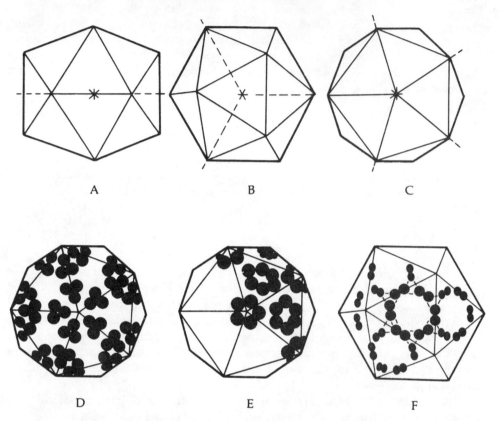

FIG. 2. Features of icosahedral structure. Above: Regular icosahedron viewed along two-fold (A), three-fold (B), and five-fold (C) axes. Various clusterings of structural subunits give characteristic appearances of capsomers in electron micrographs. With $T = 3$ the structural subunits may be arranged as $20T$ trimers (D), capsomers are then difficult to define, as in poliovirus; or they may be grouped as 12 pentamers and 20 hexamers (E) which form bulky capsomers as in *Parvovirus*, or as dimers on the faces and edges of the triangular facets (F), producing an appearance of a bulky capsomer on each face, as in *Calicivirus* (from Fenner and White, 1976).

The pattern seen on the surface of the virion need not reflect the way in which the structural units are bonded together, and gives no clue as to whether the structural units are constituted by single chemical units or are homo- or heteropolymers of the chemical units. However, the number of structural units in each capsomer can be guessed at from the arrangement and size of the capsomers (Fig. 2).

All animal viruses whose genome is DNA have isometric (or complex) capsids, as do those whose genome is double-stranded RNA (Reoviridae) and the viruses of two large families (Picornaviridae and Togaviridae) whose genome consists of a single molecule of single-stranded RNA.

1.5.3. VIRUSES WITH TUBULAR NUCLEOCAPSIDS

Tubular nucleocapsids are found in many families of viruses of vertebrates, but only among those whose genome consists of single-stranded RNA. None of these occurs 'naked';

the flexuous helical tubes are always inside lipoprotein envelopes (Fig. 1B). The diameters of the nucleocapsids of several viruses have been measured, but in only a few cases is the length or the pitch of the helix known.

1.5.4. VIRAL ENVELOPES

The term 'envelope' refers to the outer lipoprotein coat of viruses that mature by budding through cellular membranes. Except for the poxviruses, enveloped viruses contain 20–30 per cent lipid, all of which is found in the envelope. The lipid is derived from the cellular membranes through which the virus matures by budding, but all the polypeptides of viral envelopes are virus-specified. The herpesviruses are the only viruses of vertebrates that mature by budding through the nuclear membrane and their envelopes contain several virus-specified glycoproteins. All other enveloped viruses bud through cytoplasmic membranes, and their envelopes contain one or more different polypeptides. The Togaviridae have an isometric core to which a lipid layer is directly applied, and virus-specified glycoprotein peplomers project from this. All animal viruses with tubular nucleocapsids are enveloped, and in these the lipid layer from which glycoprotein peplomers project is applied to a protein shell (the membrane protein; see Fig. 1), which may be relatively rigid, as in rhabdoviruses, or readily distorted (as in the paramyxoviruses), so that in negatively stained electron micrographs the virions appear to be pleomorphic.

1.5.5. COMPLEX VIRIONS

Viruses that have large genomes have a correspondingly complex structure. Apart from the undetermined nature of the 'cores' of many of the isometric viruses (e.g. Herpesviridae and Adenoviridae), the virions of the two largest animal viruses (Poxviridae and Iridoviridae) have highly complex structures, with lipids in both the envelopes and the outer membranes of the virion. The Retroviridae also have a highly complex structure with an envelope enclosing an icosahedral capsid that, in turn, surrounds a tubular nucleocapsid.

1.6. CLASSIFICATION OF VIRUSES

In 1966 the Ninth International Congress for Microbiology established the International Committee for the Nomenclature of Viruses (ICNV). In 1974 the name, but not the responsibilities, of this committee was changed to the International Committee for the Taxonomy of Viruses (ICTV).

The ICNV and subsequently the ICTV have published reports on the current situation in viral classification and nomenclature after each International Congress for Virology (Wildy, 1971; Fenner, 1976; Matthews, 1979, 1982). Its recommendations have now been widely accepted as the basis for classification and nomenclature at the higher taxonomic levels (family and genus); the Committee has not yet addressed itself effectively to nomenclature at the species level, and it does not consider that it is the appropriate body to suggest classification at the type/subtype level. In the following pages we summarize in tabular form the names and properties of the major groups of viruses that affect vertebrate animals, following in each case the most recent (Fourth) Report of the ICTV (Matthews, 1982).

In the case of a few groups of viruses that appear to us to warrant classification as families, but whose status has not yet been decided by ICTV, we have used one of the proposed group names rather than a family name: the Birnavirus, Filovirus and Hepadnavirus groups.

1.6.1. CRYPTOGRAMS

In the descriptions of families and genera in this article the four terms of the cryptograms of Gibbs et al. (1966), somewhat modified, are shown. The data refer to the infective viral particle (the virion). The first set of terms of the cryptogram describes the type of the nucleic acid (R = RNA, D = DNA)/strandedness (1, 2 = single-, double-stranded) and the infectiousness of the purified nucleic acid (+ = infectious; − = not infectious). The second set describes the molecular weight of the nucleic acid (in millions)/nature of the genome [L = linear; C = circular; F = fragmented, with a number (3, 8, etc.) indicating the number of fragments]. Where the genome is fragmented the symbol 'Σ' indicates this fact and the figure gives the total molecular weight of the genome. The third set describes the outline of the virion and the presence of an envelope/outline of nucleocapsid [S = essentially spherical; E = elongated with parallel sides, ends not rounded; U = elongated with parallel sides, end(s) rounded; X = complex; e, in first term = presence of viral envelope]. The fourth set describes the kinds of host infected (V = vertebrate; I = invertebrate)/mode(s) of transmission (C = congenital; I = ingestion; O = contact; R = inhalation; Ve = invertebrate vector)/the kinds of vector (Di = diptera; Ac = tick or mite; Si = flea). The third term is omitted if no vector is known. An asterisk indicates that a particular property is not known.

The cryptograms constitute a useful shorthand description of the properties of viral families, as can be seen from Table 2.

TABLE 2. *The Cryptograms of Families of Viruses that Infect Vertebrates*

Poxviridae	D/2/− : 85–185/L : Xe/X : V/O, R, Ve/Ac, Di, Si
Iridoviridae	D/2/− : 130–160/L : Se/S : I, V/C, I, O, Ve/Ac
Herpesviridae	D/2/− : 80–150/L : Se/S : V/C, O, R
Adenoviridae	D/2/− : 20–30/L : S/S : V/I, O, R
Papovaviridae	D/2/+ : 3–5/C : S/S : V/O, Ve/Ac, Si
Parvoviridae	D/1/− : 1.5–2.2/L : S/S : V/C, I, O, R
Hepadnavirus group	D/2/− : 1.8/C : S/S : V/C, O
Reoviridae	R/2/− : Σ12–20/F10–11 : S/S : I, V/I, O, Ve/Ac, Di
Birnavirus group	R/2/− : Σ4.8/F2 : S/S : I, V/I, O, R
Retroviridae	R/1/− : 2 or 3 × 3 or 3.5/L : Se/* : V/C, I, O, R
Coronaviridae	R/1/+ : 6/L : Se/E : V/I, R
Paramyxoviridae	R/1/− : 5–7/L : Se/E : V/O, R
Bunyaviridae	R/1/− : Σ5–6/F3 : Se/E : I, V/C, Ve/Ac, Di
Orthomyxoviridae	R/1/− : Σ5/F6-F8 : Se/E : V/R
Arenaviridae	R/1/− : Σ5/F2 : Se/* : V/C, O
Rhabdoviridae	R/1/− : 4/L : Ue/E : V/C, O, Ve/Ap, Di
Togaviridae	R/1/+ : 4/L : Se/S : I, V/C, I, O, Ve/Ac, Di
Picornaviridae	R/1/+ : 2.6/L : S/S : V/I, O, R
Caliciviridae	R/1/+ : 2.8/L : S/S : V/O, I
Filovirus group	R/1/− : 4.2/L : Ee/E : V/O

TABLE 3. *Properties of the Virions of Families of DNA Animal Viruses*

Family	Genome*		Virion		
	Mol. wt. (× 10^6)	Nature†	Shape‡	Size (nm)	Trans-criptase
Papovaviridae	3–5	D, cyclic	Icosahedral (72)	45–55	−
Adenoviridae	20–30	D, linear	Icosahedral (252)	70–90	−
Herpesviridae	80–150	D, linear	Icosahedral (162), enveloped	Envelope 120–150; capsid 100–110	−
Iridoviridae	130–160	D, linear	Icosahedral (∼1500) enveloped	Capsid, 190	+
Poxviridae	85–185	D, linear	Brick-shaped, sometimes enveloped	300 × 240 × 100	+
Parvoviridae	1.5–2.2	S, linear	Icosahedral (32)	18–26	−
Hepadnavirus group	1.8	D(S), circular§	Spherical	42	−

*Genome invariably a single molecule.
† D, double-stranded; S, single-stranded.
‡ Figure in parentheses indicates number of capsomers in icosahedral capsids.
§ Circular molecule is double-stranded for most of its length but contains a single-stranded region of variable length.

1.6.2. CLASSIFICATION BASED ON PHYSICOCHEMICAL CRITERIA

The International Committee on Taxonomy of Viruses has agreed that classification should be based on physicochemical criteria, and not upon such properties as host range or symptomatology. Tables 3 and 10 summarize data on the morphology and chemistry of the viruses of vertebrates, and Fig. 3 illustrates their size and structure.

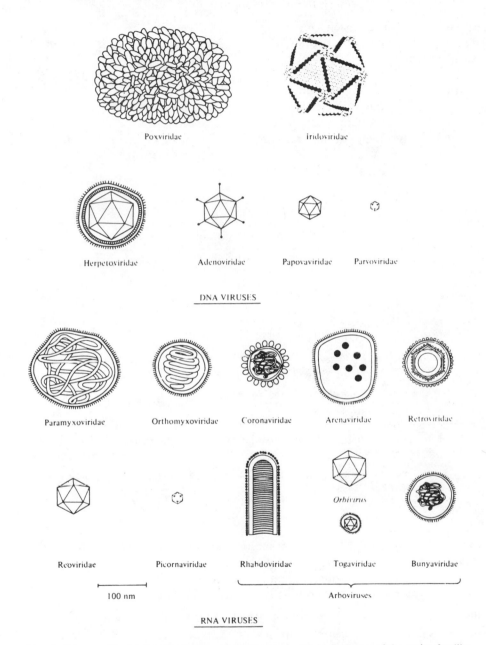

FIG. 3. Diagram illustrating the shapes and relative sizes of animal viruses of the major families (bar = 100 nm) (from Fenner and White, 1976).

1.7. SHORT DESCRIPTIONS OF THE MAJOR GROUPS OF DNA VIRUSES OF VERTEBRATES

Family: *Poxviridae* [D/2/ − : 85–185/L: Xe/X: V/O, R, Ve/Ac, Di, Si]

The poxviruses (pock = pustule) are the largest animal viruses, with a genome consisting of a single molecule of double-stranded DNA with a molecular weight (among poxviruses of vertebrates) of 85–185 million. The structure of the brick-shaped virion is complex, consisting of a biconcave DNA-containing core surrounded by several membranes of viral origin. There is a chordopoxvirus group antigen which is probably an internal component of the virion, and can be demonstrated by several kinds of serological test. Several enzymes, including a transcriptase, are found within mature virions. Multiplication occurs in the cytoplasm and the virions mature in cytoplasmic foci. Occasionally, the virion may be released within an envelope derived from cytoplasmic membranes. This is not essential for infectivity but appears to enhance the capacity for virions to spread between distant cells.

The family is divided into two subfamilies, Chordovirinae and Entomovirinae, which parasitize vertebrates and invertebrates (insects) respectively. The subfamily Chordovirinae contains six named genera (Table 4), and some chordopoxviruses have still to be classified. The virions of viruses belonging to the genera *Orthopoxvirus*, *Avipoxvirus* and *Leporipoxvirus* are morphologically indistinguishable from each other; the structure of members of the other genera is somewhat different. Species within each genus show a high degree of cross-reactivity by neutralization as well as other serological tests. Genetic recombination occurs within, but not between, genera; nongenetic reactivation (complementation) occurs between most poxviruses of vertebrates.

TABLE 4. *Family: Poxviridae; Subfamily: Chordopoxvirinae**, †

Genus	Type species	Other species
Orthopoxvirus	vaccinia	camelpox, cowpox, ectromelia, monkeypox, variola
Avipoxvirus	fowlpox	canarypox, pigeonpox, turkeypox
Capripoxvirus	sheep pox	goatpox, lumpy skin disease
Leporipoxvirus	myxoma	rabbit, squirrel and hare fibroma
Parapoxvirus	milker's node	orf, bovine papular stomatitis
Suipoxvirus	swinepox	

Unclassified poxviruses of vertebrates:
                  molluscum contagiosum

                  Yaba monkey tumor poxvirus ⎫
                                     ⎬ serologically related
                  Tanapoxvirus ⎭

* Characteristics: single linear molecule of cross-linked double-stranded DNA, molecular weight 85–185 million; most species have large brick-shaped virions 300 × 240 × 100 nm with a complex structure and an envelope in virions that are spontaneously released from cells. Capripoxviruses, parapoxviruses and suipoxviruses differ morphologically from others. Virions contain several enzymes including a transcriptase.
† Type genus: *Orthopoxvirus*.
Type species: Vaccinia virus [D/2/−: 120/L: Xe/X: V/C, O].

Poxviruses cause diseases in man, domestic and wild mammals, and birds. These are sometimes associated with single or multiple benign tumors of the skin, but are more usually generalized infections, often with a widespread vesiculo-pustular rash. Several poxviruses are transmitted in nature by anthropods acting as mechanical vectors.

Family: *Iridoviridae* [D/2/ −: 130–160/L: S or Se/S: I, V/C, I, O, Ve/Ac]

This genus (irido = iridescent) was defined on the basis of several viruses of insects whose structure and nucleic acid content had been carefully studied. However, our description is based on two groups of viruses of similar morphology that have been recovered from vertebrate animals. The family consists of five genera, two of which are viruses of insects and three are distinguishable genera of viruses of vertebrates (Table 5).

Like poxviruses, but unlike other DNA viruses, iridoviruses multiply in the cytoplasm. Their DNA consists of a single linear molecule, with a molecular weight of about 130–140 million, and the virion is a large and complex icosahedron, with an outer shell composed of about 1500 capsomers. Several enzymes are found within mature virions. Members of the three genera found in vertebrates may occur in an enveloped extracellular form.

TABLE 5. *Family: Iridoviridae**

Genera	Characteristics
Iridovirus	130 nm diameter virions ⎫ viruses of insects
Chloriridovirus	180 nm diameter virions ⎭
Ranavirus	FV3 and related viruses of amphibians; about 20 per cent of cytosine residues in FV3 are methylated
Unnamed	African swine fever virus; has virion-associated transcriptase and cross-linked DNA
Unnamed	Lymphocystis disease virus of fish; no virion-associated transcriptase

* Characteristics of vertebrate iridoviruses: single linear molecule of double-stranded DNA, molecular weight 130–140 million; complex structure with outer icosahedral capsid 130–215 nm in diameter, enveloped.

Family: *Herpesviridae* [D/2/ − : 80–150/L: Se/S: V/C, O, R]

The herpesviruses (herpes = creeping) are readily recognized by their morphology. Their icosahedral capsid is assembled in the nucleus and acquires an envelope as the virus matures by budding through the nuclear membrane. The family has been subdivided into three subfamilies: Alphaherpesvirinae, Betaherpesvirinae and Gammaherpesvirinae (Table 6).

Different herpesviruses cause a wide variety of types of infectious diseases, some localized and some generalized, often with a vesicular rash. Gammaherpesviruses proliferate in lymphocytes and may cause lymphoproliferative disease. A feature of many herpesvirus infections is prolonged latency associated with one or more episodes of recurrent clinical disease.

TABLE 6. *Family: Herpesviridae**

Subfamily:	Alphaherpesvirinae†	Betaherpesvirinae†	Gammaherpesvirinae†
Mol. wt. of DNA:	$85–110 \times 10^6$	$130–150 \times 10^6$	$85–110 \times 10^6$
Type species:	human (alpha) herpesvirus 1 (herpes simplex type 1)	human (beta) herpesvirus 5 (cytomegalovirus)	human (gamma) herpesvirus 4 (Epstein-Barr)
Other members and possible members	human (alpha) herpesvirus 2 (herpes simplex type 2)	murid (beta) herpesvirus 1 & 2	herpesvirus saimiri
		caviid (beta) herpesvirus 1	herpesvirus ateles
	human (alpha) herpesvirus 3 (varicella-zoster)	suid (beta) herpesvirus 2	gallid herpesvirus 1 (Marek's disease)
	bovid (alpha) herpesvirus 2 (bovine mammalitis)		gallid herpesvirus 2
	suid (alpha) herpesvirus 1 (pseudorabies)		leporid herpesvirus 1
	equid (alpha) herpesvirus 1 (equine abortion)		
	equid (alpha) herpesvirus 3 (coital exanthem)		
	cercopithecid (alpha) herpesvirus (B virus)		
	felid (alpha) herpesvirus 1		
	canid (alpha) herpesvirus 1		

* Characteristics: single linear molecule of double-stranded DNA, molecular weight 80–150 million; icosahedral capsid 100–110 nm in diameter, with 162 capsomers, enclosed by envelope 150 nm diameter; multiply in nucleus; mature by budding at nuclear membrane; specific antigen(s) associated with envelope.

† Members of subfamily Alphaherpesvirinae characteristically replicate rapidly, and latent infection of nerve ganglia often occurs; members of subfamily Betaherpesvirinae replicate slowly and cause cell enlargement, latent infection of salivary glands often occurs; members of subfamily Gammaherpesvirinae are specific for either B- or T-lymphocytes; latent infection of lymphoid tissue often occurs.

Family: *Adenoviridae* [D/2/ − : 20–30/L: S/S: V/I, O, R]

The adenoviruses (adeno = gland) are nonenveloped icosahedral DNA viruses which multiply in the nuclei of infected cells, where they may produce a crystalline array of particles. There are two genera; *Mastadenovirus* (mastos = breast) and *Aviadenovirus* (avis = bird), in each of which there are many species which share a common antigen(s) as well as possessing distinctive species-specific antigens. Many serotypes (species) are found in several different species of mammalian and avian host. The thirty-five species of human adenovirus have been grouped into five subgenera on the basis of a number of characters (Table 7). Allocation to the family is made primarily on the basis of the characteristic size and symmetry of the virion as seen in electron micrographs (icosahedron with 252 capsomers).

TABLE 7. *Family: Adenoviridae* *

Genus:	*Mastadenovirus*	*Aviadenovirus*
Size of virions:	70–90 nm	70–90 nm
Mol. wt. of DNA:	$20–25 \times 10^6$	30×10^6
Type species:	Human adenovirus 2	Fowl adenovirus (CELO)
Other members:	Human subgenus A (12, 18, 31)	Several species, in
	” ” B (3, 7, 11, 14, 16, 21, 34, 35)	several species of
	” ” C (1, 2, 5, 6)	birds‡
	” ” D (8, 9, 10, 13, 15, 17, 19, 20, 22,	
	23, 24, 25, 26, 27, 28, 29, 30,	
	” ” 32, 33)	
	” ” E (4)	
	Many species, in several species of mammal†	

* Characteristics: single linear molecule of double-stranded DNA, molecular weight 20 to 30 million; icosahedral capsid 80 nm in diameter, with 252 capsomers and fibers projecting from the twelve vertices; no envelope, multiply in nucleus.

† Mastadenoviruses have been recovered from many other species: cow, pig, sheep, goat, horse, mouse, opossum and dog (including canine hepatitis virus).

‡ Aviadenoviruses have been recovered from fowl, turkey, goose, pheasant and duck.

Most adenoviruses are associated with respiratory infection and many such infections are characterized by prolonged latency. Some multiply in the intestinal tract and are recovered in feces. Many adenoviruses, from both mammalian and avian sources, produce malignant tumors when inoculated into new-born hamsters, and in such situations the viral DNA is integrated into cellular chromosomes.

In the laboratory, stable hybrids have been produced between certain adenoviruses and the *Polyomavirus*, SV40.

Family: *Papovaviridae* [D/2/+: 3–5/C: S/S: V/O, Ve/Ac, Si]

The family Papovaviridae (sigla: Pa = papilloma; po = polyoma; va = vacuolating agent, SV40) encompasses two genera. *Polyomavirus* (poly = many; oma = tumor) and *Papillomavirus* (papilla = nipple; oma = tumor), which differ substantially in size and nucleic acid content of the virion (Table 8) but share many other properties.

An important property of many papovaviruses is their capacity to produce tumors. In nature, the papillomaviruses produce single benign tumors (which may undergo malignant change) and are highly host specific; many polyomaviruses cause primary malignant tumors

TABLE 8. *Family: Papovaviridae* *

Genus:	*Papillomavirus*	*Polyomavirus*
Size of virion:	55 nm	45 nm
Mol. wt. of DNA:	5×10^6	3×10^6
Type species:	Rabbit papilloma virus	Polyoma virus (mouse)
Other members:	Human (9 types)	BK & JC (human)
	Cow (5 types)	K (mouse)
	Deer	RKV (rabbit)
	Dog	HaPV (hamster)
	Goat	SV40 (rhesus monkey)
	Horse	STMV (stump-tailed macaque)
	Rat	Lymphotropic, LPV (baboon, ?human)
	Sheep	SA12 (baboon)

* Characteristics: single circular molecule of double-stranded DNA, molecular weight 5 or 3 million, isolated DNA is infectious; icosahedral capsid 55 or 45 nm diameter, with 72 capsomers; no envelope; multiply in nucleus. Two genera: *Papillomavirus* and *Polyomavirus*, in each of which there is an antigen common to the genus and species-specific surface antigens.

within a short period of their inoculation into newborn rodents. Tumor production is associated with integration of the viral genome into cellular chromosomes.

Family: *Parvoviridae* [D/1/ −: 1.5–2.2/L: S/S: V/C, I, O, R]

Parvoviruses (parvo = small) are unique among the DNA viruses of vertebrates in that their genome is a single molecule of single-stranded DNA. Three genera are recognized: *Parvovirus*, comprising several viruses of rodents which are 'normal' infectious viruses, *Dependovirus* (dependere = depending) viruses, which are able to replicate only in cells concurrently infected with an adenovirus or herpesvirus (adeno-associated viruses) and *Densovirus* (densus = thick, compact), which are parvoviruses of insects (Table 9). In the dependoviruses the single strands of DNA found in a population of virions are complementary and anneal after extraction to form a double strand.

TABLE 9. *Family: Parvoviridae**

Genus	Species
Parvovirus†·‡	rat virus
	H-1 virus
	minute virus of mice
	bovine parvovirus
	feline parvovirus (subspecies in cats, mink and dogs)
	goose parvovirus
	Aleutian mink disease virus
	lapine parvovirus
	TVX virus
	Lu III virus
	RT virus
	porcine parvovirus
Dependovirus§	Four human serotypes of adeno-associated viruses (AAV); bovine, canine, avian, equine and ovine AAVs
Densovirus	Parvoviruses of several species (and genera) of insects

* Characteristics: single linear molecule of single-stranded DNA, molecular weight 1.2 to 1.8 million; icosahedral capsid about 20 nm in diameter; no envelope; multiply in nucleus.

† Type species *Parvovirus* r-1 (rat virus) [D/1/ −: 1.5–2/L: S/S: V/C, O].

‡ HB virus and the Norwalk agents and related viruses that cause gastroenteritis in man may belong to this genus or to the family Caliciviridae.

§ Viruses of genus *Dependovirus* are defective; their multiplication depends upon concurrent infection of cells with an adenovirus or herpesvirus.

The parvoviruses of rodents cause acute fulminating disease when inoculated into newborn hamsters. The feline subspecies of the feline parvovirus causes feline panleukopenia; the canine subspecies has recently caused epidemics in dogs. The dependoviruses are not known to produce any symptoms.

Hepadnavirus Group [D/2/ −: 1.8/C: S/S: V/C, O]

Although its nomenclature has yet to be decided by ICTV, the virus that causes hepatitis B in man is now well characterized (Tiollais *et al.*, 1981). Since there are also related viruses in other animals it is appropriate to consider them as a group (Robinson, 1980), for which the name 'Hepadnavirus' has been tentatively suggested (sigla: hepa = liver; dna = DNA) (Table 10). The virion of human hepatitis B is a spherical particle 42 nm in diameter (the 'Dane particle') consisting of a 27-nm icosahedral nucleocapsid within a closely adherent envelope that contains typical cellular membrane lipids and proteins, some of which are glycosolated, plus a virus-specific surface antigen (HBs Ag). The nucleocapsid, which consists of a single polypeptide (HBc Ag), contains a circular DNA molecule 3200 nucleotides long (molecular weight 1.8 million), which consists of a long strand of fixed length and a short strand of variable length. It is the smallest genome known to occur in a vertebrate virus, and the viral DNA can be integrated into cellular DNA. The nucleocapsid also contains endogenous DNA polymerase activity.

TABLE 10. *Tentative Family: Hepadnavirus Group**·†

Members	Primary host
Hepatitis B virus	Man
Woodchuck hepatitis virus	*Marmota monax*
Ground squirrel hepatitis virus	*Spermophilus beecheyi*
Duck hepatitis virus	domestic ducks

* Characteristics: single circular double-stranded DNA molecule with length corresponding to 3200 base pairs, containing a single-stranded region of different lengths in different molecules and a nick in the long (3200 bp) strand; 27 nm nucleocapsid within 42 nm spherical particle, no envelope; characteristic surface (s), core (c) and e antigens in virion, multiply in nucleus.

† Type species: Human hepatitis B virus [D/2/ −: 1.8/C: S/S: V/C, O].

The hepadnaviruses are often associated with hepatitis, and sometimes hepatomas. They cause persistent infections with viral surface antigen and often complete virions circulating continuously in the bloodstream.

1.8. SHORT DESCRIPTIONS OF THE MAJOR GROUPS OF RNA VIRUSES OF VERTEBRATES

Family: *Reoviridae* [R/2/ −: Σ12–20/F10–F11: S/S: I, V/I, O, Ve/Ac, Au, Di]

The family Reoviridae (sigla: respiratory enteric orphan) contains three genera that infect vertebrates, *Reovirus*, *Orbivirus* (orbis = ring) and *Rotavirus* (rota = wheel), which show minor differences in morphology and the size of their genome. All are nonenveloped isometric viruses whose genome consists of ten or eleven pieces of double-stranded RNA (Table 12).

Genus: *Reovirus*. The genome is in ten pieces; the total molecular weight is 14–15 million. There are three mammalian serotypes, which contain a common antigen, which differs from the group antigen of the avian reoviruses. No association with disease has been recognized in naturally acquired infections.

Genus: *Orbivirus*. The genome is in ten pieces. This genus includes a large number of arboviruses that have several different kinds of vectors. Several species are associated with important diseases of man (Colorado tick fever) or domestic animals (bluetongue, African horse sickness).

Genus: *Rotavirus*. The genome is in eleven pieces. This genus includes viruses that cause diarrhoea in man, calves and mice (EDIM agent): other serotypes have been isolated from a wide range of mammals.

Tentative Family: *Birnavirus Group* [R/2/ −: Σ4.8/F2: S/S: I, V/I, O, R]

This family is characterized by an icosahedral virion with a single protein coat that contains two pieces of double-stranded RNA with a total molecular weight of 4.8 million (sigla: bi = two, rna).

Only a small number of viruses of these characteristics have been recovered so far, but isolations have been made from birds, fishes, molluscs and insects and three genera have been suggested on the basis of the hosts of origin (Table 1.20: avi = bird; pisci = fish; entomo = insect).

Family: *Retroviridae* [R/1/ −: 2 or 3 × 3 or 3.5/L: Se/*: V/C, I, O, R]

This large family is characterized by many viruses with virions of similar morphology, being spherical enveloped particles 80–100 nm in diameter, all with a virion-associated reverse transcriptase (retro = backwards; also a sigla relating to reverse transcriptase). It is subdivided into three subfamilies: Oncovirinae (onkos = tumor), Spumavirinae (spuma = foam) and Lentivirinae (lenti = slow). The genome varies somewhat in structure in the different subfamilies, but comprises two or three copies of a positive strand of single-stranded RNA, often associated with cell-derived genetic information for non-structural

TABLE 11. *Properties of the Virions of Families of RNA Animal Viruses*

Family	Genome		Virion				
	Mol. wt. ($\times 10^6$)	Nature*	Envelope	Shape†	Size (nm)	Trans-criptase	Symmetry of Nucleocapsid‡
Reoviridae	12–20	D,10–11	–	Icosahedral	60–80	+	Icosahedral (45–60)
Birnavirus Group	4.8	D,2	–	Icosahedral	60	+	Icosahedral (45)
Retroviridae	2×3§	S,1	+	Spherical	80–100	+ (Reverse)	Helical (?)
Coronaviridae	6	S,1	+	Spherical	75–160	–	Helical (11–13)
Paramyxoviridae	5–7	S,1	+	Spherical	100–300	+	Helical (12–17)
Bunyaviridae	5.5	S,3	+	Spherical	90–100	+	Helical (2–2.5)
Orthomyxoviridae	5	S,8	+	Spherical	80–120	+	Helical (9–15)
Arenaviridae	5	S,2	+	Spherical	110–130	+	Helical (?)
Rhabdoviridae	4	S,1	+	Bullet-shaped	170 × 70	+	Helical (5)
Togaviridae	4	S,1	+	Spherical	40–70	–	Icosahedral (25–35)
Picornaviridae	2.6	S,1	–	Icosahedral	20–30	–	Icosahedral (20–30)
Caliciviridae	2.8	S,1	–	Icosahedral	35–39	–	Icosahedral (20–30)
Filovirus Group	4.2	S,1	+	Tubular	790–970 × 80	?	Helical

* All molecules linear; S, single-stranded; D, double-stranded; number, number of molecules in genome.
† Some enveloped viruses are very pleomorphic (sometimes filamentous).
‡ Figure in brackets indicates diameter (nm) of nucleocapsids.
§ Inverted dimer.

TABLE 12. *Family: Reoviridae**

Genus	
Reovirus	Nucleic acid in 10 pieces
	Multiply only in vertebrates
	Three serotypes recovered from mammals, including man
	Several avian serotypes
Orbivirus	Nucleic acid in 10 pieces
	Multiply in both vertebrates, diptera and ticks
	There are 12 serological subgroups. The numbers in each subgroup and the vectors are indicated:
	Abadina (4) mosquitoes
	African horse sickness (9) vector unknown
	Bluetongue (20) culicoides
	Chanquinola (9) phlebotamines
	Colorado tick fever (2) ticks
	Corriparta (2) mosquitoes
	Epizootic disease of deer (4) vector unknown
	Eubenangee (3) mosquitoes
	Keremova (18) ticks
	Palyam (5) mosquitoes
	Wallal (2) vector unknown
	Warrego (2) culicoides
	And ten ungrouped viruses
Rotavirus	Nucleic acid in 11 pieces
	Multiply only in vertebrates
	Different serotypes from a wide range of mammals
Phytoreovirus	Twelve pieces of RNA in genome. Multiply in plants and insects
Fijivirus	Ten pieces of RNA in genome. Multiply in plants and insects
Cytoplasmic polyhedrosis virus group	Ten pieces of RNA in genome
	Found in many different species of insect
	Virions are occluded within a cytoplasmic inclusion body

* Characteristics: double-stranded RNA, 12–20 million, occurring as ten to twelve separate pieces; icosahedral outer capsid diameter 60–80 nm; icosahedral inner capsid 45 nm diameter; no envelope; virion contains a transcriptase; multiply in cytoplasm.

TABLE 13. *Tentative Family: Birnavirus Group**

Genus†	
Avibirnavirus	Infectious bursal disease virus of chickens and several other avian serotypes
Piscibirnavirus	Infectious pancreatic necrosis virus of trout and similar species from several other kinds of fish. Molluscs also infected.
Entomobirnavirus	Produces diseases in *Drosophila*

* Characteristics: Spherical virion 60 nm in diameter with a 45 nm core which contains a transcriptase and genome consisting of two pieces of double-stranded RNA with molecular weights of 2.5 × 2.3 million; multiply in cytoplasm.
† Tentative classification only, based solely on the kinds of host animal.

proteins. Multiplication begins with the synthesis of copy DNA, some of which, in the Oncovirinae, is integrated into the chromosomal DNA.

Subfamily: *Oncovirinae* [R/1/ −: 2 × 3/L: Se/E: V/C, O]

Because of their potential importance for the understanding of cancer, model viruses of this subfamily (Rous sarcoma virus and the mouse leukemia viruses) have been very intensively studied. Their genome consists of an inverted dimer of linear positive sense RNA, the monomers (molecular weight 3 million) being held together at the 5′ end by hydrogen bonds.

Replication occurs via a double-stranded DNA transcript of the genome which is integrated into chromosomal DNA before being transcribed by cellular RNA polymerase into virion RNA and messenger RNA. Virus matures by budding from the plasma membrane.

TABLE 14. *Family: Retroviridae** †

Subfamilies	Genera	Subgenera	Species
Oncovirinae	Type C oncovirus group	Mammalian	Distinct species in several species of mammal, including leukemia and sarcoma viruses
		Avian	Avian leukemia and sarcoma viruses
		Reptilian	Viper virus
	Type B oncovirus group	—	Mouse mammary tumor virus
	Type D retrovirus	—	Mason-Pfizer monkey
Spumavirinae	—	—	Bovine syncytial virus
			Feline syncytial virus
			Human foamy virus
			Simian foamy viruses
Lentivirinae	—	—	Visna virus ⎱
			Progressive pneumonia ⎬ sheep
			virus ⎰

* Type species: Rous sarcoma virus [R/1/−: 2 × 3/L: Se/*: V/C, O].

† Characteristics: Virion contains a virus-specified RNA-dependent DNA polymerase and other enzymes. Genome is a linear molecule of single-stranded RNA, 3–3.5 million molecular weight, consisting of two or three copies linked by hydrogen bonding, associated with tubular nucleocapsid. Structure of virion is complex, the nucleocapsid being enclosed within a capsid of cubic symmetry, which is enclosed in an envelope that carries type-specific antigens. Virion of members of subfamily Oncovirinae also contains species-specific (e.g. feline or murine) and interspecies-specific (e.g. avian or rodent) antigens.

Endogenous oncoviruses which are inherited as Mendelian genes are found in many species of vertebrates. Exogenous infection can also occur and may be associated with a variety of pathological changes including several kinds of malignancy. Transmission of endogenous oncoviruses is vertical; exogenous oncoviruses can be transmitted vertically (congenitally) or horizontally, after birth.

Subfamily: *Spumavirinae* [R/1/−: 3 × 3.5/L: Se/E: V/O]

Features that differentiate spumaviruses from oncoviruses, in addition to their inability to transform cells or produce tumors, include electron-lucent nucleoids, long peplomers projecting from the envelope, maturation by budding into intracellular vacuoles and lack of a group-specific antigen. Replication via a DNA copy of the genome occurs only in dividing cells and spumaviruses cause persistent infection without pathological effects. Infection can often be unmasked by culture *in vitro* of cells from apparently normal organs, producing foamy vacuolated cells.

Subfamily: *Lentivirinae* [R/1/−: 3 × 3.5/L: Se/E: V/O]

The three known viruses of this subfamily have a genome consisting of three linked monomers of RNA of molecular weight 3.5 million. Multiplication occurs via a double-stranded DNA intermediate. Endogenous lentiviruses are not found; infections are horizontally transmitted in sheep and give rise to slowly progressive inflammatory changes in the lungs or central nervous system.

Family: *Coronaviridae* [R/1/+: 6/L: Se/E: V/1, R]

The family Coronaviridae (corona = crown) comprises a single genus, *Coronavirus*, which consists of several enveloped RNA viruses with a tubular nucleocapsid 9 nm in diameter. The genome consists of single-stranded RNA of molecular weight 6 million, which is infectious. The envelope carries characteristic pedunculated projections. Human strains cause common colds; in other animals coronaviruses infect the respiratory or alimentary tract, or may cause systemic disease.

Family: *Paramyxoviridae* [R/1/−: 5–8/L: Se/E: V/O, R]

The paramyxoviruses (para = alongside; myxo = mucus) are enveloped viruses whose RNA occurs as a single linear molecule with a molecular weight of about 7 million (Table 16). The tubular nucleocapsid has a diameter of 18 nm and is about 1.0 m long. It is enclosed

TABLE 15. *Family: Coronaviridae; Genus: Coronavirus**, †

Avian infectious bronchitis virus (IBV)
Human respiratory coronaviruses (HCV)
Mouse hepatitis viruses (MHV)
Transmissible gastroenteritis of swine virus (TGE)
Hemagglutinating encephalomyelitis virus of pigs (HEV)
Coronaviruses of dog, turkey, calf, rat and cat

* Characteristics: genome consists of a single molecule of single-stranded RNA, which is infectious, molecular weight 6 million; tubular nucleocapsid 9 nm or 11–13 nm in diameter; pleomorphic lipoprotein envelope 75–160 nm in diameter with large pedunculated peplomers; multiply in cytoplasm and mature by budding into cytoplasmic vacuoles.
† Types species: Avian infectious bronchitis virus [R/1/+: 6/L: Se/E: V/I, R].

TABLE 16. *Family: Paramyxoviridae**

Genus	
Paramyxovirus†	Envelopes contain a homagglutinin and a neuraminidase. Includes mumps virus (human), four species of parainfluenza virus of mammals, and several parainfluenza viruses of birds, including Newcastle disease virus.
Morbillivirus	Envelope contains a hemagglutinin but not a neuraminidase. Includes four serologically related viruses: measles (human), rinderpest (cattle), distemper (dogs) and peste-despetits-ruminants (sheep) viruses.
Pneumovirus	Envelope contains neither a hemagglutinin nor a neuraminidase. Includes respiratory syncytial viruses of man and bovine, and pneumonia virus of mice.

* Type genus: *Paramyxovirus*.
Type species: Newcastle disease virus [R/1/−: 7/L: Se/E: V/O, R].
† Characteristics: single linear molecule of single-stranded RNA, molecular weight 7 million, within tubular nucleocapsid 18 nm in diameter; pleomorphic lipoprotein envelope 100–300 nm in diameter which in genus *Paramyxovirus* carries specific hemagglutinin and neuraminidase peplomers; virion contains a transcriptase; multiply in cytoplasm; mature by budding from cytoplasmic or intracytoplasmic membranes.

within a pleomorphic lipoprotein envelope 150 nm or more in diameter; long filamentous forms with the same diameter also occur.

There are three genera: *Paramyxovirus*, whose envelopes contain virus-specific hemagglutinin and neuraminidase antigens; *Morbillivirus*, comprising the related viruses that cause measles, distemper and rinderpest, and *Pneumovirus*, which includes human respiratory syncytial virus and pneumonia virus of mice. Virions of genus *Morbillivirus* contain a hemagglutinin but not a neuraminidase; those of *Pneumovirus* have neither.

Paramyxoviruses of the genera *Paramyxovirus* and *Pneumovirus* cause localized infections of the respiratory tract and morbilliviruses produce severe generalized diseases, some of which are associated with skin rashes.

Family: *Bunyaviridae* [R/1/−: Σ5.5/F3: Se/E: I, V/C, Ve/Ac, Di]

This family, named from Bunyamwera, a place in Africa in which the type species was isolated, was originally established to bring together a number of minor arbovirus groups linked by distant serological relationships. It is a very large family, comprising four named genera, *Bunyavirus* (from place name Bunyamwera), *Nairovirus* (from place name Nairobi), *Phlebovirus* (referring to phlebotomine vectors), *Uukuvirus* (from place name Uukuniemi) and some ungrouped viruses (Table 17). All are morphologically like the type species, Bunyamwera virus, and those that have been examined have a similar genome, consisting of three pieces of single-stranded RNA of molecular weights 3, 2 and 0.5 million. The ends of these RNA molecules are hydrogen-bonded, to make a circular molecule.

Most members of the *Bunyavirus* genus are mosquito-transmitted, some may be transmitted by several other kinds of arthropods. Some are transmitted transovarially by mosquitoes. Members of genus *Nairovirus* are transmitted by ticks, and *Phlebovirus* by

TABLE 17. *Family: Bunyaviridae**, †

Genus	Antigenic subgroups, number of species in brackets	
Bunyavirus	Anopheles A (11)	Koongol (2)
	Anopheles B (2)	Minatitlan (2)
	Bunyamwera (23)	Olifantsvlei (3)
	Bwamba (2)	Patois (6)
	C Group (14)	Simbu (25)
	California (14)	Tete (5)
	Capim (9)	Turlock (6)
	Guama (12)	Ungrouped (2)
Phlebovirus	At least 30 serologically related species, which are unrelated serologically to members of other genera. Members include sandfly fever and Rift Valley fever viruses.	
Nairovirus	Six serogroups (at least 27 viruses) which are serologically unrelated to members of other genera	
	Crimean-Congo hemorrhagic fever (2)	
	Dera Ghazi Khan (6)	
	Hughes (8)	
	Nairobi sheep disease (3)	
	Qalyub (2)	
	Sakhalin (6)	
Uukuvirus	A single serogroup of at least 7 viruses, serologically unrelated to members of other genera.	
Ungrouped	Four serogroups	
	Bakan (2)	
	Kaisodi (3)	
	Mapputa (4)	
	Thogoto (2)	
	Eleven unassigned viruses.	

* Characteristics: genome consists of single-stranded RNA, three pieces, with molecular weights 3, 2 and 0.5 million; tubular nucleocapsid 12–15 nm in diameter, within lipoprotein envelope 90–100 nm in diameter. All multiply in and are transmitted by arthropods; some are transmitted transovarially.

† Type genus: *Bunyavirus*.

Type species: Bunyamamwera virus [R/1/−: Σ 5–6/F3: Se/E: I, V/C, Ve/Ac, Di].

Phlebotomus, and rarely by mosquitoes and *Culicoides*. They also infect a variety of warm- and cold-blooded vertebrates. Some cause disease in man (*Phlebovirus* genus).

Family: *Orthomyxoviridae* [R/1/−: Σ5/F6-F8: Se/E: V/R]

In early classifications, some members of two very different families, now distinguished from each other as Orthomyxoviridae (ortho = correct, myxo = mucus) and Paramyxoviridae, were grouped together as *Myxovirus*. The common properties were an RNA genome, a tubular nucleocapsid, and a pleomorphic lipoprotein envelope that carried the properties of hemagglutination and enzymatic elution. The term 'myxovirus' is now only used as a vernacular expression to encompass the viruses that have these properties (viz. influenza, mumps, Newcastle disease, and parainfluenza viruses); it has no taxonomic status.

The family Orthomyxoviridae comprises two genera; one, called *Influenzavirus* (from Latin influentia = epidemic), includes two species, A and B, with their many subtypes and strains. The other genus, represented by influenza type C, has not yet been named. All members of the family have a fragmented genome consisting of six (influenza type C) or eight pieces of single-stranded RNA, which accounts for the frequent genetic reassortment found in mixed infections. The virion contains two virus-specific enzymes; a surface neuraminidase and an internal transcriptase.

Influenzavirus A has been recovered from a number of different species of animals (birds, horses and swine) as well as man; *Influenzavirus B* and influenza type C are specifically human pathogens. They are an important cause of respiratory disease in man and other animals, and some of the avian influenza viruses may cause severe generalized infections in birds.

Because of the importance of influenza A as a human disease and the secular variation in the antigenicity of its envelope antigens (hemagglutinin and neuraminidase), WHO has standardized the nomenclature of Orthopoxviridae at the strain level, by defining a certain

TABLE 18. *Family: Orthomyxoviridae**· †

Genus	
Influenzavirus	Two species, in each of which all strains share species-specific nucleo-protein and membrane protein antigens. *Influenzavirus A* causes infections in man, swine, horse and birds; *Influenzavirus B* is a specifically human virus.
Unnamed	Influenza virus type C has the major characteristics of the family but the genome consists of 6 segments rather than 8 (as in *Influenzavirus*) and the neuraminidase and hemagglutinin properties may be located on the same envelope protein. It has only been recovered from man.

* Type genus: *Influenzavirus*.

Type species: Influenza A virus [R/1/ −: Σ5/F8: Se/E: V/R].

† Characteristics: genome consists of eight (six in influenza type C virus) separate pieces of single-stranded RNA, total molecular weight 5 million; tubular nucleocapsid 6–9 nm diameter is species-specific antigen; lipoprotein envelope 80–120 nm in diameter contains strain-specific hemagglutinin and neuraminidase antigens; virion contains a transcriptase; multiply in nucleus and cytoplasm; mature by budding from the plasma membrane.

number of subtypes of both the hemagglutinin and neuraminidase antigens of *Influenzavirus A* (WHO, 1980).

Family: *Arenaviridae* [R/1/ −: Σ5/F2: Se/*: V/C, O]

The family Arenaviridae (arena = sand), which contains one genus, *Arenavirus*, was first defined by the electron microscopic appearance of the virions in thin sections, and serological cross-reactivity. The pleomorphic enveloped virions are 110–130 nm in diameter (sometimes larger) and have closely spaced club-shaped peplomers. The structure of the nucleocapsid is unknown, but in thin sections the interior of the particle is seen to contain a variable number of electron-dense granules 20–30 nm in diameter, hence the name.

Five RNA molecules have been repeatedly isolated from purified virions; two of these are virus-specific, with apparent molecular weights of 2.1–3.2×10^6, and three are of host cell origin.

TABLE 19. *Family Arenaviridae; Genus: Arenavirus**· †

Old World species:	Lymphocytic choriomeningitis (LCM), Mozambique and Lassa
New World species:	Tacaribe complex (Amapari, Junin, Latino, Machupo, Parana, Pichinide, Tacaribe, Tamiami)

* Characteristics: single-stranded RNA in two pieces, total molecular weight 5 million; virion transcriptase; lipoprotein envelope 85–300 nm in diameter; multiply in cytoplasm; mature by budding from plasma membrane. All members share a group-specific antigen. Envelope encloses 'granules' 20–30 nm in diameter; some of these are cellular ribosomes; three host RNA species are regularly recovered from purified virions.

† Type species: Lymphocytic choriomeningitis virus [R/1/ −: Σ 4–5/F2: Se/*: V/C, O].

All members of the genus are associated with chronic inapparent infections of rodents; some cause acute generalized diseases in other hosts (e.g. Lassa fever virus in man). Both vertical (including congenital) and horizontal transmission occur.

Family: *Rhabdoviridae* [R/1/ −: 4/L: Ue/E: I, V/C, O, Ve, Ap, An, Di]

The rhabdoviruses (rhabdo = rod) are enveloped RNA viruses with single-stranded RNA with a molecular weight of about 4 million. The RNA is associated with a very regular double-helical nucleocapsid 5 nm in diameter, enclosed with a bullet-shaped shell that measures about 175×75 nm (Table 20).

The family contains two named genera that infect vertebrates, *Vesiculovirus* and *Lyssavirus*, and some viruses not yet allocated to a genus; some insect and plant viruses may also belong to this family.

Family: *Togaviridae* [R/1/ +: 3.5–4/L: Se/S: I, V/C, I, O, R, Ve/Ac, Di]

During the last 30 years intensive world-wide efforts have been made to recover viruses which would multiply in both arthropods and vertebrates, and several hundred different

TABLE 20. *Family: Rhabdoviridae**· †

Genus	Species‡
Vesiculovirus	Vesicular stomatitis virus [5 serotypes (V & V, I)]
	Chandipura virus (V, I)
	Isfahan virus (I)
	Piry virus (V)
Lyssavirus	Rabies virus (V)
	Duvenhage (V)
	Kotokan (I)
	Lagos bat (V)
	Mokola (V)
	Obodhiang (I)
No genera established	Thirty-six species, recovered from vertebrates, including fishes and insects. Include bovine ephemeral fever virus
Plant rhabdoviruses (ungrouped)	Some 25 species occurring in higher plants. Also multiply in insects (aphids and leaf-hoppers) which act as vectors

* Characteristics: bullet-shaped enveloped virions measuring 170 × 70 nm and containing single-stranded RNA with molecular weight about 4 million; virion contains a transcriptase; multiply in cytoplasm and mature by budding from the plasma membrane.

† Type genus: *Vesiculovirus*.
Type species: Vesicular stomatitis virus [R/1/−: 4/L: Ue/E: I, V/C, O, Ve, Ac, Di].

‡ V = recovered from vertebrates; I = recovered from invertebrates.

agents with these biological properties are now known. They were called 'arthropod-borne viruses', a name which was shortened to 'arborviruses' and then (in order to avoid the connotation of 'tree') to 'arboviruses'. The arboviruses have been defined, on epidemiological grounds (mode of transmission), as a group comparable to the 'respiratory viruses'. Arboviruses are viruses which, in nature, can infect arthropods that ingest infected vertebrate blood, can multiply in the arthropod tissues, and can then be transmitted by bite to susceptible vertebrates.

For many years arboviruses have been recovered from vertebrate tissues and suspensions of arthropods by the intracerebral inoculation of mice, and advantage has been taken of certain chemical and physical properties found to be commonly associated with them to avoid confusion with murine picornaviruses. The property generally tested was sensitivity to lipid solvents. Many arboviruses have lipoprotein envelopes and their infectivity is destroyed by these reagents. There was thus a tendency to equate sensitivity to lipid solvents with 'arbovirus'. During the last decade it has been recognized that the epidemiologically defined arbovirus group is quite heterogeneous in its physicochemical properties. Some members are not enveloped (*Orbivirus*) and those sensitive to lipid solvents belong to at least three families (Togaviridae, Rhabdoviridae and Bunyaviridae).

This preamble has been necessary because in the past the term 'arboviruses' has been regarded as applying particularly to viruses with the physicochemical properties of what were called the 'group A' and 'group B' arboviruses. These viruses now form two genera (*Alphavirus* and *Flavivirus*) of the family Togaviridae (toga = cloak). The family also contains two other genera, *Rubivirus* and *Pestivirus*, for which no arthropod vectors are known (Table 21).

Genus: *Alphavirus* [R/1/+: 4/L: Se/S: I, V/Ve/Di]. The alphaviruses (alpha = Greek letter A), formerly known as the group A arboviruses, have the familial characteristics (Table 20) and show serological cross-reactivity by the hemagglutinin-inhibition test. The arthropod vectors are mosquitoes. In nature, they usually cause inapparent infections of birds, reptiles, or mammals, but some can cause generalized infections, sometimes associated with encephalitis, in man and in other mammals.

Genus: *Flavivirus* [R/1/+: 4/L: Se/S: I, V/C, O, Ve/Ac, Di]. This genus (flavi = yellow) comprises the group B arboviruses. All members show serological cross-reactivity. The arthropod vectors may be ticks or mosquitoes, in both of which transovarial infection may

TABLE 21. *Family: Togaviridae**,†*

Genus	Comments
Alphavirus	Type species: Sindbis virus [R/1/+ : 4/L: Se/S: V, I/Ve/Di]. All show serological cross-reactivity and all are mosquito-borne viruses.
	Members: Equine encephalitis viruses—Western, Eastern, and Venezuelan; Semliki Forest; Chikungunya; Sindbis; and sixteen other named viruses.
Flavivirus	Type species: Yellow fever virus [R/1/+: 4/L: Se/S: V, I/Ve/Di]. All show serological cross-reactivity, some are mosquito-borne and some are tick-borne viruses.
	Members: Yellow fever, St Louis encephalitis, Japanese encephalitis, dengue (four serotypes), West Nile, Murray Valley encephalitis, Russian tick-borne encephalitis and 46 other named viruses.
Rubivurus	Rubella virus.
Pestivirus	Hog cholera virus and bovine mucosal disease virus (serologically related).

* Type genus: *Alphavirus*.

† Characteristics: single linear molecule of single-stranded RNA of molecular weight 4 million, within a capsid of cubic symmetry, 20–40 nm diameter, which is enclosed within a lipoprotein envelope 40–70 nm in diameter; multiply in cytoplasm and mature by budding from cytoplasmic (*Alphavirus*, *Rubivirus*, *Pestivirus*) or intracytoplasmic (*Flavivirus*) membranes; purified RNA is infectious.

occur. Some flaviviruses may be transmitted by the ingestion of contaminated milk. They differ from the alphaviruses in that budding usually occurs into cytoplasmic vacuoles rather than from the plasma membrane. Most cause inapparent infections in mammals and less commonly in birds, but generalized infections of man may occur with visceral symptomatology (e.g. yellow fever), rashes (e.g. dengue), or encephalitis (e.g. Japanese encephalitis).

Genus: *Rubivirus* [R/1/+: 3.5/L: Se/S: V/C, R] contains only one species, rubella virus, which causes a minor generalized exanthematous disease in man, which may be associated with congenital defects in the newborn when pregnant women are infected during the first 3 months of pregnancy.

Genus: *Pestivirus* [R/1/+: 4/L: Se/S: V/C, I, R]. These are viruses recovered from cattle and swine, whose virions are physicochemically like togaviruses; but they are not transmitted by arthropods. Hog cholera virus may be transmitted congenitally.

Family: *Picornaviridae* [R/1/+: 2.3–2.8/L: S/S: V/I, O, R]

The family Picornaviridae (sigla: pico = small; rna = ribonucleic acid), which includes a very large number of viruses, has four genera: *Enterovirus* (entero = intestine), *Rhinovirus* (rhino = nose), *Cardiovirus* (cardio = heart) and *Aphthovirus* (aphtha = vesicles in the mouth) (Table 22).

Genus: *Enterovirus*. Enteroviruses have the family characteristics of the Picornaviridae. The particles are 20–30 nm in diameter, acid stable (pH 3) and have a buoyant density (in CsCl) of 1.34–1.35 g/cm³. They are primarily inhabitants of the intestines, and a large number of serotypes have been found in the feces of man and of various animals.

The enteroviruses of man have been subdivided into three major subgroups: poliovirus, three serotypes; echovirus (acronym: echo = enteric cytopathogenic human orphan), thirty-four serotypes; and coxsackievirus (Coaxsackie = town in New York State), twenty-four serotypes of type A and six of type B. The polioviruses, which show some serological cross-reactivity, are distinguished by their capacity to paralyze humans. Coxsackieviruses were originally defined in terms of their capacity to multiply in infant mice, but subsequently some echoviruses were found to do the same. It has been recommended that all future enteroviruses that are discovered should be numbered sequentially from 68, irrespective to subgroups. Most infections with enteroviruses are inapparent, a few are associated with gastrointestinal disorders or conjunctivitis and some may cause generalized infections with rash or central nervous system involvement, including poliomyelitis and aseptic meningitis, or specific damage to the heart. Human enterovirus 72 causes hepatitis A in man.

Genus: Rhinovirus. The rhinoviruses resemble the enteroviruses in several characteristics but they are acid labile (pH 3) and have a buoyant density (in CsCl) of 1.38–1.43 g/cm³. Most have a low ceiling temperature of growth and are characteristically found in the upper

TABLE 22. *Family: Picornaviridae*[*][†]

Genus	Members	Acid stability	Buoyant density in CsCl (g/cm^3)
Enterovirus	Human, including polio viruses, coxsackieviruses and echoviruses Bovine and porcine Murine encephalomyelitis virus Duck hepatitis virus Hepatitis A virus (human enterovirus 72)	Stable at pH 3	1.33–1.34
Rhinovirus	Human rhinoviruses, > 100 serotypes Bovine rhinoviruses	Labile below pH 5–6	1.38–1.42
Cardiovirus	EMC virus Mengo virus ME virus	Stable at pH 3 and pH 8 but unstable at pH 6	1.34
Aphthovirus	Foot-and-mouth disease virus (seven serotypes)	Labile below pH 5–6	1.43
—	Equine rhinovirus	Labile at pH 3	1.45

* Type genus: *Enterovirus*.
 Type species: Poliovirus type 1 [R/1/+: 2.6/L: S/S: V/I, O].
 † Characteristics: single linear molecule of single-stranded RNA, molecular weight 2.6–2.8 million; purified RNA is infectious; nonenveloped; capsid 20–30 nm in diameter, with cubic symmetry; multiply in cytoplasm.

respiratory tract of man and various animals. There are over 100 different serotypes of human rhinoviruses and several serotypes of bovine rhinovirus. Most rhinoviruses cause mild localized infections of the upper respiratory tract.

Genus: Cardiovirus. This genus comprises a single unique serotype that goes under three names. Virions are unstable at pH 5–6 in presence of 0.1 M halide.

Genus: Aphthovirus. There are seven serotypes of this virus, which causes foot-and-mouth disease in animals, and many subtypes.

Family: *Caliciviridae* [R/1/+: 2.8/L: S/S: V/O, I]

This is a small family that was initially classified as a genus of Picornaviridae, since it has a genome consisting of a single molecule of single-stranded RNA which is infectious. However, the morphology of the virion is different, with thirty-two cup-shaped surface depressions (calici = cup or goblet) arranged in icosahedral symmetry.

Different species, each consisting of several serotypes, cause vesicular exanthematous disease in swine, sea lions and cats. Norwalk agent and related viruses that cause gastroenteritis in humans, calves and swine may be members of family Caliciviridae.

Tentative Family: *Filovirus Group* [R/1/−: 4.2/L: Ee/E: V/O]

This comprises two viruses indigenous to Africa which cause hemorrhagic fever in man: Marburg virus and Ebola virus. Although initially they were regarded as possible members of the family Rhabdoviridae, it is now suggested that they belong to a distinct family from which the name Filoviridae has been proposed (filo = filament or thread) (Kiley *et al.*, 1982).

The virion contains a single linear molecule of single-stranded RNA, which is not infectious. The virions are pleomorphic, occurring as long filamentous forms, as U-shaped, '6'-shaped and circular forms, and as long rods. They have a uniform diameter of 80 nm but vary greatly in length (up to 14,000 nm). However, the peak infectivity of Marburg virus is associated with rods with rounded ends about 790 nm long and that of Ebola virus with similar rods 970 nm long. The particles are enveloped, with peplomers 7 nm long set 10 nm apart. The nucleocapsid is a complex structure with a central axis 20 nm in diameter, surrounded by a helical tubular capsid with a periodicity of 5 nm.

There is virtually no serological cross-reactivity between Marburg and Ebola viruses, but the Sudan and Zaire strains of Ebola virus, although not identical, share many antigens.

Filoviruses multiply in the cytoplasm where they produce large cytoplasmic inclusion bodies that consist mostly of nucleocapsids. Virions are produced by budding through regions of the cell membrane into which peplomers have been inserted.

Both viruses have a wide host range in experimental animals. Their natural history is unknown, but each causes severe hepatitis and hemorrhagic fever in man.

1.9. UNCLASSIFIED VIRUSES

Three groups of viruses that have not yet been classified by ICTV appear to be sufficiently distinctive and well characterized for their inclusion within the foregoing descriptions; namely the Hepadnavirus group, the Birnavirus group and the Filovirus group. There remain a number of other distinctive viruses or virus-like agents that are associated with disease in man or other animals but about which too little is yet known to allow them to be classified. Of these, the most important are the astroviruses, the agents of the subacute spongiform encephalopathies, and the virus of Korean hemorrhagic fever.

1.9.1. ASTROVIRUS GROUP

In 1975 Madeley and Cosgrove (1975) proposed the name 'Astrovirus' for 28-nm particles with a star-shaped surface configuration that were found in the feces of human neonates. Similar particles have been found in feces of lambs and calves. Human volunteer studies and experiments in gnotobiotic lambs showed that the human and lamb 'astroviruses' infected their respective hosts, sometimes causing diarrhea. No serological cross-reactivity has yet been demonstrated between the agents recovered from different species of vertebrate, nor have any of the viruses yet been cultivated. Nevertheless, the distinctive morphology and the association with enteric disease in several species suggests that these viruses do belong to a new viral family, but their classification awaits further studies on their chemistry and biology, notably their nucleic acid and strategy of multiplication.

1.9.2. AGENTS OF SUBACUTE SPONGIFORM ENCEPHALOPATHIES

Four diseases of similar nature, scrapie of sheep, transmissible encephalopathy of mink, and kuru and Creutzfeld-Jakob disease in man appear to be caused by similar agents (review: Prusiner and Hadlow, 1979), which differ from all known viruses by being nonimmunogenic. The causative agents are filtrable, highly heat-resistant, and highly resistant to ionizing radiation. It has been suggested that they may be small molecules of naked RNA, protected by being closely associated with cellular membranes (a 'viroid', Diener, 1979), or a very peculiar virus.

1.9.3. KOREAN HEMORRHAGIC FEVER VIRUS

Viral hemorrhagic fever with renal syndrome is a human disease known by numerous synonyms, among which are 'Korean hemorrhagic fever' and 'hemorrhagic nephrosonephritis'. It was shown to be caused by a virus by investigations with human volunteers as early as 1940–41 (Smorondintsev *et al.*, 1964). Subsequently it affected thousands of military personnel in the Korean War of 1950–52, and a similar milder syndrome has been reported in Sweden and Hungary. All these syndromes are caused by antigenically related viruses whose natural hosts are the rodents *Apodemus agrarius* (in Asia) and *Clethrionomys glareolus* (in northern and eastern Europe). Serological surveys suggest that infection with these viruses may also occur in southern Asia, central Africa and the Americas. The morphology and their nucleic acid suggests that they should be classified as bunyaviruses, but they are apparently not vector-borne.

REFERENCES

DIENER, T. O. (1979) *Viroids and Viroid Diseases*. Wiley, New York.
FENNER, F. (1976)*The Classification and Nomenclature of Viruses*. Second Report of the International Committee on Taxonomy of Viruses. Karger, Basel.

FENNER, F. and WHITE, D. O. (1976) *Medical Virology*. (2nd Edn) Academic Press, New York.

FENNER, F., MCAUSLAN, B. R., MIMS, C. A., SAMBROOK, J. F. and WHITE, D. O. (1974) *The Biology of Animal Viruses*. (2nd Edn.) Academic Press, New York.

GIBBS, A. J., HARRISON, B. D., WATSON, D. H. and WILDY, P. (1966) What's in a virus name? *Nature* (*Lond.*) **209**: 450.

KILEY, M. P., BOWEN, E. T. W., EDDY, G. A., ISAÄCSON, M., JOHNSON, K. M., MCCORMICK, J. B., MURPHY, F. A., PATTYN, S. R., PETERS, D., PROZESKY, O. W., REGNERY, R. L., SIMPSON, D. I. H., SLENCZKA, W., SUREAU, P., VAN DER GROEN, G., WEBB, P. A. and WULFF, H. (1982) Filoviridae: A taxonomic home for Marburg and Ebola viruses? *Intervirology* **18**: 24.

MADELEY, C. R. and COSGROVE, B. P. (1975) 28 nm particles in feces in infantile gastroenteritis. *Lancet* **ii**: 451.

MATTHEWS, R. E. F. (1979) *Classification and Nomenclature of Viruses*. Third Report of the International Committee on Taxonomy of Viruses. *Intervirology* **12**: 132.

MATTHEWS, R. E. F. (1982) *Classification and Nomenclature of Viruses*. Fourth Report of the International Committee on Taxonomy of Viruses. *Intervirology* **17**: 1.

PRUSINER, S. B. and HADLOW, W. J. (eds.) (1979) *Slow Transmissible Diseases of the Nervous System*. Academic Press, New York.

ROBINSON, W. S. (1980) Genetic variation among hepatitis B and related viruses. *Ann. N.Y. Acad. Sci.* **354**: 371.

SMORONDINTSEV, A. A., KAZBINTSEV, L. I. and CHUDAKOV, V. G. (1964) *Virus Hemorrhagic Fevers*. Israel Program for Scientific Translation, Clearing House, Springfield, Va.

TIOLLAIS, P., CHARNEY, P. and VYAS, G. N. (1981) Biology of hepatitis B virus. *Science* **213**: 406.

WHO (1980) A revision of the system of nomenclature for influenza viruses: a WHO Memorandum. *Bull. WHO* **58**: 585.

WILDY, P. (1971) Classification and nomenclature of viruses. First Report of the International Committee on Nomenclature of Viruses. *Monogr. Virol.* **5**.

CHAPTER 2

THE PATHOGENESIS AND FREQUENCY OF VIRAL
INFECTIONS IN MAN

Frank Fenner

John Curtin School of Medical Research, The Australian National University, Canberra, Australia

CONTENTS

2.1. INTRODUCTORY REMARKS

Chemotherapeutic agents are usually first tested by experiments involving viruses grown in cultured cells. Whether an agent effective in this situation is likely to be useful in human infections depends upon the properties of the chemical concerned, and also, importantly, on the nature of the disease in man. For this, pharmacologists need to have some appreciation of the pathogenesis of viral diseases. Since some chemotherapeutic agents are likely to be used for prevention rather than treatment, it is necessary to appreciate both the mode of entry of viruses into the body and their spread. Some understanding is also required of a class of infections that are particularly important targets for attack by viral chemotherapy, the persistent infections. And since chemotherapy is always used in conjunction with host defense mechanisms, pharmacologists need to appreciate what the host does to ensure that it recovers from most infections.

Finally, it is important that workers in this field should appreciate the relative frequency of different kinds of viral infection, and some data on this topic are provided.

2.2. INTRODUCTION

The pathogenesis of viral infections involves three types of interaction between viruses and their vertebrate hosts: the way in which viruses spread (or fail to spread) through the body, the immune response and its influence on viral infections, and the many non-immunological factors which affect virus–host interactions.

It is relevant here to consider the terms *pathogenicity* and *virulence* as they apply to viruses. Neither can be used without reference to the host, for they apply to the interaction between host and parasite. A virus is *pathogenic* for a particular host if it can infect that host and produce signs and symptoms of disease in it. But infection is not synonymous with disease; many infections, even with virulent viruses, may be *subclinical* or *inapparent* (see Table 9). A given strain of virus is said to be more *virulent* than another if it regularly produces more severe disease in a host in which both strains are pathogenic. Live vaccines are usually *attenuated* strains, i.e. they are less virulent than the wild-type virus. It is best not to use the word 'virulent' to describe the killing of cultured cells by viruses; the appropriate term is 'cytocidal'. Cytocidal viruses are not invariably highly virulent in intact animals; conversely, noncytocidal viruses like rubella or the leukemia viruses may cause severe disease.

Since viruses must get into susceptible cells before they can produce disease, it is necessary to consider first the important portals of entry and exit of viruses from the body (Table 1). Some viruses have a single mode of transmission, others, as the last term of the cryptograms shown in Table 2 of the previous article indicate, have several.

TABLE 1. *The Transmission of Viral Infections of Man: Routes of Entry and Exit and Modes of Transfer* (*from Evans,* 1976)

Route of exit	Routes of transmission	Examples	Factors	Routes of entry
Respiratory	Bite	Rabies	Animal	Skin
	Salivary transfer	EBV in adults	Kissing	Mouth
		? Hepatitis B	Unknown	? Mouth
	Aerosol	Influenza and other respiratory viruses	Sneeze, cough, < 2-nm particles to lung	Respiratory
	Mouth → hand or object	Herpes simplex, EBV in children, Rhinovirus, Enterovirus	Salivary contamination of hands and objects	Oropharyngeal
Gastrointestinal tract	Stool → hand	Enteroviruses— hepatitis A	Poor hygiene	Mouth
	Stool → water (or milk)	Hepatitis A	Seafood	Mouth
	Thermometer	Hepatitis A	Nurse	Rectal
Skin	Air	Poxviruses	Also via objects	Respiratory
	Skin to skin	Molluscum contagiosum, warts	Abrasions	Abraded skin
Blood	Mosquitos	Arboviruses	Extrinsic I.P.	Skin
	Ticks	Flaviviruses	Transovarial transmission	Skin
	Transfusion of blood and blood products	Hepatitis B, CMV, EBV	Carrier state, free or with leukocytes	Skin
	Needles for injection	Hepatitis B	Addicts	Skin
Urine	Rarely transmitted	CMV, measles, mumps, congenital rubella	Unknown	Unknown
Genital	Cervix	Herpes, simplex, CMV, rubella	? Venereal	Genital
	Semen	CMV	? Venereal	Genital
Placental	Vertical to embryo	CMV, rubella, smallpox	Congenital abnormalities, abortion	Blood
Eye	Tonometer	Adenovirus	Exam for glaucoma	Eye

The important portals of entry are the three major and two minor epithelial surfaces: the skin, the respiratory tract, and the alimentary tract; and the conjunctiva and genital tract (Fig. 1). Localized pathological changes may be produced when viruses breach these barriers, although invasion may also occur without the development of a local lesion. After the surface has been breached the infection may remain localized, or it may spread through the organism via the lymphatics, blood vessels, or nerves.

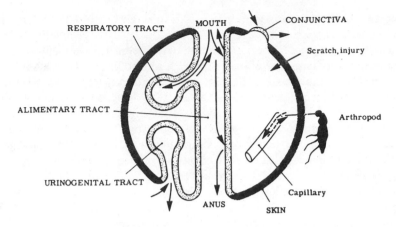

Fig. 1. Diagram illustrating the body surfaces which serve as portals of entry and exit of viruses
(from Mims, 1976).

2.3. VIRAL INFECTIONS OF THE RESPIRATORY TRACT

Man samples the environmental air about 20 times a minute during breathing, so that the respiratory tract is a very important portal of entry for viruses. Some viruses cause silent initial infection of the respiratory tract prior to systemic distribution; most remain localized in the upper or lower respiratory tract and produce disease as a result of their multiplication there. These are called the 'respiratory viruses' (Table 2), and include the rhinoviruses, orthomyxoviruses, paramyxoviruses and coronaviruses, as well as several adenoviruses and enteroviruses. Although infection is usually by inhalation of aerosols produced by coughing, sneezing or singing, high concentrations of respiratory viruses are often found on the hands, and frequent inadvertent contact of fingers with the nose and eyes may help to spread such agents.

TABLE 2. *Viral Diseases of the Respiratory Tract (from Fenner and White, 1976)*

Disease	Virus	
	Common	Less common
Upper respiratory infection (including the common cold and pharyngitis)	Rhinovirus, > 100 types Coronaviruses Parainfluenza 1–3 Respiratory syncytial Influenza A, B Herpes simplex 1	Adenovirus 1–7, 14, 21 Coxsackie A21, 24; B2-5, etc. Echovirus 11, 20, etc. Parainfluenza 4 EB virus
Croup (laryngotracheobronchitis)	Parainfluenza 1–3 Influenza A, B Respiratory syncytial	Adenoviruses Measles
Bronchiolitis	Respiratory syncytial* Parainfluenza 1, 3 (2)	Influenza A
Pneumonitis	Respiratory syncytial* Parainfluenza 1, 3, (2) Influenza A	Adenovirus 3, 4, 7 (14, 21) Measles Varicella

*In infants only.

2.3.1. INFLUENZA

As an example of the way in which these viruses produce respiratory disease, we describe the pathogenesis of influenza, the most important respiratory viral infection of man.

Infectious particles may be implanted directly on nasal surfaces from contaminated hands or from large droplets, or may reach the lower respiratory passages from aerosols. In general, aerosol particles of 3 μm in size reach the alveolus and those of 6 μm or greater are retained in the upper respiratory tract. Symptoms are produced by multiplication in the cells of the upper and lower respiratory tract; generalization via the bloodstream is a very rare event.

Virus particles alighting on the mucus film that covers the epithelium of the upper respiratory tract may undergo one of several fates. If the individual has previously recovered from an infection with that strain of influenza virus, antibody (mainly IgA) in the mucous secretion may combine with the virus and neutralize it. Mucus also contains glycoprotein inhibitors which combine with virus and prevent it from attaching to the specific receptors on the host cell; eventually these inhibitors are destroyed by the viral neuraminidase.

The successful infection of a few cells by influenza virus, and the passage of newly synthesized virions from these cells into the respiratory mucus and then into other cells, may lead to progressive infection, which is aided by the transudation of fluid that follows cellular injury and helps to disperse the virus. On the other hand, the inflammation also results in an increased diffusion of plasma constituents, including antibody and nonspecific inhibitors, which may inactivate the virus and cut short the infection. Interferon may also play a role in limiting the spread of infection.

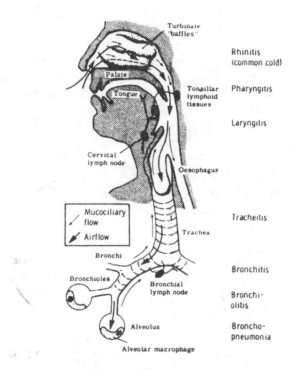

FIG. 2. Diagram of the respiratory tract of man illustrating the different anatomical structures associated with viral infection at various levels of the respiratory tract (from Mims, 1976).

Although the release of virus does not cause obvious cell damage, the end result of infection is necrosis and desquamation of the respiratory epithelium. Usually damage is confined to the epithelial cells of the upper respiratory tract, but in cases of pneumonia there are foci of infection in the epithelial cells of the bronchi, bronchioles and alveoli, and in alveolar macrophages, but not in the vascular endothelium. Destruction of the respiratory epithelium by influenza virus lowers its resistance to secondary bacterial invaders, especially pneumococci and staphylococci.

2.3.2. OTHER RESPIRATORY VIRUSES

Upper respiratory tract infection (URTI) is the most common disease of man, and most of it caused by viruses. It has been estimated to account for an average of six episodes per person per annum, up to one-third of all calls on general practitioners, and countless millions of lost working hours. Attempts have been made to assess the relative contributions of the various respiratory viruses to the total spectrum of respiratory disease (Fig. 3). The *rhinoviruses*, *coronaviruses*, *parainfluenza*, and *respiratory syncytial viruses* are the most common agents, usually producing trivial disease of the upper respiratory tract, especially when they infect adults. On the other hand, most of the respiratory infections in young children that are severe enough to require hospitalization are attributable to *respiratory syncytial*, *parainfluenza* and *influenza* viruses. In respiratory syncytial virus infections of infants, if humoral antibody is present in the absence of local antibody, a more severe reaction may occur, possibly through antigen/antibody deposition on the membrane of alveolar cells.

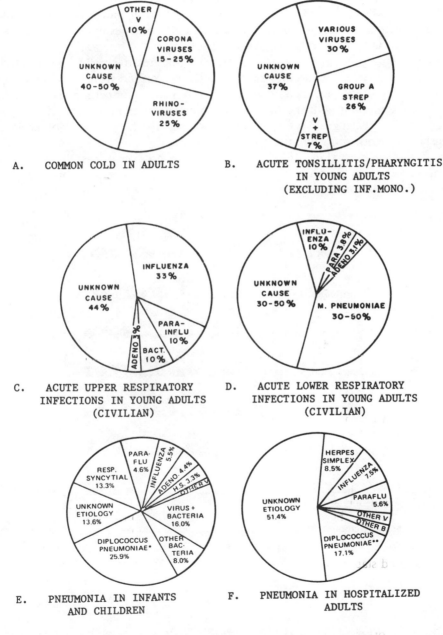

A. COMMON COLD IN ADULTS

B. ACUTE TONSILLITIS/PHARYNGITIS
IN YOUNG ADULTS
(EXCLUDING INF.MONO.)

C. ACUTE UPPER RESPIRATORY
INFECTIONS IN YOUNG ADULTS
(CIVILIAN)

D. ACUTE LOWER RESPIRATORY
INFECTIONS IN YOUNG ADULTS
(CIVILIAN)

E. PNEUMONIA IN INFANTS
AND CHILDREN

F. PNEUMONIA IN HOSPITALIZED
ADULTS

FIG. 3. Causes of respiratory infections in man. A–D. Acute respiratory syndromes in young adults. E–F. Pneumonia syndromes in infants and children and in hospitalized adults. *Based on pure throat culture. **Based on pure blood culture (from Evans, 1976).

Most of the respiratory viruses are highly infectious, spreading as droplets generated during coughing, sneezing, talking, etc. Respiratory viral infections have short incubation periods, of the order of 2–5 days. Hence they regularly produce epidemics, especially in the winter and spring. A striking example is the respiratory syncytial virus, which precipitates an abrupt epidemic in infants every winter. More widespread epidemics, which may close schools and factories, are produced every 2–3 years by influenza A and, somewhat less frequently, by influenza B. Adenovirus types 3, 4, 7, 14, 21 and parainfluenza type 1 occasionally cause limited outbreaks in military camps and other semiclosed communities of young people. The other important respiratory viruses, namely the rhinoviruses, coronaviruses, parainfluenza viruses, adenoviruses 1, 2, 5 and 6, and coxsackieviruses A21, A24, B3 and B5, tend rather to be endemic in the community, causing only sporadic cases or occasional small outbreaks. Respiratory syncytial and parainfluenza viruses are so prevalent that the first infections with them usually occur in infancy or early childhood. In contrast, some of the enteroviruses and adenoviruses may not be encountered until adult life. Subclinical infections do not occur nearly as commonly with respiratory viruses as with viruses entering the body by other routes.

Acquired immunity to the respiratory viruses tends to be relatively short-lived. Interferon confers limited protection against all viruses for a few weeks, and specific immunity against the homologous serotype, mediated principally by IgA, persists for perhaps a few years, then wanes. Hence reinfection with the same agent sometimes occurs. Even more significant, however, is the fact that a given syndrome may be caused by a large number of serologically distinguishable agents, showing little or no cross-immunity.

Many of the viruses listed in Table 2 can, on occasion, produce disease at any level in the respiratory tract – coryza, pharyngitis, laryngitis, croup, bronchitis, bronchiolitis, or pneumonia (Fig. 4). For example, respiratory syncytial virus or parainfluenza type 3 can

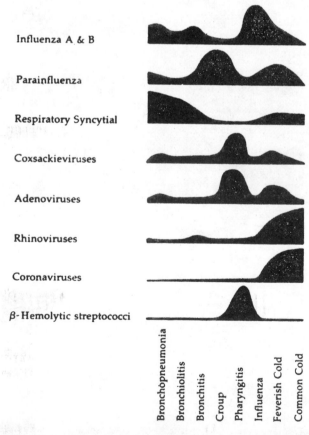

FIG. 4. Diagram showing the frequency with which particular viruses cause disease at various levels of the respiratory tract (from Fenner and White, 1976).

cause a potentially lethal pneumonitis, bronchiolitis, or croup in infants, but usually little more than a sore throat or common cold-like illness in adults. Indeed, the syndromes merge into one another as the infection moves progressively down the respiratory tract. In general, the disease becomes more serious the lower the virus goes.

2.3.3. RESPIRATORY INFECTION IN GENERALIZED DISEASES

In addition, the respiratory tract is the portal of entry for several viruses that cause generalized diseases: smallpox, measles, chickenpox, rubella, cytomegalovirus infection, mononucleosis, and sometimes various enterovirus infections. Usually no local lesion or symptoms occur during the primary infection, although there may be an exudative pharyngitis in infectious mononucleosis.

2.4. VIRAL INFECTIONS OF THE ALIMENTARY TRACT

Only nonenveloped viruses regularly cause infection of the human alimentary tract, because the infectivity of enveloped viruses is destroyed by the bile. Furthermore, the rhinoviruses are too acid-labile to pass the stomach. The main viruses that infect the gut are therefore the enteroviruses (including hepatitis A), reoviruses, and adenoviruses. Many of the same barriers that prevent cell attachment and penetration may exist there as in the respiratory tract, including local IgA antibody. Local humoral and cell-mediated immunity follows natural viral infections of the intestinal tract and forms the basis for immunity following oral administration of live vaccines, such as Sabin poliovaccines.

Most enteroviruses are parasites of the intestinal tract, but proof of the etiological role of coxsackieviruses and echoviruses in gastroenteritis has been difficult to obtain. Most infections are symptomless. Less frequently, enteroviruses (e.g. poliovirus) may spread from the alimentary tract to cause generalized infection. Important though these infections are, we know very little of their pathogenesis before they leave the gut. Adenoviruses are primarily pathogens of the respiratory tract but many serotypes can multiply asymptomatically in the alimentary tract and are excreted in the feces. The two kinds of hepatitis virus can cause infection via the alimentary tract; hepatitis A usually, hepatitis B rarely. In neither case does the initial infection of the gut cells produce symptoms. In addition, the so-called 'non-A non-B' hepatitis virus(es) are often transferred via the alimentary tract.

There are some viruses that cause gastroenteritis and diarrhea, which is second only to respiratory infection as a cause of human morbidity and in many parts of the world is a major killer of undernourished children. Symptoms include diarrhea, with a variable degree of nausea, vomiting, malaise, cramping abdominal pain and fever. The incubation period is 1– 4 days (average 2 days), the duration of illness 12–48 hours, and complete recovery is the usual outcome. The etiology of most cases remained obscure (Fig. 5) until recently, when two important new viruses were discovered by utilizing immunoelectronmicroscopy on ultra-centrifuged fecal preparations. The *Norwalk agent* is a 27-nm icosahedral virus morphologically resembling a parvovirus, and seems to be a major cause of the disease variously known as 'epidemic diarrhea and vomiting', or 'winter vomiting disease'. This agent occurs predominantly in outbreaks of acute infectious nonbacterial gastroenteritis during the colder months (September to March) in both adults and children throughout the world. It shows no serological cross-reaction with the *Hawaii agent*, which may be a member of the same family.

The *Rotaviruses* constitute a genus of the family Reoviridae. They appear to be the major cause of infantile gastroenteritis in young children throughout the world, infecting most infants in the first or second year of life with a low but significant mortality. Rotavirus infection is relatively uncommon in adults.

Additional viruses will doubtless be implicated in gastroenteritis. *Coronaviruses* and *adenoviruses*, which currently defy *in vitro* cultivation, are commonly visualized by electron microscopy in feces from patients with gastroenteritis. The role of *echoviruses* and

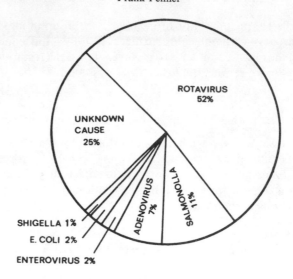

FIG. 5. Causes of acute gastroenteritis in children with enteric pathogens in feces (from Evans, 1976).

TABLE 3. *Viral Gastroenteritis* (*from Fenner and White*, 1976)

Proved	Possible
Rotavirus	Coronaviruses
Norwalk agent	Adenoviruses
Hawaii agent	Echoviruses 11, 14, 18, 22, and others
	Coxsackie A viruses
	Reoviruses

cocksackieviruses is still unclear. Certain serotypes, e.g. echoviruses 11, 14, 18 and 22, have been repeatedly recovered during epidemics, but the evidence for their causal relationship to the disease must still be regarded as circumstantial in light of the frequency with which echoviruses are excreted by well people (Table 3).

2.5. VIRAL INFECTIONS OF THE SKIN

When viruses are introduced into the skin by injection, arthropod bite, or through a breach caused by mechanical trauma, lesions may be produced at the site. The only localized viral infections of the skin in man are human warts, which are a trivial and very common hyperplasia due to a papovavirus of genus *Papillomavirus*, the recurrent vesicular eruptions of herpes simplex on skin and mucous membranes, and the proliferative inflammatory lesions produced by poxviruses: vaccinia, cowpox, orf, molluscum contagiosum and milker's nodes.

Most commonly, skin lesions occur secondarily to systemic spread, when they constitute a rash, as in the exanthemata of childhood. Rashes are more easily seen in human beings than in furred and feathered beasts, hence most of the descriptive data are derived from human infections. The individual lesions in generalized rashes are described as macules, papules, vesicles, or pustules. A lasting local dilation of subpapillary dermal blood vessels produces a macule, which becomes a papule if there is also edema and an infiltration of cells into the area. Primary involvement of the epidermis usually results in vesiculation, ulceration and scabbing, but prior to ulceration a vesicle may be converted to a pustule if there is a copious cellular exudate. Secondary changes in the epidermis may lead to desquamation. More severe involvement of the dermal vessels may lead to hemorrhagic and petechial rashes,

TABLE 4. *Viral Skin Rashes* (*from Fenner and White*, 1976)

Syndrome	Virus	
	Common	Less common
Maculopapular rash	Measles	Echovirus 2, 5, 11, 18, and others
	Rubella	Coxsackie A2, 4; B1, 3, 5, and others
	Echovirus 4, 6, 9, 16	Several arboviruses
	Coxsackie A9, 16, 23	EBV (infectious mononucleosis)
	Enterovirus 71	Reovirus 2
		Adenovirus 3, 7
Vesicular rash	Varicella-zoster	Vaccinia
	Herpes simplex	Coxsackie A4, 5, 9, 10, 16
	Smallpox*	Enterovirus 71
Hemorrhagic rash	Several arboviruses	Smallpox*
	Arenaviruses	
Localized lesions	Herpes simplex	Cowpox
	Warts	Milker's nodes
	Molluscum contagiosum	Orf

* Now extinct.

although coagulation defects and thrombocytopenia may also be important in the genesis of such lesions. Information on the occurrence of rashes in human viral infections is set out in Table 4.

2.6. GENITAL AND GENITO-URINARY INFECTIONS

Genital infection with viruses occurs commonly with herpes simplex type 2 and sometimes with human cytomegalovirus and the human wart virus.

In females, vulvovaginitis, with or without cervicitis, can be primary or recurrent. Herpes simplex type 2 infection has been closely correlated with subsequent development of cervical carcinoma but there is as yet no proof that the association is a causal one. Other viruses, notably echovirus type 4, have also been reported to be associated with cases of cervicitis.

Virus is regularly shed in the urine during generalized infections by many para-myxoviruses, herpesviruses, adenoviruses, togaviruses, arenaviruses, hepatitis viruses, rubella and the human polyomaviruses. As far as is known, however, viruria is not an indication of impairment of renal function. Only in *cytomegalovirus* infections is there clear evidence of kidney pathology. A temporary decrease in creatinine clearance has been observed in *mumps*.

Glomerulonephritis, which is an occasional feature of *hepatitis B* infection, is attributable to the accumulation of viral antigen–antibody complexes in glomeruli. Such immune complex disease is a frequent manifestation of chronic viral infections in animals and may be more common in man that we yet appreciate. A careful search for viruses, or im-munoglobulin deposits, or complement depletion in human glomerulonephritis, may reveal that some 'idiopathic' cases are in fact due to persistent infection with known or unknown viruses.

Acute hemorrhagic cystitis characterized by hematuria, frequency and dysuria has recently been associated with adenovirus types 2, 11 and 21 (Table 5).

2.7. CONJUNCTIVITIS

Adenovirus type 8 causes epidemic keratoconjunctivitis in man, the only clinical disease caused by Newcastle disease virus in man is conjunctivitis, and herpes simplex virus is one of the most common infectious causes of blindness. During the last few years *Enterovirus* 70 has emerged as the cause of epidemic hemorrhagic conjunctivitis. When smallpox vaccination was practiced, accidental transfer to the eye, causing conjunctivitis, sometimes occurred

TABLE 5. *Viruses that Initiate Infection of the Eye or Genitourinary Tract or are Excreted in Urine*

1. Ocular infections	*Mastadenovirus*: human type 8 and several others
	Enterovirus 70
	Herpesvirus: herpes simplex type 1
	Orthopoxvirus: accidental-vaccinia
	Paramyxovirus: in man, Newcastle disease virus
2. Venereal infections	*Papillomavirus*: human warts, rarely
	Herpesvirus: herpes simplex type 2
3. Excretion in urine	Papovaviridae: polyoma virus
(viruria)	Herpesviridae: cytomegalovirus
	Rubivirus: rubella
	Paramyxoviridae: measles, mumps
	Arenavirus: most species
	Mastadenovirus: human types 2, 11, 21
	Unclassified: hepatitis virus B

(Table 5). Such ocular infections are important to pharmacologists, for they present the possibility of local chemotherapy with drugs that might not be tolerated systemically, e.g. halogenated pyrimidine nucleosides in ocular herpes simplex.

When conjunctivitis occurs as part of a systemic illness, as in measles, the virus has reached the eye via the bloodstream.

2.8. THE SYSTEMIC SPREAD OF VIRUSES

Respiratory viruses, and those that cause gastroenteritis, produce symptoms, usually after a short incubation period (Table 1), referable to the respiratory or gastrointestinal tract respectively. Many other viruses that may enter via these or other portals produce symptoms only after they have spread to other parts of the body.

Systemic disease usually follows the distribution of virus via the bloodstream; the presence of virus in the bloodstream is known as *viremia*. Such a generalized infection may be inapparent, or it may produce systemic symptoms or symptoms associated with lesions in a particular organ, which differ characteristically with different viruses. The principal 'target' organs are the skin and the central nervous system; more rarely the liver, heart and certain glands may be chiefly affected. Viremia occurs in most viral infections, even though it may not be readily detectable. Rhinovirus infections and infection of the skin with warts virus may be exceptions.

In the blood, viruses may occur free in the plasma or may be characteristically associated with particular types of leukocytes, with platelets, or with erythrocytes. Leukocyte-associated viremia is a feature of several types of infection, including measles and smallpox, for example. Many viruses multiply in macrophages; others, e.g. EB virus, multiply in lymphocytes. Occasionally virus is adsorbed to erythrocytes as in Rift Valley Fever, Colorado tick fever, and lymphocytic choriomeningitis. Often virus circulates free in the plasma; all the togaviruses and the enteroviruses that cause viremia fall into this group. Finally, in some infections the viremia is mixed, i.e. the virus is partly in the plasma and partly cell-associated.

Whether virus circulates free in the plasma or is cell-associated affects its passage from the circulation to extravascular sites. Leukocytes can pass through the walls of small vessels by diapedesis, and infected leukocytes can thus initiate infection in various parts of the body. On the other hand, virus in the plasma may escape from circulation by being ingested by a cell in contact with the blood, either a macrophage or a capillary endothelial cell. Extravascular infection by such viruses may follow growth of the virus through the endothelial cells of the small blood vessels, or the virus may be transferred across the cell without growing in it.

Virus circulating in the blood is continually removed by cells of the reticuloendothelial system. Viremia can therefore be maintained only if there is a continued release of virus into the blood from cells in contact with it, or if the clearance system is grossly impaired. The circulating leukocytes could themselves constitute a source of replicating virus; indeed blood leukocytes maintained in culture (from which polymorphonuclear leukocytes are rapidly lost) support limited replication of many viruses. However, viremia is maintained primarily by organs with extensive sinusoids, like the liver, spleen and bone marrow, the endothelial cells of the blood vessels themselves, and the lymphoid tissues (via the thoracic duct). Cells of the voluntary muscles may be an important site of multiplication of some enteroviruses and togaviruses.

2.8.1. GENERALIZED INFECTIONS WITH RASH

Our understanding of the pathogenesis of systemic infections associated with a rash, such as smallpox, measles, and rubella, is based on studies with mousepox, upon which Fig. 6 is based. In each such exanthem, there is an incubation period of 10–12 days before symptoms of illness appear. After multiplication of the virus at the site of implantation and in the regional lymph nodes, a primary viremia occurs within the first few days, resulting in seeding of organs such as the liver, spleen, lymph nodes and the vascular endothelium. A secondary viremia then follows with focal involvement of the skin and mucous membranes, the appearance of a rash, and onset of symptoms. In mousepox, a primary lesion develops at the site of inoculation. Generalized symptoms and fever are probably caused by antigen–antibody complexes which are found at the end of the incubation period. In diseases like measles and rubella the rash has an immunopathologic basis; in smallpox, chickenpox, herpes simplex and herpes zoster the relevant viruses are present in the lesions in the skin and mucous membranes and this is an important mode of viral excretion.

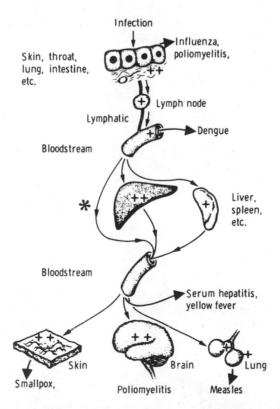

FIG. 6. Diagram illustrating the spread of infection through the body in systemic infections. + = possible sites of viral multiplication. Large arrow = possible sites for shedding virus into the environment (from Mims, 1976).

2.8.2. Generalized Infections Involving the Central Nervous System

Disease of the central nervous system (CNS) is an exceptional complication rather than the normal consequence of infection, even with the togaviruses and enteroviruses most commonly incriminated (Table 6). Some togaviruses, like Japanese encephalitis virus, involve the CNS but never produce a rash, whereas others, like dengue, do the reverse. Many of the enteroviruses occasionally produce meningitis, and polioviruses characteristically attack the anterior horn cells of the spinal cord in a small proportion of infected human beings. Several of the herpesviruses affect nerve cells; herpes simplex virus is probably the most common cause of sporadic fatal encephalitis in man, while herpes zoster is due to the activation of chickenpox virus, latent in cells of the posterior ganglia. Encephalitis occurring after measles is thought to be an autoimmune disease, possibly associated with limited viral multiplication in the neurons. The rare disease called subacute sclerosing panencephalitis is a late manifestation of CNS infection with measles virus, and another rare disease called progressive multifocal leukoencephalopathy is caused by a papovavirus.

Hematogenous spread. Viruses can spread from the blood to the brain cells by several routes. Growth through the endothelium of small cerebral vessels has been clearly demonstrated in several systems, and there is suggestive evidence that virions may sometimes be passively transferred across the vascular endothelium. The production of meningitis rather than encephalitis by enteroviruses, and the ease with which these agents are recovered from the cerebrospinal fluid, can be explained by postulating that the virus in the blood either grows or passes through the choroid plexus.

Neural spread. Spread from the periphery to the CNS is possible without generalization of viruses through the bloodstream, for the peripheral nerves and the nerve fibers of the olfactory bulb offer potential direct pathways. Although earlier workers thought in terms of spread via 'conduits' – the axon, the lymphatics, and the tissue spaces between nerve fibers – the route of spread along peripheral nerves is usually by growth within the endoneural cells,

TABLE 6. *Viral Diseases of the Central Nervous System (from Fenner and White, 1976)*

Syndrome	Virus	
	Common	Less common
Aseptic meningitis	Mumps	Other enteroviruses
	Coxsackievirus B1–6, A9	Poliovirus 1–3
		Herpes simplex
	Echovirus 4, 6, 9, 11, 14, 18, 30	Lymphocytic choriomeningitis
		Many other viruses occasionally
Paralysis	Poliovirus 1–3	Coxsackie A7, possibly others
Encephalitis	Several arboviruses	Mumps
	Herpes simplex	Rabies
	Enterovirus 71	Adenovirus 7
	Measles	Herpes B virus
Postinfectious encephalomyelitis		Vaccinia
		Varicella
		Mumps
		Influenza
		Rubella
Encephalopathy, incl. Reye's syndrome		Influenza
		Varicella-zoster
Infectious polyneuritis		Influenza
Guillain–Barré syndrome Transverse myelitis Bell's palsy Radiculomyelitis		EB virus?
Subacute sclerosing panencephalitis	Measles	
Progressive multifocal leukoencephalopathy	Human papovavirus	
Creutzfeld–Jakob disease	Viroid?	
Kuru	Viroid?	

a fact demonstrated experimentally with herpesvirus infections by fluorescent antibody staining methods. However, this cannot be the only method of neural spread, for in experiments with rabies virus, no fluorescent endoneural cells could be found, the dorsal root ganglion cells being the first cells showing specific staining.

Apart from rabies and B virus (simian herpes) infections of man after monkey bites, no examples of neural spread have been established in natural human infections. However, transmission in the reverse direction, from the dorsal root ganglia down the corresponding peripheral nerves, appears to be the most likely mode of spread of virus in herpes zoster and recurrent herpes simplex.

2.8.3. PRODUCTION OF DISEASE

Cytocidal infections of neuronal cells, whether due to poliovirus, a togavirus, or a herpesvirus, are characterized by the three hallmarks of encephalitis: cell necrosis, phagocytosis by glial cells (neuronophagia), and perivascular infiltration of inflammatory cells, which is an expression of cell-mediated immunity. The cause of symptoms in other CNS infections is more obscure. Rabies virus is noncytocidal in cultured cells; in infected animals it evokes none of the inflammatory reactions of cell necrosis found in the encephalitides, yet it is highly lethal for most species of animal. With some other viruses, infection of neurons causes no symptoms; for example, the extensive CNS infection of mice congenitally infected with lymphocytic choriomeningitis virus, readily demonstrable by fluorescent antibody staining, has no deleterious effect. Still other changes are produced by some of the viruses that cause slowly progressive diseases of the CNS (see below). In scrapie of sheep, for example, there is slow neuronal degeneration and vacuolization; in visna (another chronic disease of sheep), changes in cell membranes lead to demyelinization.

Post-infection encephalitis is most commonly seen after smallpox vaccination and measles. The pathological picture is predominantly demyelinization without neuronal degeneration – changes unlike those produced by the direct action of viruses on the CNS. Allied with the failure to recover virus from the brain, this has led to the view that post-infection encephalitis is probably an autoimmune disease.

2.8.4. CONGENITAL INFECTIONS

Oncovirus infections of chickens and rodents persist in these species by the congenital transfer of the viral genome, which is integrated into the chromosomes of the host's cells as a DNA copy of the viral RNA. In addition, viremia in the mother may be followed by congenital transfer of virions in these as well as in a variety of other infections (Table 7). Congenital infection may occur at any stage from the development of the ovum up to birth. With noncytocidal viruses, like lymphocytic choriomeningitis in mice, every cell in the embryo's body may be infected.

In severe acute viral infections (e.g. smallpox), congenital infection usually causes fetal death and abortion. More important are the viruses which do not kill the embryo but

TABLE 7. *Congenital Viral Infections (from Fenner and White, 1976)*

Syndrome	Disease	Host
Fetal death and abortion	Smallpox	Man
	Bluetongue vaccine	Sheep
Severe neonatal disease	Cytomegalovirus	Man
	Rubella	Man
Congenital defects	Rubella	Man
	Hog cholera vaccine	Pig
Inapparent, with lifelong carrier state	Lymphocytic choriomeningitis	Mouse
Inapparent, with integrated viral genome	Murine leukemia	Mouse
	Avian leukosis	Chicken

produce congenital malformations due to interference with the normal development of particular organs or tissues.

By far the most detailed observations on congenital defects are those made on human infants whose mothers were infected with rubella virus early in pregnancy. A variety of abnormalities has been recognized, of which the most severe are deafness, blindness and congenital heart and brain defects. These defects may only be recognized after the birth of an apparently healthy baby, or they may be associated with severe neonatal disease — hepatosplenomegaly, purpura and jaundice — to comprise the 'rubella syndrome'.

Little is known of the pathogenesis of congenital abnormalities in rubella. Damage occurs mainly in fetuses infected during the first trimester. Immunological tolerance does not develop; children who have contracted rubella *in utero* display high titers of neutralizing antibodies throughout their lives. Usually, in the infected human fetus, as in most types of cultured cells, rubella virus is relatively noncytocidal; few inflammatory or necrotic changes are found. The retarded growth in rubella-infected infants may be due to slowing of cell division leading to the reduced numbers of cells observed in many of their organs. Apart from rare activation of latent infections, disease due to the cytomegaloviruses usually results from infection acquired congenitally from mothers suffering an inapparent infection during pregnancy. Virus-infected cells are present in the chorionic villi. The important clinical features in neonates include hepatosplenomegaly, thrombocytopenic purpura, hepatitis and jaundice, microcephaly and mental retardation.

2.9. IMMUNOPATHOLOGY

In certain viral infections it is clear that the immune response itself is a major factor in causing pathological changes and, hence, disease. A good example is lymphocytic choriomeningitis (LCM) virus, which is lethal for untreated adult mice but nonpathogenic in the absence of an immune response. Thus, mice infected as adults can be protected by X-irradiation, neonatal thymectomy, antilymphocyte serum, or other immunosuppressive treatments, despite the fact that viral growth is similar in normal and immunosuppressed animals. In normal adult mice the cell-mediated immune response to LCM infection, though beneficial in eliminating virus from organs such as lung, liver and spleen, is also responsible for lethal inflammatory changes in the brain. Adoptive transfer of immune T cells has been shown to induce lesions in the chorioid plexus and meninges in adult mice infected with LCM virus and immunosuppressed with cyclophosphamide treatment. Recipients of immune T cells do not produce significant amounts of antibody before dying of classic LCM disease, thus suggesting that cell-mediated immunity rather than humoral factors is responsible. Further, T cells cytotoxic for LCM-infected target cells *in vitro* can be isolated from the cerebrospinal fluid of moribund mice, and levels of such T cells in the spleen are maximal at the time of onset of the lethal disease.

In other situations, the humoral immune responses to LCM virus can be pathogenic. Mice infected neonatally or *in utero* show immunological tolerance (see below) with lifelong and widespread infection of tissues, but their tolerance is incomplete. Throughout life, small amounts of antibody are produced which react with virus in the blood to form 'immune complexes', and these are precipitated out in kidney glomeruli, eventually causing glomerulonephritis. Antibody can be eluted from glomeruli, and treatments that increase or decrease antibody formation will increase or decrease the severity of glomerulonephritis. Glomerulonephritis (and arteritis) due to such immune complexes is important in several other persistent infections.

When certain classes of antibodies react with antigens on the surface of infected cells, fixation of complement can lead to cell lysis. This has been shown to occur *in vitro*, not only with LCM but with a number of other noncytopathic and cytopathic viral infections. There is no clear evidence about the part played by such reactions in the infected host, but activation of complement would result in the release of mediators of inflammation and thus cause pathological changes.

The immune response has been invoked as a major cause of pathological changes in many other viral infections, though the evidence is generally less complete than with the LCM model system. For example, there are good reasons for supposing that the T cell-mediated response to measles infection is responsible not only for recovery from the disease but also for the measles rash. On infection with measles virus, patients with a defective T cell response due to various lymphoreticular tumors with or without associated immunosuppressive chemotherapy, or with thymic aplasia, may show progressive growth of virus in the lungs leading to a fatal 'giant cell pneumonia', but no rash. Presumably the measles rash in normal children results from T cell-mediated cytolysis of virus-infected cells in the skin or capillary endothelium, and heralds recovery because these cells are destroyed immunologically before they have had time to yield large numbers of new virions.

Killed measles virus vaccines, now no longer used, were found to elicit the formation of circulating antibodies rather than cell-mediated immunity, and on subsequent infection with live virus there were unusual lesions in the skin and lungs, presumably immunopathological in nature. There was a similar experience with an experimental inactivated respiratory syncytial viral vaccine. It is likely that immunopathological mechanisms contribute to other viral diseases, such as dengue hemorrhagic fever, viral diseases of the central nervous system, and respiratory syncytial viral bronchiolitis in infants infected while they have maternal antibody.

The balance between the humoral and the cell-mediated immune responses to a viral infection (or between the numbers of immune B and T cells respectively) probably plays a key role in both recovery and pathogenesis. Recovery often depends on one, rather than the other, arm of the immune response. Elucidation of the types of experimental manipulation favouring either type of response may introduce a new era of 'immunological engineering' that will make vaccines more effective, and at the same time increase our understanding of viral immunopathology.

2.10. IMMUNODEPRESSION BY VIRUSES

It has long been known that when tuberculin-positive individuals suffer from measles, they temporarily become tuberculin-negative, and studies of Eskimos in Greenland have shown that measles exacerbates pre-existing tuberculosis. Cultured human T lymphocytes will support the growth of measles virus, and such infected cells fail to respond to tuberculin, like lymphocytes taken from individuals rendered temporarily tuberculin-negative by measles.

Direct tests for immune function have shown that several other viral infections influence the immune responses. Immunodepression is seen, for instance, in mice infected with leukemia viruses, cytomegalovirus, lymphocytic choriomeningitis virus and in chickens with Marek's disease or avian leukosis. The reduced response is to unrelated antigens, and is thus distinct from the immunologically specific effect seen in tolerance. Most reports deal with depressed antibody responses. Cell-mediated immunity is more difficult to measure, but delayed skin graft rejection has been described in mice infected with leukemia and lactic dehydrogenase viruses. Human patients with leukemia, lymphomas, or Hodgkin's disease, diseases which may be caused by viruses, usually exhibit immunodepression even in the absence of treatment with cytotoxic drugs, but one must be cautious about too facile an interpretation of this observation.

The mechanism of immunodepression is not understood, but probably results from the multiplication of virus in lymphocytes and/or macrophages. Many viruses are capable of replication in macrophages, and several viruses have now been shown to grow in T cells which have been stimulated by mitogens (concanavalin A or phytohemagglutinin) to divide *in vitro*, while a few others have been grown in cultured B cells. The immune responses are depressed, but not abolished, and individual lymphocytes infected with murine leukemia virus, for instance, can at the same time produce antibody to sheep red cells.

Immunodepression by infectious agents is not restricted to viruses; it has been demonstrated in several nonviral infections including leprosy, malaria and leishmaniasis.

2.11. NON-IMMUNOLOGICAL RESISTANCE

Many physiological responses other than the immune response affect the resistance of animals to viral infections. Our knowledge of these is sketchy; here we shall do little more than mention the existence of some factors and discuss briefly those for which there is more precise information.

2.11.1. PHAGOCYTOSIS

Polymorphs play no part in protection against viral infections, but macrophages, particularly the 'fixed' macrophages of the reticuloendothelial system, are very important in pathogenesis. Several organs (liver, spleen, bone marrow) contain blood sinuses which are partially or completely lined by macrophages and similar phagocytic cells which monitor the lymph, the pleural and peritoneal cavities, the respiratory tract, and the connective tissue throughout the body. Macrophages play an important role in clearing viruses from the bloodstream and preventing the infection of susceptible cells in target organs.

However some viruses, rather than being digested by the macrophages that ingest them, actually multiply preferentially in these cells. Indeed, circulating macrophages (the monocytes of the blood) may transport replicating viruses around the body as a cell-associated viremia, so helping to disseminate the infection. On the other hand, infected macrophages produce substantial amounts of interferon and thus protect susceptible cells from infection. They also appear to be important in the process of recovery from infection which is triggered by immune T cells, as described below.

2.11.2. INTERFERON

Interferon produced during the course of a viral infection protects some cells from infection, especially locally but perhaps also in distant target organs (Fig. 7). However, it has proved difficult to devise decisive experiments to evaluate the importance of these effects in promoting recovery, since there are no known naturally occurring diseases of man or animals in which there is a specific defect in interferon production. However, there is much circumstantial evidence that interferon is important in recovery from viral infection. Decreased interferon production caused by altered temperature, chemical inhibitors, or different viral strains has been correlated with impaired recovery, but the situation is often complex. The virulence of some viruses is associated with a weak interferon response, but in other instances there is no correlation. The responsiveness of infected cells to interferon

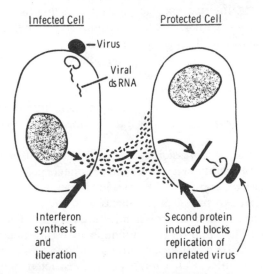

FIG. 7. Mechanisms of interferon production and action (from Mims, 1976).

action may be important. For example, mice of the C3HRV strain are much more resistant than C3H mice to flavivirus infections. Although both produce equal amounts of interferon, the cells of the resistant mice are more susceptible to the action of interferon, i.e. a genetic difference in interferon sensitivity rather than interferon production appears to determine the severity of infection. Several other 'nonspecific' factors involved in resistance may operate at least in part by their effects on interferon production; this appears to be the case with body temperature, with some types of stress, and with the effects of some hormones.

Despite the wealth of evidence (a) that interferon is produced as a by-product of most or all viral infections, and (b) that passively administered interferon can protect against certain viruses under limited experimental circumstances, there are some clinical observations which cast doubt on the primacy of the role of interferon in recovery from natural infections and at the same time temper optimism in relation to its possible therapeutic use. Neither natural infections with viruses nor immunization with live attenuated vaccines confers substantial protection against simultaneous or subsequent heterologous viral infections elsewhere in the body. Indeed, certain attenuated viruses can be combined to produce potent multivalent vaccines. Perhaps, under natural circumstances, interferon expedites recovery because transient high concentrations occur in the immediate vicinity of infected cells. It may be impossible, in terms of antiviral therapy, to produce enough interferon in the right place at the right time.

2.11.3. Body Temperature

Environmental temperature, and the level of endogenous temperature achieved during the febrile response, affect the multiplication of some viruses. Fever usually develops at the end of the incubation period, when the distribution of virus throughout the body has been completed. It may be an important protective mechanism in promoting recovery by limiting further viral multiplication.

Elevated body temperature promotes viral multiplication in the production of recurrent herpes simplex ('fever blisters') in man. Artificially induced fever precipitates an attack of herpes simplex in about 50 per cent of cases. Moreover, fever blisters are a frequent complication of some febrile diseases (malaria, influenza, streptococcal and pneumococcal infections), but are very rarely found in others (tuberculosis, smallpox, typhoid fever).

2.11.4. Other Non-immunological Factors

Several other nonspecific factors play a role in both susceptibility to viral infection and recovery. There is not space to do more than mention them: hormones (especially the corticosteriods), nutritional deficiencies, stress, trauma, concurrent infection and age of the host animal. There are also important genetic factors acting at the species level, usually associated with the presence or absence of specific cellular receptors; or within species, via the I_r (immune response) genes.

2.12. RECOVERY FROM VIRAL INFECTION

In the past, the significance of the immune response of the infected host has been largely assessed in terms of acquired immunity to reinfection, in which antibody plays the key role. Viral vaccines are designed to generate such antibodies. Less attention has been paid to the role of the immune response in *recovery* from viral infections. The coincidence in time between recovery and the appearance of circulating antibodies, and the protection conferred by 'passive immunization' with antiserum given during the incubation period of measles, originally led immunologists to believe that the humoral response was important in promoting recovery. However, the natural experiment of human dysgammaglobulinemia has cast doubt on the importance of antibodies in recovery from viral infection. Though subjects with such B cell deficiencies suffer from recurrent and intractable bacterial infections, which can be partially controlled by the administration of γ-globulin, they recover from viral infections in a normal fashion in spite of very low levels of γ-globulin and often no detectable production of specific antibodies. By contrast children with congenital or acquired T cell deficiencies are known to be extremely vulnerable to viral infections and often succumb to otherwise trivial diseases such as measles, varicella or cytomegalovirus infection.

The respective roles of antibodies, T cells, macrophages and interferon in recovery from viral infections have been the focus of much recent research in animals and cell culture.

2.12.1. Antibody

Experiments in which the immunological responsiveness of animals is totally suppressed by irradiation or cytotoxic drugs, then selectively restored by administration of antibody, reveal that viruses which produce systemic diseases with a plasma viremia can be controlled by antibody. For example, if adult mice that have been inoculated with coxsackievirus or yellow fever virus are treated with cyclophosphamide, which greatly reduces antibody production, they die from infections that cause no symptoms in untreated animals. Passive immunization with specific antibody as late as 2–4 days after infection prevents the death of such immunosuppressed mice. Neonatal thymectomy, which suppresses T cell-mediated immunity, does not increase the susceptibility of mice to enterovirus infections, suggesting that this immune response plays only a minor role in recovery from these infections. Likewise, children with severe hypogammaglobulinemia, but intact cell-mediated immunity, are more liable to develop paralytic poliomyelitis after exposure to vaccine strains than are normal children.

Restoration experiments with secretory IgA in respiratory virus infections are difficult to carry out. However, since antilymphocyte serum has no detectable effect on the pathogenicity for mice of either influenza or parainfluenza viruses, antibodies available on the epithelial surfaces (i.e. secretory antibody) probably play a role in recovery.

Although attention is usually concentrated on the effects of neutralizing antibodies in relation to recovery, other kinds of antibody may also be important. For example, antibody directed against any viral antigen present in infected tissues could, by forming immune complexes, induce the inflammatory infiltrates that lead to an antiviral effect. Conceivably antibody, cell-mediated immunity, and interferon each play a part in recovery from all viral infections, although their relative importance may vary considerably in different situations.

2.12.2. T Cell-mediated Immunity

There is ample evidence that viruses elicit 'cell-mediated' immunity (CMI). This is demonstrable by delayed hypersensitivity following intradermal injection of viral antigens into a previously infected animal, including man; the capacity to respond in this way is transferable by lymphocytes but not by serum. T cell-mediated immunity is largely abrogated by neonatal thymectomy and treatment with antilymphocyte (or better still, in mice, anti-θ serum. Such treatments greatly aggravate infections of mice due to herpesviruses and poxviruses, but have little effect on enterovirus or togavirus infections (Table 8).

Restoration experiments confirm the importance of T cell-mediated immunity in recovery from systemic infections in which viremia is cell-associated. For example, mice infected with sublethal doses of ectromelia virus (a poxvirus) died if they were treated with antilymphocyte or anti-θ serum, apparently as a result of the uncontrolled growth of virus in the liver. Antilymphocyte serum suppresses the CMI response, but not the antibody or interferon responses to ectromelia virus. Transfer of immune splenic lymphocytes to mice infected one day earlier with ectromelia virus caused striking inhibition of viral growth and a fall in viral titer in target organs, the liver and spleen. This protective effect was greatly reduced when transfused cells were first treated with anti-θ serum plus complement, which kills T, but not B,

TABLE 8. *The Effects of Depletion of T or B Lymphocytes on Recovery from Various Viral Infections (from Fenner and White, 1976)*

Animal	Immunodeficiency	Lymphocytes involved	Infections aggravated	Infections unaffected
Man	Hypogammaglobulinemia with intact CMI	B	Paralytic poliomyelitis	Smallpox vaccination
	Deficient CMI (with or without normal immunoglobulins)	T	Vaccinia Herpes simplex Varicella-zoster Cytomegalovirus Measles	
Mouse	Suppression of antibody by cyclophosphamide	B	Coxsackievirus B	
Mouse	Impairment of CMI by neonatal thymectomy or antilymphocyte (or anti-theta) serum	T	Herpes simplex Mousepox Vaccinia	Influenza Sendai Yellow fever

lymphocytes. The recipients of the immune cells did not develop detectable antibody. When mouse hyperimmune antiectromelia serum was transfused, antibody reached a high titer in recipients (far higher than that achieved in a normal primary response), and there was some inhibition of viral growth, but no fall in viral titer such as is produced by transfer of immune cells. Passively administered interferon had no effect. Prior irradiation of recipients markedly impaired the antiviral effects of immune cells or hyperimmune serum, probably by inactivating radiosensitive precursors of blood monocytes (macrophages), since in unir-radiated recipients monocyte invasion of virus-infected foci in the liver coincided with elimination of the virus. This train of experimental evidence shows that 'sensitized' (i.e. immune) T cells are the primary agents of the antiviral effect and the macrophages collaborate with them in the recovery process.

Several mechanisms have been postulated to account for the antiviral effects of sensitized T cells. By liberating lymphokines on exposure to antigens in tissues, they induce the migration and activation of macrophages which, perhaps with the help of opsonizing antibody, phagocytose and digest virions and infected cell debris. Further, sensitized T cells that encounter intact infected cells which bear virus-induced antigens on their surface kill such cells before virus is liberated; such T cell-mediated lysis has been demonstrated *in vitro* with several viruses. Finally, sensitized lymphocytes may liberate interferon on exposure to antigen, and in some infections this could have a significant local antiviral effect.

Thus, T cell-mediated immunity plays a central role in recovery from at least some viral infections, especially those generalized infections in which infected cells display virus-induced antigens on their surfaces.

2.13. PERSISTENT INFECTIONS

In the acute febrile infections that have been described so far, the causative virus enters the body, multiplies in one or more tissues, and spreads either locally or through the bloodstream. When viral multiplication has reached a critical level, after an incubation period of 2 days to 2 or 3 weeks, symptoms of disease appear, associated with localized or widespread tissue damage. Nonspecific and specific host defenses are mobilized during the incubation period and, unless the disease is fatal, the host has usually eliminated the infecting agent within 2 or 3 weeks of the onset of symptoms. Virus can ordinarily be isolated from the blood or secretions only in the short period just before and just after the appearance of symptoms. Some viruses (e.g. measles and smallpox in man) almost always cause acute disease; many others produce acute *infections* in which the pathogenic mechanisms are similar but often there is no clinical *disease*, i.e. the infection is *subclinical* (see Table 9).

Quite distinct from the acute infections, however, are those in which virus persists for months or years, i.e. *persistent viral infections*. Persistent infections are associated with a

TABLE 9. *Ratio of Subclinical to Clinical Infections in Some Viral Diseases of Man (from Evans, 1976)*

Virus	Clinical feature	Age at infection	Estimated subclinical/ clinical ratio	Percent of infection with clinical features
Poliomyelitis	Paralysis	Child	± 1000:1	0.1–1
Epstein–Barr	Heterophil-positive infectious mononucleosis	1–5	> 100:1	1
		6–15	10–100:1	1–10
		16–25	2–3:1	50–75
Infectious hepatitis	Jaundice	< 5	20:1	5
		5–9	11:1	10
		10–15	7:1	14
		Adult	2–3:1	50–75
Rubella	Rash	5–20	2:1	50
Influenza	Fever, cough	Young adult	1.5:1	60
Measles	Rash, fever	5–20	1:99	99+
Rabies	CNS symptoms	Any age	0:100	100

great variety of pathogenic mechanisms and clinical manifestations, and it is difficult to classify them satisfactorily. Because of this we shall have to draw rather heavily on experimental and natural infections in animals, as well as on observations made in human diseases. For convenience, we shall subdivide the persistent infections into three categories, recognizing that there is some overlap.

1. Persistent infections with intermittent acute episodes of disease between which virus is usually not demonstrable: *latent infections.* The important examples of these are herpes simplex and varicella-zoster, in each of which the causative virus persists in a latent state in association with sensory nerve ganglia, and may periodically, or after a long interval, be activated and produce symptoms (recurrent cold sores or shingles, respectively; see Fig. 8).

2. Persistent infections in which virus is always demonstrable and often shed, but disease is either absent, or is associated with immunopathological disturbances: *chronic infections.* Several other herpesvirus infections fall into this category, e.g. cytomegalovirus and E. B. virus; as does the virus of hepatitis B and, to some extent, rubella in infants infected *in utero.*

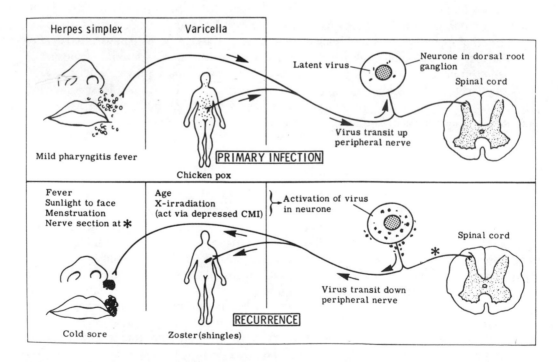

FIG. 8. Mechanisms of latent infection in man: herpes simplex and varicella-zoster (from Mims, 1976).

3. Persistent infections with a long incubation period followed by slowly progressive disease that is usually lethal: *slow infections*. This class includes three important but rare human diseases: kuru and Creutzfeld–Jacob disease, subacute sclerosing panencephalitis (measles virus) and progressive multifocal leukoencephalopathy (human papovavirus.)

The key distinctions between these three groups of persistent infections are illustrated diagrammatically in Fig. 9. In slow infections, the concentration of virus in the body builds up gradually over a prolonged period until disease finally becomes manifest. Chronic infections, on the other hand, can be regarded as acute infections (clinical or subclinical) following which the host fails to reject the virus; sometimes disease supervenes late in life as a result of an immunopathological or neoplastic complication. The distinction between chronic infections and latent infections, e.g. herpesviruses between recrudescences of endogenous disease, may be a fundamental one concerned with the state of the virus between attacks, or it may be merely a matter of the ease of demonstration of infectious virus.

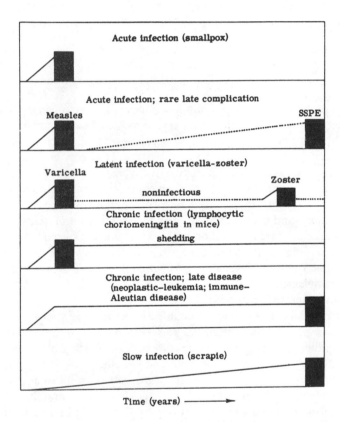

Fig. 9. Diagram illustrating acute infection, and various kinds of persistent infections. Solid line, demonstrable infectious virus; dotted line, virus not readily demonstrable; box, disease episode (from Fenner and White, 1976).

2.13.1. THE PATHOGENESIS OF PERSISTENT INFECTIONS

Several mechanisms appear to be involved in determining whether a viral infection will follow an acute course with complete recovery and immunity to re-infection, or persist. Some factors involve the virus, others the host defense mechanisms.

2.13.2. UNIQUE PROPERTIES OF THE VIRUS

Non-immunogenic "viroids". The unknown agents that cause kuru and Creutzfeld–Jacob disease seem to be completely non-immunogenic, they fail to induce interferon, and they are not demonstrably susceptible to interferon action. There appears to be no mechanism whereby the host can control the multiplication and pathological effects of these agents.

2.13.3. INTEGRATED GENOMES

RNA tumor viruses persist as DNA copies of their genomes integrated into cellular genomes. Until activated, the viral genome is only partially expressed, if at all, and it can be regarded as part of the cellular genetic material. When activated, the RNA tumor viruses multiply in lymphoid tissue and induce the production of non-neutralizing, rather than neutralizing, antibodies.

Among DNA viruses, the papovavirus of progressive multifocal leukoencephalopathy may well persist as an integrated genome until it is activated. Among the herpesviruses, those associated with or thought to be associated with malignancies probably persist as integrated, perhaps defective, genomes. The state in which herpes simplex, varicella-zoster, cytomegalovirus and EB virus persist intracellularly during prolonged latent infections is unknown, but integration (of complete genomes) is a likely possibility.

The strains of virus responsible for several of the persistent infections of animals or cultured cells with 'orthodox' viruses have turned out to be ts mutants, although most ts mutants do not cause persistent infections. The significance of this discovery has yet to be determined.

2.13.4. INADEQUATE HOST DEFENSES

Growth in protected sites. Herpes simplex virus and varicella virus avoid immune elimination by remaining within cells of the nervous system, in an occult form in the ganglion cells during the intervals between disease episodes, and within the Schwann cells of the nerve sheaths prior to acute recurrent episodes of disease. Likewise, other herpesviruses such as human cytomegalovirus and EB virus appear to bypass immune elimination, but in this instance they persist in lymphocytes. Other viruses grow in cells in epithelial surfaces, e.g. kidney tubules, salivary gland, or mammary gland, and are persistently shed in the appropriate secretions and excretions. Most such viruses are not acutely cytopathogenic and, perhaps because they are released on the lumenal borders of cells, they do not provoke an immunological inflammatory reaction, hence the cells are not destroyed by T lymphocytes or macrophages. Secretory IgA, which does have access to the infected cells, does not cause complement activation and therefore fails to induce complement-mediated cytolysis or an inflammatory response.

Growth in macrophages. In many chronic infections the virus appears to grow mainly in lymphoid tissue, especially in macrophages. This may have two effects relevant to persistence: (a) modification of the antibody response, and (b) impairment of the phagocytic and cytotoxic potential of the reticuloendothelial system.

Non-neutralizing antibodies. Viruses that cause persistent plasma-associated viremia usually multiply in lymphoid tissue and macrophages (see above) and they characteristically induce production of non-neutralizing antibodies. These antibodies combine with viral antigens and virions in the serum to form 'immune complexes' which may (a) produce 'immune complex disease' and (b) block immune cytolysis of virus-infected target cells by T lymphocytes or complement-fixing antibodies.

Tolerance. Many persistent infections are associated with a very weak antibody response, especially in congenitally infected animals. Immunological tolerance is rarely complete, but there is a severe degree of specific hyporeactivity in conditions like congenital lymphocytic choriomeningitis and retrovirus infections. Tolerance to a viral antigen may be genetically determined, and the immune response to several specific antigens has been shown to be under genetic control.

Another kind of 'tolerance', about which very little information is available, is what might be called 'interferon-tolerance'. Little or no interferon is produced in mice congenitally infected with lymphocytic choriomeningitis, lactic dehydrogenase, or murine leukemia viruses, but in each case the causative virus is sensitive to interferon. Interferon 'tolerance' appears to be specific to the virus involved, possibly involving a recognition mechanism at the messenger RNA level. Experiments with varicella cast doubt on the suggestion that low interferon production and low sensitivity are invariably characteristics of viruses that produce persistent infections, but this would hardly be expected in such a diverse group.

Defective cell-mediated immunity. Persistent infections could be caused by partial suppression of the host's CMI response, as a result of any one or combination of several factors: immunodepression by the causative virus, immunological tolerance, the presence of 'blocking' antibodies or virus–antibody complexes, failure of immune lymphocytes to reach target cells, or inadequate expression of viral antigens on the surface of the target cell. These factors are probably important in persistent infections such as visna, subacute sclerosing panencephalitis and progressive multifocal leukoencephalopathy, and in those caused by herpesviruses. Finally, we may again note that many persistent viruses multiply extensively in macrophages and lymphocytes, and thus affect several parameters of the immune response. Indeed, depressed CMI may diminish the rate of destruction of infected cells and thereby prolong the release of viral antigens. The resulting protracted immunogenic stimulus would explain the very high antibody levels found in subacute sclerosing panencephalitis and Aleutian disease of mink, for example, which may produce a cascade effect by blocking the already inadequate T cell defenses.

2.14. THE SIGNIFICANCE OF THE INCUBATION PERIOD

The incubation period of an infectious disease is the period that elapses between infection and the first manifestation of symptoms. Consideration of the mode of spread of viruses within the infected animal, set out earlier in this article, allows us to make some generalizations about the incubation period in natural infections (Table 10). It will tend to be short in diseases in which the symptoms are entirely due to viral multiplication at the portal of entry. Thus, respiratory viruses produce symptoms by virtue of their multiplication in the upper and/or lower respiratory tract and hence have short incubation periods (1–3 days). On the other hand, the incubation period will be relatively long (10–20 days) in generalized infections, like the common childhood exanthemata, measles, chickenpox and rubella, where the virus spreads in stepwise fashion through the body before reaching the target organ in which symptoms are produced.

TABLE 10. *Epidemiological Features of Some Common Human Viral Diseases (from Fenner and White,*
1976)

Disease	Mode of transmission	Incubation period* (days)	Period of communicability†	Incidence of subclinical infections‡
Influenza	Respiratory	1–2	Short	Moderate
Common cold	Respiratory	1–3	Short	Moderate
Bronchiolitis, croup	Respiratory	3–5	Short	Moderate
A.R.D. (adenovirus)	Respiratory	5–7	Short	Moderate
Dengue	Mosquito bite	5–8	Short	Moderate
Herpes simplex	Salivary	5–8	Long	Moderate
Enteroviruses	Alimentary	6–12	Long	High
Poliomyelitis	Alimentary	5–20	Long	High
Measles	Respiratory	9–12	Moderate	Low
Smallpox	Respiratory	12–14	Moderate	Low
Chickenpox	Respiratory	13–17	Moderate	Moderate
Mumps	Respiratory	16–20	Moderate	Moderate
Rubella	Respiratory	17–20	Moderate	Moderate
Mononucleosis	Salivary	30–50	? Long	High
Hepatitis A	Alimentary	15–40	Long	High
Hepatitis B	Inoculation	50–150	Very long	High
Rabies	Animal bite	30–100	Nil	Nil
Warts	Contact	50–150	Long	Low

* Until first appearance of prodromal symptoms. Diagnostic signs, e.g. rash or paralysis may not appear until 2–4 days later.

† Most viral diseases are highly transmissible for a few days before symptoms appear. Long = > 10 days; short = < 4 days.

‡ High = > 90 per cent; low = < 10 per cent.

Other factors also influence the length of the incubation period. The generalized infections produced by togaviruses may have an unexpectedly short incubation period attributable to the direct intravenous injection by an insect of a rapidly multiplying virus. Conversely, the long incubation periods of some localized infections like warts and molluscum contagiosum are presumably due to slow multiplication of the viruses concerned. An extreme, but poorly understood, case is that of the so-called *slow virus infections* and the viral leukemias, where the virus-cell interaction is initially noncytocidal and symptoms may not appear for many months or even years after infection.

REFERENCES

As in the previous chapter, this one embraces a field that is basic to planning antiviral chemotherapy but is not about chemotherapy. It is impossible to provide adequate references; instead the interested reader is referred to Mims (1976) for an excellent extended account of the subject and to Fenner *et al.* (1974) for detailed references.

FENNER, F. and WHITE, D. O. (1976) *Medical Virology.* (2nd Edn) Academic Press, New York.

FENNER, F., McAUSLAN, B. R., MIMS, C. A., SAMBROOK, J. F. and WHITE, D. O. (1974) *The Biology of Animal Viruses.* (2nd Edn) Academic Press, New York.

MIMS, C. A. (1976) *The Pathogenesis of Infectious Disease.* Academic Press, London.

EVANS, A. S. (ed.) (1976) *Viral Infections of Humans, Epidemiology and Control,* Plenum, New York.

CHAPTER 3

DIAGNOSIS OF VIRAL DISEASE AND THE ADVENT OF ANTIVIRAL DRUGS

ERNEST C. HERRMANN, Jr. and JUDITH A. HERRMANN

Department of Basic Sciences, Peoria School of Medicine, University of Illinois and Mobilab, Inc.,
Peoria, Illinois, USA

CONTENTS

3.1. INTRODUCTION

The data are substantial; there are an array of substances that inhibit viral multiplication without causing harm to the host. Antiviral drugs are widely available; therefore, it requires no great courage to predict that in the near future additional antiviral drugs will be produced and their proper use will often depend on knowledge of the virus causing the disease.

At present it may not be obvious that laboratory diagnosis should go hand in hand with the few antiviral drugs now available. Indeed, viral diagnostic laboratories are not always readily accessible to most medical practitioners. In contrast, bacteriological diagnostic laboratories were widely available even prior to the advent of antibacterial drugs. Yet, it is commonly held that there are many times more viral-induced diseases (albeit, often mild and self-limiting) than bacterial diseases. Routine diagnosis of the viral diseases seems, therefore, to be overdue; especially since such diagnosis would provide an invaluable foundation for the future rational use of antiviral drugs.

In that antiviral drugs and viral diagnostic laboratories currently seem to touch lightly on the routine practice of medicine, there is little prior experience on which to base predictions. The following discussion will, therefore, require a significant degree of conjecture about how medicine might be practiced when antiviral drugs are commonplace. It would be foolhardy to presume that in the future the use of antiviral drugs will always be based on a sound diagnosis, any more than is true today with the use of antibacterial agents. It must be acknowledged, however, that certain viral diseases can be rather firmly diagnosed on clinical and epidemiological grounds alone. We will not, therefore, take the unrealistic position that all viral disease must be diagnosed in the laboratory; indeed, it is more likely that in the foreseeable future few of the milder and self-limiting viral diseases will result in a laboratory diagnosis. We will, nonetheless, review human viral diseases and the problems of practical laboratory diagnosis. Predictions as to the nature and use of future antiviral drugs will at times require certain flights of fancy.

3.2. THE PRESENT

3.2.1. Laboratory Diagnosis of Viral Disease

Let us assume that chemotherapeutic drugs are available for all virus diseases that can presently be diagnosed in the laboratory. Would present diagnostic procedures be adequate? Let us further assume that viral diseases are handled in a manner similar to bacterial diseases; that is, an infected patient visits a physician, a hospital or a clinic, and ideally a specimen is taken and sent to the laboratory. A pathogen is isolated, a presumptive identification of the type of organism is made, confirming tests and, in some cases, a drug-sensitivity test is undertaken. In the meantime, the patient is frequently started on a course of chemotherapy based on a number of factors such as the degree of illness, some distinctive clinical signs and symptoms, or simply on whimsy or intuition. Such treatment may be stopped or altered on the basis of laboratory results. This is a one-on-one situation, one patient at a time, perhaps with slight regard for the infections that are prevalent in the general population, for such information is not always available to the physician.

In making comparisons of viral diagnostic methods to those in bacteriology, it is often assumed that the latter are very rapid and results are available within 24 hr. This is frequently not the case. When antibacterial sensitivity tests are required, results cannot be reported sooner than 48 hr after submission of the specimen. Too frequently, all bacterial diagnosis is equated with the rapid isolation of beta hemolytic streptococci, but defining whether the isolate is *Streptococcus pyogenes*, the more pathogenic streptococcus belonging to Lancefield group A, takes additional time. In bacterial diagnosis a presumptive rapid report can sometimes be made based on stained smears of specimens prior to cultivation of the organism, but it is not often appreciated that frequently cultivation and identification of a specific bacterial pathogen can take considerable time. Generally, then, how do present virological methods compare to such bacteriological methods? As will be discussed, in certain cases they compare rather well, but in many cases not so well if viewed in the classical medical situation just described.

3.2.1.1. Virus Detection

More human viruses can be detected more quickly by the use of cell cultures than by any other method and this is based on observing a viral cytopathogenic effect or virus induced adsorption to or agglutination of red blood cells. Ninety-seven per cent of virus diagnostic laboratories surveyed in the United States and Canada isolate viruses in cell cultures, and over 25 per cent use this approach exclusively (Herrmann and Herrmann, 1976a). Such a fact is not obvious from the published papers devoted to viral diagnosis that seem overwhelmingly to emphasize serological methods. But are cell-culture methods adequate if an antiviral agent is to be used?

Table 1 presents the experience in isolating more than 5000 viruses in cell culture. The data suggest that under optimal conditions, using specimens rich in virus, many viruses are detected after 1–2 days incubation, others in 3–4 days. Regrettably, conditions are rarely optimal. The quantity of virus in a specimen is often slight, so the time for isolating 50 per cent of the viruses is no less than 3 days and more frequently longer. Clearly this is not completely adequate if a physician wishes to treat a patient with a drug specific for an acute virus infection. In the overwhelming majority of viral infections, the laboratory data will be generated at a time when the patient is either well or recovering. The data in Table 1 are for the detection of a virus, the lengths of time do not include the time for specific viral identification, which could take weeks. The viral identification problem is not insurmountable, however, for in many cases the virus need not be identified as to its specific serological type. One large comprehensive viral diagnostic laboratory serotypes few viral isolates (Smith, 1979) using an approach that will be discussed. It is clear, however, that cell-culture methods for detecting human viruses require considerable improvement. Further, 80 per cent of specimens produce no viral isolate, even from patients with viral-like illnesses.

TABLE 1. *Time for Detection and Reporting of Virus Isolates after Receipt of Specimen**

Virus	Earliest detection (days)	$\geqslant$ 50 per cent detection (days)	Isolates (No.)
HSV†	1(67)‡	3	1266
Cox.B	1(26)	3	428
Cox.A, T.C.	2(14)	4	66
ECHO	2(43)	4	400
Polio	2(8)	4	87
Influenza	2(46)	4	675
Adeno	2(61)	5	681
Rhino	2(13)	6	484
V–Z	3(5)	8	43
CMV	3(3)	11	49
Mumps	3(11)	6	254
PI	4(39)	8	702
Cox.A, mice	4(11)	10	196
RSV	5(14)	10	239

* Cell cultures were read thrice weekly.
† Abbreviations: HSV—herpes simplex; Cox.B—coxsackievirus type B; Cox.A—coxsackievirus type A; T.C.—isolated in tissue culture; ECHO—echovirus (enteric, cytopathic, human orphan virus); V–Z—varicella-zoster virus; CMV—cytomegalovirus; PI—parainfluenza virus; RSV—respiratory syncytial virus.
‡ Figures in parenthesis are number of isolates reported at this time.

But what about other viral diagnostic methods, how would they fare if subjected to the logistical problem of treatment of viral disease in routine medical practice? Any test that measures a rise in specific antibody using paired sera, that is, one blood sample taken at the acute stage of illness and a second taken 2–4 weeks later, could only rarely have any pertinence to drug treatment. Further, the measurement of antibodies requires specific viral antigens and since, for example, there are at least 70 such antigens for the enteroviruses and 120 for the rhinoviruses, the cumbersome nature of this system and its limitations become obvious. A similar problem exists in using fluorescent or other labeled antibodies to detect viruses either in specimens or in cell cultures. The fluorescent method can be rapid (1–2 hr) for diagnosing herpetic infections but less sensitive than viral isolation in cell cultures (Cho and Feng, 1978). The large number of serologically distinct viruses one might find on a throat swab (Table 2), for example, makes this method impractical for general use. Despite the fact

TABLE 2. *Antigenic Types of Viruses Isolated from the Human Upper Respiratory Tract, 1962–78*

Virus	Antigenic types* (No.)	Isolates (No.)
Adeno	7	681
Cox.A, T.C.	2	66
Cox.A, mice	?†	196
Cox.B	5	428
CMV	1	10
ECHO	16‡	300
HSV	2	666
Influenza	4	675
Mumps	1	254
PI	4	702
Polio	3	52
Rhino	?§	484
RSV	1	240

* Does not count closely related subtypes of a major antigenic group as for example the various subtypes of Hong Kong influenzavirus type A (Victoria, Texas, London, etc.).

† These isolates defined by typical mouse paralysis and not serotyped, 22 human serotypes are known in addition to types 9 and 16 which were isolated in cell cultures.

‡ A total of 33 human serotypes are known.

§ Not serotyped, defined by biochemical tests (sensitivity to a pH of 3 and resistance to chloroform), about 120 human serotypes are known.

that fluorescent-labeled antibody methods have been known for well over 20 years, they have been used in a limited way in the general diagnosis of viral disease. This may be due to the difficulty in obtaining commercially produced high-quality fluorescent antiserum specific for the bulk of human viruses. There is no doubt that with a very superior effort many viruses can be detected in human specimens, very rapidly, with use of fluorescent-labeled antibody (Gardner *et al.*, 1978). It is also very likely that methods using fluorescent antiserum will be replaced with the enzyme-linked immunosorbent assay (ELISA) (Engvall *et al.*, 1971; Engvall and Perlmann, 1972; Sarkkinen *et al.*, 1981). A number of 'kits' are now commercially available for detecting certain viruses or detecting early arising IgM antibody specific for some viruses (McIntosh *et al.*, 1980). Although there is an enormous popularity in the use of a variety of antigen–antibody test methods, for rapid viral diagnosis, as suggested by the number of published reports, there is also a concern. Whether the test uses a fluorescent or enzyme-labeled antigen or antibody or it is the counter-immunoelectrophoresis test or even the radioimmunoassay, all are based on antigen–antibody specificity. Such an approach seems unlikely to be able to cope with hundreds of virus serotypes encountered by a viral diagnostic laboratory. Clearly the greatest development and use for immunodiagnostic methods has been where a virus cannot readily be grown in cell cultures. It is suggested that many immunodiagnostic methods are developed and used in association with clinical research programs with emphasis on a single or limited number of viruses. This is a far different situation than that facing a comprehensive routine diagnostic laboratory.

There has been significant interest for many years in the use of the electron microscope (EM) for rapid diagnosis of viral disease and this interest has been much enhanced by the discovery of a variety of viruses in stools of patients with gastrointestinal upsets (Middleton *et al.*, 1977). None of these viruses detected by the EM can be routinely cultured in the laboratory. In addition the EM has played an important role in defining the A and B viruses causing hepatitis (Dane *et al.*, 1970; Feinstone *et al.*, 1973). Certainly the EM is a most valuable research tool in defining the nature of viruses infecting humans but its expense of installation and operation is far in excess of what should be paid for diagnosing the average viral infection. Also in most viral disease it is difficult to obtain sufficient virus for ready detection. Use of the electron microscope can detect herpes simplex virus in fresh vesicles but it cannot distinguish these from the virus of varicella-zoster, a distinction that can be important in a clinical diagnosis. But even with such problems it would seem worthwhile for the virus laboratory to at least share some limited time with others using the EM since in a few cases its potential for rapid diagnosis might lead to effective therapy. Recent data suggest, however, that the ELISA test is more sensitive for detecting adeno and rotaviruses than is the EM (Brandt *et al.*, 1981).

The so-called 'TORCH' test for IgM antibodies to herpes simplex, cytomegalo and rubella viruses (as well as toxoplasmosis) is available in kit form using the ELISA-test method. Measuring this early arising antibody has potential for early diagnosis but cleanly separating IgM antibody from other serum proteins was not an attractive procedure for the average virus laboratory. Now, however, the use of microtiter plates coated with antihuman IgG antibody (van Loon *et al.*, 1981) has made this test more attractive but largely directed at a limited newborn population. Even though measurement of IgM specific for many human viruses can be done it would likely require hundreds of tests to resolve many cases of pharyngitis, for example, not a likely prospect. Sensitive tests for viral specific IgM exist (Baumgarten, 1980) and can give a rapid diagnosis but in virtually all cases of herpes simplex or cytomegalovirus disease (Moseley *et al.*, 1981; McIntosh *et al.*, 1980; Schmidt *et al.*, 1980) virus isolation is superior. It is suggested that such tests then be an adjunct to virus isolation (Minnich and Ray, 1980). This would hardly seem to be the direction if expense of viral diagnosis is a concern, and considering the generally mild nature of most viral disease it is a concern (Herrmann and Herrmann, 1976a). It is noteworthy that many publications presenting a 'new' immunodiagnostic test for viral disease indicate how expensive is cell-culture virus isolation when compared to serological methods. Routinely, however, no such economic comparisons are made. It would seem, therefore, that practical considerations will, as in bacteriology, dictate that most viral diagnosis will involve isolation of the pathogen at a cost that need not be greater than bacterial diagnosis. Many types of immunodiagnostic tests likely will also be used because they are superior to cell culture, less expensive, or produce earlier information (permitting chemotherapy). Likely they will not be used as an adjunct but in limited and specific ways filling a need no other test provides. This is the present status, for example, of the rubella antibody-detection tests (Dendyel *et al.*, 1981) where the virus is still isolated with some difficulty.

3.2.1.2. Virus Identification

The definitive technique for identification of a virus isolate has long been its interaction with a known, specific antibody using a wide variety of test methods. It is the need for specific antibodies that can make this a time-consuming and expensive procedure. Is this entirely necessary? In many cases, it is not. Indeed, attempting to serotype one of the 120 rhinoviruses is an impossible task for a general virus diagnostic laboratory. The emphasis on serotyping viruses goes back to the hope of vaccines for controlling most viral disease, where the antigenic nature of a virus is important. What is its importance in chemotherapy? The vast number of serotypes of pneumococci or salmonella, for example, is of little importance to a chemotherapeutic attack on these bacteria (albeit, not always successful). Some may feel that use of amantadine and rimantadine, both of which are active only against influenza type A viruses and not type B, justifies serological identification. The fact that these two types of influenza viruses differ sharply in their sensitivity to amantadine establishes they are biochemically distinct and it is only incidental that they are also serologically different. Biochemical markers would likely be more useful in virus identification. Even the sensitivity to antiviral agents may be useful as a biochemical identification test.

The present serological methods do permit, after some effort, defining that one has at least isolated a certain type of human virus and if it proved to be an echovirus, for example, then a drug specific for echoviruses could be used. It is likely that by the time one has this added information, a drug would be all but useless. Likewise, if one defined a pathogenic bacterial isolate strictly according to *Bergey's Manual*, this information also would be too late for use in applying appropriate therapy, so some compromises are in order. What is required, of course, is identification that is pertinent to therapy. If one knows they are dealing with an echo, coxsackie or even a rhinovirus, all of which are picornaviruses, which have often been shown *in vitro* to be sensitive to the similar compounds, then a single drug might well be used on infections caused by any one of them. How might one presently recognize such viruses in general?

As explained elsewhere (Herrmann, 1970) the approach of the bacteriologist can be used. Three cell-culture systems represent the virologist's differential media since certain viruses produce a cytopathic effect or hemadsorption in certain cells and not others. The distinctive nature of the cytopathic effect, or the presence of hemagglutination or hemadsorption is analogous to the bacteriologist's use of colonial morphology. And, of course, the bacteriologist's biochemical tests have counterparts in virology; some viruses are sensitive to pH 3 and lipid solvents, others are sensitive to pH 3 only and still others are resistant to both. There are also specific viral inhibitors that can be used. But biochemical tests might well take more time than seems practical in guiding the use of a drug by a single physician on a single patient.

The nature of the cytopathic or hemadsorption effect and the cell type involved when coupled with other information can often give a better indication of which type of virus one has isolated. Knowing the type of specimen helps; fecal specimens will contain only certain types of viruses, dermal specimens will contain very limited types of viruses, etc. Taking into consideration the season of the year can be helpful; certain viruses are prevalent largely during the summer, others are prevalent in the winter and fall. The clinical picture cannot, of course, be ignored; some viruses induce distinctive illnesses or lesions, in some cases distinctive enough so that laboratory diagnosis is unnecessary.

This comprehensive approach to viral diagnosis has most certainly not been fully perfected and some mistakes in naming a viral isolate are made. Yet, in many cases, one can readily detect and recognize an echo, herpes simplex, coxsackie, adeno, parainfluenza, influenza, rhino, mumps or respiratory syncytial virus in cell culture. But mistakes can occur. For example, a coxsackie A9 virus could be called an echovirus. Presently, this is of little significance clinically and since they are both picornaviruses maybe it will also have no significance in drug usage in the future; if there is a drug available for use against all picornavirus disease.

Even if one reports a virus isolate on its first detection in cell culture and correctly guesses at its proper grouping, this in most cases will still not be rapid enough so that most patients can obtain useful drug treatment, that is, of course, if we are dealing with a typical situation found in routine medical practice, such as occurs with bacterial infections. All is not hopeless, however, for a combination of clinical observations and an epidemiological approach could go far in guiding the use of antiviral therapy and this will be discussed in detail in the following sections.

In discussing general viral diagnostic methods, it should be pointed out that there are certain well established and commonly found laboratory procedures that can be used to diagnose a few viral diseases. The use of the heterophile antibody test is one such procedure. Certainly this test could be a useful guide to potential treatment of infectious mononucleosis in that detection of the Epstein–Barr virus or its specific antibody is still beyond the average virus laboratory. Also the isolation of hepatitis A and B viruses for diagnostic purposes has not been achieved, but detection of the massive amounts of a portion of the hepatitis B virus is routinely done using blood of infected persons. This latter test could aid specific antiviral drug use, especially with the more chronic or carrier cases and more will be said of this later. Rubella also can be diagnosed within one week of the onset of the disease by a serology test and certain protective drug measures might be possible if a gravid female has been exposed to a rubella case. Mosquito-borne virus infections caused by a variety of viruses, including those of the togo group, are still best diagnosed by measuring antibody in paired sera. Here the diagnosis may be too late for chemotherapy for a single patient, but establishing that such a virus outbreak has occurred can well lead to drug treatment early in the course of other similar cases prior to a definitive diagnosis.

3.2.2. ANTIVIRAL DRUGS

Once a few antibacterial drugs had reached the market there was substantial publicity regarding the 'miracle drugs' with the awarding of a number of Nobel Prizes. No similar fanfare has accompanied the advent of the antiviral drugs (Barclay, 1977), yet a close look would convince one that all the scientific data are complete. From a scientific standpoint it has been proven that synthetic chemical substances, inhibitory to viruses, can be used to cure human disease caused by both RNA and DNA viruses (Bauer, 1977). Perhaps in an age of so many 'medical miracles' we have become blasé. There are no data establishing that the advent of antiviral agents, however, so far has caused an increased demand for laboratory viral diagnosis. It is suspected that when even more such drugs are available there should, however, be an increased demand since so often one hears the complaint, 'Why diagnose viral disease, you cannot treat it anyway?' Too frequently, of course, such undiagnosed infections are then treated with antibacterial agents.

Amantadine, a compound with a well-proven effect on influenza type A disease, has been marketed in the United States since October 1966 (Oxford and Galbraith, 1980), a fact uniformly ignored by all parties to the swine influenza vaccine débâcle. Belatedly the National Institute of Allergy and Infectious Disease sponsored a consensus development conference that concluded that amantadine be used for both prevention and therapy of all types of *type A influenza* (Maugh, 1979). The trials and tribulations associated with amantadine, all unnecessary, have been described in this same article. Likely such controversy dampened progress in the antiviral field. It is noteworthy that although Sabin has made ill-advised attacks on amantadine (Sabin, 1967 and 1978), as a discussant in the above conference he made no attack on amantadine but rather took the position that no drug or vaccine would really affect influenza since most disease going by this name is not caused by the influenzavirus (Sabin, 1977). Articles in support of Dr. Sabin's positions could not be found. In addition to the above-mentioned conference a workshop on amantadine further affirmed its usefulness (LaMontagne and Galasso, 1978). Amantadine is also widely used in continuous therapy of Parkinsonism, suggesting that it is very well tolerated and would certainly be so when used for prophylaxis during an influenza type A outbreak. Amantadine is also approved for management of such viral infections, with some therapeutic benefit if used early in the course of influenza (Togo *et al.*, 1970).

Rimantadine is a close relative of amantadine but with less central nervous system effects hence not reported as an effective treatment for Parkinsonism. This compound was discovered at DuPont but not pursued further because of the amantadine controversy. Amantadine, however, which was widely used in the USSR, was replaced by rimantadine a number of years ago (Marks, 1976) without any known agreement with DuPont. Rimantadine has been found useful for influenza type A virus infections (Indulen and Kalninya, 1980). With either drug it is essential to establish if there has been an outbreak of influenza caused by the type A viruses since these compounds are inactive against the type B influenza viruses as well as other known viruses. The narrow antiviral spectrum of amantadine and rimantadine is a significant disadvantage which, hopefully, is not an indication of the nature of future antiviral drugs. If, however, this turns out to be the case, laboratory diagnosis would be significantly important in the appropriate use of antiviral drugs.

Idoxuridine (5-iodo-2'-deoxyuridine, IUdR) was the first proven therapeutic antiviral drug marketed in the United States. It has long been used in an aqueous base for treatment of herpes simplex keratitis (Bauer, 1977) and, surprisingly, surrounded by little controversy. There are convincing data that when dissolved in dimethylsulfoxide IUdR has beneficial effects on patients with zoster and may even have some effect on cold sores (Herrmann and Herrmann, 1977a). Shortly after the discovery of IUdR as an antiherpes (Herrmann, 1961) and antizoster agent (Rawls *et al.*, 1964) it was found to be somewhat inadequate for systemic application (Calabresi, 1963) a fact since rediscovered a number of times.

IUdR was the first of what now is a long list of nucleosides with inhibitory activities for certain DNA-containing viruses, most especially herpes simplex virus (Schabel and Montgomery, 1972; Shannon and Schabel, 1980) but as must be expected only very few exhibit all those numerous properties necessary to a useful drug. Adenine arabinoside (ara-A) was the next nucleoside on the market, again to treat herpes simplex virus infections of the eye and it also was in an aqueous base (Pavan-Langston et al., 1975). This seemed necessary in that IUdR was not always effective against HSV eye infections. Later ara-A was marketed for intravenous use to treat those with HSV encephalitis (Whitley et al., 1977). This has not been without controversy since: (1) accurate diagnosis requires a brain biopsy, (2) the low water solubility of this compound requires substantial intravenous fluids, and (3) the compound is rapidly deaminated in the body to the hypoxanthine derivative, which is much less an active antiviral substance. In an aqueous base neither IUdR nor ara-A have shown a usefulness in the treatment of the epidemic HSV dermal lesion. Whether use of DMSO as a carrier vehicle would solve this is, as yet, not completely clear.

Just recently trifluridine (trifluorothymidine) was marketed also to treat HSV-infected eyes (Heidelberger and King, 1979; Wellings et al., 1972). The availability of all of these drugs is encouraging and proves successful therapy but there is still some distance to go if most herpetic disease is to be properly treated. It was with this in mind that there was substantial hope for acyclovir (acycloguanidine) which might be the antiherpetic drug of choice. It had low toxicity, since it acted only on virus infected cells (Elion et al., 1977; Schaeffer et al., 1978) and it was thought, hopefully, to be active by the oral or topical routes. So far this seems to have not come to pass in human trials (Check, 1980). There are, however, a number of reports showing that acyclovir given by the intravenous route is well tolerated and helpful in managing herpetic problems in the immunocompromised patient (Selby et al., 1979; Mitchell et al., 1981; Chou et al., 1981; Saral et al., 1981). There are also indications that certain compounds related to ara-A, especially the more soluble monophosphate derivative, will be investigated for potential use in a variety of HSV infections. Unfortunately this compound is also deaminated in the primate body to the less active hypoxanthine derivative (Whitley et al., 1980). Of some interest is phosphonoacetic acid (PAA), which, although not strikingly potent in cell cultures, has shown remarkable activity when applied topically to HSV infected mice (Klein et al., 1977). Apparently this rather simple organic compound binds specifically with the DNA of herpesviruses. Although PAA may be too toxic for human use, perhaps trisodium phosphonoformate will be better tolerated (Helgstrand et al., 1978).

Of the many antiherpetic compounds reported in the literature (and many more not reported but found in industrial screening programs) (E)-5-(2-bromovinyl)-2'-deoxyuridine seems of significant interest (De Clercq et al., 1979; De Clercq et al., 1980b) and already shown to have activity in human cases of zoster (De Clercq et al., 1980a). On the other hand, using conventional cell-culture antiviral test methods, and IUdR and acyclovir as typical antiherpetic compounds as controls, we were unable to demonstrate any specific antiherpetic activity with 2-deoxy-D-glucose or zinc sulfate (unpublished data). We cannot, therefore, explain the surprising activity of 2-deoxy-D-glucose in genital herpes infection of women (Blough and Giuntoli, 1979) nor the dramatic activity of zinc sulfate in curing mice of vaginal herpetic infection (Tennican et al., 1980). The ingestion of lysine (Griffith et al., 1978) is still another claim for a cure for cold sores while zinc, urea, tannic acid and ultrasound is claimed to cure vaginal HSV infections (Fahim et al., 1980). It would seem there is substantial effort to attack the dermal herpetic lesion with venereal lesions seemingly most capturing the public's attention. The visible nature of classical herpetic lesions permits (sometimes erroneously) much clinical diagnosis with no laboratory confirmation. This will not, however, go far enough for herpes simplex virus attacks the newborn, causes encephalitis at all ages and indeed can also cause much ulcerative pharyngitis (Evans and Dick, 1964; Herrmann, 1967). Certainly, here are diseases that will require laboratory diagnosis to define which of the many potential causal agents is involved. It is, of course, possible that topical treatment with certain antiherpes drugs will be useful. More likely a systemically acting drug, taken orally, will be required. But we can be encouraged, for here is a virus rapidly isolated and recognized in the laboratory (Herrmann, 1967), causing widespread disease that is sensitive to a number of antiviral agents, so it seems likely effective treatment of these diseases is close at hand.

Despite substantial progress in treating influenza and herpesvirus diseases there are large groups of viruses that seemingly are being ignored as targets for the antiviral attack and these include the paramyxoviruses, such as the parainfluenza and respiratory syncycial viruses, the togaviruses or mosquito-borne viruses, the very large group of the picornaviruses and the coronaviruses. These latter two virus groups are responsible for much of the typical common colds but likely other viruses, even influenza, can play a role in what is commonly called 'a cold'. The picornaviruses, of course, include not only polioviruses but also the coxsackie and echoviruses as well as the rhinoviruses and together represent almost 200 known serotypes, none producing immunity to any of the others. Of the enteroviruses only polioviruses are controlled through vaccine use. The rhinoviruses, of course, have been given some attention from time to time as important causes of the common cold but the enteroviruses, with at least seventy serotypes, certain of which visit us every summer presenting a wide range of diseases, have been until recently rather neglected. No one has seriously suggested the vaccine approach to these numerous viruses so antiviral agents seem required.

Even though perhaps no more than 40 per cent of all common colds are caused by the rhinoviruses these are the viruses most studied in humans in antiviral tests. Recently it was shown that enviroxime (Phillpotts et al., 1981) had some effect on human rhinovirus-induced colds but this compound likely is as yet not the answer. This compound has upwards of 600 relatives, however, all with some activity against the picornaviruses and it is possible one or another of these benzimidazoles will be useful. It was reported that so far, of the many clinical trials against the common cold, enviroxime was the most active tested (Phillpotts et al., 1981), illustrating that with a proper effort drugs effective against the common cold are certainly probable. There, however, is very little new regarding the use of ascorbic acid beyond what was already said some years ago (Dykes and Meier, 1975) where it was not found useful for viral respiratory disease. The antihistamines have long been used for treating the common cold with little data to support such use (West et al., 1975) until recently when chlorpheniramine maleate was used in a double-blind trial against what was clinically defined as the common cold (Crutcher and Kantner, 1981). Although the authors felt they detected an effect it was not very convincing.

Until recently the coxsackie A and B and echoviruses represented a substantial challenge, or at least appeared that way, maybe through neglect. Until 1976 no confirmed data had been produced showing any effect of any compound on laboratory animals infected with these enteroviruses. Two observations may rekindle interest in chemotherapy of these viral diseases. First it was shown that combined use of guanidine HCl and hydroxybenzylbenzimidazole (HBB) produced a dramatic effect in saving infant mice from enterovirus death (Eggers, 1976). Secondly, there is the advent of the more complex benzimidazoles, as exemplified by enviroxime (DeLong et al., 1978; Wikel et al., 1980; DeLong and Reed, 1980), which is broadly active against the enteroviruses as well as the rhinoviruses. It, of course, had been long thought that neither guanidine nor HBB had any activity in animals even though there is a vast literature regarding their in vitro activities against enteroviruses. It has now been established that guanidine, HBB and enviroxime are active in mice infected with highly lethal doses of enteroviruses (Herrmann et al., 1981 a, b). Table 3 presents some representative data not only showing that the mice can be saved by treating with various compounds but treatment can be delayed until 58 hr after infection and then infant mice saved from death. There seems no scientific reason, therefore, that the generally mild human enterovirus diseases as well as rhinovirus disease cannot be treated with chemical agents. Furthermore, enteroviruses are readily isolated in the laboratory and outbreaks well established (Hable et al., 1970; Herrmann et al., 1972; Herrmann and Herrmann, 1977c). On an individual patient basis it might be difficult to define if an enterovirus were involved but on a community-wide basis the recognition of such a virus would permit ready treatment and likely the drug of choice would make no distinctions between the various enteroviruses.

In reviewing antiviral drugs that have been marketed or seem close to marketing it should not be forgotten that methisazone (1-methyl-1H-indole-2,3-dione 3-thiosemicarbazone) was for a while available in the United Kingdom for protection against smallpox and treatment of adverse smallpox vaccine reactions (Bauer, 1977). Obviously with the demise of smallpox this drug is no longer needed but it was the first (not ara-A as reported from Parke-Davis) drug marketed for a highly lethal virus infection.

Outside the United States a number of antiviral drugs are available and these include

TABLE 3. *Effect of Various Antipicornavirus Compounds on Infant Mice Infected with Enteroviruses*

Compounds	Highest concentration used (mg/k/day)*	Treatment started before (−) and after (+) virus (HR)	No. days of treatment†	Virus	LD_{50} of virus used*	Dead/total infected‡		
						Treated	Control	P value§
HBB	178	−3	8.5	Cox. A9	10–50	16/41	39/43	<.005
HBB and guanidine	178 } 253 }	,,	,,	,,	,,	4/30	36/43	<.001
Enviroxime	178	,,	,,	,,	10	8/29	29/30	<.001
HBB	89	,,	,,	Echo-9	4	3/23	17/20	<.001
HBB and guanidine	178 } 253 }	,,	,,	,,	2–4	0/33	20/45	<.001
Guanidine	253	,,	,,	,,	,,	3/19	15/20	<.001
Enviroxime	178	,,	,,	,,	1	0/39	24/45	<.001
Guanidine	253	,,	,,	Cox. A16	11–33	3/32	29/30	<.001
Enviroxime	178	,,	,,	,,	5–11	15/23	22/22	<.005
Guanidine	290	+58	2	,,	10	1/22	10/11	<.001
,,	193	,,	,,	,,	,,	11/11	11/11	NS
Guanidine and HBB	193 } 27 }	,,	,,	,,	,,	0/11	10/10	<.001
Guanidine and enviroxime	193 } 14 }	,,	,,	,,	,,	0/10	10/10	<.001

* Subcutaneous injection.
† Every 12 hr.
‡ All surviving mice healthy by 13th day.
§ Chi-square analysis, NS = not significant.

ribavirin (Smith and Kirkpatrick, 1980), inosiplex (Ginsberg and Glasky, 1977), IUdR with DMSO and prednisolone (Viruguent, Hermal-Chemiekurt, W. Germany) and tromantadine (Viru-Merz, Merz and Co., W. Germany).

Like inosiplex, levamisole (Hadden *et al.*, 1977) has been claimed to be an immunemodulator for viral disease treatment. If such agents had the promised effect on viral disease, much laboratory diagnosis would not be required. Despite some suggestive clinical studies (Waldman and Ganguly, 1977; O'Reilly *et al.*, 1977), largely unconfirmed, there are serious questions about the effectiveness of these compounds. That is not to say that other agents with similar effects might not be useful, it is just that the hypothesis of immune modulation has yet to be proven in some practical way in viral diseases.

But what of interferons? It has been over 24 years since Isaacs and Lindenmann (1957) first suggested the role of these substances in viral interference. If the often made promise of the interferons as broad-spectrum antiviral drugs were achieved, it would have a dramatic impact on the need for laboratory diagnosis. Those viral diseases that are clinically distinct would likely need no laboratory diagnosis (typical mumps, herpetic lesions, chicken pox, etc.) and with the remaining viral diseases, only determining that a virus is involved would be sufficient. Significant questions remain, however, as to whether interferons play a role in recovery from viral disease or whether they can even be used therapeutically in routine medical practice. It has also not been resolved whether much of human viral disease can be prevented by continuous use of interferons or their inducers.

Within this volume is one of the many comprehensive reviews of the interferons with a significant list of human viral diseases presumably altered by interferon use. After close study of this list one can only be impressed by the frequency of failure to confirm various interferon activities. It can be readily said that interferons are difficult to obtain, at least at the moment, to produce sufficient clinical testing, and this seems true. And yet in looking at any recent issue of *Index Medicus* it is clear much more is being published on interferons than all other antiviral agents combined. Certainly the effort has been substantial, seemingly far in excess of that expended on synthetic, chemical, antiviral drugs. Antiviral drugs are, however, on the market, have been for some years and their benefits received by many, many thousands. Based on the available data, therefore, it seems likely that viral diagnosis will respond to the available antiviral drugs, much as does bacterial diagnosis.

A limited number of drug companies have active investigations of antiviral drugs and specific antiviral activity is a common result of most of their antiviral screening programs. So far as can be determined, few such agents are antiviral to a large variety of viruses. Some compounds are active against DNA viruses, others are active against picornaviruses, and still others active against only certain influenzaviruses. As things appear now, the various virus groups are biochemically distinct enough that one would not expect specific inhibitors of viral multiplication to inhibit all viruses. This suggests that if the somewhat limited spectrum of present antiviral drugs is an indication of the future, then laboratory viral diagnosis will seemingly be an important adjunct to the use of such drugs.

It seems important to mention that certain other antiviral agents are being neglected, at least in the United States. Rimantadine is one of these that could be useful in influenza A virus infections (Wingfield et al., 1969). This drug may also have a significant impact on viral excretion and hence contagion (Schulman, 1968). Bis-benzimidazoles also are not being pursued for use in rhinovirus infections (Shipkowitz et al., 1972). Further, the use of photodynamic inactivation as a treatment for certain viral diseases continues to be controversial, based on claims by some, using only cell cultures, that such a procedure enhances virus-induced cancer (Rapp and Kemeny, 1977). Others deny and cannot confirm these data (Melnick and Wallis, 1977). Since there is as yet no proof that any virus induces cancer in humans, one wonders at the wisdom of this controversy. Preliminary clinical investigations have emphasized photodynamic treatment of herpetic mucocutaneous lesions (Melnick and Wallis, 1977). If this treatment were found useful, then laboratory diagnosis would likely not be common with most treatment based on the clinical picture. The use of dyes and ordinary light could not, of course, be used for systemic herpes simplex virus diseases.

3.3. THE FUTURE

3.3.1. LABORATORY DIAGNOSIS OF VIRAL DISEASE

What is likely to be the wave of the future? One suspects that if viral diagnosis follows the history of bacterial diagnosis it will be much like the past, that is, isolation of the organism and its identification relevant to patient care. A close look at virus detection by cell culture methods, however, suggests that little has changed since the human diploid fibroblast was introduced over 18 years ago. In some cases the inability to detect certain viruses in cell culture has encouraged the use of a number of additional methods such as those to detect hepatitis B virus antigen by radioimmunoassay. In that electron microscopy and labeled antibody methods have found only limited use (such as detection of rotaviruses in infant diarrhea) in the comprehensive virus diagnostic laboratory, these methods would likely be supplanted by cell-culture procedures that are intrinsically more sensitive, if such methods existed. It would seem the future will demand continued improvement of cell-culture procedures, to be used in such a manner that specific chemotherapy of viral diseases is possible. It is regrettable that in the last decade very little work has been done to improve cell-culture methods while substantial efforts have been made on numerous tests for viral antibody. Such a continued lag will have serious effects on the wise use of antiviral drugs in the future.

Hopefully some day there will be better cell-culture media, but most especially there is a great need for better cell types. Micro cell cultures have eliminated expense as a significant concern (Herrmann and Herrmann, 1977c) but there are still hundreds of cell lines, many derived from human and animal cancers, that as yet seem unstudied for virus-isolation purposes. Only recently has there been some hope that a number of type A coxsackieviruses, most of which are now detected only in infant mice, may be detected in a rhabdomyosarcoma cell (Schmidt et al., 1975) or a guinea-pig embryo cell (Landry, 1981). This RD cell, with its bizarre morphology, does not seem as yet completely adequate but it does illustrate that perhaps somewhere there is a cell that can detect these viruses that now are only detected expensively and inconveniently in infant mice. There is a substantial need for a substitute for primary rhesus monkey kidney cells which are so important for the detection of myxoviruses. This primary cell type, which is almost always contaminated with monkey viruses, is not always readily available due to an Indian embargo on rhesus monkeys. Perhaps the declining availability of these cells has increased interest in a substitute. Recent studies indicate that a canine kidney cell line (MDCK), with trypsin and EDTA in the medium, seems sensitive to human isolates of influenzaviruses A and B (Meguro *et al.*, 1979). But as an example of a continuing need for further cell culture development, MDCK cells are not equal to primary monkey kidney for isolation of parainfluenza viruses (Frank *et al.*, 1979) so primary rhesus or cynomolgus kidney cells seem required (Clark *et al.*, 1979). Hopefully most strains of influenzaviruses can be at least detected in cell culture so embryonated hens eggs are not also required (Monto *et al.*, 1981).

Better cell types to substitute for those now commonly used would not be enough if they only detected those viruses we already detect. The common experience in a viral diagnostic laboratory is of extensive outbreaks of what certainly appears to be viral disease but with no virus isolations. It is difficult to guess at how many viruses there must be that cannot now be detected by cell-culture procedures or, indeed, by any procedures. At present, hepatitis virus A and B, as well as non-A and non-B types, Epstein–Barr virus and a number of viruses associated with gastrointestinal upsets, cannot be cultured in a viral diagnostic laboratory. Add to this what seems an immense number of viral respiratory infections from which there are no virus isolates, and it is clear that a very comprehensive search is needed for better cell types.

There are suggestive data that some substances added to cells in culture can induce a more rapid detection of certain viruses (Herrmann, 1974). This is another neglected area of study where an organized search is needed for agents that encourage visible virus activity in cell cultures. The problem here is that such additives should be able to enhance detection of some viruses without suppressing the detection of others. Using certain halogenated pyrimidines (Staal and Rowe, 1975) to induce the detection of some viruses might be undertaken by using separate cultures. Such an approach could lead to a substantial duplication of cell cultures if it turns out that a number of substances are needed to enhance detection of many viruses. This use of multiple cell culture types, with and without inducers of viral activity, would be like the multiple media used for bacterial isolations. The number of types of cell cultures might be limited, however, by the knowledge of the nature of the specimen to be tested and perhaps even the nature of the illness. A specimen from a dermal lesion, for example, would contain far fewer classes of viruses than a throat specimen.

The methods for identifying a virus isolate using specific typing antisera are expensive and time-consuming. These techniques in the future will likely be dispensed with in many cases. HSV, from rather typical skin lesions, can be very often recognized by the type of cell culture it attacks and the nature of the cytopathic effect (Herrmann and Rawls, 1974). This is often also true for varicella-zoster and cytomegaloviruses (Benyesh-Melnick, 1974; Schmidt, 1974). In the case of a rhinovirus isolate, few laboratories even try to define its serological type. This class of virus can be defined by its cytopathic effect in certain cultures, its sensitivity to a low pH and resistance to lipid solvents. The use of differential cell cultures, the nature of the viral cytopathic effect and the use of biochemical tests would seem to be the wave of the future with only occasional need for specific typing antisera. To properly use an antiviral drug, there is a need to know the biochemical nature of a virus which may or may not be related to its serological nature. Why serotype an echovirus, if, in fact, all echovirus disease responds to the same antiviral drug? At least one comprehensive virus laboratory does not serotype its viral isolates (Smith, 1979).

Antiviral drugs themselves may become useful in defining the nature of the virus isolate. Indeed, in the future it may become necessary to define the sensitivity of a virus to antiviral drugs, as is now done in much of bacterial diagnosis. Viruses can become resistant to antiviral drugs (Herrmann and Herrmann, 1977b). What is not known is the impact this will have on the clinical use of such drugs, since laboratory observations of drug resistance are by no means directly transferable to the clinic. Antiviral drug-sensitivity tests, therefore, would seem to be part of the future both for defining the type of virus isolated and to determine the best drug to use for a specific viral disease.

There is presently a very healthy emphasis on rapid viral diagnosis (McIntosh *et al.*, 1980) which would most certainly be an adjunct to development of antiviral drugs. The methods emphasize detection of the virus particle, or a fraction of the particle, by electron microscopic or labeled antibody methods. As one might expect, their greatest use has been in detecting viruses not readily isolated in the diagnostic laboratory, and there are commercially produced 'kits' using labeled antibody methods for just this purpose.

What is not always clear is the comparison of sensitivity to rapid diagnosis. So far as can be found presently, no system of detecting herpes simplex or cytomegalovirus seems more sensitive than human fibroblast cell cultures. Varicella-zoster virus, on the other hand, is detected more frequently by using direct immunofluorescent staining (Schmidt *et al.*, 1980). In the future a substantial amount of experience will be required to define the rapidity required for diagnosis, if this justifies any loss in sensitivity and how the diagnosis relates to antiviral drug treatment.

Much, but certainly not all, virus disease occurs in sharp outbreaks. This fact can be used to alert community physicians to what virus is 'going around' and the nature of the clinical disease associated with any particular virus. This 'virus alert' program has been in existence for some years (Herrmann and Herrmann, 1977c). Publication in the news media alerts the public and the medical profession so there is at least some hope that the ill-advised use of antibacterial drugs can be avoided. Such an approach can be valuable with outbreaks of influenza, paramyxovirus, and enterovirus infections but is of little help with sporadic adeno or herpesvirus infections or other viral infections unassociated with a significant disease outbreak. Presently the approach to insect-borne (togavirus) viral disease is along the lines of a virus-alert program. Although detection of such a virus infection is largely limited to a serological diagnosis, it can alert the community to the problem; drugs, were they available, could be used on likely cases, along with improved mosquito control. It is unlikely the rapid laboratory diagnosis in cell culture will be easily achieved for insect-borne viruses because of the general inaccessibility of the virus, also a problem with HSV encephalitis. If there is no great improvement in the swiftness of viral diagnosis generally, then clinical diagnosis, along with the knowledge of the prevalence of certain types of viruses, may become the primary guide for using antiviral agents. This is not to say this is the most satisfactory approach. The exact definition of the infecting organism in each patient is always more desirable. The use of the 'virus-alert' program seems a necessary compromise and can also make serological procedures of greater pertinence where there is an outbreak of influenza, paramyxovirus, rubella and togavirus disease. Serological diagnostic procedures would still not be practical as a guide in the treatment of most sporadic viral disease, nor in outbreaks that involve virus groups with many serotypes, as is the case with the picornaviruses. With all of this, however, it is likely the use of antiviral drugs will be based most often solely on the clinical picture. Broad spectrum antiviral drugs, therefore, seem a necessity if patients are to benefit.

3.3.2. THE FUTURE OF ANTIVIRAL DRUGS

A critical study of viral disease will convince one that there are more avenues open to attack in these diseases than in bacterial disease, as suggested in Table 4. It is unlikely, for example, that one would attack bacterial disease by using drugs that produce only symptomatic relief, for the bacteria might continue to multiply, producing an unhappy outcome. With viral diseases there are only a few that are life-threatening. One could in many cases let the virus multiply, resulting in a normal immune response, and just treat the symptoms and clinical signs of the disease. This is what is so frequently promised by over-the-counter drug advertising. Only recently, however, has aspirin been studied for its worth in the common cold, and found rather unimpressive if not likely to make the patient more infectious (Stanley *et al.*, 1975). If there are little or no data to support the present nostrums' abilities to produce

TABLE 4. *Stages in Human Viral Infections Open to Attack by Drugs*

Interrupt transport to susceptible host cell
Block attachment to cell
Inhibit entrance into cell
Prevent uncoating of viral genome
Inhibit transport of viral genetic information
Inhibit synthesis of viral specific enzymes and structural proteins
Inhibit or alter viral nucleic acid
Inhibit cellular metabolic systems essential to viral multiplication but not essential to maintaining cellular integrity
Prevent assembly and maturation of viral particles
Prevent incorporation of necessary cellular substances into viral particle (lipids)
Inhibit release from cell
Prevent viral-induced cell pathology
Neutralize or block induced biochemical pathology (toxemia)
Enhance host defense mechanisms
Enhance host recovery mechanisms

symptomatic relief (West *et al.*, 1975; Crutcher and Kantner, 1981), this is far from saying it cannot be done. Even though we presently know very little of the pathogenic mechanisms of self-limiting viral diseases, one can still speculate that the part that bothers the patient most is, in fact, a virus-induced toxemia. The virus may multiply in a limited area of the body such as the upper respiratory tract, but the illness is felt throughout the body. Tests for drugs that affect this toxemia would likely best be performed on human subjects, although some studies might be undertaken in mice using influenza virus and its long neglected associated toxin (Henle and Henle, 1946 a, b). It would seem worthwhile to study those diverse drugs presently on the market, under double-blind, controlled conditions, to find if any of a variety of pharmacological actions have some effect on the most common viral respiratory diseases, those that are truly self-limiting. Do various antiinflammatory drugs, analgesics or even certain tranquilizers have some useful effect? If so, then this would give an indication of the type of drugs that might be useful. It is not suggested that the drugs that are tested necessarily be the ones of choice but rather those that have similar activity and are very well tolerated. It is most clear, however, that if such drugs were found useful, then they would have to be relatively inexpensive and readily available to have much impact on the vast number of viral ailments. One thinks, of course, mostly of the many types of human viral infections commonly lumped together as 'colds'. It is likely that there would be little viral laboratory diagnosis associated with the use of such drugs. It seems fair to say that there is almost no laboratory diagnosis of such diseases now and the majority of cases are not even seen by a physician. The physician tends to see the more severe and troublesome viral infections and these would be the ones requiring laboratory diagnosis, now and well into the future. This would be especially true when the disease was found not to respond to the hypothetical palliative measures suggested above.

Perhaps in considering the advent of antiviral drugs, viral diseases might be divided into two general classes, those that are self-limiting, never cause death or serious illness, and those that do. For the former group, well tolerated easily obtained drugs are a necessity and individual viral diagnosis perhaps not essential. It is the latter group that must be dealt with in the viral diagnostic laboratory and treated more vigorously with potent drugs. It is possible that in the future certain drugs, both specifically antiviral and palliative, will be found effective for viral diseases where it is either not possible to isolate the virus, or the diagnostic procedures are too time-consuming and expensive. It seems reasonable to assume that drugs effective against all known rhino or coronaviruses might be equally useful against their undetected relatives.

One can predict that there will be no one answer to human viral disease. Vaccines will continue to play a role in certain viral diseases just as do bacterial vaccines. Other protective measures will perhaps find a use in certain viral infections and this can be passive immunity with gamma globulin containing a high level of antiviral antibody. It seems unlikely there will be a panacea for all viral diseases and, as each new approach becomes available to clinical practice, this will determine what laboratory tests must be undertaken, just as now occurs in bacteriology. For the future, a major portion of the virus laboratory effort would be in classifying viruses according to their drug sensitivity. It must be expected that resistance to antiviral drugs will occur, inducing the search for new drugs or the use of drug combinations that do not encourage resistance development. As has been suggested, however, any drug approach to viral disease that is indirect and does not attack the specific viral-induced mechanisms would not be likely to induce drug resistance (Herrmann and Herrmann, 1977b).

The present trend is to look for specific drug inhibitors of viral-induced synthetic pathways, almost to the exclusion of other approaches, not unlike the emphasis used in the search for antibacterial agents. This approach has been productive but it will be limited since much of viral disease cannot be defeated by highly potent viral inhibitors that are expensive and must be obtained by prescription. What other approaches might one suggest for the future, new discoveries that also come from screening programs but do not involve specific viral synthetic inhibition? There are a number, as suggested in Table 4. For example, naturally occurring substances that interfere with virus infection have long been known but neglected for practical use. A variety of macromolecules that included polysaccharides (Woolley, 1954; Horsfall and McCarty, 1947; Takemoto and Spicer, 1965), mucoproteins (Li et al., 1965), tannins (Kucera and Herrmann, 1967) and lipoproteins (Clarke and Casals, 1958) will interfere with virus–cell interactions and some totally inactivate or neutralize the virus. So far as is known, none of the virus-inactivating agents have been tested as perhaps a nasal spray to attempt to protect against respiratory viruses. It may be, considering the mild nature of human viral disease, that the body needs only a slight lowering of the virus dose by some protective measure to make the difference between just an infection and disease. It may come to pass that the use of well-tolerated viral neutralizing substances, artificial antibody so to speak, are still specific enough that there has to be a general awareness of what viruses are within the community before their use would be effective. Again the virus-alert program could perform this function. One substance might be used for parainfluenza virus infections, for example, another for an influenza outbreak and perhaps still another for an echovirus outbreak. The idea would be to protect the upper respiratory tract from primary viral infection or at least decrease the magnitude of the infection.

It is widely held, without substantial proof, that the production of interferons may be one limiting factor in human viral diseases. If this were true, then inducers of interferons would indeed be chemotherapeutic and encourage recovery from viral disease. So far this has not been shown conclusively, but the concept is valid. This does not involve specific antiviral substances, which in fact interferons are not, but rather a treatment that encourages the body's recovery mechanisms, and such mechanisms could differ for different virus infections. The future should hold some further information on what permits humans to recover uneventfully from most viral disease and how this can be encouraged by chemotherapeutic measures.

3.3.3. Immune Modulators

It has been suggested that immune modulators can play a role in recovery from viral disease and this remains to be seen (see Section 3.2.2). If there are possibilities for drugs that perform this function, then what impact would it have on viral laboratory diagnosis? Barring a utopian panacea, there would seem to be some necessity at least to define the prevailing community viral problem. With sporadic viral infections, however, each case might have to be specifically diagnosed and the question remains whether this could be done rapidly enough to institute specific chemotherapeutic measures directed at hastening recovery of a patient already recovering. The inducing of higher levels of antibody or interferons most readily comes to mind, but it seems likely that other recovery mechanisms must exist to explain intrinsic immunity exhibited by those immune virgins who become infected but do not become ill. Whatever these mechanisms are, they are the ones that might also have to be enhanced. If we are so fortunate as to find that enhancement of such mechanisms decreases all viral illness or enhances recovery in virtually all viral diseases, then perhaps much viral laboratory diagnosis would become unnecessary. One should, however, not be too optimistic about this possibility.

3.3.4. ADDITIONAL ANTIVIRAL APPROACHES

There are other aspects of viral infection that seem worth attacking, such as those mechanisms by which the virus must get into the cell. Would agents that block cell receptors be useful? Long ago this was suggested by mouse experiments using receptor-destroying enzyme (neuraminidase) (Stone, 1948), but only a protective effect was shown. Would agents that influence virus entrance into the cell be useful? Presently amantadine is suggested as one such agent, although this is not likely to be its only action-mechanism. Amantadine has a chemotherapeutic effect early in the course of viral disease but, like rimantadine, it is more potent when given prophylactically. Use of drugs with such antiviral specificity would certainly seem to demand some viral laboratory diagnosis, as is now the case with the use of amantadine or rimantadine. One can perhaps safely assume that viropexis is a complex function of the cell–virus interaction, but it should not be neglected as an area open to an antiviral attack.

In addition to agents that inhibit production of nucleic acids, proteins, glycoproteins and other structural components and enzymes specific for viral synthesis, one must include the potential inhibitors of mechanisms for uncoating of virus nucleic acid, within the cell, the virus assembly mechanisms with final production of the infectious virion, and even those mechanisms of escape of virus from the cell by other than simple cell lysis. Indeed, is cell lysis itself a mechanism specific enough for attack by a chemotherapeutic drug? Drugs that inhibit specific mechanisms essential to viral multiplication would be the ones most likely to act on a relatively limited group of viruses.

Would, however, a drug that gives support to the virus-infected cell, so that cellular damage is minimal, be of a more broad spectrum type? In some cases the host cells tolerate substantial viral synthesis so well that no observable cytopathology can be observed. There certainly may be a biochemical defect in such cells that is responsible for the illness, but whatever the cellular problem, there may be drugs to aid the infected cell in its time of need and so limit the illness. This may not be considered a classical antiviral approach and it is difficult to say how specific it might be for certain viral infections. If such a hypothetical drug were beneficial in many types of viral disease, then laboratory viral diagnosis would be less essential. In all of this, one can be optimistic for certainly viral disease offers many possibilities for chemotherapeutic or chemoprophylactic approaches. In truth, of course, no one can predict the eventual role of the viral diagnostic laboratory until each new drug reaches general use. Barring the discovery of a utopian antiviral agent, it seems reasonable to predict that some viral diagnosis will be required when there are a significant number of antiviral drugs in use.

In looking at the future with all its potential for new and effective antiviral drugs a note of caution must be introduced. Well-meaning advice is being given about how antiviral agents should be sought. The term rational or logical is often used to describe the methodical approach to learning enough about the virus–cell interaction so that armed with such knowledge one can predict an antiviral structure (Cohen, 1972, 1977, 1979; Joklik, 1980). This in fact was suggested as the proper scientific approach to a search for effective antibacterial agents (Work and Work, 1948), that is before the era of effective antibacterial therapy. But, as the respected discoverer of gentamycin indicated, antibacterial agents that are to be used as drugs are discovered (but not always admitted to) by the empirical approach, most frequently via the industrial screening program. The reason this is so is because the demand that a compound inhibit a microorganism is not very difficult to achieve but to do this in a living animal, at a well-tolerated dose, is most demanding. Most leave the pharmacology out of their advice. Many antiviral compounds must be tested just to find a very few with activity in some *in vivo* system. (Note also that the cost of testing antiviral compounds in humans is presently beyond all but a few firms with enormous financial resources.) It is the demand of any *in vivo* test that make studies *in vitro* not very useful. It is true that the least expensive way to screen is using cell cultures; but the non-toxic spectrum of antiviral activity *in vitro* is about as much useful information as one obtains. Cell cultures will not indicate a compound's animal toxicity, its possible side-reactions, that is its pharmacodynamic reactions, nor anything of its pharmacokinetics. Knowing the action-mechanism of the compound will not make it more or less active *in vivo*.

3.4. VIRAL DISEASES OF THE UPPER RESPIRATORY TRACT AND ORAL CAVITY

3.4.1. THE PROBLEM

It has been estimated that in the United States there are about one billion cases (3–6 episodes per person per year) of respiratory tract disease each year (Huebner, 1963). Most of this disease is viral induced, relatively mild, self-limiting and frequently not seen by a physician. Physicians in the United States see perhaps 50 million cases of viral respiratory disease each year and the majority of these patients are children. In the practice of pediatric medicine as many as 33 per cent of the patients have respiratory disease and most of this is seemingly caused by a virus (Glezen, 1976). It is thought that overall there is likely 4–5 times more viral than bacterial respiratory tract disease (Glezen, 1976) and it is likely that ill-advised antibacterial treatment is routinely used for many such viral diseases. For the purposes of the following discussion, however, upper respiratory tract disease will obviously not include those infections of the bronchial tree and the lungs, which will be presented later.

There is a long list of known viruses that can be isolated from throat, oral and nasal specimens, as indicated in Table 2. One might guess that there are at the very least twice as many additional viruses that infect the human upper respiratory tract that cannot as yet be detected.

In discussing the known viruses that cause upper respiratory tract disease, it is common to mention those of the common cold and influenza as well as infections caused by parainfluenza, respiratory syncytial and adenoviruses. There must, however, be additional consideration given to the role of the enteroviruses and herpes simplex virus in such disease. Enteroviruses are commonly associated with childhood cases of pharyngitis and fever (Hable *et al.*, 1970; Herrmann *et al.*, 1972) but this aspect of enteroviral disease is too frequently ignored while the seemingly more serious infections, such as those associated with meningitis, are emphasized. Certainly enteroviruses, especially those of the coxsackie group, as well as herpes simplex virus, cause disease marked by oral lesions, a common problem in children. What is not so widely known is the role of herpes simplex virus in producing both pharyngitis and stomatitis in the adult (Herrmann, 1967; Sheridan and Herrmann, 1971). It was long assumed that most adults were immune to herpes simplex virus primary infections, and this was largely true for adults from a lower socioeconomic group. It is not so true of those from higher socioeconomic groups where at times as many as 50 per cent of young adults are not immune to this virus (Wentworth and Alexander, 1971). More emphasis then should be placed on the role of HSV as a common cause of oral lesions and especially its role in acute ulcerative pharyngitis in those of all ages. It is perhaps unwise always to conclude that HSV isolation from a pharyngitis is due to haphazard shedding of this virus unassociated with disease. If a drug attack on respiratory disease is to be effective then the role of enteroviruses and herpes simplex virus cannot be ignored.

Viral upper respiratory tract disease is a very demanding problem in that hundreds of serologically distinct viruses are involved. Many of these viruses contain RNA, others contain DNA and most produce rather superficial diseases, resulting in solid immunity to reinfection (enteroviruses) in some cases, or partial immunity (parainfluenza and influenza-viruses) in others. In certain cases, as with rhinoviruses, the illness is marked by no objective pathology while other viruses, such as those causing influenza, can denude the epithelium of the respiratory tract. Some infections are 'cold-like' while others are 'flu-like' and certain viruses can take their turn producing both kinds of illness. Of all viral diseases, those involving the upper respiratory tract are the most difficult to diagnose on clinical grounds and yet it will be these very diseases that will most likely be treated with little or no laboratory diagnosis.

3.4.2. POTENTIAL DRUG SOLUTIONS

With most viral upper respiratory tract disease, the pathology is very limited and sequelae rare, so what seems needed is relief from the symptoms and clinical signs. Aspirin has long been recommended to control the fever of 'colds' and 'flu' even though it is well known that adults suffering from rhinovirus infections rarely experience a fever, and as indicated before, the use of aspirin seems to make such persons more infectious. Some question should even be raised about the wisdom of suppressing a relatively mild fever with aspirin since certain viruses do not tolerate temperatures much above 37°C, or at least seem to tolerate them less well than humans. Indeed, except when there are dangers from fever, this is not an aspect of viral disease that causes great discomfort. What is really needed is a drug to produce effective relief from the cough, obstruction of the respiratory passages, sore throat, rhinorrhea, malaise, myalgias and the general toxemia that is associated with rhinoviral and other 'cold-like' viral respiratory disease. Symptomatic relief alone would not be sufficient, however, if the infection were caused by entero, herpes simplex or influenza viruses since these and a few other viruses can cause more serious disease likely requiring a potent and specific viral inhibitor.

Adenovirus disease represents a somewhat special case. Although these viruses usually produce little disease in civilian adults, they can cause a pharyngitis in children much like a 'strep throat' that is often ill-advisedly treated for lengthy periods with antibiotics. In some cases the adenoviral respiratory disease can be accompanied by a conjunctivitis; in other cases a conjunctivitis alone may occur. The problem is that these cases can be sporadic and, despite the fact adenoviruses contain DNA, they seem rather resistant to the prevalent drugs that inhibit other DNA viruses (Herrmann, 1968). What seems most needed is a drug that can inhibit adenovirus synthesis with complete safety to the patient. But again these infections can be relatively mild and in many cases effective symptomatic relief might be all that is needed.

The status of the present drug approaches to influenza has already been discussed. Clearly what is now needed are more rapid-acting chemotherapeutic drugs that influence all influenza, whether caused by the A or B virus types. Symptomatic relief should also be considered, since this virus is likely to cause a portion of the illness via a toxic mechanism. Further, the course of influenza can be of such short duration that a specific viral inhibitor may have little time to be effective. Even when the active disease is virtually over, however, some sequelae including general weakness, lethargy and even mild depression remain, sometimes for weeks, and certainly symptomatic relief seems in order in such cases. Chemoprophylactic drugs may well be life saving to high-risk patients in the absence of an effective chemotherapeutic drug for influenza, but such drugs should permit development of maximal immunity even in those who experience mild disease. Even then, when the specific influenza virus inhibitor is being sought, it best be one that is very effective chemotherapeutically in that it seems more practical to treat only those who are ill. Further, many with influenza virus infections will either not be ill or mildly so and they could be left untreated and hence acquire maximal immunity, which might not be the result if a chemoprophylactic drug were widely used. So far as is now known, antiviral chemotherapeutic drugs do not seem to prevent an immune response, likely because viral multiplication has progressed sufficiently by the time therapy is started to provide the same immunity as would normally be produced by the untreated disease.

So much progress has now been made in finding compounds active against herpes simplex virus that it is expected more antiherpes drugs will become available. Superficial and limited oral lesions might be treated topically but extensive oral lesions suggest a primary HSV infection with systemic disease, requiring something more than topical treatment. Further, infectious mononucleosis is caused by a virus from the herpes family (Epstein–Barr virus) and treatment of this disease would require a systemically active drug. There should be more concern that progress in the early treatment of herpes simplex and Epstein–Barr virus infections be swifter, for there are constant suggestions that these viruses are associated with human tumors. Chicken pox and shingles also would be expected to respond to an antiherpes drug, since they too are caused by a herpesvirus.

3.4.3. Diagnostic Needs

It is unreasonable and unrealistic to suggest that every case of viral respiratory disease be diagnosed in the laboratory. It does seem worthwhile, however, at least to define what viruses are circulating in the community, using a virus alert program. Not all virus disease outbreaks will be defined but specific antiviral drugs can be used in those outbreaks that are defined. The relatively mild viral diseases seem best treated by effective, well tolerated, symptomatic relief since a significant number of these infections will either not be seen by a physician or, if they are, will still not receive a laboratory diagnosis, even where it is readily available (Smith, 1979).

The more serious illnesses should have a laboratory diagnosis even when it fits those diseases known to be associated with a prevalent virus invasion. The more serious viral respiratory disease case could, of course, be a sporadic infection caused by a virus not known to be prevalent. It is obvious, however, that only a portion of most virus respiratory infections can now be defined by any laboratory method. Today a virus-alert program would fail on many occasions, so much still needs to be done just to define rapidly even those viruses circulating in a community at any one time.

The clinical picture of disease can at times be useful. Certainly those fairly rare cases of mumps or measles, for example, could be defined on a clinical basis. Some may feel that viral diseases of the respiratory tract can be distinguished from bacterial since the latter so often are localized and lack the generalized toxic phase common in viral disease. It would seem wiser, however, to rule out bacterial involvement by performing a throat culture. This would not, of course, define which virus is the responsible agent in the event different drugs must be used for different viruses. Perhaps what is needed is more effort in an attempt to discover those clinical signs and symptoms that are classical for certain viral infections. Certainly an outbreak of influenza is not difficult to define; it is determining whether the responsible agent is the A or B virus that poses the somewhat more difficult question. The classical clinical picture of the common cold in adults, usually without fever, would certainly suggest the use of effective and well-tolerated drugs for the rhinoviruses, if it were not for the fact these are certainly not the only viruses that can cause a classical cold. The seasonal pattern of disease could be helpful, however, in that rhinoviruses seem most prevalent in the spring, summer and fall (Person and Herrmann, 1970). Coronaviruses apparently cause many of the wintertime colds (Kaye et al., 1971). In temperate climates, as another example of seasonal prevalence, one is very unlikely to see pharyngitis cases caused by enteroviruses during the winter months. Future diagnosis of viral respiratory disease, therefore, in such a manner as to permit adequate use of specific drugs will likely require interrelating knowledge involving isolating the virus when possible, defining it serologically when this can be done along with the clinical, epidemiological and seasonal pattern of disease. Much more would be required in community–physician cooperation and communication than now seems the case, however, if antiviral drugs are to be used in a rational and effective manner.

Infections marked by lesions in the oral cavity give a clue to the possible viruses involved. Presently herpes simplex virus is a common cause of such lesions even in adults. In children, during summer months, herpangina caused by the coxsackie A viruses can be equally common. It has been found on rarer occasions, however, that intraoral lesions can also be associated with coxsackieviruses of the B type and so laboratory diagnosis may well be necessary to unravel which viruses are involved. In the winter months, with an infected child presenting with severe oral lesions and a gingivostomatitis, one would certainly think of using a well-tolerated antiherpes drug. But still some confusion can occur with cases of aphthus stomatitis which so far as known is not caused by a virus. It is claimed, however, that herpetic intraoral lesions can be distinguished from those associated with aphthus stomatitis (Weathers and Griffin, 1970), so here again is an example of the use of the clinical picture as a guide to therapy. Of course, oral lesions associated with herpes simplex virus can usually be readily defined by virus isolation in any average virus diagnostic laboratory, generally within a few days (Herrmann, 1971). But again there is the concern that this will not be swift enough to start effective therapy. Perhaps more must be done to utilize labeled specific, antibody systems for detecting HSV in oral mucosal cells, if rapid therapy based on an accurate diagnosis is to be the goal.

There can be many causes of oral lesions such as allergies and drug reactions. What does not seem so clear is the extent of viral-induced oral lesions in both children and adults and whether there are other kinds of oral lesions caused by as yet unidentified viruses. There is a substantial need to define the problem of oral lesions and, until this is done, it will be difficult to say what the diagnostic needs will be in the future. Certainly something more convenient than infant mice are needed to define coxsackie A virus-induced oral lesions. The promise of the RD cell, referred to previously as a ready aid in this diagnosis, has as yet not come to pass (Schmidt et al., 1975) but there is every hope some cell type will eventually fulfill this promise.

Infectious mononucleosis (IM), which can be a complex disease, nonetheless frequently appears to be a typical virus upper respiratory tract infection and it is certain that it is caused by the Epstein–Barr herpesvirus (Henle and Henle, 1972). It appears also that the atypical lymphocytosis and the production of the heterophile antibody are typical of E–B virus attack on the B lymphocytes (Rapp and Hewetson, 1978). The heterophile antibody determination remains, therefore, a useful tool in diagnosis, most especially in that E–B virus is usually detected with difficulty only as part of a research program. Regrettably, the younger the patient the less likely a positive heterophile test will be produced. Under 5 years of age it is all but absent. Further, at least 10 per cent of adults with what appears to be IM are both heterophile and E–B virus antibody negative (Henle et al., 1974). It is estimated that 8 per cent of IM is due in fact to cytomegalovirus (CMV) (Horwitz et al., 1979), a virus of the herpes group that too should yield to certain herpesvirus inhibitors. Certainly not all herpesvirus inhibitors are equally potent against all herpes viruses (DeClercq et al., 1980b) but yet it is not clear how potent a drug must be to give relief from IM type diseases. Some laboratories can detect E–B virus or its antibodies but these methods likely will not be so widespread as to permit an accurate use of an anti-EBV drug. Most prolonged cases are in adults and the clinical picture with atypical lymphocytes and a positive heterophile test will permit accurate drug treatment in the majority of cases once any one of many candidate drugs becomes available.

3.5. VIRUS DISEASES OF THE LOWER RESPIRATORY TRACT AND CARDIOVASCULAR SYSTEMS

3.5.1. THE PROBLEM

The extent of acute heart disease, pneumonia, bronchitis and bronchiolitis related to viral infections is not well known. One can presume that the stresses caused by viral disease, such as with influenza, likely contribute to some mortality among heart patients. There is no question that influenza virus infections, especially of the A types, produce fatal pneumonia, as well as additional disease of the lower respiratory tract (Lindsay et al., 1970). The coxsackieviruses of the B group can cause myocarditis, that is sometimes fatal in the newborn, and pericarditis and pleurodynia in those of all ages (Kibrick, 1964). What is not clear is what fraction of the total of lung and heart disease is directly caused by viral infection. Present evidence would suggest no significant role for viruses in heart disease other than that caused by the B group of coxsackieviruses, but this evidence is, of course, based on our knowledge of the presently known viruses.

In the case of viral disease of the lower respiratory tract in adults the picture is not clear. It is not uncommon to hear a diagnosis of 'viral pneumonia', frequently with reference to illnesses seemingly refractory to antibiotic treatment. In the past much 'viral pneumonia' was likely a disease caused by *Mycoplasma pneumoniae* (Denny *et al.*, 1971). Most pneumonia is still probably bacterial in origin, perhaps even bacteria not previously implicated, as exemplified by the discovery of the role of the bacterium responsible for 'Legionnaires' Disease' (Center for Disease Control, 1978). Our examination of over 800 lungs obtained from adults at autopsy produced only 35 viral isolates, mostly influenza A viruses, some cytomegaloviruses from immune compromised patients, and a few, very few, other viruses (Herrmann and Herrmann, 1976b). This suggests that severe infections of the lungs do not seem to be primarily a problem related to the known viruses. Influenza virus has been identified infrequently with severe bronchitis, and in fact bronchitis in adults, sufficiently severe to seek medical aid, has not been defined as a viral problem. Among recruits in the armed services adenoviruses can cause lower respiratory tract disease but this is a special case, rarely seen in civilian adults. These viruses do, of course, produce substantial upper respiratory disease in children but it is rarely serious if left untreated.

Childhood infections of the lower respiratory tract are, however, another matter. Influenza virus infections seem of less importance in children than in adults. Respiratory syncytial and parainfluenza viruses, on the other hand, lead the list of those important causes of childhood lower respiratory tract disease. It would now appear that the coronaviruses, and probably to a smaller extent the rhinoviruses, can also produce lower respiratory tract disease in children less than 18 months of age (McIntosh *et al.*, 1974). Respiratory syncytial virus produces the more serious diseases in pre-school children, including bronchitis, laryngialtracheal bronchitis, bronchiolitis, epiglotitis and pneumonia. Fatal viral pneumonia in children, however, seems relatively uncommon.

There seems little question that the cause of substantial amounts of lower respiratory tract infections in both adults and children have yet to be defined. Many cases of such disease suggest a viral infection but these viruses are not yet known. There is still hope, as has been suggested already, that these unknown viruses may well be relatives of known viruses, known viruses that one day will succumb to antiviral drugs. Such drugs could likely be used in a number of typical viral diseases even when no virus can be identified.

3.5.2. Potential Drug Solutions

Lower respiratory tract disease is serious enough to require specific antiviral drugs that quickly stop viral synthesis and tissue destruction. Symptomatic therapy, although perhaps beneficial, is still not enough. Treating only symptoms is perhaps also not the proper approach to cases of myocarditis and pericarditis; virus multiplication should be inhibited as early in the course of the disease as possible for it is still not known whether coxsackie B viruses can produce some sequelae, perhaps sequelae not obvious until years later. Drug treatment for infections caused by the numerous types of enteroviruses seems the only practical attack against the variety of disease problems they produce. Effective antiviral drugs also seem required for respiratory syncytial virus infections and perhaps this virus is a close enough relative to the parainfluenza viruses so they too will respond to the same therapeutic approach. Although certain drugs may be useful to treat only the symptoms of the common cold when produced by rhinoviruses and coronaviruses, this too may not be enough when these viruses produce more serious lower respiratory tract illnesses in children. Since rhinoviruses are related to the enteroviruses it could well be that drugs inhibitory for one group will work against all picornaviruses and there are a number of antiviral compounds that suggest this possibility, including HBB (Gwaltney, 1968), the bisbenzimidazoles (Schleicher *et al.*, 1972), the triazinoindoles (Gwaltney, 1970) and enviroxime (Herrmann *et al.*, 1981c).

There are substantial data supporting the concept, so far unproved, that pneumonia caused by influenza A viruses can be prevented and even treated using amantadine or rimantadine and that these drugs likely can be useful on the entire spectrum of respiratory disease caused by influenza A viruses (Hoffmann, 1973). What is needed, of course, are more potent antiviral drugs that act on infections caused by both influenza A and B viruses and this has been claimed for ribavirin (Durr *et al.*, 1975). Ribavirin, however, does not appear to be a very potent treatment for human infections and its effect is almost undetectable if the influenza case is a mild one (Togo and McCracken, 1976; Cohen *et al.*, 1976). Certainly, a broad spectrum antiinfluenzal agent, perhaps something like ribavirin, is needed, in that an outbreak of influenza is not difficult to detect on clinical grounds but it is more difficult to determine if one is dealing with influenza A or B virus, or on some occasions, both.

3.5.3. DIAGNOSTIC NEEDS

A 'virus-alert' program could aid in determining those viruses that are prevalent in the community and thus suggest what might be expected in the way of lower respiratory tract disease. Yet it would seem prudent to attempt a specific viral diagnosis in each case of lower respiratory tract disease. This should also be done at least to exclude a bacterial pathogen. Much has been said about the importance of obtaining an adequate specimen from a bacterial lower respiratory tract infection. Many believe throat swabs are not completely indicative of the bacterial flora of the lower respiratory tract while sputum frequently is little more than saliva. It is not so clear that this is a problem in viral infections, for influenza virus seems relatively easy to isolate from a throat swab from those with influenzal pneumonia (Lindsay *et al.*, 1970). Further, lower respiratory tract infections caused by respiratory syncytial and parainfluenza viruses frequently are diagnosed using only a throat swab (Smith *et al.*, 1971; Herrmann and Hable, 1970). There is some evidence, however, that throat and especially nasal washings can be more effective specimens for isolating certain viruses (Hall and Douglas, 1975) and these should be obtained, especially in the hospitalized cases. It seems valid to presume that in a lower respiratory tract infection caused by respiratory syncytial virus, where the virus is readily isolated from the nasal passages, extreme measures to sample the lower respiratory tract are not needed. It is also worth noting that even with upper respiratory viral disease a nasal swab can, at times, be more productive of a virus than is the throat swab (Bloom *et al.*, 1963).

Whatever the virus involved, superior virus detection methods are needed, and this is especially true for parainfluenza and respiratory syncytial viruses that frequently take a week or more to detect, critically depending on how much virus was contained in the specimen. In the case of influenza, it has long been suggested that labeled antibody methods can be used to detect this virus in respiratory secretions and this indeed can be a rapid and specific method, but cell-culture methods still are required additionally in the event that it was not a true case of influenza, which may be the reason so little influenza is diagnosed by labeled antibody methods. In time still more viruses associated with lower respiratory tract disease will be discovered and, as the number of virus serotypes increases, then the use of specific antibody becomes increasingly less practical; hence, better cell-culture methods are required if rapid application of a chemotherapeutic agent is to be the goal. Measurement of virus antibody in acute and convalescent sera could rarely aid in guiding therapy for the individual patient. Perhaps even detection of the virus would not be enough, for it might still have to be established that the isolated virus was sensitive to one or another drug before adequate therapy could be undertaken. It would be ideal if such viral drug sensitivity were first established, but the ideal is not always achieved and it is likely that antiviral drugs, even those with narrow antiviral spectra, will be used based solely on clinical observations. Still, a specimen should be taken prior to any therapy to confirm the clinical diagnosis so adjustment in therapy can be made when necessary. It should be reemphasized that so far as is known today, the greatest percentage of viral lower respiratory tract illness is self-limiting and not lethal, with influenza in high-risk patients the outstanding exception. So even with lower respiratory tract diseases some relief of symptoms and clinical signs by a palliative drug is also a worthwhile goal.

3.6. VIRAL DISEASES OF THE NERVOUS SYSTEM AND EYE

3.6.1. THE PROBLEM

Although viral eye infections have been recorded with smallpox, vaccinia and varicella-zoster viruses most were attributed to herpes simplex or adenoviruses, the latter causing little serious disease. Now it is clear that acute hemorrhagic conjunctivitis (AHC), associated with echovirus type 70 (Mirkovic *et al.*, 1973; Arnow *et al.*, 1977), which seemed limited to Asia, has been detected in Central and South America and now in the United States (Centers for Disease Control, 1981). Echovirus 70 disease is troublesome and can produce an explosive epidemic of AHC but it is seemingly self-limiting and not serious. This cannot be said for HSV eye infections, especially recurrent disease that seriously endangers vision. At present such disease is most treatable, with a number of agents, as will be discussed. Conjunctivitis associated with adenoviruses has yet to yield to any treatment despite the fact they, like herpesviruses, contain DNA but have long shown resistance to DNA inhibitors that are so very active against HSV (Herrmann, 1968). With the recognition of echovirus 70 as an important cause of eye infections it seems worthwhile to now restudy the role of viruses in eye disease in general.

Viral infections of the central nervous system seem far from resolution since so many diverse viruses are involved, some frequently produce relatively mild and self-limiting disease, such as mumps and enteroviruses, while others produce significant fatal encephalitides, as with herpes simplex and togaviruses. At the outset of any viral induced nervous system disease it is, of course, not clear whether one is dealing with a mild self-limiting type of CNS infection or one that will be fatal. There are many serologically distinct viruses that produce CNS disease and these include mumps, HSV, CMV, coxsackie, echo, toga, measles and varicella-zoster viruses. One must also add to this list the relatively rare human cases of rabies and a growing list of so-called 'slow virus' diseases such as subacute sclerosing panencephalitis (SSPE) (Gajdusek, 1977). The virus-induced CNS diseases can be mild with almost indetectable meningitis or can be severe meningoencephalitis, encephalitis and more rarely slow fatal degenerative disease or even peripheral nervous disorders and paralysis. There is little question that the viral-induced nervous system diseases are a major problem which has only been partially resolved by vaccines for the prevention of poliomyelitis, mumps and measles. It is also, of course, likely that some nervous system diseases involve viruses that are as yet undiscovered since there seem to be many cases that go undiagnosed but resemble viral infections.

3.6.2. POTENTIAL AND AVAILABLE DRUG SOLUTIONS

There appears to be no particular reason why eye diseases related to adenoviral infections should not in time yield to a specific antiviral drug, perhaps one that inhibits the DNA synthesis of this virus. It seems, however, with the exclusion of adenovirus type 8 and perhaps one or two other adenoviruses that cause epidemic keratoconjunctivitis, most adenovirus infections primarily involve the upper respiratory tract producing a pharyngitis that is sometimes exudative, with fever and this can include at times a conjunctivitis. Topical application of an antiadenoviral drug to the eye would, therefore, not usually be a proper drug solution but rather what is needed is a systematically active drug. In most cases adenoviral diseases would be seen in children and much less frequently in civilian adults.

As previously indicated idoxuridine, adenine arabinoside and trifluridine are all available for treatment of HSV eye disease. It is likely that these drugs are often used in the absence of any laboratory confirmation. It is also possible they are used topically for HSV infections other than of the eye. There are certain HSV eye infections that are deeper and more serious and might not be readily recognized as induced by this virus. In such cases there is much justification for laboratory confirmation of such infections. Generally, however, it is best to know early that the infection is indeed associated with HSV since, in our experience, many specimens taken from those with eye diseases produce no virus isolates, suggesting that certain eye infections may not be all that easy to diagnose by clinical observations alone. There have been occasions when varicella-zoster virus and even the poxviruses, such as the vaccine virus for smallpox, have infected the eye and in these cases the antiherpetic ophthalmic preparations seem helpful (Jones and Al-Hussaini, 1963; Jack and Sorenson, 1963; Kaufman et al., 1963). It would be hoped that with the presumed demise of smallpox neither this virus nor its vaccine strain would again be detected infecting the human eye.

Echovirus 70 pandemic eye infections represent a new challenge. Here an antipicornavirus drug is needed. Indeed, the Eli Lilly Co. has been approached to test enviroxime in Japan where AHC is widespread. It will remain to be seen whether topical treatment is required or oral dosing is needed.

Central nervous system infections require some immediate therapy because of the possibility of permanent brain damage. Yet, most cases of virus-related CNS disease will be relatively mild with no sequelae even when untreated. The greatest amount of CNS disease is produced by enteroviruses, especially the coxsackieviruses of the B type. Few communities will go through an entire year without at least some meningitis caused by one or another of these viruses; in some cases there will be a meningoencephalitis and even a few cases of encephalitis, but very rarely will it be fatal or even leave any permanent brain damage. The purpose of chemotherapy would be to shorten the course of the disease and prevent any possible potential complications. The drugs required would have to be well tolerated and rapidly halt viral synthesis. There is no reason why specific inhibitors cannot be found that are compatible with drug therapy in that inhibitors for these viruses have long been known, as pointed out earlier. Clearly, in cases of central nervous system disease, palliatives or drugs for symptomatic relief might be helpful, but still what seems needed is a specific viral inhibitor, perhaps something like enviroxime (Herrmann et al., 1981c).

The insect-borne viruses associated with central nervous system diseases are also responsible for other clinical syndromes such as yellow and hemorrhagic fevers. The greatest problem, however, is to deal with the lethal or serious sequelae that can result from infection with a number of togaviruses and certain insect-borne viruses now classified in other virus categories. These viruses contain RNA and also a lipid envelope essential to the survival of the virus. Not enough seems to have been done in the search for specific inhibitors of the RNA of these viruses or even for inhibitors of their envelope formation. Whatever the action-mechanism, specific inhibitors are required so that viral synthesis can be brought to a swift halt from the very first moment. It seems a very serious ethical problem, however, to save a life that must now spend its remaining days in an institution, a problem that still occurs in cases of bacterial meningitis no matter what the antibacterial treatment. Clearly such a chance must be taken, but the need is for a potent viral inhibitor that rapidly reaches the site of the infection. Symptomatic relief would not be adequate but a prophylactic drug might well be considered, especially in the high-risk patient groups, such as the aged, in the face of an outbreak of St. Louis encephalitis.

Even though HSV encephalitis was suggested as a serious widespread disease (Rawls et al., 1966) it has only recently been fully recognized. It is now established that HSV encephalitis produces a mortality rate upwards of 70 per cent and much brain damage among the survivors (Whitley et al., 1977). It is somewhat of a surprise that there is not much more HSV encephalitis in that this virus is likely to be one of the most widespread of all known viruses, due no doubt to the very common occurrence of the cold sore. It is the type 1 HSV that is most often isolated in both cases of the cold sore and encephalitis. The first steps have now been taken to attack HSV encephalitis with the use of araA. This is not the complete answer since more potent drugs are needed to head off the extensive sequelae that frequently occur in treated survivors (Whitley et al., 1977), but the proof is now in, potentially fatal HSV encephalitis can be altered by therapy and araA will likely be used until a more potent, less toxic or metabolically stable drug is available. It should be noted that the study of araA's use in HSV-induced encephalitis has been sharply criticized (Tager, 1977; Morris, 1977). Nonetheless, as with most viral CNS disease, the only drug to consider first is one that specifically, and rapidly, halts HSV synthesis prior to significant brain damage. In addition, extensive supportive patient care also seems important, for this was the only approach used in the apparent recovery of two persons from rabiesvirus infection (Hattwick *et al.*, 1972; Porras *et al.*, 1976). The study of the treatment of HSV encephalitis leaves little doubt that there is no fundamental reason why other viral CNS infections cannot be attacked in the same chemotherapeutic manner once there is a more aggressive search for specific viral inhibitors for all viruses causing such disease. So far, for example, there seems to have been little work done in looking for a drug to combat the rabiesvirus. Such a drug might not only be used for treatment of frank rabies cases but also could be used as a prophylactic measure, as an adjunct to the present vaccine and hyperimmune serum procedures. One would hope that harmless rabies vaccine strains could be included in the tests for antiviral activity. It is estimated that in Latin America alone some 300,000 persons receive antirabies treatment (Porras *et al.*, 1976). A drug certainly seems in order if it is recalled that a full treatment with the vaccine does not necessarily prevent a case of rabies in a human (Gomez *et al.*, 1965).

The slow-virus diseases present a considerable problem in arriving at a suggestion of how to apply antiviral chemotherapy since our present knowledge of the role of the virus is so sketchy. First, a distinction should be made between CNS diseases associated with conventional viruses and those associated with so-called unconventional viruses since so little is known about this latter type of biological entity (Gajdusek, 1977). Nonetheless, if conventional or unconventional virus production involves metabolic pathways that do not exist in normal healthy cells, then theoretically their synthesis can be halted. What is not known is whether the synthesis of either unconventional or conventional viruses is the basic cause of these serious and degenerating diseases. Whatever the process, it is clear that some drug is needed to halt whatever is going on at the very first moment when the disease is recognized. The slow pace of these diseases is such that there is some hope a drug could be applied with substantial success. SSPE is a fatal disease, and the course can extend over many months. If a drug were available to treat human measles cases then certainly it should be tried for the treatment of SSPE. Amantadine has been tried on such cases and the authors felt it was beneficial (Haslam *et al.*, 1969) even though this drug is not known to affect the measles virus. A search specifically seeking drugs to treat what, for the moment, is a rare disease seems unlikely. An antiviral drug might be found, however, that is poorly tolerated for treating the rather benign common cold, for example, but yet the toxicity would be acceptable in a degenerative, slow-virus disease, such as SSPE.

There are instances of nervous system diseases associated with shingles, chicken pox, measles (rare because of the vaccine), vaccinia viruses (rare since discontinuation of generalized smallpox vaccination) and at times other viruses such as that of infectious mononucleosis. The therapeutic approach to such complications could be just an extension of that drug treatment, were one available, that is used when the more common disease form is encountered. If the common disease is treated by an effective drug it would be expected that CNS disease caused by the same viruses would also respond, or even be aborted.

3.6.3. Diagnostic Needs

Central nervous system diseases, especially meningitis and meningoencephalitis associated with the mumps or enteroviruses, should not be difficult to diagnose. In about 60 per cent of the cases of mumpsvirus, central nervous system disease is preceded by a classical case of mumps with parotid gland swelling. Once mumps is detected in the community then mumpsvirus-associated central nervous system disease should be expected. In temperate climates, during other than the summer and early fall months, the first guess at the causal agent of CNS disease should be mumpsvirus, once a bacterial infection is excluded. In that mumps central nervous system disease frequently occurs well after infection, the virus is not easily isolated from the upper respiratory tract but it can at times be detected in the urine (Utz *et al.*, 1958; Person *et al.*, 1971). Detection of a rise in specific complement fixing antibody frequently occurs too late to be other than a retrospective diagnosis (Person *et al.*, 1971). The use of virus isolation methods, clinical observations and serology could go very far in at least determining if mumpsvirus infection is widespread in the community. The question arises if any of this would permit prompt use of a specific therapeutic antiviral drug with individual cases? With a frank case of mumps, presenting with classical salivary gland involvement, the use of an antiviral drug might well prevent development of not only CNS disease but a variety of other mumpsvirus caused problems including orchitis. With continued widespread vaccination against mumpsvirus, it is becoming far less prevalent in pediatric populations. Some adults, however, may be detected with mumpsvirus CNS disease.

Serological methods are impractical in the diagnosis of enterovirus disease because of the many serotypes that could be involved, more than 70. In tropical climates these viruses can be seen year around while in temperate climates they are primarily summertime visitors and usually can be isolated rather readily in the average virus diagnostic laboratory. Coxsackie-viruses of the B type seem to be a most common cause of CNS disease and are isolated and recognized usually in just a few days. Echoviruses take somewhat longer to isolate but can be recognized rather readily (Herrmann et al., 1972). Coxsackieviruses of the A types are not always easily isolated, requiring in many instances infant mouse inoculation, but these viruses are less commonly a cause of CNS disease.

Once certain enteroviruses are detected in the community, using either cell cultures or mice, then, of course, some cases of central nervous system disease should be viewed as likely caused by these viruses and treatment begun with a specific antiviral drug until data are produced to indicate otherwise. Enteroviruses can be readily isolated from the respiratory tract early in the course of the infection and such an isolation carries greater weight than an isolation from feces. Enterovirus isolation, however, can be achieved even many weeks after disease onset but in this case viral excretion may not be related to the disease for it is common for children to excrete these viruses unassociated with any disease. Nonetheless, any enterovirus isolation must be seriously considered. A virus-alert program for the entire community would go far in preparing physicians for the use of specific drugs to treat all types of enteroviral disease.

When herpes simplex virus infects the CNS it presents some considerable diagnostic problems since it is felt serological diagnosis can either be misleading or take too long, and virus isolation is achieved largely by using brain tissue (Johnson et al., 1968). The clinical picture of the disease can be helpful but yet there can be some confusion with other CNS problems (Rawls et al., 1966). At present isolation of the virus from a brain biopsy is thought the most accurate diagnostic method. Tissue rich in virus permits detection in 2 or 3 days in cell culture with the study of stained tissue sections also of some use if classical intranuclear inclusions are detected (which are not strictly specific for HSV but this would still be the most common virus involved). Fluorescent antibody methods are not completely reliable in such infections (Cho and Feng, 1978). In that very early treatment of HSV brain infections is best, then new, swifter, diagnostic tests will be necessary if permanent brain damage is to be avoided. Rapid treatment is very much the key to success, so diagnosis based on clinical impressions seems the most humane approach, with some type of laboratory confirmation following. A closer study, however, of typical cases of HSV encephalitis may further reveal clinical guidelines that will permit early use of antiviral drugs.

It was long thought, based on misleading serological data, that HSV was a common cause of 'aseptic meningitis'. It was found, however, that the virus was infrequently isolated from spinal fluid which is the opposite of what occurs with similar diseases caused by mumps or enteroviruses. It is still not clear if meningitis is sometimes caused by the type 2 venereal herpes simplex virus (Wolontis and Jeansson, 1977). This virus type is less prevalent when compared to the type 1 virus that is so frequently found associated with cold sores. The diagnosis of meningitis related to any type of herpes simplex virus, however, presents some problems. A brain biopsy would not seem justified. The virus should be found in the spinal fluid but this seems a rather rare occurrence (Herrmann, 1972). Again the detection of rapidly rising antibody might be a useful diagnostic method but the relative rarity of this type of meningitis could inhibit establishment of such a test on a routine basis. The use of labeled antibody methods to detect HSV antigen in infected cells in the spinal fluid and blood could be a rapid diagnostic test but it has not been shown to be as sensitive as isolation of the virus in cell cultures (Cho and Feng, 1978). Of course, the patient's medical history could be helpful if it suggests a possible recent infection with the venereal or type 2 HSV. A much closer study of the clinical picture now seems required to try and discover if there is something unique or suggestive about type 2 HSV CNS disease.

It would seem prudent to effectively treat even mild HSV-induced diseases in the hope this would abort CNS disease. It seems worth mentioning that the widespread use of antiherpes drugs on common HSV infections, such as cold sores, stomatitis, pharyngitis and a variety of dermal and mucosal lesions, might have an indirect influence on HSV induced CNS disease by limiting the huge amounts of virus being poured into the population. Some feel, of course, that latent HSV, induced to activity by some type of trauma, may be the cause of the CNS disease (Rawls et al., 1966). Even if this were proven, however, the wise course would be to effectively treat the common infections for this might also inhibit the latent infections.

Presently HSV seems our most easily detected virus, producing a cytopathic effect that is distinctive and can at times be observed within 24 hours after the culture is inoculated (Table 1). This virus isolation procedure is comparable to bacterial isolation methods and should be an example of what is needed for all viral diagnosis. Further, even in the absence of virus isolation, distinctive inclusions present in the lesions help to implicate herpesviruses. It would seem, therefore, that the combination of present diagnostic methods plus the use of known antiviral drugs should permit an effective attack on diseases caused by the herpesviruses with the possible exception of encephalitis where somewhat swifter diagnostic methods seem required.

The insect-borne virus encephalitides also present a considerable diagnostic problem. A sporadic case of something like California or St. Louis virus encephalitis would at best be diagnosed by serological methods, very late in the course of the illness. Again, however, the virus-alert concept could come into play and indeed has been to some extent already used since the news media widely announce outbreaks of mosquito-borne viral disease. A patient's history of exposure to mosquitos most certainly would be suggestive while on the other hand a CNS infection occurring during the cold months with no mosquito activity would rule out this type of viral disease (providing of course the patient had not recently been to a more tropical climate). The serological test often requires both acute and convalescent sera to detect a rise in hemagglutination inhibition antibodies. There should be some encouragement still to test the acute serum even if no convalescent serum was forthcoming, for a high antibody titer can often be suggestive of which type of mosquito-borne virus is involved. Mosquito-borne viruses can be isolated by intracerebral injection of specimens into the brains of mice. Unfortunately, the human blood stream harbors the virus very briefly leaving brain tissue the only useful specimen and this is largely an impractical specimen, especially since much of the disease produced is mild and self-limiting. Death is, however, not an uncommon result of mosquito-borne viral disease and proper treatment with antiviral drugs would have significant benefit if such drugs existed. The treatment would probably have to be prompt using clinical observations alone with later confirmation from the laboratory.

There are cases of encephalitis associated with chicken pox (varicella) where the classical skin eruption occurs first thereby permitting antiherpetic therapy at an early stage. Lymphocytic choriomeningitis (LCM) virus can also cause a relatively rare encephalitis in humans. The patient's history might in this case reveal some clues in that there should be a close association with infestations of mice and in some cases even with laboratory animals that harbor this virus. For diagnosis, specific isolation of the virus is not practical since the virus is most readily found in the brain and the disease is not so severe as to justify obtaining brain tissue. Disease caused by LCM virus has some clinical distinctiveness but the usual diagnostic procedure is to detect a rise in specific antibody in paired sera, a procedure frequently available through public health laboratories. Indeed these laboratories often perform serological tests for LCM, mumps, herpes simplex and the more prevalent mosquito-borne viruses. Unfortunately the evidence shows (Herrmann and Herrmann, 1976a) the results of these tests are much delayed and of little use as a guide to therapy for an individual patient.

Shingles, a troublesome disease caused by the chicken pox virus, can be associated with some peripheral nerve damage and even permanent paralysis. Prompt treatment, even today, with antiherpetic drugs might well prevent such nerve damage. The virus can be isolated in human fibroblast cultures from fresh vesicle fluid obtained from the vesicular lesions but very often the clinical picture alone is typical enough for an accurate diagnosis. The isolation of this virus could be time consuming so treatment might best not be delayed until a laboratory result is produced. Again a search can be made for intranuclear inclusions which would not, however, distinguish a varicella-zoster from HSV infections. Such a distinction may not be important, however, in that the same drugs seemingly could be used for both infections.

Hopefully much of the central nervous system diseases associated with polio, mumps and measles viruses will be the thing of the past with widespread use of vaccines to prevent these infections. Presently there seems little concern for even looking for drugs to use on these diseases. Regrettably, however, there are in the United States some rare cases of poliomyelitis caused by the vaccine. Antiviral agents, something like those already mentioned, active against the picornaviruses could well be used for even these rare polio cases, and, of course, for diagnosis any poliovirus can be rapidly isolated in the laboratory from both rectal and throat swabs. The vaccine strains can be distinguished from the so-called wild strains because of the failure of the vaccine strains to multiply in cell cultures at 40°C.

In the case of measles there should be some concern that the vaccine virus, as well as the wild-type strain, can be associated with those rare cases of subacute sclerosing pan-encephalitis (SSPE) (Gajdusek, 1977). As with most so-called slow-virus disease, the diagnosis is made primarily on clinical and histopathological grounds. Generally the progress of these diseases, as suggested before, is slow, hence, permitting a diagnosis with institution of proper treatment, if one existed. Certainly the earliest possible diagnosis, however, would be more desirable, especially if this could be done prior to serious illness. Presently the isolation of a measles-like virus from cases of SSPE is far from routine. The question still remains, however, would specific antiviral therapy be helpful in cases of slow-virus disease and if so at what stage in the illness?

A drug that quickly halts rabiesvirus multiplication would seem not to require a laboratory diagnosis to justify its use. Even a drug only moderately well tolerated could be used based on the clinical history alone with somewhat more freedom than now suggested for the use of the present immune antiserum and vaccine treatment. With pursuit of the responsible animal and the use of routine rabies diagnostic methods, a laboratory confirmation could follow. These laboratory methods should include fluorescent antibody to detect specific rabiesvirus as well as a search for Negri bodies and this should be further confirmed by injection of the brain tissue intracerebrally into infant mice. Even without the offending animal, however, chemotherapy could well be used when there might be greater hesitation to use vaccine and immune serum procedures which are not only rather troublesome but on occasion can produce unfortunate side reactions.

Cases of central nervous system disease have at times been associated with infectious mononucleosis (IM). Since most accept that IM is caused by the herpesvirus of Epstein and Barr (Henle et al., 1968) this disease could well be treated with one of the antiherpes drugs now under study. The heterophile antibody tests are still rather useful in diagnosing IM and these positive tests along with a classical clinical history and blood picture would be excellent guides to treatment. So far routine isolation of this virus is not possible. Of course, IM with or without CNS disease would require a systemically acting antiherpes drug and even in those cases caused by cytomegalovirus, where the heterophile antibody test is negative, an antiherpes drug could still be effective. CMV can be isolated in human fibroblast cell cultures but it is frequently time-consuming and the virus often missed. If the antiherpes drug is well tolerated there should be no reason to withhold it in infections either caused by E–B or CM virus. Certainly in those serious CMV infections occurring in infants and those that are immune deficient there should be every reason to use an antiherpes drug at the earliest moment based on the clinical picture. Later confirmation of the CMV infection can be done by detection of specific IgM antibody, the virus or the typical inclusions often seen in cells found in the urine.

3.7. VIRUS DISEASES OF THE SKIN

3.7.1. THE PROBLEM

Many viral diseases produce skin eruptions and this would include measles, rubella and infections caused by certain enteroviruses, adenoviruses and parainfluenza viruses. All of these are systemic diseases whereby the skin eruption is just one manifestation of the infection and are not considered specific skin diseases nor would they be treated topically. Rather they require treatment of the entire infected host. Measles, of course, can be adequately controlled by vaccine and this, hopefully, will also be true of rubella, which is largely a mild childhood disease that might be conveniently ignored if it were not for the attack of this virus on the human fetus.

The cold sore, whether it be on the lips or elsewhere on the body, has to be the most common of all viral skin infections. Some data are being misread giving rise to the claim that 20–40 per cent of humans have recurrent herpetic skin lesions (Spruance et al., 1977). Although considerably more data are required, the figure for those having one cold sore episode in a 6–9-month period is about 8 per cent of a study population (Young et al., 1976). But even if this lower figure is true of all human groups, in all locales, then it truly is an enormous amount of viral infection. To this must be added the problem of type 2 virus, the venereal strain, that has been suggested as having an association with cervical carcinoma (Melnick et al., 1974), and which commonly infects skin and mucosa of humans. Indeed, some claim HSV venereal disease is most common (Nahmias et al., 1969) and perhaps frequently overlooked because it is self-limiting and rarely causes any sequelae. On the other hand, it can be recurrent on the genitalia just like cold sores.

Chicken pox is, of course, a generalized disease but this is not true of zoster which is a manifestation of infection by the same virus in those who are partially immune. Zoster is localized to areas of the skin that overlay certain, specific nerves that are likewise infected. Shingles occur mostly in those over 50 years of age but it can occur at any age and it can be quite painful, persisting for months. On occasion nerve damage occurs producing persistent pain and even permanent paralysis to facial, arm and hand muscles. There seem to be no accurate data on the morbidity of shingles but it is a disease common enough that almost everyone has encountered someone who has had this troublesome problem. It should be added that pain and chronicity are not always the hallmark of this disease, for some suffer very little and get over it quickly suggesting that special immune conditions may exist in those with the more troublesome aspects of the disease.

One would hope that no need existed for a discussion of smallpox which is in fact also a systemic disease, that could be attacked by orally administered drugs (Bauer, 1977). Likewise it would seem that discussion of serious skin infections by vaccinia virus, the smallpox vaccine virus, would also not be in order since the demise of smallpox. One still hears, however, of smallpox vaccination being used to attack a cold sore problem. Such a practice cannot be condemned too strongly, most especially since smallpox vaccine is contraindicated for those with recurrent skin lesions. It seems almost unbelievable that the smallpox vaccine is still commercially available for those other than laboratory workers who use vaccinia virus (Centers for Disease Control, 1980).

3.7.2. DRUG SOLUTIONS

There is no longer any need for conjecture regarding the direction that should be taken for the treatment of herpetic skin lesions. There have long been suggestive data that IUdR in DMSO has a useful effect on HSV and zoster skin lesions (Herrmann and Herrmann, 1977a) when used topically. It is true that in an aqueous base neither IUdR or araA produced a useful effect but recent unpublished data provided by the Burroughs Wellcome Co. indicates that acyclovir in a water base is active on dermal lesions. The clinical trials of acyclovir were clearly to the disadvantage of the drug but, if nothing else, it establishes that topical treatment can be useful. Using an orally applied drug to aid a limited dermal lesion would seem to complicate the solution. Orally applied drugs may, however, be strongly supported as the debate ensues over what is a 'cure' based on the strongly held view of HSV latency in human nerves. Emphasis on curing latency rather than clinical disease establishes a demand on a drug that would be ethically unlikely to be proved. Even now clinical trials of antiherpetic drugs applied topically on well-developed lesions with frequent samplings of virus excretion cannot aid the drug in showing its full potential. More than likely if such a drug were available to those suffering from recurrent herpetic lesions it would be applied at the very first 'tingle' at onset of a recurrence. In such a case a useful drug would be most effective. Once there is an established lesion, topical therapy may well limit its extension or the formation of new lesions but have little effect on the established pathology.

The use of IUdR dissolved in DMSO on zoster suggests that topical treatment could even have an effect on the nerve pain (Herrmann and Herrmann, 1977a). Certainly DMSO aids penetration of the drug. It is understandable that drug firms might avoid the expense of obtaining a regulatory agency approval first for the drug and then for DMSO. Hopefully, however, any antiherpes drug should be effective on infections with HSV types 1 and 2 and varicella-zoster virus. With all of these infections, when severe enough, even intravenous drug use could be justified as already has been the case with acyclovir, as previously discussed. We are at the point now where there is little doubt we can treat herpesvirus disease; all that is left is to work out the details.

3.7.3. DIAGNOSTIC NEEDS

It can be hoped that an effective antiherpes virus drug would act on all herpetic skin lesions whether caused by both types of HSV or V–Z virus. This would seemingly eliminate significant laboratory diagnosis. In many cases 'cold sores' and 'shingles' can be recognized for what they are. Where viral diagnosis seems required is when there are lesions of the mucous membranes, many of which are not known to be of viral origin. Certain oral lesions are associated with HSV and coxsackieviruses of the A type and indeed, in our experience, sometimes with the B type virus. Further, the type A coxsackieviruses can produce dermal vesicles much like the vesicles produced by herpesviruses, and DNA inhibitors would have no effect on these RNA containing picornaviruses. Coxsackie A viruses tend to be summer visitors in temperate climates and with proper monitoring of the viruses in the community, one could be alerted to their presence, thus perhaps minimizing the confusion. It is worth noting that about 66 per cent of dermal specimens produced no virus isolate (Herrmann and Herrmann, 1976b). Certainly a number of factors other than viruses can cause vesicular lesions, as for example, poison ivy or other allergies. HSV is the most readily isolated and identified of all human viruses so the problem of laboratory diagnosis of these infections seems largely solved. Varicella-zoster virus is somewhat more difficult to isolate, but given fresh vesicle fluid, inoculated into cell cultures at the first possible moment, this results in a significant number of isolates even though it may take a week or more before virus activity is seen. But treatment would have largely been begun prior to a laboratory report in any event; at least that is what should, in all practicality, be expected. Generally, when confronted by a herpesvirus infection of the skin there seems no significant need for ultra-rapid viral diagnosis especially using labeled antibody methods.

3.8. VIRAL DISEASES OF THE UROGENITAL SYSTEM, THE NEONATE AND THE NEWBORN

3.8.1. THE PROBLEM

Presently the most important virus infection of the urogenital system is that caused by herpes simplex virus, frequently the type 2 venereal strain. Some of what has been said of the diagnosis and treatment of infections by this virus in previous sections applies here. Certainly these seem to be widespread infections and they can be recurrent (Nahmias *et al.*,

1969). A major concern has been suggestive data associating HSV type 2 with carcinoma of the cervix (Melnick *et al.*, 1974). A second concern, whether it be type 1 or 2 HSV, is the infection of the newborn in its travel down the infected birth canal. Although such neonatal infections can at times be limited and superficial and even subclinical, more serious disease does occur such as infections of the eye (which can, of course, be treated with presently available drugs) and a generalized infection that involves a number of organs and can produce a fatal outcome. Serious infections likely occur in about one in 10,000 births but these figures vary depending on the study population (Hanshaw, 1973), nonetheless there are enough cases to demand more rapid progress in the development of effective treatment using antiherpetic agents that are already known.

Mumpsvirus infection of the urogenital tract is common since this virus can be isolated so readily from urine even for weeks. Specific disease involving this system seems rarer, however, and usually takes the form of monolateral orchitis in post-puberty males; bilateral orchitis is rarer and hence sterility is not common. Oophoritis also occurs in some cases of mumps but sequelae from such infections is not well documented, as is the case with fetal or newborn infections. It is hoped that widespread use of the mumps vaccine will largely control these problems.

There have been claims that adenoviruses are associated with hemorrhagic cystitis, mostly in children (Manalo *et al.*, 1971). In that this work has not been fully confirmed (and in fact could not be confirmed by these authors) there is some question that this is a valid problem. It is possible that other viruses do at times infect the urogenital system, perhaps some that are still undiscovered but the problems are as yet indistinct. It is worth mentioning, however, that the very common detection of simian viruses in kidney tissue from healthy monkeys suggests that the human kidney might well also be infected with a variety of viruses. This is not to say that such infections are commonly associated with disease; probably they are not.

Cytomegalovirus, which can even be isolated at times from the urine of healthy children, is another herpesvirus that can infect the fetus, producing a devastating disease (Hanshaw, 1971). Even though the maternal urinary tract can be infected this is likely not the source of many fetal infections but it is not clear how much CMV disease occurs post-natally. The major problem is infection of the fetus and this likely occurs because of a viremia in the mother. Cytomegalovirus is presumed to infect all humans, if antibody surveys are an accurate gauge of infection, but it seems that most cases go unstudied or are mild with the possible exception of certain instances of heterophile antibody negative infectious mononucleosis and it could be such a case in the mother leads to an infected fetus. Despite what seems the more common prevalence of HSV, the more serious and frequent cases of newborn disease involve CMV infection. Like HSV and varicella-zoster, CMV takes a more serious course in the immunodeficient and immunosuppressed patient and the fetus and newborn might in a sense be considered in this category. It is estimated that CMV infections can be detected in 1–2 per cent of all newborns but there is concern that some cases of mental retardation may also be produced by this virus and even perhaps by HSV, cases that went unrecognized in the newborn (Nahmias *et al.*, 1976).

The role of rubella virus in attacks on the fetus is well known and will not be pursued further here in the hope that the rubella vaccine can in time eliminate this as a significant problem. The enteroviruses, principally those of the coxsackie B group, are of some importance in newborn infections and it is likely that echoviruses also play some role in diseases of the newborn, no doubt as a result of fecal excretion of these viruses by the mother at the time of birth. Some cases can be fatal in newborns because of a serious myocarditis while other newborns may exhibit a meningitis and even an encephalitis, although in these latter cases mortality seems rare. Considering the prevalence of enteroviruses during the summer months, infection of the newborn resulting in a serious problem seems less frequent than might be expected. Of course any viral infection, producing significant illness in the mother, might cause problems for the fetus but such problems seem rare enough that they are as yet not well defined. What has now been well defined is the role of the so-called rotaviruses in infant diarrheal disease, almost always in those under 3 years of age. It has been established that these infections can be rather serious in the infant (Carlson *et al.*, 1978).

Newborn children clearly can be subjected to those viral infections that afflict all humans but this is not as great a problem as it might seem since they have an array of antibodies from the mother that can persist for various lengths of time even up to a year after birth. One suspects that in addition there is intrinsic resistance to infection in the newborn that, however, may not be enough in the face of massive doses of virus either prior to or after birth. Again, it seems worth pointing out that many fetal and newborn problems go unexplained and a number of these, including some cases of mental retardation, could be related to infections by viruses still undetected or characterized.

3.8.2. POTENTIAL DRUG SOLUTIONS

Prior sections have discussed potential if not real drug solutions to herpesvirus infections, whether they are superficial or systemic, and this applies also to infections of the urogenital system and the newborn. How one shall prevent viral attacks on the fetus when a mother has a virus infection presents significant problems, none the least of which is the effect of the drug on the fetus. In some cases, such as with CMV or HSV, the maternal infection may not be obvious. When it is, then it should probably be treated but the benefits should outweigh the risks to the fetus and this can only be done when the cause of the viral infection is well established and any possible action of the drug on the fetus is well known. Having said this, however, antiviral drug treatment of the infected gravid female must be considered as a potentially fruitful approach to protecting the fetus and even the newborn.

In that there seems little interest in vaccines for the many enteroviruses, other than polioviruses, specific chemotherapy for these infections seems required, especially when they occur in the newborn and this would, of course, require systemic therapy, as discussed in prior sections. One should still expect that even those diseases that can be largely controlled by vaccines, such as rubella, polio or measles, in some cases will still occur and hopefully, in time, there will be adequate drugs available, perhaps those primarily for other viral diseases, that will also prove useful in the treatment of these rare cases.

3.8.3. DIAGNOSTIC NEEDS

CMV and HSV infections of the urogenital system and the newborn can in most cases be diagnosed by the clinical picture and by virus isolation so that proper drug treatment can be instituted rather promptly. There are instances when urine does not produce a positive result when from a typical case of CMV infection so there is some room for improvement in the detection of this virus in cell cultures. Also there are cases of HSV infection where no herpetic skin lesions occur or where the virus is not detected in any convenient specimen and this produces the same diagnostic problem as found with HSV encephalitis. Again the question arises whether some early rising specific antibody might aid in the diagnosis so that effective treatment might be undertaken. In some cases the clinical picture would be such that therapy could be started without a laboratory diagnosis, and continued until that time when a CMV or HSV infection is ruled out.

An epidemiological approach could be used for enterovirus infections. Coxsackieviruses of the B type cause the more serious problem in the newborn and a monitoring system would readily establish the presence of these viruses in the community. The mother might well be tested for excretion of these viruses prior to delivery even though it is not completely clear that all enterovirus infection of the newborn come from this source. Coxsackie B viruses are readily isolated in cell cultures and many times produce a recognizable cytopathic effect in 2 or 3 days. The question arises whether infections of the newborn by such viruses always permit easy access to the virus, especially in cases of myocarditis. It is not clear that all such cases shed virus in the throat or feces. Further, the cases are rare enough that some physicians may not have adequate experience to recognize the problem based on the clinical picture alone. If it is known that such viruses are in the community then treatment with a specific, systemically applied drug that is therapeutic for enterovirus infections could be used to treat a very ill newborn. It would be hard to imagine that much improvement is required in the isolation of coxsackie B viruses, that are routinely recognized and reported to the physician almost as rapidly as are bacterial isolations (Hable *et al.*, 1970). The echoviruses take somewhat longer to isolate and recognize but they seem to be less of a problem in the newborn, indeed serious illness may be rather rare (Herrmann *et al.*, 1972). Even though most enteroviruses are rather readily detected and recognized the problem has been to define the specific serotype of the over seventy that exist. The hope is that this will not be necessary in that antienteroviral drugs will be effective against all the various serotypes and identification could be a simple biochemical test even using the drug as the best indicator of the nature of the virus rather than tedious and lengthy serum neutralization tests.

Some thought must be given, of course, to the varying drug sensitivities of related viruses. For example, a newborn could well be infected with either type 1 or 2 HSV. It has been long known that these two viruses are not equally sensitive to certain antiviral drugs (Person *et al.*, 1970); hence, it might have to be determined which of the two types is infecting the child. On the other hand, it would seem prudent to promote a drug for herpes simplex virus that was equally useful on both types of infections thereby eliminating any need for typing HSV. One should be prepared, however, for the emergence of drug-resistant mutants. There are sufficient data on such mutants (Herrmann and Herrmann, 1977b) to suggest that drug-sensitivity tests will become a routine part of viral diagnosis.

3.9. VIRAL DISEASES OF THE GASTROINTESTINAL SYSTEM

3.9.1. The Problem

Substantial progress has been made in understanding the nature of hepatitis viruses and there is widespread use of methods that can detect the coat of hepatitis B virus (HBV or serum hepatitis virus) in ill patients as well as in blood donors. These methods still lack some sensitivity but are very useful. Certainly some hepatitis virus carriers still are not detected. Further, such carriers present a public health problem since there is no cure for their infection.

A vaccine for hepatitis B virus infection is now available, made from the virus coat found in the blood of carriers. Clearly this will be limited in its use, likely for those health workers most exposed to this virus. Male homosexuals are another high-risk group along with drug addicts, but it is not known if enough vaccine will be available for all at high risk. So far as the carrier state is concerned, the vaccine is not claimed to affect this condition. The problem would seem to be how can a person that has carried this virus in their bloodstream, likely for years, be made immune by injections of still more pieces of the same virus?

At least one so-called infectious hepatitis virus has been characterized, this hepatitis A virus (HAV), like the hepatitis B virus cannot be readily cultivated in cell cultures and it is recognized by concentration from feces and then visualized in electron micrographs. Work with both these viruses has led to the conclusion that they are not the only viruses that cause hepatitis in humans. Indeed, perhaps 90 per cent of post-transfusion hepatitis is neither A or B virus. There is no clear idea of how many hepatitis viruses there may be. So despite great strides the picture is complex. Something was achieved, however, when it was discovered that purchased human blood was much more likely to contain hepatitis B virus than was blood from volunteers and correcting this has lowered the rate of post-transfusion hepatitis (Holland and Alter, 1976).

The second major virus associated problem of the gastrointestinal system is just now emerging. Some had thought that the enteroviruses, such as echo and coxsackieviruses, were a common cause of gastrointestinal upsets. It is clear now that they play a minor role in these ailments. The rotaviruses are the primary cause of severe infantile diarrhea. To this can be added a number of other viruses associated with both adult and childhood bouts of vomiting and diarrhea. These include the Newport type agents, astroviruses, 'mini-reoviruses' and likely others (Middleton *et al.*, 1977). None of these viruses, usually causing a rather explosive short-term gastrointestinal upset, can as yet be cultivated in the laboratory. How many more there may be, how many types of viruses they represent, is unknown. The solution to the problem, unlike that of hepatitis, does not seem to require something as vigorous as a vaccine in that these diseases, although of substantial importance, are only life-threatening to infants who have not received proper medical care (Carlson *et al.*, 1978). Such infections might be viewed as the common cold equivalent of the G.I. tract and represent what so many for so long have incorrectly called 'intestinal flu'. So far the data suggest the morbidity from these viruses is most substantial, far in excess of what is seen with bacterial disease of the G.I. tract (Birch *et al.*, 1977).

3.9.2. POTENTIAL DRUG SOLUTIONS

Hepatitis viruses, especially the B type, cause liver damage that at times is fatal and at other times induces chronic liver problems. A vigorous application of a drug to halt virus synthesis or limit the degree of liver damage is warranted. Such a drug could also be used to protect those at risk when in contact with hepatitis cases or even to treat carriers of the virus. Further, until that time when every unit of blood for transfusion can be guaranteed free of any hepatitis virus, the same drugs might be used to protect patients receiving transfusions. Viral inhibition seems mandatory if a treatment is to be effective in halting liver damage. Unfortunately it is not known how many hepatitis viruses we are dealing with and how they may be biochemically related to each other. The A and B viruses are unrelated and each might well demand its own form of treatment. Experiments are underway in an effort to find if interferon might be useful. Here is a case where the antiviral agent is not virus specific, as certain drugs might be, and a broad spectrum drug would seem desirable. Virazole is a drug with a somewhat broad antiviral effect, part of which may not be specifically antiviral, but nonetheless it too has been considered for treatment of hepatitis. Of course, until the time all hepatitis viruses can be cultivated in some convenient laboratory system, we are not likely to be able to search for new drugs specifically active against these viruses. In assuming a specific viral inhibitor is required it must be pointed out that a recent study shows a drug that is not known to inhibit viruses (Blum *et al.*, 1977) may have some worthwhile effect on cases of hepatitis through some unknown mechanism. Hepatitis B virus is a small DNA virus, suggesting that clinical trials might well include interferon mixed with adenine arabinoside, a known inhibitor of viral DNA synthesis (Scullard *et al.*, 1981). Hepatitisvirus A, producing a much milder disease, is a small RNA virus, perhaps a picornavirus, which might be inhibited by a drug such as enviroxime, a compound known to inhibit picornaviruses (Herrmann *et al.*, 1981c).

Virus gastrointestinal disease is a different matter since most cases seem to be relatively mild, self-limiting diseases so perhaps a highly potent specific antiviral drug is not required. It seems true that certain of these viruses do produce some lesions in the G.I. tract but whether this is the direct cause of the disease problem or whether the disease is due to a toxemia is not as yet known. Nonetheless, some consideration should be given to drugs that relieve the symptoms and signs of the disease but are not specifically antiviral. Drugs that act on the toxemia or alter cellular destruction or in some manner relieve the patient's discomfort might be just what is required without making any attempt at altering the virus multiplication. The search for such drugs can be two-fold, first some attempt can be made to study various available and approved drugs for some worthwhile pharmacological effect. As mentioned before, is it possible antiinflammatory, antihistamine or even tranquilizer drugs have any worthwhile effect? Do, in fact, any of the over-the-counter drugs have any effect on human viral diseases? Animal studies could be first undertaken since virus-induced diarrhea has been established in infant mice and baby pigs and this does not involve the substantial challenge of common cold virus studies where only humans exhibit a rather subjective illness. Controlling the diarrhea would be a useful definitive criterion for the study of drugs that are not specifically antiviral.

3.9.3. Diagnostic Needs

Very substantial progress has been made in the diagnosis of both hepatitis A and B virus infections (Czaja, 1979). Tests for certain diagnostic and prognostic antigens of hepatitis B are widely available in kit form, made largely possible by the substantial amount of viral antigen found in the blood. Kits are available also for detecting, in a single blood sample, IgM antibody to hepatitis B virus infections at an early stage. Using these tests together establishes when the hepatitis is caused by a non-A, non-B virus. If, in fact, 90 per cent of today's serum hepatitis is not caused by hepatitis B virus then it is clear much still has to be done if the more dangerous 'serum-hepatitis' is to be diagnosed and then treated. Presently cell culture isolations are of little help in most hepatitis. In a few cases, however, the more common, readily isolated viruses can be associated with a hepatitis case but this is not so frequent and indicates clearly that new and more sensitive cell culture systems are needed, if all of viral hepatitis is to be accurately diagnosed and eventually treated.

The viral-induced gastrointestinal disorders present even a greater challenge since many different types are seemingly involved, none detectable presently in readily available cell cultures (Blacklow and Cukor, 1981). Rotaviruses are produced, however, in such numbers, usually seen in the EM, that an ELISA antibody labeled test for detecting virus antigen is available in kit form (Yolken and Leister, 1981). This diagnostic tool is very helpful with much gastroenteritis occurring in those under 3 years of age. For most of the viral G.I. problems in older children and adults there is complete dependence on the EM, not a widely available instrument in clinical practice which likely lacks the sensitivity a sensitive cell-culture system might have. So at present, it is not known how many serotypes of G.I. viruses there are nor even how many genera. All that is known for sure is they do not reveal their presence in the usual cell-culture systems. If the kinds of G.I. viruses are numerous then palliatives seem the only immediately useful approach to treatment.

3.10. CONCLUSIONS

There can no longer be any doubt that the era of antiviral drugs has arrived (Hahn, 1980). It is possible that antiviral drugs will find widespread use even prior to the general availability of laboratory viral diagnosis, although there is no justified reason that this should be the case. Many antiviral drugs will likely be specific inhibitors of viral infection but it is also likely there will be other types of drugs that do not influence the virus but rather have a pharmacological effect on disease symptoms and clinical signs. Some drugs may well enhance the body's own protective systems by immunmodulation or by an interferon effect. There are, in fact, many approaches to treating viral disease, a number presently neglected, but this is not likely to continue much longer as the economic potential of antiviral drugs becomes fully recognized. The advent of antiviral drugs should result in a significant decrease in the ill-advised use of antibacterial drugs for viral diseases.

The overwhelming majority of cases of viral disease involves the human respiratory tract and much of this disease looks the same even when caused by a great variety of viruses; therefore, it would seem that some type of laboratory confirmation would be required for the rational use of antiviral drugs, barring, of course, a utopian drug that inhibits many types of viruses. Even if a universal antiviral drug came into being, the need for distinguishing viral from bacterial disease would remain. The rational use of antiviral drugs based on laboratory data is not likely to come to pass, however, until it is accepted that laboratory viral diagnosis can be relatively swift, inexpensive and part of everyday, routine, medical practice. Laboratory viral diagnosis will likely follow the path of bacterial diagnosis with emphasis on isolation of the pathogen plus some indication of its drug sensitivity. In that viral diagnostic procedures may not always be useful for drug treatment of a single patient, a 'virus-alert' program should be part of medical practice. The wide transmission of information on what viruses are in the community at any one time would be an aid in the proper use of antiviral drugs. But it can still be presumed that much use of antiviral drugs will still be based solely on clinical impressions which in some cases will be correct and in other cases will be in error.

Hopefully, the degree of ill-advised use of antiviral drugs will not reach the level of what occurs with antibacterial drugs since this could cause more problems to the patient than the generally mild viral diseases. Sharp outbreaks of viral disease should be swiftly defined in an attempt to head off the wide use of an inappropriate antiviral drug.

The emphasis must be on relieving the patient's discomfort so as to produce an individual that can function in a fully effective manner. This might well be achieved with drugs that are and are not specific viral inhibitors. Of course, it would be much preferred that viral disease was prevented but there is no convincing evidence that there will be a general preventive approach to diseases produced by the hundreds of viruses that now infect humans. The future would still seem to favor specific antiviral drugs since, as indicated by antiviral studies of the past and present, it is the specific inhibitors of virus multiplication that have produced the most convincing data.

There seems little question that viral diagnosis will continue to emphasize virus isolation and identification but such an approach still seems to be lagging behind drug development. Much more needs to be done to improve virus-isolation techniques, not only for the known viruses, but for the many still unknown. The economic rewards for the successful pursuit of an antiviral drug seem obvious. The rewards for those who toil to improve viral isolation procedures is not so obvious, nor well supported financially. Until there is a dramatic change in the acceptance of laboratory viral diagnosis as part of routine, everyday, medical practice, antiviral drugs will not achieve their full potential in the relief of the patients' problems.

REFERENCES

Arnow, P. M., Hierholzer, J. C., Higbee, J. and Harris, D. H. (1977) Acute hemorrhagic conjunctivitis: a mixed virus outbreak among Vietnamese refugees on Guam. *Am. J. Epidem.* **105**: 68–74.

Barclay, W. R. (1977) Antiviral drugs. *J. Am. med. Ass.* **238**: 2531–2532.

Bauer, D. J. (1977) *The Specific Treatment of Virus Diseases.* University Park Press, Baltimore.

Baumgarten, A. (1980) Viral immunodiagnosis. *Yale J. Biol. Med.* **53**: 71–83.

Benyesh-Melnick, M. (1974) Human cytomegalovirus, Chapter 84 in *Manual of Clinical Microbiology*, 2nd edition, pp. 762–772, Lennette, E. H., Spaulding, E. H. and Truant, J. P. (eds.). American Society for Microbiology, Washington, D.C.

Birch, C. J., Lewis, M. L., Homola, M., Pritchard, H. and Gust, I. D. (1977) A study of the prevalence of rotavirus infection in children with gastroenteritis admitted to an infectious disease hospital. *J. med. Virol.* **1**: 69–77.

Blacklow, N. R. and Cukor, G. (1981) Viral gastroenteritis. *N. Engl. J. Med.* **304**: 397–406.

Bloom, H. H., Forsyth, B. R., Johnson, K. M. and Chanock, R. M. (1963) Relationship of rhinovirus infection to mild upper respiratory disease—1. Results of a survey in young adults and children. *J. Am. med. Ass.* **186**: 38–45.

Blough, H. A. and Giuntoli, R. L. (1979) Successful treatment of human genital herpes infections with 2-deoxy-D-glucose. *J. Am. med. Ass.* **241**: 2798–2801.

Blum, A. L., Doelle, W., Kortüm, K., Peter, P., Strohmeyer, G., Berthet, P., Goebell, H., Pelloni, S., Poulsen, H. and Tygstrup, N. (1977) Treatment of acute viral hepatitis with (+)-cyanidanol-3. *Lancet* **ii**: 1153–1155.

Brandt, C. D., Kim, H. W., Rodriguez, W. J., Thomas, L., Yolken, R. H., Arrobio, J. O., Kapikian, A. Z., Parrott, R. H. and Chanock, R. M. (1981) Comparison of direct electron microscopy, immune electron microscopy, and rotavirus enzyme-linked immunosorbent assay for detection of gastroenteritis viruses in children. *J. clin. Micro.* **13**: 976–981.

Calabresi, P. (1963) Current status of clinical investigations with 6-azauridine, 4-iodo-2′-deoxyuridine, and related derivatives. *Cancer Res.* **23**: 1260–1267.

Carlson, J. A. K., Middleton, P. J., Szymanski, M. T., Huber, J. and Petric, M. (1978) Fatal rotavirus gastroenteritis – an analysis of 21 cases. *Am. J. Dis. Child.* **132**: 477–479.

Centers for Disease Control (1978) Legionnaires' disease: diagnosis and management. *Ann. int. Med.* **88**: 363–365.

Centers for Disease Control (1980) Smallpox vaccine. *Morb. Mort. Wk. Rpt.* **29**: 417.

Centers for Disease Control (1981) Acute hemorrhagic conjunctivitis—Florida, North Carolina. *Morb. Mort. Wk. Rpt.* **30**: 501–502.

Check, W. A. (1980) Acyclovir for herpes: no clinical payoff yet. *J. Am. med. Ass.* **244**: 2021–2022.

Cho, C. T. and Feng, K. K. (1978) Sensitivity of the virus isolation and immunofluorescent staining methods in diagnosis of infections with herpes simplex virus. *J. infect. Dis.* **138**: 536–540.

Chou, S., Gallagher, J. G. and Merigan, T. C. (1981) Controlled clinical trial of intravenous acyclovir in heart-transplant patients with mucocutaneous herpes simplex infections. *Lancet* **i**: 1392–1394.

Clark, J., Schley, C., Irvine, K. and McIntosh, K. (1979) Comparison of cynomolgus and rhesus monkey kidney cells for recovery of viruses from clinical specimens. *J. clin. Microb.* **9**: 554–556.

Clarke, D. H. and Casals, J. (1958) Techniques for hemagglutination and hemagglutination-inhibition with arthropod-borne viruses. *Am. J. trop. Med.* **7**: 561–573.

COHEN, A., TOGO, Y., KHAKOO, R., WALDMAN, R. and SIGEL, M. (1976) Comparative clinical and laboratory evaluation of the prophylactic capacity of ribavirin, amantadine hydrochloride, and placebo in induced human influenza type A. *J. infect. Dis.* **133** supplement: A114–A120.

COHEN, S. S. (1972) On the development of programs in cancer research. *Proc. natn. Acad. Sci. USA* **69**: 1048–1051.

COHEN, S. S. (1977) A strategy for the chemotherapy of infectious disease. *Science* **197**: 431–432.

COHEN, S. S. (1979) Comparative design for infectious disease. *Science* **205**: 964–971.

CRUTCHER, J. E. and KANTNER, T. R. (1981) The effectiveness of antihistamines in the common cold. *J. clin. Pharmacol.* **21**: 9–15.

CZAJA, A. J. (1979) Serological markers of hepatitis A and B in acute and chronic liver disease. *Mayo Clin. Proc.* **54**: 721–732.

DANE, D. S., CAMERON, C. H. and BRIGGS, M. (1970) Virus-like particles in serum of patients with Australia-antigen hepatitis. *Lancet* i: 695–698.

DE CLERCQ, E., DEGREEF, H., WILDIERS, J., de JONGE, G., DROCHMANS, A., DESCAMPS, J. and DE SOMER, P. (1980a) Oral (E)-5-(2-bromovinyl)-2'-deoxyuridine in severe herpes zoster. *Br. Med. J.* **281**: 1178.

DE CLERCQ, E., DESCAMPS, J., DE SOMER, P., BARR, P. J., JONES, A. S. and WALKER, R. T. (1979) (E)-5-(2-bromovinyl)-2'-deoxyuridine: a potent and selective anti-herpes agent. *Proc. natn. Acad. Sci. USA* **76**: 2947–2951.

DE CLERCQ, E., DESCAMPS, J., VERHEIST, G., WALKER, R. T., JONES, A. S., TORRENCE, P. F. and SHUGAR, D. (1980b) Comparative efficacy of anti-herpes drugs against different strains of herpes simplex virus. *J. infect. Dis.* **141**: 563–574.

DELONG, D. C., NELSON, J. D., WU, C. Y. E., WARREN, B., WIKEL, J., CHAMBERLIN, J., MONTGOMERY, D. and PAGET, C. J. (1978) Virus inhibition studies with AR-336. I. tissue culture activity. *Abstracts of the Annual Meeting of the American Society for Microbiology*, abstract S128, p. 234.

DELONG, D. C. and REED, S. E. (1980) Inhibition of rhinovirus replication in organ culture by a potential antiviral drug. *J. infect. Dis.* **141**: 87–91.

DENDYEL, G. A., GASPAR, A. and PEYRAMOND, D. (1981) Diagnosis of recent rubella virus infection by demonstration of specific immunoglobulin M antibodies: comparison of solid-phase reverse immunosorbent test with sucrose density gradient centrifugation. *J. clin. Micro.* **13**: 698–704.

DENNY, F. W., CLYDE, W. A., Jr. and GLEZEN, W. P. (1971) *Mycoplasma pneumoniae* disease: clinical spectrum, pathophysiology, epidemiology, and control. *J. infect. Dis.* **123**: 74–92.

DURR, F. E., LINDH, H. F. and FORBES, M. (1975) Efficacy of 1-β-D-ribofuranosyl-1,2,4-triazole-3-carboxamide against influenza virus infections in mice. *Antimicrob. Agents Chemother.* **7**: 582–586.

DYKES, M. H. M. and MEIER, P. (1975) Ascorbic acid and the common cold evaluation of its efficacy and toxicity. *J. Am. med. Ass.* **231**: 1073–1079.

EGGERS, H. J. (1976) Successful treatment of enterovirus-infected mice by 2-(α-hydroxybenzyl)-benzimidazole and guanidine. *J. exp. Med.*, pp. 1367–1381.

ELION, G. B., FURMAN, P. A., FYFE, J. A., DE MIRANDA, P., BEAUCHAMP, L. and SCHAEFFER, , H. J. (1977) Selectivity of action of an antiherpetic agent, 9-(2-hydroxyethoxymethyl) guanine. *Proc. natn. Acad. Sci. USA* **74**: 5716–5720.

ENGVALL, E., JONSSON, K. and PERLMANN, P. (1971) Enzyme-linked immunosorbent assay II quantitative assay of protein antigen, immunoglobulin G, by means of an enzyme-labeled antigen and antibody coated tubes. *Biochem. Biophys. Acta* **251**: 427–434.

ENGVALL, E. and PERLMANN, P. (1972) Enzyme-linked antiimmunoglobulin assay, ELISA. III. Quantitation of specific antibodies by enzyme-linked antiimmunoglobulin in antigen-coated tubes. *J. Immun.* **109**: 129–135.

EVANS, A. S. and DICK, E. C. (1964) Acute pharyngitis and tonsillitis in University of Wisconsin students. *J. Am. med. Ass.* **190**: 699–708.

FEINSTONE, S. M., KAPIKIAN, A. Z. and PURCELL, R. H. (1973) Detection by immune electron microscopy of a virus-like antigen associated with acute illness. *Science* **182**: 1026–1028.

FAHIM, M. S., BRAWNER, T. A. and HALL, D. G. (1980) New treatment for herpes simplex virus type 2 [ultrasound and zinc, urea and tannic acid ointment] Part II: Female patients. *J. Med.* **11**: 143–167.

FRANK, A. L., COUCH, R. B., GRIFFIS, C. A. and BAXTER, B. D. (1979) Comparison of different tissue cultures for isolation and quantitation of influenza and parainfluenza viruses. *J. clin. Micro.* **10**: 32–36.

GAJDUSEK, D. C. (1977) Unconventional viruses and the origin and disappearance of kuru. *Science* **197**: 943–960.

GARDNER, P. S., GRANDIEN, M. and McQUILLIN, J. (1978) Comparison of immunofluorescence and immunoperoxidase methods for viral diagnosis at a distance: A WHO collaborative study. *Bull. WHO* **56**: 105–110.

GINSBERG, T. and GLASKY, A. J. (1977) Inosiplex: an immunomodulation model for the treatment of viral disease. *Ann. N.Y. Acad. Sci.* **284**: 128–138.

GLEZEN, W. P. (1976) Respiratory viruses and *Mycoplasma pneumoniae*. Chapter 4 In: *Viral Infections: A Clinical Approach*, pp. 69–99. DREW, W. L. (ed.). F. A. Davis Co., Philadelphia, Pa.

GOMEZ, M. R., SIEKERT, R. G. and HERRMANN, E. C., Jr. (1965) A human case of skunk rabies. *J. Am. med. Ass.* **194**: 333–335.

GRIFFITH, R. S., NORINS, A. L. and KAGAN, C. (1978) A multicentered study of lysine therapy in herpes simplex infection. *Dermatologica* **156**: 257–267.

GWALTNEY, J. M., Jr. (1968) The spectrum of rhinovirus inhibition by 2-(α-hydroxybenzyl)-benzimidazole and D-(−)-2-(α-hydroxybenzyl)-benzimidazole HCl. *Proc. Soc. exp. Biol. Med.* **129**: 665–673.

GWALTNEY, J. M., Jr. (1970) Rhinovirus inhibition by 3-substituted triazinoindoles. *Proc. Soc. exp. Biol. Med.* **133**: 1148–1154.

HABLE, K. A., O'CONNELL, E. J. and HERRMANN, E. C., Jr. (1970) Group B coxsackieviruses as respiratory viruses. *Mayo Clin. Proc.* **45**: 170–176.

HADDEN, J. W., LOPEZ, C., O'REILLY, R. J. and HADDEN, E. M. (1977) Levamisole and inosiplex: antiviral agents with immunopotentiating action. *Ann. N.Y. Acad. Sci.* **284**: 139–152.

HAHN, F. E. (1980) Virus chemotherapy: the problem, its development and nature. *Antibiotics Chemother.* **27**: 1–21.

HALL, C. B. and DOUGLAS, R. G., Jr. (1975) Clinically useful method for the isolation of respiratory syncytial virus. *J. infect. Dis.* **131**: 1–5.

HANSHAW, J. B. (1971) Congenital cytomegalovirus infection: a fifteen year perspective. *J. infect. Dis.* **123**: 555–561.

HANSHAW, J. B. (1973) *Herpesvirus hominis* infections in the fetus and the newborn. *Am. J. Dis. Child.* **126**: 546–555.

HASLAM, R. H. A., MCQUILLEN, M. P. and CLARK, D. B. (1969) Amantadine therapy in subacute sclerosing panencephalitis. *Neurology* **19**: 1080–1086.

HATTWICK, M. A. W., WEIS, T. T., STECHSCHULTE, C. J., BAER, G. M. and GREGG, M. B. (1972) Recovery from rabies a case report. *Ann. int. Med.* **76**: 931–942.

HEIDELBERGER, C. and KING, D. H. (1979) Trifluorothymidine. *Pharmac. Ther.* **6**: 427–442.

HELGSTRAND, E., ERIKSSON, B., JOHANSSON, N. G., LANNERÖ, B., LARSSON, A., MISIORNY, A., NORÉN, J. O., SJÖBERG, B., STENBERG, K., STENING, G., STRIDH, S., ÖBERG, B., ALENIUS, S. and PHILIPSON, L. (1978) Trisodium phosphonoformate, a new antiviral compound. *Science* **201**: 819–821.

HENLE, G., HENLE, W. and DIEHL, V. (1968) Relation of Burkitt's tumor-associated herpes-type virus to infectious mononucleosis. *Proc. natn. Acad. Sci. USA* **59**: 94–101.

HENLE, G. and HENLE, W. (1946a) Studies on the toxicity of influenza viruses—I. The effect of intracerebral injection of influenza viruses. *J. exp. Med.* **84**: 623–637.

HENLE, W. and HENLE, G. (1946b) Studies on the toxicity of influenza viruses—II. The effect of intra-abdominal and intravenous injection of influenza viruses. *J. exp. Med.* **84**: 639–660.

HENLE, W. and HENLE, G. (1972) Epstein–Barr virus: the cause of infectious mononucleosis. In: *Oncogenesis and Herpesviruses*, pp. 269–274. BIGGS, P. M., DE-THÉ, G. and PAYNE, L. N. (eds.). International Agency for Research on Cancer, Scientific Publications No. 2, Lyon, France.

HENLE, W., HENLE, G. E. and HORWITZ, C. A. (1974) Epstein–Barr virus specific diagnostic tests in infectious mononucleosis. *Human Path.* **5**: 551–565.

HERRMANN, E. C., Jr. (1961) Plaque inhibition test for detection of specific inhibitors of DNA containing viruses. *Proc. Soc. exp. Biol. Med.* **107**: 142–145.

HERRMANN, E. C., Jr. (1967) Experiences in laboratory diagnosis of herpes simplex, varicella-zoster and vaccinia virus infections in routine medical practice. *Mayo Clin. Proc.* **42**: 744–753.

HERRMANN, E. C., Jr. (1968) Sensitivity of herpes simplex virus, vaccinia virus and adenoviruses to deoxyribonucleic acid inhibitors and thiosemicarbazones in a plaque suppression test. *Appl. Microbiol.* **16**: 1151–1155.

HERRMANN, E. C., Jr. (1970) The tragedy of viral diagnosis. *Postgrad. med. J.* **46**: 545–550.

HERRMANN, E. C., Jr. (1971) Efforts toward a more useful viral diagnostic laboratory. *Am. J. clin. Path.* **56**: 681–686.

HERRMANN, E. C., Jr. (1972) Rates of isolation of viruses from a wide spectrum of clinical specimens. *Am. J. clin. Path.* **57**: 188–194.

HERRMANN, E. C., Jr. (1974) New concepts and developments in applied diagnostic virology. *Prog. med. Virol.* **17**: 221–289.

HERRMANN, E. C., Jr. and HABLE, K. A. (1970) Experiences in laboratory diagnosis of parainfluenza viruses in routine medical practice. *Mayo Clin. Proc.* **45**: 177–188.

HERRMANN, E. C., Jr. and HERRMANN, J. A. (1976a) Survey of viral diagnostic laboratories in medical centers. *J. infect. Dis.* **133**: 359–362.

HERRMANN, E. C., Jr. and HERRMANN, J. A. (1976b) Laboratory diagnosis of viral disease. Chapter 2 in: *Viral Infections: A Clinical Approach*, pp. 23–45. DREW, W. L. (ed.). F. A. Davis Co., Philadelphia, PA.

HERRMANN, E. C., Jr. and HERRMANN, J. A. (1977a) A neglected cure for 'cold sores' and 'shingles'. *Current Prescribing* **3**: 27–32.

HERRMANN, E. C., Jr. and HERRMANN, J. A. (1977b) A working hypothesis—virus resistance development as an indicator of specific antiviral activity. *Ann. N.Y. Acad. Sci.* **284**: 632–637.

HERRMANN, E. C., Jr., HERRMANN, J. A. and DELONG, D. C. (1981b). Antiviral activity of HBB, guanidine and LY122771–72 in mice infected with Echo 9 and coxsackie A9 viruses. Abstract A36, *Annual Meeting American Society for Microbiology 1981*, p. 7.

HERRMANN, E. C., Jr., HERRMANN, J. A. and DELONG, D. C. (1981c) Comparison of the antiviral effects of substituted benzimidazoles and guanidine *in vitro* and *in vivo*. *Antiviral Res.* **1**: 301–314.

HERRMANN, E. C., Jr., PERSON, D. A. and SMITH, T. F. (1972) Experience in laboratory diagnosis of enterovirus infections in routine medical practice. *Mayo Clin. Proc.* **47**: 577–586.

HERRMANN, E. C., Jr. and RAWLS, W. E. (1974) Herpes simplex virus. Chapter 83 in: *Manual of Clinical Microbiology* (2nd Edn), pp. 754–761. LENNETTE, E. H., SPAULDING, E. H. and TRUANT, J. P. (eds.). American Society for Microbiology, Washington, D.C.

HERRMANN, J. A. and HERRMANN, E. C., Jr. (1977c) The *mini* viral diagnostic laboratory – a necessary adjunct to the use of antiviral drugs. *Ann. N.Y. Acad. Sci.* **284**: 122–127.

HERRMANN, J. A. and HERRMANN, E. C., Jr. (1981a) Effective guanidine treatment of coxsackievirus A16 infection in mice. Abstract A35, *Annual Meeting American Society for Microbiology 1981*, p. 6.

HOFFMANN, C. E. (1973) Amantadine HCl and related compounds. In: *Selective Inhibitors of Viral Functions*, pp. 199–211. CARTER, W. A. (ed.). CRC Press, Cleveland, OH.

HOLLAND, P. V. and ALTER, H. J. (1976) Current concepts of viral hepatitis. Chapter 7 in: *Viral Infections. A Clinical Approach*, pp. 189–208. DREW, W. L. (ed.). F. A. Davis Co., Philadelphia, Pa.

HORSFALL, F. L. and MCCARTY, M. (1947) The modifying effects of certain substances of bacterial origin on the course of infection with pneumonia virus of mice (PVM). *J. exp. Med.* **85**: 623–646.

HORWITZ, C. A., HENLE, W. and HENLE, G. (1979) Diagnostic aspects of the cytomegalovirus mononucleosis syndrome in previously healthy persons. *Postgrad. Med.* **66**: 153–158.

HUEBNER, R. J. (1963) Viral respiratory disease in the Americas. *Am. Rev. resp. Dis.* **88** (Part 2): 1–13.

ISAACS, A. and LINDENMANN, J. (1957) Virus interference—I. The interferon. *Proc. R. Soc.*, B **147**: 258–267.

INDULEN, M. K. and KALNINYA, V. A. (1980) Studies on the antiviral effect and the mode of action of the antiinfluenza compound rimantadine. In: *Recent Developments in Antiviral Chemotherapy*, COLLIER, L. and OXFORD, J. S. (eds.). Academic Press, London.

JACK, M. K. and SORENSON, R. W. (1963) Vaccinial keratitis treated with IDU. *Arch Ophthal.* **69**: 730–732.

JOHNSON, R. T., OLSON, L. C. and BUESCHER, E. L. (1968) Herpes simplex virus infections of the nervous system. Problems in laboratory diagnosis. *Arch. Neurol.* **18**: 260–264.

JOKLIK, W. K. (1980) Antiviral chemotherapy, interferon, and vaccines. Chapter 68 in: *17th Edition Zinsser Microbiology*, pp. 1112–1122. JOKLIK, W. K., WILLETT, H. P. and AMOS, D. B. (eds.). Appleton-Century-Crofts, New York, N.Y.

JONES, B. R. and AL-HUSSAINI, M. K. (1963) Therapeutic considerations in ocular vaccinia. *Trans. ophthal. Soc.* **83**: 613–631.

KAUFMAN, H. E., MARTOLA, E. L. and DOHLMAN, C. H. (1963) Herpes simplex treatment with IDU and corticosteroids. *Arch Ophthal.* **69**: 468–472.

KAYE, H. S., MARSH, H. B. and DOWDLE, W. R. (1971) Seroepidemiologic survey of coronavirus (strain OC 43) related infections in a children's population. *Am. J. Epidemiol.* **94**: 43–49.

KIBRICK, S. (1964) Current status of coxsackie and echo viruses in human disease. In: *Progress in Medical Virology*, Vol. 6, pp. 27–70. MELNICK, J. L. (ed.). Hafner Publishing Co., New York, N.Y.

KLEIN, R. J., FRIEDMAN-KIEN, A. F., FONDAK, A. A. and BUIMOVICI-KLEIN, E. (1977) Immune response and latent infection after topical treatment of herpes simplex virus infection in hairless mice. *Infect. Immun.* **16**: 842–848.

KUCERA, L. S. and HERRMANN, E. C., Jr. (1967) Antiviral substances in plants of the mint family (labiatae). I. Tannin of *Melissa officinalis. Proc. Soc. exp. Biol. Med.* **124**: 865–869.

LAMONTAGNE, J. R. and GALASSO, G. J. (1978) Report of a workshop on clinical studies of the efficacy of amantadine and rimantadine against influenza virus. *J. infect. Dis.* **138**: 928–931.

LANDRY, M. L., MADORE, H. P., FONG, C. K. Y. and HSIUNG, G. D. (1981) Use of guinea pig embryo cell cultures for isolation and propagation of Group A coxsackieviruses. *J. clin. Microb.* **13**: 588–593.

LI, C. P., PRESCOTT, B., EDDY, B., CALDES, G., GREEN, W. R., MARTINO, E. C. and YOUNG, A. M. (1965) Antiviral activity of paolins from clams. *Ann. N.Y. Acad. Sci.* **130**: 374–382.

LINDSAY, M. I., Jr., HERRMANN, E. C., Jr., MORROW, G. W., Jr. and BROWN, A. L., Jr. (1970) Hong Kong influenza clinical, microbiologic, and pathologic features in 127 cases. *J. Am. med. Ass.* **214**: 1825–1832.

MCINTOSH, K., CHAO, R. K., KRAUSE, H. E., WASIL, R., MOCEGA, H. E. and MUFSON, M. A. (1974) Coronavirus infection in acute lower respiratory tract disease of infants. *J. infect. Dis.* **130**: 502–507.

MCINTOSH, K., WILFERT, C., CHERNESKY, M., PLOTKIN, S. and MATTEWS, M. J. (1980) Summary of a workshop on new and useful techniques in rapid viral diagnosis. *J. infect. Dis.* **142**: 793–802.

MANALO, D., MUFSON, M. S., ZALLAR, L. M. and MANKAD, V. N. (1971) Adenovirus infection in acute hemorrhagic cystitis. A study in 25 children. *Am. J. Dis. Child.* **121**: 281–285.

MARKS, R. G. (1976) Yes, there are antivirals. *Current Prescribing* (April) **2**: 11–19.

MAUGH, T. H. II (1979) Panel urges wide use of antiviral drug. *Science* **206**: 1058–1059.

MEGURO, H., BRYANT, J. D., TORRENCE, A. E. and WRIGHT, P. F. (1979) Canine kidney cell line for isolation of respiratory viruses. *J. clin. Microbiol.* **9**: 175–179.

MELNICK, J. L., ADAM, E. and RAWLS, W. E. (1974) The causative role of herpesvirus type 2 in cervical cancer. *Cancer* **34**: 1375–1385.

MELNICK, J. L. and WALLIS, C. (1977) Photodynamic inactivation of herpes simplex virus: a status report. *Ann. N.Y. Acad. Sci.* **284**: 171–181.

MIDDLETON, P. J., SZYMANSKI, M. T. and PETRIC, M. (1977) Viruses associated with acute gastroenteritis in young children. *Am. J. Dis. Child.* **131**: 733–737.

MINNICH, L. and RAY, C. G. (1980) Comparison of immunofluorescent staining of clinical specimens for respiratory virus antigens with conventional isolation techniques. *J. clin. Micro.* **12**: 391–394.

MIRKOVIC, R. R., KONO, R., YIN-MURPHY, M., SOHIER, R., SCHMIDT, N. J. and MELNICK, J. L. (1973) Enterovirus 70: The etiologic agent of pandemic acute haemorrhagic conjunctivitis. *Bull. WHO* **49**: 341–346.

MITCHELL, C. D., GENTRY, S. R., BOEN, J. R., BEAN, B., GROTH, K. E. and BALFOUR, H. H., Jr. (1981) Acyclovir therapy for mucocutaneous herpes simplex infections in immunocompromised patients. *Lancet* **1**: 1389–1392.

MONTO, A. S., MAASSAB, H. F. and BRYAN, E. R. (1981) Relative efficacy of embryonated eggs and cell culture for isolation of contemporary influenza viruses. *J. clin. Microb.* **13**: 233–235.

MORRIS, S. J. (1977) Correspondence to the editor. *New Engl. J. Med.* **297**: 1289.

MOSELEY, R. C., COREY, L., BENJAMIN, D., WINTER, C. and REMINGTON, M. L. (1981) Comparison of viral isolation, direct immunofluorescence, and indirect immunoperoxidase techniques for detection of genital herpes simplex virus infection. *J. clin. Micro.* **13**: 913–918.

NAHMIAS, A. J., DOWDLE, W. R., NAIB, Z. M., JOSEY, W. E., MCCLONE, D. and DOMESCIK, G. (1969) Genital infection with type 2 *Herpesvirus hominis*: a commonly occurring venereal disease. *Br. J. vener. Dis.* **45**: 294–298.

NAHMIAS, A. J., VISINTINE, A. M. and STARR, S. E. (1976) Viral infections of the fetus and newborn. Chapter 3 in: *Viral Infections. A Clinical Approach*, pp. 47–67. DREW, W. L., (ed.). F. A. Davis Co., Philadelphia, Pa.

O'REILLY, R. J., CHIBBARO, A., WILMOT, R. and LOPEZ, C. (1977) Correlation of clinical and virus-specific immune responses following levamisole therapy of recurrent herpes progenitalis. *Ann. N.Y. Acad. Sci.* **284**: 161–170.

OXFORD, J. S. and GALBRAITH, A. (1980) Antiviral activity of amantadine: A review of laboratory and clinical data. *Pharmac. Ther.* **11**: 181–262.

PAVAN-LANGSTON, D. R., BUCHANAN, R. A. and ALFORD, C. A., Jr. (Eds.) (1975) *Adenine Arabinoside: An Antiviral Agent*. Raven Press, New York, N.Y.

PERSON, D. A. and HERRMANN, E. C., Jr. (1970) Experiences in laboratory diagnosis of rhinovirus infections in routine medical practice. *Mayo Clinic Proc.* **45**: 517–526.

PERSON, D. A., SHERIDAN, P. J. and HERRMANN, E. C., Jr. (1970) Sensitivity of types 1 and 2 herpes simplex virus to 5-iodo-2'-deoxyuridine and 9-β-D-arabinofuranosyladenine. *Infect. Immun.* **2**: 815–820.

PERSON, D A., SMITH, T. F. and HERRMANN, E. C., Jr. (1971) Experiences in laboratory diagnosis of mumps virus infections in routine medical practice. *Mayo Clin. Proc.* **46**: 544–548.

PHILLPOTTS, R. J., DELONG, D. C., WALLACE, J., JONES, R. W., REED, S. E. and TYRRELL, D. A. J. (1981) The activity of enviroxime against rhinovirus infections in man. *Lancet* **1**: 1342–1344.

PORRAS, C., BARBOZA, J. J., FUENZALIDA, E., ADAROS, H. L., OVIEDO DE DIAZ and FURST, J. (1976) Recovery from rabies in man. *Ann. int. Med.* **85**: 44–48.

RAPP, C. E., Jr. and HEWETSON, J. F. (1978) Infectious mononucleosis and the Epstein–Barr virus. *Am. Dis. Child.* **132**: 78–86.

RAPP, F. and KEMENY, B. A. (1977) Oncogenic potential of *herpes simplex* virus in mammalian cells following photodynamic inactivation. *Photochem. Photobiol.* **25**: 335–337.

RAWLS, W. E., COHEN, R. A. and HERRMANN, E. C., Jr. (1964) Inhibition of varicella virus by 5-iodo-2′-deoxyuridine. *Proc. Soc. exp. Biol. & Med.* **115**: 123–127.

RAWLS, W. E., DYCK, P. J., KLASS, D. W., GREER, H. D., III and HERRMANN, E. C., Jr. (1966) Encephalitis associated with herpes simplex virus. *Ann. int. Med.* **64**: 104–115.

SABIN, A. B. (1967) Amantadine hydrochloride: analysis of data related to its proposed use for prevention of A2 influenza virus disease in human beings. *J. Am. med. Ass.* **200**: 943–950.

SABIN, A. B. (1977) Mortality from pneumonia and risk conditions during influenza epidemics. High influenza morbidity during nonepidemic years. *J. Am. med. Ass.* **237**: 2823–2828.

SABIN, A. B. (1978) Amantadine and influenza: Evaluation of conflicting reports. *J. infect. Dis.* **138**: 557–556.

SARAL, R., BURNS, W. H., LASKIN, O. L., SANTOS, G. W. and LIETMAN, P. S. (1981) Acyclovir prophylaxis of herpes-simplex-virus infections a randomized, double-blind, controlled trial in bone-marrow-transplant recipients. *N. Eng. J. Med.* **305**: 63–67.

SARKKINEN, H. K., HALONEN, P. E., ARSTILA, P. P. and SALMI, A. A. (1981) Detection of respiratory syncytial, parainfluenza type 2 and adenovirus antigens by radioimmunoassay and enzyme immunoassay on nasopharyngeal specimens from children with acute respiratory disease. *J. clin. Micro.* **13**: 258–265.

SCHABEL, F. M., Jr. and MONTGOMERY, J. A. (1972) Purines and pyrimidines. In: *Chemotherapy of Virus Diseases*, pp. 231–363. BAUER, D. J. (ed). *The International Encyclopedia of Pharmacology and Therapeutics*, Section 61, Vol. 1, Pergamon Press, Oxford.

SCHAEFFER, H. J., BEAUCHAMP, L., DE MIRANDA, P., ELION, G. B., BAUER, D. J. and COLLINS, P. (1978) 9-(2-Hydroxyethoxymethyl) guanine activity against viruses of the herpes group. *Nature (Lond)* **272**: 583–585.

SCHLEICHER, J. B., AQUINO, F., RUETER, A., RODERICK, W. R. and APPELL, R. N. (1972) Antiviral activity in tissue culture systems of *bis*-benzimidazoles, potent inhibitors of rhinoviruses. *Appl. Microbiol.* **23**: 113–116.

SCHMIDT, N. J. (1974) Varicella-zoster virus. Chapter 85 in: *Manual of Clinical Microbiology* (2nd Edn), pp. 773–781. LENNETTE, E. H., SPAULDING, E. H. and TRUANT, J. P. (eds.). American Society for Microbiology, Washington, D.C.

SCHMIDT, N. J., GALLO, D., DEVLIN, V., WOODIE, J. D. and EMMONS, R. W. (1980) Direct immunofluorescence staining for detection of herpes simplex and varicella-zoster antigens in vesicular lesions and certain tissue specimens. *J. clin. Microb.* **12**: 651–655.

SCHMIDT, N. J., HO, H. H. and LENNETTE, E. H. (1975) Propagation and isolation of group A coxsackieviruses in RD cells. *J. clin. Microbiol.* **2**: 183–185.

SCHULMAN, J. L. (1968) Effect of 1-amantanamine hydrochloride (amantadine HCl) and methyl-1-adamantanethylamine hydrochloride (rimantadine HCl) on transmission of influenza virus infection in mice. *Proc. Soc. exp. Biol. Med.* **128**: 1173–1178.

SCULLARD, G. H., POLLARD, R. B., SMITH, J. L., SACKS, S. L., GREGORY, P. B., ROBINSON, W. S. and MERIGAN, T. C. (1981) Antiviral treatment of chronic hepatitis B virus infection, I. Changes in viral markers with interferon combined with adenine arabinoside. *J. inf. Dis.* **143**: 772–783.

SELBY, P. J., POWLES, R. L., JAMESON, B., WATSON, J. G., MORGENSTERN, G., POWLES, R. L., KAY, H. E. M., THORNTON, R. and CLINK, H. M. (1979) Parenteral acyclovir therapy for herpesvirus infections in man. *Lancet* **2**: 1267–1270.

SHANNON, W. M. and SCHABEL, F. M., Jr. (1980) Antiviral agents as adjuncts in cancer chemotherapy. *Pharmac. Ther.* **11**: 263–390.

SHERIDAN, P. J. and HERRMANN, E. C., Jr. (1971) Intraoral lesions of adults associated with herpes simplex virus. *Oral Surg.* **32**: 390–397.

SHIPKOWITZ, N. L., BOWER, R. R., SCHLEICHER, J. B., AQUINO, F., APPELL, R. N. and RODERICK, W. R. (1972) Antiviral activity of a *bis*-benzimidazole against experimental rhinovirus infections in chimpanzees. *Appl. Microbiol.* **23**: 117–122.

SMITH, R. A. and KIRKPATRICK, W. (eds.) (1980) *Ribavirin A Broad Spectrum Antiviral Agent.* Academic Press, New York, N.Y.

SMITH, T. F. (1979) Specimen requirements, transport, and recovery of viruses in cell cultures. Chapter 5 in: *Diagnosis of Viral Infections*, pp. 33–47. LENNETTE, D. A., SPECTER, S. and THOMPSON, K. D. (eds.). University Park Press, Baltimore, Md.

SMITH, T. F., PERSON, D. A. and HERRMANN, E. C., Jr. (1971) Experiences in laboratory diagnosis of respiratory syncytial virus infections in routine medical practice. *Mayo Clin. Proc.* **46**: 609–612.

SPRUANCE, S. L., OVERALL, J. C., Jr., KERN, E. R., KRUEGER, G. G., PLIAM, V. and MILLER, W. (1977) The natural history of recurrent herpes simplex labialis – implications for antiviral therapy. *New Engl. J. Med.* **297**: 69–75.

STAAL, S. P. and ROWE, W. P. (1975) Enhancement of adenovirus infection in WI-38 and AGMK cells by pretreatment of cells with 5-iododeoxyuridine. *Virology* **64**: 513–519.

STANLEY, E. D., JACKSON, G. G., PANUSARN, C., RUBENIS, M. and DIRDA, V. (1975) Increased virus-shedding with aspirin treatment of rhinovirus infection. *J. Am. med. Ass.* **231**: 1248–1251.

STONE, J. D. (1948) Prevention of virus infection with enzyme of *V. cholerae*–II. Studies with influenza virus in mice. *Aust. J. exp. Biol. med. Sci.* **26**: 287–297.

TAGER, I. B. (1977) Correspondence to the Editor. *New Engl. J. Med.* **297**: 1289.

TAKEMOTO, K. K. and SPICER, S. S. (1965) Effects of natural and synthetic sulfated polysaccharides on viruses and cells. *Ann. N.Y. Acad. Sci.* **130**: 365–373.

TENNICAN, P., CARL, G., FREY, J., THIES, C. and CHVAPIL, M. (1980) Topical zinc in the treatment of mice infected intravaginally with herpes genitalis virus. *Proc. Soc. exp. Biol. Med.* **164**: 593–597.

TOGO, Y., HORNICK, R. B., FELITTI, V. J., KAUFMAN, M. L., DAWKINS, A. T., Jr. KILPE, V. E. and CLAGHORN, J. L. (1970) Evaluation of therapeutic efficacy of amantadine in patients with naturally occurring A2 influenza. *J. Am. med. Ass.* **211**: 1149–1156.

TOGO, Y. and McCRACKEN, E. A. (1976) Double-blind clinical assessment of ribavirin (Virazole) in the prevention of induced infection with type B influenza virus. *J. infect. Dis.* **133** (supplement): A109–A113.

UTZ, J. P., SZWED, C. F. and KASEL, J. A. (1958) Clinical and laboratory studies of mumps—II. Detection and duration of excretion of virus in urine. *Proc. Soc. exp. Biol. Med.* **99**: 259–261.

VAN LOON, A. M., HEESSEN, F. W. A., VAN DER LOGT, J. T. H. and VAN DER VEEN, J. (1981) Direct enzyme-linked immunosorbent assay that uses peroxidase-labelled antigen for determination of immunoglobulin M antibody to cytomegalovirus. *J. clin. Micro.* **13**: 416–422.

WALDMAN, R. H. and GANGULY, R. (1977) Therapeutic efficacy of inosiplex (isoprinosine) in rhinovirus infection. *Ann. N.Y. Acad. Sci.* **284**: 153–160.

WEATHERS, D. R. and GRIFFIN, J. W. (1970) Intraoral ulcerations of recurrent herpes simplex and recurrent aphthae: two distinct clinical entities. *J. Am. dent. Ass.* **81**: 81–88.

WELLINGS, P. C., AWDRY, P. N., BORS, F. H., JONES, B. R., BROWN, D. C. and KAUFMAN, H. E. (1972) Clinical evaluation of trifluorothymidine in the treatment of herpes simplex corneal ulcers. *Am. J. Ophthal.* **73**: 932–942.

WENTWORTH, B. B. and ALEXANDER, E. R. (1971) Seroepidemiology of infections due to members of the herpesvirus group. *Am. J. Epidem.* **94**: 496–507.

WEST, S., BRANDON, B., STOLLEY, P. and RUMRILL, R. (1975) A review of antihistamines and the common cold. *Pediatrics* **56**: 100–107.

WHITLEY, R. J., SOONG, S., DOLIN, R., GALASSO, G. J., CH'IEN, L. T., ALFORD, C. A. and the Collaborative Study Group (1977) Adenine arabinoside therapy of biopsy-proved herpes simplex encephalitis. *New Engl. J. Med.* **297**: 289–294.

WHITLEY, R. J., TUCKER, B. C., KINKEL, A. W., BARTON, N. H., PASS, R. F., WHELCHEL, J. D., COBBS, C. G., DIETHELM, A. G. and BUCHANAN, R. A. (1980) Pharmacology, tolerance, and antiviral activity of vivarabine monophosphate in humans. *Antimicrob. Ag. Chemo.* **18**: 709–715.

WIKEL, J. H., PAGET, C. J., DELONG, D. C., NELSON, J. D., WU, C. Y. E., PASCHAL, J. W., DINNER, A., TEMPLETON, R. J., CHANEY, M. O., JONES, N. D. and CHAMBERLIN, J. W. (1980) Synthesis of syn and anti isomers of 6-[[(hydroxyimino)phenyl]methyl]-1-[(1-methylethyl)sulfonyl]-1*H*-benzimidazole-2-amine. Inhibitors of rhinovirus multiplication. *J. med. Chem.* **23**: 368–372.

WINGFIELD, W. L., POLLACK, D. and GRUNERT, R. R. (1969) Therapeutic efficacy of amantadine HCl and rimantadine HCl in naturally occurring influenza A respiratory illness in man. *New Engl. J. Med.* **281**: 579–584.

WOLONTIS, S. and JEANSSON, S. (1977) Correlation of herpes simplex virus types 1 and 2 with clinical features of infection. *J. infect. Dis.* **135**: 28–33.

WOOLLEY, D. W. (1954) Inhibition of virus multiplication through considered use of antimetabolites. In: *The Dynamics of Viral and Rickettsial Infections*, pp. 421–430. HARTMAN, F. W., HORSFALL, F. L. Jr. and KIDD, J. C. (eds.). The Blakiston Co., Inc., New York, N.Y.

WORK, T. S. and WORK, E. (1948) *The Basis of Chemotherapy*, p. 32. Oliver and Boyd, Edinburgh, Scotland.

YOLKEN, R. H. and LEISTER, F. J. (1981) Evaluation of enzyme immunoassays for the detection of human rotavirus. *J. inf. Dis.* **144**: 379.

YOUNG, S. K., ROWE, N. H. and BUCHANAN, R. A. (1976) A clinical study for the control of facial mucocutaneous herpes virus infections—1. Characterization of natural history in a professional school population. *Oral Surg.* **41**: 498–507.

CHAPTER 4

THE RELATIVE ROLES OF VACCINES AND DRUGS IN PREVENTION AND TREATMENT OF HUMAN VIRUS DISEASES

Francis L. Black

Yale University School of Medicine, Department of Epidemiology and Public Health, New Haven, Connecticut, USA

CONTENTS

INTRODUCTION

At present there are too few virus control agents of any kind to pose serious problems of choice between alternative methods of treatment, but even when the range of both forms of treatment have been expanded to their full foreseeable scope, the occasions will be rare when viral vaccines and antiviral drugs will offer reasonable alternatives to each other. There is but little overlap between the two kinds of control agent either in the stage of infection when the agent may be effective or in the kind of agent which may be responsive. The two kinds of control agents generally work on distinctively different principals; the vaccines by stimulating specific immune responses and the drugs by blocking metabolic pathways. They have also been produced by distinctively different biological and organo-chemical processes; this latter difference may, however, be obscured in the future, if synthetic antigens prove out as vaccines (Lerner *et al.*, 1981b). A third distinct kind of virus-control agent is interferon and interferon inducers. This is the subject of an extensive recent review (Baron and Dianzani, 1977) and will not be covered here.

The reader of this series will have available to him other detailed descriptions of each class of antiviral drug (Prussof *et al.*, 1979; Buchanan and Hess, 1980; Rada and Doskocil, 1980; Shannon and Schabel, 1980; and Oxford and Galbraith, 1980) but it may be helpful to outline here the different classes of immunizing agents before we attempt to compare their roles with those of the drugs. The vaccines can be divided into live-virus vaccines, killed-virus vaccines and vaccines composed of specific virus subcomponents. In addition, persons may be immunized by passive transfer of immunological substances.

4.1. ANTIVIRAL IMMUNIZING AGENTS

4.1.1. LIVE-VIRUS VACCINES

Live attenuated-virus vaccines are presently the most effective class of virus-control agents. There are live vaccines against several of the most common acute virus infections of childhood (Table 1). Some of the vaccines, namely those effective against smallpox, yellow fever, poliomyelitis, measles, rubella and mumps, have been used to effect dramatic changes in world mordibity patterns. This is not to say that these vaccines do not still have problems – the smallpox vaccine often caused serious complications (Lane *et al.*, 1969); the poliomyelitis vaccine occasionally causes paralysis (Terry, 1962) and the measles vaccine is less than 100 per cent effective (Cherry *et al.*, 1973) – but they are good enough that it is highly unlikely that any drug requiring periodic doses would be chosen preferentially. Others of these vaccines, such as Venezuelan Equine encephalitis (Alvizatos *et al.*, 1967), have as yet been too little used to provide full assurance of their long-term effectiveness. However, with the successful precedence of the other products (Horstmann, 1975; Weibel *et al.*, 1980), the prospects for it seems promising. All these vaccines are, of course, prophylactic rather than therapeutic products. Drugs may be useful when it is too late to use the vaccine, but with these effective vaccines available there is no excuse for deliberately depending on drugs. An exception to this relatively favorable position of the live antiviral vaccines occurs in varicella-zoster. These two diseases are caused by the same agents, varicella as a primary infection, and zoster as a reactivation of latent virus. A live vaccine has proven useful in preventing serious complications of varicella in immuno-compromised children (Asano *et al.*, 1977). However, it will be a long time before we know if the vaccine reduces the frequency of reactivation. It could even increase it. Meanwhile, as detailed below, drugs are proving useful in the treatment of zoster.

TABLE 1. *Major Live-Virus Vaccines*

Vaccine	Source	Durability of immunity	Effectiveness	Comments
Smallpox	Calf lymph	3–5 yr	Good	Complications a problem
Yellow fever	Embryonated chicken eggs	⩾ 17 yr	Excellent	No substantial evidence of waning protection
Poliomyelitis	Primary monkey kidney Human diploid cells	⩾ 10 yr	Excellent	Type 3 retains some pathogenicity
Measles	Chick embryo T.C.	⩾ 12 yr	Excellent	Occasional inadequacies in long term immunity
Mumps	Chick embryo T.C.	⩾ 6 yr	Excellent	
Rubella	Duck embryo T.C. Human diploid cell	⩾ 5 yr	Good	Long term effectiveness is important but not established
Influenza	Chick embryo	?	Variable	Reactogenicity a problem
Adenovirus 4 & 7	Human diploid cell	?	Little tested	Enteric coated unattenuated virus
Venezuelan eq. enceph.	Guinea pig heart T.C.	Extended	Little tested	Limited to special risks

The diseases against which live-virus vaccines have had their greatest success have a number of characteristics in common. All are distinct, highly visible diseases, caused by specific agents. The public can readily identify the risk which these diseases pose, and a large proportion of the population can be persuaded to accept the discomfort and inconvenience entailed in prophylaxis by vaccination. When people are vaccinated, relatively few immunizations appear to fail, not only because these are effective vaccines, but also because few other agents, against which the vaccines offer no protection, cause similar syndromes. We may speculate, furthermore, that all of these vaccines are effective because the viruses involved, whether wild or attenuated, induce effective durable immune responses and none, except varicella-zoster virus, of the agents has the capacity of remaining in the body to become infectious again after immunity has waned.

Live-virus vaccines have not been successful in controlling infections caused by a multiplicity of antigenic types for reasons that are technical and economic as well as propagandistic. There are more than 100 antigenically distinct Rhinoviruses associated with the common cold and the Rhinoviruses are only one of several virus taxons involved in this syndrome. Experimental live vaccines against Rhinovirus have been successfully tested (Douglas et al., 1974). However, unless it develops that a few types of virus are responsible for a disproportionate share of disease, it seems unlikely that a preparation can be made, which will contain a sufficient mass, of a sufficient variety of antigenic types, to give an easily recognizable benefit, without the cost becoming prohibitively high.

In influenza, too, a major problem is multiplicity of antigenic types, but here one A and one B type predominate at any one time. There seemed to be a good possibility that virus genetic traits determining low pathogenicity could be recombined with traits determining antigenicity, to produce new influenza vaccines as needed. The search for a live vaccine against influenza was pioneered several years ago by workers in Russia (Smorodintsev et al., 1965; Zhdanov, 1967). It was revived with renewed intensity in several countries with attenuation being sought according to several theoretical principals: passage in non-human cells, cold adaptation, temperature sensitivity and recombinants of earlier strains (Mostow et al., 1973; Hobsson et al., 1973; Minor et al., 1975; Richman et al., 1977; Davenport et al., 1977). None of these candidate strains, however, possessed an appropriate balance of immunogenicity with nonpathogenicity and the intensity of research in this area has again declined.

When one comes to consider the potential for vaccination against chronic viral infections which fail to induce effective immunity in the natural course of events, the task may seem Sisyphean, but, in fact, protection may be achieved in several ways. A chronic virus infection may persist because it is poorly antigenic and induces inadequate immune response, or it may persist only inside a few sequestered cells of specialized types where it is inaccessible to attack by the immune system, or it and its subunits may be produced in many cells in such massive quantity that the immune defenses are paralyzed. It is only the first of these patterns that seems not to be amenable to immune prophylaxis and this pattern is only found in infection with agents so simplified that their identity as viruses has been questioned (Gajdusek, 1977). When persistence occurs only in sequestered cells, disease may be controlled in several ways. The critical cells can be pre-empted by an attenuated virus and thus blocked to disease-causing strains. This appears to be the basis of a successful veterinary vaccine against Marek's lymphoma of chickens (Churchill et al., 1969). Alternatively, a vaccine administered before infection with wild virus may induce immunity that will destroy the virulent agent in transit to the sequestered cells. This is the principal on which the Flury rabies vaccine works (Ajjan et al., 1980). Finally, even when there is persistent virus infection, the antigenic mass released may be too small to maintain adequate immune titers, particularly in the aging host. This seems to be the case when varicella virus erupts as herpes zoster (Hope-Simpson, 1965). A vaccine might be effective in restoring the levels of immunity. When persistence is mediated by paralyzing the immune system with excess antigen, a small primary immunization may permit the immune response to react quickly enough to prevent antigen build up. This will be discussed under subcomponent vaccines.

A number of live-virus vaccines against chronic infections are in various stages of development. As well as the aforementioned varicella vaccine which has been used quite extensively in Japan (Takahashi et al., 1974; Gershon, 1980), one against herpes simplex has been tested in rabbits (Cappel, 1976) and vaccines active against Epstein–Barr virus (Epstein, 1976) and cytomegalovirus (Stagno et al., 1977) have been proposed. In all these systems, however, there is one common problem: if a wild virus persists in a host, one may anticipate that its attenuated analog may also persist in the recipient. The long-term effects of this persisting virus may not prove to be serious, but one cannot be sure without waiting to see if the latent vaccine virus is reactivated. That could require a lifetime of testing. The vaccine cannot be considered safe until it is shown either to not persist, or, if it does persist and is reactivated, to cause no serious disease. Current research is directed toward identifying the part(s) of the viral genome associated with integration into the cell DNA, or the part which confers on the virus the capacity to grow in neurones, cells which do not themselves replicate (Channock, 1982). If this segment can be excised a safe product will be available. It must then be tested for potency. Of course the problem is circumvented by using drug therapy.

4.1.2. KILLED-VIRUS VACCINES

Development of killed vaccines is usually easier than of live vaccines because virus inactivation is easier to confirm than virus attenuation, and because adventitious agents are often eliminated in the inactivation process. The quantity of material needed for immunization with killed virus is greater than with live virus, because there is no replication of the antigen. In preparation of this larger antigenic mass, other allergenic or toxic materials may be included with the immunizing antigens in sufficient amount to cause adverse reaction. Generally, tissue culture grown products have less allergen than products grown in egg or whole animal. Killed vaccines eliminate the most serious possible sources of oncogenicity because their nucleic acids do not replicate and are, therefore, unlikely to become integrated into host cell genomes.

The immunity derived from killed vaccines is, however, commonly less durable than that derived from live vaccines and booster doses are more often needed. The reasons for this are not altogether clear and may be variable. These vaccines also have a potential of eliciting an unbalanced immunological response which may fail to protect, yet inhibit a subsequent effective response, or may actually increase the severity of disease in a subsequent infection. Every system must be evaluated independently.

Killed vaccines must be administered parentally and therefore they do not have the potential, possessed by live vaccines, of inducing local secretion of IgA at the portal of entry. For this reason they are sometimes less effective than live vaccines in preventing asymptomatic infections which can perpetuate viral endemicity. On the other hand, the killed virus does not have the potential, possessed by some live attenuated vaccines, of spreading to secondary contacts with possible reversion to virulence in the process. A summary of relative advantages of the two types of vaccine is given in Table 2.

The spectrum of successful killed vaccines is very similar to that of the live vaccines (Table 3). Killed vaccines avoid none of the problems discussed above in immunization against diseases with multiple causative agents and, while problems associated with persistence of the vaccine virus in chronic infections are avoided, other questions concerning the long-term effectiveness of the immune response are accentuated.

Rabies, poliomyelitis, Japanese B and Russian Spring–Summer Encephalitis all represent diseases caused by relatively invariant virus strains which induce lasting immunity. The killed vaccines against these diseases are all quite successful. The rabies vaccine has posed the greatest problems, because Pasteur's original experiments (Pasteur, 1885) and subsequent

TABLE 2. *Comparative Advantages of Live and Killed Vaccine*

	Live*	Killed*
1. Confer solid protection	+ + +	+ +
2. Confer durable protection	+ + +	+
3. Induce IgA active at site of initial infection	+ +	−
4. May spread to secondary contacts	+ +	−
5. Number of doses per unit virus containing material	+ + +	+
6. Immunity conferred by single dose	+ +	+
7. Able to immunize by natural portal of entry	+ +	−
8. Safety relative to freedom *from*:		
a. Potentially carcinogenic agents	+ +	+ + +
b. Adventitious infectious agents	+ +	+ + +
c. Virulent virus in vaccine	+ +	+
d. Sensitization to extraneous antigens	+ + +	+
e. Sensitization to virus antigens	+ + +	+

Key: + + + Trait regularly evident; + + Trait often manifest; + Trait little exhibited; − Trait absent.

TABLE 3. *Killed-Virus Vaccines*

Vaccine	Source	Safety	Effectiveness	Durability of protection	Comment
Rabies	Duck embryo	Low	Fair	?	Unique in being effective
	Human fibroblast	Good	Fair		after infection established
Influenza A & B	Chick embryo	Good	Poor	6 months	Problems in keeping strains
Poliovirus 1,					appropriate to current
2 & 3	Monkey kidney cells	Good	Good	> 5 yr	Does not prevent
	Human fibroblasts	Good	Good		asymptomatic infection
Japanese B	Mouse brain	Fair	Fair		Veterinary and human use
	Chick embryo	Good		2 yr	in Eastern Asia
Russian Spring–	Mouse brain	Fair	Fair		Used in epidemic situations
Summer	Chick embryo	Good		?	in USSR and India
Adenovirus	Monkey kidney cells	Good	Poor	?	Theoretical risk of
types 3, 4 & 7					oncogenicity
Herpes simplex	Rabbit kidney cells	Good	Poor	6 months	Unproven value
	Embryonated egg	Good	Questionable	?	

experience with early crude vaccines established a precedent of reasonable success which inhibited testing more refined and potent products. Only recently has a human cell grown product, free of most nonviral allergens, been put on the market in some countries (Bahmanyar *et al.*, 1976). The killed poliovirus vaccines were successful in controlling poliomyelitis in certain Scandinavian countries and earlier in the USA (Salk and Salk, 1977) but they have now been largely replaced by the less expensive live product. Use of the two arbovirus vaccines is confined to certain geographic areas where those diseases have had high incidence (Fukunaga *et al.*, 1974; Shah *et al.*, 1962).

In diseases where problems in immunization lie in the multiplicity of types, killed vaccines have had some successes but none is entirely satisfactory. A killed adenovirus vaccine has been used in the special situation where, in military populations, epidemics of specific antigenic types occur with regularity, (Pierce *et al.*, 1968) but use of this vaccine has been discontinued in the USA lest the inactivated virus DNA retain some oncogenic potential.

Killed vaccines have been the most important form of prophylaxis against influenza and large controlled studies have amply demonstrated that vaccines of the appropriate antigenic type give some protection for several months (Davenport, 1971). However, only a proportion of properly vaccinated persons are protected and the public, including much of the medical profession, has been unconvinced of the vaccine's value (Rosenstock, 1961). Furthermore, because the prevalent type is subject to continual change, appropriate strains of vaccine are often in inadequate supply. Public confidence in the killed influenza vaccine was dealt a severe blow when, in the United States in 1976, a vaccine against Swine influenza was widely distributed in anticipation of an epidemic that never came (Osborn, 1977). The fact that rare adverse effects were clearly discernible in this situation where the vaccine had no counter-balancing beneficial effect further damaged public confidence (National Influenza Immunization Program, 1977). Evidence that these side effects were specifically associated with the Swine influenza vaccine and not subsequent products (Hurwitz *et al.*, 1981) will not quickly permeate the public consciousness. Clearly, when the next major epidemic hits, much of the populace will not voluntarily use the vaccine until too late, and a drug which could provide immediate protection would have an important role (Jackson, 1977).

The persistent and recurrent virus infections have also been attacked by means of killed-virus vaccines. Particularly extensive studies have been conducted with killed vaccines against recurrent Herpes simplex stomatitis and dermatitis; yet the value of these products remains uncertain (Zur Hausen, 1979). On the one hand there is the problem that even 'killed' herpes virus DNA can cause cell transformation (Rapp and Duff, 1973), and on the other, problems with potency and effectiveness of the immune response. One product produced from type 1 virus grown in rabbit kidney tissue culture was shown in placebo controlled trials to reduce herpetic recurrences for 6 months (Hull and Peck, 1967).

However, over a 36-month period no effect could be demonstrated and further studies have been abandoned (Wise *et al.*, 1977). Other vaccines prepared in Germany from both types 1 and 2 have been shown to be associated with increasing neutralizing antibody (Remy *et al.*, 1976) and sometimes with cell mediated immunity (Jarisch and Sandor, 1977) but there is no report of a controlled field trial of the clinical effectiveness of the German products. Another killed Herpesvirus hominis vaccine is under development currently in Britain (Skinner *et al.*, 1980). The unpredictable sequence of recurrences of this disease may easily give the impression that treatment has effected a cure which, in fact, occurred by chance, and widespread utilization of these products would seem to be at least premature. In any case, the prescribed number of injections is very large and, if the choice existed, a well-tolerated drug might be preferable for personal as well as medical reasons.

Certain killed-virus vaccines, measles (Fulginiti *et al.*, 1967) and respiratory syncitial virus (Craighead, 1975) for example, have caused very serious problems of immunological sensitization. The specific immune elements involved are not well defined. These killed vaccines elicit a response in components of the immune system or against parts of the virus which does not result in adequate suppression of subsequent virus infection, but which does sensitize the host to virus antigens. The sensitized host then reacts to damage his own cells wherever the cells are associated with virus, and the severity of disease may be increased greatly. The killed vaccines which have been most associated with this problem are no longer used, but their history must be kept in mind when evaluating the potential of different modes of control.

4.1.3. Viral Sub-component Vaccines

Several technical procedures have been proposed in recent years for production of vaccines composed of selected portions of a virus. This approach would retain all the advantages of the killed vaccines with possible additional advantages in reduced chance of unbalanced immunity, with substantial reduction in exogenous allergens, and freedom from transforming DNA and other potentially dangerous virus components. The approach faces, however, increased problems in achieving adequate potency.

The most extensively tested of the subcomponent vaccines is one composed of the surface proteins separated from egg-grown influenza virus (Kasel *et al.*, 1966; Kaaden *et al.*, 1974; Laver and Webster, 1976). Although this vaccine has the above-mentioned advantages, it has been less successful than the whole virus product in its immunogenicity (Wright *et al.*, 1976). It has proven difficult to elicit with this vaccine the titers that are usually considered necessary for immunity.

A naturally occurring virus subcomponent, the hepatitis B surface antigen, HBSAg which circulates in the blood of hepatitis carriers, is a more effective immunogen. An extraordinary field trial carried out by Szmuness and his colleagues (1980) demonstrated that HBSAg collected from chronic hepatitis carriers conferred effective protection on a group at especially high risk from hepatitis, the male homosexual community. Relatively small amounts of surface antigen, when encountered before exposure to whole virus, induced sufficient immunity to block establishment of the carrier state. This antigen occurs naturally as part of a 22-nm particle with multiple polypeptide molecules sited on the particle surface.

No satisfactory method currently exists for growing the hepatitis virus, and at present the vaccine antigen must be collected from the blood of carriers. Strenuous efforts have been made to develop a bacterial clone which will produce the antigen. Success has been achieved both with the surface antigen (MacKay *et al.*, 1981) and with another hepatitis B antigen, the core protein (Pasek *et al.*, 1979). These antigens have been shown to be immunologically active and the isolated polypeptides have been shown adequate to protect chimpanzees from challenge with hepatitis when the antigen is administered as an alum precipitate (Dreesman *et al.*, 1981).

The ultimate step in this process of stripping virus vaccines down to their essential components may be represented by the work of Lerner's group (1981b) in synthesizing relatively short amino acid sequences carrying essential epitopes. This group has selected certain DNA sequences from both hepatitis B virus (Lerner *et al.*, 1981a) and retroviruses (Sutcliffe *et al.*, 1980) and produced antigenic peptide sequences coded by the DNA. This process permits further selection of antigenic epitopes in a vaccine so as to exclude all deleterious and nonessential elements from the material to be injected. Similar studies are underway with influenza antigens (Channock, 1982). This author, however, is concerned about two potential pitfalls in the process of greater and greater selectivity in the components of vaccines: inadequate potency and viral variation. Viruses, as a group, are exceptionally good antigens. This is probably due to the fact that they have multiple copies of a few biochemically active groups displayed at regular intervals on the surface of particles 20 to 200 nm in diameter. It may well be that evolution has specifically selected our immune systems to respond optimally to antigens presented in this manner. Adjuvants may be used as alternative vehicles to enhance the immune response, but the more potent adjuvants leave long-lasting traces at the injection site which would not be accepted in human use if an alternative were available. Although alum has been used in experimental and discontinued vaccines, it would not be readily accepted now. It may be that the new methods will produce so much antigen inexpensively that this problem can be overcome, but that remains to be determined.

Second, viruses, as living entities, have the power to mutate. Some do this more readily than others and some viral sequences are conserved more than others but the phenomenon is universal. To use a vaccine directed at a single epitope is comparable to using an antibiotic or antimetabolite directed at a single point in the metabolic cycle (Loddo, 1980). Resistant mutants are much more likely to develop than when combined antibiotics or chemotherapeutics are used. Rarely would mutation at a single site render a virus totally resistant to the immunity generated against the whole virion, but this problem would be encountered more often when the immunity is limited to one or a few selected epitopes.

4.1.4. PASSIVE IMMUNIZATION

Passive immunization is more likely than vaccine to be useful in situations where drugs might also be considered. Three different immune elements have been used passively: Immune serum globulin, sensitized cells and transfer factor. Serum globulin is the most important of these. Controlled trials have demonstrated the effectiveness of human gammaglobulin in prevention of measles (Karelitz, 1950), poliomyelitis (National Committee for the Evaluation. . ., 1954), varicella (Meyers and Witte, 1974), hepatitis A (Krugman, 1963) and rabies (Winkler *et al.*, 1969). It is only effective against hepatitis B if given before, or very promptly after, exposure (Prince *et al.*, 1975) and it is of no confirmed value in the treatment of rubella (Horstmann, 1976). It has been used with apparent, but unverified, success in a wide variety of rare, high risk, infections as, for instance, Lassa Fever (Monath *et al.*, 1974). It must be administered no more than a few weeks before exposure to the virus and no more than a few days after infection. It may interfere with response to vaccines, especially live-virus vaccines, administered during the time it is effective. The protection it confers can never consist of more than a part of a whole normal immune defense, but it has not been associated with adverse sensitization like the killed-virus vaccines. Because it must be obtained from human donors and because only hyperimmunized donors are suitable for treatment of some viruses, supplies will always be limited and expensive.

Immune globulin may be able to neutralize free virus in the blood of infected persons and, acting with complement, it may in some systems be capable of lysing cells with virus antigens on their surface and vegetative virus within, but the main immune defense against intracellular virus is mediated by the specifically sensitized T lymphocyte. Passive transfer of immune cells might, therefore, be a theoretically important form of therapy. Effective transfer is, however, difficult to obtain, not only because the cells are marked with highly individualistic sets of tissue antigens which render them susceptible to destruction by the recipient's immune system but also because the cells are not effective unless they share at least one tissue antigen type with the recipient (Doherty and Zinkernagel, 1975). Partial matching of donor and recipient tissue types raises the ogre of chimera formation and graft versus host reactions. This form of therapy is therefore both difficult and dangerous. Nevertheless, the literature does contain a few impressive examples of its possible usefulness in desperate situations (Kempe, 1960).

Failure of immune cell response may be due not to lack of sensitized cells but to lack of accessory 'transfer factor'. A review of this ill-defined system is beyond the scope of this paper, but several positive reports have appeared recently describing successful use of transfer factor administration in chronic virus infection (Heim *et al.*, 1976; Sano *et al.*, 1977). Persistence of virus antigen in hepatitis B may be in part due to deficiency of specific transfer factor.

4.2. RELATIVE ROLES AT DIFFERENT STAGES OF INFECTION

After infection with a virus, an incubation period follows during which disease is not manifest. This period may last anywhere from 2 days to, in the case of rabies, 1 year. During this incubation period virus multiplies and spreads through the body. Some cells are doubtless killed, but they are too few to cause more than the vaguest symptoms.

The first symptoms of disease are presumably those which are a direct result of virus damage but, unless these affect a specific tissue, they are very often insufficiently distinctive to provide a basis for diagnosis. Very often the more distinctive and more severe signs of disease result not from the virus-induced damage *per se* but from the immune response to virus antigens on cell surfaces. It is axiomatic that virus, which must grow intracellularly, can only be eliminated by rupture of the cells which harbor it, and this function of immunological cell lysis seems to be the immediate cause of erythematous rashes (Mims, 1966) and edema of virus encephalitis (Tignor *et al.*, 1974). Treatment of virus infection may, therefore, be logically directed toward suppressing the immune response as well as suppressing virus growth. The two approaches are often contradictory and the choice between them must be made with the greatest care.

4.2.1. TREATMENT PRIOR TO EXPOSURE

A vaccine can only be beneficial if it is given early enough to generate an immune response before the infecting virus has multiplied sufficiently to induce immunity by itself. A live vaccine must also have sufficient time to replicate to produce a sensitizing mass of antigen. This means that live virus vaccines must ordinarily be given before exposure to wild virus. The great advantage of these vaccines is that they may commonly be given long before exposure and thus offer long-term protection. The protection afforded by a single dose of some live-virus vaccines may actually be lifelong. There is, at present, no generally recognized necessity for revaccination with measles, mumps or rubella live vaccines. Revaccination with yellow fever vaccine is called for every 10 years by WHO regulation (World Health Org., 1977) but there is no real evidence that this is necessary (Pinheiro and Oliva, 1981). Smallpox vaccination needed be repeated every few years.

The killed vaccines are also best given before infection occurs, but because no time is needed for antigen production, the lead time needed is a little less than with live-virus vaccine (Fig. 1). An exception to the requirement for early administration exists in the case of rabies where, because of the very long incubation period of the disease, a killed vaccine given even several days after exposure may be effective. The durability of immunity induced by killed vaccines is usually less solid than that conferred by live vaccines and revaccination every year is a common practice.

Passive immunization is also most likely to succeed if it is given before the virus has a chance to become established. However, it demands no response period and it is commonly effective for several days after infection. It has even been used with apparent success after

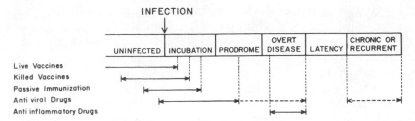

FIG. 1. Stages of disease in which various control agents may be effective. Solid lines indicate that most virus infections may be expected to be responsive; broken lines that responsiveness may be limited to certain specific infections.

onset of certain protracted diseases (Monath *et al.*, 1974). Infections, contracted (Krugman and Giles, 1973) during the period of protection, may generate enough antigen to confer lasting immunity without causing apparent disease, but if infection does not occur in this way, the treatment must be repeated on the occasion of each exposure.

It is usually impractical to administer an antiviral drug before exposure to virus because the requirement for repeated doses makes it difficult to secure necessary cooperation from the recipient, and because toxic side effects may not be tolerable over a long course. The most widely publicized situation where pre-exposure treatment has been advocated is in the use of high doses of ascorbic acid to prevent colds (Pauling, 1971). The effectiveness of this procedure has been strenuously contested (Dykes and Meier, 1975) but waning interest in this treatment seems to be determined more by popular fadism than by scientific proof. In all this dispute, little attention has been paid to possible side effects and there has been no serious study of mechanism.

Amantadine and its analogues have also been advocated as prophylactic agents in prevention of influenza A (Jackson *et al.*, 1970; Oxford and Galbraith, 1980). The problems of influenza vaccines with respect to availability of relevant types, efficacy and safety have already been mentioned, and there is considerable scope for a drug which would have broader specificity than the vaccine. Amantadine is indeed less type-specific being active against several, and possibly all, strains of influenza A (Grunnert and Hoffman, 1977). There are, however, quantitative differences in the sensitivity of different strains which make tests of efficacy desirable. Generally, its efficacy is probably less than that of the vaccine and most importantly its use may be accompanied by ill-defined personality changes (Medical Letter, 1978). It would seem to have a clear role in the protection of high-risk individuals until they can be vaccinated, in situations where vaccination has been delayed for one reason or another until an epidemic hits, but simple inertia and unfamiliarity seems to have inhibited its use, even in this role, to date.

A large number of *in vitro* and animal studies on the effect of ribovirin, as well as some clinical studies, have shown that drug to be active against a wide variety of viruses at this stage of infection (Sidwell *et al.*, 1979). None of these studies, however, suggest to this author that the drug would find practical application in such circumstances.

The great advantage of drugs over vaccines in prevention of virus disease lies in the fact that they may be immediately effective and need no response period. This consideration gives them a role in situations where an epidemic cannot be anticipated far enough in advance to make vaccination practical. However, where there is adequate warning the vaccine will usually be preferred because a single course of treatment provides extended protection.

4.2.2. THE INCUBATION PERIOD

The value of vaccines administered after infection has occurred is very limited. Measles vaccine may be effective up to 2 days after exposure. The intramuscular route of injection accelerates the course of virus progression by about that amount of time, allowing the attenuated virus to take precedence over a wild agent acquired through the respiratory tract

(Black, 1962). The same may hold true for mumps and rubella, but it has not been demonstrated. Killed vaccine, too, may be effective for a short time after exposure to wild virus. This is especially true for rabies vaccine which may be helpful several days after exposure (World Health Organization, 1973). Even with rabies vaccine, however, as preparations which are freer of extraneous allergens and less prone to cause allergic encephalitis are developed, recommendations have been progressively modified to advocate prompter vaccine use in instances of progressively less well defined exposure. The fact that rabies vaccine is effective at all several days after infection is evidence that the antigenic mass of the replicating virus increases slowly and does not exceed the mass contained in a dose of vaccine for several days.

Passive immunization has had its greatest value during the incubation period. The effect of immune serum administered during the measles incubation period has been well defined (Black and Yannet, 1960), but seldom used since the advent of the more attenuated vaccines. The greatest roles of immune globulin now are in control of rarer infections for which no alternative method of control exists and in treatment of virus infections in immuno-suppressed individuals who cannot respond normally to vaccine (Orenstein et al., 1981).

In as much as the studies with immune serum globulin demonstrate that an attack on a virus infection which is begun after the infection has been initiated, but before symptoms appear, may not be too late to have beneficial effects, this period may well be the time when drugs will ultimately prove to have their greatest values. A course of drug treatment, initiated after the infection has been established, needs be maintained for less time than one given in anticipation of infection and the toxic effects, as well as the cost, are thus minimized. The best studied instance in which a drug has been recommended for use during this period is the treatment of smallpox with the β-thiosemicarbazone (Bauer, 1965). The toxicity of this drug is such that it would not be tolerated for extended periods prior to infection, but it may be effective when it is too late to vaccinate. In this particular instance, however, disease-control procedures, based almost entirely on vaccination, have totally eliminated the disease smallpox, and the need for this therapy has disappeared. Methisazone may still have some role to play in treatment of vaccinia complications (McLean, 1977). There will be fewer vaccinia immunizations performed in the future, but those which are continued will be mostly in military personnel, an age group which may manifest more adverse reactions to primary immunization.

Experimental studies with a wide variety of antiviral substances have suggested beneficial effects in humans and animals during the incubation period (Salido-Rengell et al., 1977; Overby et al., 1977; Lopez and Giner-Sorolla, 1977). However, few of these systems have been pursued vigorously with controlled studies in humans. It seems that early chemotherapy offers limited incentive to the commercial market and unless governmental agencies supplement more vigorously the developmental work of the drug houses, research emphasis will remain on drugs useful for treatment of disease at a stage when the symptomatology has brought the patient to a physician.

4.2.3. Prodromal Period

There is no evidence of any vaccine being effective once symptoms have appeared. By this time the infecting virus will usually have produced a sufficient antigenic mass that injection of more antigen has no effect. Even immune serum globulin is usually ineffective at this stage. We may presume, therefore, that elimination of circulating virus has little effect at this stage, and that the only way to reduce the disease would be to limit virus production from already infected cells. In attempting to do this we face the same problems as were encountered in using drugs during the incubation period. Specific diagnoses are difficult, and the patient may not yet be sufficiently sick to seek medical help. In addition, the virus has had more time to replicate and chances of controlling it before severe damage is done have been reduced. A number of popular nostrums call for treatment in this period – alcohol administered topically for incipient herpes gingivostomatitis, orange juice for the common cold – but none of these have been proven efficaceous in controlled trials.

4.2.4. Overt Disease and Recurrence

It is during periods of overt disease that demand for chemotherapy is greatest. The patient knows he is sick and it is too late for any preventive measure. It seems probable that it is also too late to treat any acute self-limited infection with antiviral agents. In diseases such as measles and the common cold, symptomatology seems to result from the reaction of the immune system with infected tissues and virus replication ceases rapidly without treatment. However, in semiacute and chronic diseases, such as most notably the infections with agents of the Herpesvirus genus, continuing virus replication plays an important role in pathogenesis; some of the most notable successes of chemotherapy have been achieved in treating these infections. These will be discussed in Section 4.3.

Because so much of the damage occurring in overt disease is due to the immune reaction, it is reasonable to suppose that immuno-suppressive drugs might modulate the response and improve the condition of the patient. Obviously, this is a delicate proposition which would have to be closely tailored to the nature and the stage of the infection. Probably the only system that has been adequately studied to provide a reasonable understanding of these complexities is lymphocytic-chorio-meningitis in mice (Nathanson *et al.*, 1975). It has also been observed that immuno-suppression can extend the survival time of mice infected with rabies (Tignor *et al.*, 1974). In general, however, even in animal model systems it has been difficult to achieve a marked reduction in long-term mortality. In humans, steroids have been advocated in treatment of severe infectious mononucleosis pharyngitis (Andiman and Miller, 1977) and there is an inadequately confirmed report of a beneficial effect of steroids in herpes encephalitis (Ilis and Merry, 1972). In addition, cerebral decompression by drainage or by treatment with mannitol has been found effective in treatment of Reye's syndrome, a severe systemic disease associated with Influenza B infection (Shaywitz *et al.*, 1977).

4.2.5. Latent Period

It would be very desirable if drugs could be designed to eliminate latent virus. If the latent agent is in the form of a provirus, i.e. virus nucleic acid under cell replicative control, this would be difficult to achieve, but when the latent agent is simply replicating at a low rate in a few cells, it may be subject to attack. Drugs seem a more promising agent for this purpose than vaccines, as the immune system will commonly have been stimulated during the primary phases of the infection. In some instances it might be possible to eliminate the virus by local administration of a drug, thus avoiding systemic toxic effects. No substantial work has, however, been done in this area as yet.

Meanwhile, although it has yet not been possible to eliminate viral latency with drugs, an important role of drugs has been demonstrated in preventing reactivation of latent virus during periods of immune suppression. Saral *et al.* (1981) have demonstrated that it is possible to reduce greatly the frequency of Herpesvirus hominis activation during bone marrow transplantation by initiating therapy with acyclovir prior to the transplantation.

4.3. RELATIVE ROLES IN DIFFERENT TYPES OF INFECTION

Viruses may be classified in many different ways. Certainly the standard taxonomic criteria, which reflect different metabolic systems, are highly relevant to the type of drugs that may be effective. This will doubtless be covered in other papers on individual drugs. Here, a broader, more disease-oriented classification seems relevant. Many viruses cause an acute disease, elicit an immune response, and then either kill the host or are themselves eliminated terminating the illness – 'acute infections'. Other viruses cause pathology that may persist and even worsen in the face of a full immunological reaction – 'chronic infection'. Still others cause no direct pathology but interfere with normal cell replicative control mechanisms and may ultimately induce tumor formation – 'transforming infections'. The roles of vaccines and drugs can profitably be examined in terms of these classifications.

4.3.1. Acute Infections

The acute virus infections are those which are limited by a prompt effective immune response. These are therefore the natural target for control by immunizing agents. Some successes have also been scored in this area by drugs such as methisazone and amantadine, but these successes are pallid beside the successes of the vaccines. Current control methods are now dependent on the vaccines, and this control is very effective, except in instances where the causative virus occurs in a multiplicity of antigenic types. Here, as epitomized by the popular interest in Vitamin C prophylaxis of the common cold, a large field awaits the development of appropriate drugs.

Two drugs, guanidine and 2-(a-hydroxybenzyl)-benzimidazole (HBB) exhibit highly specific anti-picornavirus activity. Both were developed early in the course of research on antiviral drugs (Tamm and Eggers, 1963). However, drug-resistant strains of virus arose quickly, adequate *in vivo* drug concentrations were not easily attained (Eggers, 1976), and the work has progressed slowly. Studies on guanidine analogues which do not so easily induce resistance (Swallow *et al.*, 1977) and studies capitalizing on the synergistic effects of these two types of drug (Eggers, 1976) have kept alive hopes for successful therapy. This work might be expected to proceed faster if we had a better idea of the mode of action of these drugs. The whole replicative process of these viruses seems to be extraordinarily difficult to dissect (Sergiescu *et al.*, 1972). Whereas guanidine-sensitivity maps with the coat protein (Cooper *et al.*, 1971) its most pronounced effect is on RNA synthesis (Baltimore, 1969). HBB presumably acts at some point in the RNA synthetic process (Tamm and Eggers, 1963), but because it has never been possible to isolate the RNA polymerase(s) of picornaviruses in pure form, it has not been possible to identify a specific point of action.

Less progress has been made in the chemotherapy of the Togaviruses (Arbovirus groups A and B in old terminology) than the Picornaviruses, but their mode of replication is similar and the multiplicity of antigenic types represented is analogous. In terms of lives to be saved, the potential usefulness of drugs for treatment of dengue, the viral encephalitides and the less well-defined arthropod-borne virus diseases may be as great as the potential for treatment of the common cold and other picornavirus caused diseases.

4.3.2. Chronic Infections

The relative importance of acute virus infections as causes of human disease is probably over-emphasized due to the fact that these include most of the syndromes familiar to each of us from childhood. The various human herpes-group viruses, the hepatitis viruses, the spongiform encephalopathies, the common wart and the as yet unidentified agents associated with multiple sclerosis (Black, 1975) and Paget's disease of bone (Rebel *et al.*, 1976) all cause chronic diseases. Of all this diverse group, vaccines have been extensively investigated only against Herpes simplex.

The herpes-group viruses commonly cause protracted acute diseases at the time of primary infection as well as recurrent episodes following reactivation of latent viruses. Even the primary infections tend to be localized to one part of the anatomy: the face, the genitalia, or the brain. Although most primary infections are not serious, they are often troublesome and, when the brain is involved, they are life threatening. Whitley *et al.* (1977, 1981) have demonstrated that it is possible to identify herpes virus encephalitis in time to offer effective treatment with vidarabine. Delayed treatment may save the life, but fail to prevent irreparable brain damage. This work is not only important in the treatment of herpes encephalitis, but it also suggests that, when we have a drug which does no lasting damage by toxicity or immune suppression, it may be practical to treat the much more frequently recurring skin and mucous membrane lesion of the herpes viruses.

Although progress with vaccines against chronic virus diseases has been very slow, it is against them that the greatest successes have been achieved with drugs. Kaufman's initial success in treating herpes keratitis with Idoxuridine (Idurd) (Kaufman, 1962) encouraged clinical studies on a wide variety of pyrimidine analogues in a corresponding variety of disease situations. The report of successful treatment of herpes encephalitis with vidarabine (ara-A) (Whitley *et al.*, 1977) is but one of the encouraging developments. These studies are the subject of several other chapters in this series and cannot be adequately covered here. The use of methisazone in treatment of persistent complications of smallpox vaccine represents another instance of effective chemotherapy of chronic virus infection (McLean, 1977).

4.3.3. TRANSFORMING INFECTIONS

It is very difficult to conceive of any vaccine against a tumor virus, other than a subunit product, being accorded general medical acceptance in the foreseeable future. The problems of testing and proving freedom from long delayed adverse effects are too difficult. A subunit vaccine devoid of nucleic acid might be acceptable but the precedent we have from work with other vaccines (Wright *et al.*, 1976) suggests that these might not confer the durable immunity that would be needed. Mention has already been made of the live-virus vaccine made from a turkey agent for protection of chickens against Marek's lymphoma (Churchill *et al.*, 1969) but this is an animal vaccine and does not require the same safety standards.

The retroviruses, which are associated with many leukemia and lymphoma syndromes in animals, offer a tempting target for chemotherapy because they depend on a process of transcription of DNA off an RNA template, a process which has no known role in mature host cells.

It is too soon to expect very much from chemotherapy of tumor viruses in man because, in spite of the many animal models, few human cancers have been clearly associated with a virus etiology. Until an agent is known, attempts at chemotherapy must be stabs in the dark. Nevertheless, in the instance where a virus has been best established as a major etiologic factor, Burkitt's lymphoma (Miller *et al.*, 1977), chemotherapy has played a major role in inducing remission and possible cure (Nkrumah and Perkins, 1976). Cyclophosphamide by itself has produced a large proportion of long-term remissions. It seems probable, however, combinations of several drugs used with radiotherapy in a coordinated vigorous attack on the cancer may be most effective. This has been the case in Hodgkin's disease, another cancer which has many of the hallmarks of a virus infection (Kaplan and Rosenberg, 1975). If these two examples are representative of virus-caused cancers, we hope that other cancers with virus etiology may be more responsive to drugs than cancers in which viruses play little or no role in determining differential prevalence rates.

4.4. SUMMARY

A safe effective vaccine will usually be preferred to a drug active against the same disease, because side effects are likely to be fewer and the required number of doses less. However, a vaccine must ordinarily be administered before infection and when this is difficult to do, either because the infecting virus may vary or because a very large number of different viruses may each be responsible for a small fraction of all cases of a disease, drugs may provide a very important alternative. Furthermore, it seems probable that a fully stimulated immune mechanism may be inadequate to protect against certain chronic virus infections and that drugs may offer the only satisfactory opportunity for control of these infections. Virus-induced tumors may fall in this category.

Acknowledgement—I wish to thank Dr. William H. Prusoff for his help in surveying literature and evaluating statements made in this paper.

REFERENCES

AJJAN, N., SOULEBOT, J. P., TRIAU, R. and BIRON, G. (1980) Intradermal immunization with rabies vaccine. *J. Am. Med. Ass.* **244**: 2528–2531.

ALEVIZATOS, A. C., McKINNEY, R. W. and FEIGIN, R. D. (1967) Live attenuated Venezuelan equine encephalomyelitis virus vaccine. I. Clinical effects in man. *Am. J. Trop. Med. Hyg.* **16**: 762–768.

ANDIMAN, W. A. and MILLER, G. (1977) Infectious mononucleosis, pp. 539–542. In: *Pediatrics*, RUDOLF, A. M., BARNETT, H. L. and EINHORN, A. H. (eds.). Appleton-Century-Crofts, New York.

ASANO, Y., NAKAYAMA, H., YAZAKI, T., KATO, R., HIROSE, S., TSUZUKI, K., ITO, S., ISOMURA, S. and TAKAHASHI, M. (1977) Protection against varicella in family contacts by immediate inoculation with live varicella vaccine. *Pediatrics* **59**: 3–7.

BAHMANYAR, M., FAYAZ, A., NOUR-SALELI, S., MOHAMMADI, M. and KOPROWSKI, H. (1976) Successful protection of humans exposed to rabies infection. Post-exposure treatment with new human diploid cell rabies vaccine and antirabies serum. *J. Am. Med. Ass.* **236**: 2751–2754.

BALTIMORE, D. (1969) The replication of picornaviruses. In: *The Biochemistry of Viruses*, pp. 101–176. LEVY, H. B. (ed.). Dekker, New York.

BARON, S. and DIANZANI, F. (eds.) (1977) The interferon system. A current review to 1978. *Texas Rpts. Biol. and Med.* **35**: 1–573.

BAUER, D. J. (1965) Clinical experience with the antiviral drug Marboran (1-methylisatin B-thiosemicarbazone). *Ann. N.Y. Acad. Sci.* **130**: 110–117.

BLACK, F. L. (1975) The association between measles and multiple sclerosis. *Prog. med. Virol.* **21**: 158–164.

BLACK, F. L. (1962) Measles: its spread from cell to cell and person to person. *Can. J. Pub. Hlth.* **56**: 517–520.

BLACK, F. L. and YANNET, H. (1960) Inapparent measles after gammaglobulin administration. *J. Am. Med. Ass.* **173**: 1183–1188.

BUCHANAN, R. A. and HESS, F. (1980) Vidarabine: Pharmocology and clinical experience. *Pharmacol. Ther.* **10**: 143–172.

CAPPEL, R. (1976) Comparison of the humoral and cellular immune responses after immunization with live, UV inactivated Herpes simplex virus and a subunit vaccine and efficacy of these immunizations. *Archiv. of Virology* **56**: 29–35.

CHANNOCK, R. M. (1982) Vaccines – new developments. In: *Viral Diseases in South-East Asia and the Western Pacific*, pp. 139–155. MACKENZIE, J. (ed.). Academic, Sydney.

CHERRY, J. D., FEIGIN, R. D., SHACKELFORD, P. G., HINTHORN, D. R. and SCHMIDT, R. R. (1973) A clinical and serological study of 103 children with measles vaccine failure. *J. Pediat.* **82**: 802–809.

CHURCHILL, A. E., PAYNE, L. N. and CHUFF, R. C. (1969) Immunization against Marek's Disease using a live attenuated virus. *Nature* **221**: 744–747.

COOPER, P. D., GEISSLER, E., SCOTTI, P. D. and TANNOCK, G. A. (1971) Further characterization of the genetic map of poliovirus temperature-sensitive mutants. In: *Strategy of the Viral Genome*, pp. 75–95, WOLSTENHOLME, G. E. W. and O'CONNER, M. (eds.). Livingstone, Edinburgh.

CRAIGHEAD, J. E. (1975) Report of a workshop: Disease accentuation after immunization with inactivated microbial vaccines. *J. Infec. Dis.* **131**: 749–754.

DAVENPORT, F. M. (1971) Killed influenza vaccines: Present status, suggested use, desirable developments. *PAHO Sci. Pub.* **226**: 85–95.

DAVENPORT, F. M., HENNESSY, A. V., MAASAAB, H. F., MINUSE, E., CLARK, L. C., ABRAMS, G. D. and MITCHELL, J. R. (1977) Pilot studies on recombinant cold-adapted live type A and B influenza vaccines. *J. Infec. Dis.* **136**: 17–25.

DOHERTY, P. C. and ZINKERNAGEL, R. M. (1975) A biological role for the major histocompatibility antigens. *Lancet* **1**: 1406–1409.

DOUGLAS, R. G., COUCH, R. B., BAXTER, B. D. and GOUGH, M. (1974) Attenuation of rhinovirus type 15: relation of illness to plaque size. *Infec. Immun.* **9**: 519–523.

DYKES, M. H. M. and MEIER, P. (1975) Ascorbic acid and the common cold. Evaluation of efficacy and toxicity. *J. Am. Med. Ass.* **231**: 1073–1079.

DREESMAN, G. R., HOLLINGER, F. B., SANCHEZ, Y., OEFINGER, P. and MELNICK, J. L. (1981) Immunization of chimpanzees with Hepatitis B derived polypeptides. *Infec. Immun.* **32**: 62–67.

EGGERS, H. J. (1976) Successful treatment of enterovirus infected mice by 2(d-hydroxybenzyl)-benzimidazole and guanidine. *J. Exper. Med.* **143**: 1367–1381.

EPSTEIN, M. A. (1976) Epstein–Barr Virus – is it time to develop a vaccine program? *J. Nat. Canc Inst.* **56**: 697–700.

FUKUNAGA, T., ROJANSUPHOT, S., WUNGKORBKIAT, S., THAMMANICHON, A., KAN, T., OTSU, K., TUCHINDA, P., JATANASEN, S. and CHIOWANICH, P. (1974) Japanese encephalitis vaccination in Thailand. *Biken J.* **17**: 21–31.

FULGINITI, V. A., ELLER, J. J., DOWNIE, A. W. and KEMPE, C. H. (1967) Altered reactivity to measles virus: Atypical measles in children previously immunized with inactivated measles virus vaccines. *J. Am. Med. Ass.* **202**: 1075–1080.

GAJDUSEK, D. C. (1977) Unconventional viruses and the origin and disappearance of Kuru. *Science* **197**: 943–960.

GERSHON, A. A. (1980) Live attenuated varicella-zoster vaccine. *Rev. Infec. Dis.* **2**: 393–407.

GRUNNERT, R. R. and HOFFMAN, C. E. (1977) Sensitivity of influenza A/New Jersey/8/76 (Hsw1N1) Virus to Amantadine HCl. *J. Infec. Dis.* **136**: 297–300.

HEIM, L. R., BERNHARD, G., GOLDMAN, A. L., DORFF, G. and RYTEL, M. (1976) Transfer factor treatment of viral diseases in Milwaukee. In: *Transfer Factor Basic Properties and Clinical Applications*, pp. 457–464. ASHER, M. S., GOTTLIEB, A. A. and KIRKPATRICK, C. H. (eds.). Academic, New York.

HOBSSON, D., BAKER, F. A., CURRY, R. L., BEARE, A. S. and MASSEY, P. M. D. (1973) The efficacy of live and inactivated vaccines of Hong Kong influenza virus in an industrial community. *J. Hyg. (Camb.)* **71**: 641–647.

HOPE-SIMPSON, R. E. (1965) The nature of Herpes-Zoster: A long-term study and a new hypothesis. *Proc. Roy. Soc. Med.* **58**: 9–20.

HORSTMANN, D. M. (1975) Controlling rubella: Problems and perspectives. *Ann. Int. Med.* **83**: 412–417.

HORSTMANN, D. M. (1976) Rubella. In: *Viral Infections of Humans. Epidemiology and Control*, pp. 409–427. EVANS, A. S. (ed.). Plenum, New York.

HULL, R. N. and PECK, F. B. (1967) Vaccination against herpes-virus hominis. In: *Proceedings of the 1st*

International Conference on Vaccines Against Viral and Rickettsial Disease of Man, PAHO Sci. Pub. 147, PAHO, Washington, D.C.

HURWITZ, E. S., SCHONBERGER, L. B., NELSON, D. B. and HOLMAN, R. C. (1981) Guillaim–Barre' syndrome and the 1978–79 influenza vaccine. *New Engl. J. Med.* **304**: 1557–1561.

ILIS, L. S. and MERRY, R. T. G. (1972) Treatment of herpes simplex encephalitis. *J. Roy. Coll. Phys. Lond.* **7**: 34–44.

JACKSON, G. G. (1977) Sensitivity of influenza A virus to amantadine. *J. Infec. Dis.* **136**: 301–302.

JACKSON, G. G., STANLEY, E. D. and MULDOON, R. L. (1970) Prospects for the control of viral diseases with chemical substances. *PAHO Sci. Pub.* **226**: 588–601.

JARISCH, R. and SANDOR, I. (1977) MIF in der Therapiekontrolle von Herpes simplex recidivans: Behandlung mit Leviamisole, BCG, Urushiol and Herpes Antigen Vaccine. *Arch. Derm. Res.* **258**: 151–159.

KAADEN, O-R., DIETZSCHOLD, B. and UEBERSCHAER, S. (1974) Vaccination against Marek's disease: Immunizing effect of purified turkey herpes virus and cellular membranes from infected cells. *Med. Microbiol. Immunol.* **159**: 261–269.

KAPLAN, H. S. and ROSENBERG, S. A. (1975) The management of Hodgkin's disease. *Cancer* **36**: 796–803.

KARELITZ, S. (1950) Does modified measles result in lasting immunity. *J. Pediat.* **36**: 697–703.

KASEL, J. A., ALFORD, R. H., LEHRICH, J. R., BANKS, P. A., HUBER, M. and KNIGHT, V. (1966) Adenovirus soluble antigens for human immunization. *Am. Rev. Resp. Dis.* **94**: 170–174.

KAUFMAN, H. E. (1962) Clinical cure of herpes simplex keratitis by 5-iodo-2' deoxyuridine. *Proc. Soc. Exptl. Biol. Med.* **109**: 251–252.

KEMPE, C. H. (1960) Studies on smallpox and complications of smallpox vaccination. *Pediatrics* **26**: 176–189.

KLEID, D. G., YANSURA, D., SMALL, B., DOWBENCO, D., MOORE, D. M., GRUBMAN, M. J., MCKERCHER, P. D., MORGAN, D. O., ROBERTSON, B. H. and BACHRACH, H. L. (1981) Cloned viral protein vaccine for foot-and-mouth disease: Responses in cattle and swine. *Science* **214**: 1125–1129.

KRUGMAN, S. (1963) The clinical use of gammaglobulin. *N. Engl. J. Med.* **269**: 195–201.

KRUGMAN, S. and GILES, J. P. (1973) Viral hepatitis, type B (MS-2 strain). Further observations on natural history and prevention. *New Engl. J. Med.* **288**: 755–760.

LANE, J. M., RUBEN, F. L., NEFF, J. M. and MILLAR, J. D. (1969) Complications of smallpox vaccination. *New Engl. J. Med.* **281**: 1201–1208.

LAVER, W. G. and WEBSTER, R. G. (1976) Preparation and immunogenicity of an influenza virus hemagglutinin and neuraminidase subunit vaccine. *Virology* **69**: 511–522.

LERNER, R. A., GREEN, N., ALEXANDER, H., LIU. F-T., SUTCLIFFE, J. G. and SHINNICK, T. M. (1981a) Chemically synthetized peptides predicted from the nucleotide sequence of hepatitis B virus genome elicit antibodies reactive with native envelope proteins of Dane particles. *Proc. Natl. Acad. Sci. (Washington)* **78**: 3403–3407.

LERNER, R. A., GREEN, N., OLSON, A., SHINNICK, T. and SUTCLIFFE, J. G. (1981b) The development of synthetic vaccines. *Hosp. Pract.* **16**: 55–62.

LODDO, B. (1980) Development of drug resistance and dependence in viruses. *Pharmacol. Ther.* **10**: 431–460.

LOPEZ, C. and GINER-SOROLLA, A. (1977) Arabinosyl-N^6-hydroxyadenine: A new potent antivirus drug. *Ann. N.Y. Acad. Sci.* **284**: 351–357.

MACKAY, P., PASEK, M., MAGAZIN, M., KOVACIC, R. T., ALLET, B., STAHL, S., GILBERT, W., SCHALLER, H., BRUCE, S. A. and MURRAY, K. (1981) Production of immunologically active surface antigens of hepatitis B virus by *Escherichia coli. Proc. Natl. Acad. Sci. (Washington)* **78**: 4510–4514.

MCLEAN, D. M. (1977) Methisazone therapy in pediatric vaccinia complications. *Ann. N.Y. Acad. Sci.* **284**: 118–121.

The Medical Letter on Drugs and Therapeutics, Unsigned, 1978, **20**: 25–26.

MEYERS, J. D. and WITTE, J. J. (1974) Zoster immune globulin in high risk children. *J. Infec. Dis.* **129**: 616–618.

MILLER, G., SHOPE, T., COOPE, D., WATERS, L., PAGANO, J., BORNKAMM, G. W. and HENLE, W. (1977) Lymphoma in cotton top marmosets after inoculation with Epstein–Barr virus: tumor incidence, histologic spectrum, antibody responses, demonstration of viral DNA and characterization of viruses. *J. Exper. Med.* **145**: 948–967.

MIMS, C. A. (1966) Pathogenesis of rashes in virus diseases. *Bact. Rev.* **30**: 739–760.

MINOR, T. E., DICK, E. C., DICK, C. R. and INHORN, S. L. (1975) Attenuated influenza A vaccine (Alice) in an adult population: Vaccine-related illness, serum and nasal antibody production and intrafamilial transmission. *J. Clin. Microbiol.* **2**: 403–409.

MONATH, T. P., MAHER, M., CASALS, J., KISSLING, R. E. and CACIAPUOTI, A. (1974) Lassa fever in the eastern province of Sierra Leone 1970–72. II. Clinical observations and virological studies on selected hospital cases. *Am. J. Trop. Med. Hyg.* **23**: 1140–1149.

MOSTOW, S. R. and TYRRELL, D. A. J. (1973) The behavior *in vitro* of attenuated recombinant influenza virus. *Arch. gesamte Virusforsch* **43**: 385–392.

NATHANSON, N., MONJAN, A. A., PANITCH, H. S., JOHNSON, E. D., PETURSSON, G. and COLE, G. A. (1975) Virus-induced cell-mediated immunopathological disease. In: *Viral Immunity and Immunopathology*, pp. 357–391. NOTKINS, A. L. (ed.). Academic, New York.

National Committee for the Evaluation of GammaGlobulin in the Prophylaxis of Poliomyelitis (1954) An evaluation on the efficacy of gammaglobulin the prophylaxis of paralytic poliomyelitis as used in the United States. *Publ. Hlth. Monogrs.* 20.

National Influenza Immunization Program 1977. Follow-up on Guillaum-Barre' Syndrome – United States. *Morbidity and Mortality Weekly Report* **26**: 7.

NKRUMAH, F. K., and PERKINS, I. V. (1976) Burkitt's lymphoma. A clinical study of 110 patients. *Cancer* **37**: 671–676.

ORENSTEIN, W. A., HEYMANN, D. L., ELLIS, R. J., ROSENBERG, R. L., NAKANO, J., HALSEY, N. A., OVERTURF, G. D., HAYDEN, G. F. and WITTE, J. J. (1981) Prophylaxis of varicella in high risk children. Dose-response effect of zoster immune globulin. *J. Pediat.* **98**: 368–373.

OSBORN, J. (1977) Epilogue – The costs and benefits of the National Immunization Program of 1976. In: *Influenza in America 1918–1976*. OSBORN, J. (ed.). Prodist, New York.

OVERBY, L. R., DUFF, R. G. and MAO, J. C-H. (1977) Antiviral potential of phosphonoacetic acid. *Ann. N.Y. Acad. Sci.* **284**: 310–320.

OXFORD, J. S. and GALBRAITH, H. (1980) Antiviral activity of amantadine: A review of laboratory and clinical data. *Pharmacol. Ther.* **11**: 181–262.

PASEK, M., GOTO, T., GILBERT, W., ZINK, B., SCHALLER, H., MACKAY, P., LEADBETTER, G. and MURRAY, K. (1979) Hepatitis B virus genes and their expression in *E. coli. Nature* **282**: 575–579.

PASTEUR, L. (1885) Methode pour prevenir la rage après morsure. *C. R. Acad. Sci.* **101**: 765–772.

PAULING, L. (1971) The significance of the evidence about ascorbic acid and the common cold. *Proc. natn. Acad. Sci. USA* **63**: 2678–2681.

PIERCE, W. E., ROSENBAUM, M. J., EDWARDS, E. A., PECKINPAUGH, R. O. and JACKSON, G. G. (1968) Live and inactivated adenovirus vaccines for the prevention of acute respiratory illness in naval recruits. *Am. J. Epidemiol.* **87**: 237–246.

PINHEIRO, F. P. and OLIVA, O. (1981) Antibody to yellow fever forty years after vaccination with the 17D strain of attenuated virus (unpublished).

PRINCE, A. M., SZMUNESS, W., MANN, M. K., VYAS, G. N., GRADY, G. F., SHAPIRO, F. L., SUKI, W. N., FRIEDMAN, E. A. and STENZEL, K. H. (1975) Hepatitis B 'immune' globulin: effectiveness in prevention of dialysis associated hepatitis. *N. Engl. J. Med.* **293**: 1063–1067.

PRUSSOF, W. H., CHEN, M. S., FISHER, P. H., LIN, T. S., SHIAU, G. T., SCHINAZI, R. F. and WALKER, T. (1979) Antiviral iodinated deoxyribonucleosides: 5-iodo-2′ deoxyuridine; 5-iodo-2′-deoxycytidine; 5-iodo-5-amino-2′5′dideoxyuridine. *Phamocol. Ther.* **7**: 1–34.

RADA, B. and DOSKOCIL, J. (1980) Azapyrimidine nucleosides. *Phamocol. Ther.* **10**: 171–218.

RAPP, F. and DUFF, R. (1973) Transformation of hamster embryo fibroblasts by herpes simplex viruses 1 and 2. *Cancer Res.* **33**: 1527–1534.

REBEL, A., MALKANI, K., BASLE, M. and BERGEON, C. (1976) Osteoclast ultrastructure in Paget's disease. *Calc. Tiss. Res.* **20**: 187–199.

REMY, W., ANTONIADIS, G., BOCKENDAHL, H. and REMY, B. (1976) Antikorpertiter -Verlaufe bei Patienten mit recidivierenden Herpes simplex Virus -Infectionen unter Vakzination mit hitzeinaktivierten Herpes-viren. *Z. Hautkrankh* **51**: 103–107.

RICHMAN, D. D., MURPHY, B. R., BELSHE, R. B., RUSTEN, H. M., CHANNOCK, R. M., BLACKLOW, N. R., PARRINO, T. A., ROSE, F. B., LEVINE, M. M. and CAPLAN, E. (1977) Temperature sensitive mutants of Influenza A Virus. XIV. Production and evaluation of Influenza A/Ga/74-ts-1E. Recombinant viruses in human adults. *J. Infec. Dis.* **136**: 256–262.

ROSENSTOCK, I. M. (1961) Public acceptance of influenza vaccination programs. Int. Conf. on Asian Influenza. *Am. Rev. Resp. Dis.* **83** (pt. 2): 171–174.

SALIDO-RENGELL, F., NASSER-QUINONES, H. and BRISENO-GARCIA, B. (1977) Clinical evaluation of 1-β-D-ribofuranosyl-1,2,4-triazole-3-carboximide (Ribavirin) in a double-blind study during an outbreak of influenza. *Ann. N.Y. Acad. Sci.* **284**: 272–277.

SALK, J. and SALK, D. (1977) Control of influenza and poliomyelitis with killed virus vaccines. *Science* **195**: 834–847.

SANO, M., TAKEUCHI, T., ADACHI, M., TAMI, Y. and ITO, K. (1977) Transfer factor in treating hepatitis B (cont.). *N. Engl. Med.* **296**: 53–54.

SARAL, R., BURNS, W. H., LASKIN, O. L., SANTOS, G. W. and LERTMAN, P. S. (1981) Acyclovir prophylaxis of herpes-simplex virus infection. A randomized double blind, controlled trial – bone-marrow-transplant recipients. *New Engl. J. Med.* **305**: 63–67.

SERGIESCU, D., HORODNICEANU, F. and AUBERT-COMBIESCU, A. (1972) The use of inhibitors in the study of picornavirus genetics. *Prog. Med. Virol.* **14**: 123–199.

SHAH, K. V., ANIKER, S. P., NARASIMHA MURTHY, D. P., RODRIGUES, F. M., JAYADEVIAH, M. S. and PRASANNA, H. A. (1962) Evaluation of the field experience with formalin-inactivated mouse brain vaccine of Russian Spring–Summer encephalitis virus against Kyasanur Forest disease. *Ind. J. Med. Res.* **50**: 163–174.

SHANNON, W. M. and SCHABEL, F. M., Jr. (1980) Antiviral agents as adjuncts in cancer chemotherapy. *Phamocol. Ther.* **11**: 263–390.

SHAYWITZ, B. A., LEVENTHAL, J. M., KRAMER, M. S. and VENES, J. L. (1977) Prolonged continuous monitoring of intracranial pressure Reye's syndrome. *Pediatrics* **59**: 595–605.

SIDWELL, R. W., ROBINS, R. K. and HILLYARD, I. W. (1979) Ribavirin: an antiviral agent. *Phamacol. Ther.* **6**: 123–146.

SKINNER, G. R. B., BUCHAN, A., HARTLEY, C. E., TURNER, S. P. and WILLIAMS, D. R. (1980) The preparation, efficacy and safety of 'Antigenoid' vaccine NFU (5L) MRC toward prevention of *herpes simplex* virus infections in human subjects. *Med. Microb. Immunol.* **169**: 39–51.

SMORODINTSEV, A. A., ALEXANDROVA, G. A., CHALKINA, O. M. and SELIVANOV, A. A. (1965) Experiences in the development of live vaccines against influenza and influenza-like respiratory infections. In: *1st Annual Symposium on Applied Virology*, pp. 166–181. SANDERS, M. and LENNETTE, E. H. (eds.). Olympic, Sheboygan.

STAGNO, S., REYNOLDS, D. W., HUANG, E-S., THAMES, S. D., SMITH, R. J. and ALFORD, C. A. (1977) Congenital cytomegalovirus infection. Occurrence in an immune population. *New Engl. J. Med.* **296**: 1254–1258.

SUTCLIFFE, J. G., SHINNICK, T. M., GREEN, N., LIU, F.-T., NIMAN, H. L. and LERNER, R. A. (1980) Chemical synthesis of a polypeptide predicted from nucleotide sequence allows detection of a new retroviral gene product. *Nature* **287**: 801–805.

SWALLOW, D. L., BUCKNALL, R. A., STANIER, W. E., HUTCHINSON, A. and GASKIN, H. (1977) A new antivirus compound ICI73602: Structure, properties and spectrum of activity. *Ann. N.Y. Acad. Sci.* **284**: 305–309.

SZMUNESS, W., STEVENS, C. E., HARLEY, E. J., ZANG, E. A., OLESZKO, W. R., WILLIAM, D. C., SADOVSKY, R., MORRISON, J. M. and KELLNER, A. (1980) Hepatitis B vaccine. Demonstration of efficacy in a controlled clinical test in a high-risk population in the United States. *New Engl. J. Med.* **303**: 833–841.

TAKAHASHI, M., OTSUKA, Y., ASANO, Y., YAZAKI, T. and ISOMURA, S. (1974) Live vaccine used to prevent the spread of varicella in children in hospital. *Lancet* **2**: 1288–1290.

TAMM, I. and EGGERS, H. J. (1963) Specific inhibition of replication of aminal viruses. *Science* **142**: 24–33.

TERRY, L. L. (Sept. 20, 1962) Association of cases of poliomyelitis with the use of Type III vaccines: With the use of Type III oral poliomyelitis vaccine. A technical report. U.S. Dept. of Health, Education and Welfare.

TIGNOR, G. H., SHOPE, R. E., GERSHON, R. K. and WAKSMAN, B. H. (1974) Immunopathological aspects of infection with Lagos Bat virus of the rabies group. *J. Immunol.* **112**: 260–265.

WEIBEL, R. E., BUYNAK, E. B., McLEAN, A. A., ROEHM, R. R. and HILLEMAN, M. R. (1980) Persistence of antibody in human subjects for 7 to 10 years following administration of combined attenuated measles, mumps and rubella virus vaccines. *Proc. Soc. Exptl Biol. Med.* **165**: 260–263.

WHITLEY, R. J., SOONG, S.-J., DOLIN, R., GALASSO, G. J., CH'IEN, L. T., ALFORD, C. A. and Collaborative Study Group (1977) Adenine arabinoside therapy of biopsy-proved herpes simplex encephalitis. *New Engl. J. Med.* **297**: 289–294.

WHITLEY, R. J., SOONG, S.-J., HIRSCH, M. S., KARCHINER, A. W., DOLAN, R. D., GALASSO, G., DUNNICK, J. K., ALFORD, C. A. and the NIAID Collaborative Antiviral Study Group (1981) Herpes simplex encephalitis. Vidarabine therapy and diagnostic problems. *New Engl. J. Med.* **304**: 313–318.

WINKLER, W. G., SCHMIDT, R. G. and SIKES, R. K. (1969) Evaluation of human rabies immune globulin and homologous and heterologous antibody. *J. Immunol.* **102**: 1314–1320.

WISE, T. G., PAVAN, P. R. and ENNIS, F. A. (1977) Herpes simplex virus vaccines. *J. Infec. Dis.* **136**: 706–711.

World Health Organization (1973) *Technical Report series* No. 523. WHO Expert Committee on Rabies. 6th Report, Geneva.

World Health Organization (1977) Vaccination certificate requirements for international travel situation as on 1 January 1977. WHO, Geneva.

WRIGHT, P. F., DOLIN, R. and LAMONTAGNE, J. R. (1976) Summary of clinical trials of influenza vaccine. II. *J. Infec. Dis.* **134**: 633–638.

ZHDANOV, V. M. (1967) Present status of live influenza virus vaccines. *Proc. 1st Conf. on Vaccines against Viral and Rickettsial Diseases of Man.* PAHO, Washington.

ZUR HAUSEN, H. (1979) Herpes simplex virus: benefit versus risk factors in immunization. *Dev. Biol. Stand.* **43**: 373–379.

CHAPTER 5

THE REPLICATION OF ANIMAL VIRUSES

Luis Carrasco

*Departamento de Microbiología de la U.A.M. Centro de Biología Molecular
Canto Blanco, Madrid-34, Spain*

and

Alan E. Smith

*National Institute for Medical Research, Medical Research Council,
The Ridgeway Mill Hill, London NW7 1AA*

SUMMARY

The knowledge of viral replication for simple viruses is very complete and the main features of more complex animal viruses are also relatively well understood. The different steps in the viral replicative cycle are discussed as potential targets for antiviral chemotherapy. In particular the modification of membrane permeability by viral infection and its exploitment to design more selective antiviral agents is presented. Finally, we review the different theories that try to explain the shut-off of several cellular functions after viral infection.

CONTENTS

5.1. INTRODUCTION

The understanding of animal virus molecular biology has greatly increased during the last few years. The actual knowledge of viral development for small, simple viruses is very complete and the main features in molecular terms of larger, more complex animal virus biology are also relatively well understood. Animal viruses have been and still are largely studied, for two principal reasons. First, they are etiological agents in several human and domestic animal diseases, probably including cancer. Second, they serve as model systems for the study of gene expression in eukaryotes. It is obvious that a deeper knowledge of all aspects of viral development in molecular terms will provide us, in many instances, with a rationale for the design of specific antiviral agents.

The aim of the present review is to give a general picture of the biology of the different groups of animal viruses. This chapter begins by analyzing the steps in viral development and discussing in each step examples of antiviral agents. The bulk of the review is devoted to an analysis of gene expression in some of the more representative and better known members of animal viruses. We then concentrate on the modifications that viral infection produces on host cell metabolism and try to correlate these modifications with the changes that occur in the plasma membrane after infection. We finish by discussing a new rationale for the design of antiviral agents based on the permeability changes induced by viral development.

5.2. STEPS IN THE VIRAL LIFE-CYCLE, POTENTIAL TARGETS FOR ANTIVIRAL CHEMOTHERAPY

The viral life-cycle can be divided into several steps, any one of which could be a potential target for an antiviral agent (for reviews see Osdene, 1970; Bauer, 1972a; Prusoff and Goz, 1973; Shugar, 1974; Hoffmann, 1976; Diana and Pancic, 1976).

5.2.1. EXTRACELLULAR PHASE

When a virus first enters an animal, or when it is transmitted from one cell to another, it can be inactivated by specific antibody molecules. The immune response to viral infection constitutes the basis for vaccination and has been considered in detail in many recent reviews. To date this is the phase in which a virus is most susceptible to medical treatment.

A different mechanism of antiviral chemotherapy is the direct inactivation of the virus particles by some compounds. Glycyrrhicic acid seems to exert its antiviral properties by the direct inactivation of lipid-enveloped virus particles (Pompei et al., 1979). The reported antiherpes properties of some fatty acids is based in part on a similar direct inactivation of the herpesvirus particles (Kohn et al., 1980).

5.2.2. ATTACHMENT AND PENETRATION

The recognition by a virus of its host cell involves membrane receptors (Dales, 1973). There are regions of the cell surface that serve as virus attachment sites, located on rigid and very differentiated regions of the membrane as well as on flexible portions (Dales, 1973). The recognition step also involves some viral protein components. Generally, in enveloped viruses, the lipidic bilayer is necessary for attachment (Bose and Sagik, 1970) although in some instances, such as herpesviruses (Dales and Silverberg, 1969) and rhabdoviruses (Cartwright et al., 1970) treatment with detergents does not totally inhibit attachment and infection. Some capsid proteins of the non-enveloped viruses are directly involved in attachment, for example protein VP4 of picornaviruses (Crowell and Philipson, 1971) and the penton capsomer of adenoviruses (Sussenbach, 1967).

Attachment often involves two steps. One is temperature independent and can occur at 4°C; this is normally reversible and is followed by an irreversible step for which a raised temperature is necessary (Dales, 1973). Although it has been shown that in some instances viruses can enter the cell by phagocitosis, this may only be the case when a large inoculum of virus is used.

It still remains unclear how viruses actively penetrate into cells. One interesting theory is that some viral proteins, or the virion itself, complex relatively large quantities of calcium ions. These are passed into the infected cell and as there is a very low concentration of calcium ions in the cytoplasm, this process releases energy. This energy, at least in part, could account for the driving force that pushes the virus into the cell (Durham, 1978).

Alternatively, some animal viruses could use the membrane potential and enter the cell by a mechanism similar to that proposed for some bacteriophages (Labedan and Golberg, 1979; Kalasavskaite *et al.*, 1980). Another mechanism suggested for the entry of Semliki Forest virus involves the formation of coated pits and their fusion with lysosomes (Helenius *et al.*, 1980). This mechanism has recently been questioned (Coombs *et al.*, 1981). Adamantadine is an example of an antiviral compound that blocks viral development by inhibiting attachment and penetration and is effective against influenza A-2 virus. However, this compound may affect other later stages in the infectious cycle of other viruses such as lymphocytic choromeningitis virus (Welsh *et al.*, 1971).

On theoretical grounds antiviral therapy directed against virus adsorption does not seem very appropriate. If, as is likely, the virus is able to survive in the body longer than the antiviral agent, viral infection would only be delayed, but not prevented. Thus, therapy based on inhibition of attachment would be mainly prophylactic rather than curative.

A drastic modification in membrane permeability is observed during virus entry. Such modification allows the entry into the infected cell of several antibiotics and protein toxins (Fernandez-Puentes and Carrasco, 1980. These compounds are transported into the cell along with the infecting virus particle. These substances are pernicious to viral development since they act at a key point in cellular metabolism that is essential for the viral infection cycle. This mechanism is the basis of the antiviral action of the plant lectin extracted from *Phytolacca americana* known as PAP (Wyatt and Shepherd, 1969; Irvin, 1975). It was first suggested that this protein binds to viral particles and is transported to the cytoplasm of the infected cell (Ussery *et al.*, 1977). However, our results suggest that viral entry induces an unspecific increase in permeability to a number of protein toxins and low molecular weight antibiotics (Fernandez-Puentes and Carrasco, 1980). The molecular target of PAP is the ribosomal GTPase center, causing inhibition of protein synthesis (Fernández-Puentes and Vázquez, 1977; Fernández-Puentes and Carrasco, 1980) and therefore also virus production. Similarly, the abrin or ricin A chains, alpha-sarcin, mitogillin and restrictocin (Olsnes and Pihl, 1976; Vázquez, 1979) are inhibitors of virus production. In addition to their specificity in killing only infected cells, they are very potent since it has been shown that a single molecule of ricin or abrin A chain is enough to kill a cell (Olsnes and Pihl, 1976).

5.2.3. Uncoating

In many cases the whole virion particle does not penetrate into the cell, instead only the nucleocapsid enters the cytoplasm. In other instances, an almost complete virion enters and then loses its protein shell before the synthesis of viral macromolecules begins. As mentioned above many virions bind considerable amounts of calcium ions that upon entry into the cytoplasm becomes dissolved. This process, in addition to providing energy for penetration, also favors uncoating, since the loss of the calcium ions tends to destabilize the virion structure (Durham, 1978). Rhodamine has been shown to interfere with the process of uncoating (Eggers *et al.*, 1970). Unfortunately, this compound seems to be highly specific in its action and is only active against echovirus type 12.

5.2.4. Viral Macromolecular Synthesis

We can broadly consider three different kinds of viral macromolecular synthesis: (a) genome replication, (b) transcription and (c) translation. These three aspects of viral molecular biology will be considered in detail in Sections 5.3 and 5.4 of this article.

Many nucleoside and nucleotide analogs that block nucleic acid metabolism have been developed as antiviral agents (Prusoff and Goz, 1973; Shugar, 1974; Hoffmann, 1976; Diana and Pancic, 1976; Kusmierek and Shugar, 1979). In the case of herpesviruses several compounds such as 5-iodo-5'-amino-2',5'-dideoxyuridine (Chen, *et al.*, 1976), acyclo-guanosine (Schaeffer *et al.*, 1978), (E)-5-(2-bromovinyl)-2'-deoxyuridine (BVdUrd) (De

Clercq *et al.*, 1979) and phosphonoacetic acid (Gerstein *et al.*, 1975) have proved to be potent antiviral agents. Some of those compounds possess a low toxicity, although their antiviral spectrum is narrow.

Much less is known about antiviral agents that primarily block translation. Although some translation inhibitors such as cycloheximide or puromycin have been recorded as antiviral agents (Prusoff and Goz, 1973), they are very toxic and show no specificity against normal or virus-infected cells (Contreras and Carrasco, 1979). We have suggested an approach to the design of antiviral agents that interferes with the translation machinery of the cell, but this is selective in that it depends on agents that are not permeable for normal cells (Carrasco, 1978) (see Section 5.6.1).

5.2.5. SPECIFIC VIRAL ENZYMES

As viruses have specific, unique requirements in order to express their genome, they often contain in their virion or code for specific enzymes that are essential for the viral life-cycle, but are not normally found in uninfected cells. Retroviruses, for instance, have in their virion an enzyme known as reverse transcriptase that synthesizes DNA by copying the virion RNA template (Tooze, 1973; Aaronson and Stephenson, 1976). In other instances, such as with RNA viruses, specific replicases and polymerases are required to synthesize RNA using as template a ssRNA or dsRNA molecule. Poxviruses are dsDNA viruses that develop in the cytoplasm of the infected cells and they contain a specific RNA polymerase which transcribes the viral genome in the cellular cytoplasm. Generally complex viruses such as herpesviruses, poxviruses and iridoviruses code for a great many other specific viral enzymes. Acycloguanosine (Schaeffer *et al.*, 1978; Datta *et al.*, 1980) and BVdUrd (Allaudeen *et al.*, 1981) are antiherpes agents that show a selective inhibition of viral enzymes as compared to the cellular counterparts. Based on these considerations it should be possible to search for agents that could specifically inhibit such viral enzymes or even cellular enzymes induced during viral development, which are necessary for virus replication but dispensable for the cell. It has been suggested (Cohen, 1977) that chemotherapy and in particular antiviral chemotherapy, could be based on an understanding of the specific enzymic activities of viruses and parasites in general. Such a hypothesis is based on the idea that if we knew the primary structure of the enzymes in question and more precisely the conformation of the active site, specific inhibitors of such enzymes could be designed. However, this approach is unlikely to produce broad spectrum antiviral agents. Furthermore, it should be emphasized that the most powerful and useful chemotherapeutic agents in use today are based on naturally occurring compounds, which have a high affinity for their specific targets. Often there are few clues in the structure of an inhibitor that tell us *a priori* what its target is, unless of course it is an obvious substrate analog. Conversely, knowing the active site of an enzyme, it may still not be obvious what a suitable inhibitor might be. We must also bear in mind that in many instances inhibitors do not bind to the active site of a molecule, but act at a distant region via an allosteric effect.

5.2.6. ASSEMBLY AND RELEASE

Once the viral genome and sufficient coat proteins have been synthesized in the infected cell, the assembly process takes place. Assembly of new virion particles occurs by discrete additions of the viral components in a defined series of steps (Eiserling and Dickson, 1972; Casjens and King, 1975). Although early experiments on *in vitro* assembly led to the idea that assembly was a spontaneous and straightforward process, it seems now that the formation of new virions is a rather complicated phenomenon. In some instances several proteins, that are not present in the mature virion, participate in the formation of new viral particles (Persson *et al.*, 1979). Assembly is also frequently accompanied by proteolytic cleavages of some precursors to produce the mature virion proteins; these cleavages probably induce conformational changes that facilitate the entrance of the genome into the subviral particle.

In addition, modifications in the genome such as cleavage might also happen at the moment of entry of the genome into the empty capsids. The last step in the assembly of enveloped animal viruses occurs by the interaction of the nucleocapsid with portions of the plasma membrane containing clusters of some viral proteins, and results in the occlusion of the lipid bilayer of their envelope from the host membrane (Kääriäinen and Renkonen, 1977; Morrison and McQuain, 1978). The release of these enveloped viruses occurs by budding off from the cell.

Very little is known about specific inhibitors of the assembly process. Interferon primarily blocks translation and transcription in a number of virus-cell systems (Friedman, 1977): however, it is now established that inhibition by interferon in the development of RNA tumor viruses is precisely located in the assembly process, during the budding off of new viral particles (Friedman, 1977; Dolei et al., 1979). The exact mechanism by which interferon blocks the release of new RNA tumor viruses is still very poorly understood.

5.3. DNA CONTAINING VIRUSES

5.3.1. PAPOVAVIRUSES

Polyoma and SV40 are included in the papovaviruses group; they are amongst the most intensively studied and best understood animal viruses in molecular terms. They have also been used as models of eukaryotic gene expression and have attracted the attention of many laboratories, because of their oncogenic potential (Tooze, 1973; Salzman and Khoury, 1974). The 50 nm icosahedral SV40 virion (Fig. 1) (Finch and Crawford, 1975) contains

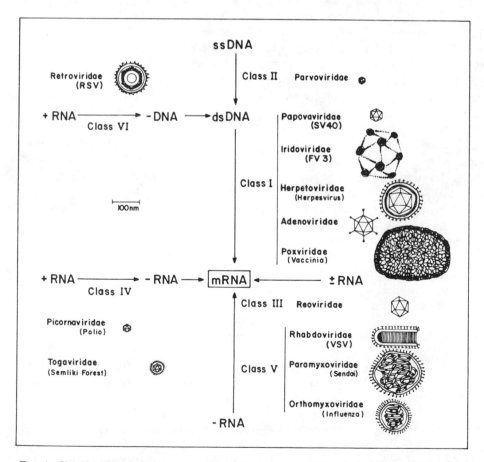

FIG. 1. Classification of animal viruses according to the expression of their genome (Baltimore, 1971). In each family the names of the most representative members are given. The relative sizes and shapes of the different virions are also represented.

dsDNA of 5224 base pairs as genome (Fiers *et al.*, 1978; Reddy *et al.*, 1978), associated with host histones H2A, H2B, H3 and H4. It is surrounded by the capsid, composed of a major protein VP1 (mol. wt. 39,000) and two minor components, VP2 (mol. wt. 38,000) and VP3 (mol. wt. 27,000) (Fiers *et al.*, 1978; Reddy *et al.*, 1978). VP3 contains sequences in common with VP2, whereas VP1 is structurally unrelated to the other two capsid proteins. Papovaviruses are capable of a lytic cycle of replication or a latent infection that leads to transformation of the infected cell. SV 40 infection of monkey cells results in a lytic cycle, but infection of mouse or human cells, for instance, leads, in a small percentage of cells, to the stable integration of the viral DNA into the host genome, resulting in cellular transformation (Salzman and Khoury, 1974; Levine, 1976; Tooze, 1980).

The supercoiled, circular duplex SV40 DNA is replicated bidirectionally. The initiation point is located in the position 0.67 of the SV40 map (Fig. 2) and termination occurs on the opposite side of the genome, where the two replication forks meet. Half of the genome, from positions around 0.67–0.17, are expressed early during the infectious cycle and are transcribed from the E strand of viral DNA. An integral TATA box in the early promotor region functions to fix the initiation of transcription (Mathis and Chambon, 1981).

The other half of the genome is transcribed from the L strand DNA and is expressed in the late phase of the lytic cycle (Acheson, 1976; Kelly and Nathans, 1977). At least two different mRNAs that code for two different proteins known as large T (mol. wt. 90,000) and small t antigen (mol. wt. 20,000) (Prives and Beck, 1977; Prives *et al.*, 1978; Crawford *et al.*, 1978; Paucha *et al.*, 1978) are present in the cytoplasm of transformed or lytic infected cells during the early phase of infection. In addition, a third middle T antigen (mol. wt. 55,000) is present in polyoma infected cells (Hutchinson *et al.*, 1978; Hunter *et al.*, 1978; Smart and Ito, 1978). The existence of an analogous middle T antigen in SV 40 infected cells seems unlikely (Carroll *et al.*, 1978; Lane and Crawford, 1979; Renart *et al.*, 1979).

Gene expression in the early region of SV40 genome is schematically represented in Fig. 2. Large T antigen mRNA is encoded by the region between 0.65–0.59 and 0.54–0.17 map units. Both small t and large T antigen contain identical amino termini, and share a segment of 82 amino acids whereas the sequences between 0.59–0.54 map units on SV40 DNA contain a unique coding region for small t antigen (Fiers *et al.*, 1978; Paucha and Smith, 1978). These two proteins are responsible for full transformation, although the exact mechanisms, in molecular terms, by which they transform is unknown (Martin and Chou, 1975; Weinberg, 1977; Bouck *et al.*, 1978; Sleigh *et al.*, 1978). The expression of small t in productive infection is dispensable (Cole *et al.*, 1977; Sleigh *et al.*, 1978), but large T is essential. Its function is related to the initiation of replication of viral and cellular DNA (Chou *et al.*, 1974; Tjian *et al.*, 1978; Mueller *et al.*, 1978).

In polyoma virus there are viable deletion mutants that synthesize normal large T but not middle T antigen. Such mutants are unable to transform cells (Lania *et al.*, 1979). Mutants that synthesize normal small t, but a deficient middle t antigen are also impaired in transformation (Novak and Griffin, 1981). Several polyoma virus-transformed cell lines analyzed indicated that all contained middle and small t antigens, but not all of them possessed a full-sized large T antigen (Ito *et al.*, 1980). More recently a polyoma virus genome that encodes the middle T antigen, but not the large T or small t antigen has been constructed (Treisman *et al.*, 1981). Transfection of this viral DNA efficiently induced the formation of transformed cells that grew as tumors after injection into rats (Treisman *et al.*, 1981). These data indicate that the middle t antigen plays an essential role in transformation. This protein has been found in association with the plasma membrane (Ito *et al.*, 1977) and a protein kinase activity that phosphorilates tyrosine residues has been reported associated with this protein (Smith *et al.*, 1979; Eckhart *et al.*, 1979). However, the exact molecular mechanism by which the middle t antigen transform cells is still unknown. A protein kinase activity associated with SV40 large T antigen was also reported (Griffin *et al.*, 1979).

Large T antigen is also involved in the regulation of viral DNA transcription and the switch from early to late (Alwine *et al.*, 1977; Mueller *et al.*, 1978). The binding of large T to the origin of viral DNA replication could serve to explain its function at the molecular level (Tjian, 1978; J. Renart; personal communication).

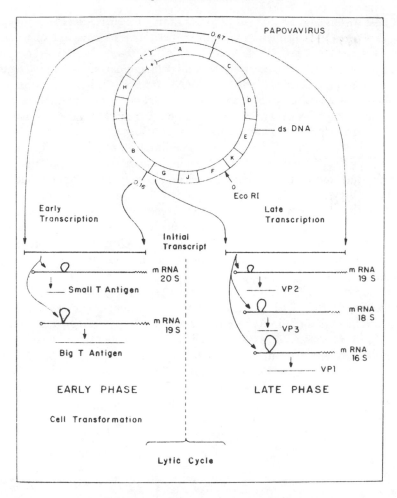

F𝖨𝖦. 2. Schematic representation of SV40 gene expression. During the early phase the E strand on the circular SV40 dsDNA is transcribed, giving rise to two early mRNAs that are processed by splicing of some internal sequences. These early mRNAs code for large and small T antigens, involved in the establishment and maintenance of the transformed state. After DNA synthesis, the late phase begins and the L strand of the dsDNA is transcribed. The splicing of the transcripts produces three mRNAs, each of which directs the synthesis of a different virion protein: VP1, VP2 and VP3.

During the lytic cycle, viral DNA replication is followed by transcription of the sequences that code for late proteins. The initiation of late transcription starts at coordinate 0.67 ± 0.02 on the conventional SV40 map (Laub *et al.*, 1979). The post-transcriptional modifications of SV40 mRNAs include 5′-end capping, polyadenylation at the 3′ end and splicing (Ziff, 1980). Unspliced late 19S RNAs are found in the nucleus whereas the spliced 19S SV 40 RNAs are mainly located in the cytoplasm (Villareal and Jovanovich, 1980). The cytoplasmic RNAs have lost a 32 nucleotide intervening sequence located between 0.760 and 0.765 map units.

Three different late mRNAs are found in lytically infected cells, each one directs the synthesis of a single coat protein. The 19 S mRNA codes for all three coat proteins VP 1, VP 2 and VP 3, but only directs the synthesis of VP 2, the other two internal initiation sites remain closed (Smith *et al.*, 1976). VP 3 is synthesized from a different 18 S mRNA (Siddell and Smith, 1978; Hunter and Gibson, 1978), whereas VP 1 is made from the most abundant mRNA species present in the cytoplasm of infected cells, with a sedimentation coefficient of 16 S (Prives *et al.*, 1974a, b; Wheeler *et al.*, 1977). This cytoplasmic 16 S mRNA contains a leader sequence of about 210 nucleotides, that map at positions 0.72–0.76 and they are spliced to the coding sequences (Lai *et al.*, 1978). The 3′ ends of all three late mRNA species hybridize to regions located around position 0.17 and they also have a common 5′ leader sequence. These results suggest that the synthesis of papovavirus mRNAs involves the direct transcription of the DNA sequences and the subsequent splicing out of the intervening segment of RNA (Aloni *et al.*, 1977; Lai *et al.*, 1978). Moreover, the long primary transcripts made in the nucleus hybridize to positions beyond 0.28, indicating that a long segment at the 3′ end of the transcript is deleted before poly (A) addition (Lai *et al.*, 1978).

As SV40 has been completely sequenced, the primary structures of all three coat proteins are known. The VP2 gene starts at nucleotide number 543 and the VP3 gene at 897; both end at nucleotide number 1599. VP3 contains 234 aminoacids, all of which are present in VP2, because both genes are translated in the same reading frame. The VP2/VP3 gene overlaps with the VP1 gene for 122 nucleotides, although in this case they are translated in a different reading frame. The amino terminal region of VP2 is very hydrophobic and it has been suggested that it may be involved in the interaction of this protein with membranes (Fiers *et al.*, 1978). Another interesting aspect of the SV40 genome is that only 15 per cent of it does not code for protein; this noncoding region is mainly located at the origin of replication and contains information for the initiation of DNA replication, the promoters for early and late transcription, the signals for mRNA processing and the ribosome binding-site (Jay *et al.*, 1976; Fiers *et al.*, 1978).

The late region of the SV40 genome contains between map positions 0.72–0.76 an open nucleotide reading frame of 62 codons that code for the agnogene so called because its product was not identified until very recently (Jay *et al.*, 1981; Jackson and Chalkley, 1981). In cells lytically infected by SV40 a basic protein Mr 7900 is identified late in infection. This protein is associated with viral nucleoprotein and might be involved with the assembly or maturation of the SV40 virion, although the protein itself is not present in the mature virion particle.

Even though many of the structural features of SV40 and polyoma virus are already known, there are still many puzzling aspects in their biology. Particularly intriguing is the mechanism by which the T antigens induce and maintain the transformation state.

5.3.2. ADENOVIRUSES

Adenoviruses are similar to papovaviruses in that they also have a dsDNA as genome and can also produce two types of response after infection: transformation or productive infection (Philipson and Lindberg, 1974). Since the discovery of adenoviruses as potential causative agents of tumors, they have attracted the attention of many workers. Adenoviruses have been divided in four serological subgroups: A, B, C and D. Subgroup A comprises highly oncogenic viruses.

Adenoviruses are much more complex than papovaviruses as they have a linear genome of $20–29 \times 10^6$ mol. wt. and a coding capacity for about 25 proteins (Philipson and Lindberg, 1974; Winnacker, 1978). The genome also contains a protein covalently attached to the 5′ ends (Robinson and Bellett, 1974; Rekosh *et al.*, 1977). The protein is linked to DNA via a phosphodiester bond joining a serine residue to the 5′-OH of the terminal deoxycytidine residue (Challberg *et al.*, 1980). This protein has a molecular weight of 55,000 and originates from an 80,000 precursor polypeptide (Challberg and Kelly, 1981; Stillman *et al.*, 1981). This protein is involved in the replication of viral DNA (Stillman and Bellett, 1979; Enomoto *et al.*, 1981).

The nonenveloped virion with a diameter of 65–80 nm is composed of the dsDNA genome surrounded by the icosahedral capsid, containing 252 capsomers. 240 are called hexons, whereas the other twelve capsomers located in the vertex are called pentons. Each penton is composed of a penton base and a projection called fiber. At least fifteen different polypeptides form the virion (Everitt *et al.*, 1973; Anderson *et al.*, 1973) and they have been localized in the different structural constituents of the particle. The hexon is the major capsid protein of the adenovirion and is composed of three identical large polypeptide chains, each containing approximately 1000 residues. The primary structure of the adenovirus hexon polypeptide has been determined by amino acid sequence studies of peptides from all regions of the molecule combined with sequence analysis of areas of its gene (Jornvall *et al.*, 1981). The penton base has been isolated and the amino acid composition determined. (Boudin *et al.*, 1979). The DNA-protein core consists of double-stranded viral DNA and at least four core proteins: Polypeptide V (45,000), polypeptide X (40,000), polypeptide VII (17,000) and the 55,000 protein covalently attached to the DNA. A chromatin-like organization has been proposed for the viral core (Corden *et al.*, 1976). After infection the virus is established in the nucleus of the cell, where the viral DNA is first transcribed and later replicated. Transcription of the viral DNA produces large RNA molecules that are later cleaved into the mature mRNA species (Bachenheimer and Darnell, 1975). The adenovirus RNA synthesis and processing has provided a suitable model system to study eukaryotic mRNA synthesis and biogenesis. Before the onset of viral DNA replication a limited portion of the viral genome, about 25 per cent, is transcribed into mRNA (Green *et al.*, 1970; Petterson *et al.*, 1976; Berk and Sharp, 1978). This RNA is complementary to four distinct regions of the genome, two from each DNA strand (Sharp *et al.*, 1974; Philipson *et al.*, 1974) and includes at least five mRNA species (Craig *et al.*, 1975; Buttner *et al.*, 1976) that have been separated by hybridization to specific restriction DNA fragments. The different viral mRNAs have thus been purified, separated from cellular mRNA and translated in a cell-free protein synthesizing system (Lewis *et al.*, 1976). Six early polypeptides of mol. wt. 72,000, 44,000, 19,000, 15,500, 15,000 and 11,000 were identified in this way. The largest polypeptide (of 72,000 daltons) was shown to be the DNA binding protein present in adenovirus infected cells (Van der Vliet and Levine, 1973). The mRNAs from adenovirus transformed cells have also been purified using this procedure and shown to synthesize polypeptides of 44,000 and 15,000 daltons. These two proteins could be of great interest as they are possibly involved in the initiation and maintenance of cell transformation. The two left-end transcription units E1A and E1B encode functions capable of cell transformation (Flint *et al.*, 1975; Esche *et al.*, 1980; Ross *et al.*, 1980). The products of region E1A are involved in the production of mRNA from other early regions (Ziff, 1980; Philipson and Petterson, 1980). Region E2 encodes the 72,000 molecular weight DNA binding protein. The E3 region encodes three proteins with molecular weights of 16,000, 14,500 and 14,000 (Persson *et al.*, 1980). The 16,000 protein is the precursor to a 19,000 glycoprotein which is associated with the cell membrane (Persson *et al.*, 1979). Region E1A constitutes a class of pre-early viral genes since its expression is required for the transcription of all other early viral mRNAs (Berk *et al.*, 1979). Recently some immediate early viral mRNAs independent for their expression of the pre-early mRNAs have been described (Lewis and Mathews, 1980) (Fig. 3).

The late phase starts 8–10 hr post-infection and is characterized by the synthesis of large amounts of viral DNA. At the same time transcription changes drastically, both quantitatively and qualitatively, giving rise to large amounts of viral RNA transcripts (Parsons *et al.*, 1971; Lindberg *et al.*, 1972; McGuire *et al.*, 1972). Approximately 10–20 per cent of the total nonribosomal RNA synthesized late in infection corresponds to viral RNA. However, there is a preferential exit of the viral mRNA to the cytoplasm and thus more than 90 per cent of the mRNA transported from the nucleus to the cytoplasm late in infection is

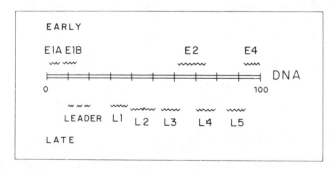

FIG. 3. Adenovirus genome map. The early transcripts are represented on top of the DNA. Late transcripts are represented below the viral DNA.

viral RNA (Lindberg *et al.*, 1972). The rate of synthesis of cellular mRNA sequences remains constant throughout the course of adenovirus type 2 infection. Poly (A) is also added normally to cellular mRNA and is metabolized with kinetics similar to those observed in uninfected cells. However, 16 hr after infection all the newly synthesized mRNA reaching the cytoplasm is virus-specific (Beltz and Flint, 1979). The mRNA present in the cytoplasm late in infection is able to hybridize to the whole adenovirus genome, indicating that all the early mRNAs are also present during the late phase (Sharp *et al.*, 1974; Tibbetts *et al.*, 1974). Analysis of the mRNA sequences present exclusively at late times indicates that it is derived from several locations, but that it mostly hybridizes with a major block in the 1 strand that corresponds to about 60 per cent of the total genome length (Petterson *et al.*, 1976; Flint and Sharp, 1976; Miller *et al.*, 1980).

Transcription from the adenovirus genome late in infection initiates predominantly at the promotor located at map position 16.3 and proceeds in a rightward direction for about 28,000 base pairs (Ziff, 1980). This long transcript is processed into five families of mRNAs, each family having co-terminal 3′ ends and each family containing a tripartite leader, encoded at coordinates 16.6, 19.6 and 26 (Nevins and Darnell, 1978; Chow *et al.*, 1977). These findings on adenovirus transcription have changed our ideas about the mechanism by which the mature mRNAs are generated. It was found by electron microscopy and biochemical studies that a leader sequence from the 5′ end of several adeno late mRNAs hybridizes with three different regions of the genome that map at positions 16.8, 19.8 and 26.9, whereas the coding portion of the mRNA maps at a distant region between positions 51.9 and 62.2 on the genome (Berget *et al.*, 1977; Chow *et al.*, 1977; Klessig, 1977). Of the several theoretical possibilities that could explain these results, it now seems most probable that these mRNAs originate from higher mol. wt. precursor RNA molecules. We can envisage the mechanism of mRNA synthesis in the following steps. (1) The RNA polymerase attaches to specific promotors on the genome and synthesizes a large RNA molecule. (2) This RNA molecule is processed or spliced to remove several internal sequences thereby creating an appropriate leader sequence attached to the mRNA sequences that code for the protein. (3) In addition this mRNA molecule is modified in the 5′ end to generate a cap structure (Wold *et al.*, 1976; McGuire *et al.*, 1976) and poly (A) is added to the 3′ end. The major late adenovirus is also active early in infection at a rate equal to that of the other early transcription units. However, these transcripts terminate early in infection near map position 60–70 in contrast to late in infection (Nevins and Wilson, 1981; Akusjarvi and Persson, 1981). Those events of transcriptional termination, poly (A) site selection and splicing can change depending on the conditions of the cell and therefore can participate in the regulation of gene expression.

Cellular protein synthesis drastically declines during the late phase of adenovirus infection (Ginsberg *et al.*, 1967; Russell and Skehel, 1972; Anderson *et al.*, 1973) and the mRNA found in polysomes is mostly of viral origin. This phenomenon cannot exclusively be explained by the reduced transport of cellular mRNAs to the cytoplasm, because there is a very slow turnover of cellular mRNAs and these still remain intact in the cytoplasm late in infection. Analysis of the proteins synthesized late in infected cells indicates a complicated pattern of polypeptides. In addition to the virion proteins, other polypeptides are present; some of these are precursors to the structural proteins (Russell and Skehel, 1972; Walter and Maizel, 1974; Westphal, 1976). At least 22 viral proteins could be detected late in infection, each of them is translated from a monocistronic mRNA molecule, although some limited proteolytic cleavage of the primary products occurs to render some of the mature virion components (Anderson *et al.*, 1973). The structural proteins are synthesized in large excess and only 5–10 per cent are incorporated into mature virions (Philipson and Lindberg, 1974). Once synthesized they are assembled and rapidly transported to the nucleus where the assembly process is completed. It is now established that mature virions are formed from empty capsids into which the viral DNA is packed (Sundquist *et al.*, 1973).

Other aspects of the molecular biology of adenovirus development, such as abortive infection in monkey cells and adeno-SV40 hybrids have been recently reviewed and will not be considered here (Smith and Carrasco, 1978).

5.3.3. Herpesviruses

Herpesviruses have a dsDNA as genome with a mol. wt. of 100×10^6 (Roizman and Furlong, 1974; Roizman *et al.*, 1977). The virion has a diameter of 100 nm and is composed of a core surrounded by the capsid, the tegument and the envelope. The genome is localized in the core, whereas the capsid and the tegument are built up by several species of viral proteins. The envelope of the virion is composed of cell-derived lipids and viral glycoproteins (Roizman and Furlong, 1974; Honess and Watson, 1977). Herpesviruses are able to transform cells in tissue culture and possess a clear oncogenic potential (Rapp and Duff, 1972).

The genome of herpes simplex virus 1 (HSV-1) is a linear double-stranded DNA molecule of 96×10^6 and consists of two covalently linked components, L and S. The orientation of L and S components relative to one another can vary, giving rise to four equimolar populations of molecules. This hetereogeneity is reflected in the restriction endonuclease maps (Hayward *et al.*, 1975). In addition, HSV DNA has terminal and internal redundancy (Sheldrick and Berthelot, 1975; Wadsworth *et al.*, 1975). Each L and S component consists predominantly of unique sequences, bracketed by large inverted repeats. The L component is bracketed by the sequence ab and its inversion b'a' and the S component is bracketed by the sequences a'c' and ca. The a sequence is in the same orientation at both ends of the genome (Roizman, 1979) (see Fig. 4). The single a sequence consists of two 20 base pairs direct repeats bracketing a region that contains 19 tandem direct repeats of a 12 base pairs sequence adjacent to three direct repeats of a 37 base pairs sequence, in addition to short stretches of unique sequences (Mocarski and Roizman, 1981).

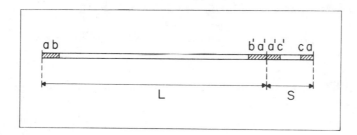

Fig. 4. Herpesvirus genome organization.

The virion contains at least 24 proteins (Spear and Roizman, 1972) widely differing in mol. wt. A large number of them are bigger than 100,000 dalton (Strnad and Aurelian, 1978) and several others are modified by glycosylation (Spear and Roizman, 1972) or are phosphorylated (Gibson and Roizman, 1974). Many of those polypeptides have now been localized in the different structural components of the virion (Gibson and Roizman, 1974). Associated with the capsid-tegument structures there is a virion protein kinase activity. This enzyme *in situ* phosphorilates a number of virion structural proteins (Lemaster and Roizman, 1980).

During infection, the envelope of herpesvirus fuses with the cellular plasma membrane allowing the release of the viral nucleocapsid into the cytoplasm (Morgan *et al.*, 1968; Iwasaki *et al.*, 1973). Immediately after entry, the nucleocapsid migrates to the nucleus, where the viral DNA is freed after uncoating. The transcription of this parental viral DNA produces the early mRNAs. The relative concentration of early mRNA and the portion with the genome to which it hybridizes has not yet been determined with precision. In the late phase there are sequences in the cellular cytoplasm that hybridize with 48–50 per cent of the viral genome (Frenkel *et al.*, 1973). It is likely that transcription of the viral DNA is carried out by host enzymes, although there is not yet overwhelming evidence for this conclusion. After synthesis the RNA transcripts are processed and transported to the cytoplasm. The processing includes polyadenylation (Rakusanova *et al.*, 1972; Bachenheimer and Roizman, 1972; Bartkoski and Roizman, 1978) and capping (Bartkoski and Roizman, 1978). The possibility that some internal regions of the transcripts are spliced out, as occurs with other viral mRNAs, has not yet been established.

The replication of viral DNA starts at about 3 hr after infection and continues until about 8–10 hr. Inhibition of protein synthesis blocks the initiation of viral DNA replication, but once the synthesis of DNA is initiated, protein synthesis is no longer required. Herpesvirus DNA synthesis occurs in a semiconservative fashion (Frenkel and Roizman, 1972), like cellular DNA synthesis. Once the viral DNA is synthesized, it is relatively quickly found in mature virions (Olshevsky *et al.*, 1967). Herpes simplex virus DNA is apparently replicated by a rolling circle mechanism that gives long concatemers; these are cleaved to generate unit-length DNA (Roizman, 1979). A model of HSV DNA replication was proposed to account for the mechanism of inversion of L and S components relative to each other (Roizman, 1979).

The analysis of herpesvirus proteins synthesized in infected cells has given a complicated picture of around 50 polypeptides (Powell and Courtney, 1975; Roizman *et al.*, 1974; Strnad and Aurelian, 1978) with mol. wt. ranging from 280,000 to 15,000. Evidence that these polypeptides are virus coded comes from analysis of viral proteins produced by mutant viruses, by different strains of herpes viruses (Schaffer *et al.*, 1973; Pereira *et al.*, 1976; Marsden *et al.*, 1976) and also from the immunological specificity of antisera raised against disrupted virus-infected cells (Watson and Wildy, 1969; Honess and Watson, 1974). About 23 of the polypeptides detected in this way are related to virion structural proteins, as judged by migration on polyacrylamide gels (Strnad and Aurelian, 1976). Approximately 30 polypeptides have been mapped from analyses of DNA sequences and polypeptides specified by HSV1 × HSV2 recombinants (Marsden *et al.*, 1978; Morse *et al.*, 1977; Ruyechan *et al.*, 1979).

The different viral proteins have been divided into four groups according to the time at which they are synthesized. They have also been divided into three groups on the basis of factors which regulate their synthesis, the three groups being designated α, β, and γ, (Honess and Roizman, 1974; Roizman *et al.*, 1974). Polypeptides of group α include predominantly nonstructural components. Once synthesized they migrate to the nucleus. Their synthesis is necessary for the appearance of the second group of proteins: the β polypeptides. These include some minor structural and nonstructural components. All the viral enzymes involved in viral DNA synthesis belong to the β group of proteins, their rate of synthesis is maximal between 5–7 hr post-infection. The β proteins are also responsible for killing the host cell and causing the shut-off of host macromolecular synthesis. They are also needed to stop the synthesis of the α polypeptides and trigger the synthesis of the γ polypeptides. The γ polypeptides are structural proteins of the virus which once they are synthesized, migrate to the nucleus for assembly. Clearly, during herpesvirus development there are complicated mechanisms that regulate the type and the amount of each protein synthesized. Some of those mechanisms operate at the translational level and are not yet well understood (Honess and Roizman, 1975a).

Many of the herpesvirus proteins undergo several post-translational modifications such as phosphorylation (Gibson and Roizman, 1974) and glycosylation (Honess and Roizman, 1975b; Spear, 1976) that normally modify their apparent molecular weight as analyzed by polyacrilamide gel electrophoresis. Several of the glycosylated proteins are localized in the nuclear and plasma membranes (Rodriguez and Dubois-Dalq, 1978).

During the assembly process of herpesvirus the core and the capsid are formed in the nucleus of the infected cell, the nucleocapsid buds through the nuclear membrane and moves to the plasma membrane in which several viral glycoproteins are already localized in clusters (Ben-Porat and Kaplan, 1972; Rodriguez and Dubois-Dalcq, 1978).

At present antiviral chemotherapy against herpesvirus development is mainly based on several nucleoside and nucleotide analogs (Shugar, 1974; Schaeffer *et al.*, 1978). In addition, phosphonoacetic acid has also proved to be effective against HSV growth in tissue culture and experimental animals.

5.3.4. POXVIRUSES

Poxviruses are still poorly understood in molecular terms because of their complexity. The genome is dsDNA with a molecular weight of $120–130 \times 10^6$ (Geshelin and Berns, 1974; Cabrera and Esteban, 1978) with crosslinked ends (Geshelin and Berns, 1974) and inverted terminal repeats (Garon et al., 1978; Schumperli et al., 1980) enough to code for about 200 proteins of a medium size. The 10 K base pairs inverted terminal repetition is divided into transcribed and nontranscribed regions (Wittek et al., 1980a).

A fragment of 6.3×10^6 of the long inverted terminal repeat has been cloned in phage λ and used to isolate RNAs from virus-infected cells. There is now evidence that some early RNAs are transcribed from the repeated sequence (Wittek et al., 1980b). The terminal 3 Kbp nontranscribed region is of special interest because it contains a set of 13–17 direct tandem repeats of a 70 base pair sequence on each side of a 435 base pair intervening region (Wittek and Moss, 1980). The virion has a complex structure and measures approximately 250 nm in diameter (Fig. 1). It contains a core in which the genome is located, two lateral bodies and an envelope (Moss, 1974). Analysis of the virion proteins by polyacrilamide gel electrophoresis in one dimension yields around 30 polypeptide bands (Sarov and Joklik, 1972). Analysis of the virion proteins by two-dimensional gel electrophoresis renders at least 111 spots, of which seven or more were basic proteins (Essani and Dales, 1979). A glycoprotein of molecular weight 34,000 and a phosphorylated basic protein of 11,000 were identified in this way (Essani and Dales, 1979).

The development of vaccinia virus in cultured cells takes place in about 12 hr, producing a clear cytopathic effect and inhibition of host macromolecular synthesis within 2–4 hr after infection (Bablanian, 1972a, 1975; Bablanian et al., 1978). Poxvirus development occurs in the cytoplasm of the infected cell and can even take place in enucleated cells, indicating that replication and transcription of the viral DNA is carried out by virus coded enzymes.

The first step in infection is the attachment of the virus to the cellular membrane, the virion then enters into the cell by phagocytic vacuoles or by fusion (Granados, 1973). A partial uncoating leaves the virion core, containing the DNA in a DNAase resistant state, in the cytoplasm. This is followed by transcription of the parental DNA, carried out by a virion RNA polymerase, to produce early viral mRNA. In addition, the core contains several other enzymic activities such as a poly(A) polymerase, protein kinase, etc. (Moss, 1974). It has been suggested that the synthesis of early mRNAs is involved in the shut-off of host protein synthesis (Bablanian et al., 1978). This contrasts with results showing that shut-off still occurs even if viral RNA synthesis is inhibited (Person and Beaud, 1978). Nevertheless, this inhibition of host protein synthesis facilitates the detection of specific viral proteins. Studies on the synthesis of these early viral products indicate that there are around 20–30 viral proteins synthesized before DNA replication takes place (Esteban and Metz, 1973; Pennington, 1974). Among these early proteins there are several enzymes involved in the metabolism of viral nucleic acid, such as the viral DNA polymerase, thymidine kinase and some structural proteins (McAuslan and Kates, 1967; Holowczak and Joklik, 1967). Viral DNA synthesis takes place in the cytoplasm of infected cells (Hruby et al., 1979) within discrete foci designated as virosomes. Both initiation and termination of DNA synthesis occur at the ends of the molecule (Esteban et al., 1977; Pogo et al., 1981). Newly synthesized virosomal DNA consists of concatemers wherein unit length molecules are joined by fusion of two left or right ends resulting in genomes aligned in alternating head to head and tail to tail mirror image arrays (Moyer and Graves, 1981). The concatemeric molecules serve as substrates from which unit length DNA molecules are excised during morphogenesis.

After viral DNA replication, the synthesis of late viral mRNA takes place. This mRNA codes for most of the virion structural components and some virion enzymes, such as the viral RNA polymerase (Pennington, 1974, Moss, 1974). During the late phase the synthesis of early proteins ceases, even though early viral mRNA is still present and continues to be synthesized (Oda and Joklik, 1967).

Vaccinia virions can be partially disrupted and the core thus formed is very active in in vitro RNA synthesis. The mRNAs synthesized in this way have been translated giving rise to many early viral proteins, in addition to several unidentified products (Beaud *et al.*, 1972; Pelham *et al.*, 1978). The mRNAs formed have poly (A) at the 3′ end and contain capped 5′ termini (Kates and Beeson, 1970; Moss *et al.*, 1976). Many of the vaccinia primary products translated *in vivo* undergo several postranslational modifications such as cleavage, glycosylation and phosphorylation, but it seems unlikely that more than one mature viral protein arises by proteolytic cleavage of a primary precursor polypeptide, as is the case in several plus-stranded RNA viruses (see Section 5.4). Some ribosomal proteins are modified after infection of HeLa cells with vaccinia virus. Three 40 S ribosomal proteins S2, S6 and S16 are phosphorylated after infection. S6 is also phosphorylated in uninfected cells but the degree of phosphorylation is enhanced after infection (Kaerlein and Horak, 1976; 1978).

The morphogenesis of new poxviruses begins with the *de novo* formation of virus envelope and continues with the formation of nucleoprotein core beneath the plasma membrane (Moss, 1974). Once the mature particles are formed most of them do not exit from the infected cell.

Some specific inhibitors of poxvirus development have been described. Isatin 3-thiosemicarbazone blocks poxvirus growth (Bauer, 1972b) affecting a late step in replication: Early viral functions, including DNA replication, appear to proceed normally in the presence of isatin-β-thiosemicarbazone whereas the synthesis of late proteins is severely inhibited. However, the amount of viral RNA that is capped, properly methylated and polyadenylated is only reduced to about 50 per cent (Pennington, 1977; Cooper *et al.*, 1979). Rifampicin also inhibits vaccinia development (Subak-Sharpe *et al.*, 1969) and leads to an interruption of morphogenesis at a unique step in the formation of virus envelope (Nagayama *et al.*, 1970). This has been used to study the virion proteins that undergo maturational processing (Moss and Rosenblum, 1973).

5.4. RNA CONTAINING VIRUSES

5.4.1. Picornaviruses

The picornaviruses are the simplest RNA containing viruses. They have been divided into five different subgroups (Rekosh, 1977). Representative members in this family are poliovirus, encephalomyocarditis virus and foot and mouth disease virus (Rekosh, 1977; Levintow, 1974; Brown, 1981). The virion particle of icosahedral symmetry is very small with a diameter of 28–30 nm (Fig. 1). The genome is composed of a single-stranded RNA molecule of approximately 2.5×10^6 (Granboulan and Girard, 1969; Tannock *et al.*, 1970; Brown *et al.*, 1970; Nair and Lonberg-Holm, 1971) which is surrounded by a protein capsid containing four viral polypeptides designated VP1, VP2, VP3 and VP4 (Maizel and Summers, 1968; Stoltzfuz and Rueckert, 1972). There are 60 copies of each polypeptide per virion (Rekosh, 1977; Hordern *et al.*, 1979; Dunker, 1979).

The primary structure of the polio virus genome is known (Kitamura *et al.*, 1981; Racaniello and Baltimore, 1981). The RNA genome is 7433 nucleotides long and contains a reading frame of 6621 nucleotides that codes for the polyprotein NCVPOO (see below). The 3′ end consists of a stretch of adenylic residues with an average length of 15–90 residues (Miller and Plagemann, 1972; Yogo and Wimmer, 1972). In contrast to the postranscriptional origin of the poly(A) in cellular mRNAs, the poly(A) in the picornavirus genome originates by transcription of a poly(U) stretch in minus strand RNA (Dorsch-Häsler *et al.*, 1975). EMC and foot and mouth disease RNA contain a poly(C) region of variable length near the 5′ end around 70 nucleotides long (Brown *et al.*, 1974; Pérez-Bercoff and Gander, 1977; Rowlands *et al.*, 1978). The function of such a region is not yet known. Another unusual feature in the picornaviral RNA is that, unlike cellular mRNAs, the 5′ end does not terminate in a cap structure (Shatkin, 1976). Although it was first reported that polio RNA has pA at the 5′ end (Wimmer, 1972) it is now well established that the last nucleotide is pUp (Hewlett *et al.*, 1976; Nomoto *et al.*, 1976; Fernandez-Muñoz and Darnell, 1976). An unusual feature is the finding of a protein covalently attached by an O^4-(5′-Uridylyl) tyrosine bond (Rothberg *et al.*, 1978) to the 5′ end of the virion RNA (Wieges *et al.*, 1976; Sangar *et al.*, 1977; Flanegan *et al.*, 1977; Petterson *et al.*, 1978). This protein known as VPg is not found in polysomic viral mRNA, and is cleaved off from poliovirion RNA by an enzyme activity present in uninfected cells (Ambros *et al.*, 1978). The enzyme has a molecular weight of 27,000 and cleaves the tyrosine–phosphate bond between VPg and poliovirus RNA, even if VPg or the RNA have been partially degraded (Ambros and Baltimore, 1980). The VPg–RNA complex is able to form an initiation complex of translation *in vitro* (Golini *et al.*, 1980).

The role of the protein is still obscure, but it may act as a primer for RNA replication and also as a signal to indicate the portion of the total population of viral RNA to be encapsidated into virions.

Picornavirus development takes place in the cytoplasm of the infected cell (Levintow, 1974; Rekosh, 1977). Soon after entry into the cytoplasm and decapsidation of the virion, the viral genome functions as mRNA to direct the synthesis of viral proteins (Fig. 5). Amongst these proteins is a subunit of the viral replicase which is necessary to replicate the genome (Shatkin, 1974; Agol, 1980). This finding is consistent with the observation that the isolated virion RNA is infectious by itself when added to susceptible cells (Wilson *et al.*, 1979) and

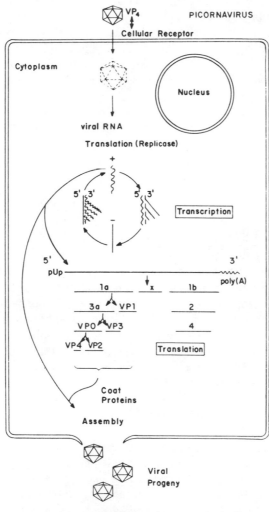

Fig. 5. Schematic representation of picornavirus development. The interaction of the virion with membrane receptors is followed by entry and decapsidation of the virion. The free virion RNA directs the synthesis of viral proteins formed by proteolytic cleavage of a larger precursor. The +RNA also serves as template to make −RNA that, in turn, will direct the synthesis of more +RNA. This RNA will be used in the infected cell in three different ways: (a) as mRNA to direct the synthesis of viral proteins, (b) as template to direct the synthesis of −RNA and (c) after covalent attachment of the protein VPg, it will become encapsidated into new virions that leave the cell.

that the virion particle does not contain replicase activity (Bishop and Levintow, 1971; Spector and Baltimore, 1974). The viral replicase is insensitive to actinomycin D (Baltimore *et al.*, 1963) and is composed of several subunits, only one of which is virus-coded (Dasgupta *et al.*, 1979).

This is also the case with bacteriophage $Q\beta$. Once the replicase subunit has been made and the whole enzyme formed, the genomic RNA serves as a template to synthesize negative stranded RNA molecules (Baltimore and Girard, 1966; Levintow, 1974). The paradox of how a single RNA molecule, which is being translated in the 5′–3′ direction, stops making proteins, to allow attachment and transcription by the RNA polymerase in the 3′–5′ direction, has not yet been resolved. It may be that circularization of the RNA template is the event that stops the attachment of further ribosomes and is the signal that starts transcription. Alternatively, the attachment of the RNA template to membranes may signal transcription. It is known that the replication complex is tightly associated with the membranes of the smooth endoplasmic reticulum (Girard *et al.*, 1967; Traub *et al.*, 1976).

The replicative form (RF) of picornavirus RNA is a double-helical molecule made up of two complementary strands of RNA (Bishop and Koch, 1967; Bishop *et al.*, 1967). The 3′ terminal sequence of the minus strand is an exact complement to the 5′ end of polio RNA. In addition to the genetically coded poly(A) tract of the plus strand in RF, a single-stranded poly(A) tail protrudes beyond the double-stranded RNA (Larsen *et al.*, 1980) (see Fig. 6).

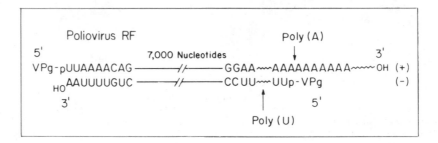

FIG. 6. Poliovirus replicative form. Adapted from Larsen *et al.* (1980).

The replicative intermediate (RI) is composed of a portion of dsRNA, with several ssRNA tails of variable length (Bishop *et al.*, 1967; Savage *et al.*, 1971). RF accumulates in the infected cell along the course of infection. This does not happen with RI, which is an intermediate in the transcription of minus strands of RNA. About 5–10 per cent of the RNA produced during infection is minus-stranded (Baltimore and Girard, 1966). The predominant form of RNA in the cell at mid-cycle is ssRNA. A quantitative estimate of the RNA molecules in HeLa cells infected by poliovirus indicates that there are a maximum of 3.7×10^5 molecules of ssRNA per cell and about 7×10^4 molecules of dsRNA. The molar ratio of poliovirus mRNA to cellular mRNA 3 hr after infection, is only about 0.04–0.1 (Hewlett *et al.*, 1977). The availability of these amounts of viral plus-stranded RNA molecules in the cytoplasm of the infected cell is sufficient to direct the synthesis of considerable quantities of viral proteins.

Analysis of the proteins synthesized in infected cells gives rise to a large variety of products of very different mol. wt., the sum of all their mol. wt. greatly exceeds the coding capacity of the genomic RNA (Summers *et al.*, 1965) (see Fig. 7). This finding led Summers and Maizel (1968) and Jacobson and Baltimore (1968b) to suggest that the viral proteins are synthesized as a large precursor that is subsequently cleaved via a series of intermediates to produce the mature virion proteins. The large precursor, the so-called 'polyprotein', is not normally seen *in vivo*, but under some experimental conditions in which the cleavage is prevented by means of inhibitors, for example zinc ions or amino-acids analogs, a large protein of 214,000 mol. wt. is detected (Jacobson and Baltimore, 1968b; Jacobson *et al.*, 1970; Butterworth and Korant, 1974).

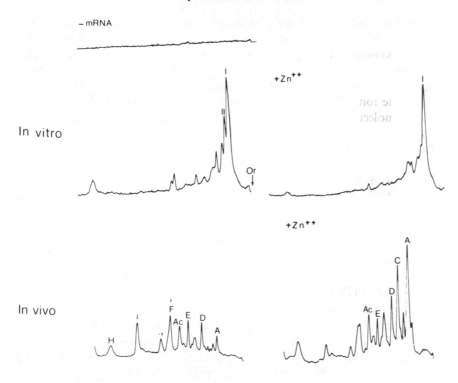

FIG. 7. Picornavirus protein synthesis, effect of Zn^{2+} ions. The three upper densitometries represent *in vitro* protein synthesis carried out in a S-30 cell-free system from L cells (for conditions see Carrasco and Smith, 1976). The products synthesized by the addition of EMC RNA were labeled with (^{35}S) methionine and run in a 15 per cent polyacrylamide gel. The autoradiogram of the dried gel was analyzed in a densitometer. The origin (Or) is on the right hand side of the densitograms. The proteins labeled *in vivo* after the infection of a mouse 3T6 cell by EMC are represented in the two lower densitograms. It can be observed that the addition of 1 mM Zn^{2+} ions inhibits some of the proteolytic steps shown in Fig. 2, and hence, the amount of larger products increases, whereas the production of low mol. wt. components diminishes.

Although the enzymology of the cleavage process is still poorly understood, it appears that several enzymes are involved (Korant, 1975; Hershko and Fry, 1975) and they could probably be of viral origin (Pelham, 1978a; Shih *et al.*, 1978; Agol, 1980). A nonstructural 40,000 dalton protein from poliovirus (Korant *et al.*, 1979) and the EMC coded protein p22 (Gorbalenya *et al.*, 1979) are involved in proteolytic processes.

Three different kinds of cleavages can be distinguished in the whole process of the formation of viral mature proteins (Hershko and Fry, 1975). Polysomal cleavages occur when the ribosome is still translating the viral mRNA, and hydrolize the nascent peptide chain. Two such cleavages occur in the case of polio, giving rise to the precursor polypeptides 1a, 3b and 1b. These proteins are further processed by cytoplasmic cleavages, the precursor 1a generates the capsid proteins VP1, VP3 and VP0 (Levintow, 1974; Rekosh, 1977; Smith and Carrasco, 1978). A further cleavage of VP0 to render VP2 and VP4 takes place during the morphogenesis process, at the same time as the viral RNA is encapsidated. The precursor of the replicase subunit is the protein 1b; this undergoes two cleavages as shown in Fig. 5. Keeping in mind that the synthesis of the polyprotein occurs from the 5′ to the 3′ end of the viral RNA, and that a single initiation site operates on this messenger, it is possible to map the different mature proteins by means of translation inhibitors that block initiation, such as pactamycin (Summers and Maizel, 1971; Taber *et al.*, 1971; Rekosh, 1972; Butterworth and Rueckert, 1972; Paucha *et al.*, 1974), or hypertonic medium (Saborio *et al.*, 1974). The conclusion from these studies is that the virion capsid proteins are coded near the 5′ end, whereas the replicase is coded by the 3′ portion of the genome. These results are in agreement with the genetic studies (Cooper, 1969). On the other hand, VPg is coded by an internal region of the genome that codes for non-structural proteins. In EMC virus it is perhaps derived by proteolytic cleavage from protein H (Pallansch *et al.*, 1980).

The *in vitro* translation of picornavirus RNA has been studied since the earliest developments of eukaryotic cell-free systems (Smith *et al.*, 1970; Smith and Carrasco, 1978); the products in these early systems were not adequately characterized. More recently, with the improvement of cell-free systems the complete translation of the genome has been accomplished (Villa-Komaroff *et al.*, 1975; Hunt, 1976). In some of these systems many of the cleavages that occur *in vivo* have been reproduced (Esteban and Kerr, 1974; Pelham, 1978a; Svitkin and Agol, 1978). A single initiation site in the picornavirus RNA has been characterized *in vitro* (Öberg and Shatkin, 1972; Smith, 1973). The significance of an additional initiation site that functions under some ionic conditions remains unclear (Celma and Ehrenfeld, 1975). A characteristic of the translation of picornavirus RNA is the high concentration of monovalent ions required for efficient translation (Mathews and Osborn, 1974; Carrasco and Smith, 1976). This feature may correlate with the shut-off of host protein synthesis by these viruses (Carrasco and Smith, 1976; Carrasco, 1977).

The mechanism of the expression of the picornavirus genome is reasonably well understood. Nevertheless, much less is known about the regulation of the replicative cycle of these viruses. As mentioned above, it is not yet known how translation on the parental viral RNA is blocked to allow it to be used as a template to direct the synthesis of new minus-stranded RNA molecules. A further unanswered question about the synthesis of viral proteins concerns the amount of different proteins synthesized. If all the mature viral proteins are derived from a common precursor they should be synthesized in equimolar amounts. However, it has been found in some instances that although this applies early in infection, later the synthesis of capsid proteins is favored and twice as much capsid proteins are made as compared to replicase (Paucha *et al.*, 1974; Lucas-Lenard, 1974). This phenomenon has been referred to as premature termination, but the exact molecular mechanism by which it occurs *in vivo* remains to be elucidated.

Another instance of the regulation of translation is observed when picornaviruses infect their host cell; there is a specific inhibition of cellular protein synthesis (Carrasco, 1977). We proposed that such specific inhibition is brought about through an interaction between the viral proteins and the host cell plasma membrane that induces an increase of ions in the infected cell. No role for the virion capsid proteins is known other than to protect the genome and interact with the cellular surface. However, it is possible that a capsid protein is involved in such an inhibition (Steiner-Pryor and Cooper, 1973). VP4 is a good candidate because of its affinity to bind to the membrane (Crowell and Philipson, 1971; Lonberg-Holm and Korant, 1972).

Some compounds selectively block poliovirus development (Caliguiri and Tamm, 1972). For instance, guanidine interferes with poliovirus RNA synthesis (Loddo *et al.*, 1962; Tamm and Eggers, 1963), morphogenesis (Jacobson and Baltimore, 1968a), incorporation of choline into membranes (Penman and Summers, 1965), cytopathic lesions (Bablanian *et al.*, 1965) and coat protein (Korant, 1977). The amounts of guanidine used to prevent virus production are rather high (0.5–1 m) and although under these concentrations guanidine does not influence cell metabolism, it is not considered useful for chemotherapy in animals.

5.4.2. TOGAVIRUSES

This group of viruses was originally named arboviruses and they have been divided in two groups: Alphaviruses (group A) and Flaviviruses (group B) (Casals, 1971; Pfefferkorn and Shapiro, 1974). The virion particle is of 40–70 nm in diameter, consists of a nucleocapsid formed by the genome bound to a core protein (protein C) (Strauss *et al.*, 1968) plus a lipid containing envelope in which projections formed by the viral glycoproteins can be distinguished. Three different glycoproteins form the envelope of Semliki Forest virus (SFV) and are named E1, E2 and E3 (Simons *et al.*, 1973). The genome is a single and plus stranded RNA molecule with a molecular weight of $4–4.5 \times 10^6$ daltons (Dobos and Faulkner, 1970; Simmons and Strauss, 1972a).

As with picornaviruses the reproductive cycle of SFV starts by the interaction with surface receptors which are the histocompatibility antigens HLA-A and HLA-B in man and H-2K and H-2D in mouse (Helenius *et al.*, 1978). After entry the genome is released into the cytoplasm. This ssRNA is translated to yield the virus coded components of the RNA polymerase. Once the polymerase has been synthesized, the synthesis of viral RNA begins. The exact details of viral RNA replication are still obscure, although several ts replication mutants have been isolated (Keranen and Kääriäinen, 1974; Sawicki *et al.*, 1978).

Two phases can be distinguished in the replicative cycle of togaviruses. During the early phase the only viral mRNA present in the cell is the virion 42S RNA. This RNA is capped (Dubin *et al.*, 1977) and has a poly(A) sequence at the 3′ end. It contains information for structural and non-structural proteins. The RNA has at least two different sites at which sequences coding for protein begin but only the site nearer to the 5′ end of 42S RNA is functional in protein synthesis (Cancedda *et al.*, 1975; Glanville *et al.*, 1976b). The translation of this mRNA only produces several nonstructural proteins. Some difficulties exist in their characterization because (a) They are made in minute amounts and (b) Cellular protein synthesis is unabated during their synthesis. Special manipulations such as addition of hypertonic medium and infection with a high multiplicity of infection have been used and indicate that two thirds of the 42 S RNA are translated to give rise to a large precursor of about 300,000 daltons (Fig. 8). This is cleaved through a series of nonstable intermediates to give rise to the mature proteins (Kaluza, 1976; Lachmi and Kääriäinen, 1976; Brzeski and Kennedy, 1977) which are involved in early events such as the replication of viral RNA. The *in vitro* translation of 42 S RNA has recently been reported, and indicates that a single functional initiation site exists on this RNA (Glanville *et al.*, 1976a, b). Some of the products encoded by this mRNA *in vitro* have also been characterized (Simmons and Strauss, 1974; Glanville and Lachmi, 1977).

During the late phase of infection a subgenomic 26 S RNA appears in the cytoplasm. This

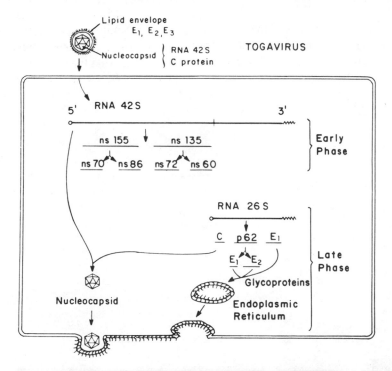

FIG. 8. Schematic representation of Semliki Forest virus development. Once the genomic 42S RNA is freed in the cytoplasm it directs the synthesis of nonstructural proteins, that are probably involved in replicating the genome and in the synthesis of the late 26S mRNA. The translation of this mRNA produces structural proteins that are synthesized in the late phase of the viral life cycle. The morphogenesis of the virus occurs in tight association with membranes and new virions originate by budding.

mRNA is capped and is similar to the terminal 3′ one-third of 42 S RNA (Kennedy, 1976; Wengler and Wengler, 1976a). Both the 42 S and the 26 S mRNAs are transcribed from a 42 S minus stranded RNA (Bruton and Kennedy, 1975). Synthesis of 26 S mRNA starts at an internal position around 8000 nucleotides from the 3′ end of the 42 S minus stranded RNA (Petterson *et al.*, 1980).

The termination site is common for both RNAs (Sawicki and Gomatos, 1976). The two RNAs are synthesized on two types of replicative intermediates, RIa for the 42 S RNA and RIb for the 26 S RNA (Sawicki *et al.*, 1978). Three different replicative forms have been isolated from group A togavirus infected cells: RF I, RF II and RF III. RF I is the ds 42 S RNA; treatment of RFI with RNAase gives rise to RF II and RF III. The latter is ds 26 S RNA wheras RF II represents the double-stranded form of the remaining two-thirds of the total 42 S RNA sequence (Simmons and Strauss, 1972b). The total nucleotide sequence of the 26 S mRNA of Sindbis virus has been determined (Rice and Strauss, 1981). Hence, the amino acid sequences of the encoded structural proteins are also known.

During the late phase of arbovirus infection, host protein synthesis is inhibited (Wengler and Wengler, 1976b; Lachmi and Kääriäinen, 1977) and only the 26 S RNA species of viral mRNA is translated. The translation of this mRNA produces all the virus structural proteins. A single initiation site has been detected in this mRNA (Cancedda *et al.*, 1975; Glanville *et al.*, 1976b). The production of all the mature structural proteins occurs by cleavage of a precursor of 130,000 mol. wt., in the steps indicated in Fig. 8 (Clegg, 1975; Söderlund, 1976). The *in vitro* translation of this mRNA in classic S-30 systems, almost exclusively produces the core protein (Clegg and Kennedy, 1974; Glanville *et al.*, 1976a). More recently, with the development of improved cell-free systems, the synthesis of proteins associated with membranes is achieved. Thus it has been possible to synthesize togavirus glycoproteins, as well as to determine with more precision the molecular mechanisms by which they are inserted in the membrane (Wirth *et al.*, 1977; Garoff *et al.*, 1978) (see Fig. 9). The initiation AUG codon is located around 175 nucleotides towards the 5′ end of the 26 S mRNA.

Once the ribosome attaches to the 5′ end of the 26 S mRNA, it starts to synthesize the p130 precursor. This is not normally found in infected cells, because the nascent peptide chain is cleaved whilst the ribosome is still translating the mRNA. This first cleavage, releases the

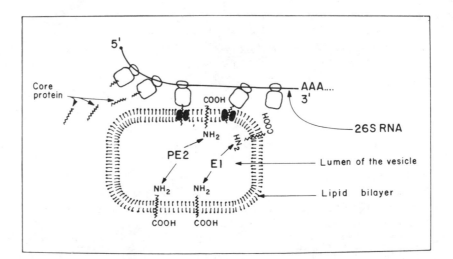

FIG. 9. The translation of the Togavirus 26S mRNA takes place in connection with the endoplasmic reticulum membranes (Wirth *et al.*, 1977). The ribosomes bind to the 5′ end of the mRNA and direct the synthesis of the capsid protein C, that originates by a polysomal cleavage. The nascent peptide chain is then inserted into the membrane and grows into the lumen of the endoplasmic reticulum. Further cleavages, that most probably occur at the membrane level, generate the structural glycoproteins, which remain inserted in the membrane and migrate to the plasma membrane where the morphogenesis of new virions takes place.

core protein and the amino terminus of the remaining peptide constitutes what has been called the 'signal peptide'. This peptide binds to membranes of the endoplasmic reticulum and the translation of the mRNA continues. The NH_2-terminus of the peptide now synthesized is extruded in the lumen of the vesicles of the endoplasmic reticulum. Further cleavage at the polysomal level generates the precursor pE_2 which remains attached to the membranes and continued synthesis produces E1. Subsequently pE_2 is cleaved to E_3 and E_2, and the vesicle containing all three glycoproteins fuses with the plasma membrane, leaving the two amphiphilic membrane proteins E1 and E_2 attached to the lipid bilayer by their COOH- terminal ends (Garoff and Söderlund, 1978). The E3 glycoprotein of Sindbis virus, unlike the E3 glycoprotein of Semliki Forest virus, is not present in the mature viral particle. Instead, it is predominantly found in the medium of infected cells (Welch and Sefton, 1979). The genomic 42 S RNA synthesized in the cytoplasm associates with the nascent core protein to form the nucleocapsid. The 264 amino acid long capsid protein has clusters of basic aminoacids in the NH_2-terminal half which are perhaps involved in the interaction with the genomic RNA to form the nucleocapsid (Rice and Strauss, 1981; Garoff et al., 1980). This associates with the membrane bound glycoproteins and finally buds off, taking with it lipid from the host cell. This lipid membrane together with the glycoproteins constitutes the viral envelope (Renkonen et al., 1971; Sefton et al., 1973).

5.4.3. RETROVIRUSES

This group of enveloped lipid-containing viruses have as a common characteristic a virion RNA dependent DNA polymerase, which is commonly known as reverse transcriptase (Bader, 1975; Temin, 1974; Verma, 1977). Retroviruses have been classified in four subgroups: A, B, C and D. Type C viruses are the best characterized in molecular terms. Type C viruses are divided into two groups: the sarcoma viruses, which are able to transform fibroblasts in vitro, and the leukemia viruses which cannot.

The size of the virion is around 80–150 nm and is composed of an outer envelope containing lipids and the virion glycoproteins, gp85 and gp37. The core of the virion is formed by the group specific (gs) antigens: p27, p19, p15, p10 and p12 for the avian group, the latter is tightly associated with the genomic RNA forming the nucleoid (Fig. 10). The genome of retroviruses consists of two identical subunits of single-stranded RNA (King, 1976) held together presumably by regions of complementarity and by specific tRNAs. (Fig. 11). The function of one of these tRNA molecules (tRNA Trp or tRNA Pro) is to serve as a primer for reverse transcriptase (Taylor and Illmensee, 1975; Haseltine et al., 1976) 35 S RNA is terminally redundant and has the sequence 5′ GCCAUUUUACCAUUCACCACA poly(A)3, (Schwartz et al., 1977). This same sequence, except for the poly (A) tail, is also present at the 5′ end of Rous sarcoma virus RNA (Haseltine et al., 1977; Shine et al., 1977). It has been suggested that this sequence might be involved in circularizing the RNA molecule to allow its transcription into DNA.

Two different ways of transmission can be distinguished in retroviruses: (a) Horizontal infection happens when virus produced in a given host cell infects another cell by direct contact (exogenous viruses) and (b) genetic transmission occurs when the integrated viral genome (provirus) passes from the parents to the offspring through the germinal line (endogenous viruses). The provirus can stay in the host genome in an unexpressed form or it may be activated spontaneously, thereby producing new virus particles (Aaronson and Stephenson, 1976; 1977). Several agents such as halogenated pyrimidines (Lowry et al., 1971) or inhibitors of protein synthesis (Aaronson and Dunn, 1974) can induce the production of new viruses. On the basis of their host range and serological tests, three different classes of endogenous mouse type C viruses are distinguished (Aaronson and Stephenson, 1977).

The fact that retrovirus development does not kill, but instead induces the host cell to proliferate, led to the suggestion that retroviruses are etiologically involved in the induction of tumors. Although this belief has received some support from studies with experimental

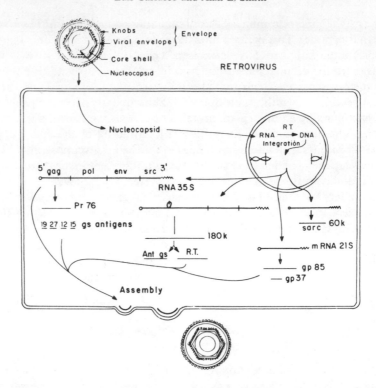

FIG. 10. Schematic representation of retrovirus development. The retrovirus virion passes through the plasma membrane to the cell nucleus where its +RNA is converted to dsDNA that becomes integrated in the cellular genome. Once integrated, it directs the synthesis of several viral mRNAs that are originated by splicing mechanisms. These mRNAs direct the synthesis of the structural and non-structural viral proteins. Some of the mature viral products e.g. the gs antigens, are formed by a proteolytic mechanism, as detailed in the figure. The new virions arise by budding-off through the plasma membrane.

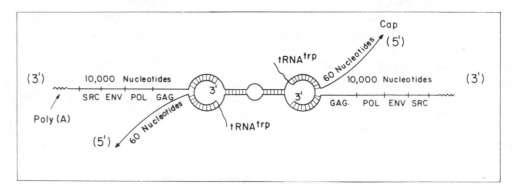

FIG. 11. Retrovirus genome organization. Adapted from Haseltine *et al.* (1977).

animals, it still remains a matter of controversy as to whether human cancer is caused by the stimulation of an integrated provirus (the provirus theory) (Temin, 1974) or even the derepression of a gene from a defective virus or of cellular origin that makes the cell cancerous (the oncogene theory) (Huebner and Todaro, 1969).

Infection of a cell by an exogenous virus starts by attachment of the virus to specific cellular receptors (Fig. 10). The virus then passes to the nucleus where the RNA is released (Dales and Hanafusa, 1972). Infection is established only if the cell is dividing (Nakata and Bader, 1968), indicating that some cellular activities present in the cell when it is in the S phase of the cell cycle are required early in retrovirus infection. Once the genomic RNA is freed in the nucleus, the synthesis of complementary DNA catalyzed by the virion DNA polymerase begins. The input virion RNA is then degraded from the RNA-DNA hybrid by RNAse H activity present in the reverse transcriptase. Circular dsDNA is then synthesized and integrated in the host genome. The integrated virion dsDNA genome is replicated concomitantly with the cellular genome in each round of cell division. Inhibition of DNA synthesis by nucleoside analogs during the early stages of infection blocks the production of new viruses (Bishop, 1978).

The ends of retroviral RNA are different from the ends of retroviral DNA. A small terminal repeat is present in the RNA, while the DNA has a large terminal repeat (LTR) (Hsu *et al.*, 1978; Majors and Varmus, 1981; Temin, 1981). These structural features make retroviruses similar to bacterial transposons (Temin, 1980; Swanstrom *et al.*, 1981). The small repeat in the RNA is important in the synthesis of DNA, whereas the LTR is important for integration of viral DNA into the host genome. The closed circular species of viral DNA can contain one or two copies of LTR (Hsu *et al.*, 1978; Shank *et al.*, 1978; Swanstrom *et al.*, 1981). The integration of viral DNA into the host genome can occur in a wide variety of sites in the host DNA.

Four genes have been detected in Rous sarcoma virus (Stephenson *et al.*, 1978; Eisenman and Vogt, 1978). Their order from the 5′ to the 3′ end of the virion RNA is *gag, pol, env* and *src* (see Figs. 10, 12).

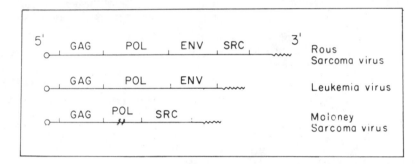

FIG. 12. Genome organization of some retrovirus genomes.

Virion RSV RNA is plus stranded because it has the same sense as viral mRNA from infected cells. Furthermore, virion RNA is able to function as mRNA *in vitro* (Von der Helm and Duesberg, 1975; Pawson *et al.*, 1976). Its translation *in vivo* and *in vitro* produces a protein of 76 K which is the precursor of the *gs* antigens (Vogt and Eisenman, 1973; Naso *et al.*, 1975; Okasinski and Velicer, 1977). This precursor is cleaved *via* intermediates to produce the mature *gs* antigens (Vogt *et al.*, 1975; Barbacid *et al.*, 1976; Von der Helm, 1977). The order of these antigens on Pr76 from amino to carboxy terminus is p19-p27-p12-p15 (Vogt *et al.*, 1975) for avian viruses, the order in murine viruses is p15-p12-p30-p10 (Barbacid *et al.*, 1976). The processing of the 76K has been achieved *in vitro* catalyzed by one of the mature cleavage products, p15. Its presence leads to the specific cleavage of 76K (Von der Helm, 1977). A minor compound of high mol. wt. (200,000) has also been found, that is precipitated by antisera against the *gag* protein and reverse transcriptase (Arcement *et al.*, 1976). A similar component has also been found in the avian system (Oppermann *et al.*, 1977). The mechanism by which this putative precursor of the reverse transcriptase originates is still uncertain. It has been proposed that in murine viruses it may be a translation product of the 35 S RNA by the read-through of a termination codon (Kopchick *et al.*, 1978; Murphy *et al.*, 1978; Philipson *et al.*, 1978). The read-through product would contain the *gag* precursor plus the reverse transcriptase; mature reverse transcriptase would then originate by the processing of this product. This model could explain the finding that *gs* antigens and reverse transcriptase are synthesized in very different amounts in the host cell (Stephenson *et al.*, 1978) and indeed a leaky termination codon has been described in tobacco mosaic virus RNA (Pelham, 1978b) and the Qβ A1 protein is also formed by this mechanism (Weiner and Weber, 1971). Another possible model not excluded by the above experiments is illustrated in Fig. 10. This alternative proposes that the reverse-transcriptase precursor originates from a different 35 S RNA that is produced by splicing out (Fan and Verma, 1978; Krzyzek *et al.*, 1978) a small region of the *gag* gene including the termination sequence. This model is also in agreement with most recent findings and, in addition, explains why isolated virion RNA is not infectious by itself, but needs to carry the reverse transcriptase in the virion for the infection to be established.

Analysis of the mRNAs from the cytoplasm of infected cells indicates that, in addition to a 35 S mRNA directing the synthesis of the *gag* precursor (Eisenman and Vogt, 1978), a smaller mRNA of 20-22 S directs the synthesis of the glycoprotein encoded in the *env* gene (Pawson *et al.*, 1977; Van Zaane *et al.*, 1977). An elegant approach has been used by Stacey *et al.* (1977) to identify the glycoprotein mRNA. They separated the mRNAs by gradient centrifugation and microinjected the fractionated mRNAs into chick embryo fibroblasts transformed by a RSV strain deficient in viral envelope glycoproteins. It was found that injection of the 21 S mRNA fraction induces the production of virus. A similar glycoprotein mRNA probably exists in cells infected with B type viruses. Certainly, a 75K *gag* precursor has been found in MMTV infected cells (Racevskis and Sarkar, 1978) and the use of the hypertonic shock technique favors the idea that two independent mRNAs synthesize the *gs* antigens and the glycoproteins in these cells (Schochetman and Scholm, 1976).

The model that can be derived from these findings is that each of the genes in the retrovirus genome is translated from a different mRNA. The 35 S RSV RNA then, has a single functional initiation site for the *gag* gene, which is the one closest to the 5′ end (Pawson *et al.*, 1976), and several 'closed' initiation sites for the other three genes. The possibility that all the retrovirus proteins originate from a huge precursor which is then cleaved, similar to picornavirus protein synthesis, seems very unlikely because of two reasons: (a) subgenomic mRNAs have been identified and (b) the proportions in which the viral proteins are made is very different.

A fourth gene exists in sarcoma viruses, the *src* gene which is involved in initiating and maintaining transformation of the cells and codes for a product called *sarc*. This gene is absent in leukemia viruses (Tooze, 1973; Wyke, 1975). Cells infected by *ts src* mutants and shifted at the permissive temperature in the presence of protein synthesis inhibitors do not get transformed, arguing that *sarc* is a protein (Martin, 1970; Kawai and Hanafusa, 1971; Ash *et al.*, 1976).

Indeed, a 60 K protein has been identified as the putative *sarc*, in avian sarcoma virus transformed chicken cells (Brugge and Erikson, 1977). It was detected by immunoprecipitation of labeled cell extracts, using serum from newborn rabbits bearing retrovirus induced tumors. In chicken cells transformed by a *ts* mutant in the *src* gene, the expression of this antigen was temperature dependent. The *in vitro* translation of virion RSV RNA indicated the existence of two small size products of 25 K and 18 K, that were absent when virion RNA from a *td* mutant in the *src* gene was used (Kamine and Buchanan, 1977; Beemon and Hunter, 1977). Further analysis indicated that the synthesis of these two products was directed by 18 S RNA. More recently an additional 60 K product synthesized *in vitro* was found (Kamine *et al.*, 1978), in agreement with Brugge and Erikson (1977). The 60 K protein shares common peptides with the 25 K and 18 K products. This presumed *sarc* protein is synthesized from a discrete 18 S mRNA that probably represents a degradation product of the 35 S virion RNA (Kamine *et al.*, 1978). In any case, the 25 K and 18 K will more likely represent degradation products of the 60 K protein. *In vivo* the *src* gene is transcribed into a 21 S polyadenylated mRNA, that represents about the 3′ one-third of the viral genome and directs the synthesis of the 60 K protein (Puchio *et al.*, 1978).

Very little is known about the molecular mechanism of action of this *sarc* protein, (Erikson *et al.*, 1980). A protein kinase associated with *sarc* has been described (Collett and Erikson, 1978) but its target remains unknown. As transformation involves the alteration of so many cellular functions, the sarc product would probably act in a central element controlling cellular metabolism, possibly at the genome or membrane level (Weiss, 1976; Durham, 1978). More recently, the sarc protein has been identified anchored in the cytoplasmic membrane (Willingham *et al.*, 1979; Courtneidge *et al.*, 1980). The protein kinase activity of this protein phosphorylates tyrosine residues exclusively and the cells transformed by RSV contain more phosphotyrosine than do uninfected cells (Hunter *et al.*, 1980; Erikson *et al.*, 1980). The complete nucleotide sequence of RSV oncogene and hence the aminoacid sequence of the sarc protein have been accomplished (Czernilofsky *et al.*, 1980). Src encodes a single hydrophobic protein of 530 amino acids (Mr 58,449). The gene is flanked by a repeated nucleotide sequence that could facilitate the deletion of the gene from the viral genome (Czernilofsky *et al.*, 1980).

Murine sarcoma viruses have also been extensively studied (Bishop, 1978; Tooze, 1980). Several lines of evidence indicate that they originate from recombination of a leukemia virus with cellular sequences that code for a gene involved in transformation (Goff *et al.*, 1980; Gelmann *et al.*, 1981). This event renders the transforming virus defective for replication and as a consequence they need a helper virus (leukemia virus) for further propagation. A number of sarc proteins have been identified in the different murine sarcoma viruses (Barbacid *et al.*, 1980; Cremer *et al.*, 1980; Witte *et al.*, 1980; Hunter and Sefton, 1980; Ellis *et al.*, 1981). Most of these sarc proteins now identified are also protein kinases that phosphorylate tyrosine residues. The whole nucleotide sequence of the genome of Moloney murine sarcoma virus is known (Van Beveren *et al.*, 1981a). It contains two LTR, the total gag gene, portions of the pol gene and the entire transforming gene (see Fig. 12). The cleavage of the gag polyprotein (538 aminoacids) NH_2-p15-p12-p30—10-COOH originates the mature core proteins and does not involve the loss of any amino acids. The viral transforming gene codes for a protein of 374 amino acids (Van Beveren *et al.*, 1981b; Della Favera *et al.*, 1981; Parker *et al.*, 1981). A great effort has concentrated to identify and isolate the cellular oncogenes homologous to src, since they could be involved in tumorigenesis. It seems possible that the protein sarc is also present in uninfected cells at low levels and its concentration is elevated in virus-transformed cells (Karess *et al.*, 1979; Oppermann *et al.*, 1979; Collett *et al.*, 1979).

In a RSV-infected cell with the continuous supply of 35 S RNA and viral protein in the cell, new virions are formed which are secreted to the medium. The assembly of retroviruses occurs in association with the plasma membrane in which several viral proteins are localized (Bader, 1975; Bolognesi *et al.*, 1978). The new virions bud from the cell surface taking the envelope from the plasma membrane. As these viruses do not kill their host, continuous production of viruses occurs and the cells become chronically infected. Once the virus is exported into the medium, further maturation has to occur before infection of a new host cell is possible. Treatment of retrovirus-infected cells with interferon specifically blocks budding of new virus particles (Friedman, 1977).

The search for compounds that specifically interfere with retrovirus development has been extensive, especially because they could be involved in causing tumors. Part of this effort was directed to find specific inhibitors of reverse transcriptase. A large list of such compounds now exists (Chandra *et al.*, 1979). However, it has to be pointed out that such inhibitors will only block the integration of the genome early in infection. Once the viral genome has been integrated in the host chromosomes, no effect of such compounds would then be expected. Their use will only be for profilaxis rather than as a cure, furthermore, they could not be used against endogenous viruses. A therapy directed against possible diseases produced by retrovirus which exploits the different susceptibilities to drugs that may exist between normal and virus-transformed cells may be more profitable.

5.4.4. RHABDOVIRUSES

Rhabdoviruses belong to class V in the Baltimore classification (Fig. 1). Two other families of viruses are also included in this class: myxoviruses and paramyxoviruses. The characteristics of these three families is to possess negative single stranded RNA as genome. We will only consider in this article the rhabdovirus family. Typical of this group are vesicular stomatitis virus (VSV), rabies virus and Kern Canyon virus (Wagner, 1975). The virion (70 × 180 nm) has a characteristic rod-shaped morphology (see Fig. 13). The virus has an

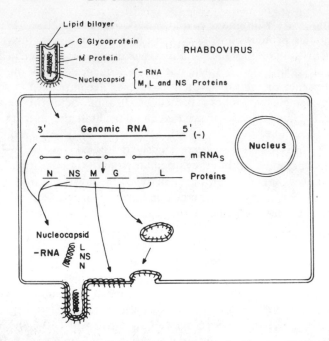

FIG. 13. Schematic representation of vesicular stomatitis virus development. The lipid bilayer of the virion fuses with the plasma membrane leaving the nucleocapsid in the cellular cytoplasm. This virion nucleocapsid contains a transcriptase activity that synthesizes the five virion mRNAs, using as template the negative RNA genome. Each mRNA directs the synthesis of a single virion protein. The glycoprotein G is synthesized on membrane-bound polysomes, following much the same mechanism shown in Fig. 5. After the synthesis of the M protein it is positioned just beneath the plasma membrane. The morphogenesis of new virions starts by assembly of the nucleocapsids in the cytoplasm. These migrate to specific areas of the plasma membrane, where M and G are located and budd-off, taking a portion of the lipid bilayer containing the M and G viral proteins.

external lipid envelope containing a glycoprotein (G) which projects as spikes. Underneath the envelope there is a matrix protein, called M protein. The envelope surrounds the virion nucleocapsid which is made up of the genomic RNA associated with three proteins, namely N, NS and L. Protein N, the major protein in the nucleocapsid, is closely associated with the genomic RNA and is uniformly distributed along it. There is about one protein molecule per 10–20 nucleotides (Wagner *et al.*, 1969). The other two proteins of the nucleocapsid are present in lower quantities and are involved in an RNA-dependent RNA polymerase activity (Naito and Ishihama, 1976). The genomic RNA of rhabdoviruses is composed of a single molecule of molecular weight of $3.6–4.0 \times 10^6$ (Schincariol and Howatson, 1972; Kiley and Wagner, 1972) and comprises only 1.3 per cent of the total virion mass (Cartwright *et al.*, 1972). The 5′ terminal sequence of this genomic RNA is complementary to the 3′ sequence (Keene *et al.*, 1979) (see Fig. 14).

The total coding capacity of this RNA molecule approximately corresponds to the sum of all five virion proteins (Smith and Carrasco, 1978). The isolated RNA is not infectious by itself (Huang and Wagner, 1966) but partially disrupted VSV virions containing the

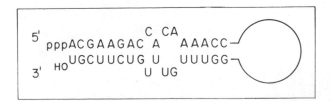

FIG. 14. 5′ and 3′ terminal sequences of vesicular stomatitis virus genome. Adapted from Keene *et al.* (1979).

polymerase activity are infectious (Szilagyi and Uryvayev, 1973), indicating that virion enzymes are necessary for infectivity. In addition to the virion associated RNA-dependent RNA polymerase, purified vesicular stomatitis virus contains a capping enzyme that blocks the 5′ termini of VSV mRNAs (Abraham et al., 1975). Two methyltransferase activities (Testa and Banerjee, 1977) a polyadenylating enzyme that adds around 200 A residues at the 3′ end of VSV mRNAs (Banerjee and Rhodes, 1973) and an enzyme activity that synthesizes cytidylyl (5′-3′) guanosine 5′-triphosphate (Chanda and Banerjee, 1981).

The first event in rhabdovirus development is the interaction of the virus with a susceptible cell, followed by fusion of the virion lipid bilayer with the plasma membrane. Endocytosis is not essential for the infection by vesicular stomatitis virus (Coombs et al., 1981). This leaves the naked nucleocapsid in the cellular cytoplasm. The next step in the infection cycle is transcription of the genomic negative stranded RNA molecule. In the Wagner–Emerson model (Wagner, 1975) it is assumed that the L protein acts first as the polymerase that makes the different mRNAs. The mRNAs originate by cleavage of a precursor RNA indicating that there is a single promotor site on the virion RNA (Breindl and Holland, 1976; Banerjee and Rhodes, 1976). The genome serves as a template for the synthesis of two types of RNA products. One is a full-length positive copy that is an intermediate of genome replication, while the other comprises the five viral mRNAs and a short leader RNA that is encoded at the 3′ end of the genome (Colonno and Banerjee, 1976; 1978). The RNA polymerase can gain access to its template in two ways: by initiation at internal sites and by sequential read-through from the 3′ end (Testa et al., 1980; Ball and Wertz, 1981). All five mRNA molecules have the common 5′ terminal sequence of G(5′) ppp (5′)-ApApCpApGp (Banerjee and Rhodes, 1976; Rose, 1977) and to explain this finding, it has been proposed that the sequence UpUpGpUpCp is located in five different positions along the genome including the promotor site. Indeed, the complete intergenic and flanking gene sequences from the genome of vesicular stomatitis virus are now known and they contain that sequence (Rose, 1980).

Once the mRNA has a pppAp . . . 5′ sequence, it is capped, possibly by a virion enzyme (Abraham et al., 1975), rendering the structure GpppAp . . . . Once the mRNAs are cleaved, a poly(A) tract is added to the 3′ end (Soria and Huang, 1975), the enzyme responsible for this also being a virion protein, possibly the NS protein (Naito and Ishihama, 1976). It has been suggested that polyadenylation could be blocked by alteration of NS, resulting in the synthesis of complete plus strand RNA complementary to the genome. Such a putative molecule would have the sequence pppApCpUp . . . at the 5′ end (Banerjee and Rhodes, 1976). Subsequently, the positive strand of the replicative form serves as template to synthesize the progeny negative stranded virion RNA molecules. The L protein acts as the replicase in such a reaction. As suggested by Perlman and Huang (1973) transcription and replication of the VSV genome should be interchangeable processes. The model above also predicts the mechanism of formation of defective interfering (DI) particles, which are common in rhabdovirus infections (Huang and Baltimore, 1970). In such a model the messenger like RNA species serve as template for the polymerase to make smaller progeny negative stranded RNA molecules, that will be encapsidated to make defective virions.

Early studies on the proteins synthesized in cells infected with VSV identified all five virion proteins (Mudd and Summers, 1970; Wagner, 1975), and it is now agreed that all the viral proteins synthesized in infected cells are also found in virions. Their identification is greatly facilitated by the rapid and complete shut-off of host protein synthesis after infection when high multiplicities of virus are used. Five different viral mRNAs exist in the infected cells, each of them is monocistronic, i.e. each directs the synthesis of a single protein. It has now been established that the L protein is synthesized from a 28 S mRNA fraction, a 17 S mRNA fraction directs the synthesis of P63, a precursor to G, the 14.5 S RNA codes for N and a 12 S RNA fraction directs the synthesis of M and NS (Ghosh et al., 1973; Grubman et al., 1974; Morrison et al., 1974; Moyer et al., 1975; Banerjee et al., 1977). Disrupted virions have a high in vitro transcriptase activity. This has been utilized to synthesize all five classes of viral mRNAs (Breindl and Holland, 1976) for use in in vitro translation (Preston and Szilágyi, 1977).

The sequence of the ribosome binding sites of the VSV mRNAs has been now determined

(Rose, 1977; Rose, 1978) (see Fig. 15) and shows an homology of nine nucleotides in the first eleven nucleotide tract at the 5′ end of N and NS mRNAs. In contrast to procaryotic mRNAs, these mRNAs do not have significant regions of complementarity with the 3′ end of the 18 S rRNA from the smaller ribosomal subunit. The complete nucleotide sequences of the mRNAs encoding the N and NS proteins have been reported (Gallione *et al.*, 1981). The mRNA encoding the N protein is 1326 nucleotides plus the polyadenylic acid tail and contains an open reading frame that codes for 422 amino acids. The mRNA encoding the NS protein is 815 nucleotides long and encodes a 222 amino acid protein. The molecular weight of the NS protein is around 25,110, which is only one-half of that predicted from the mobility of NS in polyacrylamide gels (Gallione *et al.*, 1981).

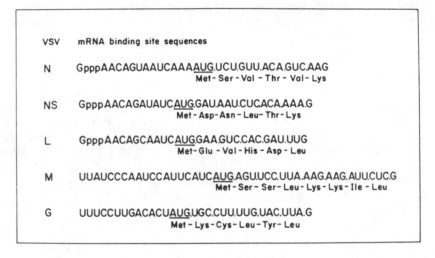

FIG. 15. Vesicular stomatitis virus mRNA ribosome binding site sequences. Data are taken from Rose, 1977; 1978.

The rates of initiation and elongation both *in vivo* and *in vitro* is the same for the mRNAs encoding the N and G proteins (Lodish and Froshaver, 1977). These results contrast with the finding that hypertonic salt treatment of cells infected with VSV results in a preferential inhibition of the synthesis of G (Nuss and Koch, 1976). The synthesis of the G glycoprotein occurs almost exclusively on membrane-bound polysomes (Ghosh *et al.*, 1973; Grubman *et al.*, 1974; Toneguzzo and Ghosh, 1977) and the molecular mechanism of its synthesis is in accord with the signal sequence model (Blobel and Dobberstein, 1975; Lingappa *et al.*, 1978). Indeed, it has been shown that trypsin digestion of VSV G protein synthesized *in vitro* in the presence of membranes, only removes 50 amino acid residues from the protein, indicating that upon synthesis, most of the molecule is extruded into the lumen of a membrane vesicle. DOC treatment of the vesicles renders all the G protein sensitive to the proteolytic activity of trypsin (Rothman and Lodish, 1977).

The synthesis of VSV proteins *in vitro* in the presence of membranes produces, in addition to other viral proteins, two polypeptides designated G_1 and G_2 with mol. wt. 63,000 and 67,000 respectively. Both have identical tryptic peptide maps as G protein. Only the synthesis of G_2 required the presence of membranes *in vitro*. These results suggest that G_2 is the desialated form of G, whereas G_1 is the nonglycosylated protein (Toneguzzo and Ghosh, 1977; 1978). Two regions on the nascent G protein have now been identified as targets for glycosylation at positions 178 and 335 (Rose and Gallione, 1981).

The evidence now available indicates that the G protein is synthesized on membrane bound polysomes and the NH_2 terminus contains a signal sequence of 15 amino acids (Lingappa *et al.*, 1978) to insert the protein into the membranes of the rough endoplasmic reticulum. From the RER the protein migrates to the Golgi apparatus via clathrin-coated vesicles that finally fuse with the membrane (Strous and Lodish, 1980; Rothman *et al.*, 1980;

Bergmann *et al.*, 1981). Recently, the VSV G protein has been cloned and it has been synthesized by *E. coli* (Rose and Shafferman, 1981).

Once synthesized the M protein positions itself beneath the lipid bilayer and is possibly associated with the carboxy terminus of G. By contrast N, NS and L proteins associate with the genomic RNA to form the nucleocapsid. This migrates to the regions of the plasma membrane rich in M and G proteins and forms a new virion by budding through the membrane in a process in which the envelope is taken from the cellular membrane. Curiously enough, there is a polarized distribution of the G protein, that preferentially concentrates in the basolateral region of epithelial cells (Rodriguez-Boulan and Pendergast, 1980). The viral nucleocapsid migrates there and budding occurs in that region of the cell.

5.4.5. Reovirus

The characteristic of this class of viruses is that they contain double-stranded RNA as genome (Gomatos and Tamm, 1963), the RNA is fragmented in ten different pieces (Shatkin *et al.*, 1968) that can be grouped into three classes according to their mol. wt.: 3L (large) RNAs of mol. wt. $\sim 2.4 \times 10^6$, 3 M (medium) RNAs, mol. wt. $\sim 1.4 \times 10^6$ and 4 S (small RNAs, mol. wt. $\sim 0.8 \times 10^6$ (Joklik, 1974). The virion, of icosahedral symmetry, has a diameter of 60–80 nm and contains at least nine different proteins encapsidating the genome. These proteins can also be classified into three groups according to their size, viz. $\lambda 1, \lambda 2, \lambda 3$ are large, $\mu 1, \mu 1C, \mu NS, \mu 2$ are medium and $\sigma 1, \sigma 2, \sigma 3$ and NS are small proteins. μNS and σNS are nonstructural proteins (Joklik, 1981). Reovirus contains about 1500 molecules of oligoadenylic acid encapsidated in the virion. A portion of these oligomers are covalently bound to structural proteins of the virus (Carter, 1979). Adenosine residues are found in two types of structures, oligo (A) bound through its 3'-terminus and ADP-ribose bound through the ribose moiety. The major adenylated protein is $\mu 1C$, that forms part of the outer shell (Carter *et al.*, 1980).

The coding assignment of each dsRNA fragment has been elucidated by means of studies on the genetic reassortment between different strains of reovirus (Mustoe *et al.*, 1978) and also by translation of the individual denatured dsRNA fragment in an *in vitro* protein synthesizing system (McCrae and Joklik, 1978) (see Fig. 16).

Associated with the core is a virion transcriptase which synthesizes mRNA from the

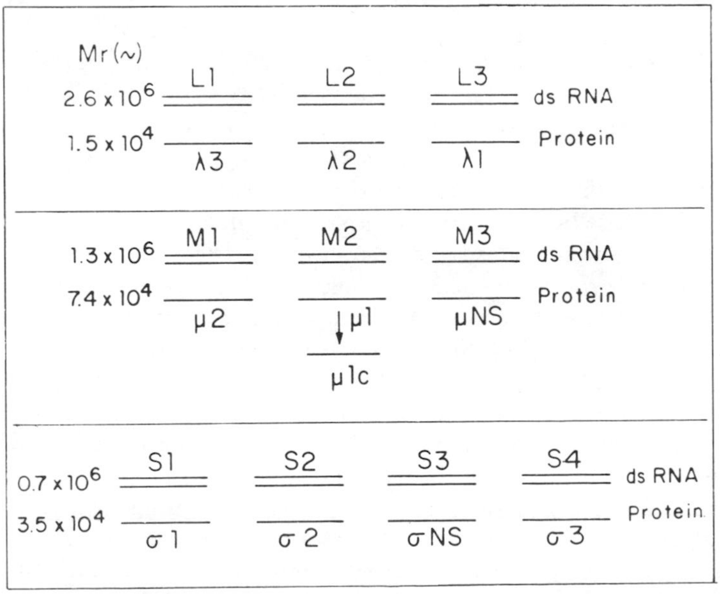

Fig. 16. Reovirus ds RNA genomic fragments and proteins coded by them.

dsRNA genome. This transcriptase is activated by removal of the outer capsid. This process occurs during uncoating when the polypeptide $\sigma 3$ is degraded and polypeptide $\mu 2$ is cleaved (Silverstein et al., 1972; Shatkin and La Fiandra, 1972). Although the proteins that form part of the transcriptase activity have not yet been accurately characterized, it seems that the polypeptides of the core particle are involved, namely $\lambda 1$, $\lambda 2$, $\mu 1$ and $\sigma 2$ (Joklik, 1974).

Two phases can be distinguished during the reproductive cycle of reoviruses (Watanabe et al., 1967; Shatkin and Rada, 1967). During the early phase, early mRNA is transcribed directly from the parental genome catalyzed by the virion transcriptase. This early transcription occurs even in the presence of translation inhibitors. The late phase begins when the dsRNA is replicated. This is accompanied by an increase in the transcription of late mRNA from immature progeny virus particles (Joklik, 1974). The enzymes involved in both processes need to be synthesized de novo (Watanabe et al., 1967; Shatkin and Rada, 1967).

Since the transcriptase is active in vitro, it is possible to produce large quantities of mRNA from activated virions (Borsa and Graham, 1968; Shatkin and Sipe, 1968; Skehel and Joklik, 1969; Levin and Samuel, 1977). This transcription is assymetric and all ten dsRNA segments produce a mRNA species. The ten different mRNAs formed are grouped into three size classes designated: l, m and s.

In the absence of S-adenosyl-L-methionine the 5′ termini of these mRNAs is (p) ppGp . . . (11, 12) and G (5′) ppp (5′) Gp, whereas in the presence of SAdoMet the complete cap structure is synthesized (Both et al., 1975a). This has served to analyse the requirements of methylation of the 5′ terminus of mRNA for activity; the results indicate that methylation of the 5′ end of these mRNAs does not affect transcription, whereas the unmethylated mRNAs are much less efficiently translated than methylated ones (Levin and Samuel, 1977). Like some histone mRNAs, reovirus mRNAs do not contain a poly(A) sequence in their 3′ end (Stoltzfus et al., 1973).

The relative transcription frequencies of the ten different mRNAs vary and is inversely proportional to their mol. wt. (Skehel and Joklik, 1969), i.e. there are twice as many copies of mRNAs from the s class than from the m class and 20 times as much as from the l class size mRNAs. Moreover, the transcription frequencies are also different in cells and in cell-free systems. In vitro they are highly dependent on the nucleoside triphosphate and magnesium concentrations (Nichols et al., 1972). The coding properties and translational efficiencies of the four S class reovirus RNAs indicate that ssRNA S1 encodes polypeptide $\sigma 1$; S2 encodes $\sigma 2$; S3 encodes σNS and S4 encodes $\sigma 3$. The relative translation efficiency varies from one mRNA to another, with S4 being the most efficient and S1 the least efficient mRNA (Levin and Samuel, 1980). An excellent correlation between relative translational efficiency in vitro and the amount of polypeptide synthesized in vivo was found.

The function of reovirus plus strand RNA in the infected cell is to serve as mRNA and to function as template for the transcription of minus RNA. Transcribed minus-strand RNA can remain associated with its template, thereby generating the progeny dsRNA (Schonberg et al., 1971; Zweerink et al., 1972). The enzyme that catalyzes the formation of plus strands is the transcriptase, whereas the replicase catalyzes the formation of minus strands of RNA.

During the late phase of infection the synthesis of cellular proteins is inhibited (Zweerink and Joklik, 1970). This facilitates the detection of virus products in infected cells. At least sixteen different viral proteins are detected in reovirus infected cells (Both et al., 1975b; Cross and Fields, 1976). Ten of them correspond to the primary translation products, whereas polypeptides P_{135}, P_{73}, P_{69}, P_{66}, P_{40} and P_{36} are derived by cleavage from the primary translation proteins. There is no correlation between the amount of each protein synthesized and the abundance of each mRNA species, either in vivo or in vitro (Zweerink et al., 1972; Ward et al., 1972). Thus, mRNA S1 has the lowest translation frequency among the s class mRNAs, whereas polypeptide $\mu 3$ is by far the major product synthesized from the m class mRNAs (Both et al., 1975b). This clearly indicates that reovirus gene expression is regulated at the translational level, this regulation most probably reflects differences in the efficiency with which reovirus mRNAs bind to ribosomes. It has been shown that some of the reovirus mRNAs, or even the ribosome protected fragments of mRNAs, bind with very different efficiencies to ribosomes in vitro (Kozak and Shatkin, 1976). The 40 S ribosome protected initiation regions from six different reovirus mRNAs have been sequenced (Kozak, 1977; Kozak and Shatkin, 1976, 1977a, b). These are shown in Fig. 17. The 40 S nuclease protected region contains the 5′ cap structure and the AUG codon that presumably operates *in vivo*. The 80 S protected fragments of mRNAs are considerably smaller and do not contain the cap region, although they still retain the AUG initiation codon. These fragments can be isolated and tested to rebind to ribosomes. It is then observed that only the fragments containing both the 5′ cap region and the AUG initiation codon are able to reassociate efficiently and stably with ribosomes (Kozak and Shatkin, 1978).

Reovirus mRNA binding site sequences

m52 GpppGCUAAUCUGCUGACCGUUACUCUGCAAAG*AUG*GGGAACG
  Met - Gly - Asn

m44 GpppGCUAAAGUGACCGUGGUC*AUG*GCUUCAUUCAAGGGAUUCUCCG
  Met - Ala - Ser - Phe - Lys - Gly - Phe - Ser

m30 GpppGCUAUUCGCGGUC*AUG*GCU
  Met - Ala

S54 GpppGCUAUUUUGCCUCUUCCCAGACGUUGUCGCA*AUG*GAGGUGUGCUUGCCCAACG
  Met - Glu - Val - Cys - Leu - Pro - Asn

S45 GpppGCUAAAGUCACGCCUGUCGUCGUCACU*AUG*GCUUCCUCACUCAG
  Met - Ala - Ser - Ser - Leu

S46 GpppGCUAUUCGCUGGUCAGUU*AUG*GCU
  Met - Ala

Fig. 17. Reovirus mRNA ribosome binding site sequences. Data are taken from Kozak and Shatkin, 1978.

A model has been advanced to account for the inhibition of host protein synthesis in reovirus-infected cells. It was found that the reovirus mRNAs transcribed early in infection, which are capped, are efficiently translated in extracts of uninfected cells, but not in extracts of reovirus-infected cells, whereas uncapped reovirus mRNAs are translated poorly in extracts of uninfected cells, but efficiently in extracts of infected cells (Skup and Millward, 1980). This claim is not in agreement with the finding that the mRNAs made in infected cells between 5–11 hr post-infection all have a cap structure (Desrosiers *et al.*, 1976). This suggests that although the reovirus progeny subviral particles *in vitro* synthesize uncapped mRNAs (Zarbl *et al.*, 1980) the molecules synthesized *in vivo* are all capped (Desrosiers *et al.*, 1976).

Large quantities of viral proteins are made during the late phase and their relative proportions closely resemble their abundance in virions. The morphogenesis of new virions starts by the formation of immature particles containing the ten different dsRNA molecules bound to some proteins, mainly $\lambda 1$, $\lambda 2$, $\mu 1$ and $\sigma 2$. The final step is probably the association of $\sigma 3$, accompanied by the loss of transcriptase activity (Astell *et al.*, 1972). A puzzling point in the morphogenesis of reoviruses is how the ten different dsRNA molecules recognize each other and become encapsidated in the correct molar proportions. It is, however, known that assortment of RNA molecules occurs at the stage of ssRNA (Joklik, 1981), and that the dsRNA fragments are arranged in the virion connected at a common focus (Kavenoff *et al.*, 1975).

5.5. INTERFERENCE OF VIRAL DEVELOPMENT WITH HOST METABOLISM

Viral infection has profound effects on host cell metabolism, and although these effects generally adapt the cell for efficient virus production, in many cases they are detrimental to the cell itself. We can broadly distinguish two kinds of alterations induced by viral infection: (a) Stimulation of host metabolism which is produced by infection with retroviruses and during transformation or in the early phase of the replicative cycle of papovaviruses and adenoviruses infection and, (b) inhibition of host metabolism, the so-called shut-off phenomenon, induced by the infection of susceptible cells with cytocidal viruses.

The stimulation of host metabolism is related to cellular transformation and to an increase in the rate of cell proliferation (Tooze, 1973; Aaronson and Stephenson, 1976). The molecular mechanism by which viruses are able to induce those effects are still poorly understood. As discussed above the *sarc* protein from retroviruses, and the T antigens from papovaviruses and adenoviruses, are in some way involved in initiating and maintaining the transformed state. The genome or the membrane or even both (Durham, 1978) are possible targets of those viral proteins involved in the stimulation of cell proliferation.

The inhibition of cell functions by viral infection has been intensively studied and most work has concentrated on four viral systems: picornaviruses, adenoviruses, poxviruses and rhabdoviruses (for reviews Roizman and Spear, 1969; Bablanian, 1972a; Bablanian, 1975; Carrasco, 1977; Kohn, 1979; Agol, 1980).

Attention in the picornavirus system has been concentrated on protein synthesis mainly because this is more easy to study. The most striking fact of the inhibition is its specificity. Viral infection causes a specific block in host cell macromolecular synthesis, whereas viral macromolecules are still synthesized (Ackermann *et al.*, 1959; Martin and Work, 1961; Franklin and Baltimore, 1962; Holland, 1965). The analysis of polysomal profiles in poliovirus infected cells showed a breakdown to monosomes, indicating that the initiation step on translation was the target of the shut-off following viral infection (Willems and Penman, 1966; Ehrenfeld and Manis, 1979).

The inhibition appeared to be an inactivation of the host mRNA (Willems and Penman, 1966) but, although at first a decreased activity in the cellular mRNA fraction from infected cells was reported (Lawrence and Thach, 1974), it is now accepted that after infection, cellular mRNA is not degraded (Leibowitz and Penman, 1971; Colby *et al.*, 1974; Fernández-Muñoz and Darnell, 1976; Kaufmann *et al.*, 1976).

Poliovirus mutants which are unable to shut-off host protein synthesis map in the region of the genome that codes for viral coat proteins (Steiner-Pryor and Cooper, 1973). This is in agreement with the findings that input virions alone, when added at a very high multiplicity of infection, are able to cause shut-off, and that shut-off still occurs in cells infected in the presence of inhibitors of viral multiplication (Holland, 1964; Bablanian *et al.*, 1965; Bablanian, 1972b; Collins and Roberts, 1972) and by u.v. inactivated virions (Bablanian, 1972a, b; Collins and Roberts, 1972).

In addition, cell-free systems derived from normal or mengovirus-infected cells were equally effective in translating both cellular and viral mRNAs *in vitro* (Abreu and Lucas-Lenard, 1976; Hackett *et al.*, 1978a). This indicated that the specificity that existed *in vivo* is lost during cell breakage and the subsequent preparation of the cell free system.

In 1971 it was suggested (Ehrenfeld and Hunt, 1971) that the production of dsRNA during viral infection might be responsible for the specific inhibition of host protein synthesis observed *in vivo*. However, that suggestion did not account for the previous observations that shut-off occurred in the absence of virus replication and hence in the absence of viral dsRNA. Indeed, later work tended to rule out any direct role of dsRNA in the shut-off phenomenon (Celma and Ehrenfeld, 1974), because it was found that it inhibited equally the *in vitro* translation of both viral and cellular mRNAs. More recent results indicate that viral mRNA can outcompete *in vitro* cellular mRNA in binding to ribosomes (Golini *et al.*, 1976). This seems only to occur under some particular conditions (Abreu and Lucas-Lenard, 1976) and these experiments have not been reproduced by others (Hackett *et al.*, 1978b). It should be emphasized that competition alone cannot explain the shut-off phenomenon, because it does not explain why there is an inhibition in total protein synthesis after infection and why there is shut-off even in the absence of viral mRNA production (Steiner-Pryor and Cooper, 1973; Holland, 1964; Bablanian, 1972b; Collins and Roberts, 1972).

An impairment in the activity of initiation factors after poliovirus infection has been reported (Kaufmann *et al.*, 1976; Helentjaris and Ehrenfeld, 1978; Rose *et al.*, 1978). The factor inactivated in cell-free extracts from poliovirus-infected cells was first identified as eIF-

4B (Rose et al., 1978). It was claimed that the factor was inactivated after poliovirus infection and that it was specifically required for the translation of capped mRNAs. It was then surprising to find that this factor has a strong affinity to bind to picornavirus uncapped mRNA (Baglioni et al., 1978). In a subsequent report the activity that restores the capacity to translate capped mRNAs of cell-free systems from poliovirus-infected cells was identified by electrophoretic mobility and triptic peptide pattern with a Mr 24,000 polypeptide, so-called cap binding factor (Trachsel et al., 1980). This protein differentially stimulates the translation of capped mRNAs in cell-free systems (Sonnerberg et al., 1980). However, more recent evidence suggests that the cap binding factor is also present in poliovirus-infected cells (Hansen and Ehrenfeld, 1981) and that the restoring activity is not the Mr 24,000 cap binding factor (Tahara et al., 1981). It still remains to be established whether these results are simply artefacts of the preparation of cell-free systems or are reflections of physiological processes. Cell-free systems from virus-infected cells or from cells in which translation has been inhibited are less active than control cells. Their activity is enhanced by addition of different initiation factors and other components that participate in translation (Hackett et al., 1978a; Rose et al., 1978). In fact HeLa cells double-infected with poliovirus and Semliki Forest virus simultaneously translate the poliovirus uncapped mRNA and the 26S mRNA from SFV that possess a cap structure (Alonso and Carrasco, 1982b). This also occurs in cells double infected with EMC virus and SFV, suggesting that the factor necessary to translate capped mRNAs is not inactivated after infection (Alonso and Carrasco, 1982a).

Recent experiments indicate that enteroviruses (poliovirus) and cardioviruses (EMC virus; mengovirus) could inhibit cellular protein synthesis by different mechanisms (Jen et al., 1980; Lacal and Carrasco, 1982). We have proposed a model to explain the shut-off phenomenon in EMC virus-infected cells (Carrasco, 1977) that we think is in agreement with many of the classic observations and has also been supported by new experimental evidence (Carrasco and Smith, 1976; Carrasco, 1978; Carrasco et al., 1979). The model indicates that a viral protein (in some instances a virion protein) is able to modify the plasma membrane of the infected cell and that this modification of the membrane leads to gradual changes in the intracellular conditions, such as the concentration of ions within the cell. The change in these conditions in the cell causes a parallel interference with a variety of cellular functions, some being affected more than others, depending on their requirement for membrane integrity. The model supposes that the modifications which are in general harmful to the host cell are less detrimental to viral functions and in some cases even stimulate them.

If changes in the concentration of ions are the cause of the specificity seen *in vivo* then no modifications of the protein synthesizing machinery would be expected in cell-free systems isolated after viral infection (Abreu and Lucas-Lenard, 1976), as ions would have been removed during the preparation of the system. However, it is possible that the damage of membranes and lysosomes occurring after infection could modify or confer a greater fragility to some components that participate in protein synthesis and they could then become more easily inactivated during the purification procedures (Rose et al., 1978).

What is the present evidence that supports the membrane-leakage model? To prove such a model one needs *in vitro* evidence and this *in vitro* evidence must be consistent with *in vivo* results. The model predicted that the translation of cellular mRNAs should be inhibited by ions, whereas viral protein synthesis would be resistant or even stimulated by such conditions. This was the case for the translation of picornavirus mRNA (Carrasco and Smith, 1976). More recently, we have extended these observations and shown that many viral mRNAs which are translated in the cell when shut-off occurs, have a higher monovalent ion optimum for their *in vitro* translation, whereas the viral mRNAs that are translated when cellular protein synthesis is unabated, show the same ionic requirement for *in vitro* translation than the cellular mRNAs (Carrasco et al., 1979). Penman's group have provided evidence (Willems and Penman, 1966; Leibowitz and Penman, 1971) that the modifications in translation that occur after picornavirus infection act at the level of polypeptide chain initiation. Indeed, this is the site of action of the inhibition seen with an elevated concentration of ions (Fig. 18). A high ionic concentration *in vitro* inhibits initiation on cellular mRNAs, whereas initiation of viral mRNA is stimulated.

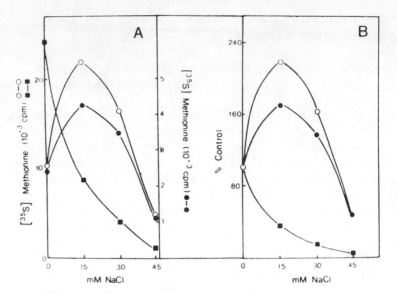

FIG. 18. Initiation of translation on globin mRNA and EMC RNA under different concentrations of NaCl, as studied by the sparsomycin technique (Smith, 1973). (■——■) Globin dipeptide synthesized. (●——●) EMC dipeptide and ○——○ EMC tripeptide.

It has been found in experiments using intact cells that the plasma membrane becomes leaky to ions at the same time as viral protein synthesis is occurring in the infected cell (Farnham and Epstein, 1963; Carrasco and Smith, 1976); these changes in the membrane lead to a redistribution of ions in the cytoplasm (Egberts *et al.*, 1977). As small molecules are also able to cross the membrane (Carrasco, 1978; Contreras and Carrasco, 1979), leading to a decrease in the pool of low molecular weight compounds (Genty, 1975) an increase in the concentration of ions has to occur in the cytoplasm, to maintain the isotonicity. Figure 19 shows the parallelism that exists between the inhibition of cellular protein synthesis in EMC virus-infected cells and the modification of membrane permeability to monovalent ions (Muñoz and Carrasco, 1981; Lacal and Carrasco, 1982).

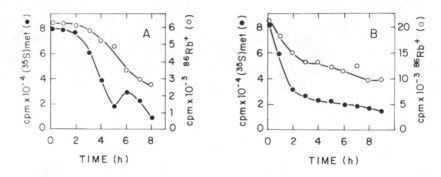

FIG. 19. Relationship between protein synthesis (●——●) and ionic content (○——○) in EMC-infected HeLa cells (panel A) and Semliki Forest virus-infected BHK cells (panel B).

It has been argued (Helentjaris and Ehrenfeld, 1978) that although changes in the membrane occur, they 'appear to occur late in infection' and may not be relevant for shut-off. In the case of the EMC-3T6 system, using low multiplicities of infection, shut-off starts to occur at about 4 hr p.i. and viral protein synthesis extends until 7 hr p.i. (Fig. 20). What the membrane leakage model predicts in this system is that the membrane will be altered beginning at about 4 hr after infection and, from then on, a gradual change of the intracellular conditions in the cytoplasm will occur, producing a gradual inhibition of total protein

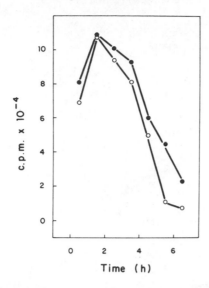

FIG. 20. Time course of protein synthesis in EMC infected 3T6 cells in the absence (●——●) and in the presence (○——○) of 0.1 mM gougerotin. Protein synthesis was studied by giving 1-hr pulses with (^{35}S)methionine at different times after infection. The inhibition of host protein synthesis in this system (3T6 cells grown in monolayer and 3 PFU/cell) started at about 4 hr after infection; at that time viral protein synthesis started to be detected on gels and the leakiness of the membrane, as measured by protein synthesis inhibitors impermeable to normal cells, commenced (Contreras and Carrasco, 1979).

synthesis and favoring the translation of viral mRNAs (Lacal *et al.*, 1980). Direct evidence has been provided recently (Carrasco, 1978) that indicates two important points in the model: (a) That a cell which is actively synthesizing viral proteins has a membrane not only leaky to ions but also to small molecules and (b) That this occurs with many different viruses, for example picornaviruses, togaviruses, papovaviruses, herpesviruses, rhabdoviruses and paramyxoviruses (see Section 5.6.1).

Some years ago Saborio *et al.* (1974) reported that a hypertonic medium induced a preferential inhibition of host protein synthesis in picornavirus-infected cells. More recently we have been able to reverse the shut-off by means of a hypotonic medium (Alonso and Carrasco, 1981a). When HeLa cells infected by EMC virus are placed in a hypotonic medium, a selective inhibition of viral protein synthesis is observed, the cells could even recuperate and translate only cellular mRNAs. Then, simply by the modification of the external ionic conditions the relative translation of viral versus cellular mRNAs can be modulated (Alonso and Carrasco, 1981a). Moreover, amphotericin B, a known poliene ionophore that modifies membrane permeability, induces a selective inhibition of host protein synthesis as compared with viral translation (Alonso and Carrasco, 1981b). This result indicates that modification of membrane permeability has a selective effect on cellular versus viral mRNA translation.

Adenoviruses cause a drastic inhibition of macromolecular synthesis during the late phase of infection (Bablanian, 1975; Bello and Ginsberg, 1967). At that time viral coat proteins are synthesized. The purified fiber antigen is able to produce by itself the shut-off phenomenon (Levine and Ginsberg, 1967), although the mechanism by which the fiber protein is able to do so has not been investigated in detail. Late in infection when cellular protein synthesis is blocked the transcription of the host genome continues at control levels; however there is a preferential transport of viral mRNAs to the cytoplasm (Beltz and Flint, 1979). On the other hand, the translation of viral mRNAs both *in vivo* and *in vitro* is more resistant to hypertonic medium than cellular mRNAs (Cherney and Wilhelm, 1979). Whether this phenomenon is connected with a modification of membrane permeability to ions during infection remains to be established. Papovaviruses also inhibit the synthesis of host proteins during the late phase of infection (see Fig. 21), and after 50 hr p.i. virtually only viral coat proteins are synthesized in the cytoplasm of the infected cell. It should be noted that both the translation of adenovirus late mRNAs (Westphal *et al.*, 1974; Cherney and Wilhelm, 1979) and the polyoma

146 Luis Carrasco and Alan E. Smith

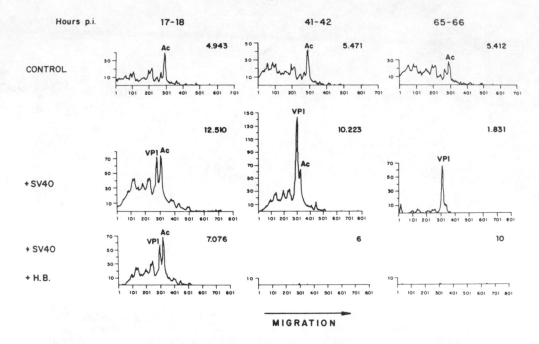

FIG. 21. Protein synthesis in normal and SV40 infected CV1 cells at different times after infection. The cells were pulsed with (^{35}S)methionine for 2 hr at different times as indicated in the figure. It is obvious that, as occurs in other systems, only the synthesis of viral proteins is detected late in infection. A parallelism between the inhibition of host protein synthesis and membrane leakiness is also observed.

16 S RNA (Carrasco et al., 1979) require a high concentration of ions for translation. Figure 22 illustrates the synthesis of proteins directed by the population of mRNAs that exist in a polyoma infected mouse cell in the late phase of the infection. The synthesis of cellular or viral proteins is differentially dependent on the concentration of potassium chloride in the reaction mixture. Similarly, the related papovavirus SV40 causes membrane leakiness at the time when synthesis of VP1 is maximal (Carrasco, 1979; Contreras and Carrasco, 1979) (Fig. 21).

Rhabdovirus development drastically inhibits nucleic acid and protein synthesis a few hours after infection (Huang and Wagner, 1965; Wertz and Youngner, 1972). As all the viral proteins present in infected cells are also virion proteins (see Section 5.4.4.) it seems reasonable to suppose that the isolated virions could induce shut-off, provided a high moi is used. This seems to be the case, since heavily irradiated viruses (Huang and Wagner, 1965; Wertz and Youngner, 1972; Yaoi et al., 1970; Yaoi and Amano, 1970), the presence of inhibitors of viral development, or even defective interfering particles which lack the transcriptase activity (Baxt and Bablanian, 1976a, b), are all able to produce shut-off in the infected cells. Moreover, the isolated virion glycoprotein G produced inhibition of nucleic acid synthesis in BHK cells (McSharry and Choppin, 1978). VSV infection also produces changes in cell membrane activity such as an inhibition in the capacity of cells to take up uridine (Genty, 1975; Genty, 1978); the uptake of uridine by simple diffusion was not affected after VSV infection. Analyses with ts mutants suggest that the M protein is involved in the modification of uridine transport. This inhibition will also contribute to a decrease in the labeling of RNA, at the time of studying the shut-off of nucleic acid synthesis by viral infection (Simonsen et al., 1979). Recent work suggests that competition of viral mRNAs for ribosomes plays an important role in the inhibition of translation in VSV-infected cells (Lodish and Porter, 1980; 1981). It is obvious that when different populations of mRNAs are present in excess in the cytoplasm, there is a competition for the components that participate in translation. The amount of each protein synthesized will depend, among other factors, on the concentration of each mRNA and their relative affinity to initiate translation. However, it still remains unexplained the cause of the drastic decrease of total protein synthesis during VSV infection.

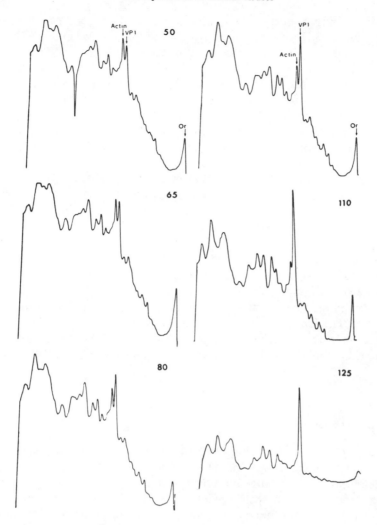

FIG. 22. *In vitro* translation of the mRNA present late in infection in polyoma-infected 3T6 cells. 1 μg of the poly (A)-containing RNA fraction was translated in a wheat germ cell-free system under different concentrations of KCl. Optimal synthesis of the cellular protein actin is observed at 80 mM KCl. It has to be pointed out that this is observed with a mixed population of the different mRNAs present in the same test tube. A similar effect was observed under different concentrations of potassium acetate. (Carrasco *et al.*, 1979).

Togaviruses do also induce a profound inhibition of host protein synthesis soon after infection (Alonso and Carrasco, 1982). We observed that the late 26 S mRNA from SFV had a higher monovalent ion optimum for *in vitro*, translation as compared to the early 42 S mRNA (Carrasco *et al.*, 1979). Also the membrane of SFV-infected cells becomes leaky to low molecular weight compounds at the time when the shut-off of protein synthesis occurs (Lacal *et al.*, 1980). Direct measurement of sodium and potassium ions in Sindbis virus-infected cells has shown a correlation with the changes in protein synthesis that take place during infection (Garry *et al.*, 1979). All together, these results suggest that the membrane-leakage model perfectly fits for togavirus-infected cells (Carrasco, 1977). The possibility that SFV-infection inactivates an initiation factor activity necessary to translate capped mRNAs (Van Stoeg *et al.*, 1981) seems very unlikely, since cells double-infected with VSV and SFV preferentially translate the VSV mRNAs (Alonso and Carrasco, unpublished results).

A detailed study on the translation of reovirus mRNAs *in vivo* and *in vitro* and competition studies with host mRNAs has been published (Walden *et al.*, 1981; Brendler *et al.*, 1981a; 1981b; Godefroy-Colburn and Thach, 1981). This competition is strongly influenced by the ionic conditions present in the assay system. A kinetic model of protein synthesis has been proposed in which mRNA must bind to a 'discriminatory factor' prior to its recognition by the native 40 S subunit. This factor selects against those messengers for which its affinity is lowest, when it is present in limiting amounts. Whereas if the factor is present in excess all the messengers are translated at maximum efficiency (Godefroy-Colburn and Thach, 1981). A different model has been proposed for the switch from cellular to viral protein synthesis in reovirus-infected cells (Skup and Millward, 1980). Cell-free extracts from reovirus-infected L cells translate capped but not uncapped reovirus mRNAs when they are prepared early in infection, whereas if the extracts are obtained late in infection exclusively translate the uncapped mRNAs. On this basis a change in the protein synthesizing machinery during reovirus infection has been claimed.

Poxvirus infection produces a very early shut-off in the cell (Kit and Dubbs, 1962; Shatkin, 1963; Salzman and Sebring, 1967). The inhibition of host translation by vaccinia virus has been correlated with the synthesis of viral RNA (Bablanian et al., 1978; Schröm and Bablanian, 1979). When cells are infected with UV-irradiated virus there is a correlation between viral RNA synthesis and the shut-off of protein synthesis (Bablanian et al., 1981a). Evidence has been obtained that the viral RNA involved in the inhibition is of low molecular weight and is about 50–100 nucleotides long (Bablanian et al., 1981b). In contrast, early reports suggested that the input virions can cause shut-off (Moss, 1968; Shatkin, 1963). More recently, shut-off by vaccinia virus has been observed in the presence of cordycepin (Person and Beaud, 1978; Drillien et al., 1978). The relevance of the finding that purified vaccinia cores are able to inhibit protein synthesis in vitro is still unclear, because no mRNA specificity of such an inhibition has yet been shown (Ben-Hamida and Beaud, 1978).

5.6. MEMBRANE CHANGES PRODUCED BY VIRAL INFECTION

During the development of any kind of virus there are interactions between some viral components and the cellular membrane. There are at least four ways during the viral cycle in which the membrane could become modified: (1) During attachment, (2) by the insertion into the membrane of some specific viral components, (3) by interference with the metabolism or the turnover of membrane components and (4) during the exit of the virus from the infected cell to the surrounding medium.

The attachment of several viruses such as EMC, West Nile, polyoma, Sendai and vesicular stomatitis virus produces changes in the fluidity of the lipids in the host cell membranes (Levanon et al., 1977; Levanon and Kohn, 1978; Lyles and Landsberger, 1977; Moore et al., 1978; Kohn, 1979; Pasternak and Micklem, 1981). These changes in membrane fluidity induce the redistribution of some membrane proteins (Bächi et al., 1973) and lead to profound alterations in several membrane functions, including redistribution of ions and transport of metabolites (Farnham and Epstein, 1963; Genty, 1975; Carrasco and Smith, 1976; Micklem and Pasternak, 1977). In the case of Sendai virus the F protein is involved in the induction of these changes in membrane fluidity, and it was suggested that they are produced by alterations in the interactions between lipids and protein structures, e.g. microtubules which interact at the interior surface of the membrane (Lyles and Landsberger, 1977; Wyke et al., 1980).

During viral infection changes in the proteins localized in the plasma membrane are observed with almost any kind of virus-cell system (for reviews see Rifkin and Quigley, 1974; Burns and Allison, 1977). These changes correspond in many cases to the insertion in the membrane of some viral proteins. As discussed in the sections above, many viral proteins are synthesized in close association with membranes. During this process the protein grows through the membrane into the lumen of a vesicle which later fuses with the plasma membrane (see Section 5.4.2). Probably, all viral glycoproteins are synthesized in this way.

A large number of virus-specific surface antigens have been detected on virus-infected cells (Burns and Allison, 1977). However, it has to be remembered that in some cases these antigens have a cellular origin and their synthesis is induced, or they become exposed on the surface, only after viral infection. In addition to the changes in the membrane antigens, there are also modifications in the interaction of the cell surface with lectins (Nicolson, 1974), and a redistribution of receptors and transplantation antigens on a variety of cell types after viral infection has been described (Burns and Allison, 1977).

The G protein of rhabdoviruses is localized in the membrane of the cell during infection (Wagner et al., 1971; David, 1976; Toneguzzo and Ghosh, 1977) and, curiously, the isolated protein is able to produce drastic changes in the cellular metabolism when added to the medium of susceptible cells (McSharry and Choppin, 1978). On the other hand, the M protein is localized just beneath the plasma membrane and might be involved in the inhibition of the transport of several nucleosides (Genty, 1975; 1978). Paramixoviruses, or even some isolated proteins, also produce drastic effects in the membranes of infected cells (Dubois-Dalcq and Reese, 1975; Hosaka and Shimizu, 1977; Pasternak and Micklem, 1981) infected cells contain at least seven structural proteins associated with the membrane (Lazarowitz et al., 1971) including the hemaglutinin (HA) and the neuraminidase (NA) proteins (Burns and Allison, 1977). Togaviruses also insert some structural and non-structural proteins into the plasma membrane of infected cells (Stohlman et al., 1975), and a similar situation is found with retroviruses (Yoshiki et al., 1974; Ikeda et al., 1974) and picornaviruses (Gschwender and Traub, 1979). Unfortunately, there is little information about how these structural modifications of the cellular membrane could produce any alteration on host cell metabolism.

DNA-containing viruses also induce changes in the cell membranes following infection. It is well known that cells transformed by papovaviruses contain a cell surface antigen known as TSTA (Bustel, 1975); an analogous antigen has been described in adenoviruses transformed cells (Allison, 1964; Berman, 1967). The presence of herpesvirus proteins in the plasma membrane has also been recognized (Spear et al., 1970; Keller et al., 1970; Heine and Roizman, 1973; Rodriguez and Dubois-Dalcq, 1978). Among the modifications observed in the membranes of herpesvirus-infected cells, there is an electrokinetic alteration of the surface, indicating that there is a change in its ionic composition (Thompson et al., 1978). The transmembrane potential also varies (Fritz and Nahmias, 1972), suggesting that leakiness of the membrane occurs after infection. Indeed, several enzymes and even RNA molecules leak out from herpesvirus-infected cells beginning at about 6–8 hr post-infection (Kamiya et al., 1964; Zemla et al., 1967; Wagner and Roizman, 1969; Benedetto et al., 1980).

Cytocidal viruses also alter the lipid metabolism of their host. Picornavirus infection increases the synthesis of lipids and this phenomenon is accompanied by a great proliferation of intracellular membranes (Penman, 1965; Plagemann et al., 1970). A similar situation is observed for adenoviruses (McIntosh et al., 1971), paramixoviruses (Gilbert, 1963), poxviruses (Gaush and Yougner, 1963) and papovaviruses (Norkin, 1977). In the case of SV 40 infection, the increase in phospholipid synthesis reaches a peak at about 32 hr p.i., and is followed by a decline in membrane synthesis, that correlates in time with the release of lactic dehydrogenase into the medium. What is the reason for this increase in membrane proliferation so common in viral infection? One could speculate that the infection by cytolytic viruses damages the membrane at a given time during the course of the infection, and this damage serves as a signal to increase the synthesis of lipids. An increase in membrane proliferation could be useful to the virus, as the synthesis of many viral macromolecules takes place in close association with membranes. Furthermore, such membrane structures might also provide the necessary architecture for viral assembly.

The last step in the morphogenesis of the lipid-containing viruses is the budding through the cellular membrane. During this process a nucleocapsid recognizes specific regions on the membrane in which some virion proteins are already localized and distributed forming some special structures (Dubois-Dalcq and Reese, 1975; Brown and Riedel, 1977; Bolognesi et al., 1978; Rodriguez and Dubois-Dalcq, 1978). The lipids of the viral envelope are always of cellular origin. However, they do not always reflect the same composition as the membrane from which they have budded (Rifkin and Quigley, 1974). Budding also modifies the structure and the composition of the cell membranes.

150   Luis Carrasco and Alan E. Smith

5.6.1. MEMBRANE LEAKINESS AND ANTIVIRAL AGENTS

As mentioned in the preceding section, viruses alter the membranes of infected cells both structurally and functionally. We have recently shown that the permeability properties of the plasma membrane to a number of compounds changes during infection. We first observed that the GTP analog GppCH$_2$p which is an inhibitor of protein synthesis in *in vitro* systems, was unable to block translation in normal cells, probably because it is unable to cross the plasma membrane. However, when added to virus-infected cells it readily inhibited protein synthesis in the infected cells, indicating that the permeability barrier to that compound was altered after infection (Carrasco, 1978, 1981b). In a thorough analysis, using 24 inhibitors of translation it was found that several inhibitors which are impermeable to normal cells such as gougerotin, edeine, blasticidin S and hygromycin B, act as specific inhibitors of protein synthesis in picornavirus-infected cells (Contreras and Carrasco, 1979; Lacal *et al.*, 1980) (Fig. 23). The appearance of membrane leakiness in virus-infected cells was concomitant with the bulk of synthesis of picornavirus proteins and some evidence that a viral gene product was involved in making the membrane leaky to those compounds, was obtained.

The induction of membrane leakiness was not specific for picornavirus, as it was also observed after infection with togaviruses (Carrasco, 1978; Contreras and Carrasco, 1979), papovaviruses (Carrasco, 1979; Contreras and Carrasco, 1979), herpesviruses, rhabdo-viruses and paramyxoviruses (Benedetto *et al.*, 1980) and poxviruses (Carrasco and Esteban, 1982). It is probable that many if not all cytolytic viruses induce membrane leakiness in their host cell during their life-cycle. The use of the inhibitors reduced by more than 99 per cent the production of new virus in cells grown in culture. Furthermore, the presence of hygromycin B in the agar used in a typical plaque assay reduced the size of the plaques formed by VSV when plated on L cells (Benedetto *et al.*, 1980).

These findings have led us to suggest a new approach to develop antiviral agents (Carrasco, 1978; Carrasco *et al.*, 1981). This approach is based on the use of inhibitors of any viral function that takes place after membrane leakiness, irrespective of whether the viral function uses cellular enzymes or not. The only new parameter to consider is that such an inhibitor must be impermeable to uninfected cells. The results we have obtained to date, using picornavirus-infected cells, suggest that the inhibitors should not exceed a given size,

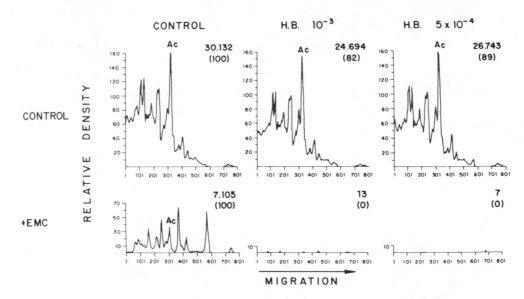

FIG. 23. Effect of hygromycin B on protein synthesis in normal and EMC infected 3T6 cells. 3T6 cell monolayers were mock or infected with EMC at a moi of 3 PFU/cell. At 4 hr after infection the medium was replaced by methionineless medium and the indicated amounts of hygromycin B were added to the medium. Labeling with (^{35}S)methionine was done between $4\frac{1}{2}$–$5\frac{1}{2}$ hr after infection. The proteins were analyzed by polyacrylamide gel electrophoresis. In this figure we represent the densitograms of the autoradiograms obtained. We want to emphasize the specific inhibition of protein synthesis which hygromycin B exerts on EMC-infected cells.

probably around 1500 daltons. In addition, such an inhibitor must be highly inhibitory *in vitro* and it must be heavily charged; this latter property being directly related to its impermeability for normal cells.

This new rationale for the design of antiviral agents is encouraging in that it predicts that one can even use classic inhibitors of cellular functions as antiviral agents, providing they can be rendered impermeable to uninfected cells by chemical modification, and provided the modifications do not lead to a decrease in their inhibitory activity. Modification of membrane permeability to antibiotics by viruses has also been found very early during infection, when the virus enters to the cell (Fernández-Puentes and Carrasco, 1980; Carrasco, 1981b; Carrasco and Esteban, 1982). Not only low molecular weight compounds but also macromolecules can enter in virus-infected cells (Fernández-Puentes and Carrasco, 1980). Curiously enough, some ionophores such as nigericin also render mammalian cells permeable to low molecular weight compounds and macromolecules (Alonso and Carrasco, 1980, 1981).

Acknowledgements—Comision asesora de investigacion científica y tecnica is acknowledged for financial support.

REFERENCES

AARONSON, S. A. and DUNN, C. Y. (1974) High-frequency C-type virus induction by inhibitors of protein synthesis. *Science* **183**: 422–424.

AARONSON, S. A. and STEPHENSON, J. R. (1977) Intracellular and systemic regulation of biologically distinguishable encogenous type C RNA viruses of mouse cells. In: *Contemporary Topics in Immunology*, vol. 6, pp. 107–126, HANNA, M. G. and RAPP, F. (eds.). Plenum Press, New York.

AARONSON, S. A. and STEPHENSON, J. R. (1976) Endogenous type-C RNA viruses of mammalian cells. *Biochim. Biophys. Acta* **458**: 323–354.

ABRAHAM, J., RHODES, D. P. and BANERJEE, A. K. (1975) Novel initiation of RNA synthesis *in vitro* by vesicular stomatitis virus. *Nature* **255**: 37–40.

ABREU, S. L. and LUCAS-LENARD, J. (1976) Cellular protein synthesis shut-off by mengovirus: Translation of nonviral and viral mRNA's in extracts from uninfected and infected Ehrlich ascites tumor cells. *J. Virol.* **18**: 182–194.

ACHESON, N. H. (1976) Transcription during productive infection with polyoma virus and simian virus 40. *Cell* **8**: 1–12.

ACKERMANN, W. W., LOH, P. C. and PAYNE, F. E. (1959) Studies of the biosynthesis of protein and ribonucleic acid in HeLa cells infected with poliovirus. *Virology* **7**: 170–183.

AGOL, V. I. (1980) Structure, translation and replication of picornaviral genomes. *Prog. Med. Virol.* **26**: 119–157.

AKUSJÄRVI, G. and PERSSON, H. (1981) Controls of RNA splicing and termination in the major late adenovirus transcription unit. *Nature* **292**: 420–426.

ALLAUDEEN, H. S., KOZARICH, J. W., BERTINO, J. R. and DE CLERCQ, E. (1981) On the mechanism of selective inhibition of herpesvirus replication by (E)-5-(2-bromovinyl)-2'-deoxyuridine. *Proc. Natn. Acad. Sci. USA* **78**: 2698–2702.

ALLISON, A. C. (1964) Relationship of cellular and humoral immunity in virus carcinogenesis. *Life Sci.* **3**: 1415–1422.

ALONI, Y., DHAR, R., LAUB, O., HOROWITZ, M. and KHOURY, G. (1977) Novel mechanism for RNA maturation: The leader sequences of simian virus 40 mRNA are not transcribed adjacent to the coding sequences. *Proc. Natn. Acad. Sci. USA* **74**: 3686–3690.

ALONSO, M. A. and CARRASCO, L. (1980) Action of membrane active compounds on mammalian cells. Permeabilization of human cells by ionophores to inhibitors of translation and transcription. *Eur. J. Biochem.* **109**: 535–540.

ALONSO, M. A. and CARRASCO, L. (1981a) Reversion by hypotonic medium of the shut-off of protein synthesis induced by encephalomyocarditis virus. *J. Virol.* **37**: 535–540.

ALONSO, M. A. and CARRASCO, L. (1981b) Selective inhibition of cellular protein synthesis by amphotericin B in EMC virus-infected cells. *Virology* **114**: 247–251.

ALONSO, M. A. and CARRASCO, L. (1981) Permeabilization of mammalian cells to proteins by the ionophore nigericin. *FEBS Letters* **127**: 112–114.

ALONSO, M. A. and CARRASCO, L. (1982a) Translation of capped viral mRNA in encephalomyocarditis virus-infected cells. *J. gen. Virol.* **60**: 315–325.

ALONSO, M. A. and CARRASCO, L. (1982b) Translation of capped viral mRNAs in poliovirus-infected HeLa cells. *EMBO Journal* **1**: 913–917.

ALWINE, J. C., REED, S. I. and STARK, G. R. (1977) Characterization of the autoregulation of simian virus 40 gene A. *J. Virol.* **24**: 22–27.

AMBROS, V. and BALTIMORE, D. (1980) Purification and properties of a HeLa cell enzyme able to remove the 5' terminal protein from poliovirus RNA. *J. Biol. Chem.* **255**: 6739–6744.

AMBROS, V., PETTERSSON, R. F. and BALTIMORE, D. (1978) An enzymatic activity in uninfected cells that cleaves the linkage between poliovirion RNA and the 5' terminal protein. *Cell* **15**: 1439–1446.

ANDERSON, C. W., BAUM, S. G. and GESTELAND, R. F. (1973) Processing of adenovirus 2-induced proteins. *J. Virol.* **12**: 241–252.

ARCEMENT, L. J., KARSHIN, W. L., NASO, R. B., JAMJOON, G. and ARLINGHAUS, R. B. (1976) Biosynthesis of

Rauscher leukemia viral proteins: Presence of p30 and envelope p15 sequences in precursor polypeptides. *Virology* **69**: 763–774.

ASH, J. F., VOGT, P. K. and SINGER, S. J. (1976) Reversion from transformed to normal phenotype by inhibition of protein synthesis in rat kidney cells infected with a temperature sensitive mutant of Rous sarcoma virus. *Proc. Natn. Acad. Sci. USA* **73**: 3603–3607.

ASTELL, C., SILVERSTEIN, S. C., LEVIN, D. H. and ACS, G. (1972) Regulation of the reovirus transcriptase by a viral capsomere protein. *Virology* **48**: 648–654.

BABLANIAN, R. (1972a) Mechanisms of virus cytopathic effects. *Symp. Soc. Gen. Microb.* **22**: 359–381.

BABLANIAN, R. (1972b) Depression of macromolecular synthesis in cells infected with guanidine-dependent poliovirus under restrictive conditions. *Virology* **47**: 255–259.

BABLANIAN, R. (1975) Structural and functional alterations in cultured cells infected with cytocidal viruses. *Prog. Med. Virol.* **19**: 40–83.

BABLANIAN, R., COPPOLA, G., SCRIBANI, S. and ESTEBAN, M. (1981a) Inhibition of protein synthesis by vaccinia-virus. III. The effect of ultraviolet irradiated virus on inhibition of protein synthesis. *Virology* **111**: 1–12.

BABLANIAN, R., COPPOLA, G., SCRIBANI, S. and ESTEBAN, M. (1981b) Inhibition of protein synthesis by vaccinia virus. IV. The role of low molecular weight viral RNA in the inhibition of protein synthesis. *Virology* **111**: 13–24.

BABLANIAN, R., EGGERS, H. J. and TAMM, I. (1965) Studies on the mechanism of poliovirus-induced cell damage. I. The relation between poliovirus-induced metabolic and morphological alterations in cultured cells. *Virology* **26**: 100–113.

BABLANIAN, R., ESTEBAN, M., BAXT, B. and SONNABEND, J. A. (1978) Studies on the mechanisms of vaccinia virus cytopathic effects. I. Inhibition of protein synthesis in infected cells is associated with virus-induced RNA synthesis. *J. Gen. Virol.* **39**: 391–402.

BACHENHEIMER, S. and DARNELL, J. E. (1975) Adenovirus 2 mRNA is transcribed as part of a high-molecular weight precursor RNA. *Proc. Natn. Acad. Sci. USA* **72**: 4445–4449.

BACHENHEIMER, S. L. and ROIZMAN, B. (1972) Ribonucleic acid synthesis in cells infected with herpes simplex virus. VI. Polyadenylic acid sequences in viral messenger ribonucleic acid. *J. Virol.* **10**: 875–879.

BACHI, T., AGUET, M. and HOWE, C. (1973) Fusion of erythrocytes by Sendai virus studied by immuno-freeze-etching. *J. Virol.* **11**: 1004–1012.

BADER, J. P. (1975) Reproduction of RNA tumor viruses. In: *Comprehensive Virology*, vol. 4, pp. 253–332, FRAENKEL-CONRAT, H. and WAGNER, R. R. (eds.). Plenum Press, New York.

BAGLIONI, C., SIMILI, M. and SHAPRITZ, D. A. (1978) Initiation activity of EMC virus RNA, binding to initiation factor eIF-4B and shut-off of host cell protein synthesis. *Nature* **275**: 240–243.

BALL, L. A. and WERTZ, G. W. (1981) VSV RNA synthesis: How can you be positive? *Cell* **26**: 143–144.

BALTIMORE, D. (1971) Expression of animal virus genomes. *Bacteriol. Rev.* **35**: 235–241.

BALTIMORE, D., EGGERS, H. J., FRANKLIN, R. M. and TAMM, I. (1963) Poliovirus-induced RNA polymerase and the effects of virus-specific inhibitors on its production. *Proc. Natn. Acad. Sci. USA* **49**: 843–849.

BALTIMORE, D. and GIRARD, M. (1966) An intermediate in the synthesis of poliovirus RNA. *Proc. Natn. Acad. Sci. USA* **56**: 741–748.

BANERJEE, A. K. and RHODES, D. P. (1973) *In vitro* synthesis of RNA that contains polyadenylate by virion-associated RNA polymerase of vesicular stomatitis virus. *Proc. Natn. Acad. Sci. USA* **70**: 3566–3570.

BANERJEE, A. K. and RHODES, D. F. (1976) 3′-terminal sequence of vesicular stomatitis virus genome RNA. *Biochem. Biophys. Res. Commun.* **68**: 1387–1394.

BANERJEE, A. K., ABRAHAM, G. and COLONNO, R. J. (1977) Vesicular stomatitis virus: Mode of transcription. *J. Gen. Virol.* **34**: 1–8.

BARBACID, M., BEEMON, K. and DEVARE, S. G. (1980) Origin and functional properties of the major gene product of the Snyder-Theilen strain of feline sarcoma virus. *Proc. Natn. Acad. Sci. USA* **77**: 5158–5162.

BARBACID, M., STEPHENSON, J. R. and AARONSON, S. A. (1976) Gag gene of mammalian type-C RNA tumor viruses. *Nature* **262**: 554–559.

BARTKOSKI, M. J. JR and ROIZMAN, B. (1978) Regulation of herpesvirus macromolecular synthesis. VII. Inhibition of internal methylation of mRNA late in infection. *Virology* **85**: 146–156.

BAUER, D. J. (1972a) Introduction to antiviral chemotherapy. In: *Chemotherapy of Virus Diseases*, vol. 1, pp. 1–33, BAUER, D. J. (ed.). Pergamon Press, Oxford.

BAUER, D. J. (1972b) Thiosemicarbazones. In: *Chemotherapy of Virus Diseases*, vol. 1, pp. 35–113. BAUER, D. J. (ed.). Pergamon Press, Oxford.

BAXT, B. and BABLANIAN, R. (1976a) Mechanisms of vesicular stomatitis virus-induced cytopathic effects. I. Early morphologic changes induced by infectious and defective-interfering particles. *Virology* **72**: 370–382.

BAXT, B. and BABLANIAN, R. (1976b) Mechanisms of vesicular stomatitis virus-induced cytopathic effects. II. Inhibition of macromolecular synthesis induced by infectious and defective-interfering particles. *Virology* **72**: 383–392.

BEAUD, G., KIRN, A. and GROS, F. (1972) *In vitro* protein synthesis directed by RNA transcribed from vaccinia DNA. *Biochem. Biophys. Res. Commun.* **49**: 1459–1466.

BEEMON, K. and HUNTER, T. (1977) *In vitro* translation yields a possible Rous sarcoma virus src gene product. *Proc. Natn. Acad. Sci. USA* **74**: 3302–3306.

BELLO, L. J. and GINSBERG, H. S. (1967) Inhibition of host protein synthesis in type 5 adenovirus-infected cells. *J. Virol.* **1**: 843–850.

BELTZ, G. and FLINT, S. J. (1979) Inhibition of HeLa cell protein synthesis during adenovirus infection. Restriction of cellular messenger RNA sequences to the nucleus. *J. Mol. Biol.* **131**: 353–373.

BENEDETTO, A., ROSSI, G. B., AMICI, C., BELARDELLI, F., CIOÉ, L., CARRUBA, G. and CARRASCO, L. (1980) Inhibition of animal virus production by means of translation inhibitors impermeable to normal cells. *Virology* **106**: 123–132.

BEN-HAMIDA, F. and BEAUD, G. (1978) *In vitro* inhibition of protein synthesis by purified cores from vaccinia virus. *Proc. Natn. Acad. Sci. USA* **75**: 175–179.

BEN-PORAT, T. and KAPLAN, A. S. (1972) Studies on the biogenesis of herpesvirus envelope. *Nature* **235**: 165–166.

BERGET, S. M., MOORE, C. and SHARP, P. A. (1977) Spliced segments at the 5′ terminus of adenovirus 2 late mRNA. *Proc. Natn. Acad. Sći. USA* **74**: 3171–3175.

BERGMANN, J. E., TOKUYASU, K. T. and SINGER, S. J. (1981) Passage of an integral membrane protein, the vesicular stomatitis virus glycoprotein, through the Golgi apparatus en route to the plasma membrane. *Proc. Natn. Acad. Sci. USA* **78**: 1746–1750.

BERK, A. J., LEE, F., HARRISON, T., WILLIAMS, J. and SHARP, P. A. (1979) Pre-early adenovirus 5 gene product regulates synthesis of early viral messenger RNA. *Cell* **17**: 935–944.

BERK, A. J. and SHARP, P. A. (1978) Structure of the adenovirus 2 early mRNAs. *Cell* **14**: 695–711.

BERMAN, L. D. (1967) On the nature of transplantation immunity in the adenovirus tumor system. *J. Exp. Med.* **125**: 983–999.

BISHOP, J. M. (1978) Retroviruses. *Ann. Rev. Biochem.* **47**: 35–88.

BISHOP, J. M. and KOCH, G. (1967) Purification and characterization of poliovirus-induced infectious double-stranded RNA. *J. Biol. Chem.* **242**: 1736–1743.

BISHOP, J. M., KOCH, G., EVANS, B. and MERRIMAN, M. (1967) Poliovirus replicative intermediate: structural basis of infectivity. *J. Mol. Biol.* **46**: 235–249.

BISHOP, J. M. and LEVINTOW, L. (1971) Replicative forms of viral RNA. Structure and function. *Prog. Med. Virol.* **13**: 1–82.

BLOBEL, G. and DOBBERSTEIN, B. (1975) Transfer of proteins across membranes. I. Presence of proteolytically processed and unprocessed nascent immunoglobulin light chains on membrane-bound ribosomes of murine myeloma. *J. Cell. Biol.* **67**: 835–851.

BOLOGNESI, D. P., MONTELARO, R. C., FRANK, H. and SCHÄFER, W. (1978) Assembly of type C oncornaviruses: a model. *Science* **199**: 183–186.

BORSA, J. and GRAHAM, A. F. (1968) Reovirus: RNA polymerase activity in purified virions. *Biochem. Biophys. Res. Commun* **33**: 895–901.

BOSE, H. R. and SAGIK, B. P. (1970) The virus envelope in cell attachment. *J. Gen. Virol.* **9**: 159–161.

BOTH, G. W., FURUICHI, Y., MUTHUKRISHNAN, S. and SHATKIN, A. J. (1975a) Ribosome binding to reovirus mRNA in protein synthesis requires 5′ terminal 7 methylguanosine. *Cell* **6**: 185–195.

BOTH, G. W., LAVI, S. and SHATKIN, A. J. (1975b) Synthesis of all the gene products of the reovirus genome *in vivo* and *in vitro*. *Cell* **4**: 173–180.

BOUCK, N., BEALES, N., SHENK, T., BERG, P. and DI MAYORCA, G. (1978) New region of the simian virus 40 genome required for efficient viral transformation. *Proc. Natn. Acad. Sci. USA*. **75**: 2473–2477.

BOUDIN, M. L., MONCARY, M., D'HALLUIH, J. C. and BOULANGER, P. A. (1979) Isolation and characterization of adenovirus type 2 vertex capsomer (Penton base). *Virology* **92**: 125–138.

BREINDL, M. and HOLLAND, J. J. (1976) Studies on the *in vitro* transcription and translation of vesicular stomatitis virus mRNA. *Virology* **73**: 106–118.

BRENDLER, T., GODEFROY-COLBURN, T., CARLILL, R. D. and THACH, R. E. (1981a) The role of mRNA competition in regulating translation. II. Development of a quantitative *in vitro* assay. *J. Biol. Chem.* **256**: 11, 747–11, 754.

BRENDLER, T., GODEFROY-COLBURN, T., YU, S. and THACH, R. E. (1981b) The role of mRNA competition in regulating translation. III. Comparison of *in vitro* and *in vivo* results. *J. Biol. Chem.* **256**: 11, 755–11, 761.

BROWN, D. T. and RIEDEL, B. (1977) Morphogenesis of vesicular stomatitis virus: electron microscope observations with freeze-fracture techniques. *J. Virol.* **21**: 601–609.

BROWN, F. (1981) Foot-and-mouth disease virus. *TIBS* **6**: 325–327.

BROWN, F., NEWMAN, J. F. E. and STOTT, E. J. (1970) Molecular weight of rhinovirus ribonucleic acid. *J. Gen. Virol.* **8**: 145–148.

BROWN, F., NEWMAN, J., SCOTT, J., CARTER, A., FRISBY, D., NEXTON, C., COREY, N. and FELLNER, P. (1974) Poly (C) in animal viral RNAs. *Nature* **251**: 342 344.

BRUGGE, J. S. and ERIKSON, R. L. (1977) Identification of a transformation-specific antigen induced by an avian sarcoma virus. *Nature* **269**: 346–348.

BRUTON, C. J. and KENNEDY, S. I. T. (1975) Semliki Forest virus intracellular RNA: properties of the multistranded RNA species and kinetics of positive and negative strand synthesis. *J. Gen. Virol.* **28**: 111–127.

BRZESKI, H. and KENNEDY, S. I. T. (1977) Synthesis of Sindbis virus nonstructural polypeptides in chicken embryo fibroblasts. *J. Virol.* **22**: 420–429.

BURNS, W. H. and ALLISON, A. C. (1977) Surface antigens of virus-infected cells. In: *Virus Infection and the Cell Surface*, pp. 213–247, POSTE, G. and NICOLSON, G. L. (eds.). North-Holland Publ. Comp.

BUSTEL, J. S. (1975) The role of SV40 genes in cellular transformation. *Prog. Med. Virol.* **21**: 88–102.

BUTTERWORTH, B. E. and KORANT, B. D. (1974) Characterization of the large picornaviral polypeptides produced in the presence of zinc ion. *J. Virol.* **14**: 282–291.

BUTTERWORTH, B. E. and RUECKERT, R. R. (1972) Gene order of encephalomyocarditis virus as determined by studies with pactamycin. *J. Virol.* **9**: 823–828.

BÜTTNER, W., VERES-MOLNAR, Z. and GREEN, M. (1976) Preparative isolation and mapping of adenovirus 2 early messenger RNA species. *J. Mol. Biol.* **107**: 93–114.

CABRERA, C. B. and ESTEBAN, M. (1978) Procedure for purification of intact DNA from vaccinia virus. *J. Virol.* **25**: 442–445.

CALIGUIRI, L. A. and TAMM, I. (1972) Guanidine. In: *Chemotherapy of Virus Diseases*, vol. 1, pp. 181–230, BAUER, D. J. (ed.). Pergamon Press, Oxford.

CANCEDDA, R., VILLA-KOMAROFF, L., LODISH, H. F. and SCHLESSINGER, M. (1975) Initiation sites for translation of Sindbis virus 42 S and 26 S messenger RNAs. *Cell* **6**: 215–222.

CARRASCO, L. (1977) The inhibition of cell functions after viral infection. A proposed general mechanism. *FEBS Letters* **76**: 11–15.

CARRASCO, L. (1978) Membrane leakiness after viral infection and a new approach to the development of antiviral agents. *Nature* **272**: 694–699.

CARRASCO, L. (1979) The development of new antiviral agents based on virus-mediated cell modification. In:

154   Luis Carrasco and Alan E. Smith

Antiviral Mechanisms for the control of neoplasia, pp. 623–631, CHANDRA, P. (ed.). Plenum Press, New York.
CARRASCO, L. (1981a) Action of nucleotide derivatives on translation in encephalomyocarditis virus-infected
    mouse cells. *J. Gen. Virol.* **54**: 125–134.
CARRASCO, L. (1981) Modification of membrane permeability induced early in infection by animal viruses. *Virology*
    113: 623–629.
CARRASCO, L. and ESTEBAN, M. (1982) Modification of membrane permeability in vaccinia virus-infected cells.
    Virology **117**: 62–69.
CARRASCO, L., FERNÁNDEZ-PUENTES, C., ALONSO, M. A., LACAL, J. C., MUÑOZ, A., FERNÁNDEZ-SOUSA, J. M. and
    VÁZQUEZ, D. (1981) New approaches to antivirual agents. In: *Medicinal Chemistry Advances*, pp. 211–224. DE
    LAS HERAS, F. and VEGA, S. (eds.). Pergamon Press. Oxford.
CARRASCO, L., HARVEY, R., BLANCHARD, C. and SMITH, A. E. (1979) Regulation of translation of eukaryotic virus
    mRNAs. In: *Modern Trends in Human Leukemia III*, pp. 189–192, NETH, R., HOFSCHENEIDER, P. and
    MANNWEILER, K. (eds.). Springer Verlag.
CARRASCO, L. and SMITH, A. E. (1976) Sodium ions and the shut-off of host cell protein synthesis by picornavirus.
    Nature **264**: 807–809.
CARROLL, R. B., GOLDFINE, F. M. and MELERO, J. A. (1978) Antiserum to polyacrylamide gel-purified simian virus
    40 T antigen. *Virology* **87**: 194–198.
CARTER, C. A. (1979) Polyadenylation of proteins in reovirus. *Proc. Natn. Acad. Sci. USA* **76**: 3087–3091.
CARTER, C. A., LIN, B. Y. and METLAY, M. (1980) Polyadenylation of reovirus proteins. *J. Biol. Chem.* **255**:
    6479–6485.
CARTWRIGHT, B., SMALE, C. J. and BROWN, F. (1970) Dissection of vesicular stomatitis virus into the infective
    ribonucleo-protein and immunizing components. *J. Gen. Virol.* **7**: 19–32.
CARTWRIGHT, B., SMALE, C. J., BROWN, F. and HULL, R. (1972) A model for vesicular stomatitis virus. *J. Virol.* **10**:
    256–260.
CASALS, J. (1971) Arboviruses: incorporation into a general system of virus classification. In: *Comparative Virology*,
    pp. 307–333, MARAMOROSCH, K. and KURSTAK, E. (eds.). Academic Press, New York.
CASJENS, S. and KING, J. (1975) Virus assembly. *Ann. Rev. Biochem.* **44**: 555–611.
CELMA, M. L. and EHRENFELD, E. (1974) Effect of poliovirus double-stranded RNA on viral and host-cell protein
    synthesis. *Proc. Natn. Acad. Sci. USA* **71**: 2440–2444.
CELMA, M. L. and EHRENFELD, E. (1975) Translation of poliovirus RNA *in vitro*: detection of two different
    initiation sites. *J. Mol. Biol.* **98**: 761–780.
CHALLBERG, M. D., DESIDERIO, S. V. and KELLY, T. J. (1980) Adenovirus DNA replication *in vitro*:
    Characterization of a protein covalently linked to nascent DNA strands. *Proc. Natn. Acad. Sci. USA* **77**:
    5105–5109.
CHALLBERG, M. D. and KELLY, T. J. (1981) Processing of the adenovirus terminal protein. *J. Virol.* **38**: 272–277.
CHANDA, P. K. and BANERJEE, A. K. (1981) Purified vesicular stomatitis virus contains an enzyme activity that
    synthesizes cytidylyl (5′–3′) guanosine 5′-triphosphate *in vitro*. *J. Biol. Chem.* **256**: 11, 393–11, 396.
CHANDRA, P., EBENER, U. and GERICKE, D. (1979) Molecular mechanisms for control of RNA tumor viruses. In:
    Antiviral Mechanisms in the Control of Neoplasia, pp. 523–537, CHANDRA, P. (ed.). Plenum Press, New York.
CHEN, M. S., WARD, D. C. and PRUSSOFF, W. H. (1976) Specific herpes simplex virus-induced incorporation of
    5-iodo-5′-amino-2′,5′,-dideoxyuridine into deoxyribonucleic acid. *J. Biol. Chem.* **251**: 4833–4838.
CHERNEY, C. S. and WILHELM, J. M. (1979) Differential translation in normal and adenovirus type 5-infected
    human cells and cell-free systems. *J. Virol.* **30**: 533–542.
CHOU, J. Y., AVILA, J. and MARTIN, R. G. (1974) Viral DNA synthesis in cells infected by temperature-sensitive
    mutants of simian virus 40. *J. Virol.* **14**: 116–124.
CHOW, L. T., GELINAS, R. E., BROKER, T. R. and ROBERTS, R. J. (1977) An amazing sequence arrangement at the 5′
    ends of adenovirus 2 messenger RNA. *Cell* **12**: 1–8.
CLEGG, C. and KENNEDY, I. (1974) Translation of Semliki-Forest virus intracellular 26 S RNA. Characterization of
    the products synthesized *in vitro*. *Eur. J. Biochem.* **53**: 175–183.
CLEGG, J. C. S. (1975) Sequential translation of capsid and membrane proteins in alphaviruses. *Nature* **254**: 454–
    455.
COHEN, S. (1977) A strategy for the chemotherapy of infectious disease. *Science* **197**: 431–432.
COLBY, D. S., FINNERTY, V. and LUCAS-LENARD, J. (1974) Fate of mRNA of L-cells infected with mengovirus.
    J. Virol. **13**: 858–869.
COLE, C. N., LANDERS, T., GOFF, S. P., MANTEVIL-BRUTLAG, S. and BERG, P. (1977) Physical and genetic
    characterization of deletion mutants of simian virus 40 constructed *in vitro*. *J. Virol.* **24**: 277–294.
COLLETT, M. S. and ERIKSON, R. L. (1978) Protein kinase activity associated with the avian sarcoma virus src gene
    product. *Proc. Natn. Acad. Sci. USA* **75**: 2021–2024.
COLLETT, M. S., ERIKSON, E., PURCHIO, A. F., BRUGGE, J. S. and ERIKSON, R. L. (1979) A normal cell protein
    similar in structure and function to the avian sarcoma virus transforming gene product. *Proc. Natn. Acad. Sci.
    USA* **76**: 3159–3163.
COLLINS, F. D. and ROBERTS, W. R. (1972) Mechanism of mengovirus-induced cell injury in L cells: Use of
    inhibitors of protein synthesis to dissociate virus-specific events. *J. Virol.* **10**: 969–978.
COLONNO, R. J. and BANERJEE, A. K. (1976) A unique RNA species involved in initiation of vesicular stomatitis
    virus RNA transcription *in vitro*. *Cell* **8**: 197–204.
COLONNO, R. J. and BANERJEE, A. K. (1978) Complete nucleotide sequence of the leader RNA synthesized *in vitro*
    by vesicular stomatitis virus. *Cell* **15**: 93–101.
CONTRERAS, A. and CARRASCO, L. (1979) Selective inhibition of protein synthesis in virus-infected mammalian
    cells. *J. Virol.* **29**: 114–122.
COOMBS, K., MANN, E., EDWARDS, J. and BROWN, D. T. (1981) Effect of chloroquine and cytochalasis B on the
    infection of cells by Sindbis virus and vesicular stomatitis virus. *J. Virol.* **37**: 1060–1065.
COOPER, P. D. (1969) The genetic analysis of poliovirus. In: *Biochemistry of Viruses*, pp. 177–218. LEVY, H. B. (ed.).
    Marcel Dekker, New York.

COOPER, J. A., MASS, B. and KATZ, E. (1979) Inhibition of vaccinia virus late protein synthesis by isatin-B-thiosemicarbazone: characterization and *in vitro* translation of viral mRNA. *Virology* 96: 381–392.

CORDEN, J., ENGELKING, H. M. and PEARSON, G. D. (1976) Chromatin-like organization of the adenovirus chromosome. *Proc. Natn. Acad. Sci. USA* 73: 401–404.

COURTNEIDGE, S. A., LEVINSON, A. D. and BISHOP, J. M. (1980) The protein encoded by the transforming gene of avian sarcoma virus (pp60[src]) and a homologous protein in normal cells (pp60[proto-src]) are associated with the plasma membrane. *Proc. Natn. Acad. Sci. USA* 77: 3783–3787.

CRAIG, E. A., ZIMMER, S. and RASKAS, H. J. (1975) Analysis of early adenovirus 2 RNA using Eco R1 viral DNA fragments. *J. Virol.* 15: 1202–1213.

CRAWFORD, L. V., COLE, C. N., SMITH, A. E., PAUCHA, E., TEGTMEYER, P., RUNDELL, K. and BERG, P. (1978) Organization and expression of early genes of simian virus 40. *Proc. Natn. Acad. Sci. USA* 75: 117–121.

CREMER, K., REDDY, E. P. and AARANSON, S. A. (1980) Translational products of Moloney murine sarcoma virus RNA: Identification of proteins encoded by the murine sarcoma virus src gene. *J. Virol.* 38: 704–711.

CROSS, R. K. and FIELDS, B. N. (1976) Reovirus-specific polypeptides: analysis using discontinuous gel electrophoresis. *J. Virol.* 19: 162–173.

CROWELL, R. L. and PHILIPSON, L. (1971) Specific alterations of coxsackievirus B3 eluted from HeLa cells. *J. Virol.* 8: 509–515.

CZERNILOFSKY, A. P., LEVINSON, A. D., VARMUS, H. E., BISHOP, J. M., TISHER, E. and GOODMAN, H. M. (1980) Nucleotide sequence of an avian sarcoma virus oncogene (src) and proposed amino acid sequence for gene product. *Nature* 287: 198–203.

DALES, S. (1973) Early events in cell-animal virus interactions. *Bacteriol. Rev.* 37: 103–135.

DALES, S. and HANAFUSA, H. (1972) Penetration and intracellular release of the genomes of avian RNA tumor viruses. *Virology* 50: 440–458.

DALES, S. and SILVERBERG, H. (1969) Viropexis of herpes simplex virus by HeLa cells. *Virology* 37: 475–480.

DASGUPTA, A., BARON, M. H. and BALTIMORE, D. (1979) Poliovirus replicase: a soluble enzyme able to initiate copying of poliovirus RNA. *Proc. Natn. Acad. Sci. USA* 76: 2679–2683.

DATTA, A. K., COLBY, B. M., SHAW, J. E. and PAGANO, J. S. (1980) Acyclovir inhibition of Epstein–Barr virus replication. *Proc. Natn. Acad. Sci. USA* 77: 5163–5166.

DAVID, A. E. (1976) Control of vesicular stomatitis virus protein synthesis. *Virology.* 71: 217–229.

DE CLERCQ, E., DESCAMPS, J., DE SOMER, P., BARR, P. J., JONES, A. S. and WALKER, R. T. (1979) (E)-5-(2-Bromovinyl)-2′-deoxyuridine: A potent and selective anti-herpes agent. *Proc. Natn. Acad. Sci. USA* 76: 2947–2951.

DELLA FAVERA, R., GELMANN, E. P., GALLO, R. C. and WONG-STAALS, E. (1981) A human onc gene homologous to the transforming gene (v-sis) of simian sarcoma virus. *Nature* 292: 31–35.

DESROSIERS, R. C., SEN, G. C. and LENGYEL, P. (1976) Difference in 5′ terminal structure between the mRNA and the double-stranded virus RNA of reovirus. *Biochem. Biophys. Res. Commun.* 73: 32–39.

DIANA, G. D. and PANCIC, F. (1976) Chemotherapy of virus diseases. *Angew. Chem. Int. Ed. Engl.* 15: 410–416.

DOBOS, P. and FAULKNER, P. (1970) Molecular weight of Sindbis virus ribonucleic acid as measured by polyacrylamide gel electrophoresis. *J. Virol.* 6: 145–147.

DOLEI, A., CAPOBIANCHI, M. R., CIOÉ, L., COLLETTA, G., VECCHIO, G., ROSSI, G. B., AFFABRIS, E. and BELARDELLI, F. (1979) Effects of interferon on the expression of cellular and integrated viral genes in Friend erythroleukemic cells. In: *Antiviral Mechanisms in the Control of Neoplasia*, pp. 729–739, CHANDRA, P. (ed.). Plenum Press, New York.

DORSCH-HÄSLER, K., YOGO, Y. and WIMMER, E. (1975) Replication of picornaviruses. I. Evidence from *in vitro* RNA synthesis that poly (A) of the polyovirus genome is genetically coded. *J. Virol.* 16: 1512–1527.

DRILLIEN, R., SPEHNER, D. and KIRN, A. (1978) Host range restriction of vaccinia virus in chinese hamster ovary cells: Relationship to shut-off of protein synthesis. *J. Virol.* 28: 843–850.

DUBIN, D. T., STOLLAR, V., HSUCHEN, C. C., TIMKO, K. and GUILD, G. M. (1977) Sindbis virus messenger RNA: The 5′-termini and methylated residues of 26 and 42 S RNA. *Virology* 77: 457–470.

DUBOIS-DALCQ, M. and REESE, T. S. (1975) Structural changes in the membrane of Vero cells infected with a paramyxovirus. *J. Cell. Biol.* 67: 551–565.

DUNKER, A. K. (1979). The structure of picornaviruses: Classification of the bonding networks. *Virology* 97: 141–150.

DURHAM, A. (1978) A single protein key to cancer. *New Scientist* 77: 860–862.

ECKHART, W., HUTCHINSON, M. A. and HUNTER, T. (1979) An activity phosphorylating tyrosine in polyoma T antigen immunoprecipitates. *Cell* 18: 925–933.

EGBERTS, E., HACKETT, P. B. and TRAUB, P. (1977) Alteration of the intracellular energetic and ionic conditions by mengovirus infection of Ehrlich Ascites tumor cells and its influence on protein synthesis in the midphase of infection. *J. Virol.* 22: 591–597.

EGGERS, H. J., KOCH, M. A., DAVES, G. D., WILCZYNSK, J. J. and FOLKERS, K. (1970) Rhodamine: A selective inhibitor of the multiplication of echovirus 12. *Science* 167: 294–297.

EHRENFELD, E. and HUNT, T. (1971) Double-stranded poliovirus RNA inhibits initiation of protein synthesis by reticulocyte lysates. *Proc. Natn. Acad. Sci. USA* 68: 1075–1078.

EHRENFELD, E. and MANIS, S. (1979) Inhibition of 80 S initiation complex formation by infection with poliovirus. *J. gen. Virol.* 43: 441–445.

EISENMAN, R. N. and VOGT, V. M. (1978) The biosynthesis of oncovirus proteins. *Biochim. Biophys. Acta* 473: 187–239.

EISERLING, F. and DICKSON, R. (1972) Assembly of viruses. *Ann. Rev. Biochem.* 41: 467–502.

ELLIS, R. W., DE FEO, D., SHIH, T. Y., GONDA, M. A., YOUNG, H. A., TSUCHIDA, N., LOWRY, D. R. and SCOLNICK, E. M. (1981) The p21 src genes of Harvey and Kirsten sarcoma viruses originate from divergent members of a family of normal vertebrate genes. *Nature* 292: 506–511.

ENOMOTO, T., LICHY, J. J., IKEDA, J. E. and HURWITZ, J. (1981) Adenovirus DNA replication *in vitro*: Purification of the terminal protein in a functional form. *Proc. Natn. Acad. Sci. USA* 78: 6779–6783.

ERIKSON, R. L., PURCHIO, A. F., ERIKSON, E., COLLETT, M. S. and BRUGGE, J. S. (1980) Molecular events in cells transformed by Rous sarcoma virus. *J. Cell Biol.* **87**: 319–325.

ESCHE, H., MATHEWS, M. B. and LEWIS, J. R. (1980) Proteins and messenger RNAs of the transforming regions of wild type and mutant adenovirus. *J. Mol. Biol.* **142**: 399–417.

ESSANI, K. and DALES, S. (1979) Biogenesis of vaccinia: Evidence of more than 100 polypeptides in the virion. *Virology* **95**: 385–394.

ESTEBAN, M., FLORES, L. and HOLOWCZAK, J. (1977) A model for vaccinia virus DNA replication. *Virology* **83**: 467–473.

ESTEBAN, M. and KERR, K. M. (1974) The synthesis of encephalomyocarditis virus polypeptides in infected L-cells and cell-free systems. *Eur. J. Biochem.* **45**: 567–576.

ESTEBAN, M. and METZ, D. H. (1973) Early virus protein synthesis in vaccinia virus-infected cells. *J. Gen. Virol.* **19**: 201–216.

EVERITT, E., SUNDQUIST, B., PETTERSON, V. and PHILIPSON, L. (1973) Structural proteins of adenoviruses X. Isolation and topography of low-molecular-weight antigens from the virion of adenovirus type 2. *Virology* **52**: 130–147.

FAN, H. and VERMA, I. M. (1978) Size analysis and relationship of murine leukemia virus specific mRNA's: Evidence for transposition of sequences during synthesis and processing of subgenomic mRNA. *J. Virol.* **26**: 468–478.

FARNHAM, A. E. and EPSTEIN, W. (1963) Influence of encephalomyocarditis (EMC) virus infection on potassium transport in L cells. *Virology* **21**: 436–447.

FERNÁNDEZ-MUÑOZ, R. and DARNELL, J. (1976) Structural difference between the 5' termini of viral and cellular mRNA in poliovirus-infected cells: Possible basis for the inhibition of host protein synthesis. *J. Virol.* **18**: 719–726.

FERNÁNDEZ-PUENTES, C. and CARRASCO, L. (1980) Viral infection permeabilizes mammalian cells to protein toxins. *Cell* **20**, 769–775.

FERNÁNDEZ-PUENTES, C. and VÁZQUEZ, D. (1977) Effects of some proteins that inactivate the eukaryotic ribosome. *FEBS Letters* **78**: 143–146.

FIERS, W., CONTRERAS, R., HAEGEMAN, G., ROGIERS, R., VAN DE VOORDE, A., VAN HEUVERSWYN, H., VAN HERREWEGHE, J., VOLCKAERT, G. and YSEBAERT, M. (1978) Complete nucleotide sequence of SV40 DNA. *Nature* **273**: 113–120.

FINCH, J. T. and CRAWFORD, L. V. (1975) Structure of small DNA-containing animal viruses. In: *Comprehensive Virology*, vol. 5, pp. 119–154, FRAENKEL-CONRAT, H. and WAGNER, R. R. (eds). Plenum Press, New York.

FLANEGAN, J. B., PETTERSON, R. F., AMBROS, V., HEWLETT, M. J. and BALTIMORE, D. (1977) Covalent linkage of a protein to a defined nucleotide sequence at the 5'-terminus of virion and replicative intermediate RNAs of poliovirus. *Proc. Natn. Acad. Sci. USA* **74**: 961–965.

FLINT, S. J., GALLIMORE, P. H. and SHARP, P. A. (1975). Comparison of viral RNA sequences in adenovirus 2-transformed and lytically infected cells. *J. Mol. Biol.* **96**: 47–68.

FLINT, S. J. and SHARP, P. A. (1976) Adenovirus transcription. V. Quantitation of viral RNA sequences in adenovirus 2-infected and transformed cells. *J. Mol. Biol.* **106**: 749–771.

FRANKLIN, R. M. and BALTIMORE, D. (1962) Patterns of macromolecular synthesis in normal and virus-infected mammalian cells. *Cold. Spring. Harbor Symp. Quant. Biol.* **27**: 175–198.

FRENKEL, N. and ROIZMAN, B. (1972) Separation of the herpesvirus deoxyribonucleic acid on sedimentation in alkaline gradients. *J. Virol.* **10**: 565–572.

FRENKEL, N., SILVERSTEIN, S., CASSAI, E. and ROIZMAN, B. (1973) RNA synthesis in cells infected with herpes simplex virus VII. Control of transcription and of transcript abundances of unique and common sequences of herpes simplex 1 and 2, *J. Virol.* **11**: 886–892.

FRIEDMAN, R. M. (1977) Antiviral activity of interferons. *Bacteriol. Rev.* **41**: 543–567.

FRITZ, M. E. and NAHMIAS, A. J. (1972) Reversed polarity in transmembrane potential of cells infected with herpes virus. *Proc. Soc. Exp. Biol. Med.* **139**: 1159–1161.

GALLIONE, C. J., GREENE, J. R., IVERSON, L. E. and ROSE, J. K. (1981) Nucleotide sequences of the mRNA's encoding the vesicular stomatitis virus N and NS proteins. *J. Virol.* **39**: 529–535.

GAROFF, H., FRISCHAUF, A. M., SIMONS, K., LEHRACH, H. and DELIUS, H. (1980) The capsid protein of Semliki Forest virus has clusters of basic amino acids and prolines in its amino-terminal region. *Proc. Natn. Acad. Sci. USA* **77**: 6376–6380.

GAROFF, H., SIMONS, K. and DOBBERSTEIN, B. (1978) Assembly of the Semliki Forest virus membrane glycoproteins in the membrane of the endoplasmic reticulum *in vitro*. *J. Mol. Biol.* **124**: 587–600.

GAROFF, H. and SÖDERLUND, H. (1978) The amphiphilic membrane glycoproteins of Semliki Forest virus are attached to the lipid bilayer by their COOH-terminal ends. *J. Mol. Biol.* **124**: 535–549.

GARON, C. F., BARBOSA, E. and MOSS, B. (1978) Visualization of an inverted terminal repetition in vaccinia virus DNA. *Proc. Natn. Acad. Sci. USA* **75**: 4863–4867.

GARRY, R. F., BISHOP, J. M., PARKER, S., WESTBROOK, K., LEWIS, G. and WAITE, M. R. F. (1979) Na^+ and K^+ concentrations and the regulation of protein synthesis in Sindbis virus-infected chick cells. *Virology* **96**: 108–120.

GAUSH, C. R. and YOUGNER, J. S. (1963) Lipids of virus infected cells. II. Lipid analysis of HeLa cells infected with vaccinia virus. *Proc. Soc. Exp. Biol. Med.* **112**: 1082–1085.

GELMANN, E. P., WONG-STAAL, F., KRAMER, R. A. and GALLO, R. C. (1981) Molecular cloning and comparative analyses of the genomes of simian virus and its associated helper virus. *Proc. Natn. Acad. Sci. USA* **78**: 3373–3377.

GENTY, N. (1975) Analysis of uridine incorporation in chicken embryo cells infected by vesicular stomatitis virus and its temperature-sensitive mutants: Uridine transport. *J. Virol.* **15**: 8–15.

GENTY, N. (1978) Modifications induced by VSV and ts mutants in chick embryo cell permeation. In: *Negative Strand Viruses and the Host Cell*. MAHY, B. W. and BARRYODS, R. D. Academic Press, London.

GERSTEIN, D. C., DAWSON, C. R. and OH, J. O. (1975) Phosphonoacetic acid in the treatment of experimental herpes simplex keratitis. *Antim. Agents and Chemoth.* **7**: 285–288.

GESHELIN, P. and BERNS, K. I. (1974) Characterization and localization of the naturally occurring cross-links in vaccinia virus DNA. *J. Mol. Biol.* **88**: 785–796.

GHOSH, H. P., TONEGUZZO, F. and WELLS, S. (1973) Synthesis *in vitro* of vesicular stomatitis virus proteins in cytoplasmic extracts of L cells. *Biochem. Biophys. Res. Commun.* **54**: 228–233.

GIBSON, W. and ROIZMAN, B. (1974) Proteins specified by herpes simplex virus. A. Staining and radiolabeling properties of B-capsid and virion proteins in polyacrylamide gels. *J. Virol.* **13**: 155–165.

GILBERT, V. E. (1963) Enzyme release from tissue cultures as an indicator of cellular injury by viruses. *Virology* **21**: 609–616.

GINSBERG, H. S., BELLO, L. J. and LEVINE, A. J. (1967) Control of biosynthesis of host macromolecules in cells infected with adenovirus. In: *The Molecular Biology of Viruses*, pp. 547–572, COLTER, J. S. and PARANCHYCH, W. (eds.). Academic Press, New York.

GIRARD, M., BALTIMORE, D. and DARNELL, J. E. Jr. (1967) The poliovirus replication complex: site for synthesis of poliovirus RNA. *J. Mol. Biol.* **24**: 59–74.

GLANVILLE, N. and LACHMI, B. E. (1977) Translation of proteins accounting for the full coding capacity of the Semliki Forest virus 42 S RNA genome. *FEBS Letters* **81**: 399–402.

GLANVILLE, N., MORSER, J., VOMALA, P. and KÄÄRIÄINEN, L. (1976a) Simultaneous translation of structural and nonstructural proteins from Semliki Forest virus RNA in two eukaryotic systems *in vitro*. *Eur. J. Biochem.* **64**: 167–175.

GLANVILLE, N., RANKI, M., MORSER, J., KÄÄRIÄINEN, L. and SMITH, A. E. (1976b) Initiation of translation directed by 42 S and 26 S RNAs from Semliki Forest virus *in vitro*. *Proc. Natn. Sci. USA.* **73**: 3059–3063.

GODEFROY-COLBURN, T. and THACH, R. E. (1981) The role of mRNA competition in regulating translation. IV. Kinetic model. *J. Biol. Chem.* **256**: 11.762–11.773.

GOFF, S. P., GILBOA, E., WITTE, O. N. and BALTIMORE, D. (1980) Structure of the Abelson murine leukemia virus genome and the homologous cellular gene: studies with cloned viral DNA. *Cell* **22**: 777–785.

GOLINI, F., SEMLER, B. L., DORNER, A. J. and WIMMER, E. (1980) Protein-linked RNA of poliovirus is competent to form an initiation complex of translation *in vitro*. *Nature* **287**: 600–603.

GOLINI, F., THACH, S. A., BIRGE, C. H., SAFER, B., MERRICK, W. C. and THACH, R. E. (1976) Competition between cellular and viral mRNAs *in vitro* is regulated by a messenger discriminatory initiation factor. *Proc. Natn. Acad. Sci. USA* **73**: 3040–3044.

GOMATOS, P. J. and TAMM, I. (1963) The secondary structure of reovirus RNA. *Proc. Natn. Acad. Sci. USA* **49**: 707–714.

GORBALENYA, A. E., SVITKIN, Y. V., KAZACHKOV, Y. A. and AGOL, V. I. (1979) Encephalomyocarditis virus-specific polypeptide p22 is involved in the processing of the viral precursor polypeptides. *FEBS Letters* **108**: 1–5.

GRANADOS, R. R. (1973) Entry of an insect poxvirus by fusion of the virus envelope with the host cell membrane. *Virology* **52**: 305–309.

GRANBOULAN, N. and GIRARD, M. (1969) Molecular weight of poliovirus ribonucleic acid. *J. Virol.* **4**: 475–479.

GREEN, M., PARSONS, J. Y., PIÑA, M., FUJINAGA, K., CAFFIER, H. and LANDGRAF-LEURS, I. (1970) Transcription of adenovirus genes in productively infected and in transformed cells. *Cold Spring Harbor Symp. Quant. Biol.* **35**: 803–813.

GRIFFIN, J. D., SPANGLER, G. and LIVINGSTON, D. M. (1979) Protein kinase activity associated with simian virus 40 T antigen. *Proc. Natn. Acad. Sci. USA* **76**: 2610–2614.

GRUBMAN, M. J., EHRENFELD, E. and SUMMERS, D. F. (1974) *In vitro* synthesis of proteins by membrane-bound polyribosomes from vesicular stomatitis virus-infected HeLa cells. *J. Virol.* **14**: 560–571.

GSCHWENDER, H. H. and TRAUB, P. (1979) Mengovirus-induced capping of virus receptors on the plasma membrane of Ehrlich ascites tumor cells. *J. Gen. Virol.* **42**: 439–442.

HACKETT, P., EGBERTS, E. and TRAUB, P. (1978a) Translation of ascites and mengovirus RNA in fractionated cell-free systems from uninfected and mengovirus-infected Ehrlich-ascites-tumor cells. *Eur. J. Biochem.* **83**: 341–352.

HACKETT, P. B., EGBERTS, E. and TRAUB, P. (1978b) Selective translation of mengovirus RNA over host mRNA in homologous, fractionated, cell-free translational systems from Ehrlich-ascites-tumor cells. *Eur. J. Biochem.* **83**: 353–361.

HANSEN, J. and EHRENFELD, E. (1981) Presence of the cap binding protein in initiation factor preparations from poliovirus-infected HeLa cells. *J. Virol.* **38**: 438–445.

HASELTINE, W. A., KLEID, D. G., PANET, A., ROTHENBERG, E. and BALTIMORE, D. (1976) Ordered transcription of RNA tumor virus genomes. *J. Mol. Biol.* **106**: 109–131.

HASELTINE, W. A., MAXAM, A. M. and GILBERT, W. (1977) Rous sarcoma virus genome is terminally redundant: The 5′ sequence. *Proc. Natn. Acad. Sci. USA* **74**: 989–993.

HAYWARD, G. S., FRENKEL, N. and ROIZMAN, B. (1975) The anatomy of herpes simplex virus DNA: Strain difference and heterogeneity in the location of restriction endonuclease cleavage sites. *Proc. Natn. Acad. Sci. USA* **72**: 1768–1772.

HEINE, J. W. and ROIZMAN, B. (1973) Proteins specified by herpes simplex virus. IX Contiguity of host and viral proteins in the plasma membrane of infected cells. *J. Virol.* **11**: 810–813.

HELENIUS, A., KARTENBECK, J., SIMONS, K. and FRIES, E. (1980) On the entry of Semliki Forest virus into BHK-21 cells. *J. Cell Biol.* **84**: 404–420.

HELENIUS, A., MOREIN, B., FRIES, E., SIMONS, K., ROBINSON, P., SCHIRRMACHER, V., TERHORST, C. and STROMINGER, J. L. (1978) Human (HLA-A and HLA-B) and murine (H-2K and H-2D) histocompatibility antigens are cell surface receptors for Semliki Forest virus. *Proc. Natn. Acad. Sci. USA* **75**: 3846–3850.

HELENTJARIS, T. and EHRENFELD, E. (1978) Control of protein synthesis in extracts from poliovirus-infected cells. 1 mRNA discrimination by crude initiation factors. *J. Virol.* **26**: 510–521.

HERSHKO, A. and FRY, M. (1975) Post-translational cleavage of polypeptide chains: role in assembly. *Ann. Rev. Biochem.* **44**: 775–797.

HEWLETT, M. J., ROSE, J. K. and BALTIMORE, D. (1976) 5' Terminal structure of poliovirus polyribosomal RNA is pUp. *Proc. Natn. Acad. Sci. USA* **73**: 327–330.

HEWLETT, M. J., ROZENBLATT, S., AMBROS, V. and BALTIMORE, D. (1977) Separation and quantitation of intracellular forms of poliovirus RNA by agarose gel electrophoresis. *Biochemistry.* **16**: 2763–2767.

HOFFMANN, C. E. (1976) Anviral agents. *Ann. rep. Med. Chem.* **11**: 128–137.

HOLLAND, J. J. (1964) Inhibition of host cell macromolecular synthesis by high multiplicities of poliovirus under conditions preventing virus synthesis. *J. Mol. Biol.* **8**: 574–581.

HOLLAND, J. J. (1965) Depression of host-controlled RNA synthesis in human cells during poliovirus infection. *Proc. Natn. Acad. Sci. USA* **49**: 23–28.

HOLOWCZAK, J. A. and JOKLIK, W. K. (1967) Studies of the structural proteins of vaccinia virus. II. Kinetics of the synthesis of individual groups of structural proteins. *Virology* **33**: 726–739.

HONESS, R. W. and ROIZMAN, B. (1974) Regulation of herpesvirus macromolecular synthesis. I. Cascade regulation of the synthesis of three groups of viral proteins. *J. Virol.* **14**: 8–19.

HONESS, R. W. and ROIZMAN, B. (1975a) Regulation of herpesvirus macromolecular synthesis: Sequential transition of polypeptide synthesis requires functional viral polypeptides. *Proc. Natn. Acad. Sci. USA* **72**: 1276–1295.

HONESS, R. W. and ROIZMAN, B. (1975b) Proteins specified by herpes simplex virus. XIII. Glycosilation of viral polypeptides. *J. Virol.* **16**: 1308–1326.

HONESS, R. W. and WATSON, D. H. (1974) Herpes simplex virus-specific polypeptides studied by polyacrylamide gel electrophoresis of immune precipitates. *J. Gen. Virol.* **22**: 171–183.

HONESS, R. W. and WATSON, D. H. (1977) Unity and diversity in the Herpesvirus. *J. gen. Virol.* **37**: 15–37.

HORDERN, J. S., LEONARD, J. D. and SCRABA, D. G. (1979) Structure of the mengo virion. VI. Spatial relationships of the capsid polypeptides as determined by chemical cross-linking analyses. *Virology* **97**: 131–140.

HOSAKA, Y. and SHIMIZU, K. (1977) Cell fusion by Sendai virus. In: *Virus Infection and the Cell Surface*, pp. 129–156, POSTE, G. and NICOLSON, G. L. (eds.). North-Holland Publ. Comp.

HRUBY, D. E., GUARINO, L. A. and KATES, J. R. (1979) Vaccinia virus replication. I. Requirement for the host–cell nucleus. *J. Virol.* **29**: 705–715.

HSU, T. W., SABRAN, J. L., MARK, G. E., GUNTAKA, R. V. and TAYLOR, J. M. (1978) Analysis of unintegrated avian RNA tumor virus double-stranded DNA intermediates. *J. Virol.* **28**: 810–818.

HUANG, A. S. and BALTIMORE, D. (1970) Defective viral particles and viral disease processes. *Nature* **226**: 325–327.

HUANG, A. S. and WAGNER, R. R. (1965) Inhibition of cellular RNA synthesis by non-replicating vesicular stomatitis virus. *Proc. Natn. Acad. Sci. USA* **54**: 1579–1584.

HUANG, A. S. and WAGNER, R. R. (1966) Comparative sedimentation coefficients of RNA extracted from plaque-forming and defective particles of vesicular stomatitis virus. *J. Mol. Biol.* **22**: 381–384.

HUEBNER, R. J. and TODARO, G. J. (1969) Oncogenes of RNA tumor viruses as determinants of cancer. *Proc. Natn. Acad. Sci. USA* **64**: 1087–1094.

HUNT, L. A. (1976) *In vitro* translation of encephalomyocarditis viral RNA: Synthesis of capsid precursor-like polypeptides. *Virology* **70**: 484–492.

HUNTER, T. and GIBSON, W. (1978) Characterization of the mRNA's for the polyoma virus capsid proteins VP1, VP2 and VP3, *J. Virol.* **28**: 240–253.

HUNTER, T., HUTCHINSON, M. A. and ECKHART, W. (1978) Translation of pólyoma virus T antigens *in vitro. Proc. Natn. Acad. Sci. USA* **75**: 5917–5921.

HUNTER, T. and SEFTON, B. M. (1980) Transforming gene product of Rous sarcoma virus phosphorylates tyrosine. *Proc. Natn. Acad. Sci. USA* **77**: 1311–1315.

HUTCHINSON, M. A., HUNTER, T. and ECKHART, W. (1978) Characterization of T antigens in polyoma infected and transformed cells. *Cell* **15**: 65–77.

IKEDA, H., PINCUS, T., YOSHIKI, T., STRAND, M., AUGUST, Y., BOYSE, E. and MELLORS, R. C. (1974) Biological expression of antigenic determinants of murine leukemia virus proteins gp 69/71 and p 30. *J. Virol.* **14**: 1274–1280.

IRVIN, J. D. (1975) Purification and partial characterization of an antiviral protein from *Phytolacca americana* which inhibits eukaryotic protein synthesis. *Arch. Biochem. Biophys.* **169**: 522–528.

ITO, Y., BROCKLEHURST, J. R. and DULBECCO, R. (1977) Virus-specific proteins in the plasma membrane of cells lytically infected or transformed by polyoma virus. *Proc. Natn. Acad. Sci. USA* **74**: 4666–4670.

ITO, Y., SPURR, N. and GRIFFIN, B. E. (1980) Middle T antigen as primary inducer of full expression of the phenotype of transformation by polyoma virus. *J. Virol.* **35**: 219–232.

IWASAKI, Y., FURUKAWA, T., PLOTKIN, S. and KOPROWSKI, H. (1973) Ultrastructural study on the sequence of human cytomegalo-virus infection in human diploid cells. *Arch. Ges. Virusforsch.* **40**: 311–324.

JACKSON, V. and CHALKLEY, R. (1981) Use of whole-cell fixation to visualize replicating and maturing simian virus 40: Identification of new viral gene product. *Proc. Natn. Acad. Sci. USA* **78**: 6081–6085.

JACOBSON, M. F., ASSO, J. and BALTIMORE, D. (1970) Further evidence on the formation of poliovirus proteins. *J. Mol. Biol.* **49**: 657–669.

JACOBSON, M. F. and BALTIMORE, D. (1968a) Morphogenesis of poliovirus. I. Association of the viral RNA with the coat protein. *J. Mol. Biol.* **33**: 369–378.

JACOBSON, M. F. and BALTIMORE, D. (1968b) Polypeptide cleavage in the formation of poliovirus proteins. *Proc. Natn. Acad. Sci. USA* **61**: 77–84.

JACQUEMONT, B., GRANGE, J., GAZZOLO, L. and RICHARD, M. H. (1972) Composition and size of Shope fibroma virus deoxyribonucleic acid. *J. Virol.* **9**: 836–841.

JAY, G., NOMURA, S., ANDERSON, C. W. and KHOURY, G. (1981) Identification of the SV40 agnogene product: a DNA binding protein. *Nature* **291**: 346–349.

JAY, E., ROYCHOUDHURY, R. and WU, R. (1976) Nucleotide sequence with elements of an unusual two-fold rotational symmetry in the region of origin of replication of SV40 DNA. *Biochem. Biophys. Res. Commun.* **69**: 678–686.

JEN, G., DETJEN, B. M. and THACH, R. E. (1980) Shut-off of HeLa cell protein synthesis by encephalomyocarditis virus and poliovirus: a comparative study. *J. Virol.* **35**: 150–156.

JOKLIK, W. K. (1974) Reproduction of reoviridae. In: *Comprehensive Virology*, Vol. 2, pp. 231–334, FRAENKEL-CONRAT, H. and WAGNER, R. R. (eds.). Plenum Press, New York.

JOKLIK, W. K. (1981) Structure and function of the reovirus genome. *Microbiological Rev.* **45**: 483–501.

JÖRNVALL, H., AKUSJÄRVI, G., ALESTRÖM, P., VON BAHR-LINDSTRÖM, H., PETTERSON, U., APPELLA, E., FOWLER, A. V. and PHILIPSON, L. (1981) The adenovirus hexon protein. The primary structure of the polypeptide and its correlation with the hexon gene. *J. Biol. Chem.* **256**: 6181–6186.

KÄÄRIÄINEN, L. and RENKONEN, O. (1977) Envelopes of lipid-containing viruses as models for membrane assembly. In: *The Synthesis, Assembly and Turnover of Cell Surface Components*, pp. 741–801, POSTE, G. and NICHOLSON, G. L. (eds.). Elsevier, North-Holland Biomedical Press.

KAERLEIN, M. and HORAK, I. (1976) Phosphorylation of ribosomal proteins in HeLa cells infected with vaccinia virus. *Nature* **259**: 150–151.

KAERLEIN, M. and HORAK, I. (1978) Identification and characterization of ribosomal proteins phosphorylated in vaccinia virus-infected HeLa cells. *Eur. J. Biochem.* **90**: 463–469.

KALASAVSKAITÉ, E., GRINIUS, L., KADISAITE, D. and JASAITIS, A. (1980) Electrochemical H^+ gradient but not phosphate potential is required for *Escherichia coli* infection by phage T4. *FEBS Letters* **117**: 232–236.

KALUZA, G. (1976) Early synthesis of Semliki Forest virus-specific proteins in infected chicken cells. *J. Virol.* **19**: 1–12.

KAMINE, J. and BUCHANAN, J. M. (1977) Cell-free synthesis of two proteins unique to RNA of transforming virions of Rous sarcoma virus. *Proc. Natn. Acad. Sci. USA* **74**: 2011–2015.

KAMINE, J., BURR, J. G. and BUCHANAN, J. M. (1978) Multiple forms of sarc gene proteins from Rous sarcoma virus RNA. *Proc. Natn. Acad. Sci. USA* **75**: 366–370.

KAMIYA, T., BEN-PORAT, T. and KAPLAN, A. S. (1964) The role of progeny viral DNA in the regulation of enzyme and DNA synthesis. *Biochem. Biophys. Res. Commun.* **16**: 410–415.

KARESS, R. E., HAYWORD, W. S. and HANAFUSA, H. (1979) Cellular information in the genome of recovered avian sarcoma virus directs the synthesis of transforming protein. *Proc. Natn. Acad. Sci. USA* **76**: 3154–3158.

KATES, J. R. and BEESON, J. (1970) Ribonucleic acid synthesis in vaccinia virus. II. Synthesis of polyriboadenylic acid. *J. Mol. Biol.* **50**: 19–33.

KAUFMANN, Y., GOLDSTEIN, E. and PENMAN, S. (1976) Poliovirus-induced inhibition of polypeptide initiation *in vitro* on native polyribosomes. *Proc. Natn. Acad. Sci. USA* **73**: 1834–1838.

KAVENOFF, R., TALCOVE, D. and MUDD, J. A. (1975) Genome-sized RNA from reovirus particles. *Proc. Natn. Acad. Sci. USA* **72**: 4317–4321.

KAWAI, S. and HANAFUSA, H. (1971) The effects of reciprocal changes in temperature on the transformed state of cells infected with a Rous sarcoma virus mutant. *Virology* **46**: 470–479.

KEENE, J. D., SCHUBERT, M. and LAZZARINI, R. A. (1979) Terminal sequences of vesicular stomatitis virus RNA are both complementary and conserved. *J. Virol.* **32**: 167–174.

KELLER, J. M., SPEAR, P. G. and ROIZMAN, B. (1970) The proteins specified by herpes simplex virus III. Viruses differing in their effects on the social behavior of infected cells specify different membrane glycoproteins. *Proc. Natn. Acad. Sci. USA* **65**: 865–871.

KELLY, T. J. and NATHANS, D. (1977) The genome of simian virus 40. In: *Advances in Virus Research*, Vol. 21. pp. 85–174, LAUFFER, M. A., BANG, F. B., MARAMOROSCH, R. and SMITH, K. M. (eds.). Academic Press, New York.

KENNEDY, S. I. T. (1976) Sequence relationships between the genome and the intracellular RNA species of standard defective-interfering Semliki Forest virus. *J. Mol. Biol.* **108**: 491–511.

KERANEN, S. and KÄÄRIÄINEN, L. (1974) Isolation and basic characterization of temperature sensitive mutants from Semliki Forest virus. *Acta Pathol. Microbiol. Scand. Sect. B*, **82**: 810–820.

KILEY, M. P. and WAGNER, R. R. (1972) Ribonucleic acid species of intracellular nucleocapsids and released virions of vesicular stomatitis virus. *J. Virol.* **10**: 244–255.

KING, A. M. Q. (1976) High molecular weight RNAs from Rous sarcoma virus and Moloney murine leukemia virus contain two subunits. *J. Biol. Chem.* **251**: 141–149.

KIT, S. and DUBBS, D. R. (1962) Biochemistry of vaccinia-infected mouse fibroblasts (strain L-M) I. Effects on nucleic acid and protein synthesis. *Virology* **18**: 274–285.

KITAMURA, N., SEMLER, B. L., ROTHBERG, P. G., LARSEN, G. R., ADLER, C. J., DORNER, A. J., EMINI, E. A., HANECAK, R., LEE, J. J., VAN DER WERF, S., ANDERSON, C. W. and WIMMER, E. (1981) Primary structure gene organization and polypeptide expression of poliovirus RNA. *Nature* **291**: 547–553.

KLESSIG, D. G. (1977) Two adenovirus mRNAs have a common 5′ terminal leader sequence encoded at least 10 Kb upstream from their main coding regions. *Cell* **17**: 9–21.

KOHN, A. (1979) Early interactions of viruses with cellular membranes. *Adv. Virus. Res.* **24**: 223–276.

KOHN, A., GITELMAN, J. and INBAR, M. (1980) Interaction of polyunsaturated fatty acids with animal cells and enveloped viruses. *Antim. Agents Chemoth.* **18**: 962–968.

KOPCHICK, J. J., JAMJOON, G. A., WATSON, K. F. and ARLINGHAUS, R. B. (1978) Biosynthesis of reverse transcriptase from Rauscher murine leukemia virus by synthesis and cleavage of a gag-pol read-through viral precursor polyprotein. *Proc. Natn. Acad. Sci. USA* **75**: 2016–2020.

KORANT, B. D. (1975) Regulation of animal virus replication by protein cleavage. In: *Proteases and Biological Control*, pp. 621–644. Cold Spring Harbor, New York.

KORANT, B. D. (1977) Poliovirus coat protein as the site of guanidine action. *Virology* **81**: 25–36.

KORANT, B., SHOW, N., LIVELY, M. and POWERS, J. (1979) Virus-specified protease is poliovirus-infected HeLa cells. *Proc. Natn. Acad. Sci. USA* **76**: 2992–2995.

KOZAK, M. (1977) Nucleotide sequences of 5′ terminal ribosome-protected initiation regions from two reovirus messages. *Nature* **269**: 390–394.

KOZAK, M. and SHATKIN, A. J. (1976) Characterization of ribosome protected fragments from reovirus messenger RNA. *J. Biol. Chem.* **251**: 4259–4266.

KOZAK, M. and SHATKIN, A. J. (1977a) Sequences of two 5'-terminal ribosome-protected fragments from reovirus messenger RNAs. *J. Mol. Biol.* **112**: 75–96.

KOZAK, M. and SHATKIN, A. J. (1977b) Sequences and properties of two ribosome binding sites from the small size class of reovirus messenger RNA. *J. Biol. Chem.* **252**: 6895–6908.

KOZAK, M. and SHATKIN, A. J. (1978) Identification of features in 5' terminal fragments from reovirus mRNA.

KRZYZEK, R. A., COLETT, M. S., LAV, A. F., PERDUE, M. L., LEIS, J. P. and FARAS, A. J. (1978) Evidence for splicing of avian sarcoma virus 5'-terminal genomic sequences onto viral-specific RNA in infected cells. *Proc. Natn. Acad. Sci. USA* **75**: 1284–1288.

KUSMIEREK, J. and SHUGAR, D. (1979) Nucleotides, nucleoside phosphate diesters and phosphonates as antiviral antineoplastic agents. An overview. In: *Antiviral Mechanisms in the Control of Neoplasia*, pp. 481–498, CHANDRA, P. (ed.). Plenum Press, New York.

LABEDAN, B. and GOLBERG, E. B. (1979) Requirement for membrane potential in injection of phage T4 DNA. *Proc. Natn. Acad. Sci. USA* **76**: 4669–4673.

LACAL, J. C. and CARRASCO, L. (1982) Relationship between membrane integrity and the inhibition of host translation in virus-infected mammalian cells. Comparative studies between encephalomyocarditis virus and poliovirus. *Eur. J. Biochem.* **127**: 359–366.

LACAL, J. C., VAZQUEZ, D., FERNANDEZ-SOUSA, J. M. and CARRASCO, L. (1980) Antibiotics that specifically block translation in virus-infected cells. *J. Antibiotics* **33**: 441–447.

LACHMI, B. E. and KÄÄRIÄINEN, L. (1976) Sequential translation of nonstructural proteins in cells infected with a Semliki Forest virus mutant. *Proc. Natn. Acad. Sci. USA* **73**: 1936–1940.

LACHMI, B. E. and KÄÄRIÄINEN, L. (1977) Control of protein synthesis in Semliki Forest virus-infected cells. *J. Virol.* **22**: 142–149.

LAI, C. J., DHAR, R. and KHOURY, G. (1978) Mapping the spliced and unspliced late lytic SV 40 RNAs. *Cell* **14**: 971–982.

LANE, D. P. and CRAWFORD, L. V. (1979) T antigen is bound to a host protein in SV 40-transformed cells. *Nature* **278**: 261–263.

LANIA, L., GRIFFITHS, M., COOKE, B., ITO, Y. and FRIED, M. (1979) Untransformed rat cells containing free and integrated DNA of polyoma nontransforming (Hr-t) mutant. *Cell* **18**: 793–802.

LARSEN, G. R., DORNER, A. J., HARRIS, T. J. R. and WIMMER, E. (1980) The structure of poliovirus replicative form. *Nucleic Acids Res.* **8**: 1217–1229.

LAUB, O., BRATOSIN, S., HOROWITZ, M. and ALONI, Y. (1979) The initiation of transcription of SV40 DNA at late time after infection. *Virology* **92**: 310–323.

LAWRENCE, C. and THACH, R. E. (1974) Encephalomyocarditis virus infection of mouse plasmocytoma cells. *J. Virol.* **14**: 598–610.

LAZAROWITZ, S. G., COMPANS, R. W. and CHOPPIN, P. W. (1971) Influenza virus structural and nonstructural proteins in infected cells and their plasma membranes. *Virology* **46**: 830–843.

LEIBOWITZ, R. and PENMAN, S. (1971) Regulation of protein synthesis in HeLa cells. Inhibition during poliovirus infection. *J. Virol.* **8**: 661–668.

LEMASTER, S. and ROIZMAN, B. (1980) Herpes simplex virus phosphoproteins. II. Characterization of the virion protein kinase and of the polypeptides phosphorylated in the virion. *J. Virol.* **35**: 798–811.

LEVANON, A. and KOHN, A. (1978) Changes in cell membrane microviscosity associated with adsorption of viruses. *FEBS Letters* **85**: 245–248.

LEVANON, A., KOHN, A. and INBAR, M. (1977) Increase in lipid fluidity of cellular membranes induced by adsorption of RNA and DNA virions. *J. Virol.* **22**: 353–360.

LEVIN, K. H. and SAMUEL, C. E. (1977) Biosynthesis of reovirus-specified polypeptides. Effect of methylation on the efficiency of reovirus genome expression *in vitro*. *Virology* **77**: 245–259.

LEVIN, K. H. and SAMUEL, C. E. (1980) Biosynthesis of reovirus-specified polypeptides. Purification and characterization of the small-sized class mRNAs of reovirus type 3: coding assignments and translational efficiencies. *Virology* **106**: 1–13.

LEVINE, A. J. (1976) SV40 and adenovirus early functions involved in DNA replication and transformation. *Biochem. Biophys. Acta* **458**: 213–241.

LEVINE, A. J. and GINSBERG, H. S. (1967) Biochemical studies on the mechanism by which the fiber antigen inhibits multiplication of type 5 adenovirus. *J. Virol.* **1**: 747–759.

LEVINTOW, L. (1974) The replication of picornaviruses. In: *Comprehensive Virology*, Vol. 3, pp. 109–169, FRAENKEL-CONRAT, H. and WAGNER, R. R. (eds.). Plenum Press, New York.

LEWIS, J. B., ATKINS, J. F., BAUM, P. R., SOLEM, R., GESTELAND, R. F. and ANDERSON, C. W. (1976) Location and identification of the genes for adenovirus type 2 early polypeptides. *Cell* **7**: 141–151.

LEWIS, J. B. and MATHEWS, M. B. (1980) Control of adenovirus early gene expression: a class of immediate early products. *Cell* **21**: 303–313.

LINDBERG, U., PERSSON, R. and PHILIPSON, L. (1972) Isolation and characterization of adenovirus mRNA in productive infection. *J. Virol.* **10**: 909–919.

LINGAPPA, V. R., KATZ, F. N., LODISH, H. F. and BLOBEL, G. (1978) A signal sequence for the insertion of a transmembrane glycoprotein. *J. Biol. Chem.* **253**: 8667–8670.

LODDO, B., FERRARI, W., SPANEDDA, A. and BROTZU, G. (1962) *In vitro* guanidino resistance guanidino-dependence of poliovirus. *Experientia* **18**: 518–519.

LODISH, H. F. and FROSHAVER, S. (1977) Rates of initiation of protein synthesis by two purified species of vesicular stomatitis virus messenger RNA. *J. Biol. Chem.* **252**: 8804–8811.

LODISH, H. F. and PORTER, M. (1980) Translational control of protein synthesis after infection by vesicular stomatitis virus. *J. Virol.* **36**: 719–733.

LODISH, H. F. and PORTER, M. (1981) Vesicular stomatitis virus mRNA and inhibition of translation of cellular mRNA. Is there a P function in vesicular stomatitis virus? *J. Virol.* **38**: 504–517.

LONBERG-HOLM, K. and KORANT, B. D. (1972) Early interactions of rhinoviruses with host cells. *J. Virol.* **9**: 29–40.

LOWRY, D. R., ROWE, W. P., TEICH, N. and HARTLEY, J. W. (1971) Murine leukemia virus high-frequency activation *in vitro* by 5-iododeoxy-uridine and 5-bromodeoxyuridine. *Science* **174**: 155–156.

LUCAS-LENARD, J. (1974) Cleavage of mengovirus polyproteins *in vivo*. *J. Virol.* **14**: 261–269.

LYLES, D. A. and LANDSBERGER, R. F. (1977) Sendai virus-induced homolysis: Reduction in heterogeneity of erthrocyte lipid bilayer fluidity. *Proc. Natn. Acad. Sci. USA* **74**: 1918–1922.

MAIZEL, J. V. JR. and SUMMERS, D. F. (1968) Evidence for differences in size and composition of the poliovirus-specific polypeptides in infected HeLa cells. *Virology* **36**: 46–54.

MAJORS, J. E. and VARMUS, H. E. (1981) Nucleotide sequences at host-proviral junctions for mouse mammary tumour viruses. *Nature* **289**: 253–258.

MARSDEN, H. S., CROMBIE, I. K. and SUBAK-SHARPE, J. H. (1976) Control of protein synthesis in herpesvirus-infected cells: Analysis of the polypeptides induced by wild type and sixteen temperature-sensitive mutants of HSV strain 17. *J. gen. Virol.* **31**: 347–372.

MARSDEN, H. S., STOW, N. D., PRESTON, V. G., TIMBURY, M. C. and WILKIE, N. M. (1978) Physical mapping of herpes simplex virus induced polypeptides. *J. Virol.* **28**: 624–642.

MARTIN, G. S. (1970) Rous sarcoma virus: A function required for maintenance of the transformed state. *Nature* **227**: 1021–1023.

MARTIN, R. G. and CHOU, J. Y. (1975) Simian virus 40 function required for the establishment and maintenance of malignant transformation. *J. Virol.* **15**: 599–612.

MARTIN, E. and WORK, T. (1961) Studies on protein synthesis and nucleic acid metabolism in virus infected mammalian cells. 4. The localization of metabolic changes within cellular subfractions of Krebs II mouse ascites-tumor cells infected with encephalomyocarditis virus. *Biochem. J.* **81**: 514–520.

MATHEWS, M. B. and OSBORN, M. (1974) The rate of polypeptide chain elongation in a cell-free system from Krebs II ascites cells. *Biochem. Biophys. Acta* **340**: 147–152.

MATHIS, D. J. and CHAMBON, P. (1981) The SV40 early region TATA box is required for accurate *in vitro* initiation of transcription. *Nature* **290**: 310–315.

McAUSLAN, B. R. and KATES, J. R. (1967) Poxvirus-induced acid deoxyribonuclease: Regulation of synthesis: Control of activity *in vivo*; purification and properties of the enzyme. *Virology* **33**: 709–718.

McCRAE, M. A. and JOKLIK, W. K. (1978) The nature of the polypeptide encoded by each of the 10 ds RNA segments of reovirus type 3. *Virology* **89**: 578–593.

McGUIRE, P. M., PIATAK, M. and HODGE, L. D. (1976) Nuclear and cytoplasmic adenovirus RNA. Differences between 5'-termini of messenger and non-messenger transcrips. *J. Mol. Biol.* **101**: 379–396.

McGUIRE, P. M., SWART, C. and HODGE, L. D. (1972) Adenovirus messenger RNA in mammalian cells: Failure of polyribosome association in the absence of nuclear cleavage. *Proc. Natn. Acad. Sci. USA* **69**: 1578–1582.

McINTOSH, K., PAYNE, S. and RUSSEL, W. C. (1971) Studies on lipid metabolism in cells infected with adenovirus. *J. Gen. Virol.* **10**: 251–265.

McSHARRY, J. J. and CHOPPIN, P. W. (1978) Biological properties of the VSV glycoprotein. I. Effects of the isolated glycoprotein on host macromolecular synthesis. *Virology* **84**: 172–182.

MICKLEM, K. J. and PASTERNAK, C. A. (1977) Surface components involved in virally mediated membrane changes. *Biochem. J.* **162**: 405–410.

MILLER, J. S., RICCIARDI, R. P., ROBERTS, B. E., PATERSON, B. M. and MATHEWS, M. B. (1980) Arrangement of messenger RNAs and protein coding sequences in the major late transcription unit of adenovirus 2. *J. Mol. Biol.* **142**: 455–488.

MILLER, R. L. and PLAGEMANN, P. W. G. (1972) Purification of mengovirus and identification of an A-rich segment in its ribonucleic acid. *J. Gen. Virol.* **17**: 349–353.

MOCARSKI, E. and ROIZMAN, B. (1981) Site-specific inversion sequence of the herpes simplex virus genome: Domain and structural features. *Proc. Natl. Acad. Sci. USA* **78**: 7047–7051.

MOORE, N. F., PATZER, E. J., SHAW, J. M., THOMPSON, T. E. and WAGNER, R. R. (1978) Interaction of vesicular stomatitis virus with lipid vesicles: Depletion of cholesterol and effect on virion membrane fluidity and infectivity. *J. Virol.* **27**: 320–329.

MORGAN, C., ROSE, H. M. and MEDNIS, B. (1968) Electron microscopy of herpes simplex virus. I. Entry. *J. Virol.* **2**: 507–516.

MORRISON, T. G. and McQUAIN, C. O. (1978) Assembly of viral membranes. Nature of the association of vesicular stomatitis virus proteins to membranes. *J. Virol.* **26**: 115–125.

MORRISON, T., STAMPFER, M., BALTIMORE, D. and LODISH, H. F. (1974) Translation of vesicular stomatitis messenger RNA by extracts from mammalian and plant cells. *J. Virol.* **13**: 62–72.

MORSE, L. S., BUCHMAN, T. G., ROIZMAN, B. and SCHAFFER, P. A. (1977) Anatomy of herpes simplex virus DNA. IX. Apparent exclusion of some parental DNA arrangements in the generation of intertypic (HSV1 × HSV2) recombinants. *J. Virol.* **24**: 231–149.

MOSS, B. (1968) Inhibition of HeLa protein synthesis by the vaccinia virion. *J. Virol.* **2**: 1028–1037.

MOSS, B. (1974) Reproduction of poxviruses. In: *Comprehensive Virology*, Vol. 3, pp. 405–474. FRAENKEL-CONRAT, H. and WAGNER, R. R. (eds.). Plenum Press, New York.

MOSS, B., GERSHOWITZ, A., WEI, C. M. and BOONE, R. (1976) Formation of the guanylylated and methylated 5'-terminus of vaccinia mRNA. *Virology* **72**: 341–351.

MOSS, B. and ROSENBLUM, E. N. (1973) Protein cleavage and poxviral morphogenesis: Triptic peptide analysis of core precursors accumulated by blocking assembly with rifampicin. *J. Mol. Biol.* **81**: 267–269.

MOYER, R. W. and GRAVES, R. L. (1981) The mechanism of cytoplasmic orthopoxvirus DNA replication. *Cell* **27**: 391–401.

MOYER, S. A., GRUBMAN, M. J., EHERENFELD, E. and BANERJEE, A. R. (1975) Studies on the *in vivo* and *in vitro* messenger RNA species of vesicular stomatitis virus. *Virology* **67**: 463–473.

MUDD, J. A. and SUMMERS, D. F. (1970) Protein synthesis in vesicular stomatitis virus-infected HeLa cells. *Virology* **42**: 328–340.

MUELLER, C., GRAESMANN, A. and GRAESMANN, M. (1978) Mapping of early SV40-specific functions by microinjection of different early viral DNA fragments. *Cell* **15**: 579–585.

MUÑOZ, A. and CARRASCO, L. (1981) Protein synthesis and membrane integrity in interferon-treated HeLa cells infected with encephalomyocarditis virus. *J. Gen. Virol.* **56**: 153–162.

MURPHY, E. C., KOPCHICK, J. J., WATSON, K. F. and ARLINGHAUS, R. F. (1978) Cell-free synthesis of a precursor polyprotein containing both gag and pol gene products by Rauscher murine leukemia virus 35 S RNA. *Cell* **13**: 359–369.

MUSTOE, T. A., RAMIG, R. F., SHARPE, A. H. and FIELDS, B. N. (1978) Genetics of reovirus; Identification of the dsRNA segments encoding the polypeptides of the mu and sigma size classes. *Virology* **89**: 594–604.

NAGAYAMA, A., POGO, B. G. T. and DALES, S. (1970) Biogenesis of vaccinia: Separation of early stages from maturation by means of rifampicin. *Virology* **40**: 1039–1051.

NAIR, C. N. and LONBERG-HOLM, K. K. (1971) Infectivity and sedimentation of rhinovirus ribonucleic acid. *J. Virol.* **7**: 278–280.

NAITO, S. and ISHIHAMA, A. (1976) Function and structure of RNA polymerase from vesicular stomatitis virus. *J. Biol. Chem.* **251**: 4307–4314.

NAKATA, Y. and BADER, J. P. (1968) Transformation by murine sarcoma virus: Fixation (deoxyribonucleic and synthesis) and development. *J. Virol.* **2**: 1255–1261.

NASO, R. B., ARCEMENT, L. J. and ARLINGHAUS, R. B. (1975) Biosynthesis of Rauscher leukemia viral proteins. *Cell* **4**: 31–36.

NEVINS, J. R. and DARNELL, J. E. (1977) Groups of adenovirus type 2 mRNA's derived from a large primary transcript probable nuclear origin and possible common 3′ ends. *J. Virol.* **25**: 811–823.

NEVINS, J. R. and WILSON, M. C. (1981) Regulation of adenovirus-2 gene expression at the level of transcriptional termination and RNA processing. *Nature* **290**: 115–118.

NICHOLS, J. L., HAY, A. J. and JOKLIK, W. K. (1972) 5′-terminal nucleotide sequence in reovirus mRNA synthesized *in vitro*. *Nature New Biol.* **235**: 105–107.

NICOLSON, G. L. (1974) The interactions of lectins with animal cell surfaces. *Int. Rev. Cytol.* **39**: 89–190.

NOMOTO, A., LEE, Y. F. and WIMMER, E. (1976) The 5′ end of poliovirus mRNA is not capped with m⁷G(5′)ppp (5′)Np. *Proc. Natn. Acad. Sci. USA* **73**: 375–380.

NORKIN, L. C. (1977) Cell killing by simian virus 40: Impairment of membrane formation and function. *J. Virol.* **21**: 872–879.

NOVAK, U. and GRIFFIN, B. E. (1981) Requirement for the C-terminal region of middle T-antigen in cellular transformation by polyoma virus. *Nucleic Acids Res.* **9**: 2055–2073.

NUSS, D. L. and KOCH, G. (1976) Differential inhibition of vesicular stomatitis virus polypeptide synthesis by hipertonic initiation block. *J. Virol.* **17**: 283–286.

ÖBERG, B. F. and SHATKIN, A. J. (1972) Initiation of picornavirus protein synthesis in ascites cell extracts. *Proc. Natn. Acad. Sci. USA* **69**: 3589–3593.

ODA, K. and JOKLIK, W. K. (1967) Hybridization and sedimentation studies on early and late vaccinia messenger RNA. *J. Mol. Biol.* **27**: 395–419.

OKASINSKI, G. F. and VELICER, L. F. (1977) Analysis of intracellular feline leukemia virus proteins II. Generation of feline leukemia virus structural proteins from precursor polypeptides. *J. Virol.* **22**: 74–85.

OLSNES, S. and PIHL, A. (1976) Abrin, Ricin and their associated agglutinins. In: *Receptors and Recognition Series: The Specificity and Action of Animal, Bacterial and Plant Toxins*, pp. 130–173, CUATRECASAS, P. (ed.). Chapman and Hall, London.

OLSHEVSKY, U., LEVITT, J. and BECKER, Y. (1967) Studies on the synthesis of herpes simplex virions. *Virology* **33**: 323–334.

OPPERMANN, H., BISHOP, J. M., VARMUS, H. E. and LEVINTOW, L. (1977) A joint product of the genes gag and pol of avian sarcoma virus: a possible precursor of reverse transcriptase. *Cell* **12**: 993–1005.

OPPERMANN, H. D., LEVINSON, A., VARMUS, H. E., LEVINTOW, L. and BISHOP, J. M. (1979) Uninfected vertebrate cells contain a protein that is closely related to the product of the avian sarcoma virus transforming gene. *Proc. Natn. Acad. Sci. USA* **76**: 1804–1808.

OSDENE, T. S. (1970) Antiviral Agents. In: *Medical Chemistry*, pp. 662–679, BURGER, A. (ed.). Wiley Interscience, New York, London, Sidney, Toronto.

PALLANSCH, M. A., KEW, O. M., PALMENBERG, A. C., GOLINI, F., WIMMER, E. and RUECKERT, R. R. (1980) Picornaviral VPg sequences are contained in the replicase precursor. *J. Virol.* **35**: 414–419.

PARKER, R. C., VARMUS, H. E. and BISHOP, J. M. (1981) Cellular homologue (c-src) of the transforming gene of Rous sarcoma virus: Isolation, mapping and transcriptional analysis of c-src and flanking regions. *Proc. Natn. Acad. Sci. USA* **78**: 5842–5846.

PARSONS, J. T., GARDNER, J. and GREEN, M. (1971) Biochemical studies on adenovirus multiplication XIX. Resolution of late viral RNA species in the nucleus and cytoplasm. *Proc. Natn. Acad. Sci. USA* **68**: 557–560.

PASTERNAK, C. A. and MICKLEM, K. J. (1981) Virally induced alterations in cellular permeability: A basis of cellular and physiological damage. *Biosc. Reports* **1**: 431–448.

PAUCHA, E., HARVEY, R. and SMITH, A. E. (1978) Cell-free synthesis of simian virus 40 T-Ag. *J. Virol.* **28**: 154–170.

PAUCHA, E. and SMITH, A. E. (1978) The sequences between 0.59 and 0.54 mp units on SV40 DNA code for the unique region of small t antigen. *Cell* **15**: 1011–1020.

PAUCHA, E., SEEHAFER, J. and COLTER, J. S. (1974) Synthesis of viral-specific polypeptides in mengo virus-infected L cells: evidence for asymmetric translation of the viral genome. *Virology* **61**: 315–326.

PAWSON, T., HARVEY, R. and SMITH, A. E. (1977) The size of Rous sarcoma virus mRNAs active in cell-free translation. *Nature* **268**: 416–420.

PAWSON, T., MARTIN, G. S. and SMITH, A. E. (1976) Cell-free translation of virion RNA from nondefective and transformation-defective Rous sarcoma virus. *J. Virol.* **19**: 950–967.

PELHAM, H. R. B. (1978a) Translation of encephalomyocarditis virus RNA *in vitro* yields an active proteolytic processing enzyme. *Eur. J. Biochem.* **85**: 457–462.

PELHAM, H. R. B. (1978b) Leaky UAG termination codon in tobacco mosaic virus RNA. *Nature* **272**: 469–471.

PELHAM, H. R. B., SYKES, J. M. M. and HUNT, T. (1978) Characteristics of a coupled cell-free transcription and translation system directed by vaccinia cores. *Eur. J. Biochem.* **82**: 199–209.

PENMAN, S. (1965) Stimulation of the incorporation of choline in poliovirus-infected cells. *Virology* **25**: 148–152.

PENMAN, S. and SUMMERS, D. (1965) Effects on host cell metabolism following synchronous infection with poliovirus. *Virology* **27**: 614–620.

PENNINGTON, T. H. (1974) Vaccinia virus polypeptide synthesis: sequential appearance and stability of pre- and post-replicative polypeptides. *J. Gen. Virol.* **25**: 433–444.

PENNINGTON, T. H. (1977) Isatin-β-thiosemicarbazone causes premature cessation of vaccinia virus-induced late post-replicative polypeptide synthesis. *J. Gen. Virol.* **35**: 567–571.

PEREIRA, L., CASSAI, E., HONESS, R. W., ROIZMAN, B., TERNI, M. and NAHMIAS, A. (1976) Variability in the structural polypeptides of herpes simplex virus 1 strains: Potential application in molecular epidemiology. *Infection and Immunity* **13**: 211–220.

PÉREZ-BERCOFF, R. and GANDER, M. (1977) The genomic RNA of mengovirus I. Location of the poly(C) tract. *Virology* **80**: 426–429.

PERLMAN, S. M. and HUANG, A. S. (1973) RNA synthesis of vesicular stomatitis virus. V. Interactions between transcription and replication. *J. Virol.* **12**: 1395–1400.

PERSON, A. and BEAUD, G. (1978) Inhibition of host protein synthesis in vaccinia virus infected cells in the presence of cordycepin (3'-Deoxyadenosine). *J. Virol.* **25**: 11–18.

PERSSON, H., JÖRNVALL, H. and ZABIELSKI, J. (1980) Multiple mRNAs species for the precursor to an adenovirus-encoded glycoprotein: Identification and structure of the signal sequence. *Proc. Natn. Acad. Sci.* **77**: 6349–6353.

PERSSON, H., MATHISEN, B., PHILIPSON, L. and PETTERSSON, U. (1979) A maturation protein in adenovirus morphogenesis. *Virology* **93**: 198–208.

PERSSON, H., SIGNÄS, C. and PHILIPSON, L. (1979) Purification and characterization of an early glycoprotein from adenovirus type 2-infected cells. *J. Virol.* **29**: 938–948.

PETTERSON, R. F., AMBROS, V. and BALTIMORE, D. (1978) Identification of a protein linked to nascent poliovirus RNA and to the polyuridylic acid of negative-strand RNA. *J. Virol.* **27**: 357–365.

PETTERSON, R. F., SÖDERLUND, H. and KÄÄRIÄINEN, L. (1980) The nucleotide sequences of the 5'-terminal T1 oligonucleotides of Semliki Forest virus 42S and 26S RNAs are different. *Eur. J. Biochem.* **105**: 435–443.

PETTERSON, V., TINNETTS, C. and PHILIPSON, L. (1976) Hybridization maps of early and late messenger RNA sequences on the adenovirus type 2 genome. *J. Mol. Biol.* **101**: 479–502.

PFEFFERKORN, E. R. and SHAPIRO, D. (1974) Reproduction of togaviruses. In: *Comprehensive Virology*, Vol. 2, pp. 171–230, FRAENKEL-CONRAT, H. and WAGNER, R. R. (eds.). Plenum Press, New York.

PHILIPSON, L., ANDERSSON, P., OLSHEVSKY, U., WEINBERG, R., BALTIMORE, D. and GESTELAND, R. (1978) Translation of Mu LV and MSV RNAs in nuclease-treated reticulocyte extracts: Enhancement of the gag-pol polypeptide with yeast suppressor tRNA. *Cell* **13**: 189–199.

PHILIPSON, L. and LINDBERG, U. (1974) Reproduction of adenoviruses. In: *Comprehensive Virology*, Vol. 3, pp. 143–227, FRAENKEL-CONRAT, H. and WAGNER, R. R. (eds.). Plenum Press, New York.

PHILIPSON, L., PETTERSON, U., LINDBERG, V., TIBBETTS, C., VENN-STRÖM, B. and PERSSON, T. (1974) RNA synthesis and processing in adenovirus-infected cells. *Cold Spring Harbor. Symp. Quant. Biol.* **39**: 447–456.

PHILIPSON, L. and PETTERSON, U. (1980) Control of adenovirus gene expression. *TIBS 5*, 135–137.

PLAGEMANN, P. G. W., CLEVELAND, P. H. and SHEA, M. A. (1970) Effect of mengovirus replication on choline metabolism and membrane formation in Novikoff hepatoma cells. *J. Virol.* **6**: 800–812.

POGO, B. G. T., O'SHEA, M. and FREIMUTH, P. (1981) Initiation and termination of vaccinia virus DNA replication. *Virology* **108**: 241–248.

POMPEI, R., FLORE, O., MARCCIALIS, M. A., PANI, A. and LODDO, B. (1979) Glycyrrhicic acid inhibits virus growth and inactivates virus particles. *Nature* **281**: 689–690.

POWELL, K. L. and COURTNEY, R. J. (1975) Polypeptides synthesized in herpes virus type 2 infected HEp-2 cells. *Virology* **66**: 217–228.

PRESTON, C. M. and SZILÁGYI, J. F. (1977) Cell-free translation of RNA synthesized *in vitro* by a transcribing nucleoprotein complex prepared from purified vesicular stomatitis virus. *J. Virol.* **21**: 1002–1009.

PRIVES, C. L., AVIV, H., GILBOA, E., REVEL, M. and WINOCOUR, E. (1974a) The cell-free translation of SV40 messenger RNA. *Cold Spring Harbor Symp. Quant. Biol.* **39**: 309–316.

PRIVES, C. L., AVIV, H., PATERSON, B. M., ROBERTS, B. E., ROZENBLATT, S., REVEL, M. and WINOCOUR, E. (1974b) Cell-free translation of messenger RNA of simian virus 40: synthesis of the major capsid protein. *Proc. Natn. Acad. Sci. USA* **71**: 302–306.

PRIVES, C. and BECK, Y. (1977) Characterization of simian virus 40 T-antigen polypeptides synthesized *in vivo* and *in vitro*. *INSERM Colloquium* **69**: 175–187.

PRIVES, C., GLUZMAN, Y. and WINOCOUR, E. (1978) Cellular and cell-free synthesis of simian virus 40 T-antigens in permissive and transformed cells. *J. Virol.* **25**: 587–595.

PRUSOFF, W. H. and GOZ, B. (1973) Potential mechanisms of action of antiviral agents. *Fed. Proceedings* **32**: 1679–1687.

PUCHIO, A. F., ERIKSON, E., BRUGGE, J. S. and ERIKSON, R. L. (1978) Identification of a polypeptide encoded by the avian sarcoma virus src gene. *Proc. Natn. Acad. Sci. USA* **75**: 1567–1571.

RACANIELLO, V. R. and BALTIMORE, D. (1981) Molecular cloning of poliovirus cDNA and determination of the complete nucleotide sequence of the viral genome. *Proc. Natn. Acad. Sci. USA* **78**: 4887–4891.

RACEVSKIS, J. and SARKAR, N. H. (1978) Synthesis and processing of precursor polypeptides to murine mammary tumor virus structural proteins. *J. Virol.* **25**: 374–383.

RAKUSANOVA, T., BEN-PORAT, T. and KAPLAN, A. S. (1972) Effect of herpes virus infection on the synthesis of cell specific RNA. *Virology* **49**: 537–548.

RAPP, F. and DUFF, R. (1972) *In vitro* cell transformation by herpesviruses. *Fed. Proc.* **31**: 1660–1668.

REDDY, V. B., THIMMAPPAYA, B., DHAR, R., SUBRAMANIAN, K. N., ZAIN, B. S., PAN, J., GHOSH, P. K., CELMA, M. L. and WEISSMAN, S. M. (1978) The genome of simian virus 40. *Science* **200**: 494–502.

RENART, J., REISER, J. and STARK, G. R. (1979) A method for studying antibody specificity and antigen structure: Transfer of proteins from gels to diazobenzyloximethyl-paper and detection with antisera. *Proc. Natn. Acad. Sci. USA* **76**: 3116–3120.

REKOSH, D. (1972) The gene order of the poliovirus capsid proteins. *J. Virol.* **9**: 479–487.

REKOSH, D. M. K. (1977) Molecular biology of picornaviruses. In: *The Molecular Biology of Animal Viruses.* NAYAK, D. (eds.). Marcel Dekker, New York.

REKOSH, D. M. K., RUSSELL, W. C., BELLETT, A. J. D. and ROBINSON, A. J. (1977) Identification of a protein linked to the ends of adenovirus DNA. *Cell* **11**: 283–295.

RENKONEN, O., KÄÄRIÄINEN, L., SIMONS, K. and GAHMBERG, C. G. (1971) The lipid class composition of Semliki Forest virus and of plasma membranes of the host cells. *Virology* **46**: 318–326.

RICE, C. M. and STRAUSS, J. H. (1981) Nucleotide sequence of the 26S mRNA of Sindbis virus and deduced sequence of the encoded virus structural proteins. *Proc. Natn. Acad. Sci. USA* **78**: 2062–2066.

RIFKIN, D. B. and QUIGLEY, J. P. (1974) Virus-induced modification of cellular membranes related to viral structure. *Ann. Rev. Microbiol.* **28**: 325–351.

ROBINSON, A. J. and BELLETT, A. J. D. (1974) A circular DNA-protein complex from adenoviruses and its possible role in DNA replication. *Cold Spring Harbor Symp. Quant. Biol.* **39**: 523–531.

RODRÍGUEZ, M. and DUBOIS-DALCQ, M. (1978) Intramembrane changes occurring during maturation of herpes simplex virus type 1: Freeze-fracture study. *J. Virol.* **26**: 435–447.

RODRÍGUEZ-BOULAN, E. and PENDERGAST, M. (1980) Polarized distribution of viral envelope proteins in the plasma membrane of epithelial cells. *Cell* **20**: 45–54.

ROIZMAN, B. (1979) The structure and isomerization of herpes simplex virus genomes. *Cell* **16**: 481–494.

ROIZMAN, B., FRENKEL, N., KIEFF, E. D. and SPEAR, P. G. (1977) The structure and expression of human herpes virus DNAs in productive infection and in transformed cells. In: *Origins of Human Cancer*, pp. 1069–1111. Cold Spring Harbor Laboratory.

ROIZMAN, B. and FURLONG, D. (1974) The replication of herpes virus. In: *Comprehensive Virology*, Vol. 3, pp. 229–403, FRAENKEL-CONRAT, H. and WAGNER, R. R. (eds.). Plenum Press, New York.

ROIZMAN, B., KOZAK, M., HONESS, R. W. and HAYWARD, G. S. (1974) Regulation of herpesvirus macromolecular synthesis: Evidence for multilevel regulation of herpes simplex 1 RNA and protein synthesis. *Cold Spring Harbor Symp. Quant. Biol.* **39**: 687–701.

ROIZMAN, B. and SPEAR, P. G. (1969) Macromolecular biosynthesis in animal cells infected with cytolytic viruses. *Current Topics develop. Biol* **4**: 79–108.

ROSE, J. K. (1977) Nucleotide sequences of ribosome recognition sites in messenger RNAs of vesicular stomatitis virus. *Proc. Natn. Acad. Sci. USA* **74**: 3672–3676.

ROSE, J. K. (1978) Complete sequences of the ribosome recognition sites in vesicular stomatitis virus mRNAs: recognition by the 40 S and 80 S complexes. *Cell* **14**: 345–353.

ROSE, J. K. (1980) Complete intergenic and flanking gene sequences from the genome of vesicular stomatitis virus. *Cell* **19**: 415–421.

ROSE, J. K. and GALLIONE, C. (1981) Nucleotide sequences of the mRNA's encoding the vesicular stomatitis virus G and M proteins determined from cDNA clones containing the complete coding regions. *Virol.* **39**: 519–528.

ROSE, J. K. and SHAFFERMAN, A. (1981) Conditional expression of the vesicular stomatitis virus glycoprotein gene in *Escherichia coli. Proc. Natn. Acad. Sci. USA* **78**: 6670–6674.

ROSE, J. K., TRACHSEL, H., LEONG, K. and BALTIMORE, D. (1978) Inhibition of translation by poliovirus: inactivation of a specific initiation factor. *Proc. Natn. Acad. Sci. USA* **75**: 2732–2736.

ROSS, S. R., FLINT, S. J. and LEVINE, A. J. (1980) Identification of the adenovirus early proteins and their genomic map positions. *Virology* **100**: 419–432.

ROTHBERG, P. G., HARRIS, T. J. R., NOMOTO, A. and WIMMER, E. (1978) O^4 (5'-Uridyl) tyrosine is the bond between the genome-linked protein and the RNA of poliovirus. *Proc. Natn. Acad. Sci. USA* **75**: 4868–4872.

ROTHMAN, J. E., BURSZTYN-PETTEGREW, H. and FINE, R. E. (1980) Transport of the membrane glycoprotein of vesicular stomatitis virus to the cell surface in two stages by clathrin-coated vesicles. *J. Cell Biol.* **86**: 162–171.

ROTHMAN, J. and LODISH, H. F. (1977) Synchronized transmembrane insertion and glycosylation of a nascent membrane protein. *Nature* **269**: 775–780.

ROWLANDS, D. J., HARRIS, T. J. and BROWN, F. (1978) More precise location of the polycytidylic acid tract in foot and mouth disease virus RNA. *J. Virol.* **26**: 335–343.

RUSSELL, W. C. and SKEHEL, J. J. (1972) The polypeptides of adenovirus-infected cells. *J. Gen. Virol.* **15**: 45–57.

RUYECHAN, W. T., MORSE, L. S., KNIPE, D. M. and ROIZMAN, B. (1979) Molecular genetics of herpes simplex virus. II. Mapping of the major viral glycoproteins and of the genetic loci specifying the social behaviour of infected cells. *J. Virol.* **29**: 677–697.

SABORIO, J. L., PONG, S. S. and KOCH, G. (1974) Selective and reversible inhibition of initiation of protein synthesis in mammalian cells. *J. Mol. Biol.* **85**: 195–211.

SALZMAN, N. P. and KHOURY, G. (1974) Reproduction of papovaviruses. In: *Comprehensive virology*, vol. 3. pp. 63–141, FRAENKEL-CONRAT, H. and WAGNER, R. R. (eds.). Plenum Press, New York.

SALZMAN, N. P. and SEBRING, E. D. (1967) Sequential formation of vaccinia virus proteins and viral deoxyribonucleic acid replication. *J. Virol.* **1**: 16–23.

SANGAR, D. V., ROWLANDS, D. J., HARRIS, T. J. R. and BROWN, F. (1977) Protein covalently linked to foot and mouth disease virus RNA. *Nature* **268**: 648–650.

SAROV, I. and JOKLIK, W. K. (1972) Studies on the nature and location of the capsid polypeptides of vaccinia virions. *Virology* **50**: 579–592.

SAVAGE, T., GRANBOULAN, N. and GIRARD, M. (1971) Architecture of the poliovirus replicative intermediate RNA. *Biochimie* **53**: 533–543.

SAWICKI, D. L. and GOMATOS, P. J. (1976) Replication of Semliki Forest virus: polyadenylate in plus-strand RNA and polyuridylate in minus-strand RNA. *J. Virol.* **20**: 446–464.

SAWICKI, D. L., KÄÄRIÄINEN, L., LAMBEK, C. and GOMATOS, P. J. (1978) Mechanism for control of synthesis of Semliki Forest virus 26 S and 42 S RNA. *J. Virol.* **25**: 19–27.

SCHAFFER, P. A., ARON, G. M., BISWAL, N. and BENYESH-MELNICK, M. (1973) Temperature-sensitive mutants of herpes simplex virus type 1: Isolation, complementation and partial characterization. *Virology* **52**: 57–71.

SCHAEFFER, H. J., BEAUCHAMP, L., DE MIRANDA, P., ELION, G. B., BAUER, D. J. and COLLINS, P. (1978) 9-(2-Hydroxyethoxymethyl) guanine activity against viruses of the herpes group. *Nature* **272**: 583–585.

SCHINCARIOL, A. L. and HOWATSON, A. F. (1972) Replication of vesicular stomatitis virus. II. Separation and characterization of virus-specific RNA species. *Virology* **49**: 766–768.

SCHOCHETMAN, G. and SCHOLM, J. (1976) Independent polypeptide chain initiation sites for the synthesis of different classes of proteins for an RNA tumor virus: mouse mammary tumor virus. *Virology* **73**: 431–441.

SCHONBERG, M., SILVERSTEIN, S. C., LEVIN, D. H. and ACS, G. (1971) Asynchronous synthesis of the complementary strands of the revovirus genome. *Proc. Natn. Acad. Sci. USA* **68**: 505–508.

SCHRÖM, M. and BABLANIAN, R. (1979) Inhibition of protein synthesis by vaccinia virus. II. Studies on the role of virus-induced RNA synthesis. *J. Gen. Virol.* **44**: 625–638.

SCHUMPERLI, D., MENNA, A., SCHWENDIMANN, F., WITTEK, R. and WYLER, R. (1980) Symmetrical arrangement of the heterologous regions of rabbit poxvirus and vaccinia virus DNA. *J. Gen. Virol.* **47**: 385–398.

SCHWARTZ, D. E., ZAMECNIK, P. C. and WEITH, H. L. (1977) Rous sarcoma virus genome is terminally redundant: The 3′ sequence. *Proc. Natn. Acad. Sci. USA* **74**: 994–998.

SEFTON, B. M., WICKUS, G. G. and BURGE, B. W. (1973) Enzymatic iodination of Sindbis virus proteins. *J. Virol.* **11**: 730–735.

SHANK, P. R., HUGHES, S. H., KUNG, H. J., MAJORS, J. E., QUINTRELL, N., GUNTAKA, R. V., BISHOP, J. M. and VARMUS, H. E. (1978) Mapping unintegrated avian sarcoma virus DNA.

SHARP, P. A., GALLIMORE, P. H. and FLING, S. J. (1974) Mapping of adenovirus 2 RNA sequences in lytically infected cells and transformed cell lines. *Cold Spring Harbor Symp. Quant. Biol.* **39**: 457–474.

SHATKIN, A. (1963) Actinomycin D and vaccinia virus infection of HeLa cells. *Nature* **199**: 357–358.

SHATKIN, A. J. (1974) Animal RNA viruses: Genome structure and function. *Ann. Rev. Biochem.* **43**: 643–665.

SHATKIN, A. J. (1976) Capping of eukaryotic mRNAs. *Cell* **9**: 645–653.

SHATKIN, A. J. and LA FIANDRA, A. J. (1972) Transcriptions by infections subviral particles of reovirus. *J. Virol.* **10**: 698–706.

SHATKIN, A. J. and RADA, B. (1967) Reovirus-directed ribonucleic acid synthesis in infected L cells. *J. Virol.* **1**: 24–35.

SHATKIN, A. J. and SIPE, J. D. (1968) RNA polymerase activity in purified reovirus. *Proc. Natn. Acad. Sci. USA* **61**: 1462–1469.

SHATKIN, A. J., SIPE, J. D. and LOH, P. C. (1968) Separation of ten reovirus genome segments by polyacrylamide gel electrophoresis. *J. Virol.* **2**: 986–991.

SHELDRICK, P. and BERTHELOT, N. (1975) Inverted repetitions in the chromosome of herpes simplex virus. *Cold Spring Harbor Symp. Quant. Biol.* **39**: 667–678.

SHIH, D. S., SHIH, C. T., KEW, O., PALLANSCH, M., RUECKERT, R. and KAESBERG, P. (1978) Cell-free synthesis and processing of the proteins of poliovirus. *Proc. Natn. Acad. Sci. USA* **75**: 5807–5811.

SHINE, J., CZERNILOFSKY, A. P., FRIEDRICH, R., BISHOP, J. M. and GOODMAN, H. M. (1977) Nucleotide sequence at the 5′ terminus of the avian sarcoma virus genome. *Proc. Natn. Acad. Sci. USA* **74**: 1473–1477.

SHUGAR, D. (1974) Progress with antiviral agents. *FEBS Letters* **40**: S 48–S 62.

SIDDELL, S. G. and SMITH, A. E. (1978) Polyoma virus has three late mRNAs: one for each virion protein. *J. Virol.* **27**: 427–431.

SILVERSTEIN, S. C., ASTELL, C., LEVIN, D. H., SCHONBEG, M. and ACS, G. (1972) The mechanisms of reovirus uncoating and gene activation *in vivo*. *Virology* **47**: 797–806.

SIMMONS, D. T. and STRAUSS, J. H. (1972a) Replication of Sindbis virus. I. Relative size and genetic content of 26 S and 49 S RNA. *J. Mol. Biol.* **71**: 599–613.

SIMMONS, D. T. and STRAUSS, J. A. (1972b) Replication of Sindbis virus. II. Multiple forms of double-stranded RNA isolated from infected cells. *J. Mol. Biol.* **71**: 615–631.

SIMMONS, D. T. and STRAUSS, , J. H. (1974) Translation of Sindbis virus 26 S RNA in lysates of rabbit reticulocytes. *J. Mol. Biol.* **86**: 397–409.

SIMONS, K., KERÄNEN, S. and KÄÄRIÄINEN, L. (1973) Identification of a precursor for one of the Semliki Forest virus membrane proteins. *FEBS Letters* **29**: 87–91.

SIMONSEN, C. C., BATT-HUMPHRIES, S. and SUMMERS, D. F. (1979) RNA synthesis of vesicular stomatitis virus-infected cells: *In vivo* regulation of replication. *J. Virol.* **31**: 124–132.

SKEHEL, J. J. and JOKLIK, W. K. (1969) Studies on the *in vitro* transcription of reovirus RNA catalyzed by reovirus cores. *Virology* **39**: 822–831.

SKUP, D. and MILLWARD, S. (1980) Reovirus-induced modification of cap-dependent translation in infected cells. *Proc. Natn. Acad. Sci. USA* **77**: 152–156.

SLEIGH, M. J., TOPP, W. C., HANICH, R. and SAMBROOK, J. F. (1978) Mutants of SV40 with an altered small t protein are reduced in their ability to transform cells. *Cell* **14**: 79–88.

SMART, J. E. and ITO, Y. (1978) Three species of polyoma virus tumor antigens share common peptides probably near the amino termini of the proteins. *Cell* **15**: 1427–1437.

SMITH, A. E. (1973) The initiation of protein synthesis directed by the RNA from encephalomyocarditis virus. *Eur. J. Biochem.* **33**: 301–303.

SMITH, A. E. and CARRASCO, L. (1978) Eukaryotic viral protein synthesis. In: *Amino Acid and Protein Biosynthesis II*, pp. 261–311, ARNSTEIN, H. R. V. (ed.). (*Intern Rev. Biochem.* Vol. 18). University Park, Press, Baltimore.

SMITH, A. E., KAMEN, R. I., MANGEL, W. F., SHURE, H. and WHEELER, T. (1976) Location of the sequences coding for capsid proteins VP1 and VP2 on polyoma virus DNA. *Cell* **9**: 481–487.

SMITH, A. E., MARCKER, K. A. and MATHEWS, M. B. (1970) Translation of RNA from encephalomyocarditis virus in a cell-free system. *Nature* **225**: 184–187.

SMITH, A. E., SMITH, R., GRIFFIN, B. E. and FRIED, M. (1979) Protein kinase activity associated with polyoma virus middle T antigen *in vitro*. *Cell* **18**: 915–924.

SÖDERLUND, H. (1976) The post-translational processing of Semliki Forest virus structural polypeptides in puromycin treated cells. *FEBS Letters* **63**: 56–58.

SONNERBERG, N., TRACHSEL, H., HECHT, S. and SHATKIN, A. J. (1980) Differential stimulation of capped mRNA translation *in vitro* by cap binding protein. *Nature* **285**: 331–333.

SORIA, M. and HUANG, A. S. (1975) Association of polyadenylic acid with messenger RNA of vesicular stomatitis virus. *J. Mol. Biol.* **77**: 449–455.

SPEAR, P. G. (1976) Membrane proteins specified by herpes simplex viruses. I. Identification of four glycoprotein precursors and their products in type 1-infected cells. *J. Virol.* **17**: 991–1008.

SPEAR, P. G., KELLER, J. M. and ROIZMAN, B. (1970) The proteins specified by herpes simplex virus. II. Viral glycoproteins associated with cellular membranes. *J. Virol.* **5**: 123–131.

SPEAR, P. G. and ROIZMAN, B. (1972) Proteins specified by herpes simplex virus. V. Purification and structural proteins of the herpesvirion. *J. Virol.* **9**: 143–159.

SPECTOR, D. H. and BALTIMORE, D. (1974) Requirement of 3'-terminal poly (adenylic acid) for the infectivity of poliovirus RNA. *Proc. Natn. Acad. Sci. USA* **71**: 2983–2987.

STACEY, D. W., ALLFREY, V. G. and HANAFUSA, H. (1977) Microinjection analysis of envelope-glycoprotein messenger activities of avian leukosis viral RNAs. *Proc. Natn. Acad. Sci. USA* **74**: 1614–1618.

STEINER-PRYOR, A. and COOPER, P. (1973) Temperature sensitive mutants defective in repression of host protein synthesis are also defective in structural protein. *J. Gen. Virol.* **21**: 215–225.

STEPHENSON, J. R., DEVARE, S. G. and REYNOLDS, F. H. JR. (1978) Translational products of type-C RNA tumor viruses. In: *Advances in Cancer Res.*, Vol. 27, pp. 1–53. Academic Press, New York.

STILLMAN, B. W. and BELLETT (1979) An Adenovirus protein associated with the ends of replicating DNA molecules. *Virology* **93**: 69–79.

STILLMAN, B. W., LEWIS, J. B., CHOW, L. T., MATHEWS, M. B. and SMART, J. E. (1981) Identification of the gene and mRNA for the adenovirus terminal protein precursor. *Cell* **23**: 497–508.

STOHLMAN, S. A., WISSEMAN, C. L., EYLAR, O. R. and SILVERMAN, D. J. (1975) Dengue virus-induced modifications of host cell membranes. *J. Virol.* **16**: 1017–1026.

STOLTZFUS, C. M. and RUECKERT, R. (1972) Capsid polypeptides of mouse Elberfeld virus I. Aminoacid compositions and molar rations in the virion. *J. Virol.* **10**: 347–355.

STOLTZFUS, C. M., SHATKIN, A. J. and BANERJEE, A. K. (1973) Absence of polyadenylic acid from reovirus messenger RNA. *J. Biol. Chem.* **248**: 7993–7998.

STRAUSS, J. H., JR., BURGE, B. W., PFEFFERKORN, E. R. and DARNELL, J. E. JR. (1968) Identification of the membrane protein and 'core' protein of Sindbis virus. *Proc. Natn. Acad. Sci. USA* **59**: 533–537.

STRNAD, B. C. and AURELIAN, L. (1976) Proteins of herpesvirus type 2: 1. Virion, nonvirion and antigenic polypeptides in infected cells. *Virology* **69**: 438–452.

STRNAD, B. C. and AURELIAN, L. (1978) Proteins of herpesvirus type 2 III: Isolation and immunologic characterization of a large molecular weight viral protein. *Virology* **87**: 401–415.

STROUS, G. and LODISH, H. F. (1980) Intracellular transport of secretory and membrane proteins in hepatoma cells infected by vesicular stomatitis virus. *Cell* **22**: 709–717.

SUBAK-SHARPE, J. H., TIMBURY, M. C. and WILLIAMS, J. F. (1969) Rifampicin inhibits the growth of some mammalian viruses. *Nature* **222**: 341–345.

SUMMERS, D. F. and MAIZEL, J. V. JR. (1968) Evidence for large precursor proteins in poliovirus synthesis. *Proc. Natn. Acad. Sci. USA* **59**: 966–971.

SUMMERS, D. F. and MAIZEL, J. V. (1971) Determination of gene sequence of poliovirus with pactamycin. *Proc. Natn. Acad. Sci. USA* **68**: 2852–2856.

SUMMERS, D. F., MAIZEL, J. V. JR. and DARNELL, J. E. JR. (1965) Evidence for virus-specific noncapsid proteins in poliovirus-infected HeLa cells. *Proc. Natn. Acad. Sci. USA* **54**: 505–513.

SUNDQUIST, B., EVERITT, E., PHILIPSON, L. and HÖGLUND, S. (1973) Assembly of adenoviruses. *J. Virol.* **11**: 449–459.

SUSSENBACH, J. S. (1967) Early events in the infection process of adenovirus type 5 in HeLa cells. *Virology* **33**: 567–574.

SVITKIN, Y. V. and AGOL, V. I. (1978) Complete translation of encephalomyocarditis virus RNA and faithful cleavage of virus-specific proteins in a cell-free system from Krebs-2 cells. *FEBS Letters* **87**: 7–11.

SWANSTROM, R., DE LORBE, W. J., BISHOP, J. M. and VARMUS, H. E. (1981). Nucleotide sequence of cloned unintegrated avian sarcoma virus DNA: viral DNA contains direct and inverted repeats similar to those in transposable elements. *Proc. Natn. Acad. Sci. USA* **78**: 124–128.

SZILÁGYI, J. F. and URYVAYEV, L. (1973) Isolation of an infectious ribonucleoprotein from vesicular stomatitis virus containing an active RNA transcriptase. *J. Virol.* **11**: 279–286.

TABER, R., REKOSH, D. and BALTIMORE, D. (1971) Effect of pactamycin on synthesis of poliovirus proteins: a method for genetic mapping. *J. Virol.* **8**: 395–401.

TAHARA, S. M., MORGAN, M. A. and SHATKIN, A. J. (1981) Two forms of purified m⁷ G-cap binding protein with different effects on capped mRNA translation in extracts of uninfected and poliovirus infected HeLa cells. *J. Biol. Chem.* **256**: 7691–7694.

TAMM, I. and EGGERS, H. J. (1963) Specific inhibition of replication of animal viruses. *Science* **142**: 24–33.

TANNOCK, G. A., GIBBS, A. J. and COOPER, P. D. (1970) A re-examination of the molecular weight of poliovirus RNA. *Biochem. Biophys. Res. Commun.* **38**: 298–304.

TAYLOR, J. M. and ILLMENSEE, R. (1975) Site on the RNA of an avian sarcoma virus at which primer is bound. *J. Virol.* **16**: 553–558.

TEMIN, H. M. (1974) On the origin of RNA tumor viruses. *Ann. Rev. Genetics* **8**: 155–177.

TEMIN, H. M. (1980) Origin of retroviruses from cellular moveable genetic elements. *Cell* **21**: 599–600.

TEMIN, H. M. (1981) Structure, variation and synthesis of retrovirus long terminal repeat. *Cell* **27**: 1–3.

TESTA, D. and BANERJEE, A. K. (1977) Two methyltransferase activities in the purified virions of vesicular stomatitis virus. *J. Virol.* **24**: 786–793.

TESTA, D., CHANDA, P. K. and BANERJEE, A. K. (1980) Unique mode of transcription *in vitro* by vesicular stomatitis virus. *Cell* **21**: 267–275.

THOMPSON, C. J., DOCHERTY, J. J., BOLTZ, R. C., GAINES, R. A. and TODD, P. (1978) Electrokinetic alteration of the surface of herpes simplex virus infected cells. *J. Gen. Virol.* **39**: 449–461.

TIBBETTS, C., PETTERSSON, U., JOHANSSON, K. and PHILIPSON, L. (1974) Relationship of messenger ribonucleic acid from productively infected cells to the complementary strands of adenovirus type 2 deoxyribonucleic acid. *J. Virol.* **13**: 370–377.

TJIAN, R. (1978) The binding site on SV 40 DNA for a T antigen related protein. *Cell* **13**: 165–179.

TJIAN, R., FEY, G. and GRAESSMANN, A. (1978) Biological activity of purified simian virus 40 T antigen proteins. *Proc. Natn. Acad. Sci. USA* **75**: 1279–1283.

TONEGUZZO, F. and GHOSH, H. P. (1977) Synthesis and glycosylation of glycoprotein of vesicular stomatitis virus. *Proc. Natn. Acad. Sci. USA* **74**: 1516–1520.

TONEGUZZO, F. and GHOSH, H. R. (1978) *In vitro* synthesis of vesicular stomatitis virus membrane glycoprotein and insertion into membranes. *Proc. Natn. Acad. Sci. USA* **75**: 715–719.

TOOZE, J. (1973) The molecular biology of tumor viruses. Cold Spring Harbor, New York.

TOOZE, J. (1980) Molecular biology of animal tumor viruses. Cold Spring Harbor.

TRACHSEL, H., SONENBERG, N., SHATKIN, A. J., ROSE, J. K., LEONG, K., BERGMANN, J. E., GORDON, J. and BALTIMORE, D. (1980) Purification of a factor that restores translation of vesicular stomatitis virus mRNA in extracts from polio-virus-infected cells. *Proc. Natn. Acad. Sci. USA* **77**: 770–774.

TRAUB, A., DISKIN, B., ROSENBERG, H. and KALMAR, E. (1976) Isolation and properties of the replicase of encephalomyocarditis virus. *J. Virol.* **18**: 375–382.

TREISMAN, R., NOVAK, U., FAVALORO, J. and KAMEN, R. (1981) Transformation of rat cells by an altered polyoma virus genome expressing only the middle T protein. *Nature* **292**: 595–600.

USSERY, M. A., IRVIN, J. D. and HARDESTY, B. (1977) Inhibition of polio-virus replication by a plant antiviral peptide. *Ann. N.Y. Acad. Sci.* **284**: 431–440.

VAN BEVEREN, C., GALLESHAW, J. A., JONAS, V., BERNS, A. J. M., DOOLITTLE, R. F., DONOGHUE, D. J. and VERMA, I. M. (1981a) Nucleotide sequence and formation of the transforming gene of a mouse sarcoma virus. *Nature* **289**: 258–262.

VAN BEVEREN, C., VAN STRAATEN, F., GALLESHAW, J. A. and VERMA, I. M. (1981b) Nucleotide sequence of the genome of a murine sarcoma virus. *Cell* **27**: 97–108.

VAN DER VLIET, P. C. and LEVINE, A. J. (1973) DNA binding proteins specific for cells infected with adenovirus. *Nature New Biol.* **246**: 170–174.

VAN STOEG, H., THOMAS, A., VERBEEK, S., KASPERATIS, M., VOORMA, H. O. and BENNE, R. (1981) Shut off of neuroblastoma cell protein synthesis by Semliki Forest virus: loss of ability of crude initiation factors to recognize early Semliki Forest virus and host mRNA's. *J. Virol.* **38**: 728–736.

VAN ZAANE, D., GIELKENS, A. L. J., HESSELINK, W. G. and BLOEMERS, H. P. J. (1977) Identification of Rauscher murine leukemia virus-specific mRNAs for the synthesis of gag- and env-gene products. *Proc. Natn. Acad. Sci. USA* **74**: 1855–1859.

VÁZQUEZ, D. (1979) Inhibitors of protein biosynthesis. *Molec. Biol. Biochem. and Biophys.*, Vol. 30. Springer-Verlag.

VERMA, I. M. (1977) The reverse transcriptase. *Biochem. Biophys. Acta* **473**: 1–38.

VILLA-KOMAROFF, L., GUTTMAN, N., BALTIMORE, D. and LODISH, H. (1975) Complete translation of poliovirus RNA in a eukaryotic cell-free system. *Proc. Natn. Acad. Sci. USA* **72**: 4157–4161.

VILLAREAL, L. P. and JOVANOVICH, S. (1980) Leakage of nuclear transcripts late in simian virus 40-infected CV1-cells: quantitation of spliced and unspliced late 19S RNAs. *J. Virol.* **36**: 595–600.

VOGT, V. M. and EISENMAN, R. (1973) Identification of a large polypeptide precursor of avian oncornavirus proteins. *Proc. Natn. Acad. Sci. USA* **70**: 1734–1738.

VOGT, V. M., EISENMAN, R. and DIGGELMAN, H. (1975) Generation of avian myeloblastosis virus structural proteins by proteolytic cleavage of a precursor polypeptide. *J. Mol. Biol.* **96**: 471–493.

VON DER HELM, K. (1977) Cleavage of Rous sarcoma viral polypeptide precursor into internal structural protein involves viral protein p. 15. *Proc. Natn. Acad. Sci. USA* **74**: 911–915.

VON DER HELM, K. and DUESBERG, P. H. (1975) Translation of Rous sarcoma virus RNA in cell-free systems from ascites Krebs II cells. *Proc. Natn. Acad. Sci. USA* **72**: 614–618.

WADSWORTH, S., JACOB, R. J. and ROIZMAN, B. (1975) Anatomy of herpes simplex virus DNA. II. Size, composition and arrangement of inverted terminal repetitions. *J. Virol.* **15**: 1487–1497.

WAGNER, R. R. (1975) Reproduction of rhabdoviruses. In: *Comprehensive Virology*, Vol. 4, pp. 1–93. FRAENKEL-CONRAT, H. and WAGNER, R. R. (eds.). Plenum Press, New York.

WAGNER, R. R., SCHNAITMAN, T. C., SNYDER, R. M. and SCHITMAN, C. A. (1969) Protein composition of the structural components of the vesicular stomatitis virus. *J. Virol.* **3**: 611–618.

WAGNER, R. R., HEINE, J. W., GOLSTEIN, G. and SCHNATTMUN, C. A. (1971) Use of antiviral-antiferritin hybrid antibody for localization of viral antigen in plasma membrane. *J. Virol.* **7**: 274–277.

WAGNER, E. K. and ROIZMAN, B. (1969) RNA synthesis in cells infected with herpes simplex virus. I. The patterns of RNA synthesis in productively infected cells. *J. Virol.* **4**: 36–46.

WALDEN, W. E., GODEFROY-COLBURN, T. and THACH, R. E. (1981) The role of mRNA competition in regulating translation. I. Demonstration of competition *in vivo*. *J. Biol. Chem.* **256**: 11.739–11.746.

WALTER, G. and MAIZEL, J. V. (1974) The polypeptides of adenovirus IV. Detection of early and late-induced polypeptides and their distribution in cellular fractions. *Virology* **57**: 402–408.

WARD, R. L., BANERJEE, A. K., LA FIANDRA, A. and SHATKIN, A. J. (1972) Reovirus specific ribonucleic acid from polysomes of infected L cells. *J. Virol.* **9**: 61–69.

WATANABE, Y., KUDO, H. and GRAHAM, A. F. (1967) Selective inhibition of reovirus ribonucleic acid synthesis by cycloheximide. *J. Virol.* **1**: 36–44.

WATSON, D. H. and WILDY, P. (1969) The preparation of monoprecipitin antisera of herpes-specific antigens. *J. Gen. Virol.* **4**: 163–168.

WEINBERG, R. A. (1977) How does T antigen transform cells? *Cell* **11**: 243–246.

WEINER, A. M. and WEBER, K. (1971) Natural read-through at the UGA termination signal of Qβ coat protein cistron. *Nature New Biol.* **234**: 206–209.

WEISS, R. (1976) Molecular analysis of the oncogene. *Nature.* **260**: 93.

WELCH, W. J. and SEFTON, B. (1979) Two small virus-specific polypeptides are produced during infection with Sindbis virus. *J. Virol.* **29**: 1186–1195.

WELSH, R. M., TROWBRIDGE, R. S., KOWALSKI, J. B., O'CONELL, C. M. and PFAU, C. J. (1971) Amantadine hydrochloride inhibition of early and late stages of Lymphocytic choriomeningitis virus-cell interactions. *Virology* **45**: 679–686.

WENGLER, G. and WENGLER, G. (1976a) Localization of the 26 S RNA sequence on the viral genome type 42 S RNA isolated from SFV-infected cells. *Virology* **73**: 190–199.

WENGLER, G. and WENGLER, G. (1976b) Protein synthesis in BHK-21 cells infected with Semliki Forest virus. *J. Virol.* **17**: 10–19.

WERTZ, G. W. and YOUNGNER, J. S. (1972) Inhibition of protein synthesis in L cells infected with vesicular stomatitis virus. *J. Virol.* **9**: 85–89.

WESTPHAL, H. (1976) *In vitro* translation of adenovirus messenger RNA. *Current Topics in Immunol. and Microbiol.* **73**: 124–140.

WESTPHAL, H., ERON, L., FERDINAND, F. J., CALLAHAN, R. and LAI, S. P. (1974) Analysis of adenovirus type 2 gene functions by cell-free translation of viral messenger RNA. *Cold Spring Harbor Symp. Quant. Biol.* **39**: 575–579.

WHEELER, T., BAYLEY, S. T., HARVEY, R., CRAWFORD, L. V. and SMITH, A. E. (1977) Cell-free synthesis of polyoma virus capsid proteins VP1 and VP2. *J. Virol.* **21**: 215–224.

WIEGES, K. J., YAMAGUCHI-KOLL, U. and DRZENIEK, R. (1976) A complex between poliovirus RNA and the structural polypeptide VP1. *Biochem. Biophys. Res. Commun.* **71**: 1308–1312.

WILLEMS, M. and PENMAN, S. (1966) The mechanism of host cell protein synthesis inhibition by poliovirus. *Virology* **30**: 355–367.

WILLINGHAM, M. C., JAY, G. and PASTAN, I. (1979). Localization of the avian sarcoma virus src gene product to the plasma membrane of transformed cells by electron microscopic immunocytochemistry. *Cell* **18**: 125–134.

WILSON, T., PAPAHADJAPOULOS, D. and TABER, R. (1979) The introduction of poliovirus RNA into cells via lipid vesicles (liposomes). *Cell* **17**: 77–84.

WIMMER, E. (1972) Sequence studies of poliovirus RNA 1. Characterization of the 5′-terminus. *J. Mol. Biol.* **68**: 537–540.

WINNACKER, E. L. (1978) Adenovirus DNA: Structure and function of a novel repliron. *Cell* **14**: 761–773.

WIRTH, D. F., KATZ, F., SMALL, B. and LODISH, H. F. (1977) How a single Sindbis virus mRNA directs the synthesis of one soluble protein and two integral membrane glycoproteins. *Cell* **10**: 253–263.

WITTE, O. N., DASGUPTA, A. and BALTIMORE, D. (1980). Abelson murine leukemia virus protein is phosphorylated *in vitro* to form phosphotyrosine. *Nature* **283**: 826–831.

WITTEK, R., BARBOSA, E., COOPER, J. A., GARON, C. F., CHAN, H. and MOSS, B. (1980b). Inverted terminal repetition in vaccinia virus DNA encodes early mRNAs. *Nature* **285**: 21–25.

WITTEK, R., COOPER, J. A., BARBOSA, E. and MOSS, B. (1980a) Expression of the vaccinia virus genome: analysis and mapping of mRNAs encoded within the inverted terminal repetition.

WITTEK, R. and MOSS, B. (1980) Tandem repeats within the inverted terminal repetition of vaccinia virus DNA. *Cell* **21**: 277–284.

WOLD, W. S. M., GREEN, M. and MUNNS, T. W. (1976) Methylation of late adenovirus 2 nuclear and messenger RNA. *Biochem. Biophys. Res. Commun.* **68**: 643–649.

WYATT, S. D. and SHEPHERD, R. J. (1969) Isolation and characterization of a virus inhibitor from *Phytolaca americana. Phytopathology* **59**: 1787–1794.

WYKE, J. A. (1975) Temperature sensitive mutants of avian sarcoma viruses. *Biochim. Biophys. Acta* **417**: 91–121.

WYKE, A. M., IMPRAIM, C. C., KNUTTON, S. and PASTERNAK, C. A. (1980) Components involved in virally mediated membrane fusion and permeability changes. *Biochem. J.* **190**: 625–638.

YAOI, Y. and AMANO, M. (1970) Inhibitory effect of ultraviolet-inactivated vesicular stomatitis virus on initiation of DNA synthesis in cultured chick embryo cells. *J. Gen. Virol.* **9**: 69–75.

YAOI, Y., MITSUI, H. and AMANO, M. (1970) Effect of U.V.-irradiated vesicular stomatitis virus on nucleic acid synthesis in chick embryo cells. *J. Gen. Virol.* **8**: 165–172.

YOGO, Y. and WIMMER, E. (1972) Polyadenylic acid at the 3′-terminus of poliovirus RNA. *Proc. Natn. Acad. Sci. USA* **69**: 1877–1882.

YOSHIKI, T., MELLORS, R. C., HARDY, W. D. and FLEISSNER, F. (1974) Common cell surface antigen associated with mammalian C-type RNA viruses. *J. Exp. Med.* **139**: 925–942.

ZARBL, H., SKUP, D. and MILWARD, S. (1980) Reovirus progeny subviral particles synthesize uncapped mRNA. *J. Virol.* **34**: 497–505.

ZEMLA, J., COTO, D. and KAPLAN, A. S. (1967) Correlation between loss of enzymatic activity and of protein from cells infected with pseudorabies virus. *Virology* **31**: 736–738.

ZIFF, E. B. (1980) Transcription and RNA processing by the DNA tumor viruses. *Nature* **287**: 491–499.

ZWEERINK, H. J., ITO, Y. and MATSUHISA, T. (1972) Synthesis of reovirus double-stranded RNA within virion like particles. *Virology.* **50**: 349–358.

ZWEERINK, H. J. and JOKLIK, W. K. (1970) Studies on the intracellular synthesis of reovirus-specified proteins. *Virology.* **41**: 501–518.

CHAPTER 6

ANTI-INFLUENZA VIRUS ACTIVITY OF AMANTADINE: A SELECTIVE REVIEW OF LABORATORY AND CLINICAL DATA

JOHN S. OXFORD

Division of Virology, National Institute for Biological Standards and Control, Holly Hill, London NW3

ALAN GALBRAITH

Pharmaceuticals Division, Ciba-Geigy (UK), Horsham, Sussex

CONTENTS

6.1. INTRODUCTION

Influenza A virus has been recognized as a disease entity for several hundred years and world-wide outbreaks or pandemics have been recorded in England since the seventeenth century (Table 1). The causative virus was not isolated from man and grown successfully in the laboratory, however, until 1933, when C. Andrewes and W. Smith in the Hampstead Laboratories of the Medical Research Council described infection of ferrets and later virus transmission from experimentally infected ferrets to man (Andrewes *et al.*, 1934 (reviewed by Stuart-Harris, 1984)). At that stage studies commenced on the development of inactivated vaccines and, a little later, on the search for specific inhibitors of virus replication. For the last 40 years research into methods of control of the disease has intensified but, compared to other virus infections such as measles, rubella, polio and smallpox, which have meanwhile been successfully controlled, in at least some parts of the world, with vaccine, apparently little progress has been achieved with influenza. Particular features of the replication of the virus and the epidemiology of the virus may have contributed strongly to this apparent lack of success. Thus, as we shall discuss in more detail below, influenza virus has a segmented RNA genome composed of 8 or 9 single stranded RNA pieces (McGeoch *et al.*, 1976; Palese and Schulman, 1976), each acting as template for the transcription of one or more messenger RNA species (Lamb *et al.*, 1980; Allen *et al.*, 1980). Perhaps as a result of the genome structure, recombination or gene reassortment can occur with unusually high frequency between different influenza viruses infecting the same cell. Thus, the potential for genetic change is considerable, unlike other RNA viruses such as measles, rubella or polio where, even if antigenic types occur, they are genetically stable and genetic recombination is a rare event. Epidemiological and ecological studies have indicated that many influenza A viruses co-exist in animal, avian and human groups (reviewed by Stuart-Harris and Schild, 1976). Thus, a large genetic pool of influenza A virus genes occurs in nature, and one hypothesis to explain the emergence of new pandemic strains of influenza A virus invokes the intervention of gene reassortment between avian and human viruses to give a novel antigenic subtype with mixed genes from both parents which can then infect man (Webster and Laver, 1975; Webster *et al.*, 1982).

It is against this background of knowledge about the virus that a method of prevention of the disease must be formulated. Unlike empirical methods used to successfully control outbreaks of other RNA viruses mentioned above, a particular strategy may have to be devised for influenza. It must be admitted that to date little consideration has been given to such a strategic plan. Planning has usually been uncoordinated, depending on the immediate epidemiological situation. Also, to date, understandably, particular emphasis has been placed on the use of vaccines to prevent influenza virus infection in man, because of the successful experiences with vaccines against other viruses. However, the epidemiological pattern of the influenza A virus indicates that the virus is able to circumvent any herd immunity—at least immunity which is naturally induced. It would be unlikely, therefore, that an artificial immunogen, such as an inactivated influenza vaccine, would provide any better protection on a large scale although small groups may be protected. The potential of chemoprophylaxis or chemotherapy should be considered, therefore, in conjunction with vaccination. National policies, where they exist, have tended to emphasise the use of vaccine for the protection of groups in the population at special risk. Groups such as the very young (under 5 years old), old (over 60 years old) chronic bronchitics, asthmatics and persons with pre-existing heart disease have a relatively high mortality following an outbreak of influenza A virus (reviewed by Stuart-Harris, 1977; Tillett *et al.*, 1980). Apart from this group, vaccine has often been given to persons involved in public transport, armed forces and hospitals. In this group the risk of influenza illness in epidemics may reach 20 per cent and the risk of fatal influenza 0.2 per cent. Only one country to date has even attempted to prevent an actual epidemic of influenza—namely America. With the circumscribed outbreak of the swine-like virus A/New Jersey/8/76 (H1N1) in the military camp Fort Dix in 1976, and the evidence of man-to-man transmission of the swine virus, a mass vaccination campaign was initiated. Approximately 50 million persons in the US were immunized with inactivated A/NJ/76 virus

TABLE 1. *History of Influenza 'Pandemics'*

Year	Virus
1658	?
1688	?
1710	?
1743	?
1762	?
1782	?
1803	?
1831	?
1833	?
1837	?
1889	?
1918	H1N1
1948	H1N1
1957	H2N2 'Asian' era
1968	H3N2 'Hong Kong' era
1977	H3N2
1978	H3N2 and H1N1 (possibly 'frozen' since 1950 in nature or a laboratory escape)
1980	H3N2 and H1N1 (possibly 'frozen' since 1950 in nature or a laboratory escape)
1981	,, ,,
1982	,, ,,

Influenza A viruses are designated as type A, B or C. Influenza A viruses alone are able to cause world-wide epidemics or pandemics. Influenza B and C viruses are responsible for more localised outbreaks. Clinically they are not distinguishable. For influenza A viruses an index in the virus description describes the antigenic character of the haemagglutinin (H) and neuraminidase (N).

vaccines containing either whole virus or detergent disrupted virus. Although not completely successful as a total mass vaccination exercise, it did provide considerable data as regards vaccine composition, antibody responses and side-reactions of vaccine.

The only other countries to attempt immunization on a large scale have been the USSR and China. In both these countries, live attenuated influenza vaccine strains have been used in doses probably greater than 10 million per year. Success has been claimed but some of the studies, because of their size, have been difficult to control. Studies using live attenuated viruses are continuing both in the USSR, Europe and China and appear promising. But the problem of almost yearly antigenic drift (Schild *et al.*, 1974) and variation is still unsolved and may negate any efforts to prevent influenza on a large scale with live or inactivated vaccine. We shall discuss in more detail the recent concepts and future possibilities of influenza vaccines later in this review (also reviewed by Belyavin, 1976; Selby, 1976; Schild, 1979; Stuart-Harris, 1981; Lennette, 1981; Oxford and Oberg, 1984; Stuart-Harris, 1984).

Following the successful use of specific inhibitors of bacterial and protozoal replication investigators have searched for specific inhibitors of influenza virus replication (reviewed by Bauer, 1973; Collier and Oxford, 1980). Thousands of molecules have been examined, but to date only a single class of compounds has been shown unequivocally useful in preventing influenza in man. The parent compound, a cyclic primary amine, 1-aminoadamantane hydrochloride (amantadine or Symmetrel), was discovered in the laboratories of Du Pont in the early 1960s (Davies *et al.*, 1964). The compound* (Fig. 1) is used at present on a rather limited scale in England, Europe and the United States but a derivative, α-methyl-1-adamantane methylamine, or rimantadine, is being used more widely in the USSR as a therapeutic agent (M. Indulen, personal communication; Blyuger *et al.*, 1970; Maikovskiy *et al.*, 1970; Smorodintsev *et al.*, 1970a,b; Indulen and Kalninya, 1980; Zlydnikov *et al.*, 1981) against influenza. Since amantadine is the first clinically useful inhibitor of influenza A virus, much can be learned from a study of the mode of action of the compound, of useful experimental models and finally of application in man. This review will consider each of these aspects in more detail below. Fortunately, good correlation exists between the *in vitro*,

---

* Amantadine is licensed in the USA and the UK for use as a prophylactic agent for influenza A infections.

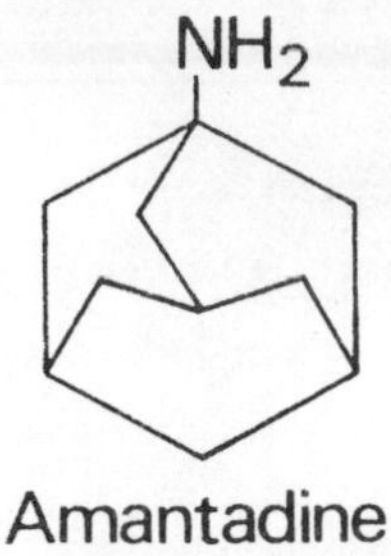

$$NH_2$$

Amantadine

FIG. 1. Molecular structure of 1-aminoadamantane (amantadine or Symmetrel). The molecule is thermostable, low molecular weight and water soluble. It is administered as the hydrochloride, (see also Hoffmann, 1980).

in vivo and clinical data for this compound. The toxicology and pharmacology of amantadine have been well studied and, for example, following oral administration, the compound is known to be present in the upper respiratory tract at concentrations which would inhibit virus replication ($\sim 2\,\mu g/ml$). Nevertheless, the clinical use of the compound is still not widespread enough to have any impact on the spread of virus in the community (Editorial, Maugh, 1980). We will examine below the prospects of using a combined approach of immuno and chemo prophylaxis for the prevention of inter pandemic or pandemic influenza viruses (Jackson, 1977). Also, to place amantadine in some perspective as an inhibitor of influenza virus replication, we shall first consider details of the replication of the virus at the molecular level. It is not surprising that the precise mode of action of the compound is not clear, since little is known about the early events of influenza virus penetration and uncoating *per se*. Recent studies have indicated the complex control mechanisms at both the transcriptional and translational level which the virus must initiate to ensure correct synthesis and packaging of 8 proteins and 8–9 RNA fragments into an infectious virion (reviewed by Mahy and Barry, 1978; Schild, 1979; McCauley and Mahy, 1983). This could encourage a search for further compounds which could upset this presumably delicate balance and hence abort virus infection.

Influenza is not a life-threatening disease in healthy adults—mortality only becomes significant in elderly persons and chronic bronchitics, asthmatics and persons with pre-existing heart disease. Therefore, any antiviral should be without significant toxic side-reactions. To prevent influenza in 100 people (assuming a 70 per cent protective efficacy and a 10 per cent attack rate) amantadine would have to be given to 1428 persons (Douglas, 1980).

An optimum situation is to inhibit virus replication sufficiently to abort or prevent clinical signs of the disease but, at the same time, to allow some synthesis of influenza virus glycoproteins so that the infected person can develop protective antibodies to prevent subsequent reinfection when drug therapy ceases. One problem with chemoprophylaxis is that persons must take the drug continuously and immediately become susceptible to infection when drug treatment stops. This is another reason why combined use of drugs and vaccines should be given more careful consideration than in the past.

6.2. RECENT CONCEPTS OF THE MOLECULAR BIOLOGY OF INFLUENZA VIRUS REPLICATION, AND APPLICATION TO THE DEVELOPMENT OF A STRATEGY FOR VIRUS CONTROL

A unique feature of the life cycle of the influenza virus was described as early as 1940—the very high rate of recombination between different strains (Fig. 2). Recombination rates of 5–20 per cent are not uncommon between different influenza A viruses (Simpson and Hirst, 1968). The implications are most important since recombination in this manner can extend the genetic pool of the virus and lead, under the influence of selection, to rapid emergence of new strains with different virulence characteristics and antigenicity. Indeed, as mentioned

GENETIC INTERACTIONS

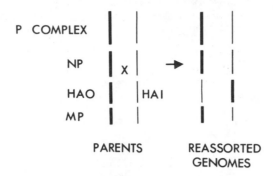

FIG. 2. Genetic recombination and reassortment between influenza A viruses. The RNA genome is segmented with 8 genes. Following mixed infection of a cell with two parental viruses with different genome fragments, 254 offspring with mixed genes can theoretically be produced. The process is illustrated with the P complex as a single gene for simplicity. NP—nucleoprotein. MP—Matrix protein. HAO—HA from parent A/PR/8/34 (H1N1). HA1—HA from parent A/FM1/47 (H1N1).

above, this problem of antigenic 'shift' and 'drift' is an important reason for the absence of preventative measures against this virus. Vaccines rapidly become outdated, while virus sub-types may vary somewhat in susceptibility to anti-viral drugs. Recent work has provided an explanation at the molecular level of the earlier biological observations of recombination. The RNA genome of influenza A, B and C viruses is in the form of 8 or 9 fragments (Palese and Schulman, 1976). Transcripts of the fragments, with the exception of fragments 7 and 8, then act as a series of monocistronic messenger RNAs (Allen et al., 1980; Briedis et al., 1981; Lamb et al., 1980). Thus, each fragment codes for a virus protein, which may be structural or non-structural. Figure 3 illustrates the size range of virion RNA pieces from influenza A viruses. Eight or nine distinct RNA bands are found for influenza A or B viruses with a total molecular weight of $5-6 \times 10^6$ daltons. A minimum value of 4.7×10^6 daltons was also obtained for influenza C virus. Table 2 indicates the individual virus proteins, and the RNA fragments which code for them, and it is apparent that the total genome of the virus is almost accounted for. Figure 4 illustrates the morphology of influenza virus and the correlation with the different proteins coded by the virus RNA.

Studies have shown differences in the RNA patterns of different influenza A viruses. It may be possible to identify which gene, or most likely which genes, are responsible for virulence of influenza viruses (reviewed by Rott, 1979). As regards chemoprophylaxis, studies have demonstrated transfer of resistance to amantadine by recombination between influenza viruses (Appleyard and Maber, 1976). Some studies have indicated that gene 7, coding for the virus matrix protein, carries the property of amantadine resistance (Lubeck, Schulman and Palese, 1978) although more recent work indicates that the genetic basis of resistance is more complex (Scholtissek and Faulkner, 1979; Hay, A. J., personal communication). Further, it may prove possible to synthesize or select inhibitors of the transcription of particular segments of the influenza genome. If such inhibitors had a dual specificity, involving both the virus RNA and the RNA transcriptase enzyme, then they would be highly selective inhibitors of the virus, with a lesser chance of acting as generalised inhibitors of cell transcription processes.

Detailed immunochemical studies are in progress on the surface haemagglutinin (HA) antigen of the virus and these are important to understand the mechanism of antigenic drift. The HA can be selectively cleaved off the virion using proteolytic enzymes such as bromelain (Brand and Skehel, 1972). The resultant HA spikes are purified in sucrose gradients in sufficient quantities for amino acid sequence studies. Studies have indicated common short amino acid sequences in the HA of a range of influenza A and B viruses and these studies have now been confirmed using gene cloning techniques (Porter et al., 1979). X-ray crystallography of an influenza A virus HA molecule at 3 Å resolution has established that

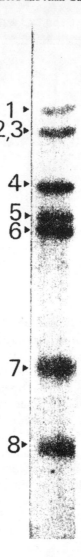

F<small>IG</small>. 3. Fragmented RNA genome of influenza A viruses. Influenza virus was grown for 24 hr in MDCK cells labelled with 1 mCi per 60 mm petri dish of ^{32}P. Virus was purified from the supernatant fluid, ^{32}P-RNA extracted using phenol-SDS and analysed on a 2.5 per cent polyacrylamide gel containing 6M urea. Numbers show gene allocation (see Table 2). Eight genes are detected on the autoradiograph.

the molecule is a trimer of two structurally distinct regions. The first is a triple-stranded coded coil and extends 76 Å from the virus membrane. The second area is a globular region of anti-parallel B-sheet which contains the receptor binding site and the variable antigenic determinants on the top of the stem (Wilson, Skehel and Wiley, 1981). Details of the three-dimensional configuration, and sequence of amino acids, at the tip of the HA spike, may lead to the development of short peptide inhibitors of virus adsorption to cells (Richardson *et al.*, 1980). Similar studies have now been reported for NA (Colmon *et al.*, 1983).

Influenza virus probably absorbs to glycoprotein receptors (Fig. 5) on the plasma membrane of the cell. A suitable model for studies of receptor sites is the major sialoglycoprotein of the red cell membrane, glycophorin, which has been isolated and purified in a homogenous water-soluble form (Marchesi *et al.*, 1972). Glycophorin represents approximately 10 per cent of the total protein of the red cell ghost. It has blood-group antigens and most of the membrane-bound sialic acid and is the major receptor for influenza virus. Future detailed analysis of the exact virus-binding sites could lead to

TABLE 2. *Correlation between RNA Segments and virus-Induced Proteins of Influenza A virus*

M-Wt of RNA segment	Possible protein coded for	M-Wt of protein (daltons)	Function of protein
10.7×10^5	Pl	100×10^3	RNA polymerase?
9.5×10^5	P2*	90×10^3	RNA polymerase?
8×10^5	HA	80×10^3	spike glycoprotein
6.5×10^5	NA	72×10^3	spike glycoprotein
6×10^5	NP	60×10^3	RNA polymerase?
4.7×10^5	M + unidentified protein (M2)	35×10^3	internal structure protein
3.9×10^5	NSI and	26×10^3	non-structural
2.1×10^5	NS2	$10-15 \times 10^3$	non-structural

An RNA transcript of the virus RNA acts as a messenger RNA and, with the exception of genes 7 and 8, which code for two polypeptides, each mRNA is monocistronic and codes for a single virus protein.

In this scheme the RNA segment coding for P3 polypeptide is not identified. (For additional details see Webster *et al.*, 1982).

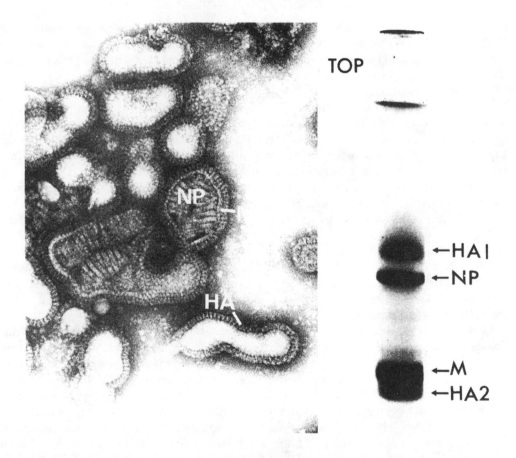

FIG. 4. Morphology of influenza virions. A single particle is partially disrupted showing internal components. The virus polypeptides were analysed on a discontinuous slab gel of 20 per cent w/v polyacrylamide (Oxford and Schild, 1977) and stained with Coomassie blue. Polymerase proteins P1, P2 and P3 polypeptides were not resolved in this gel. Neuraminidase (NA) co-migrates with nucleoprotein (NP).

production of antibodies or synthesis of analogs capable of specifically inhibiting influenza virus adsorption in this model system. Present knowledge indicates that glycophorin is composed of a single polypeptide chain to which multiple oligosaccharides of varying composition and length are attached, mainly to the N-terminal half of the molecule. More

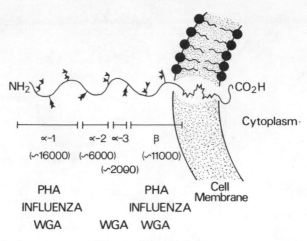

FIG. 5. Glycophorin receptor on red blood cell membrane. PHA—phytohaemagglutinin. WGA—wheat germ agglutinin. Two portions of the molecule have receptor sites for influenza virus, the alpha-1 chain and the beta chain.

detailed analysis of the glycoprotein is based on tryptic digestion, resulting in production of at least four unique glycopeptides. One of the glycopeptides is partially associated with the lipid bilayer. The α-1 (16,000 daltons) and the β polypeptides (11,000 daltons) have receptor sites for influenza virus.

The virus probably enters the cell by viropexis, although some role of fusion is not excluded at present (Dourmashkin and Tyrrell, 1974; White *et al.*, 1981). Virus particles were found in direct contact with the cell surface 10 min after inoculation: at 20 min particles were observed within cytoplasmic vacuoles. Particles within vacuoles often appeared ruptured, suggesting that partial uncoating might occur within the vesicle. Recent electron microscope studies indicate that the adsorption and penetration of influenza virus is an energy-independent process (Patterson, Oxford and Dourmashkin, 1979). Cells were treated with 10^{-4} M sodium azide, cytochalasin B or colchicine, but virus was able to penetrate and initiate infection, as indicated by subsequent production of virus-specified polypeptides.

Under certain conditions of low pH, influenza viruses, in which the HA has been a proteolytically cleaved into HA1 and HA2 polypeptides, can fuse to the plasma membrane of BHK-21 cells (White *et al.*, 1981). The physiological significance of this observation is not clear at present but allows reasonable speculation about intracellular events following virus penetration. Thus fusion may occur intracellularly, so allowing penetration of virus RNA through the cytoplasmic membrane to the cell nucleus for transcription.

Little conclusive data is available on virus uncoating, but cytoplasmic proteases and lipases presumably disrupt the virus envelope and activate the virion transcriptase enzyme. Observations of these early events by electron microscopy show that the outer spike layer of the virus particles in the vacuoles become less distinct approximately 10–20 min post-adsorption (Patterson, Oxford and Dourmashkin, 1979). A fusion event could occur at this stage. The transcriptase enzyme is known to transcribe a copy (complementary strand RNA) of the virus RNA, which is then processed and used as a virus message (summarized in Fig. 6). Studies indicate that all of the eight viral RNA segments are copied. Under conditions where primary transcription is permitted, but protein synthesis is inhibited by cycloheximide, almost all the viral polypeptides could be detected immediately after reversal of the block in protein synthesis. There is regulation of the amounts of each protein synthesized as shown, for example, by differences in the relative amounts of M and NS proteins synthesized, depending on the duration of the cycloheximide block (Lamb and Choppin, 1976). Control is exerted at both the levels of translation and transcription. It is now apparent that the virus mRNA is shorter than full length viral RNA transcripts (Hay and Skehel, 1978). Indirect evidence to date indicates that transcriptase activity requires a combination of P1, P2 and P3, and NP polypeptides (McCauley and Mahy, 1983; Kawakami and Ishihama, 1983).

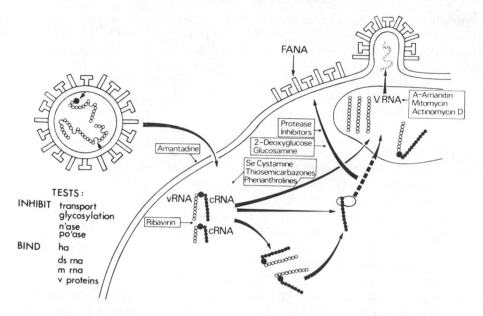

FIG. 6. Life cycle of influenza virus. Following a high multiplicity of virus infection, most events illustrated are completed by 4 hr. Inhibitors are illustrated at their proposed site of action. Tests which can be used to select new antivirals are listed. n'ase—neuraminidase. p'ase—RNA polymerase. ha—haemagglutinin. v proteins—viral proteins. ds RNA—double-stranded RNA. mRNA— messenger RNA. FANA—2-deoxy-2,3-dehydro-N-trifluoroacetyl-neuraminic acid Se-cystamine-selenocystamine, α amanitin. (See àlso McCauley and Mahy, 1983).

Studies in several laboratories have indicated that primary transcription i.e. transcription not inhibited by cycloheximide or puromycin, and carried out using infecting virus RNA as template, occurs first in the nucleus as early as 10 min after infection, and subsequently in the cytoplasm (reviewed by Mahy and Barry, 1978). Parental virus RNA is detected in the nucleus immediately after adsorption of virus to cells, even in cells kept at 4°C. Secondary transcription (i.e. transcription from progeny viral-like RNA templates) probably occurs in the cell cytoplasm. Certainly secondary transcription starts before 1-hr post-infection, which means that the earliest rounds of replication also start before 1-hr post-infection.

It is of importance to determine the exact location of RNA polymerase enzyme activity in the virus-infected cell. Certain inhibitory compounds may more easily reach the cell cytoplasm than the nucleus and this could lead to selectivity if the cell polymerases are restricted mainly to the nucleus, whereas virus-induced polymerases have activity in the cell cytoplasm. Obviously, specific inhibitors of the RNA transcriptase enzyme would act at a theoretically important stage in the life cycle of the virus. We have studied the inhibitory activity of thiosemicarbazones, phenanthrolines and selenocystamine on the virion associated RNA-dependent RNA transcriptase of influenza A and B viruses (Oxford and Perrin, 1977; Perrin and Stunzi, 1980). Although these molecules inhibit the virus enzyme activity *in vitro*, we have been unable to demonstrate *in vivo* activity. Technical details of the test are given, in the Appendix. At some stage the virus-induced complementary RNA also enters the nucleus to become the template for the synthesis of virion RNA. It is not clear if a further RNA replicase enzyme is required or whether the existing transcriptase is modified. Inhibition of this stage would presumably halt the replication of the virus in the cell. Chemicals binding to the enzyme itself, or the enzyme and template together, rather than the virus RNA alone, would appear to be more useful because of the previously demonstrated lack of specificity of antibiotics binding to nucleic acid. Detailed knowledge of the binding or initiation site of the polymerase to the RNA template would also be of great interest.

Inhibitors of virus replication control factors, such as the postulated 'equestron' of polio virus, would be expected to interfere specifically with virus multiplication. Cooper (1977) proposed the equestron regulator because such a multi-functional complex with affinities for 45S ribosomal subunits and 5' of viral RNA would explain the suppression of host protein synthesis of viral RNA and protein, and the timing of maturation. Host cell factors probably are required for influenza virus replication. The virus is inhibited by actinomycin D (Barry, 1964) and α-amanitin, and these compounds as inhibitors of DNA transcription on RNA polymerase II may act by stopping synthesis of capped RNA primers (Krug *et al.*, 1981).

6.3. EARLY SEARCHES FOR AN INFLUENZA VIRUS INHIBITOR

Compounds with a wide range of chemical structures have been shown to inhibit influenza virus growth in eggs and mice (reviewed by Hoyle, 1968; Oxford, 1977; Swallow, 1978). The compounds studied included inhibitors of protein synthesis such as *p*-phenylserine and *p*-fluorophenylalanine; inhibitors of nucleic acid synthesis such as thiouracil and proflavine; and derivatives of natural products, including eucalyptus leaf extracts, streptothricins. Studies of the antiviral activity of natural products are continuing and some interesting molecules have been isolated (Becker, 1980).

More interestingly Eaton *et al.* (1962) described the inhibition of influenza A viruses by ammonium ions. These studies were confirmed and extended by Oxford and Schild (1967, 1968). Ammonium acetate was shown to inhibit both A and B viruses in tissue culture (Table 3). Amantadine, a primary amine, and other amines and ammonium salts, may inhibit virus replication by a common mechanism.

TABLE 3. *Inhibition of Influenza A and B Viruses by Amantadine and Ammonium Ions*

Virus	Reduction in virus end point titre ($\log_{10}$ TCID$_{50}$/ml)		
	amantadine (25 μg/ml)	ammonium acetate (100 μg/ml)	rimantadine (25 μg/ml)
A/NWS (H1N1)	2.0	1.7	1.5
A/Singapore/1/57 (H2N2)	2.5	3.5	not tested
A/Scotland/49/57 (H2N2)	6.0	4.5	5.5
B/England/13/65	0.5	2.6	0.5

MK cell cultures were infected with influenza viruses and incubated in the presence or absence of drugs for 3–4 days. Virus infectivity endpoints were determined by haemadsorption. A reduction of 1.0 $\log_{10}$ TCID$_{50}$/ml or 90 per cent inhibition of virus growth is considered significant in this test. (Data from Oxford and Schild, 1967).

A sensitive immunofluorescence technique (Table 4) was used to compare the antiviral effects of amantadine, ammonium acetate and n-butylamine (Oxford and Schild, 1968). Of particular interest is the inhibition of influenza B virus by certain amines. We shall refer to this observation in more detail below, since it may be possible to synthesize amantadine molecules which inhibit influenza B virus.

The prospect of prevention of influenza in man only became possible with the discovery of the colourless, low molecular weight, water-soluble amphiphilic primary amine, amantadine by Davies *et al.* (1964) as a result of a random screen, and early clinical studies demonstrated clinical efficacy (Jackson *et al.*, 1963).

Up to the present most laboratories searching for new antivirals have used a random screening procedure in tissue cultures and mice. These tests are usually biological in that they investigate any inhibition by compounds of virus formation or virus growth in tissue culture cells. The advent of easily applied biochemical techniques (see Appendix) may lead to a change in emphasis on antiviral screening procedures and more reliance could be placed on specific virus enzymes such as the RNA replicase (reviewed in Stuart-Harris and Oxford, 1983).

TABLE 4. *Antiviral Effect of Amines and Ammonium Ions on Influenza A and B Viruses*

Compound	conc (μg/ml)	% BHK-21 cells fluorescing 24 hr post-infection		
		A/Scotland/57/(H2N2)	A/NWS(H1N1)	B/England/59
none	—	100	100	100
amantadine	25	0.6	—	—
ammonium acetate	200	16.6	89.9	96.0
methylamine	150	39.3	49.0	100
n-propylamine	100	19.2	—	38.1
n-butylamine	120	38.6	10.0	36.2

Note that the maximum non-toxic concentration of compound was used in each case.

Fluorescing cells contained virus-synthesized antigens, and the degree of decrease of Nos. of fluorescing cells indicated the relative antiviral effect of the compounds. (Data from Oxford and Schild, 1968).

6.4. ANTIVIRAL ACTIVITY OF AMANTADINE IN TISSUE CULTURE

The initial report of the antiviral activity of amantadine (Davies *et al.*, 1964) described the inhibition of influenza A viruses in tissue culture and mice (Table 5). These results were rapidly confirmed in many laboratories, and agreement has since been reached on most aspects of the inhibition of influenza A virus by this group of molecules. Tissue culture studies were carried out subsequently in a variety of systems including plaque, haemadsorption inhibition, egg piece, quantitative haemadsorption, S^{35}-methionine labelling, virus HA release from tissue culture cells, and organ cultures, with essentially identical results. A variety of cells, including monkey kidney, Vero, MDCK (canine kidney) chick fibroblast and human amnion have given similar results, and there is no evidence of a host cell restriction of antiviral activity. Pseudo rabies virus (Neumayer *et al.*, 1965) Semliki Forest virus (Helenius *et al.* 1980) and rubella virus (Cochran *et al.*, 1965; Oxford and Schild, 1967) have been shown to be inhibited in tissue culture by amantadine, but to a lesser degree than most influenza A (H3N2) viruses. Most other RNA and DNA viruses are not inhibited (Table 6).

However, some disagreement continues in the literature about the sensitivity of different sub-types of influenza A virus to inhibition by amantadine. This is an important point

TABLE 5. *Viruses Inhibited by 25 μg/ml or Less of Amantadine in Tissue Culture*

Viruses	Host cell system	Test method[a]
Influenza		
A/PR8	CE	HaI,HA
A/Swine/S15	CE	HaI,HA
	MK	CPE
A/WS	CE	HaI,HA
A/WSN	CE	HaI,HA,PI,PAF
	CK,MK,HK	CPE
A/FM-1/47	CE	HaI,HA
A/Japan/305	CE	HaI,HA
/57	HK	CPE
A/Jp	CE	PI
A/AA/2/60	CE	HaI,HA
C/1233	MK	CPE
Parainfluenza	MK	CPE
I/Sendai	CE	HA
Pseudorabies,	HuA	CPE
Aujeszky	CE	PAF

A number of influenza A viruses as well as other RNA containing viruses were initially tested *in vitro* for any sensitivity to the inhibitory effects of amantadine.

[a]Abbreviations: MK, monkey kidney; CK, canine kidney; CE, chick embryo; HK, hamster kidney; HuA, human amnion; HaI, Haemadsorption inhibition; HA, haemagglutination titre; CPE, cytopathic effects; PI, plaque inhibition; PAF, plaque assay of fluid.

TABLE 6. *Organisms Found Insensitive to Amantadine in Tissue Culture or* in ovo

Organism	Host system	Test method
Adeno 2 & 4	HeLa	CPE
Coxsackie A-9 & B-2	MK,HeLa	CPE,PI
ECHO 4 & 22	MK	CPE
Herpes simplex, HF	MK	PI
Influenza B/Lee & GL	CE[a]	PI
	Chick embryo	HA
Canine hepatitis, Led.255	CK	CPE
Mouse hepatitis, MHV-3	CE	PI
Myxoma	CE	PI
NDV, Bonney & Roakin	CE	PI
	Chick embryo	HA
Parain- 1/C35 fluenza 2/Greer 3/C243	MK	CPE
Polio, Type 2, Lansing	HeLa	PI
Reo, Type 1, Lang	MK	CPE
Respiratory syncitial Long	HeLa	CPE
Rhinovirus, HFP	MK	CPE
Semliki Forest	CE	PI
Vaccinia, Lederle[b]	CE	PI
Vesicular stomatitis	CE	PI
Yellow Fever, 17-D	CE	PI
Feline pneumonitis	Chick embryo	MDD + % survivors[c]
Laryngotracheitis	Chick embryo	Pock count on CA membrane
Lymphogranuloma venereum	Chick embryo	MDD + % survivors
Rickettsia, akari & prowazekii	Chick embryo	MDD + % survivors
Rous sarcoma	Chick embryo	Count on CA membrane

Amantadine base at 25 μg/ml in tissue culture and 500 μg/embryo *in ovo* administered 15 min and 30 min prior to infection.
[a]CE—chick embryo cell monolayer.
[b]Variable results.
[c]Mean day of death.

because, if it can be demonstrated that all influenza A virus subtypes from 1918 (H1N1) to the present day (H3N2) are inhibited equally well by amantadine, then it is reasonable to conclude that future antigenic variants, including new pandemic viruses, would be more likely to be inhibited by the compound. Thus amantadine could be used to control an initial outbreak of a new pandemic virus during the period when vaccine was still being produced. Most evidence at present indicates that older laboratory strains of different subtypes of influenza A virus are inhibited to a different extent by amantadine or derivatives. Table 7 gives results obtained in two tissue systems—recent viruses of the A/Hong Kong/1/68 (H3N2) subtype are well inhibited by amantadine (2.5–4.0 $\log_{10}$ inhibition). However, older laboratory viruses of the H1N1 subtypes are less well inhibited (1.0 $\log_{10}$ inhibition approximately) (Schild and Sutton, 1965). Additional data indicating a possible variation in the inhibitory effects of amantadine-type molecules on different influenza A viruses have been reported by Appleyard and Maber (1976). The inhibitory effect of cyclooctylamine, a compound similar to amantadine, varied greatly according to the virus strain. The concentration of cyclooctylamine required to reduce the plaque count to 50 per cent of the control value varied from 0.1 μg/ml for (H2N2) viruses to 20 μg/ml for A/PR/8/34 (H1N1), A/WSN/34 (H1N1) and B/LEE/40 viruses. Viruses which became resistant to cyclooctylamine by passage were also

TABLE 7. *Inhibition of Human and Animal Influenza A Viruses by Amantadine*

Human	Virus	Log_{10} reduction in virus titre
A/PR/8/34	(H1N1)	0.5
A/NWS	(N1N1)	1.3
A/FM1/47	(H1N1)	1.3
A/Singapore/57	(H2N2)	2.4
A/Tokyo/62	(H2N2)	4.0
A/HK/1/68	(H3N2)[a]	2.5 ± 0.5
A/Port Chalmers/73	(H3N2)[a]	2.3
A/Hannover/1/74	(H3N2)[a]	4.0
A/Puerto Rico/74	(H3N2)[a]	2.2
A/Victoria/3/75	(H3N2)[a]	3.6
A/England/75	(H3N2)[a]	4.3
A/NJ/8/76	(Hsw1N1)[a]	2.6
A/Swine/Iowa/15/30	(Hsw1N1)[a]	3.0
A/Swine/Mannitoba/67	(Hsw1N1)[a]	3.0
A/Swine/Wisconsin/61	(Hsw1N1)[a]	2.2

Monkey kidney cells were infected with virus in the presence and absence of 25 μg/ml amantadine and virus growth estimated by haemadsorption after 72 hr incubation. Reduction in virus titre of 1.0 log_{10} TCID_{50}/ml or greater is significant in this test. In some experiments (designated a) the egg piece system of Fazekas de St. Groth and White (1958) was used.

resistant to amantadine, indicating the molecular similarity of the two compounds. By contrast, Grunert and Hoffmann (1977) have presented data indicating that influenza A viruses are very similar in their sensitivity to inhibition by amantadine (Table 8).

A recent study has shown that certain viruses may appear to be resistant or sensitive depending on the assay system (Scholtissek and Faulkner, 1979). In addition, mutations are induced by virus passage which may affect biological properties (Brand and Palese, 1981).

In practical terms, however, a new pandemic virus can be quickly isolated and tested in tissue culture for any degree of inhibition by amantadine. The correlation in the past with amantadine between *in vitro*, *in vivo* and inhibitory effects in man would enable an accurate assessment of antiviral potential with any new influenza A virus. It should not be necessary to repeat clinical trials with every new influenza A virus.

In this context it was of interest to investigate the *in vitro* inhibition of the virus A/New Jersey/8/76 (H1N1) by the compound in detail as a model system. This virus was isolated from an outbreak of influenza at Fort Dix, New Jersey, and is of considerable epi-

TABLE 8. *Relative Sensitivities of Influenza A Viruses to Amantadine Tested in Rhesus Monkey Kidney Cells*

Strain	Serologic type	ED_{50} (μg/ml)
PR/8/34	H0N1	5.7 ± 3.6
FM/1/47	H1N1	4.1 ± 4.5
Japan/305/57	H2N2	5.5 ± 4.7
Hong Kong/50/68	H3N2	3.1 ± 2.4
England/42/72	H3N2	5.0 ± 3.4
Port Chalmers/1/73	H3N2	7.5 ± 5.7
Scotland/840/74	H3N2	6.3 ± 6.2
Georgia/1/75	H3N2	4.1 ± 4.0
Victoria/3/75	H3N2	6.1 ± 3.9
New Jersey/8/76	Hsw1N1	<1

Rhesus monkey kidney cells were infected with 2–10 TCID_{50} of virus and treated with 1, 5 or 25 μg of drug/ml; calculations were done by the method of Reed and Muench, with SD values based on evaluations showing a positive response. ED_{50} is the concentration of amantadine that prevented the appearance of HA in 50 per cent of the cultures. (Data from Grunert and Hoffmann, 1977).

demiological interest because of its close antigenic relationship to the virus which was the presumptive causative agent of the 1918 influenza pandemic. Influenza A/NJ/8/76 (H1N1) virus was kindly supplied by Dr W. Dowdle, Communicable Diseases Centre, Atlanta, Georgia. It was passaged twice at terminal dilutions by conventional techniques in 10-day-old embryonated hens eggs and the infective allantoic fluid stored at $-70°C$. The techniques of virus infection, isotopic labelling and analysis of the polypeptides are described in detail in the Appendix. Briefly, Vero cells were infected with 10 EID_{50} (egg infectious doses) virus per cell in the presence or absence of 25 $\mu g/ml$ amantadine. After virus adsorption the cultures were incubated for 6 hr at 37°C and then pulsed for 30 min with 20 μc of S^{35} methionine (specific activity 445 ci/mmol, Radiochemical Centre, Amersham) per 60 mm plastic petri dish. The cell monolayers were lysed with 0.2 ml of a mixture of 2 per cent w/v SDS, 5 per cent v/v B-mercaptoethanol in 0.06 M Tris buffer at pH 6.8 and analysed by polyacrylamide gel electrophoresis using the discontinuous buffer system of Laemmli (1970), followed by autoradiography of the gel slab.

As early as 6 hr after infection, influenza A/New Jersey/76 virus coded nucleoprotein (NP), nonstructural (NS1) and matrix (M) polypeptides were detected in infected cells (Fig. 7, channels 1 and 3). In infected cells incubated with 100, 50 or 25 $\mu g/ml$ amantadine, virus-induced polypeptide synthesis was almost completely inhibited by 100 $\mu g/ml$ amantadine and partially inhibited by 25 $\mu g/ml$ (Fig. 7, channels 4 and 6). The same concentrations of amantadine (25 $\mu g/ml$) also inhibited the production of haemagglutinin (HA) polypeptides, which were detected intracellularly at 9 hr post-infection, using the above isotopic labelling methods. The production of all virus proteins was inhibited to an equivalent degree by amantadine and there was no selective blockage of a particular polypeptide. The technique has been applied to recent isolates including A/Brazil/11/78 (H1N1) and A/Alaska/78 (H3N2) and these are well inhibited by amantadine (Oxford, 1981).

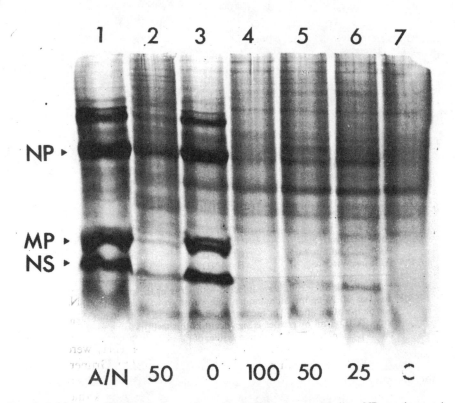

FIG. 7. Inhibition of A/NJ/76 virus polypeptide synthesis by amantadine. NP—nucleoprotein. MP—matrix protein. NS—virus nonstructural protein No. 1. Autoradiograph of S^{35} methionine labelled polypeptides separated on 20 per cent acrylamide slab gel (Oxford and Schild 1977). 100, 50 and 25 $\mu g/ml$ amantadine. C—control, uninfected cells.

6.5. INHIBITION OF INFLUENZA VIRUS HAEMAGGLUTININ PRODUCTION

Vero cell cultures infected in the presence or absence of 25 µg/ml amantadine were incubated for 144 hr and virus replication determined by titration of the supernatant fluids for virus haemagglutinin. Virus HA production of A/NJ/76 and of A/England/864/75 (H3N2), an example of a recently isolated influenza variant, was inhibited by amantadine (Fig. 8, a and b), thus confirming the findings from the intracellular labelling experiments that virus HA synthesis was blocked.

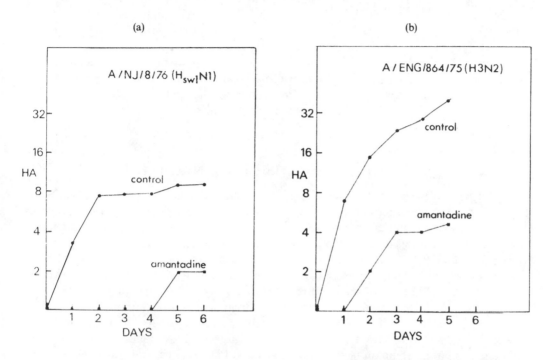

Fig. 8a and b. Inhibition of virus haemagglutinin production and release by amantadine. a A/New Jersey/8/76 (H1N1) virus. b A/England/864/75 (H3N2) virus. Vero or MDCK cells were infected with viruses in the presence or absence of amantadine and incubated for 6 days at 37° C. Virus HA released was quantitated daily using standard haemagglutination techniques.

In further experiments we compared the inhibitory effect of amantadine for a number of influenza A viruses using the egg-piece method of Fazekas de St. Groth and White (1958), which allows a more quantitative estimate of antiviral activity. Influenza A viruses were titrated in 10-fold dilution steps and, after 2 days incubation, egg pieces were removed and virus production estimated by haemagglutination patterns using 0.5 per cent fowl red blood cells. Table 7 indicates that the current influenza subtypes such as A/England/75 (H3N2) and A/Victoria/75 (H3N2) viruses were highly sensitive to the inhibitory effects of amantadine (4.3 and 3.6 $\log_{10}ID_{50}$ reduction in virus end point titre, respectively). A/NJ/8/76 virus was inhibited to the same extent as the sensitive A/HK/68 viruses (2.6 $\log_{10}ID_{50}$ inhibition). The antigenically related influenza A viruses of swine origin A/Swine/Iowa/15/30 (H1N1), A/Swine/Manitoba/67 (H1N1) and A/Swine/Wisconsin/61 (H1N1) were inhibited to a similar degree by amantadine. Similar results have been reported by Grunert and Hoffmann (1977). The response of influenza A/New Jersey/8/76 virus to amantadine was determined by Grunert and Hoffmann (1977) in microcultures of rhesus monkey kidney cells with the maximal well-tolerated concentration (25 µg/ml) of the drug, which was continuously present from 2 hr before infection. This concentration of amantadine significantly reduced the number of infected cultures up to an infection level of 76 $TCID_{50}$.

6.6. GENETIC AND BIOLOGICAL VARIABILITY OF INFLUENZA VIRUSES

A considerable degree of genetic and phenotypic diversity is now known to exist within influenza A and B viruses of a single antigenic subtype (Young *et al.*, 1979; Hinshaw *et al.*, 1978; Sriram *et al.*, 1980; Oxford *et al.*, 1981; Hugentobler *et al.*, 1981). At present, viruses of two antigenic subtypes are co-circulating in the community (Kendal *et al.*, 1979). In addition, recombination has been detected between certain naturally occurring influenza A viruses of the H1N1 and H3N2 subtypes (Young and Palese, 1979). Certain of the influenza A viruses of epidemiological importance vary considerably in the biological properties of plaquing (Oxford *et al.*, 1981) and temperature sensitivity. This variation may result from random mutations or from recombination. Thus influenza viruses, even within a single antigenic subtype, appear to constitute a heterogeneous population and it is of some importance to determine if recent influenza A viruses vary in the susceptibility to inhibition by amantadine. In preliminary studies an analysis of recent virus isolates has detected naturally occurring amantadine-resistant viruses (Oxford and Potter, unpublished data), but the study will now have to be extended to include many more viruses (see also Heider *et al.*, 1981).

6.7. MODE OF ACTION OF AMANTADINE

It must be made clear that the precise point of action on influenza virus replication of amantadine in molecular terms is not known. The details of the early stages of influenza virus infection of cells are unclear and therefore the point of action of an inhibitor acting, as amantadine does, at this early stage remains unestablished. The initial biological studies of Hoffmann *et al.* (1965) suggested that amantadine specifically blocked or slowed down virus penetration into cells. Thus, exposure of infected amantadine-treated cells to viral antiserum for 15 min from $1\frac{3}{4}$–2 hr after infection resulted in a delay in the appearance of HA and a reduction in total HA produced compared to treatment with compound alone. This suggested that, in the presence of amantadine, adsorbed infectious virus remained at the cell surface. The effect, however, was minimal. Kato and Eggers (1969) could only detect a very slight effect of amantadine on penetration of A/Fowl Plague virus, and concluded that the compound affected virus uncoating. The data indicated that two-thirds of neutral red labelled virus in amantadine-treated cultures remained photosensitive even after 3 hr incubation. The rationale of the experiment is that neutral red incorporated into a virion renders it photosensitive but the virus loses this photosensitivity shortly after infecting cells and this loss of photosensitivity can be used as an indicator of uncoating. Thus, at the end of the virus adsorption period, 10 per cent of the infective centres in control cultures had become photoresistant, increasing to 90 per cent after 1 hr at 37°C. By contrast, in amantadine-treated cultures, the number of photoresistant infective centres increased to only 30 per cent after 1 or 2 hr. Hence, in cultures not treated with amantadine, nearly all virus which adsorbed to cells was uncoated within 1 hr at 37°C, whereas in amantadine-treated cultures, even after 3 hr, only one-third of virus was uncoated, suggesting that amantadine inhibits uncoating in this system.

Electron microscope studies by Dourmashkin and Tyrrell (1974) indicated that influenza A virus penetrated cells and appeared in cytoplasmic vacuoles in the presence of amantadine. We have confirmed these results (Patterson, Oxford and Dourmashkin, unpublished) and extended them to determine the inhibitory effect of the compound on subsequent virus-induced polypeptide synthesis (Figs. 9 and 10). The studies demonstrated that in amantadine-treated cultures where influenza A/Hong Kong/1/68 (H3N2) penetrated normally, as observed by electron microscopy, virus-induced polypeptide synthesis was inhibited, indicating that the point of action of amantadine is post-penetration. Furthermore, amantadine has no effect on the virion-associated RNA-dependent RNA polymerase activity of influenza A viruses (Table 9) and hence its point of action appears to be at the stage of virus uncoating or shortly thereafter (see also Bukrinskaya *et al.*, 1980).

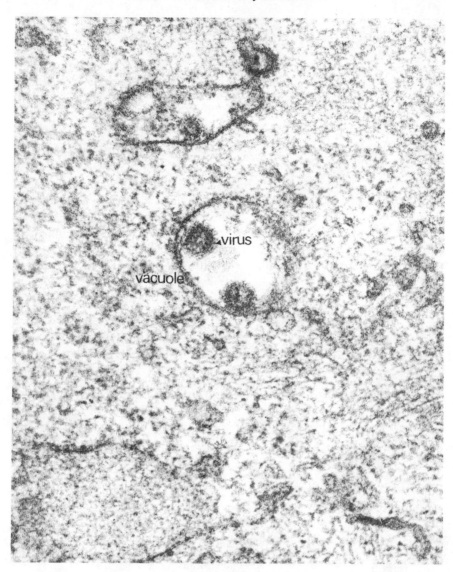

Fig. 9. Adsorption and penetration of A/HK/1/68 virus in the presence of amantadine. Cells were treated with 50 μg/ml amantadine, infected, and examined for penetrated virus 15 min later. Virus has penetrated and uncoated in the presence or absence of the compound. (Patterson and Oxford, 1980).

Skehel *et al.* (1978) examined the effect of amantadine on the synthesis of virus messenger RNA early in infection, in the presence of [H^3]-uridine. After $1\frac{1}{2}$ hr incubation at 37°C, total cell RNA (H^3-labelled) was extracted and hybridized to unlabelled viral RNA. After incubation with RNAase to eliminate residual single-stranded RNA, the hybridized double-stranded RNA was analysed by polyacrylamide gel electrophoresis and autoradiography. In the presence of amantadine no virus specific RNAs were detected. As for the polypeptide studies described above, it was concluded that amantadine has to be added within $1\frac{1}{2}$ hr of infection to be effective. Therefore amantadine does not inhibit transcription of the virus genome directly. Skehel *et al.* (1978) further investigated any effect of amantadine on primary transcription by infecting cells in the presence of cycloheximide, which gave complete transcription of all 8 gene segments. In cells infected in the presence of cycloheximide and amantadine, no transcription of any virus gene was detected. Therefore amantadine appears to have no direct effect on the translation or the synthesis of influenza messenger RNA. Recent analysis of amantadine-resistant viruses has indicated that gene 7, coding for matrix

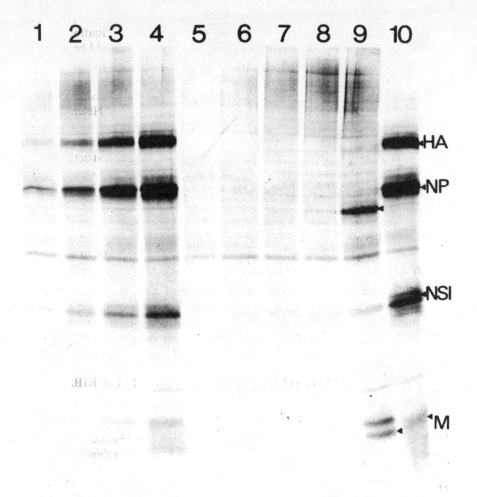

FIG. 10. Effect of amantadine on polypeptide synthesis induced by A/Hong Kong/68 (H3N2) and B/HK/73 viruses. 1–4: B/HK/73 + amantadine (200, 100, 50 and 25 μg/ml respectively). 5–8: A/HK/68 (H3N2) + amantadine (200, 100, 50 and 25 μg/ml respectively). 9: A/HK/68 control. 10: B/HK/73 control. M—matrix protein. NSI—nonstructural protein No. 1. HA—haemagglutinin. NP—nucleoprotein. Virus induced polypeptides are resolved clearly in control infected cultures but no virus polypeptide synthesis is detectable in cultures treated with 50 μg/ml amantadine and infected with the influenza A virus. In contrast amantadine has no effect on influenza B virus induced polypeptide synthesis, except at very high concentrations of 200 μg/ml.

TABLE 9. *Absence of Inhibition of Influenza A Virion-Associated RNA-Dependent RNA Polymerase Activity by Amantadine*

Concentration of compound (mM)		H^3-UMP incorporated dpm/mg virus protein/hour $\times 10^{-3}$
amantadine	100	96.1
	10	84.2
	1	80.0
selenocystamine	0.1	0
control (no drug)		97.1

RNA polymerase enzyme activity, estimated as described previously (Oxford, 1977), is proportional to cpm incorporated into acid precipitable RNA. Thus in the test, virus was incubated for 30′ at 37°C with or without the compounds. The reaction was stopped by the addition of trichloracetic acid. Selenocystamine had been shown previously to inhibit influenza A virus RNA transcriptase (Oxford and Perrin, 1977) and therefore acted as a positive control.

protein, may transfer drug resistance by recombination (Lubeck, Schulman and Palese, 1978). This could suggest that the matrix protein interacts with amantadine at an early stage of virus infection to prevent late uncoating or transcription. It should be noted that other studies indicate a more complex derivation of resistance involving additional virus genes (Scholtissek and Faulkner, 1979).

Amantadine and other amines are known to be lysomotropic agents since they accumulate in the lysosomes and tend to increase the intra lysosomal pH (Helenius et al., 1980). Ammonium chloride increases the pH of mouse peritoneal macrophages from pH 4.5 to pH 6.2 whilst amantadine raises the pH to pH 5.5 (Ohkuma and Poole, 1978). Fusion of influenza membrane with plasma membranes occurs in vitro and is strictly pH dependent, fusion only occurring at pH 6.0 or lower. Thus, in theory, amantadine could prevent this fusion in the lysosome by increasing the pH and hence result in abortion of virus infection. The problem with this hypothesis is that low pH fusion is mediated by the virus HA and experiments with recombinants have failed to establish any role for gene 4 coding for HA in amantadine resistance or sensitivity.

Some derivatives of amantadine affect the fluidity of the membrane in artificial liposome spherules (Jain et al., 1976) and this property may affect virus fusion events at uncoating. A recent study suggests that amantadine may protect cells by interacting with the external surface of the plasma membrane. Of course this conflicting data could be resolved if amantadine had several points of action.

6.8. TISSUE CULTURE STUDIES OF THE ANTIVIRAL EFFECTS OF COMBINED AMANTADINE AND INTERFERON OR RIBAVIRIN

To date the antiviral activity of most inhibitors of influenza virus has been examined independently. However, precedent from antibacterials suggest that in certain clinical circumstances combinations of drugs could be used with benefit. Since amantadine inhibits only influenza A viruses, it may be of advantage to initiate combined therapy with an inhibitor of influenza B viruses which are important causes of morbidity in non-influenza A years. In addition, the use of combinations of inhibitors acting at different stages of the infectious cycle would be expected to reduce the chances of emergence of drug-resistant strains of virus. One of the few experimental papers reporting data on drug combinations is that of Lavrov et al. (1968, 1969). The experiments indicated that combinations of amantadine with 5-fluorouracil (an inhibitor of nucleic acid synthesis), or with D, L-ethionine (an inhibitor of protein synthesis), produced an additive-inhibitory effect on the replication of A/FPV in chick cells. In addition, and of more importance for future practical applications, interferon and amantadine had an additive antiviral effect on the replication of A/WSN (H1N1) virus in chick embryo cells. In the presence of both inhibitors, infectious virus was not detected in cells and medium. The inhibitor produced only a marginal effect when added

TABLE 10. *The Proportion of Influenza A Infected Cells in the Presence of Interferon and Amantadine*

Inhibitor	Ratio of the infectious centres number: the number of cells in chick embryo cell culture (per cent) Time after inoculation (h)		
	1	24	48
None	0.04	100.0	100.0
Interferon	0.04	1.5	1.7
Amantadine	0.004	8.5	77.0
Interferon plus amantadine	0.005	0.013	0.031

Cells treated with interferon or amantadine were infected at a multiplicity of infection 10^{-2}PFU virus/cell. At different times after inoculation the No. of infectious centres was determined and compared to the No. of cells in the culture. (Data from Lavrov et al., 1968).

24 hr post-infection, as expected. An additive effect of interferon and amantadine was also noted on the accumulation of haemagglutinin in cultures infected at high multiplicity of 2 $\times 10^2$ PFU per cell. When the proportion of infected cells in the culture was quantitated, the rate of cumulative inhibition was approximately 10 times higher in double-treated cultures than could be expected from the product of separate effects of interferon and amantadine (Table 10).

Recent studies have indicated a synergistic effect of α-methyl-1-adamantane methylamine and the nucleoside analogue, ribavirin (Zlydnikov et al., 1981). Ribavirin had been shown previously to inhibit replication of influenza A and B viruses in mice and tissue cultures (Sidwell et al., 1972, Oxford, 1975a,b). The antiviral activity of Ribavirin is discussed in more detail below, and has been the subject of an excellent review (Smith and Kirkpatrick, 1980; Knight et al., 1981; Hillyard, 1980; McClung et al., 1983).

6.9. DERIVATIVES OF AMANTADINE WITH ANTIVIRAL ACTIVITY

Many hundreds of derivatives of 1-amino adamantane have now been synthesized and tested for anti-influenza virus activity. Studies of molecular variants are still continuing (Indulen and Kalninya, 1973, 1980). One object of further screening is to synthesize amantadine molecules which inhibit influenza B viruses (Table 3). Molecules have not yet been obtained which have any marked advantage compared to 1-aminoadamantane. Rimantadine, or α-methyl-1-adamantane methylamine, has been widely used in the USSR but its virus inhibitory effects in tissue culture are the same (Table 3) or only marginally better than amantadine, although toxicity in man may be less than amantadine. Addition of side chains to delay the excretion rate of amantadine would appear promising (Zlydnikov et al., 1981). Jain et al. (1976) described the effect of 34 amantadine derivatives on the phase transition characteristics of artificial liposomes but no details were given of relative antiviral effects.

A typical series of amantadine derivatives was described by Vaczi et al. (1973), who screened the compounds against A/Singapore/1/57 (H2N2) virus. The N-methylene aryl derivatives proved to be less active than 1-aminoadamantane hydrochloride itself. The activity of these derivatives was differently modified by the different aryl radicals. As compared to the N-benzyl derivative (compound 1 in Table 11), substitution in the ortho position by an OH (2) or NO_2 (4) resulted in a 4-fold and 15-fold increase in activity, respectively. The activity index of the ortho Cl derivative (3) was low owing to its high toxicity. The activity index of the 2-hydroxybenzyl derivative (2) was reduced by substitution with a methoxy group at the ortho position (5). The dimethoxy derivatives (6, 7 and 8) were even less active. The activity of the Cl-substituted benzyl derivatives (9, 3, 10) was considerably influenced by the position of the substituent(s), and by their relative position if more than one Cl is substituted in a molecule. The 2,6-dichlorobenzyl derivative had the highest activity index because of its low toxicity. Substitution on the para position of the benzyl group resulted in reduced activity as compared to 1. An increase in the length of the chain linking the benzyl ring with the amino group resulted in an increased toxicity and thus a low activity index. Derivatives containing a heteroaromatic group in place of the phenyl group were more active than the phenyl derivative (1). The 4-pyridyl derivative was 16 times as active as 1. The activity index of the compound containing cyclohexyl (2) instead of the adamantyl skeleton, but the same N-substituent (N-ortho-hydroxy-benzyl), was very low.

The thioglycolate of 1-aminoadamantane was found to be as active as its hydrochloride. The activity of the mercaptopropionate, on the other hand, was twice as high as that of the hydrochloride. Noradamantane has been synthesized (Nickon et al., 1967; Vogt and Hoover, 1967).

6.10. SYNTHESIS OF ADAMANTANE SPIRO COMPOUNDS

The discovery of a method for the synthesis of 2-adamantanone encouraged chemists to investigate substitution at a bridge atom of the adamantane nucleus and made synthesis of

TABLE 11. *Chemical and Antiviral Characterization of a Series of Amantadine Compounds*

—NH—CH$_2$—R

Designation	R	Molecular weight	Activity index
1	(phenyl)	277.85	100
2	(phenyl, HO)	293.84	400
3	(phenyl, Cl)	312.28	25
4	(phenyl, O$_2$N)	322.84	1500
5	(phenyl, HO, OCH$_3$)	323.86	50
6	(phenyl, CH$_3$O, OCH$_3$)	337.89	< 37.5
7	(phenyl, OCH$_3$, CH$_3$O)	337.89	< 12.5
8	(phenyl, OCH$_3$, CH$_3$O)	337.89	37.5
9	(phenyl, Cl)	312.28	12
10	(phenyl, Cl, Cl)	346.73	10
24	HS—CH—COO with CH$_3$	257.39	6000
25	Cl	187	3000

Amantadine derivatives were synthesized and compared for antiviral activity against influenza A viruses. (Data from Vaczi *et al.*, 1973).

secondarily substituted adamantanes, including spiro compounds, possible (Lundahl *et al.*, 1972; Van Hes *et al.*, 1972). The *N*-methyl derivative was 3 times more active than 1-aminoadamantane *in vivo*. The adamantane spiro-3^1-pyrolidines, which have smaller alkyl substituents, are comparable to the *N*-methyl derivative in level and spectrum of activity. Increasing size of the substituents at the N atom tended to diminish *in vivo* activity. Activity was highest for a molecule structurally most closely related to amantadine.

The cyclohexane derivative had no detectable antiviral activity. The diamantane spiro-3^1-pyrrolidine and its *N*-methyl derivative were less active *in vivo* than the *N*-methyl derivative. Finally none of the spiro compounds had antiviral activity against influenza B strains.

Further syntheses were carried out by the same group of 6- and 7-membered ring analogues of the pyrrolidine molecule. Most compounds were cytotoxic except for piperidine derivatives with activity comparable to 1-aminoadamantane.

The antiviral activity of 1-(*p*-(methylnitrosamino)-benzylideneamino)-adamantane has been described by Tonew *et al.* (1973, 1974).

6.11. WATER-SOLUBLE POLYMERS

Holt and Thadani (1973) investigated the possibility of copolymerisation of *N*-vinylpyrrolidone and *N*-allylamino-adamantane to enhance antiviral action (Fig. 11). Attempts were made to synthesize water soluble polymers by attaching the antiviral molecule by a grouping unlikely to be degradable *in vivo* and by condensation of the amino group with a group on a polymer to give a linkage likely to be hydrolysed in a cell, there to liberate free aminoadamantane. To date no details have been published on the antiviral activity of these compounds.

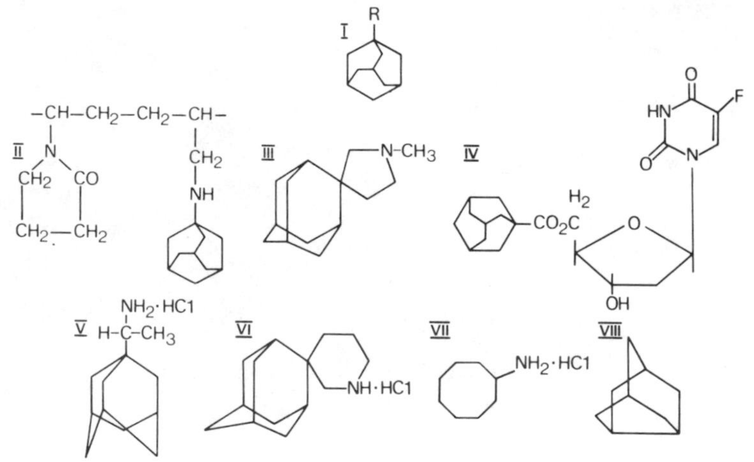

FIG. 11. Some typical molecular derivatives of amantadine. I—aminoadamantane, amantadine or Symmetrel. II—poly-(1,2′-oxo-1′pyrrolidinyl-4-(-*N*-1′adamantylamino methyl) butylene. III—1′-methyl spiro-(adamantane-2,3′pyrrolidine)-maleate. IV—5′adamantoyl-2′-deoxy-5-fluorouridine. V—α-methyl-1-adamantane methylamine. VI—adamantane spiro-3′-piperidine. VII—cyclo octyl-amine. VIII—noradamantane (see also Swallow, 1978).

6.12. ANTIVIRAL EFFECT OF AMANTADINE IN ANIMAL MODELS

6.12.1. MOUSE MODEL

The various animal model infections used in the laboratory with influenza are discussed in more detail in the Appendix. Some examples will be given here to illustrate the degree of antiviral activity noted in animals. Most laboratories searching for new inhibitors of influenza A virus use amantadine as a positive control in animal studies.

The early studies of Davies *et al.* (1964) described the ameliorating effect of amantadine on influenza pneumonia in mice. Doses of the compound as low as 2.5 mg/kg had detectable antiviral effects and this would approximate to the drug dosage in man (see below) and to a tissue level of 2.5 μg/ml which is known to inhibit most sensitive influenza A viruses. In these initial experiments, A/Swine, A/WS (H1N1) and A/AA/60 (H2N2) viruses were inhibited to the same extent *in vivo*. Grunert and Hoffmann (1977) also investigated the *in vivo* effects of amantadine against the A/NJ/76 (H1N1) virus and the results are presented in Table 12.

TABLE 12. In vivo *Inhibition of A/NJ/76 Virus by Amantadine*

Infection LD$_{50}$	Positive infections (%)		p
	control	amantadine	
50	100	8	<0.001
5	83	0	<0.001
0.5	42	0	0.007

Amantadine was provided in the drinking water of mice (0.25 mg/ml) starting on day 1 through day 14.

Animals were infected intranasally with A/NJ/76 virus and examined daily for deaths. (Data from Grunert and Hoffmann, 1977).

Schulman (1968) investigated the effect of amantadine and rimantadine on the transmission of influenza A virus in mice (Table 13). This model infection was of particular interest because subsequently amantadine was investigated by Galbraith *et al.* (1969a and b) for ability to prevent intrafamilial virus spread in General Practice in the UK (see below).

TABLE 13. *Effect of Amantadine and Rimantadine on Virus Spread in the Mouse Model*

Drug treatment (20 mg/kg)	No. of contact mice infected	
	No.	%
Saline	35/60	58.3
amantadine	28/60	48.3
rimantadine	5/60	8.3

Amantadine or rimantadine were given intraperitoneally 0.5 hr before and 12, 24 and 36 hr post-infection of mice with influenza A virus. Spread of virus could be estimated by virus isolation procedures. (Data from Schulman, 1968).

Rabinovich (1972) examined the effect of rimantadine on weight loss and water uptake in mice infected with A/Jap/305/57 (H2N2) virus. Virus infection resulted in weight loss and decrease in water consumption—treatment with rimantadine (24 mg/kg/day) partially reversed the decline (Fig. 33, below).

6.12.2. THERAPEUTIC EFFECT OF AMANTADINE *IN VIVO*

Studies of the pathology of influenza in the mouse and ferret model infections (see Appendix) have been interpreted to indicate that symptoms of virus infection occur at the time of maximum viral replication and cell destruction. It was considered unlikely therefore that amantadine or any other inhibitor of influenza virus would have detectable therapeutic effects. Nevertheless studies in animal models, and in man, have now demonstrated quite conclusively some mild therapeutic effect of amantadine and rimantadine. At present this is attributed to the specific antiviral activity of amantadine. Immunofluorescence studies of post-mortem tracheas (Mulder and Hers, 1972) from persons dying of influenza pneumonia have indicated that only a proportion of potentially susceptible cells have intracellular influenza antigens. Thus, even at a time of apparent maximum virus replication, virus spread is still occurring. Amantadine may limit virus spread even at this late stage in the infection and so initiate faster resolution of the clinical effects of the disease. However, an alternative explanation—some effect of amantadine on the immunological response or virus induced immunopathology—is not completely discounted. Amantadine has been reported to have mild immunosuppressive activity and this may influence the host's response to the infection (Bredt and Mardiney, 1969a and b).

McGahen and Hoffmann (1968) used an objective measure of influenza infection in the mouse—a decrease in water consumption which occurs as an early disease symptom—to quantitate the degree of therapeutic activity of amantadine. Female white mice 28 to 30 days old (t. 18 ± 2 g), first caged on wire in continuous light for 5 days, were used throughout. Such mice, under light ether anaesthesia, were infected intranasally with 0.05 ml of a mouse lung preparation of influenza A/Bethesda/10/63 (H2N2) diluted to a concentration calculated to cause 85 per cent mortality on the tenth day after infection ($3-5LD_{50}$). The water consumption of virus-infected and sham-infected mice was measured to the nearest 1 ml at 4-hr intervals beginning 4 hr after infection. The data were analysed as the cumulative millilitres of water consumed by groups of 60–80 mice. Amantadine was administered 12 hr after the first measurement period of significant water-consumption difference. With influenza A/Bethesda/10/63, amantadine was dosed by two methods, singly and in combination: ad libitum in the drinking water as a 0.5 mg/ml solution from 48 hr through 240 hr after infection, and by oral intubation at 100 mg/kg in 0.2 ml of water as a single dose at 48 hr, as two doses at 48 and 72 hr and as three doses at 48, 72 and 96 hr after infection.

As shown in Table 14, significant ($p = 0.05$) increases of both percentage of survivors and survival time occurred only in those groups of mice which received amantadine in the drinking water; a significant increase in survival time, but not in survivors, occurred in the group of mice given three oral doses of amantadine at 48, 72 and 96 hr after infection. The single 48-hr oral dose was not additive to the drinking water treatment, while two doses at 48 and 72 hr were additive and the third oral dose at 96 hr caused no additional effects. Significant reduction in disease severity and increase in the number of healthy animals occurred among those groups of mice which received amantadine in the drinking water, and in the group which received three oral doses. The oral dosing afforded no additional protection when given with the drinking-water treatment.

TABLE 14. *Survival and Disease Severity Ratings of Mice Infected with Influenza A/Bethesda/10/63 (H2N2) and Treated with Amantadine*

Drinking water[a]	Oral intubation[b]	No. in group	% Survival at day 10	Mean survival day	Healthy animals (%)
Control		77	14.3	6.2	2.6
48–240	None	78	42.3[d]	7.9[c]	25.6[d]
48–240	48	76	44.8[d]	8.0[c]	27.6[d]
48–240	48, 72	76	52.6[d]	10.2[d]	26.3[d]
48–240	48, 72, 96	79	50.6[d]	10.2[d]	26.6[d]
None	48	80	17.5	7.0	10.0
None	48, 72	76	23.7	7.5	5.3
None	48, 72, 96	78	27.0	7.7	14.3[c]

Mice were infected and then treated with amantadine by different routes at varying times post infection.

[a]Dose: 0.5 mg/ml in water.

[b]Dose: 100 mg/kg in 0.2 ml of water.

[c]$p = 0.05$.

[d]$p = 0.01$.

(Data from McGahen and Hoffmann 1968).

6.12.3. AVIAN MODEL INFECTIONS

An interesting model infection which indicated the marked prophylactic effect of amantadine was described by Lang *et al.* (1970) and used turkeys exposed to A/Turkey/Ontario/7732/66 virus (Table 15). The virus was highly pathogenic for turkeys and lethal by any route. The increasing number of antigenic subtypes isolated from domestic birds in recent years means that control of avian influenza by vaccines has become increasingly difficult. Initially 3-week-old birds were placed together and 6 were given 15 mg/kg amantadine for 7 days before, and 23 days after, infection. All untreated birds died between 3 and 7 days after intranasal infection. In contrast, only one of the amantadine-treated birds died on day 9. Similar results were obtained when the birds were infected orally. In a dose-response experiment birds were infected with 2500 EID_{50}/ml of virus and mortality was 5/5 for the control untreated group, 0/4 at 10 mg/kg, 1/5 at 5 mg/kg and 4/7 at 1 mg/kg amantadine. All survivors had detectable antibody after infection, suggesting sub-clinical infection. Amantadine was also shown to protect birds against infection with a massive dose of virus approximating to 10^5 LD_{50}. Amantadine administration (10 mg/kg) was delayed to 20-hr post-infection. All 5 untreated birds were dead 2 days p.i. but only one-quarter of the treated birds died. Amantadine incorporated in the feed pellets at 0.025 per cent offered full protection against challenge with virus. Overall the experiments indicated 80 per cent protection of turkeys from signs of disease. An important variable was the dosage with amantadine. The compound is rapidly absorbed in birds and rapidly excreted and therefore a dosage regimen which assures a constant level of compound in the tissue was necessary. In domestic birds a feed formulation was the most satisfactory method of administration. Since influenza A virus is a natural infection in many domestic birds (Easterday, 1975), this model system for prophylaxis may have wider application for the study of anti-influenza compounds.

TABLE 15. *Prophylactic Effect of Amantadine in Turkeys Infected with A/Turkey/Ontario/66 Virus*

Infection	Treatment	Deaths	HI titre day 14	Re-exposure day 14	Deaths	HI titre day 23
contact	amantadine	1/6	< 8	3 im 2 in	0	10, 160, 2560, 0, 160
	control	5/5	ND	ND	ND	ND
virus in drinking water	amantadine	1/5	< 8	2 in 2 im	0	320, 160, 640, 1280
	control	5/5	ND	ND	ND	ND

Turkeys were given 15 mg/kg amantadine per day from—7 days to 23–28 days post-infection, infected, and then examined daily for deaths.

HI haemagglutination inhibition antibody titre. (Data from Lang, Narayan and Rouse, 1970).

6.13. SELECTION OF AMANTADINE-RESISTANT INFLUENZA VIRUSES IN THE LABORATORY

In a series of early experiments we demonstrated that the passage of an influenza A virus in mice, in the presence of a high concentration of amantadine, resulted in the selection of virus variants which required a 100-fold increase in amantadine concentration for inhibition. In practical terms the variants were completely drug resistant (Oxford *et al.*, 1970; Tuckova *et al.*, 1973).

The 36 virus pools from the control mice passage series were all inhibited by 0.02 to 0.2 μg/ml of amantadine in the QH test. In contrast, influenza viruses resistant to inhibition by amantadine were detected in a proportion of the 36 virus pools from drug-treated mice. Drug-resistant viruses were detected in the lungs of 1 of 12 mice on the first passage of virus in drug-treated animals. After three passages in drug-treated mice, the proportion of amantadine-resistant viruses increased, and resistant viruses were present in 8 of the 12 passage series. A single virus strain showed partial resistance to inhibition by amantadine after one passage in mice: before passage in mice, growth of the virus in tissue culture was inhibited by 0.1 μg/ml of the compound and, after one pass in drug-treated mice, 1.3 μg/ml was required for inhibition (Table 16). After two and three passes in drug-treated mice, 5 and 12.5 μg/ml of amantadine respectively, were required for inhibition. Three virus strains required two passages in drug-treated mice before showing any resistance to inhibition by the compound, while in four strains drug resistance became apparent only after three passages in treated mice. Thus, strains of A/Singapore/1/57 virus, resistant to inhibition by amantadine, could be obtained with relatively high frequency after several passages of virus in mice treated with high concentrations of the compound.

In a second series of experiments, influenza A/Singapore/1/57 virus was passed four times in groups of mice treated with varying concentrations of amantadine. Drug-resistant viruses were recovered only from mice treated with very large doses (150 mg/kg/day) of drug; no drug-resistant viruses were recovered from mice treated with 15 or 1.5 mg/kg/day of the compound.

We have attempted, without success, to recover drug-resistant variants from persons infected with influenza and undergoing treatment with amantadine. However, the experiments involved very few persons, and similar experiments are required in future trials of this and any other anti-influenza compounds to monitor the possible emergence of drug-resistant viruses. Continuing studies of amantadine-resistant influenza viruses are important practically; the variants may also be helpful in establishing the precise mode of action of the compound. Some field viruses have now been shown to be drug resistant (Heider *et al.*, 1981).

TABLE 16. *Selection of Amantadine Resistant Influenza A Viruses* in vivo

Passage in drug-treated mice	No. of passages	IC$_{50}$ conc. of amantadine range	(μg/ml)[a] mean
O	3	0.04–0.43	0.3
O	4	0.03–0.85	0.4
+	1	1.5–6.3	3.4
+	3	—	25
+	6	10–50	25.3
+	6[b]	—	25

Mice were treated with amantadine at a dosage of 150 mg/kg/day. This is the maximum tolerated dose of compound and caused drug-induced illness in approximately 25 per cent of mice. Mice were then infected with influenza A/Singapore/57 (H2N2) virus and at intervals lungs removed and ground to a 10 per cent suspension. Virus was then used to infect further amantadine-treated mice.

[a]IC$_{50}$ concentration of amantadine (μg/ml) causing 50 per cent inhibition of virus haemadsorption in infected cells.

[b]Passaged in amantadine-treated mice and subsequently passaged allantoically 4 times at terminal dilutions in untreated eggs.

6.14. RECOMBINATION BETWEEN DRUG-RESISTANT AND DRUG-SENSITIVE INFLUENZA VIRUSES

Appleyard and Maber (1976) investigated whether COA (cyclooctylamine, a compound related to amantadine) resistance could be used as a genetic marker for influenza viruses, and whether COA-resistance was dependent upon either of the surface antigens of the virus. A group of eggs was inoculated with a mixture of 8×10^6 p.f.u. A2 virus (COA-sensitive) and 5×10^6 p.f.u. BEL/CR virus (COA-resistant). After incubation at 36°C for 24 hr, the allantoic fluids were harvested and pooled, and the total content of infective virus was determined by plaque assay. The yields of A2, BEL, A2-BEL and BEL-A2 viruses were estimated individually by plaque assay in the presence of rabbit antisera prepared against

BEL, A2, BEL-A2 and A2-BEL viruses, respectively, the antiserum concentrations necessary to select for the appropriate viruses having been established in previous tests. Each titration was also performed in the presence of 15 μg/ml COA to determine the amount of each virus that was COA-resistant. The results (Table 17) indicated that there was a high frequency of recombination between the two parent viruses: at least 10 per cent of the progeny were of mixed antigenic type, the BEL-A2 recombinant being commoner than A2-BEL. About 7 per cent of the yield of A2 virus was resistant to COA. This was far more than the proportion of about 0.01 per cent found in other experiments for the input virus, showing that COA-resistance could be transferred without a simultaneous change in surface antigenic structure. Some, but probably not all, of the BEL-A2 and the A2-BEL recombinants were resistant to COA, again suggesting that COA-resistance was independent of the nature of the surface antigens. To confirm that the BEL-A2 and A2-BEL recombinants included some viruses that were sensitive to COA and others that were resistant, 36 plaques of each recombinant type were picked from the assay plates. Their sensitivities to inhibition by COA were determined by plating in the absence and in the presence of COA. Of the BEL-A2 recombinants, 17/36 (47 per cent) were resistant to COA, and of the A2-BEL recombinants, 23/36 (64 per cent) were resistant. Amantadine resistance was transferred along with gene 7 coding for virus matrix protein in a series of recombinants (Lubeck, Schulman and Palese, 1978). Studies by other groups have indicated a more complex gene involvement in amantadine resistance (Scholtissek and Faulkner, 1979) and further studies are required with larger series of recombinant viruses.

TABLE 17. *Genetic Transfer of Amantadine Resistance*

| Antigenic type | Virus yield (p.f.u./ml × 10^{-6}) | |
	Total	COA-resistant
Total	49	16
A2	8.4	0.62
BEL	8.5	9.0
A2-BEL	0.32	0.11
BEL-A2	4.4	2.6

COA—cyclooctylamine, an amantadine derivative.

An amantadine-sensitive virus (A2 subtype) was recombined with an amantadine-resistant virus (A/BEL) and the progeny 'recombinants' or reassorted genome viruses examined for the degree of amantadine resistance or susceptibility. (Data from Appleyard and Maber, 1976).

6.15. PHARMACOLOGY AND TOXICOLOGY OF AMANTADINE

Studies of the toxicology, metabolism and phamacology of potential antiviral compounds are of particular importance for the correlation of *in vitro* with clinical activity. The half-life and general pharmacological properties of amantadine were established early and proved of considerable use for interpretation of the antiviral activity *in vivo*. Some of the data are discussed below but, in summary, it has been established that, following oral administration of the compound to man or mice, concentrations of amantadine could be attained in the tissues which would be expected to have influenza virus inhibitory effects (around 1 μg amantadine/g tissue). However, what does *not* appear to be clearly established is the exact intracellular localization of administered amantadine. The studies of the mode of action of amantadine in inhibiting influenza A virus replication would suggest an action of the compound at late uncoating (see above). However, some earlier experiments using (H^3)-labelled amantadine appeared to indicate that, although the compound was associated with the plasma membrane of cells, treatment of cells with trypsin, after addition of amantadine removed amantadine from the cells. This suggested binding of the compound to an *external* layer of the cell which was removed by mild trypsin treatment. The studies of Skehel *et al.* (1978) using (H³)-amantadine, which suggested rapid cellular uptake of the compound, but slow release, do not establish if the compound was intracellular or only bound to the outside of the plasma membrane.

More recent studies demonstrated that amantadine was rapidly concentrated in the lysosomes and in the cytosol of MDCK cells, and the cells were able to attain an intracellular concentration 100-fold higher than in the external medium. A considerable portion of the amantadine taken up by the cells was also shown to be resistant to subsequent elution. In contrast, the antiviral effect of the drug was lost immediately upon its removal from the medium. Thus most of the cell associated amantadine may not contribute to the antiviral action of the drug. The portion of the amantadine which does account for its antiviral activity is rapidly exchanged with the extracellular medium and may actually be amantadine in the extracellular medium. Amantadine may protect cells from influenza A virus infection by its interaction with the external surface of the cell plasma membrane.

It is possible that, when influenza adsorbs to the plasma membrane and, as a result of viropexis, enters the cytoplasm in vacuoles, the amantadine is taken up at the same time in the intracytoplasmic vacuole. This could explain the apparent intracellular antiviral activity of the drug even if the compound remains predominantly on the cell surface. Amantadine has been shown to increase the pH of cellular lysosomes (Ohkuma and Poole, 1978).

A recent study has investigated interaction between amantadine and the specific subcellular organelles in which biogenic amines are stored. Amantadine was shown to distribute across the membrane of chromaffin granules and the author suggested that *in vivo* amantadine may be concentrated and stored as a pharmacologic agent in amine containing granules (Johnson *et al.*, 1981).

Some derivatives of amantadine affect the fluidity of the membrane in artificial liposome spherules and this is worthy of further investigation. Jain *et al.* (1976) studied 34 proto and homo adamantane derivatives on phase transition characteristics of bilayers and the compound derivatives modified the phase properties. Minor modifications in the structure of amantadine can alter its influence on the phase transition temperature. If amantadine alters the rigidity of lipid bilayers, either of the virus itself or the plasma membrane of the cell, then this might be expected to influence virus uncoating or release of RNA and this should be the subject of further investigation.

6.15.1. Assay of Amantadine

Amantadine can be assayed in biological samples by a sensitive method based on vapour phase chromatography (Bleidner *et al.*, 1965). In brief, chromatographic isolation of amantadine is achieved isothermally or in a combination of programmed temperature and isothermal operations using a column of 10 per cent Carbowax 20 M on base-treated Chromosorbs W.

6.15.2. Mouse Model—Excretion of Amantadine

The total percentage of unchanged amantadine recovered in the urine of treated mice was high and reasonably constant over a range of single oral doses of the hydrochloride from 1 mg/kg to 100 mg/kg (average 63 per cent, range 51–75). Excretion was largely complete in about 12 hr. A semilogarithmic plot of excretion rate at a representative dose level, using the mid-points of the urinary collection intervals, indicated that excretion did not reach its maximum rate for periods up to 6 hr after treatment. Only about 2 per cent of the dose was found in the faeces of two mice given 496 mg/kg orally.

The low level of the compound in the faeces and the regularity of the excretion data over a wide range of doses indicated that amantadine hydrochloride was well adsorbed orally in the mouse following oral administration. A very satisfactory level was found in the lung (Table 18). The absence of total recovery, and the appearance of dose-related extraneous

TABLE 18. *The Distribution of Amantadine in Mouse Tissues*

| Hours after dose | Concentration of amantadine | | |
	Lung (μg/g)	Heart (μg/g)	Blood (μg/ml)
0.25	59	18	4
0.50	35	14	8
1	33	7	1
2	33	9	0.5
4	7	1	0.2
8	3	0.5	0.2
16	0.9	0.2	0.1

Groups of 10 to 13 mice were given a single oral dose of 25 mg/kg amantadine. At given time intervals organs were removed and examined for the presence of amantadine. (Data from Bleidner *et al.*, 1965).

peaks in certain chromatograms, were evidence that amantadine was metabolized to some extent.

6.15.3. MAN

Following single oral doses of amantadine hydrochloride, an average of 86 per cent of the dose was recovered from the urine in five different subjects on nine occasions when urine collections were continued for 4 days or more. The average excretion in 24 hr was 56 per cent of the dose based on 21 determinations in 16 subjects (Table 19).

The pattern of excretion in one individual was determined (Bleidner *et al.*, 1965). The cumulative amount of amantadine recovered from the urine approached a value of 93 per cent of the dose and it was still possible to detect the compound in the urine 1 week after this single dose. A saliva sample taken at 30 hr showed the compound to be present at a concentration approximating that in blood. Amantadine is excreted in man according to regular first-order kinetics. Blood levels of amantadine in man as a function of dose and time were investigated. The maximum blood level was generally reached in 1 to 4 hr after an oral dose (Table 20). There was no evidence of acetylated or methylated forms of amantadine in any of the human urine samples examined in spite of efforts to demonstrate their presence, and no extraneous peaks have been observed that can be attributed to metabolites of the drug.

Aoki *et al.* (1979) investigated the disposition of doses of 25, 100 and 150 mg amantadine taken every 12 hr for 15 days in thirteen healthy young adults. The authors detected a rather slower absorption of the drug compared to previous studies. The average time to peak plasma concentrations was 3–4 hr. Almost complete oral bioavailability of amantadine was indicated by the recovery of approximately 80 per cent of a single

TABLE 19. *Urinary Excretion of Amantadine in Human Subjects*

Time after dose (hr)	Dose range (mg/kg)	Recovery (% of dose)	Recovery range (% of dose)
0–24	2–7	56 $\pm$ 13[a]	27–78[b]
0–96	2–4	86 $\pm$ 9	62–93[c]

Human volunteers were given a single oral dose of amantadine and levels of amantadine in the urine were determined at various times thereafter.

[a] $\pm$ standard deviation.
[b] 21 determinations in 16 subjects.
[c] 9 determinations in 5 subjects.
(Data from Bleidner *et al.*, 1965).

TABLE 20. *Blood Levels of Amantadine in Human Subjects Following Single-Oral Doses of the Hydrochloride*

	Blood level (μg/ml) Dose		
Time after dose	2.5 mg/kg	4.0 mg/kg	5.0 mg/kg
0	0	0	0
0.5	0	0.1	0.1
1	0.1	0.3	0.6
2	0.2	0.3	0.6
4	0.3	0.5	0.4
6	0.2	0.3	0.3
8	0.2	0.3	0.5
24	0.1	0.1	

(Data from Bleidner *et al.*, 1965).

oral dose. The median ratio of plasma to renal clearance of amantadine approximated unity which suggested that the compound was not extensively metabolized.

Distribution of an amantadine derivative (1-amino-3,5-dimethyl adamantane) was established in post-mortem tissues of a 77-year-old woman with Parkinson's disease The patient had been treated with 2×10 mg of the amantadine molecule daily for 53 days. Levels of the compound (μg/g) in the tissues were as follows: kidney (0.18), lung (0.17), spleen (0.1), blood (0.07), cerebellum (0.22). Thus relatively high levels of the molecule were found in the lung and kidney.

Levels of amantadine in tissue specimens were determined in a 5-month-old girl with influenza A virus pneumonia (Fishaut and Mostow, 1980). 2.5 mg/kg each 12 hr of amantadine was administered and tissue specimens obtained $4\frac{1}{2}$ hr after the final dose. Serum concentrations ranged from 0.8 to 1.64 μg/ml whilst higher concentrations of amantadine were found in the lung (21.4 μg/ml). This level of compound would significantly inhibit the replication of recent H3N2 and H1N1 influenza A viruses. Since amantadine is apparently preferentially sequestered in respiratory tissues, future studies could usefully investigate the antiviral effect of lower dosages.

In other studies volunteers were given aerosols of amantadine (Knight *et al.*, 1979, Hayden *et al.*, 1979). One hour after aerosol treatments with 1.0 g amantadine per 100 ml of solution in the glass nebulizer, amantadine levels in nasal wash samples (mean 30.3 μg/ml) greatly exceeded blood and nasal wash levels following oral administration. This may be of significance in certain therapeutic applications of amantadine and is discussed in more detail later.

TABLE 21. *Acute Toxicity of Amantadine in Animals*

	LD$_{50}$ and 95% confidence limits (values in brackets)		
Species, sex	Oral (mg/kg)	Intraperitoneal (mg/kg)	Intravenous (mg/kg)
Mouse, F	700 (621, 779)	205 (194, 216)	97 (88, 106)
Rat, F	890 (761, 1019)	223 (167, 279)	
Rat, M	1275 (1095, 1455)		
Rat, neonatal, M, F		150 (111, 189)	
Guinea pig, F	360 (316, 404)		
Dog, M, F	> 372[a]		> 37
Monkey, rhesus, M	> 500[a]		
Monkey, African green, F	> 75		
Horse, M, F	> 96		

Animals were given doses of amantadine by different routes and followed for signs of toxicity or death. (Data from Vernier *et al.*, 1969).

6.15.4. ACUTE AND CHRONIC TOXICITY STUDIES

A central nervous stimulant effect of amantadine has been described (Vernier et al., 1969) in acute and chronic toxicity studies in animals, but only at concentrations around 30 mg/kg orally, which is about 10 times the dosage in man. The predominant signs of central nervous stimulation were increased motor activity, tremors, anorexia, increased sensitivity to environmental stimuli or convulsions in some cases. The stimulant effects have also been described in volunteers given high doses of the compound (Council on Drugs, 1967). At relatively high doses in animals, other effects were transient vasodepressor effects, cardiac arrhythmias, weak ganglionic blocking effect, increase of myocardial contractile force or blocks of phenethylamine vasopressor response (Vernier et al., 1969).

Any anti-influenza compound to be used in man must be non-toxic and with no serious side effects. Most studies with amantadine administered at 200 mg per person per day have not detected significant side effects of the compound (Table 22). Our own experience in carefully controlled trials in general practice in the UK (Galbraith et al., 1969a, 1969b, 1970) has been satisfactory, with no evidence of more side effects in amantadine-treated persons compared to placebo-treated persons.

Trials with the compound as an anti-Parkinson's disease drug have detected some side effects at 200 mg per day, after 3–4 months continuous daily dosage (Timberlake and Vance, 1978). Over one million patient doses have now been administered (Douglas, 1980). Ankle oedema is noted in some elderly patients and a recent report described possible induced heart failure in a man of 65 years who had received the compound for the preceding 4 years (Vale and Maclean, 1977). Investigators should continue to examine the possible side effects of amantadine after long-term dosage. Isolated reports have raised the question of possible teratogenicity in pregnant women and further definitive studies are required before the compound is used on a large scale (Coulson, 1975; Nora et al., 1975). Rimantadine has even fewer side effects (Galasso et al., 1984).

TABLE 22. *Summary of Reported Side Effects of Amantadine (Early Studies)*

Reference	Dose (mg/day)	No. of subjects Treated	No. of subjects Placebo	No. with side effects[a] Treated	No. with side effects[a] Placebo
Wendel et al. (1966)	200	469	380	8(1.7%)	7(1.8%)
Togo et al. (1968)	200	29	29	0	0
Wingfield et al. (1969)	100	23	48	0	0
Galbraith et al. (1969a)	200	94	82	2	0
Galbraith et al. (1969b)	200	102	100	3	0
Hornick et al. (1969)	200	94	103	0	0
Knight et al. (1969)	200	13	16	0	0
Togo et al. (1970)	200	54	48	0	0
Smorodintsev et al. (1970a)	100, 200	206	198	0	0
Smorodintsev et al. (1970b)	100	1313	512	94(7.1%)	26(5.2%)
Oker-Blom et al. (1970)	200	192	199	–(8.7%)	–(3.4%)
Kitamoto (1971)	200	182	173	18(9.9%)	21(12.1%)
				9(4.9%)	9(5.2%)
				5(2.7%)	6(8.5%)
O'Donoghue et al. (1973)	200	50	61	0	0

[a]Side effects in treated or placebo groups included insomnia, headache, nausea, vomiting and diarrhea.

6.15.5. AMANTADINE HAS NO ANTI-PYROGENIC EFFECT

Grossgebauer and Langmaack (1970) investigated amantadine for any modifying effect on drug or influenza-induced temperature response in the rabbit model. This is an important consideration, especially when extrapolated to therapeutic studies of the drug in man, where it has been shown that amantadine reduced the temperature, among other symptoms, following influenza infection (see below). Presumably this effect in man results from an antiviral effect of the compound rather than a simple antipyretic effect *per se*. In brief, rabbits were pretreated with saline, or saline containing 60 mg of amantadine and, after 10, 20, 120 min or 24 hr, were given a pyrogen in the form of a crude allantoic fluid containing influenza virions. Two hours after the administration of pyrogen the rabbits showed elevated temperature responses between 0.4 and 1.6°C. Pretreatment with amantadine had no effect on the development of the temperature. Also amantadine itself was not pyrogenic.

6.15.6. Effects of Amantadine on Pregnancy in Animal Models

In a study by Kyo *et al.* (1970) amantadine hydrochloride was administered orally in two separate doses of 120 mg/kg (larger dose group) and 40 mg/kg once a day for 6 successive days from the 9th to the 14th day of pregnancy to nullipara rats of Wistar strain at the age of 3–4 months, in order to examine its effects upon the foetus during the final stage of pregnancy and their post-natal growths. The results indicated a slight retardation of increase in the body weight of dams in the larger dose group, but amantadine had no effect on the number of nidations at the end of the final stage of pregnancy. In the larger dose group, however, the mortality rate of the foetus and the drop in body weight of surviving littermates showed a significant difference from those of the control group, although no deformation was observed in the group. Finally, observations on the growth of the littermates up to the end of the 6th post-natal week in the spontaneous parturition group indicated that the parturition rate was significantly lower in the larger amantadine dose group than in the control group. Amantadine at the doses tested had no effect on suckling rate, external differentiation, survival rate, auditory senses, motility and development of gonadal functions or skeletal structure.

In a study of Lamar *et al* (1970), Holtzman rats and New Zealand white rabbits were dosed orally with amantadine (0, 50, 100 mg/kg) from 5 days prior to mating until day 6 of pregnancy. In rats, but not in rabbits, results of autopsies performed on day 14 of gestation showed significant decreases in the number of implantations and increases in the number of resorptions at 100 mg/kg. Teratology studies were performed in rats (0, 37, 50 and 100 mg/kg) by administering the drug orally on days 7–14 of gestation. Autopsy was just before expected parturition. Increases in resorption and decreases in the number of pups per litter were noted at 50 and 100 mg/kg. Gross examination of rat pups at these dose levels revealed no malformations at 37 mg/kg. Malformations at 50 and 100 mg/kg included edema, malrotated hindlimbs, missing tail, stunting and brachygnatha. Examination of cleared and alizarin-stained skeletal preparations of foetuses revealed cases of absent ribs and absence of the lumbar and sacral portions of the spinal column in the 50 and 100 mg/kg groups. Thus, in rats but not in rabbits, amantadine seems to be embryotoxic and teratogenic. Teratogenicity in rats occurs at 50 mg/kg/day, or about 12 times the usual human dose.

Data from Vernier *et al* (1969) are summarized in Table 23. Doses of amantadine below 32 mg/kg had no effect on rat reproduction or lactation or number of live births. Unfortunately, the effect of high amantadine doses was not examined.

6.15.7. Amantadine has no Inhibitory Effect on Antibody Response

Maciag and Hoffmann (1968) were unable to detect any inhibitory effect of amantadine on antibody formation in mice to bacteriophage T2. Groups of ten female Huntingdon D mice, weighing 17–19 g, were injected once intraperitoneally with 0.2 ml of sterile water containing amantadine HCl to provide a dose of 100 mg/kg. Bacteriophage T2 from a single preparation was injected intravenously to give 20 μg of protein in 0.2 ml sterile saline per mouse. There was no significant difference between amantadine-treated and control mice in the titres of neutralizing antibody and this was confirmed by an analysis of variance (confidence limit 95 per cent). The effect of amantadine given by continual oral administration was also determined. Female Huntingdon D mice received 1 mg/ml of compound in their drinking water for 24 hr prior to phage injection and continuously until the time of bleeding. Groups of five animals were bled by heart puncture up to 24 days after phage injection, and the pooled sera were titred. Water-compound consumption and body

TABLE 23. *Effects of Amantadine on Rat Reproduction and Lactation*

Drug	Control			Amantadine		
Dose (mg/kg):	0	0	0	10	10	32
Mating cycle:	1	2	3	1	2	3
1 Fertility index[a]	95	95	85	95	90	77
2 Gestation index[b]	95	100	88	95	88	100
3 Viability index[c]	93	98	97	91	95	99
4 Lactation index[d]	65	91	84	63	97	65
5 Number of matings	20	20	20	20	19	17
6 Number of pregnancies	19	19	17	19	17	13
Number of litters						
7 Alive at 4 days	18	19	15	18	15	13
Number of pups						
8 Cast alive	181	198	138	157	130	122
9 Cast dead	5	3	25	8	15	8
10 Alive at 4 days	169	193	134	143	124	121
11 Alive at 21 days	109	176	112	90	121	79
Number of pups/litter						
12 Cast	9.6	10.4	9.2	8.3	8.7	11.1
13 Alive	5.7	9.3	7.5	4.7	8.0	7.2
Mean body weight of pups						
14 Cast	6.1	6.4	6.2	6.0	6.6	5.9
15 Alive at 21 days	34.4	39.8	43.0	36.4	41.9	37.3

Amantadine was given daily orally to pregnant rats.
[a] Percent matings resulting in pregnancies (line 6/line 5).
[b] Percent of pregnancies resulting in litters cast alive (line 7/line 6).
[c] Percent of pups cast alive that survived at 4 days (line 10/line 8).
[d] Percent of pups alive at 4 days survived to weaning at 21 days (line 11/line 10).
(Data from Vernier et al., 1969).

weight gains were normal during the test period. The mean daily intake per group was 197 ± 48.6 mg of amantadine per kilogram whole body weight. Again, no significant differences were found between the two groups of animals in the titres of neutralizing antibody to the phage. These results indicated that amantadine administered either by single intraperitoneal injection or by continuous oral supply had no effect on the rate and the level of antibody response to phage T2 antigen. The only qualification is the relative lack of precision of the phage neutralization test, particularly when the results of phage neutralization of a single pooled serum dilution are compared and one finds nearly 100 per cent neutralization from day 18 onwards.

6.15.8. EFFECTS OF AMANTADINE ON ASPECTS OF CELL-MEDIATED IMMUNITY

In vitro studies utilizing (H^3)-thymidine uptake indicated that amantadine suppressed the reactivity of normal sensitized human lymphocytes to tetanus toxoid and purified protein derivative but *enhanced* the proliferative response to phytohaemagglutinin (Bredt and Mardiney, 1969a and b). This suggests that amantadine has some mild immunosuppressive activity, at least *in vitro*. Dent *et al.* (1968) investigated the effect of amantadine on the PHA and graft versus host response to chicken peripheral leukocytes. Stimulation of chicken peripheral leukocytes with phytohaemagglutinin (PHA) was inhibited completely by 100 μg/ml amantadine and partially by 1 μg/ml amantadine. Peripheral leukocytes were incubated with amantadine *in vitro* for 30 min prior to i.v. injection in 13-day embryos and splenomegaly measured 5 days later. 1000 μg/ml amantadine inhibited the graft versus host response but no effect was noted with lower concentrations of the compound. Inhibition was attributed to an effect of amantadine on the donor cells, and it was concluded that concentrations of amantadine which caused inhibition of PHA and graft versus host response may also interfere with cell functions. Other studies have noted very mild or no immunosuppressive activity of amantadine (Killen *et al.*, 1969). In conclusion, despite somewhat conflicting data, it appears that any immunosuppressive activity is mild enough to be of no practical importance in antiviral chemoprophylaxis.

6.16. OTHER INFLUENZA VIRUS INHIBITORY COMPOUNDS

Many laboratories worldwide are searching for compounds with influenza virus inhibitory activity. To date only amantadine derivatives and a nucleoside analogue 1-β-D ribofuranosyl 1,2,4-triazole-3-carboxamide (ribavirin) have been tested *in vitro*, *in vivo* and in man (Sidwell *et al.*, 1972; Oxford 1975a; reviewed by Smith and Kirkpatrick, 1980). Ribavirin has undergone only limited clinical testing to date with influenza and marked prophylactic activity has not been demonstrated following oral administration (Cohen *et al.*, 1976). The compound inhibits DNA synthesis in replicating cells and has some immunosuppressive activity *in vitro* and *in vivo* (Smith and Kirkpatrick, 1980). Clinical and toxicological studies are continuing with the compound, which may yet prove useful when applied as an aerosol. Thus, a small group of fourteen students ill with influenza A (H1N1) virus were treated by inhalation of a small particle aerosol of ribavirin for relatively long periods each day and a mild but significant therapeutic effect was detected. When admitted to the trial, the drug and placebo groups had systemic illness of nearly equal severity. However, within 24 hr ribavirin-treated patients were much improved compared to a slight improvement in the placebo group ($p = 0.004$). In addition, there was a rapid reduction in the mean virus titre for treated patients (Knight *et al.*, 1981). Similar results have been reported with influenza B infections (McClung *et al.*, 1983).

To date only a few clinical trials have been carried out with low yields of relatively impure interferon and these gave relatively poor or no protection against influenza virus (Galasso *et al.*, 1979). However, following the cloning and insertion of interferon genes in *E. coli* (Nagata *et al.*, 1980) and other organisms very rapid expansion in investigations of purified high yield interferon can now be anticipated. It might be expected that the interferon molecule or reconstructed hybrid molecules would have broad antiviral effects.

Experimental studies are in progress in several laboratories with inhibitors of the virus RNA transcriptase, as discussed above (reviewed by Perrin, 1977), but to date these compounds have not been reported to have antiviral activity *in vivo* or in man.

It may be possible to synthesize different amantadine molecules with greater antiviral activity or with inhibitory effects on influenza B virus. This would be a considerable advance—the selectivity of amantadine for influenza A viruses has not been explained.

At present 12–15 laboratories worldwide are searching for new anti-influenza compounds, mainly using random screening techniques in tissue cultures or egg pieces, followed by *in vivo* testing in mice. These methods have not yielded enough potent anti-influenza molecules and different approaches may now have to be used. The marked increase in our knowledge of viral events at the molecular level, and the use of easily applied techniques for the analysis of virus specific RNA, DNA and polypeptides, could lead to the application of such methodology for screening for antiviral compounds. Biological approaches used up to the present time attempt to obtain compounds which reach the correct point in the virus-infected cell to inhibit virus replication—therefore the screening method has to contend with at least two problems simultaneously—pharmacological and virological. More extensive use of virus specific enzyme tests, for example, should enable compounds with a precise mode of action to be selected (reviewed by Stuart-Harris and Oxford, 1983).

6.17. INFLUENZA VACCINES

Inactivated influenza virus vaccines are used in the UK, Europe and the USA to provide some immunity to persons at special risk of mortality from influenza (Smith *et al.*, 1976; Stuart-Harris, 1981; Lennette, 1981). At present it is generally accepted that a protection rate of around 70 per cent can be achieved with inactivated vaccines (reviewed by Selby, 1976). Inactivated influenza vaccines are composed of a suspension of purified virus particles containing approximately 100 μg/ml virus protein, and inactivated with β-propiolactone or formalin. The virus is propagated initially in embryonated hens eggs and precipitated or partially purified from the allantoic fluid and then purified further by rate zonal centrifugation in continuous flow rotors. Vaccines may be contaminated with low quantities of egg proteins and so are not given to persons with egg allergy. In addition, a high reaction rate is noted in children given these vaccines, including fever and headache. Studies are in progress with detergent split virus vaccines or purified subunit (HA or NA) vaccines (reviewed by Perkins and Regamey, 1977; Schild, 1979). These vaccines are less reactogenic in children but are also less immunogenic. Two doses of a vaccine containing a new virus sub-type are required to give protective levels of antibody. Studies are also in progress with adjuvants in attempts to stimulate higher levels of protective anti-HA antibody and to increase the duration of immunity to beyond a year. In the USA approximately 2 million doses of inactivated vaccine can be produced per week if a high-yield recombinant virus is available. However, a minimum of several weeks is required to produce and distribute suitable virus recombinants for vaccine production. A 2–3-month period is required therefore before sizeable amounts of tested and standardized vaccine become available.

Alternatively, live attenuated influenza vaccines may provide rapid and more easily admin-istered protection (reviewed by Stuart-Harris, 1981, 1984). However, the main problem at present is the requirements for extended clinical testing of new candidate vaccine strains—such viruses have to be carefully analysed to ensure that clinical effects are minimal and that no spread occurs from vaccinated to unvaccinated persons. Many candidate live vaccine strains are produced by recombination between a well-tested laboratory virus attenuated for man and the 'wild' virulent virus causing the influenza outbreak. Viruses with the HA and NA genes of the wild virus and the remaining 6 genes of the laboratory virus are screened—but the recombinants still have to be tested in volunteers. Live vaccines have the advantage that as many as 100 doses can be cultivated in a single embryonated hens egg, whilst with inactivated vaccine only a single dose is commonly obtained from 1 egg. Administration of live vaccines by spray can also be rapid on a large scale. However, much time is lost at the safety and clinical testing stages. Several months commonly elapse between the time of the first isolation of a new virus and the production of an attenuated vaccine virus. At present, attenuated vaccine viruses are used extensively in the USSR and China. Smaller scale studies are continuing in UK, Europe and the USA. (Stuart-Harris, 1984; Tyrrell and Smith, 1979).

In summary, inactivated influenza vaccines have been used in man on a small scale for 40 years, although technological advances, particularly in the last 10 years, have led to more pure, standardized and potent vaccines. The efficacy of such preparations (70 per cent protective effect) is rather disappointing and the search continues for more immunogenic preparations. As discussed above, the recent large-scale immunization programme in the USA against the swine influenza virus provided extensive data on side reactions and complications of vaccination, including Guillain–Barré syndrome (Keenlyside et al., 1980) but, on the other hand, indicated that modern methods can produce the very large quantities of inactivated vaccine needed to vaccinate an entire population. Genetic engineering techniques will undoubtedly produce high yields of HA for vaccine (Chanock, 1982; Gething and Sambrook 1982; Green et al., 1982; Oxford and Oberg, 1984).

6.18. ECONOMIC ASPECTS OF MASS VACCINATION OR CHEMOPROPHYLAXIS PROGRAMMES

At present no country, with the exception of the US, has attempted a mass vaccination campaign with the intention of preventing an influenza outbreak. The policy in most countries has been to use the limited quantities of available vaccine to protect persons considered to be at special risk, e.g. diabetics, bronchitics, asthmatics, persons with heart disease, etc. It should be realised that some vaccine is used for persons who are not at any special risk. Also a proportion of old persons' homes and geriatric hospitals, where a high morbidity and mortality might be expected, do not immunize at all or wait until there is evidence of influenza infection—at this late stage immunization is not effective. Vaccine is also used industrially in attempts to prevent economic disruption during an influenza outbreak (Smith et al., 1976). It is with the latter group that economic projections are of value. A study on post-office employees in the UK has shown that, over an extended 5-year period, vaccine administration resulted in a saving in economic terms. The rationale behind the trials is treated below and in Table 24.

TABLE 24. *Theoretical Projections of Cost-Benefits of Influenza Vaccines*

| | Epidemic Year (15% attack rate) | | Ordinary Year (2% attack rate) | |
	No vaccination	Vaccination	No vaccination	Vaccination
Cases	150	120	20	15
Influenza days	1,500	1,200	200	150
Other sick days	15,000	15,000	15,000	15,000
Cost of vaccination	—	£600	—	£600
Cost of total sickness	£165,000	£162,000	£152,000	151,500
Savings	—	+£2,400	—	−£100
Lost time	6.6%	6.4%	6.1%	6.1%

An attempt to estimate cost-benefits of influenza vaccination in a factory group. (Data from Geigy Symposium on Influenza, Banbury, 1976. For additional data see Tillett *et al.*, 1980; Tyrrell and Smith, 1979).

6.18.1. ASSUMPTIONS

A factory population of 1000 with a 'Normal' absence level of 6 per cent, i.e. 15 days per employee per year. Vaccine protects 70 per cent recipients and the acceptance rate is 30 per cent. Vaccination costs £2 per head. A case of influenza takes 10 days off and such absence costs £10 per day. (These are reasonable assumptions based on published studies.)

If epidemics occur once in 5 years, the overall saving would be 200 days out of a total assumed absence of 77,300 days. However, if *all* employees were immunized (highly unlikely) the days saved would then be about 1500 days in the 5-year period, because only 45 cases would occur in the epidemic year and 5 cases in an ordinary year. Vaccine cost would then be £2000 each year. (There is some preliminary evidence to suggest that savings may be greater than those given in these calculations since there may also be a reduction in absence outside the immediate influenza season. If confirmed, the cost-benefit analysis would become more favourable.)

On the other hand, to be sure of adequate protection, amantadine might have to be administered throughout the influenza season, i.e. December to March (Muldoon *et al.*, 1976). The current cost of this treatment would be approximately £40, although presumably this would be reduced if the compound were widely used. The alternative would be to wait for epidemiological signs of virus spread and then take the antiviral compound for the period of the outbreak, commonly 2–6 weeks of peak activity (this has been recommended now by a WHO group). An important consideration is that savings would be made in *non-epidemic years*, whereas at present similar numbers of persons are immunized each year. Also, regardless of the fact that little influenza may circulate, amantadine could be of use in preventing *spread* in a closed community like a factory, school or family group. The early studies of Galbraith *et al.* (1969a) illustrated quite clearly the effect of amantadine in preventing spread of influenza in the family. There are many possibilities for application of an effective anti-influenza compound which can be explored in future studies. Not least important is the combination of live or inactivated vaccine and amantadine, so avoiding the apparent dilemma of a choice between vaccines and antiviral compounds (Chanin, 1977). Trials in the USSR (see below) have shown some additive protective effect.

The problems of mass immunization (or, alternatively chemoprophylaxis) in large urban populations are considerable and the Swine Influenza Immunization Programme in the USA has provided useful data. For example, in New York City, which covers 300 square miles and has a population of 7.9 million, the health services are provided by two major groups—public and private sectors. The latter constitutes 35,000 doctors, 224 nursing homes and 102 voluntary and proprietary hospitals. The public sector has 16 municipal hospitals with 15,000 beds and an annual budget of 1 billion dollars. For the influenza immunization programme Congress approved $107 million for vaccine production and $28 million for vaccine administration. Influenza immunization was carried out in schools in district health centres. The core of the staff was provided by the State Health Department with assistance from volunteers. Vaccine was also made available to private physicians, nursing homes, hospitals and industrial medical units. The programme commenced on 15th October 1976 and was planned during April to August. In New York 90 new personnel were recruited and trained in the use of jet guns, as well as 75 sanitary inspectors and 150 nursing assistants; 500–600 volunteers per day were recruited to help and 45 clinics were established throughout the city. Furthermore, 15 mobile teams were used for nursing homes, old people's homes, etc. The department itself provided 60 teams of six persons. The Federal grant to New York City for the programme was $3.4 million, but extra costs to the city's Department of Health amounted to $1 million, mainly in salaries of extra staff. Of course no comparable large-scale use of an anti-influenza compound has been attempted to date. Assuming the use of a safe, cheap and readily available non-toxic compound, very rapid administration in the face of an influenza pandemic should be possible via clinics and doctors in much the same way as vaccine. Administration would be easier if no injections are involved.

6.19. RECURRENCE OF H1N1 VIRUSES AS EPIDEMIC VIRUSES

In May 1977, a virus with surface HA and NA antigens similar to those viruses which circulated worldwide between 1947 and 1957 (namely, H1N1 viruses) re-emerged in North China and spread into eastern parts of the Soviet Union. By December 1977 the virus had reached Finland and by January 1978 was causing extensive outbreaks in England, particularly in young persons under the age of 20, who would not be expected to have antibody to H1N1 viruses. A most interesting epidemiological situation therefore has occurred recently with three viruses circulating simultaneously—A/USSR/90/77 (H1N1), A/Texas/77 (H3N2) and A/Victoria/75 (H3N2) (Kendal et al., 1979). All three viruses are well inhibited by amantadine (Oxford, 1979). Recent clinical trials in the US have demonstrated good prophylactic activity of amantadine against currently circulating viruses antigenically related to A/USSR/92/77 (H1N1). It is of interest that the H1N1 virus is well inhibited by the compound because, as described above, laboratory-adapted strains of 'older' H1N1 viruses isolated in the 1950s are less well inhibited. This gives extra substance to the speculation that future pandemic influenza A viruses may be inhibited by amantadine. Clinical trials in the USA with viruses of the H1N1 antigenic subtype established an efficacy of prevention by amantadine of serologically confirmed influenza of 70.7 per cent (Monto et al., 1979; Dolin et al., 1982; Galasso et al., 1984).

6.20. CLINICAL STUDIES WITH AMANTADINE

Following satisfactory safety testing of amantadine in animals, and clearance by the Food and Drug Administration in the United States of America, human volunteer studies were begun using attenuated strains of influenza A virus as a challenge. We have not attempted to analyse the data from all clinical trials reported in the literature—rather, the review is selective. We shall consider artificial and natural challenge studies of amantadine as a prophylactic and therapeutic agent.

6.20.1. ARTIFICIAL CHALLENGE STUDIES

The advantages of this method, involving as it does the challenge of human subjects with a known virus, are two-fold. The first is administrative convenience in that results of such clinical investigations are generated immediately, as compared with the delay involved when waiting for a naturally occurring outbreak, or epidemic of influenza. The second concerns the use of a virus of known virulence to the host and sensitivity to the chemoprophylactic or chemotherapeutic agent. The design can be planned in meticulous detail, including the screening of all volunteers for resting antibody to the challenge or related viruses. It is thus possible to involve groups of volunteers with low or absent antibody to the challenge virus, and to compare the response seen in volunteers who already possess a significant level of antibody to the virus at the time of challenge. A possible objection to this method of investigation of an anti-influenza agent may be its dissimilarity to the infection as it occurs in natural epidemic form.

In an infection which demonstrates such a variable clinical picture, while retaining an essentially typical pattern, it is essential to employ a placebo-controlled design, preferably double-blind.

Initially, following the discovery by the Du Pont Company of the antiviral activity of amantadine, in the United States, clinical studies were confined to America. However, as evidence of prophylactic action in influenza was disseminated, investigations were set up in Europe and the Far East. In general, the dosage used was 100 mg every 12 hr, but some studies, notably that by Smorodintsev in 1969, employed 100 mg daily. Clinical studies in the Soviet Union using rimantadine have been reviewed recently (Indulen and Kalninya, 1980; Zlydnikov *et al.*, 1981; Galasso *et al.*, 1984) and therefore will not be discussed here in detail.

In initial challenge studies, Jackson *et al.* (1963) selected volunteers from amongst 735 college students who submitted blood specimens for determination of the influenza antibody titre. Two-thirds (497) of the students were considered to have a high serum antibody titre, 1:20 or greater. Subjects for placebo challenge were randomly selected from the high antibody group; 21 subjects served as placebo controls, and 18 were observed for drug toxicity. Among the 735 initial subjects, 199 were in the low antibody group (1:10 or less). These subjects, who were challenged with influenza virus, were placed in groups which received either placebo or 100 mg amantadine (also called EXP 105-1). One-half of each group was given the capsule as pretreatment, beginning 18 hr before virus challenge. The other half received treatment beginning 4 hr after challenge. All treatment was continued for the next 6 days. After challenge, illness, virus recovery, exfoliative cytology and serology were studied. The rate of infection was strongly affected by the prechallenge antibody status of the volunteers (Fig. 12). Among the 199 volunteers challenged with influenza virus, 89 (45 per cent) had a four-fold or greater rise in the convalescent sera, indicating infection with the challenge virus. This represented an infection rate of 70 per cent among subjects with a prechallenge antibody titre of 1:10 or less. Volunteers who had a prechallenge antibody titre of 1:20 had an infection rate of only 22 per cent. Among those with a higher serum level of antibody, only 9 per cent became infected. The effect of the drug in comparison with placebo is shown in Fig. 13. Among the two placebo groups, 66 per cent and 73 per cent of the subjects with a low antibody titre became infected as judged by a serological rise in titre. Among those with higher antibody, 14 per cent and 26 per cent were infected. The differences are not significant. Similarly, among subjects treated with amantadine therapeutically, *after* challenge with the virus, 72 per cent of subjects with a low antibody titre, and 10 per cent of those with a titre of 1:20 or more, became infected. Thus the compound had no *therapeutic* effect in

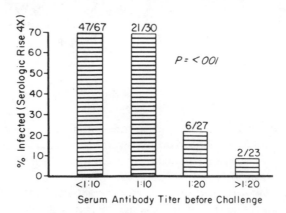

FIG. 12. Incidence of influenza viral infection according to prechallenge antibody status in prophylactic study. Volunteers were tested for the level of antibody to influenza virus HA. A relationship between titre and resistance to challenge with virus was demonstrated. (From Jackson *et al.*, 1963; with permission of the publisher).

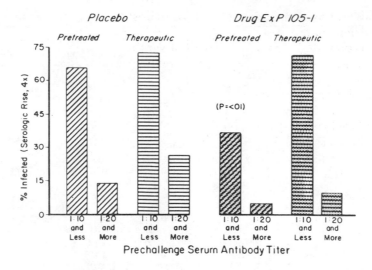

FIG. 13. Effect of amantadine prophylaxis and therapy on influenza virus infection in volunteers. Exp 105-1 = Amantadine. Volunteers were given amantadine prophylactically or after infection with a laboratory strain of influenza A virus. (Data from Jackson *et al.*, 1963; with permission of the publisher).

volunteers with little or no antibody. The reduction of infection among volunteers with antibody was 50 per cent in the drug-treated group as compared with the combined placebo groups with prechallenge antibody, and, this was not statistically significant. It is clear, however, that the therapeutic effect of the drug, if any, occurred only in conjunction with pre-existing antibody. In contrast, among subjects pretreated with the drug, a considerable reduction in infection was observed in volunteers of either antibody status. Low antibody subjects given amantadine had an infection rate of only 37 per cent, which was a statistically significant reduction ($p < 0.01$) compared with the combined placebo groups. However, an early challenge study, carried out at the Common Cold Research Centre in England, using an attenuated strain of influenza A sensitive to amantadine in *in vitro* laboratory studies (Table 3), demonstrated the absence of prophylactic action of the drug clinically and serologically (Tyrrell *et al.*, 1965). It is conceivable that the virus infection produced in the human subjects was materially different from that *in vitro*. Large doses of egg-adapted virus were used in the volunteers (Table 25) and the numbers involved were small (Table 26).

In another challenge study, Bloomfield *et al.* (1970) evaluated amantadine in a matched pairs design involving eighteen susceptible volunteers. The subjects were healthy young adult male inmates of a state correctional institution. About one-third of the prison population, 412 inmates, were considered suitable candidates for the study by prison officials. Three months before the actual study, sera were collected from these men and tested for the presence or absence of HI antibody to the challenge virus, influenza A/Rockville/1/65 (H2N2) strain. Eighteen of the volunteers, who were fully fit prior to the actual challenge, and whose antibody status was unchanged (HI titre ≤ 1:2), took part. They were matched in pairs on the basis of age, weight and HI titres and subjects were unaware of the pairing. Nine volunteers received amantadine and their concurrently treated partners an indistinguishable lactose placebo, the allocation determined by random numbers. Subjects entered isolation 2 days prior to administration of the challenge virus. Amantadine (300 mg) or placebo was given in two divided doses on the day before, and on the day of, viral challenge; for the next 8 days 100 mg was given twice daily. A challenge dose of 64,000 $TCID_{50}$ virus was administered to all subjects by intra-oral spray and by intranasal drip. The clinical and serological responses were followed meticulously for 11 days. HI titres were measured at the start of the study, 14 and 21 days following virus challenge.

Four cases of typical influenza-like illness occurred among the nine placebo-treated subjects. Illness began on the second day after viral challenge and lasted 48–72 hr. In three of

TABLE 25. *Amantadine Prophylaxis Experiments in Human Volunteers (Salisbury Trials)*

Virus strain given	Dose EID_{50}	Drug mg/day	Proportion of volunteers showing	
			Illness	Laboratory evidence of infection
A/Eng/443/57	?	400	1/4[a]	1/4
		0	1/3	1/3
None		400	1/3[a]	—
		0	0/3	—
A/Scot/49/57	10^6	400	0/3	2/3
A/Scot/49/57	10^6	0	1/3	1/3
A/Scot/49/57	10^7	400	3/4	4/4
A/Scot/49/57	10^7	0	1/4	3/4
A/Scot/49/57	10^7	200	1/3	2/3
A/Scot/49/57	10^7	0	1/3	1/3
A/Scot/49/57	10^6 or 10^7	200 or 400	4/10	8/10
	10^6 or 10^7	0	3/10	5/10

Volunteers were given amantadine and then infected with an influenza A virus of known *in vitro* sensitivity to amantadine.

[a] Malaise, tremors and insomnia—other subjects developed upper respiratory tract symptoms but some of those given drug had insomnia from time to time.

(Data from Tyrrell, Bynoe, Hoorn, 1965).

TABLE 26. *Prophylactic Experiments in Volunteers With Amantadine (Salisbury Trials)*

Virus given	Drug given	Proportion of volunteers showing		
		Virus in throat	Rising antibody titre by	
			HI.	Neutralization[a]
A/Eng/443/57	Yes	1/4	0/3	1/3
	No	1/3	0/3	0/2
A/Scot/49/57	Yes	2/10	6/10	3/8
	No	1/10	4/10	5/6

Volunteers were given amantadine and then infected with an influenza A virus of known *in vitro* sensitivity to amantadine.

[a] Not all sera were tested.

(Data from Tyrell, Bynoe and Hoorn, 1965).

these four cases, influenza A virus was recovered from throat washings on the third and fourth days after virus challenge (Table 27). Influenza-like illness and viral shedding were not observed in the amantadine-treated subjects. Comparison of peak illness scores between members of each of the matched treatment pairs revealed that illness score was suppressed in the amantadine-treated member in six of the nine pairs (Table 27). Eight of the nine placebo-treated subjects had a four-fold or greater rise in antibody titre 14 days after virus challenge. A similar rise in titre occurred in only three of the amantadine-treated partners although one additional amantadine-treated subject exhibited a rise in titre 21 days after virus inoculation. Comparison of rises in HI titres 14 days after viral inoculation, between members of each of the treatment pairs, revealed that the average difference in fold rise between placebo-treated subjects and amantadine-treated partners was 13.7 ± 3.3 (Table 27). Twenty-one days after challenge, the mean difference in fold rise in HI titre within treatment pairs was 12.7 ± 3.0 ($p < 0.01$). However, despite the lowered antibody response to virus challenge associated with the administration of amantadine, a significant increase in antibody titre from 2 to 5.8 ± 2.1 did occur 21 days after challenge ($p < 0.05$). Thus amantadine reduced, but did not

TABLE 27. *Prophylactic Trial of Amantadine and Placebo-Treated Paired Subjects after Challenge with Influenza A virus. (Prison Study)*

| Matched treatment pairs | Peak illness score | | Fold rise in HI antibody titre | | | | Virus shedding[b] | |
| | | | 14 days after challenge | | 21 days after challenge | | | |
	Placebo	Amantadine	Placebo	Amantadine	Placebo	Amantadine	Placebo	Amantadine
1	36[a]	9	32	4	16	8	+	0
2	8	4	2	2	2	1	0	0
3	31[a]	1	32	4	32	16	+	0
4	5	8	8	2	16	2	0	0
5	15[a]	3	32	16	32	16	0	0
6	45[a]	0	16	2	32	2	+	0
7	6	2	16	1	16	2	0	0
8	3	4	4	2	4	4	0	0
9	4	5	16	2	16	1	0	0
Means of paired differences	13.0		13.7 ± 3.3		12.7 ± 3.0		—	
T or t	−6.0		4.1		4.2		—	
P (2 tailed)	−0.05		< 0.01		< 0.01		—	

Pairs of volunteers were given amantadine or placebo and then infected with influenza A virus. Illness scores were recorded as were parameters of virus shedding and HI antibody response.

[a] Subjects with typical influenza-like illness.

[b] In + subjects virus was recovered from throat washings on the 3rd and 4th days after viral challenge.

(Data from Bloomfield *et al.*, 1970).

abolish, the immunologic response to influenza A viral challenge. As discussed above, it is most useful if anti-influenza compounds allow the development of natural immunity, but suppress clinical reactions to the virus.

Togo *et al.* (1968) reported a study performed with the cooperation of volunteers at the Maryland House of Correction. Sixty-five men with titres of 1:2 or less of neutralizing antibodies were enrolled and, after full baseline evaluation, were housed in the research ward at the prison. Oral temperature, pulse rate and respiration rates were recorded at 4-hourly intervals. Follow-up specimens were collected at 7, 14, 21 and 28 days post-challenge. Seven trials were conducted. In the preliminary potency-testing of the inoculum, seven men were challenged. In the following six drug-evaluation studies, viral challenge was performed on a total of 58 men, volunteers in each group numbering 14, 6, 12, 6, 8 and 12. Amantadine and lactose-containing placebo capsules were administered by double-blind technique from randomly numbered bottles. The drug was given in 100 mg doses twice daily for 8 days in the first two studies and for 9 days in the following four studies, starting about 26 hr prior to the viral challenge. The drug-treated group received a total of 300 mg of amantadine before the virus dose of 64,000 $TCID_{50}$ was given nasopharyngeally. The virulence of the virus inoculum was examined in 7 men who received undiluted virus fluid containing 64,000 $TCID_{50}$. Clinical illness observed was classified according to the severity of signs and symptoms. The following criteria applied:

2 + = moderately ill with temperature above 38.3 C and occasional respiratory tract signs.

1 + = mild illness, significant symptomatology and temperature 37.8 C.

± = questionable illness, no fever, but comprising of pertinent symptoms.

○ = no suspected illness.

Subsequent experience with the 18 volunteers enrolled in the drug-evaluation study showed similar clinical responses and the impression was gained that the induced illness was generally milder than naturally occurring influenza. The prophylactic effectiveness of amantadine in volunteers with experimentally induced influenza A infection was assessed in six separate but consecutive double-blind trials. The cumulative results of clinical findings in a total of 58 subjects are graphically depicted in Fig. 14. The rating of the clinical illness of

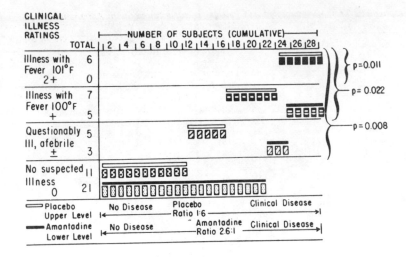

Fig. 14. Prophylactic study of amantadine in a prison population. Antibody-free volunteers were given amantadine or placebo and challenged with an influenza A virus (H2N2 antigenic subtype). Clinical examination was at 4 hourly intervals. Distribution of types of clinical responses occurring in amantadine-treated and placebo-treated volunteers exposed to influenza virus is illustrated. Men receiving placebo mediation (blocks in upper half of each classification). Those given amantadine (in lower half) (from Togo *et al.*, 1968; with permission of the publisher).

each subject is listed. The 29 blocks in the upper half of each of the four disease classifications represent placebo-treated individuals. Those with prophylactic amantadine treatment are represented by the 29 lower blocks in each level. It was observed that the most severe illnesses (24) occurred only in the placebo-treated subjects. The occurrence of six instances of 2 + illnesses in the placebo-treated subjects compared with none in the drug-treated group is a statistically significant difference ($p = 0.011$). There was a striking disparity in the overall incidence of clinical illness between the two groups. A total of 18 cases was observed in the 29 amantadine-treated subjects for an attack rate of 28 per cent ($p = 0.008$). Febrile illness, with ratings of 1 + or 2 + were observed in thirteen patients in the placebo-treated group, compared with five patients with 1 + febrile illness in the amantadine group. This is statistically significant ($p = 0.022$).

In an interesting challenge study, Russian workers (Smorodintsev *et al.*, 1970a) evaluated amantadine in A and B influenza. A total of 404 male and female medical student volunteers participated in the various sub-studies in which 206 received amantadine and 198 received identical-appearing placebos. Table 28 describes the various groups as to their purpose and composition. Partially attenuated viruses A/Moscow/21/65 (H2N2), A/Leningrad/133/65 (H2N2) and B/Leningrad/95/67 were inoculated into each volunteer by nasal inhalation into the upper and lower respiratory tract of an aerosol produced by an atomizer. Deep inspirations assured droplet dispersal into the bronchiolar-alveolar air passages. At the time of the studies the A/Hong Kong/68 (H3N2) virus variant had been isolated but, since the strain A/Hong Kong/1/68 (H3N2) had not been attenuated, it was introduced by intra-nasal spray in the volunteer experiments. Amantadine (100 mg) or placebo capsules were administered double-blind, either in a single daily dose of two capsules or in two daily doses of one capsule each. The twice-daily dosage was utilised in all studies except that 57 of the 122 subjects challenged with influenza A virus in groups 1 and 2 received the drug once daily and some volunteers in group 4 received 100 mg once daily. Medication was begun 24 hr prior to virus challenge and continued daily for 11 days. In the clinical trials designed to evaluate the effects of amantadine as a therapeutic agent, the capsules were administered twice daily, double-blind, after symptoms of influenza developed.

The prophylactic studies on influenza A virus were conducted prior to the emergence of the influenza A/Hong Kong/68 strains in the autumn of 1968 (Table 28, groups 1 and 2). One hundred and thirty-two of the 146 placebo subjects (90.4 per cent) in groups 1, 2, 3 and 5

TABLE 28. *Summary of Russian Prophylactic Studies with Amantadine*

Group no.	Purpose	Challenge virus	No. of subjects		
			Amantadine	Placebo	Total
1	Prophylaxis, influenza A	A/Moscow/21/65 (H2N2)	102	95	197
2	Prophylaxis, influenza A	A/Leningrad/133/65 (H2N2)	20	21	41
Subtotal, prophylaxis, influenza A with pre-Hong Kong strains (groups 1–2)			122	116	238
3	Prophylaxis, Hong Kong influenza	A/Hong Kong/1/68 (H3N2)	17	16	33
Subtotal, prophylaxis, influenza A (groups 1–3)			139	132	271
4	Prophylaxis, A2 influenza, 100-vs 200 mg dosage	A/Moscow/21/65 (H2N2)	38	31	67
5	Prophylaxis, B influenza	B/Leningrad/95/67 (H2N2)	10	14	24
6	Treatment, A2 influenza	A/Moscow/21/65 (H2N2)	19	21	40
Total, all studies (groups 1–6)			206	198	404

(Data from Smorodintsev *et al.*, 1970a,b).

(Fig. 15) developed clinical influenza after virus challenge. As shown in Figs. 15 and 16, the use of amantadine resulted in significant reduction in the incidence of induced influenza when compared with that in subjects receiving placebo. Febrile disease and serological response were also significantly reduced in the drug-treated groups. In the A/Hong Kong/68 (H3N2) prophylactic studies (Table 28, group 3) who received amantadine were protected to a degree

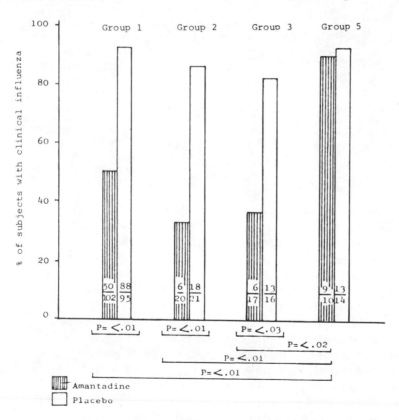

FIG. 15. Prophylactic challenge study of amantadine in Russian medical students. Partially attenuated influenza A viruses of the H2N2 and H3N2 antigenic subtype were inoculated intranasally into volunteers. Amantadine or placebo was given in a double-blind protocol twice daily for 11 days beginning 1 day prior to virus challenge. (Modified from Smorodintsev *et al.*, 1970a; with permission of the publisher).

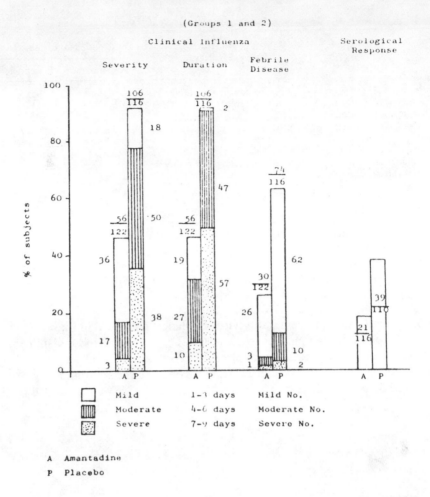

FIG. 16. Prophylactic artificial challenge studies with amantadine and influenza A in Russian medical students. Partially attenuated influenza A viruses of the H2N2 antigenic subtype were inoculated intranasally into volunteers. Amantadine or placebo was given in a double-blind protocol twice daily for 11 days beginning 1 day prior to virus challenge. (Modified from Smorodintsev *et al.*, 1970a,b; with permission of the publisher).

equivalent to that observed among those described who were challenged with the H2N2 subtype viruses (Fig. 17). The total incidence of induced clinical influenza was 35 per cent among amantadine subjects but 82 per cent in the controls. Febrile disease occurred at the rate of 29 per cent and 75 per cent, respectively. Further data on the relationships between the serum influenza A antibody titres prior to virus challenge and patient responses can be seen in Fig. 18. Dose frequency (100 mg twice daily or 200 mg daily) was without significance, as was total daily dose (200 mg daily or 100 mg daily). The drug was without effect in B influenza challenge, as anticipated, because influenza B virus is not inhibited *in vitro* (see above), and no therapeutic effect of amantadine was observed in those volunteers whose medication was withheld until symptoms of influenza developed (Table 28, group 6).

Another challenge study involving the A/Hong Kong/68 (H3N2) virus and amantadine was performed in Yugoslavia by Likar (1970). Healthy, predominantly male, steel workers, ranging in age from 17 to 54 years, were selected after passing a medical examination and also shown to have no CF or HI antibodies to A/Hong Kong/68 (H3N2) virus. Of the 280 original volunteers, 141 were selected as meeting all the criteria for the study. Volunteers were inoculated intranasally by means of a Wilby's aerosol, with 0.1 ml of a virus suspension containing 10^5 50 per cent EID. Amantadine (200 mg daily) or placebo was administered double-blind to 65 and 75 volunteers, respectively, for 14 days beginning on the day of

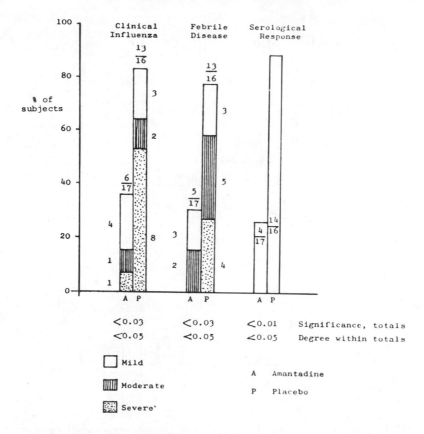

FIG. 17. Prophylactic challenge studies with amantadine and influenza A/HK/68 (H3N2) in Russian medical students. Partially attenuated influenza A/HK/68 (H3N2) virus was inoculated intranasally into volunteers. Amantadine or placebo was given in a double-blind protocol twice daily for 11 days beginning 1 day prior to virus challenge. (Modified from Smorodintsev *et al.*, 1970a,b with permission of the publisher).

infection. Each volunteer was seen at least once daily by a nurse over the 15-day trial period. In the analysis of results, taking only those volunteers with clinical symptoms and laboratory confirmation of influenza infection, there was a significant difference between the placebo group and those treated with amantadine ($p < 0.01$), in favour of the drug-treated group. Twelve cases of proven influenza occurred amongst those volunteers on placebo while only two individuals developed the infection amongst the amantadine-treated volunteers (Table 29).

6.20.2. Conclusions Concerning Artificial Challenge Studies

The majority of trials of the drug showed a protective effect when compared with placebo, which was highly significant, provided amantadine was administered 4–6 hr prior to virus inoculation (summarized in Table 30). These studies opened the way to full-field trials of amantadine during naturally occurring epidemics of influenza.

6.20.3. Field Studies on the Prophylactic Effect of Amantadine

One of the problems in relation to the study of amantadine during a naturally occurring outbreak of influenza was demonstrated by Peckinpaugh *et al.* (1970) during a study performed in 1967 amongst American navy recruits. One hundred and sixty-two men entered the dose finding and tolerance study in which amantadine, rimantadine and placebo were administered from two 20-day phases on a cross-over basis. Seventy-one men received

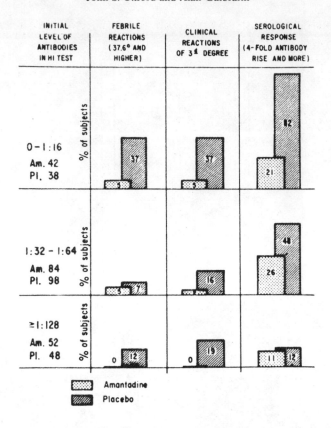

FIG. 18. Prophylactic challenge studies with amantadine and influenza A virus in Russian medical students. The figure analyses the relationship between serum antibody titres prior to virus challenge and the subsequent patients' response in the double-blind trial. (Modified from Smorodintsev *et al.*, 1970a; with permission of the publisher).

TABLE 29. *Prophylactic Trial of Amantadine in a Factory Population in Yugoslavia*

Treatment groups	No. of cases of influenza confirmed by laboratory tests		Total no. of influenza cases
	yes	not	
Placebo	12	63	75
Amantadine	2	64	66
Total	14	127	141

Volunteers given amantadine were challenged with A/Hong Kong/68 (H3N2) virus and examined daily for clinical signs of influenza. The trial was double-blind.
(Data from Likar 1970).

amantadine. The drugs were well tolerated and a study to assess the effect of amantadine or placebo in the face of a naturally occurring outbreak of influenza A was conducted between December 1968 and May 1969 amongst a total of 2650 recruits (1329 took amantadine, 1321 placebo). Each man received 100-mg capsules twice daily for 20 days. Figure 19 shows the percentage of men in the two treatment groups. There was no significant difference between any of the hospitalization rates. Only 6 per cent of 416 individual's sera tested seroconverted to influenza A and 2 per cent to influenza B which demonstrated the absence of clinical influenza in the community studied. This illustrates one of the hazards of field studies of influenza prophylaxis in which a great deal of time and effort are expended, and, with lack of clinical spread of infection, the generation of results is rendered fruitless.

TABLE 30. *Summary of Double-Blind Prophylactic Artificial Challenge Studies in Volunteers*

Investigators	Location	Strain	No. of patients treated with amantadine	Date of clinical trial	Significant effect
Tyrrell, Bynoe, Hoorn	GB	A(H2N2) (Asian)	27	1965	0
Jackson, Muldoon, Akers	US	A(H2N2) (Asian)	32	1963	+
Togo, Hornick, Dawkins	US	A(H2N2) (Asian)	29	1968	+
Smorodintsev et al.	USSR	A(Asian) (H2N2)	139	1970	+
		A/HK/68 (H3N2)	17	1970	
Likar	Yugoslavia	A/HK/68 (H3N2)	65	1970	+

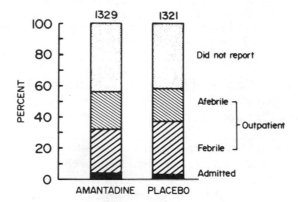

FIG. 19. Effect of amantadine on acute respiratory disease in field trials (Navy study). Volunteers received 100 mg amantadine twice daily for 20 days. However a very low seroconversion rate in both groups was detected illustrating the difficulties of field studies. (From Peckinpaugh *et al.*, 1970; with permission of the publisher).

Subsequent successful trials were conducted during naturally occurring influenza A infection. A double-blind procedure was employed, volunteers receiving either amantadine (100 mg) or placebo capsules, randomly allocated, the duration of administration varied but generally volunteers took the capsules for about 10 days. It must be remembered that prophylaxis is effective only whilst amantadine is being taken and it is estimated that it ceases once the half-life of the final capsule has expired.

One of the early studies was performed by Finklea *et al.* (1967), the 299 subjects in this instance being boarding-school student volunteers for mentally retarded but educable children. Each child received an oral dose of amantadine or placebo twice daily for 1 week and once daily thereafter from February 10 to June 10, 1965. Pre-pubertal children received a 60-mg dose and post-pubertal children a 100-mg dose. This resulted in a dosage range of 1.0–2.5 mg/kg. All subjects who were ill during the study period were admitted to the clinic. Paired sera, throat swabs and full clinical history were obtained from each child reported ill during the trial. All paired sera were titrated by haemagglutination inhibition and complement fixation tests. The results showed that over 97 per cent of the 36,725 prescribed doses were properly dispensed. In this study, assay of oxalated blood or urine for amantadine showed 2 of 124 specimens in the drug-treated group to be negative and 6 of 108 specimens from the placebo group positive. These eight errors among 232 specimens indicated a failure rate of 3.4 per cent. The authors also drew the interesting conclusion from their assay that blood amantadine levels of subjects receiving comparable amantadine dosages did not differ among groups of individuals who were acutely ill, convalescent or well.

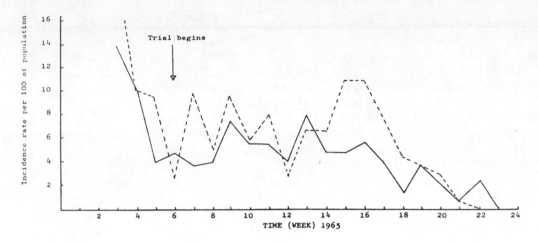

FIG. 20. Prophylactic effect of amantadine on incidence of illness in children (Boarding school trial). Volunteers were given amantadine or placebo twice daily for 1 week and once daily thereafter from February to June 1965. Paired sera, throat swabs and clinical history were obtained from each child ill during the trial. Dotted line is the placebo group. (From Finklea *et al.*, 1967; with permission of the publisher).

Weekly incidence rates of illness are shown in Fig. 20. When influenza A is considered, 12 clinical illnesses were identified as Influenza A and 3 as influenza B. Significantly more influenza A occurred in the placebo group (Table 31). This is a highly significant difference ($p = 0.0016$).

The authors remarked on the higher incidence of non-streptococcal illness amongst the placebo group and suggest that amantadine might have an effect on a respiratory agent not yet described and considered this to be more likely than the result occurring by chance. Whatever the true explanation, the study demonstrated the careful attention to detailed technique during a relatively long trial in which the incidence of influenza A was not large. Nevertheless, by accurate measurement, a statistically highly significant difference in favour of the drug treated group was revealed.

In another study amongst mentally retarded children, Quilligan *et al.* (1966) administered amantadine or placebo for 64 days from January to March 1964, then again from April until the study finished in July 1964. The drug was given as a syrup in single oral doses of O (placebo) 70, 105 or 35 to 140 mg, depending on the weight of the child. When the code was examined, it was found that the children in the three amantadine groups had received average mg/kg per day doses that were approximately the same, so the authors felt justified in combining the groups for statistical analysis. A four-fold or greater rise in titre between acute

TABLE 31. *Prophylactic Study of Amantadine in a Boarding School Field Study*

Trial group	Group[a] population	Sera pairs tested	Four-fold rises Against A/AA/ 1/65	Against B/Md/ 1/59
Placebo	139	133	11[b]	1
Amantadine	154	104	1[b]	2
Totals	293	237	12	3

Boarding school children were given amantadine or placebo prophylactically from February to June. Illness incidence was recorded and serological data enabled identification of influenza A infections.

[a]In residence at least 10 of the first 12 weeks of trial.

[b]$p = 0.0016$ (Fisher exact probability test).

(Data from Finklea *et al.*, 1967).

and convalescent serum pairs was used as the criterion of influenzal infection. The number of children with confirmed influenza A infection in the amantadine and placebo groups is listed in Table 32. The difference is highly significant. An interesting finding noted by the authors was that the presence of pre-existing antibody did not influence the percentage of children in the placebo group who developed febrile influenza plus a four-fold rise in CF titre. By contrast, no child in any of the amantadine groups who had a pre-existing HI titre of 1:160 or more developed influenza A.

The first study of amantadine in the family environment was performed by Galbraith *et al.* (1969a) with the co-operation of family doctors, the majority of whom were members of the epidemic observation unit of the Royal College of General Practitioners. Each doctor, many of whom had experience in the conduct of serologically controlled clinical trials, was asked to include in the study the families of up to five index cases and five contact cases. In the study, 'the family' was defined as all occupants of a household over 2 years of age living in daily contact with each other. The 'index case' was defined as the first person over the age of 2 years to contract clinical influenza in a household, and 'contact cases' were defined as individuals living in the household and having contact with the index case. All index cases received placebo medication in order not to influence the possible spread of influenza, while the families of index or contact cases received drug or placebo by random allocation. All the members of one family except the index case received the same treatment (drug or placebo). The diagnosis of influenza in the index case was made on clinical and epidemiological grounds. At the doctor's first visit, blood was taken from the index case and from as many of the other members of the family as practicable. A second blood sample was taken 2 or 3 weeks later. The blood specimens were sent by post to the University of Sheffield Virus Research Laboratory and tests for HI and CF antibody were performed. Daily records were kept of body temperature and the presence of a cough. A cough, accompanied by a rise of temperature to 37.8°C or higher, was taken as the criterion for a diagnosis of clinical influenza.

Twenty-two family doctors studied 52 families comprising 208 contacts who were divided between treated and placebo groups. Of the 52 index cases, 35 (67 per cent) showed serological evidence of influenza A infection. In the thirty-five families in which there was serological evidence of influenza A infection in the index case, two of 55 (3.6 per cent) contacts in the amantadine-treated group developed clinical symptoms of influenza, whilst 12 of 85 (14.1 per cent) contacts in the corresponding placebo group developed an influenza-like illness. The difference in incidence in these two groups was of marginal significance ($p = 0.07$). However, there was no serological evidence of infection with influenza A virus in the two individuals of the amantadine group who developed clinical illness. In contrast, in the placebo group, 10 of the 69 contacts from whom paired sera were available developed antibody rises to influenza A (Table 33). When serologically confirmed cases of influenza are considered, the difference between the drug and placebo-treated groups is significantly different statistically ($p = 0.05-0.01$). The authors also observed that when the proportion of contacts with serological evidence of influenza A infection, irrespective of clinical illness, was compared for the placebo and drug-treated groups (Table 34), the difference between the groups was highly significant ($p = 0.001-0.01$).

The following winter, the investigators repeated the family study in the face of an epidemic of Hong Kong influenza—A/HK/1/68 (H3N2). Seventy-two general practitioners volunteered to take part but, due to the patchy nature of the epidemic, only 29 actually contributed results. Nevertheless, 58 families were included, comprising 176 individuals.

The only difference in design between this study and the previous year's was that the index case in each family received amantadine or placebo in keeping with the rest of the family. As before, the results of cases suffering from clinical influenza and those with serological proof of influenza A infection, were submitted to statistical analysis. In this instance, the drug and placebo-treated individuals behaved similarly and amantadine failed to protect persons receiving the compound from influenza (Table 35). The virus itself was equally sensitive to amantadine as the previous year's strain and the authors sought to explain this reversal by considering the initial antibody status of those cases under study. It was seen that during the

TABLE 32. *Prophylactic Study of Amantadine in Schools—Clinical Influenza in the Placebo and Amantadine-Treated Groups (Field Trial)*

| Patient group | No. observed | No. of patients with temperature of 101°F or more with four-fold or more increase in titre of CF plus HI antibody | | | | | | | |
| | | Medication 9th Jan.–12th Mar. | | Medication 13th Mar.–9th April | | Medication 10th April–15th July | | Total influenza 9th Jan.–15th July | |
		No.	%	No.	%	No.	%	No.	%
Placebo	43	5	11.0[a]	6	14.0	2	4.7	13	30.2[a]
Amantadine	126	2	1.6[a]	10	7.9	0	0	12	9.5[a]

[a] Significant difference at 0.01 level.
Mentally retarded children were given amantadine or placebo daily.
In this study a four-fold increase in antibody titre was accepted as evidence of influenza virus infection. (Data from Quilligan et al., 1966).

TABLE 33. *General Practice (UK) Study: Effect of Amantadine on Incidence of Clinical Influenza in Contacts of Index-Cases*

| Laboratory evidence of influenza A infection in index case | Treatment | No. of families | Contacts who developed clinical influenza within 10 days of entering the study | | | | | |
| | | | All cases | | | Confirmed serologically[a] | | |
			No.	%	P	No.	%	P
Present	Amantadine	13	2/55	3.6		0/48	0	
	Placebo	22	12/85	14.1	0.07	10/69	14.5	0.05–0.04
Absent	Amantadine	11	1/45	22.2		0/43	0	
	Placebo	6	3/23	13.0	0.3–0.2	2/21	9.5	0.10

The study examined the prophylactic effect of amantadine by determining the effect of the compound on spread of influenza from an initial index case (which was left untreated) to the rest of the family.
[a] A four-fold or greater rise in antibody titre in either or both haemagglutination-inhibition tests with A/England/10/67'(H2N2) virus, or in complement-fixation tests with influenza A 'S' antigen, was taken as serological evidence of influenza A infection. (Data from Galbraith et al., 1969a).

TABLE 34. *General Practice (UK) Study: Effect of Amantadine on the Incidence of Clinical and Subclinical Influenza A infections*

Laboratory evidence of influenza A infection in index cases	Treatment	Contacts with serological evidence of influenza infection					
		Clinical and subclinical infections			Subclinical infections only		
		No.	%	P	No.	%	P
Present	Amantadine	7/48	14.6		7/48	14.6	
	Placebo	27/69	39.1	0.001–0.01	17/69	24.6	0.2
Absent	Amantadine	7/43	16.3		7/43	16.3	
	Placebo	5/21	23.8	0.7	3/21	14.3	0.8

The study examined the prophylactic effect of amantadine by determining the effect of the compound on spread of influenza from an initial index case (which was left untreated) to the rest of the family.

A four-fold or greater rise in antibody titre in either or both haemagglutination-inhibition tests with A/England/10/67 (H2N2) virus, or in complement-fixation tests with influenza A 'S' antigen, was taken as serological evidence of influenza A infection.

(Data from Galbraith *et al.*, 1969a).

1967/68 study, the initial level of HI antibody to the current strain of influenza A was higher (40 per cent with initial HI antibody below 1:12) compared with the 1968/69 study when 90 per cent of the contacts studied possessed initial HI titres below 1:12 (Table 36). This may have been responsible for the difference but the administration of amantadine to half the number of index cases could have influenced the infectivity of these individuals so that a direct comparison of these two trials is not possible.

In another study of amantadine used prophylactically in the face of an epidemic of Hong Kong influenza, Nafta *et al.* (1970) included 215 subjects from the Stejaris Tuberculosis Preventorium, the Bradeful tuberculosis preventorium, the emergency treatment and blood transfusion centre and the Public Health Inspectorate, Brasov. Blood samples were collected before the administration of amantadine from 298 subjects between 3 and 50 years of age. Haemagglutination-inhibition titres against A/Hong Kong/68 virus were found not to exceed 1:14 in 192 sera. The 192 donors of these sera were distributed at random in two groups, and 99 subjects forming one group were given amantadine, while 93 forming the other group were given placebo. In addition, 23 subjects from whom blood was not collected before treatment were also included in the study; 13 of these received amantadine, 10 placebo. Treatment was given for 20 days, tablets being administered twice daily. The tablet content of amantadine was 100 mg, the placebo tablets were identical in constitution although containing no active compound. At the end of tablet administration, blood was taken for antibody estimation. The results were analysed by grouping individuals with or without clinical symptoms of influenza, with or without serological evidence of infection (Table 37). The incidence rate for 'clinical influenza' (irrespective of serological findings (Table 38)) in the amantadine-treated group was considerably lower than in the control group and, when only serologically confirmed influenza cases were considered (Table 39), the differences were more striking. The authors concluded that amantadine was as efficient in preventing influenza caused by the A/Hong Kong/68 virus as it was in preventing influenza caused by pre-Hong Kong variants.

After the relatively small-scale studies described above, the Russian experiences with amantadine demonstrate the size of trials that can be organized given the necessary co-operation and co-ordination. Smorodintsev *et al.* (1970a) included 8169 subjects in their evaluation of the drug during prophylactic administration prior to an epidemic caused by viruses related to A/Hong Kong/68 variants. The population studied consisted of adult males between the ages of 18 and 30 years at semi-isolated engineering schools. The subjects were divided into three groups, namely, amantadine dosed, placebo dosed and 'internal control'. While the dosed subjects lived at the institutions and had little outside contact, those in the internal control groups did not receive medication and lived at home. The students in another engineering school made up a fourth group, the 'external control'. The

TABLE 35. General Practice (UK) Study: Incidence of Clinical Influenza and Serological Evidence of Influenza A Infection[a] in Amantadine Treated and Placebo Groups—A*Hong Kong*68 (H3N2) outbreak

Laboratory evidence of influenza A infection in the index case	No. of families	Treatment of contacts	No. treated	Proportion of contacts who developed clinical influenza within 10 days of entering study						Proportion of contacts with serological evidence of influenza A infection (clinical + subclinical)		
				All cases			Serologically proven cases					
				No.	%	P	No.	%	P	No.	%	P
Present	36	Amantadine	58	9/58[b]	15.5	0.9	5/44	11.4	0.7–0.5	21/44	47.7	0.3–0.2
		Placebo	49	8/49[c]	16.3		6/42	14.3		14/42	33.3	
Absent	22	Amantadine	36	4/36[d]	11.1	0.8–0.9	0/21	0		2/21	9.5	0.7–0.5
		Placebo	33	4/33[e]	12.1		0/23	0		3/23	13.0	

The trial was organized as described in Table 33 except that the index case was now given amantadine or placebo in keeping with the rest of the family.
A four-fold or greater rise in antibody titre in either HI or CF tests or both was taken as evidence of influenza infection.
[a] No serological results in 4 of the 9.
[b] No serological results in 1 of the 8.
[c] No serological results in 2 of the 4.
[d] No serological results in 2 of the 4.
(Data from Galbraith et al., 1969b).

TABLE 36. Distribution of Initial Serum HI Titres in the Consecutive Prophylactic General Practitioner Trials in the UK

Studies	% of persons with following serum HI titres:					
	titre of 1:12 or less		titre of 1:12–1:60		titre of 1:96 or greater	
	amantadine	placebo	amantadine	placebo	amantadine	placebo
1967/68 Study	43	38	45	51	12	11
1968/69 Study	88	92	5	8	8	0

A serum of 1:40 or greater is considered to confer immunity to infection with influenza virus.
(Data from Galbraith 1975).

TABLE 37. *Prophylactic Studies of Amantadine in Hospitals—Clinical and Serological Findings*

Local group	Treatment group	Clinical symptoms present Antibody increase				No clinical symptoms Antibody increase				Combined total
		Present	Absent	Not tested	Total	Present	Absent	Not tested	Total	
Stejaris preventorium	Amantadine	0	0	—	0	6	27	10	43	43
	Placebo	7	1	—	8	2	23	10	35	43
Bradetul preventorium	Amantadine	0	1[a]	—	1	1	26	—	27	28
	Placebo	5	1[b]	—	6	0	23	—	23	29
Emergency-treatment centre	Amantadine	0	0	—	0	1	15	—	16	16
	Placebo	1	0	—	1	0	11	—	11	12
PH1, Brasov	Amantadine	—	—	1	1	—	—	24	24	25
	Placebo	—	—	5	5	—	—	14	14	19
All 4 groups combined	Amantadine	0	1	1	2 (1.8%)	8	68	34	110 (93.2%)	112
	Placebo	13	2	5	20 (19.4%)	2	57	24	83 (80.6%)	103
	Total	13	3	6	22 (10%)	10	125	58	193 (90%)	215

[a] = Catarrhal symptoms and diarrhoea.
[b] = Diarrhoea with bloody stools.
Persons were distributed at random in two groups and were given amantadine or placebo prophylactically for 20 days. Natural infection with A/HK/68(H3N2) virus occurred during this period.
(Data from Nafta *et al.*, 1970).

TABLE 38. *Clinical Influenza, Irrespective of Serological Findings in Hospital Prophylactic Studies*

Treatment group	Clinical influenza		
	Present	Absent	Total
Amantadine	2	110	112
Placebo	19	83	102
Total	21	193	214
$X^2 = 15.26$; Degree of freedom = 1: $p < 0.001$			

Persons were distributed at random in two groups and were given amantadine or placebo prophylactically for 20 days. Natural infection with A/HK/68 (H3N2) virus occurred during this period.
(Data from Nafta *et al.*, 1970).

TABLE 39. *Serologically   Confirmed   Influenza   in Amantadine Hospital Prophylaxis Study*

Treatment group	Serologically confirmed influenza		
	Present	Absent	Total
Amantadine	0	68	68
Placebo	13	57	70
Total	13	125	138
Fischer's exact test (2-tail): $p = 0.002$			

Persons were distributed at random in two groups and were given amantadine or placebo prophylactically for 20 days. Natural infection with A/HK/68 (H3N2) virus occurred during this period.
(Data from Nafta *et al.*, 1970).

distribution of the study population is shown in Fig. 21. Of the total of 10,053 subjects, 50.7 per cent received amantadine, 31.6 per cent placebo, 10 per cent were in the internal control group and 7.7 per cent in the external control group. Unfortunately, a proportion of subjects either contracted influenza before dosing began or did not take the medication regularly, leaving 3885 and 2498 in the amantadine and placebo groups, respectively, to be included in the analysis. The dose of amantadine was 100 mg administered orally once daily after the evening meal. Placebo capsules were given in a similar manner. Dosing of five of the seven populations was continued for 30 days, two populations were dosed for 12 days. Individuals reporting sick with clinical influenza were hospitalized and a record kept of the illness. Paired sera were taken and CF and HI tests performed. On analysing the results, the authors used an index of effectiveness based on the relative frequencies of influenza diagnoses confirmed by laboratory tests in the respective group (Fig. 22). On this basis they calculated that the effectiveness of amantadine in the group which regularly received the drug was almost twice as high (1.95) as in the placebo group. When only those with serologically confirmed influenza A are considered, the effectiveness of amantadine (2.7) is even more striking. When the amantadine-treated group is compared with the non-medicated, non-isolated internal group, the index of effectiveness was 5.34. Morbidity from influenza A/Hong Kong/68 in the three subgroups is illustrated in Fig. 22. An additional finding from this extensive study was that there was an increase of 1.14 per cent in complaints of various sleep disturbances, but that these did not interfere with the working capacity of the students. The authors conclude that the general use of the drug amongst high-risk groups for the prophylaxis of influenza A is desirable and the once daily administration of 100 mg amantadine is a well-tolerated and effective dose.

Aksenov *et al.* (1971) performed a study of amantadine and an interferon stimulator amongst troops of the Moscow garrison during an influenza epidemic in 1969. A tablet of 100 mg amantadine or placebo was administered each evening in combination with an intranasal application by atomizer of interferon stimulator or placebo equivalent. The

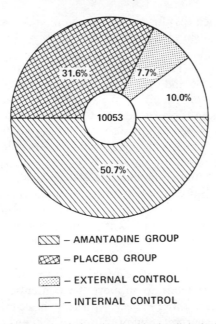

- ▨ – AMANTADINE GROUP
- ▨ – PLACEBO GROUP
- ▨ – EXTERNAL CONTROL
- ☐ – INTERNAL CONTROL

FIG. 21. Distribution of the study populations involved in the clinical trials of the effectiveness of amantadine as a prophylactic in influenza epidemics (Russian field trials). In this study amantadine (100 mg) or placebo was administered orally once daily after the evening meal, for 12 days or 30 days depending on the student group under study. Individuals reporting sick with influenza were hospitalized and paired sera were taken for serological testing. (Data from Smorodintsev et al., 1970a; with permission of the publisher).

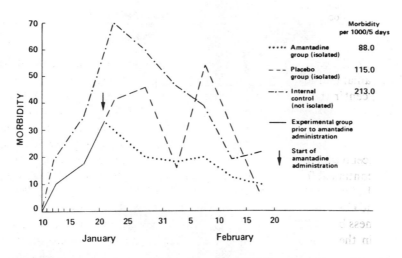

FIG. 22. Morbidity from influenza A/Hong Kong/68 (H3N2) among subjects of 3 subgroups of population No. 6 during January and February (Russian student trials). In this study amantadine (100 mg) or placebo was administered orally once daily after the evening meal, for 12 days or 30 days depending on the student group under study. Individuals reporting sick with influenza were hospitalized and paired sera were taken for serological testing. (Modified from Smorodintsev et al., 1970a with permission of the publisher).

troops studied numbered 4952 and were divided into five groups. One group received amantadine and interferon stimulator, group 2 amantadine placebo and the interferon stimulator, the third group amantadine and the placebo stimulator, group 4 placebo amantadine and placebo stimulator and group 5 was untreated. Administration and observation continued for up to 25 days. The conclusions reached by the authors were that amantadine used prophylactically reduced the sickness rate during an influenza epidemic as compared with control, and that the combined use of amantadine with the interferon stimulator rendered an assessment of the effect of the latter in epidemic influenza difficult.

Nevertheless, it was suggested that further experimental and epidemiological studies of the prophylactic effectiveness during influenza of combinations of different antiviral preparations, should continue.

During an A/Hong Kong/68 (H3N2) influenza epidemic, Mate *et al.* (1970) administered amantadine or placebo to 2435 and 2127 subjects respectively. The drug failed to influence the morbidity of the disease (6.0 per cent in the placebo group and 7.1 per cent in the drug-treated group) but did reduce the peak fever ($p < 0.01$), the duration of fever by $0.7-1.1$ days ($p < 0.001$) and the period of bed-care by $0.9-1.6$ days ($p < 0.001$). Although statistically significant, it is debatable whether a clinician would be persuaded to prescribe amantadine prophylactically on such evidence of efficacy.

Oker-Blom *et al.* (1970) offered amantadine 100 mg twice daily, or a similar placebo capsule, to 391 medical student volunteers during the influenza A/Hong Kong/68 epidemic in Helsinki during the winter of 1969. Serologically confirmed influenza occurred in 27 of 192 students in the amantadine group against 57 of 199 in the placebo group, giving a protection rate of 52 per cent. An observation by these workers was that students with pre-epidemic complement fixation titres greater than 1:16, when taking amantadine, had a highly significant protection against influenza (the infection rate being 1 per cent against 17 per cent in the placebo group). This tends to support the contention that high protection by amantadine is obtained only in those subjects with some basic immunity. Such a suggestion would lend support for concurrent administration of influenza vaccine and amantadine. Preliminary trials of this combination have been performed in the USSR (Slepushkin, personal communication and Table 49) and it is likely that such a study could generate data which might influence future programmes for influenza prophylaxis. The above prophylactic trials of amantadine are summarized in Table 40.

TABLE 40. *Summary of Early Double-Blind Prophylactic Field Studies in Volunteers*

Investigators	Location	Strain	Number of patients treated with amantadine	Reduction in influenza[a]	Date of clinical trial
Finklea	US Hospital	A (Asian)	154	8.8	1965
Keating, Harris	US	A	211	?	1966
Quilligan, Hirayama & Baernstein	US Hospital	A (Asian)	126	3.3	1964
Galbraith, Oxford, Schild, Watson	GB	A (Asian)	102	4.6	1967
Aksenov, *et al.*	USSR	A/HK/68(H3N2)	1967	?	1969
Galbraith, Oxford, Schild, Watson	GB	A/HK/68(H3N2)	58	none	1969
Natfa, *et al.*	Roumania	A/HK/68(H3N2)	112	10.9	1969
Smorodintsev, *et al.*	USSR	A/HK/68(H3N2)	3885	2.0	1969
Mate, *et al.*	Hungary	A/HK/68	2440	none	1969
Oker, Blom, *et al.*	Sweden	A/HK/68	192	2.0	1969
O'Donoghue, Ray, Terry, Beaty	US	A/HK/68(H3N2) variant	50	> 7.0	1972

[a] $\dfrac{\text{case incidence in control group}}{\text{case incidence in treated group}}$.

6.20.4. THERAPEUTIC STUDIES

While investigations were proceeding with amantadine prophylaxis, it was suggested that should a patient with established influenza be given drug, the length and severity of the infection would be reduced (Togo *et al.*, 1970). This was based on laboratory studies (Grunert *et al.*, 1965) and experimental infections in mice (McGahen and Hoffmann, 1968; McGahen *et al.*, 1970).

Hornick *et al.* (1970) studied prisoners with an influenza-like illness during 1968. In addition, a small number of patients in a Masonic home were also enrolled. Febrile men who, by history, were ill less than 48 hr, were asked to volunteer. Drug was assigned in a double-blind fashion; each volunteer received either 100 mg amantadine or lactose placebo twice a day for 10 days. Body temperature and symptom-complex were recorded regularly. Serum specimens were obtained on entry to the study and on day 21. The figures represent only those men with confirmed influenza infection. Amongst the participants, there was no significant difference between the drug and placebo-treated groups as regards mean time of start of medication from first sign of illness, nor did the groups differ concerning mean admission temperatures. Subsequent clinical response demonstrated to the authors that patients made either a rapid clinical improvement or the response was delayed. Three categories were established entitled slow, medium or rapid resolvers. Figure 23 lists the criteria for the three categories; analysis demonstrated a statistically significant effect in favour of amantadine in the slow and rapid resolvers. Fifty-one per cent of the patients receiving the drug had a rapid response compared with 13.6 per cent of the placebo group. The rate of defervescence of fever amongst the patients in the treatment and placebo groups is demonstrated in Fig. 24, which shows the flowing mean temperature in the groups in the six locations. Throughout the investigations, no toxic effects of amantadine were demonstrated.

In another study of amantadine performed during a naturally occurring outbreak of influenza in the Virginia State Penitentiary, Wingfield *et al.* (1969) reported a double-blind controlled trial. Volunteers who developed symptoms and signs of 'influenzal' illness within 24 hr were admitted to the trial and received either amantadine (100 mg), rimantadine (150 mg) or placebo in identical capsules distributed by random number. Oral temperature, symptoms and signs of severity of illness were reported on a scale of 0–4 (absent, mild, moderate, severe and very severe) for a total of 10 days. Concurrent medication was prescribed as needed but antipyretics were not administered. All of the patients with confirmed influenza A illness were used to evaluate the symptoms and signs data. Those with oral temperatures of 37.8°C or greater on the first day of the study were used to evaluate the temperature data. From a total population of 1400 inmates, ninety-five patients who met the necessary criteria were admitted to the study. After the code was broken at the end of the study, it was found that forty-eight patients received placebo, twenty-three amantadine and twenty-four had received rimantadine. The effect of the active drugs on the rate of overall clinical improvement is shown in Fig. 25, revealing a significant advantage of the drug-treated groups over that receiving placebo ($p = 0.05$ and $p = 0.01$). The effect of amantadine and rimantadine on the duration of fever was also significantly demonstrated (Fig. 26) when the median time for the temperatures of the former group to fall to less than 37.8°C was

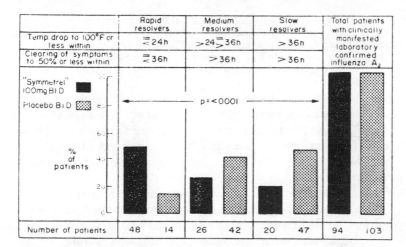

Fig. 23. Therapeutic effect of amantadine in clinical field trials (prison trial). Composite of 6 double-blind, placebo controlled clinical trials. Febrile men who were ill for less than 48 hr volunteered and were assigned amantadine or placebo in a double-blind protocol for 10 days. Infected persons were divided into 3 groups depending on the rapidity of the resolution of clinical symptoms. (From Hornick *et al.*, 1970; with permission of the publisher).

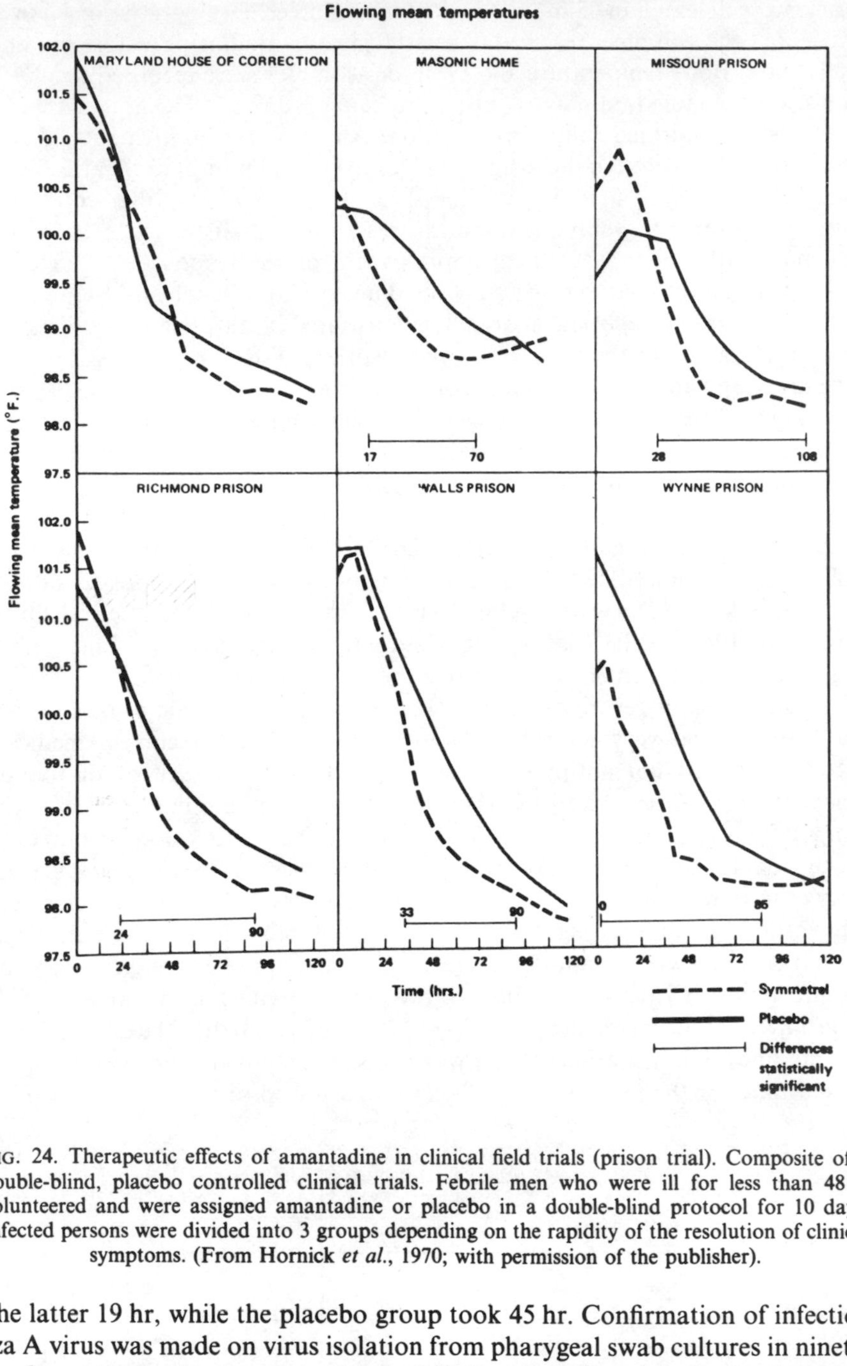

Flowing mean temperatures

FIG. 24. Therapeutic effects of amantadine in clinical field trials (prison trial). Composite of 6 double-blind, placebo controlled clinical trials. Febrile men who were ill for less than 48 hr volunteered and were assigned amantadine or placebo in a double-blind protocol for 10 days. Infected persons were divided into 3 groups depending on the rapidity of the resolution of clinical symptoms. (From Hornick *et al.*, 1970; with permission of the publisher).

23 hr, the latter 19 hr, while the placebo group took 45 hr. Confirmation of infection with influenza A virus was made on virus isolation from pharygeal swab cultures in ninety-three of ninety-five patients, the two patients who failed to shed virus were in the placebo group. There were no differences between the virus-shedding patterns of the drug and placebo-taking patients. No complaint attributable to amantadine or rimantadine was observed during the 10 days of dosing.

In another State Penitentiary, in Missouri, Baker *et al.* (1969) carried out an evaluation of amantadine, double-blind, during a naturally-occurring influenza A outbreak. Inmates who had had symptoms of influenza for less than 48 hr, and who volunteered, were admitted to the study. No patient had been vaccinated for influenza during the previous year. Amantadine (100 mg) or inert placebo capsules were administered twice daily. Patients entering the study in the evening received 2 capsules immediately. Blood samples were drawn on the first and twenty-first days for diagnostic CF and HI serology. Oral temperature signs and symptoms of illness were recorded regularly each day. Thirteen of the 14 amantadine-

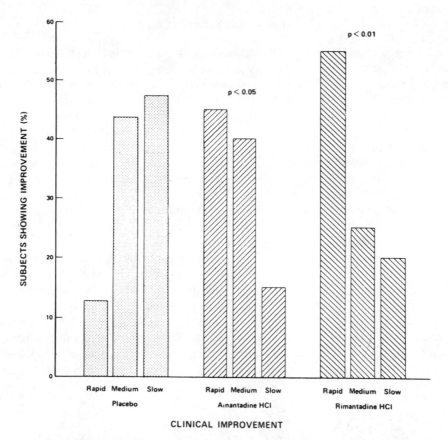

FIG. 25. The therapeutic effect of amantadine and rimantadine in influenza outbreak (prison trial). Volunteers who developed symptoms and signs of influenza within 24 hr were admitted to the trial and received amantadine (100 mg), rimantadine (150 mg) or placebo for 10 days. All of the patients with confirmed influenza A illness were used to evaluate the symptoms and signs data. (From Wingfield *et al.*, 1969; with permission of the publisher).

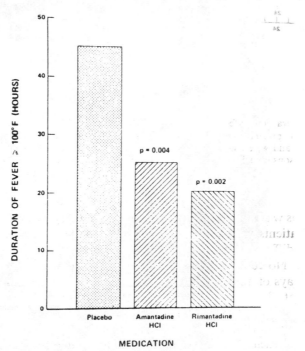

FIG. 26. Therapeutic effects of amantadine and rimantadine on temperature duration—prison trial. Volunteers who developed symptoms and signs of influenza within 24 hr were admitted to the trial and received amantadine (100 mg), rimantadine (150 mg) or placebo for 10 days. All of the patients with confirmed influenza A illness were used to evaluate the symptoms and signs data. (From Wingfield *et al.*, 1969; with permission of the publisher).

treated patients and 8 of the 13 placebo-treated patients had serologically confirmed influenza. Only these patients are considered in the analysis of the results. Before the drug code was broken, the resolution of the disease in each patient was classified as being rapid, medium or slow. A 'rapid improver' was a patient whose temperature dropped to less than 37.8°C in less than 24 hr and who had a 50 per cent reduction in total severity scores of signs and symptoms in less than 36 hr. If the temperature dropped in this manner, but the time required for 50 per cent reduction in symptom-complex was more than 36 hr, the patient was considered as a 'medium improver'. A 'slow improver' was one whose temperature dropped to less than 37.8°C only after 36 hr. The advantage to the amantadine-treated patients is seen in Fig. 27 as representing a significant difference ($p = 0.05$) over those receiving placebo. When fever is considered, moving 24-hr mean body temperature curves demonstrate a significantly more rapid resolution of those receiving amantadine ($p = 0.05$) (Fig. 28). No side effects attributable to the drug were observed.

A study of the therapeutic effect of amantadine amongst patients in the family environment was carried out by general practitioners in the United Kingdom and reported by Galbraith *et al.* (1971). Fifty-seven doctors took part and included 203 patients with clinically diagnosed influenza. Amantadine was provided in capsule form (100 mg) or as a syrup (50 mg in 5 ml) and patients received active or placebo medication by random number allocation on a double-blind basis. Adults received 100 mg every 12 hr and children aged 10–15 years 100 mg daily, younger children (2–10) a proportional dose of syrup. Medication was started from the time the patient was first seen by the doctor and was continued for 7

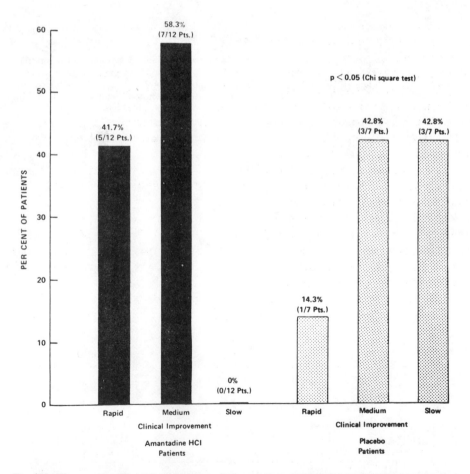

FIG. 27. Therapeutic effect of amantadine—Missouri State Penitentiary trial. Inmates who had symptoms of influenza for less than 48 hr were admitted to the study and were given amantadine (100 mg) or placebo twice daily. Only persons with serologically confirmed influenza were analysed. Persons were divided into rapid, medium or slow resolvers on clinical criteria. (Data from Baker *et al.*, 1969; with permission of the publisher).

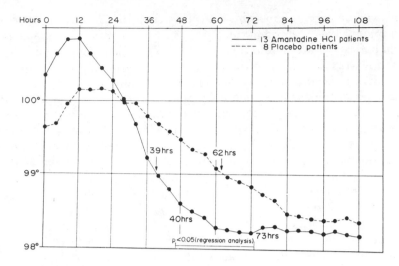

Fig. 28. Therapeutic trial of amantadine at Missouri State Penitentiary. Flowing means of body temperature. Temperatures for 4 hr through 20 hr are means from beginning of treatment period indicated by zero (0). Temperature for 24 hr through 108 hr are 24 hr means. Inmates who had symptoms of influenza for less than 48 hr were admitted to the study and were given amantadine (100 mg) or placebo twice daily. Only persons with serologically confirmed influenza were analysed. Persons were divided into rapid, medium or slow resolvers on clinical criteria. (Data from Baker *et al.*, 1969; with permission of the publisher).

days. A blood sample was taken at the doctor's first visit and a second 2–3 weeks later. These were tested for HI antibody with A/Hong Kong/68 virus and for CF antibody. A four-fold or greater rise in either or both these tests was taken as evidence of influenza A infection. Of the 203 patients entered, only 153 provided results which satisfied the criteria for analysis. Of the 153, 72 received amantadine and 81 placebo. The mean duration of fever is shown in Table 41 where the differences between drug- and placebo-treated patients were significantly different. When symptomatology was considered, no differences were demonstrated between the two groups, but this may have been due to the lack of sensitivity in the method of recording clinical illness. There was no evidence of reduction in the levels of serum antibody in infected individuals who received amantadine, so it would appear from this study that amantadine does not have the disadvantage of inhibiting the development of natural immunity when used therapeutically.

Subsequently, further evaluation of amantadine amongst patients ill at home with influenza was carried out and reported by Galbraith (1975). The design of the trials was similar to that described previously. Family doctors were provided with all the necessary equipment, record cards and randomized treatment (amantadine or placebo medication) to include the number of patients they wished, following clinical progress during the influenzal illness. The studies were performed during the winters of 1972/73 and 1973/74. (The influenza A viruses circulating during this time were inhibited by amantadine *in vitro*.) The

TABLE 41. *Therapeutic Trial of Amantadine in General Practice (UK Study)*

	Duration of temperature (hrs)			
	Amantadine	Placebo	Difference	*p*
Males	55.1	71.5	16.4	$0.05 > p > 0.02$
Females	37.7	80.6	42.8	< 0.01
Both Sexes	46.6	75.1	28.5	< 0.01

In this double-blind placebo-controlled trial, medication with amantadine was initiated within 24 hr of onset of symptoms and continued for 7 days. A blood sample was taken at the time of the doctor's first visit and 2–3 weeks later for serological studies. This table analyses the effect of amantadine on the duration of temperature. (Data from Galbraith *et al.*, 1971).

former study yielded thirty-nine patients with proven influenza A and completed records and the latter a total of 104. The serology in the 1973/74 study proved most interesting in that twenty-eight patients showed a four-fold or greater rise in antibody titre to influenza A and 30 patients showed a four-fold or greater rise in titre to influenza B. Forty-six patients had no titre rise to either influenza A or B. The infection groups are shown in Table 42. When considering fever amongst those with A influenza in the 1972/73 trial, the mean duration in those receiving the drug was 45 hr compared with 62.5 hr in those on placebo—a difference bordering on the significant $(0.1 > p > 0.05)$. In the 1973/74 trial, the mean duration of fever in those receiving the drug was 60.5 hr compared with 92.1 hr in those on placebo, a difference again bordering on the significant $(0.1 > p > 0.05)$. As the influenza A viruses responsible for the infection during both winters had essentially the same sensitivity *in vitro* to amantadine (J. S. Oxford, unpublished data), the author considered it appropriate to combine the results of the two trials (see Table 42). Thus with larger numbers, the mean duration of fever in the drug-treated group was 51.4 hr and in the controls it was 74.3 hr, a significant difference $(0.02 > p > 0.01)$. In those patients who were subsequently discovered to have suffered from influenza B, the mean duration of fever in those receiving the drug was 80.9 hr, compared with 82.4 hr in those on placebo, a difference of no significance $(p = 0.9)$. Influenza B virus is not inhibited *in vitro* by amantadine. The time taken for the symptoms to clear was calculated for each symptom separately and for all symptoms combined. In the 1973/74 trial, when considering the clearance of all symptoms combined, 53 per cent of patients with influenza A receiving amantadine did so in 4 days compared with only 23 per cent of their controls. This result borders on the significant. The number of days spent in bed by each patient was also recorded (Table 43). The trials separately give a difference bordering on the significant in favour of the amantadine-treated groups but combined show a statistically significant difference. Those patients with influenza B showed no difference. In these studies, the appearance of influenza B infection in patients, confirmed only after the clinical recording was completed, illustrated the sensitivity of the trial design, for it had been demonstrated previously (Davies *et al.*, 1964) that this virus was insensitive to amantadine.

TABLE 42. *Therapeutic Trial of Amantadine in General Practice (UK Study)*

| Influenza A | Duration of fever (hr) | | | |
	Amantadine	Control	Difference	Significance
1972/73	45.0 (21)	62.5 (18)	17.5	$0.1 > p > 0.05$
1973/74	60.5 (15)	92.1 (12)	31.6	$0.1 > p > 0.05$
Combined	51.4 (36)	74.3 (30)	22.9	$0.2 > p > 0.01$
Influenza B	80.9 (14)	82.4 (14)	1.5	$p > 0.9$

Medication with amantadine was initiated within 24 hr of onset of symptoms and continued for 7 days. A blood sample was taken at the time of the doctor's first visit and 2–3 weeks later for serological studies. Data analysed of effect of amantadine on duration of virus-induced fever (hr).
(Data from Galbraith, 1975).

TABLE 43. *Therapeutic Trial of Amantadine (UK Study)*

| Influenza A | No. of days in bed | | |
	Amantadine	Control	Significance
1972/73	2.13	2.95	$0.1 > p > 0.05$
1973/74	3.27	4.15	$0.2 > p > 0.1$
Combined	2.58	3.44	$p > 0.01$
Influenza B	3.45	3.67	$0.9 > p > 0.8$

Medication with amantadine was initiated within 24 hr of onset of symptoms and continued for 7 days. A blood sample was taken at the time of the doctor's first visit and 2–3 weeks later for serological studies. This table analyses the effect of amantadine on the number of days in bed.
(Data from Galbraith, 1975).

One would therefore have predicted that those patients with influenza B, receiving amantadine, would respond similarly to those on placebo.

In an interesting study with members of two units of the Hungarian People's Army, Mate *et al.* (1971) used amantadine hydrochloride in early 1970 in a double-blind, placebo-controlled trial (Fig. 29). The patients were aged 18–21 years, and amantadine or placebo was administered within 24 hr of symptoms of influenza. Proof of infection was by virus isolation and four-fold antibody titre rise. The causative virus was identified as influenza A/Hong Kong/68 in Unit I, while both influenza A and influenza B infections occurred in Unit II. The clinical course of the patients was recorded and it became apparent that individual responses varied, some being quick, some slower and some slow responders. Patients with not more than 4 nursing days were grouped in category I, those with 4–6 nursing days in category II and those requiring more than 6 days for recovery as members of category III. 'Nursing days' included the duration of pyrexia, the existence of clinical manifestations of the illness and 24 hr of convalescence. Figure 29 shows the distribution of patients in those categories statistically; the difference was significantly ($p < 0.01$) in favour of the amantadine-treated group. When fever alone was considered, in Unit I, the drug-treated group had fever for an average of 2.5 days while in the placebo-treated group, it lasted for an average of 4.1 days. The difference is significant ($p < 0.01$). When Unit II was considered, the difference is not significant, a not surprising result as influenza B virus is known to be insensitive to amantadine (see above). The duration of fever in the two Units is shown in Fig. 30. In their discussion, Mate *et al.* (1970a) stress that, as the frequency of immune response to influenza A virus was 81 per cent, the infection could be regarded as being exclusively caused by this virus in Unit I, while that in Unit II was mixed A and B. The significantly shorter duration of illness amongst patients in Unit I who received amantadine, compared with those taking placebo, is explained by the effect of the active drug while the compound had no effect on the members of Unit II with non-influenza A infections.

A study in Japan, reported by Kitamoto (1968), during the winter of 1967/68, in which amantadine was compared with placebo medication in double-blind fashion, again demonstrated the effectiveness of the drug when used therapeutically. The infection was prevalent in many parts of Japan and was confirmed as influenza A (H2N2). Children were included in this study receiving amantadine syrup in a dose depending on age.

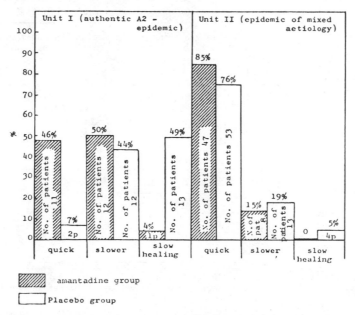

FIG. 29. Therapeutic trial of amantadine in the Hungarian army. Persons were admitted to the trial within 24 hr of onset of influenza symptoms. Virus isolation and serology confirmed influenza A/HK/68 (H3N2) infection. Volunteers were analysed in three groups, fast, medium or slow resolvers depending on clinical criteria. (Modified from Mate *et al.*, 1971; with permission of the publisher).

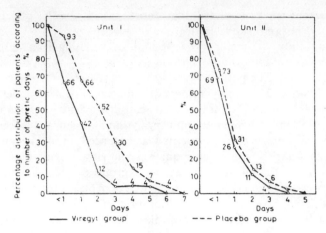

FIG. 30. Therapeutic trial of amantadine in the Hungarian army. Persons were admitted to the trial within 24 hr of onset of influenza symptoms. Virus isolation and serology confirmed influenza A/HK/68 (H3N2) infection. Volunteers were analysed in three groups, fast, medium or slow resolvers depending on clinical criteria. (Modified from Mate *et al.*, 1971; with permission of the publisher).

Administration of capsules or syrup was begun within 2 days of illness and continued for 7 days. Fever and symptoms were recorded daily. HI and CF tests were carried out to confirm infection with influenza A virus. A total of 182 patients with clinical influenza received amantadine and 173 placebo. Of these patients, 35 and 56, respectively, had proven influenza A infection. The duration of fever was significantly shorter in the amantadine treated groups both for children and adults (see Table 44). In this study, the maximum body temperature achieved by patients in whom the infection was confirmed serologically, was also recorded. An analysis demonstrated that drug-treated patients had statistically significantly lower maximum temperatures than those in the placebo group (Table 45).

Kitamoto (1971) repeated the study during the nationwide epidemic of A/Hong Kong/68 influenza which occurred in the winter of 1968–69 in Japan. A total of 737 patients entered the study, 226 cases had influenza A and 158 influenza B. In 155 cases out of 226, medication was started within 2 days of the onset of symptoms and of these, 79 received amantadine and

TABLE 44. *Therapeutic Effect of Amantadine (Japanese Trial)*

Group		0^b	1	2	3	4	5	6	7	8	Total	Mean (days)
		Duration of fever[a] after the 2 days of drug administration (days)										
Children	amantadine	4	11	1	3	1	1				21	1.48
	placebo	7	5	3	7	5	2	3	1		33	2.64
Adults	amantadine	5	4	1	2					2	14	2.00
	placebo	7	2	7	4	3					23	2.74

Duration of fever	AD	P1	Total
0–1	24	19	43
2–	11	37	48
Total	35	56	91
$X^2 = 10.37 \; p < 0.01$			

This double-blind placebo-controlled trial demonstrated therapeutic effects of amantadine against influenza variants of the H2N2 antigenic subtype. Capsules were given within two days of onset of illness and continued for 7 days. Fever and symptoms were recorded daily.

AD = amantadine.
Pl = placebo.
[a]Over 37.5°C in children and over 37.0°C in adults.
[b]0 day means no fever on the day following drug administration.
(Data from Kitamoto, 1968).

TABLE 45. *Therapeutic Effect of Amantadine on Maximum Temperature*

The day of illness in which treatment was started			Maximum temperature after the 2nd day of drug administration (°C) 36–	37–	38–	39–	40–	Total	Mean temperature (°C)
Children	1st day	A	1	5	4	3	1	14	38.4
		P	1	4	6	10	3	24	38.9
	2nd day	A			7			7	38.5
		P		5	2	2		9	38.2
	3rd day	A	1	2				3	
		P							
	4th day	A	1					1	
		P	1					1	
	1st +	A	1	5	11	3	1	21	38.4
	2nd day	P	1	9	8	12	3	33	38.7
Adults	1st day	A	1	2	1	2		6	38.2
		P		2	8	2		12	38.5
	2nd day	A	4	2	2			8	37.3
		P		4	6	1		11	38.2
	3rd day	A	1	4	1	1		7	37.7
		P	5					5	36.5
	4th day	A						0	
		P		1				1	
	1st +	A	5	4	3	2		14	37.6
	2nd day	P		6	14	3		23	38.4

High fever: 39°C or more in children, 38°C or more in adults

high fever	amantadine	placebo	total	
+	9	32	41	
–	26	24	50	$X^2 = 7.37\ p < 0.01$
total	35	56	91	

This double-blind placebo-controlled trial demonstrated therapeutic effects of amantadine against influenza variants of the H2N2 antigenic subtype. Capsules were given within 2 days of onset of illness and continued for 7 days. Fever and symptoms were recorded daily.

(Data from Kitamoto, 1968).

TABLE 46. *Therapeutic Trial of Amantadine Versus A/HK/68 (H3N2) Virus (Japanese Study)*

Group	Treatment	No. of patients	Maximum temperature after the 2nd day of treatment (°C) 36.0–36.9	37.0–37.9	38.0–38.9	39.0–39.9	40.0–	Mean
Children	amantadine	30	9	11	9	1	0	37.30
	placebo	20	3	7	8	2	0	37.80
Adults	amantadine	38	11	15	9	3	0	37.38
	placebo	46	9	15	14	6	2	37.83

Comparison of the occurrence of high fever in Hong Kong influenza patients treated with amantadine or placebo and receiving no concomitant antipyretics

Treatment	High fever[a] +	–	Total
amantadine	13	55	68
placebo	24	42	66
Total	37	97	134

$X^2 = 4.93$ ($p < 0.05$).

[a] High fever: 39.0°C or more in children and 38.0°C or more in adults.

This double-blind placebo-controlled trial demonstrated therapeutic effects of amantadine against influenza A/HK/68. Capsules were given within 2 days of onset of illness and continued for 7 days. Fever and symptoms were recorded daily.

(Data from Kitamoto, 1971).

76 placebo. Fever was evaluated in the same way, as was maximum body temperature. The group receiving amantadine had a shorter duration of fever (Table 46) and a lower mean maximum temperature. This was demonstrable also in patients receiving no antipyretics (Table 47). In both studies no adverse reactions to amantadine were observed.

In conclusion, for the therapeutic studies described above, a demonstrable reduction in the duration of fever and maximum temperature has been reported in the majority of studies performed, all of which were double-blind and placebo-controlled, in those groups receiving amantadine, provided treatment was begun within 2 days of the onset of symptoms caused by influenza A virus (summarized in Table 48). The severity of symptoms of influenza vary widely from one patient to another and, while the trend has been for drug-treated patients to improve symptomatically more quickly than those on placebo, the difference has not always reached significance. The benefit of such reduction in duration of fever or rate of amelioration of symptoms to a community stricken with influenza, or even to individuals

TABLE 47. *Therapeutic Effect of Amantadine on Duration of Fever (Japanese Study)*

| Group | Treatment[b] | No. of patients | Duration of fever[a] after the start of treatment (days) | | | | | | | | | Mean |
			1[c]	2	3	4	5	6	7	8	9	
Children	Amantadine	30	16	12	1	0	0	1	—	—	—	0.63
	Placebo	20	6	8	5	0	1	0	—	—	—	1.10
Adults	Amantadine	38	9	11	11	5	2	0	0	—	0	1.47
	Placebo	46	9	7	6	11	5	4	3	—	1	2.57

Comparison of the duration of fever in Hong Kong influenza patients
receiving no concomitant antipyretics

| Duration (days) | No. of patients with fever | | |
	Amantadine	Placebo	Total
0–1	48	30	78
2–	20	36	56
Total	68	66	134

[a] 37.5°C or more in children and 37.0°C or more in adults.
[b] Treatment was started within the 2nd day of illness.
[c] Fever disappeared the day after start of treatment.
$X^2 = 8.70 (p < 0.01)$.
This double-blind placebo-controlled trial demonstrated therapeutic effects of amantadine against influenza A/HK/68. Capsules were given within 2 days of onset of illness and continued for 7 days. Fever and symptoms were recorded daily.
(Data from Kitamoto, 1971).

TABLE 48. *Summary of Early Double-Blind Therapeutic Studies in Volunteers*

Investigators	Location	Virus strain	Number of patients treated with amantadine	Significant effect	Date of clinical trial
Baker, Paulshock, Iezzoni	US	A(H2N2) Asian	13	+	1968
Galbraith, Oxford, Schild, Potter, Watson	GB	A/HK/68(H3N2) variant	72	+	1969/70
Galbraith, Schild, Potter, Watson	GB	A/HK/68(H3N2)	34	+	1971/72 1972/73
Galbraith	GB	A/HK/68(H3N2) variant	36	+	1973/74
Hornick, Togo, Mahler, Iezzoni	US	A(H2N2) Asian	94	+	1968
Wingfield, Pollock, Grunert	US	A(H2N2) Asian	23 (24 rimantadine)	+	1968
Mate, Simon, Juranez	Hungary	A/HK/68(H3N2) variant	24	+	1970
Kitamoto	Japan	A(N2N2) variant	35	+	1968
Kitamoto	Japan	A/HK/68(H3N2)	79	+	1969

anxious to return to work quickly, may be debatable. The decision, whether to administer amantadine to early cases of clinical influenza or not, will depend in the final analysis on the physician's assessment of the risk to the patient of allowing the infection to run its natural course. In the young and healthy, symptomatic treatment may be all that is required; in the older patient, or in those with chronic disease, it may well be advisable to prescribe amantadine as early as possible in the infection.

6.20.5. PRESENT AND FUTURE CLINICAL USE OF AMANTADINE

At present amantadine (or derivatives) has not found widespread use as an anti-viral compound except in the USSR. As the first clinically useful anti-influenza compound, new concepts have had to be expounded and developed and the early use of the compound was hampered by criticism from Sabin (1978) much of which was shown subsequently to have been unfounded.

Jackson (1977) has suggested several venues for the clinical use of amantadine and a number of these have been emphasised in a recent WHO report (Galasso *et al.*, 1984). Some of these have been discussed above but are usefully summarized here:

1. Households contacts of an index case of influenza. The UK trials organized by Galbraith *et al.* (1969a, 1969b, 1970, 1971) have established the usefulness of this approach both prophylactically and therapeutically.
2. Hospital patients and personnel, to prevent hospital spread when patients with influenza A virus infections are admitted. This would mainly be prophylactic use of the compound.
3. Persons in institutions, such as old persons' homes.
4. Unvaccinated adults, who nevertheless have serious underlying disease which place them in a potentially high mortality group following an attack of influenza, e.g. persons with pulmonary, cardiac, metabolic or immunological deficiencies. Amantadine could be used prophylactically and persons vaccinated at the same time.
5. Vaccinated adults who are at high risk from an attack of influenza. Amantadine-supplemented protection would be expected to raise the basic 70 per cent protective effect of vaccine alone. Single non-reactogenic doses of vaccine against a new pandemic virus subtype would not be expected to give significant protection—two doses of vaccine would be required—particularly with subunit or split virus vaccines. Therefore amantadine could be administered prophylactically during the 3-week period of development of vaccine induced immunity.
6. Adults, such as hospital workers, public transport personnel, etc., in the face of an epidemic when insufficient vaccine is available, or when contraindications exist to vaccine.
7. Persons presenting with clinical influenza within 48 hr of the onset of clinical signs. The therapeutic activity of amantadine, although mild, is now established in clinical trials in several countries. Future clinical trials may establish if amantadine used therapeutically can reduce mortality in persons at special risk, or reduce the rate of complications such as pneumonia.

In the face of a new pandemic influenza A virus, it is quite possible that a suitable vaccine, either live or inactivated, could not be produced in sufficient quantities for rapid general administration in the first wave of infection. Prophylaxis with amantadine would be an alternative possibility. Such a widespread use of an antiviral compound would give doctors and epidemiologists a unique opportunity to conduct large-scale trials and would provide the necessary data for the development of future plans for the control of influenza as one of the last pandemic diseases of man.

A consensus development panel convened in the USA to examine the usefulness of amantadine for the prevention or treatment of influenza A virus infections concluded that the compound should be used prophylactically in combination with influenza vaccines in patients at high risk of morbidity and also in certain low risk unvaccinated persons including hospital or nursing home patients, policemen and firemen. Three groups for which amantadine *therapy* was strongly recommended were:

1. The same high-risk patients identified for prophylaxis, i.e. persons with underlying diseases, including pulmonary, cardiovascular, metabolic, neuromuscular or immuno-deficiency diseases.
2. Patients with diagnosed life threatening influenza or infants with influenza-associated croup.
3. Essential community personnel in whom shortening a symptomatic illness by as little as 24 hr is judged important.

The panel considered that side effects of the compound were transient and subsided with continued use of the compound (reviewed by Elliott, 1979). It was also considered that further studies were required to investigate the efficacy of amantadine in elderly patients and children and in cases of primary influenzal pneumonia. Optimum regimens of dosage and duration of treatment and the safety of amantadine in pregnancy were also areas for future investigation. As a result of recent studies a WHO group has been able to recommend the use of amantadine or rimantadine as a therapeutic agent but rimantadine only for prophylaxis (Galasso et al., 1984).

6.20.6. COMBINED VACCINE AND AMANTADINE

Studies in the USSR have commenced with vaccine–rimantadine combinations (Table 49). In this trial, in an army camp, carried out by Slepushkin and co-workers (personal communication), persons were given live attenuated vaccine alone, rimantadine (200 mg/day) alone or combinations of the two. The influenza outbreak was, in fact, caused by the current H1N1 virus and the mild (37 per cent) protective effect given by the antigenically unrelated H3N2 vaccine was attributed to virus interference or induction of interferon by the vaccine virus. But the interesting data from the trial is the 60 per cent protection noted in the group given combined vaccine and rimantadine. Combinations of vaccines and anti-influenza compounds may find an important application in the overall strategy for the future control of influenza in the community.

TABLE 49. *Prophylactic Effects of Rimantadine and Influenza Vaccine Combinations (Moscow Study)*

Groups	No. of persons	No. of illnesses	% illness	% protection	Mean duration (days) of: Temperature	Illness
Vaccine + rimantadine	400	34	8.5	60	2.6	4.8
Placebo + rimantadine	277	40	14.4	32.4	3.6	5.8
Vaccine + placebo	378	51	13.4	37	4.2	6.0
Placebo only	408	87	21.3	—	4.5	6.2

The prophylactic study was carried out in an army camp near Moscow. A live attenuated vaccine containing virus of the (H3N2) antigenic subtype was administered to certain groups. Protection elicited by this vaccine was attributed to interferon production since no antigenic relationship was present between the vaccine virus and the virus actually causing the outbreak (H1N1) antigenic subtype.
37 H1N1 viruses isolated from 49 samples.
Vaccine—live attenuated H3N2 given 2 days prior to outbreak.
Data from A Slepushkin, Ivanovsky Institute of Virology, Moscow (personal communication).
(See also Zlydnikov et al., 1981).

6.20.7. RECENT CLINICAL STUDIES WITH AMANTADINE AEROSOLS

As described above, amantadine has been shown to have a good degree of prophylactic and therapeutic activity in man against influenza A virus of three subtypes (H2N2, H3N2, H1N1) but its possible role in the management of more severe illness such as primary influenza virus pneumonia remains undefined. Animal studies have shown greater therapeutic activity when the compound is administered as an aerosol (Schmidt-Ruppin and Poncioni, 1979). Topical application into the respiratory tract attempts to provide local high concentrations of drug and concomitantly to minimize drug toxicity. Studies have been undertaken using volunteers to establish safety and acceptability of delivery of amantadine by small particle aerosol (Hayden *et al.*, 1979; 1980). After aerosol administration, drug concentrations in the upper respiratory tract greatly exceeded blood and nasal wash levels found after oral administration. This is a most useful and significant finding. An aerosol mist was generated with a Devilbis glass nebulizer with an aerodynamic mass median diameter of 3 μm. The mist was directed to the face with a large bore plastic tube which served as a face mask and reservoir. Thirty-minute treatments were given twice daily for 12 days. One hour after aerosol treatments with a 1.0 g/100 ml solution, amantadine levels in nasal wash samples (mean 30.3 μg/ml) greatly exceeded blood and nasal wash levels following oral administration. Thus following 200 mg/day amantadine orally, blood levels of less than 1 μg/ml were detected. With a plaque inhibition test 0.3 μg/ml amantadine is required for inhibition of virus. Aerosol delivery was followed by rapid appearance of the drug in the urine. Nasal irritation, rhinorrhea and disagreeable taste occurred in all subjects receiving 2.5 g/100 ml solution concentration. However, a qualification here is that inhalation of water mist is known to provoke broncho constriction in persons with bronchopulmonary disease for example.

In studies by another group of workers, seven well volunteers and three persons with influenza were given amantadine by small particle aerosol (Knight *et al.*, 1979). A continuous flow modified Collison nebulizer was used and inhalations were given intranasally through a rubber aviator mask. The mass median diameter of aerosol particles was about 1.2 μm. Varying inhalation periods from 15 min to 6 hr were used and estimates of retained doses in 9 hr were 74–149 mg. About two-thirds of the dose was recovered in the urine and approximately 4 μg/ml amantadine was detected in the urine within 45 min of the start of the aerosol, indicating rapid absorption of the drug. Experimental studies of small particle aerosols in humans have indicated that 36 per cent of particles will deposit in the nose, 1 per cent in the pharynx and bronchi, 25 per cent in tertiary bronchi and respiratory bronchioles and 21 per cent in alveolar ducts. Such a retention, assuming similar absorption of amantadine at all sites, would be very suitable since influenza infection involves cells at all levels of the respiratory tract. Pulmonary function studies found no evidence of abnormalities after amantadine inhalation with five normal volunteers although two persons, one an asthmatic, had mild episodes of bronchospasm after prolonged inhalation. The authors concluded that although normal subjects tolerated amantadine inhalation extremely well, the compound may irregularly produce mild abnormalities in susceptible patients with reactive airways. In the three young adults with influenza, amantadine aerosol was started at 6, 24 and 36 hr in 2–4 hr courses 10–11 hr daily for 3 days. Recovery was rapid in all cases. Despite acute influenza there was no evidence of irritation of the respiratory tract by the inhalations. Further studies are now required to determine precise dosages, and time schedules in normal volunteers.

6.20.8. Recent Prophylactic and Therapeutic Clinical Studies with H1N1 and H3N2 Influenza A Viruses

Although the earlier studies described above established unequivocally the prophylactic and therapeutic efficacy of amantadine, certain questions remained unanswered. Thus, is rimantadine more effective than amantadine and are recent strains of influenza A virus also susceptible to inhibition by the compound?

Quarles *et al.* (1981) compared the efficacy of 200-mg doses of amantadine and rimantadine for the prophylaxis of A/USSR/77 virus in a double-blind placebo-controlled trial in students. The study was begun late in the epidemic and thus a precise efficacy of the two compounds was not possible. A statistically significant protective effect against infection was noted for younger students taking amantadine. A lower frequency of seroconversions occurred among the antibody negative 18–21-year-olds given amantadine than among the students given placebo (12 of 61 persons versus 21 of 60 persons in the placebo group, $p = 0.06$). When divided into two age groups the protective effect was significant among

18–19-year-olds ($p = 0.01$). Sixty-five per cent fewer seroconversions occurred among those with the highest attack rate. In addition, although the numbers were small, illness with cough was also reduced among 18–19-year-olds given amantadine. When illness among seroconverters was compared, illness tended to be less common and severe among those given rimantadine ($p < 0.01$).

An interesting recent trial compared the potential therapeutic effect of amantadine and rimantadine in a group of students ill with A/USSR/77 (H1N1) virus (Van Voris et al., 1981). Students were admitted to the trial if they were feverish with malaise and myalgia of less than 48 hr duration. A complete history was taken and respiratory examinations performed at 24, 48, 72 hr and 7 days and 3 weeks. Drug (100 mg) or placebo was taken twice daily. Forty-five of the 54 volunteers who entered the study had proven influenza. Total symptom and sign scores were calculated for each group and compared with pretreatment scores to assess the resolution of illness. A level of 50 per cent improvement was reached in the amantadine and rimantadine groups at 48 hr whereas this was not reached until 72 hr in the placebo group ($p < 0.025$). The greatest therapeutic effect was on generalized symptoms but relative improvement was noted in all clinical categories. Mean temperatures for the treated groups were significantly reduced compared to placebo ($p < 0.01$). A temperature of less than 37.2°C at 48 hr was noted in 13 of 14 amantadine and all 19 rimantadine persons compared to 6 of 12 persons in the placebo group. At 48 hr and 72 hr after initiation of the study significantly more students from both the drug-treated groups attended classes than students in the control group. Finally at 48 hr the proportion of students shedding virus was significantly lower in groups treated with amantadine or rimantadine. Side effects appeared limited and transient, and were confined almost exclusively to the amantadine group. The study therefore compares well with previous therapeutic studies with H3N2 viruses in which the duration of illness was reduced by 1–2 days from the usual 3–5 days (see above). The authors concluded that the differences in therapeutic effectiveness between amantadine and rimantadine was small. Of particular interest is the demonstration of reduced virus shedding because this would be expected to reduce the frequency of transmission of virus. The authors concluded 'the 24–48 hour benefit appears to justify the therapeutic use of amantadine, especially if one considers the current widespread use of unproved and potentially harmful measures such as antibiotics, antihistamines and cough suppressants'.

(Dolin et al., 1982) reported the first well-controlled comparison in the USA of the prophylactic effects of rimantadine and amantadine in an area where an active influenza surveillance indicated early that an influenza A outbreak had commenced caused by H3N2 (20 per cent of cases) and H1N1 viruses (80 per cent of cases). A total of 450 volunteers enrolled with a mean age of 25.0 ± 0.5 years and with no significant differences in age, race, male : female ratios or level of pre-existing HI antibody. Throat swabs for virus isolation were taken 2 times per week and volunteers were assigned to amantadine, rimantadine and placebo groups. A 100 mg tablet was taken twice daily for 7 days and any symptoms were recorded. Each week the volunteers returned the symptoms diary to the co-ordinating centre and received a further 7 days' supply of tablets. If any respiratory illness occurred, volunteers were asked to return at once to the centre, and were examined by a physician. Influenza-like illness was defined as a cough and/or fever greater than 37.7°C and two or more of the following symptoms: sore throat, headache and myalgia. The trial lasted 6 weeks and a serum sample was obtained at the beginning and again at the end of the study for serological analysis. Significantly more placebo recipients (40.9 per cent) developed influenza-like illness compared to amantadine (8.9 per cent) or rimantadine (14.3 per cent) groups giving a reduction in the rate of illness of 78.2 per cent and 65.0 per cent respectively.

Because the above study was carried out in healthy young adults, the important question remained as to whether rimantadine would be equally effective and free of side effects when employed in prophylaxis against influenza A in elderly, high-risk individuals. Because of the lack of reactogenicity observed with rimantadine in the above study, Dolin et al., (personal communication) concluded that risk/benefit ratio of the drug was sufficiently favourable to conduct a trial of prophylaxis in elderly individuals residing in nursing homes. Rimantadine at a dose of 100 mg twice a day or placebo was administered to 105 elderly subjects (mean age:

83) in a double-blind, randomised trial lasting 6–7 weeks during which time an outbreak of influenza A was occurring at Rochester, New York. Subjects were followed for the development of respiratory illness or potential side effects in a manner similar to that described in the study in young adults. Influenza-like illness occurred in 12/44 (27.3 per cent) placebo recipients compared to 4/39 (10.3 per cent) rimantadine recipients ($p < 0.05$). The efficacy rate for rimantadine in the prevention of influenza-like illness was 62.3 per cent, which was similar to that described previously for rimantadine in the reduction of influenza-like illness in young adults.

In another recent controlled study, 100 mg/day amantadine was shown to be as effective as 200 mg/day amantadine in terms of therapeutic efficacy, and both were superior to aspirin in relief of fever and other symptoms (Younkin, 1983).

Further studies on the side effects of amantadine and rimantadine.

Millet et al., (1982) carried out a controlled comparison of amantadine and rimantadine on cns side effects and included a commonly used antihistamine compound (chlorpheniramine). The study was carried out at the University of California and 52 adult volunteers participated, with a mean age of 25 years. There was no significant difference among treatment groups with respect to age or sex of the subjects. Mild symptoms occurred with approximately equal frequency in all groups and therefore were excluded from further analysis. The frequency of reported symptoms was low in the amantadine and placebo groups. Antihistamine-like side effects, such as drowsiness and dry mouth, were less frequent and severe in the amantadine group than in the chlorpheniramine group. However, moderate to severe inability to concentrate, dizziness, and fatigue were reported more frequently by subjects who received the combination of amantadine and chlorpheniramine. Two subjects who received this combination reported additional symptoms of confusion and distorted depth perception as well as nausea and chills. There were no significant differences between the group mean scores on the second practice trial and the pretreatment trial of the Critical Tracking Test among all treatment groups.

The effects of amantadine or rimantadine on higher central nervous system functions, such as memory and attention, become more important when considering its use for prophylaxis of large populations. This data of Millet et al., (1982) shows that neither of these drugs had a significant effect upon performance of tasks which involved attention, cognition, and memory.

The early clinical studies of rimantadine in the USSR (Smorodintsev et al., 1970 a, b) and more recently in the USA have apparently indicated that the rimantadine molecule is less toxic (Dolin et al., 1982) and fewer cns side effects are noted (although these effects are very mild with amantadine and are detected in no more than 10 per cent of patients as described above). In a recent study Hayden et al., (1983) found that at similar plasma concentrations amantadine and rimantadine did not differ in the frequency severity of their side effects. Oral dosing of volunteers with the same concentration (200 mg/day) of amantadine and rimantadine resulted in two-fold different plasma levels (4 hrs after the initial dose of drug) of 300 ± 98 ng amantadine and 140 ± 68 ng rimantadine. Moreover the plasma drug concentrations correlated significantly with total symptom score. Thus an important conclusion was that amantadine and rimantadine appeared to differ in their pharmacokinetics but not in their potential for side effects at comparable plasma concentrations.

As a result of these more recent comparative studies of toxicity and antiviral effects, rimantadine is now recommended for prophylactic use and either compound for therapeutic use (Galasso et al., 1984) during epidemics of influenza A virus.

APPENDIX

IN VITRO AND *IN VIVO* METHODS SUITABLE FOR STUDIES OF INFLUENZA AND INHIBITING COMPOUNDS

INTRACELLULAR LABELLING METHODS WITH [S^{35}]-METHIONINE

High resolution slab gels of polyacrylamide containing sodium dodecyl sulphate (SDS) can be used to analyse the newly synthesized polypeptides induced intracellularly by a number of RNA and DNA viruses including influenza (Skehel, 1972; Oxford, 1975a), herpes virus (Watson and Honess, 1977) and picornaviruses. The method can give rapid results since with influenza virus some virus polypeptides are detected as early as 2 hr post-infection. In brief, virus-infected cells in 60-mm plastic petri dishes are pulsed at suitable times post-infection for 20 min at 37°C with approximately 20 μc of [S^{35}]-methionine (445 ci/m mol Radiochemical Centre, Amersham). The whole cell monolayer is disrupted with 0.2 ml of SDS and β-mercaptoethanol mixture in buffer at pH 6.8 and approximately 50 μl aliquots boiled for 2 min and used for subsequent electrophoresis (Fig. 7). The high resolution gel system described by Laemmli (1970) with a discontinuous buffer system is used, as modified by the Cambridge virology laboratory (J. Almond, personal communication). Samples to be analysed include uninfected cells, virus-infected cells, drug-treated cells and virus-infected drug-treated cells. Any effect of a compound on virus-induced protein synthesis can then be accurately assessed.

TECHNICAL DETAILS

SDS Acrylamide gels for total of 36 ml. Main gel

per cent Gel:	5%	7.5%	10%	12.5%	15%	17.5%	20%
30% Acrylamide	6.0	9.0	12	15	18	21	24
1% Bisacrylamide	9.4	7.0	4.7	3.7	3.1	2.64	2.4
1.5 M Tris pH 8.7	9.0	9.0	9.0	9.0	9.0	9.0	9.0
Water	10.9	10.3	9.4	7.5	5.1	2.8	0.12
10% SDS (μl)	360	360	360	360	360	360	360
10% Ammonium persulphate (μl)	120	120	120	120	120	120	120
TEMED (μl)	12	12	12	12	12	12	12

Stacking Gel 5%

30% acrylamide	3.2 ml
1% bis	2.6 ml
1 M Tris pH 6.8	2.5 ml
20% SDS	50 μl
Water	6.8 ml
Amm persulphate 10%	100 μl

Usually the slabs have 60 ml of main gel and 6 ml of stacking gel

Sample Buffer

β-mercaptoethanol	0.3 ml
20% SDS	5 ml
1.5 M Tris pH 6.8	0.83 ml
Sucrose	10 g
0.2% BPB	0.3 ml
dilute to 50 ml	

PREPARATION OF GEL

Make a watertight former with plastic spacers and silicone grease, mix the main gel components except the SDS, TEMED and AMPS, add the remaining components and, after thorough but ungassy mixing, pour into the mould. Overlay with water and wait for it to set (15 min). Then remove overlay, wash with water and dry with tissues and pour on spacer gel, and insert 'comb'. Allow to set, remove comb, place gel in apparatus, load and run. Usually we warm reagents to 37°C before addition of catalyst to speed polymerisation.

Running Buffer (5X concentrated)

Glycine	144 g
Tris	30 g
10 % SDS	50 ml
Water → 1 litre	

Dilute five-fold before use with water

At the end of the run, signalled by the dye-marker nearing the end of the gel. Stain in 0.3 per cent Coomassie blue in water : methanol : acetic acid (5 : 5 : 1) for 3 hr. Destain in the same solvent for 2 days with several changes. The gels can then be dried on a sheet of porous plastic and preserved or autoradiographed.

If the label in the proteins is tritium, rather than 14_C, 35_S, 32_P or 125_I, impregnate the gel with a scintillant before drying.

Modifications of the electrophoresis system whereby the acrylamide concentration is lowered from 15–20 per cent to 2.8 per cent allow examination of virus-induced RNA species using a label of H^3 or C^{14}-uridine (Palese and Schulman, 1976). These methods have wide applicability for investigating points of action of virus inhibitory compounds.

TISSUE CULTURE METHODS WITH INFLUENZA VIRUSES

A feature of the virology of influenza is the great variability among the influenza A strains of human, avian, and equine origin regarding the growth of the viruses in tissue cultures. The embryonated hen's egg can be used successfully to propagate and quantitate all known influenza A and B viruses, but tissue culture experiments are required for some studies; the egg-piece method of Fazekas de St. Groth and White (1958) is used successfully in our laboratory. More recently plaque methods suitable for recent isolates of influenza virus have been developed.

INFLUENZA VIRUS PLAQUE FORMATION IN TISSUE CULTURES

Falcon tissue culture dishes, 5 cm in diameter, are seeded with 5 ml of 2×10^5 per ml of canine kidney cells (MDCK) in minimal essential medium (MEM, GIBCO F-15) with 0.088 per cent sodium bicarbonate and 5 per cent foetal bovine serum; and incubated at 34°C in 3 per cent in air. When confluent cell sheets are obtained, usually after 4 days, the culture medium is removed from the dishes by aspiration and the diluted virus inoculated 0.1 ml per dish and left to adsorb at room temperature for 30 min. The cultures are then overlaid with an agar medium comprising MEM, sodium bicarbonate 0.176 per cent, bovine serum albumin 0.14 per cent, DEAE-Dextran 100 μg/ml, trypsin TPCK (Worthington) 0.6 u/ml (Appleyard and Maber, 1976; Oxford et al., 1980b), Oxoid Ionagar No. 2 0.5 per cent and antibiotics. The agar is prepared at 1 per cent in distilled water to half the total volume of medium required, autoclaved and cooled at 56°C. The remainder of the medium is prepared in a half volume using MEM × 5 concentrated. Two parts are mixed thoroughly and used immediately. The overlay is allowed to set and the dishes are then inverted and incubated at 34°C in 3 per cent CO_2 in air for 3 days. The dishes are then further overlaid with 2 ml of the above medium containing 0.005 per cent neutral red. The plaques are counted. Alternatively the dishes can be stained by removing the agar overlay, rinsing in saline and staining with 0.1 per cent Naphthalene black, 6 per cent v/v glacial acetic and 1.36 per cent sodium acetate and destaining in tap water (Fig. 31).

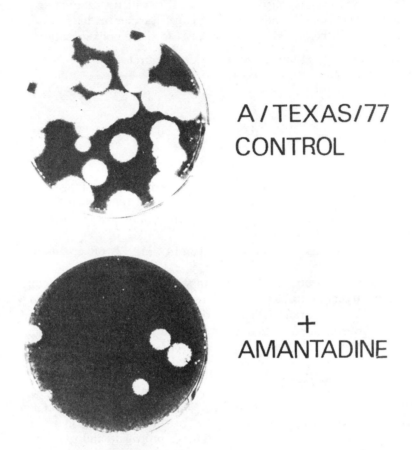

A / TEXAS/77 CONTROL

+ AMANTADINE

FIG. 31. Influenza A virus plaques in MDCK cells with trypsin. Amantadine at 5 μg/ml was incorporated in the overlay in the experimental dishes. The overlay contained trypsin to enhance plaque formation (see Appendix). Control and treated MDCK cells were infected with virus, overlaid with agar with or without amantadine and examined for plaques after 3 days incubation at 34°C.

VIRION-ASSOCIATED RNA-DEPENDENT RNA POLYMERASE ENZYME ASSAY

The influenza virion-associated RNA-dependent RNA transcriptase enzyme has to be activated by incubation of the virus with mild detergent. With a supply of nucleoside triphosphates, one of them labelled with H^3 or C^{14} and the correct cations (Mg^{2+}), the enzyme can transcribe the influenza virion RNA into an RNA copy, precipitable by trichloracetic acid. For the test, therefore, enzyme activity is proportional to the radioactive counts incorporated into TCA precipitable material. It is easily possible to screen twenty compounds a day at varying compound concentrations (Oxford and Perrin, 1977). The results from the scintillation counter can be directly printed on tape and fed into a computer to enable detailed analysis of the results. The test is technically simple, care being required to eliminate reagents contaminated with RNAse, an extremely heat-stable enzyme. The presence of very low quantities of RNAse would result, of course, in the digestion of newly synthesized single-stranded RNA; therefore the virus sample would appear to have little or no RNA polymerase activity. It is particularly important to ensure that any inhibition of RNA polymerase activity by a particular chemical 'inhibitor' is not, in fact, simply due to contamination of the compound with RNAse.

Influenza virus purified from infected egg allantoic fluids has proven satisfactory for this test. Approximately 50 mg of virus protein would be purified from 1000 eggs and can be used for 2000 enzyme reaction tubes (Oxford, 1977). Several different virus preparations are screened in the RNA polymerase test to select a preparation with high enzyme activity and low RNAse contamination.

RNA Polymerase Assay

The reaction mixture is prepared to the following composition and can be frozen at $-80°C$ in aliquots without addition of virus and used for different experiments.

1. 50 mM tris-HCl pH 8.0
2. 5 mM $MgCl_2$
3. 2 mM $MnCl_2$
4. 0.5 mM GTP
5. 0.5 mM ATP
6. 0.5 mM CTP
7. 0.005 mM H^3-UTP
8. 0.2 % v/v Nonidet P40
   (500 μg/ml influenza virus protein to be added separately).

The mixture is kept in ice and water, and influenza virus is added last. Small aliquots are then distributed (usually 60 μl) to Dreyer tubes for the actual experiment. A small volume (10 μl) of varying dilutions of the inhibitor under test can then be added to the appropriate Dreyer tubes. (Separate experiments can be carried out to check that the 'inhibitor' compound under test contains no RNAse. A simple test is to incubate different concentrations of the compound with H^3-uridine-labelled ribosomal RNA for 30 min at 37°C and then to examine the mixture for any decrease in TCA precipitable counts.) Samples (20 μl) are removed from the polymerase reaction mixture at zero time using a 'microcap' pipette (Drummond Scientific Co., USA) and pipetted onto small numbered filter paper discs. The Dreyer tubes are incubated at 37°C for 30 min, cooled to 4°C, and further 20-μl samples are pipetted onto filter discs. Duplicate discs are used. The discs are air dried and then washed in 6 per cent TCA containing 0.1 M pyrophosphate (approximately 200 discs can be washed in 500 ml of 6 per cent TCA), ethanol, and finally ether. The discs are air dried for 20 min at 37°C, placed in vials containing 10 ml of toluene solution containing 0.5 per cent PPO (2,5-diphenyloxazole) and 3 per cent POPOP, 1,4-bis 2-(4-methyl-5-phenoxazolyl)-benzene, and counted for radioactivity in a liquid scintillation spectrometer.

In a typical experiment sample discs at time zero would have around 50 cpm; after incubation at 37°C a five- to ten-fold increase in TCA precipitable counts would be expected with an influenza virus preparation which possessed an active polymerase enzyme.

Compounds causing 50 per cent inhibition of enzyme activity at low molarity are of interest. Further tests can then be set up to examine any differential effect on host DNA-dependent DNA polymerase or DNA-dependent RNA polymerase enzymes and also any effect on influenza B RNA polymerase.

In Vivo Methods with Influenza

It is likely that no single animal species will prove to be a completely adequate model for human influenza; the extremes of convenience provided by mice and the similarity to influenza infection of man which is shown by ferrets may provide two models that should be used in parallel (reviewed by Potter and Oxford, 1977).

The Ferret Model for Influenza

Ferrets are susceptible to infection by all human influenza A and B strains that have been tested. Virus strains do not require adaptation to grow to high titre in this species, and virus infection can easily spread to other ferrets or to man. The results of infection can be studied using a number of parameters, and the effect of chemotherapeutic compounds on influenza virus infection in ferrets can be assessed both quantitatively and qualitatively by measuring one or more of these responses in control and drug-treated ferrets.

Virus can be given to ferrets by nose drops (Fig. 32); anaesthetics can be used for this procedure, but this is not always necessary for ferrets that have become used to handling. The animals are simply suspended by holding them by the head and neck with one hand, and the inoculum is applied dropwise directly into the nose. The inoculum must be given to nonanaesthetized animals slowly in small drops or the animal will blow back.

Unlike any other animal species, ferrets infected with influenza A virus develop a sharp, febrile response; this is a measurable reaction similar to that found in man and is one of the most important reasons why the ferret is considered a good model system for the study of chemotherapeutic drugs against influenza. Ferrets should be housed in individual cages for at least 1 week prior to any critical assessment of the temperature response to influenza virus infection. During this time, a routine of feeding and cleaning should be used, and the temperature should be taken by a single operator at a fixed time or times each day. This is necessary since ferrets are highly excitable, and their temperature can be made to rise by banging on the cage or otherwise exciting the animals. During the period of 1 week, however, ferrets become tolerant to the routine of feeding, cleaning and handling. The temperature can be taken per rectum using a clinical thermometer or a thermocouple probe—the temperatures are recorded daily for 4 days and subsequently once daily for 3 days after virus infection. The criteria by which a febrile response is measured in virus-infected animals given antiviral compounds are arbitrary, depending on the response seen in control ferrets; either the evaluation of the temperature response above the mean preinfection level and/or the maximum temperature can be used. Two temperature readings of over 40°C measured in the period 24 to 72 hr after infection can usually be taken to indicate a significant temperature response, and two temperature readings of 1°C or more above the mean pre-infection temperature can usually be taken to indicate a significant rise in temperature.

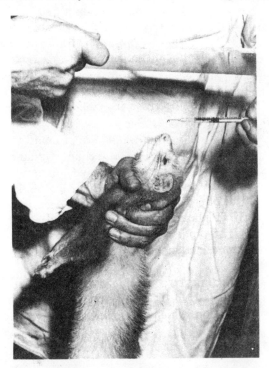

FERRET
INNOCULATION
TECHNIQUE

FIG. 32. Inoculation of ferrets with influenza A virus. Virus in the form of infected egg allantoic fluid is diluted in tryptose phosphate broth to contain approximately $10^6 EID_{50}$/ml and inoculated dropwise into the nose of anaesthetized ferrets. A transparent perspex plate helps prevent direct droplet spread to handlers from the inoculated ferret by sneezing (see Appendix). Temperatures are taken twice daily, as are throat washings. Animals look ill approximately 48 hr post-infection.

Virus isolation and quantitation is also carried out from nasal washes taken at 24, 48 and 72 hours post-infection.

THE MOUSE MODEL FOR INFLUENZA

Usually, laboratories involved in the search for inhibitors of influenza virus use virus-infected mice as a primary or secondary screening procedure. Compared to ferrets, for example, mice are inexpensive, and large numbers can be handled with relative ease to give statistically significant results; usually, groups of 10–20 mice are used with a single concentration of inhibitor under test. Most mouse models of influenza infection use highly mouse-adapted viruses which cause acute infection of the lower respiratory tract; the animals die of virus pneumonia. Human influenza on, the other hand, is predominantly an acute infection of the upper respiratory tract, only rarely producing pneumonia and death. It might be anticipated that such mouse models present a rigorous test to the efficacy of any anti-influenza compound.

RESPONSE OF MICE TO INFECTION WITH INFLUENZA

Since influenza virus strains adapted to grow in mouse lungs frequently produce death, this has been one of the most commonly used parameters of assaying the effects of virus infection in this species. Influenza virus-infected animals are examined for 14 days for sickness, and the number of daily deaths is recorded. The results are expressed both as the percentage of mice surviving the infection at the end of the experiment and the mean day of death of the nonsurvivors. In studies of influenza virus inhibitors, only low doses of virus, in the region 5 to 10 LD_{50}/mouse, are commonly used to infect mice. Under these conditions, most mice would appear ill, with rapid breathing and ruffled fur about 3 to 4 days post-infection; they would die at about 7 to 9 days after virus infection.

In the case of most influenza virus infections of mice, the response is quantal; the animals either die or survive. The results are statistically evaluated by comparing (by means of the t test) the mean survival time of drug-treated, virus-infected animals dying on, or before day 14 with the mean survival time of the virus control animals.

LUNG CONSOLIDATION

A further method of evaluating influenza virus infection of mice is based on the degree of lung consolidation; this is carried out by scoring each lung on a 'blind' basis, i.e. the scorers do not know the history of the donors of the lungs. The lungs are graded according to the following scale: 5, death with consolidation; 4, 100 per cent consolidation; 3, 75 per cent consolidation; 2, 50 per cent consolidation, 1, 25 per cent consolidation, 0, no consolidation. An average lung-consolidation score is calculated by dividing the total grade of consolidation by the number of lungs graded. Mice which have been exposed only to virus diluent are treated with identical drug dosages at the same time as the test animals. These animals are held 30 days after the end of treatment and serve as drug toxicity controls.

VIRUS HAEMAGGLUTININ IN MOUSE LUNGS

It is of particular importance to demonstrate that a potential influenza virus inhibitor actually reduced the titre of virus in the lung, rather than exerting some effect on the immunopathology of influenza infection in lung cells, indirectly resulting in animal survival. A useful technique, particularly applicable to mouse-adapted strains of virus, is to remove infected mouse lungs 48 to 72 hr post-infection, grind up the lung in a pestle and mortar with sand, centrifuge at 1500 g (10 min), and titrate the supernatant fluid for virus haemagglutinin (HA) using 0.5 per cent chicken red blood cells. This method can be quantitative and avoids the delay and expense of titrating lung extracts for infective virus.

FOOD AND WATER INTAKE AND BODY WEIGHT

Two interesting developments seen in studies of amantadine in influenza virus-infected mice are the observations of changes in the food and water intake. Thus, virus infection causes a decrease in both water and food intake and a subsequent weight loss; however, the late administration of amantadine and derivatives to infected mice restored their weight gain and water uptake to almost normal levels. These extended models of *in vivo* infection will undoubtedly prove to be useful for the assessment of other antiviral compounds against influenza virus. In experiments in Swiss white mice infected intranasally with 30 LD_{50} of A/Japan/305/57 (H2N2) virus, the mice appeared ill about 36 hr post-infection; water and food consumption decreased, and weight reduction was easily quantitated. Infected and nontreated mice lost weight progressively until death. Infected mice treated with 24 mg/kg/day of rimantadine (α-methyl-1, -adamantane methylamine) had an initial decrease in weight followed by an increase in weight at a rate parallel to that of the controls. By the end of the experiment, however, they had not reached the same weight as the noninfected animals. Mice given rimantadine and not infected continued to gain weight, drink and eat the same as the controls (Fig. 33).

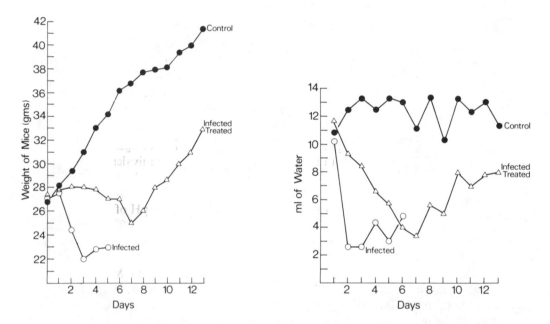

FIG. 33. Ameliorating effect of amantadine on influenza virus induced weight loss and decrease in water consumption in mice. Mice were infected intranasally with 30LD_{50} of A/Jap/57 (H2N2) virus and appeared ill 36 hr post infection when water and food consumption decreased. These were easily and accurately quantitated. Infected mice treated with rimantadine (24 mg/mg/day) responded by an increase in weight parallel to the control group. a—weight loss in influenza infected mice. b—decrease in water consumption in influenza infected mice (data from Rabinovich 1972; with permission of the publisher).

CHANGES IN LUNG WEIGHT

A refinement of the method of measuring the effect of virus infection on mice is to measure the lung weight increase in infected animals; these weight increases are a result of pneumonic changes that occur in the lungs of mice infected with lethal virus challenge levels.

NEW SEROLOGICAL METHODS WITH INFLUENZA VIRUS

It is of particular importance that detailed serological studies should accompany any clinical trials with antiviral agents and influenza virus. Particularly in non-epidemic years many other respiratory viruses can cause symptoms which resemble true influenza and can be thus mis-diagnosed. The trials organized by Galbraith *et al.* (1969a; 1969b) in the UK have indicated quite clearly that in some years only 50 per cent of cases diagnosed by experienced general practitioners as influenza fulfil serological and virus isolation criteria. Particularly in large-scale trials serological testing of acute and convalescent sera may be a considerable task. Methods utilizing the principle of single radial diffusion have been applied to studies with influenza viruses by Schild (reviewed by Schild, 1977). Thus, methods employing virus (SRD) or virus-red blood cells and complement (single radial haemolysis, SRH) immobilized in agarose gel have been developed. As many as 56 sera can be tested on a single SRD plate measuring approximately 2.4 × 7.3 cm. Sera do not have to be treated with receptor-destroying enzyme, as in the haemagglutination-inhibition test, which effects a considerable monetary saving. In addition the method is rapid, accurate (with a coefficient of variation of 2–3 per cent compared to 200–300 per cent for the HI test) and can be carried out with small volumes (10–20 μl) of sera which need not be diluted.

PREPARATION OF SINGLE-RADIAL-HAEMOLYSIS IMMUNOPLATES

Ten per cent (v/v) suspensions of freshly washed sheep erythrocytes were made up in phosphate buffered saline. Influenza virus was added to the erythrocytes in the form of purified virus or crude allantoic fluid at a 'standard' concentration of 10,000 haem-agglutinating units (HAU) of virus per 1.0 ml of 10 per cent erythrocyte suspension. The suspensions were held at 4°C for 10 min to allow the virus to adsorb to the erythrocytes. A half volume of freshly prepared diluted $CrCl_3$ solution (diluted 1:400 in saline from a 2.25 M stock solution) is added and the mixture left for 10 min at 4°C. Cells were then washed to remove unadsorbed virus by two cycles of sedimentation by low-speed centrifugation and resuspended in saline containing 0.2 per cent w/v bovine serum albumin. Immunoplates were prepared by incorporating 0.3 ml of virus-treated erythrocytes together with 0.1 ml complement (undiluted guinea-pig serum) in 2.6 ml volumes of melted agarose held at 45°C in a water bath. The final concentration complement in the gel was equivalent to 2.5 minimal haemolytic doses in a standard assay system with sheep erythrocytes. The agarose employed was A-37 agarose (Indubiose) from l'Industrie Biologique Francais S.A., Genevilliers, France, made up to contain 1.5 per cent agarose in PBSA at a final pH of 7.0; 0.1 per cent sodium azide was added as preservative. The agarose was melted at 100°C and cooled to 42°C before use. The 3.0-ml volumes of erythrocyte suspension in agarose were shaken vigorously to distribute the erythrocytes evenly and poured into empty plastic immunoplates (microscope slide-sized chambers from Hyland Laboratories, Costa Mesa, California, USA). Wells of 2 mm diameter were cut in the gel after standing the plates for 30 min to allow the agarose to set. Prepared immunoplates may be stored at 4°C for several weeks before use.

Before testing, sera were heated at 60°C for 20 min before addition to the SRH immunoplates and the plates transferred to a moist environment and incubated at 37°C for 16 hr before reading (Fig. 34). The diameters of the zones of complete or partial haemolysis developing around the wells were measured using a micrometer eyepiece scale calibrated in 0.1 ml divisions (Matchless Machines Ltd., Horsham, Sussex).

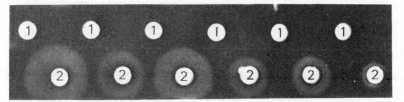

FIG. 34. SRH plate used for serological investigations in clinical trials with amantadine. Acute (1) and convalescent (2) human sera are tested in pairs. Approximately 10 μl of antiserum is placed in the well and the plates incubated overnight at 37°C. Area of haemolysis zone is directly proportional to number of antivirus HA antibodies (see Appendix). The latter antibodies cause lysis of the virus-coated RBC in the presence of the excess complement present in the agarose.

REFERENCES

AKSENOV, V. A., SELIDOVKIN, D. A., AKSENOR, L. A., FEDOROVE, G. I., HADEZHDIN, A. S., GALEGOV, G. A., FADEYERA, L. L. and SLEPUSHKIN, A. M. (1971) Comparative evaluation of the efficacy of amantadine, An interferon stimulant, and a combination of both in the prevention of influenza. *Vopr. Virusol.* **16**: 189–94.

ALLEN, H., McCAULEY, J., WATERFIELD, M. and GETHING, M. J. (1980) Influenza virus RNA segment 7 has the coding capacity for two polypeptides. *Virology* **107**: 548–551.

ANDREWES, C. H., LAIDLAW, P. P. and SMITH, W. (1934) The susceptibility of mice to the viruses of human and swine influenza. *Lancet* **ii**: 859.

AOKI, F. Y., SITAR, D. S. and OGILVIE, M. D. (1979) Amantadine kinetics in healthy young subjects after long term dosing. *Clin. Pharmacol. Ther.* **26**: 729–736.

APPLEYARD, G. and MABER, H. B. (1976) A plaque assay for the study of influenza virus inhibitors. In: *Chemotherapy of Influenza Virus.* OXFORD, J. S. and WILLIAMS, D. (eds.), London. Academic Press.

BAKER, L. M., PAULSHOCK, M. and IEZZONI, D. G. (1969) The therapeutic efficacy of symmetral (amantadine hydrochloride) in naturally occurring influenza A2 Respiratory illness. *J. Am. Osteopath. Ass.* **68**: 1244–1250.

BARRY, R. D. (1964) The effects of actinomycin D and UV irradiation on the production of FPV. *Virology* **24**: 563–569.

BAUER, D. J. (1973) Antiviral chemotherapy: The first decade. *Br. Med. J.* **iii** 275–279.

BECKER, Y. (1980) Antiviral agents from natural sources. *Pharmac. Ther.* **10**: 119–159.

BELYAVIN, G. (1976) Experience in the control of influenza by vaccination: a brief review. Chemotherapy of influenza virus. OXFORD, J. S. and WILLIAMS, D. (eds.). Academic Press.

BLEIDNER, W. E., HARMON, J. B., HEWES, W. E., LYNES, T. E. and HERMANN, E. C. (1965) Absorption, distribution and excretion of amantadine hydrochloride. *J. Pharmacol. Exper. Ther.* **150**: 484–490.

BLOOMFIELD, S. S., GAFFNEY, T. E. and SCHIFF, G. M. (1970) A design for the evaluation of anti-viral drugs in human influenza. *Am. J. Epidem.* **91**: 568–574.

BLYUGER, A. F., KRUPNIKOVA, E. Z., GINSKAYA, YE. V., DZEGUZE, D. R., INDULIN, M. K., MASTRYUKOVA, V. A., RINGA, I. K., KHVATOV, P. P. and YAVAYST, E. YU. (1970) Use of midantane for the prevention of influenza. *Zh. Mikrobiol.* (Mosk.) **47**: 134.

BRAND, C. M. and PALESE, P. (1980) Sequential passage of influenza virus in embryonated eggs or tissue culture: emergence of mutants. *Virology* **107**: 424–433.

BRAND, C. M., SKEHEL, J. J. (1972) Crystalline antigen from the influenza virus envelope. *Nature (New Biology)* **238**: 145–147.

BREDT, A. B. and MARDINEY, M. R. (1969a) Suppression of sensitized lymphocyte reactivity to specific antigens. *Immunol. Fed. Proc.* **28**: 693.

BREDT, A. B. and MARDINEY, M. R. (1979b) Effects of amantadine on the reactivity of human lymphocytes stimulated by allogenic lymphocytes and phytohaemagglutinin. *Transplantation* **8**: 763–773.

BRIEDIS, D. J., LAMB, R. A. and CHOPPIN, P. W. (1981) Influenza B RNA Segment 8 codes for two non structural proteins. *Virology* **112**: 417–425.

BUKRINSKAYA, A. G., VORKUNOVA, N. K. and NARMANBETOVA, R. A. (1980) Rimantadine hydrochloride blocks the second step of influenza virus uncoating. *Archives of Virology* **66**: 275–282.

CHANIN, A. (1977) Influenza: vaccines or amantadine? *J. Am. Med. Ass.* **237**: 1445.

CHANOCK, R. M. (1982) New opportunities for development of safe effective live virus vaccines. *Yale J. Biol. Med.* **55**: 361–367.

COCHRAN, K. W., MAASSAB, H. F., TSUNODA, A. and BERLIN, B. S. (1965) Studies on the antiviral activity of amantadine hydrochloride. *Ann. N.Y. Acad. Sci.* **130**: 432.

COHEN, A., TOGO, Y., KHAKOO, R., WALDMAN, R. and SIGEL, M. (1976) Comparative clinical and laboratory evaluation of the prophylactic capacity of Ribavirin, amantadine HCl and placebo in induced human influenza type A. *J. Infect. Dis.* **133**: 114 120.

COLMAN, P. M., VARGHESE, J. N. and LAVER, W. G. (1983) Structure of the catalytic and antigenic sites in influenza virus neuraminidase *Nature* **303**: 41–44.

COOPER, P. D. (1977) In: *Chemoprophylaxis and Virus Infections of the Respiratory Tract.* Volume II. CRC Press, Cleveland.

COULSON, A. S. (1975) Amantadine and teratogenesis. *Lancet* **ii**: 1044.

COUNCIL ON DRUGS (1967) Evaluation of a new antiviral agent—amantadine hydrochloride (Symmetrel). *J. Am. Med. Ass.* **201**: 374–375.

DAVIES, W. L., GRUNERT, R. R., HAFF, R. F., McGAHEN, J. W., NEUMAYER, E. M., PAULSHOCK, M., WATTS, J. C., WOOD, T. R., HERMANN, E. C. and HOFFMAN, C. E. (1964) *Science* **144**: 862–863.

DENT, P. P., OLSON, G. B. and RAWLS, W. F. (1968) The effect of amantadine-HCl on the graft-versus-host response of chicken peripheral leukocytes. *Fed. Proc.* **27**: 474.

DOLIN, R., REICHMAN, R. C., MADORE, H. P., MAYNARD, R., LINTON, P. M. and WEBBER-JONES, J. (1982) A controlled trial of amantadine a rimantadine in the Prophylaxis of influenza A infection. *The New England . Journal of Medicine* **307**: 580–584.

DOUGLAS, R-G. (1980) Amantadine: should it be used as an antiviral? In *Controversies in Therapeutics*, p. 271. LASAGNE, L. (ed.), W. B. Saunders Co.

DOURMASHKIN, R. and TYRRELL, D. A. J. (1974) Electron microscopic observations on the entry of influenza virus into susceptible cells. *J. gen. Virol.* **24**: 129–141.

EASTERDAY, B. C. (1975) Animal influenza. In *The Influenza Viruses and Influenza.* KILBOURNE, E. D. (ed.), Academic Press, New York.

EATON, M. D., LOW, I. E., SCALA, A. R. and URETSKY, S. (1962) Inhibition by ammonium ion of the growth of influenza virus in chorio allantoic tissue. *Virology* **18**: 102–108.

ELLIOTT, J. (1979) Consensus on amantadine use in influenza A. *JAMA* **242**: 2383–2384.

FAZEKAS DE ST. GROTH, S. and WHITE, D. O. (1958) An improved assay for the infectivity of influenza viruses. *J. Hyg.* **56**: 151.

FINKLEA, J. F., HENNESSY, A. V. and DAVENPORT, F. M. (1967) A field trial of amantadine chemoprophylaxis in acute respiratory disease. *Am. J. Epidem.* **85**: 403–12.

FISHAUT, M. and MOSTOW, S. R. (1980) Amantadine for severe influenza A pneumonia in infancy. *Am. J. Dis. Children.* **134**: 321–322.

GALASSO, G. J., MERIGAN, T. C. and BUCHANAN, R. A. (eds.). (1979) *Antiviral Agents and Viral Disease of Man.* Raven Press, New York.

GALASSO, G. J., OXFORD, J. S., DOLIN, R., DOUGLAS, R. G., KRYLOV, V. F. and BEKTIMIROV, T. (1984) Clinical use of amantadine and rimantadine in influenza. *Bull. WHO* (in press).

GALBRAITH, A. W. (1975) Therapeutic trials of amantadine (Symmetrel) in general practice. *J. Antimicrob. Chem.* **1**: 81.

GALBRAITH, A. W., OXFORD, J. S., SCHILD, G. C., POTTER, C. W. and WATSON, G. I. (1971) Therapeutic effect of 1-adamantanamine hydrochloride in naturally occurring influenza A2/Hong Kong infection. *Lancet* **ii**: 113–115.

GALBRAITH, A. W., OXFORD, J. S., SCHILD, G. C. and WATSON, G. I. (1969a) Protective effect of 1-adamantanamine hydrochloride on influenza A2 infections in the family environment. *Lancet* 1026–1028.

GALBRAITH, A. W., OXFORD, J. S., SCHILD, G. C. and WATSON, G. I. (1969b) Study of 1-adamantanamine hydrochloride used prophylactically during the Hong Kong influenza epidemic in the family environment *Bull. Wld. Hlth. Org.* **41**: 677–682.

GALBRAITH, A. W., OXFORD, J. S., SCHILD, G. C. and WATSON, G. I. (1970) Protective effect of amino-adamantane on influenza A2 infections in the family environment. *Ann. N.Y. Acad. Sci.* **173**: 29–43.

GETHING, M. J. and SAMBROOK, J. (1982) Construction of influenza haemagglutinin genes that code for intracellular and secreted forms of the protein. *Nature* **300**: 598–603.

GREEN, N., ALEXANDER, H., OLSON, A., ALEXANDER, S., SHINNICK, T. M., SUTCLIFFE, J. G., LERNER, R. A. (1982) Immunogenic structure of the influenza virus haemagglutinin. *Cell,* **28**: 477–487.

GROSSGEBAUER, K. and LANGMAACK, H. (1970) Failure of 1-adamantanamine (Symmetrel) to modify influenza virus-induced pyrogenicity. *Archiv fur die gesamte Virusforschung* **31**: 385–486.

GRUNERT, R. R. and HOFFMANN, C. E. (1977) Sensitivity of influenza A/New Jersey/8/76 (Hsw1N1) virus to Amantadine HCl. *J. Infect. Dis.* **136**: 297–300.

GRUNERT, R. R., McGAHAN, J. W. and DAVIES. W. L. (1965) The *in vivo* antiviral activity of 1-adamantanamine (amantadine). 1. Prophylactic and therapeutic activity against influenza viruses. *Virology* **26**: 262–269.

HAY, A. SKEHEL, J. J. (1978) In: *Negative Strand Viruses and the Host Cell.* BARRY, R. D. and MAHY, B. W. J. (eds.). Academic Press, London.

HAYDEN, F. G., GWALTNEY, J. M., Jr., VAN DE CASTLE, R. L., ADAMS, K. F., and GIORDANI, B. (1981) Comparative toxicity of amantadine hydrochloride and rimantadine hydrochloride in healthy adults. *Antimicrob. Agents Chemother.* **19**: 226–233.

HAYDEN, F. G., HALL, W. J., DOUGLAS, R. G., Jr. (1980) Therapeutic effects of aerosolized amantadine in naturally acquired infection due to influenza A virus. *J. Inf. Dis.* **141**: 535–542.

HAYDEN, F. G., HOFFMAN, H. E. and SPYKER, D. A. (1983) Differences in side effects of amantadine hydrochloride and rimantadine hydrochloride relate to differences in pharmacokinetics. *Antimicrobial Agents and Chemotherapy,* **23**: 458–464.

HAYDEN, F. G., HALL, W. J., DOUGLAS, R. G. JR. and SPEERS, D. M. (1979) Amantadine aerosols in normal volunteers: pharmacology and safety testing. *Antimicrob. Ag. Chem.* **16**: 644–650.

HEIDER, H., ADAMCZCK, B., PRESBER, H. W., SCHROEDER, C., FELDBLUM, R. and INDULEN, M. K. (1981) Occurrence of amantadine and rimantadine resistant influenza A virus strains during the 1980 epidemic. *Acta Virologica* **25**: 395–400.

HELENIUS, A., KARTENBECK, J., SIMONS, K. and FRIES, E. (1980) On the entry of Semliki Forest Virus into BHK-21 cells. *J. Cell. Biol.* **84**: 404–420.

HILLYARD, I. W. (1980) The preclinical toxicology and safety of ribavirin. In: SMITH, R. A., KIKPATRIC, W., (eds.) *Ribavirin: a broad spectrum antiviral agent.* New York, Academic Press, pp. 59–71.

HINSHAW, V. S., BEAN, W. J., WEBSTER, R. G. and EASTERDAY, B. C. (1978) The prevalence of influenza viruses in swine and the antigenic and genetic relatedness of influenza viruses from man and swine. *Virology* **84**: 51–62.

HOFFMANN, C. E. (1980) Amantadine HCI and related compounds, pp. 199–211. In: W. A. CARTER, (ed.) *Selective Inhibitors of Viral Functions.* CRC Press, Cleveland Ohio.

HOFFMANN, C. E., NEUMAYER, E. M., HAFF, R. F. and COLDSBY, R. A. (1965) Mode of action of the antiviral activity of amantadine in tissue culture. *J. Bact.* **90**: 623–8.

HOLT, P. and THADANI, C. (1973) Water-soluble polymers containing adamantylamino and other amino residues. *Die Makromolekulare Chemie* **169**: 55–58.

HOPE-SIMPSON, R. E. (1979) Epidemic mechanisms of Type A influenza. *J. Hyg.* **83**: 11–26.

HORNICK, R. B., TOGO, Y., MAHLER, S. and IEZZONI, D. (1969) Evaluation of amantadine hydrochloride in the treatment of A2 influenzal disease. *Bull. WHO* **41**: 641–646.

HORNICK, R. B., TOGO, Y., MAHLER, S. and IEZZONI, D. G. (1970) Evaluation of amantadine hydrochloride in the treatment of A2 influenzal disease. *Ann. N.Y. Acad. Sci.* **173** (1): 10–19.

HOYLE, L. (1968) In: *The Influenza Virus. Virology Monograph,* Karger, Basle.

HUGENTOBLER, A. L., SCHILD, G. C. and OXFORD, J. S. (1981) Differences in the electrophoretic migration rates of polypeptides and RNAs of recent isolates of influenza B viruses. *Archiv. Virol.* **69**: 197–207.

IEZZONI, D. (1970) Evaluation of amantadine hydrochloride in the treatment of A2 influenza disease. *Ann. N.Y. Acad. Sci.* **173**: 10–19.

INDULEN, M. K. and KALNINYA, V. A. (1973) Study on the mechanism of inhibiting action of aminoadamantane on the reproduction of fowl plaque virus. *Acta Virol.* **17**: 273–280.

INDULEN, M. K. and KALNINYA, V. A. (1980) Studies on the antiviral effect and the mode of action of the anti-influenza compound rimantadine. In: *Recent Developments in Antiviral Chemotherapy.* COLLIER, L. and OXFORD, J. S. (eds.). Academic Press, London.

JACKSON, G. G. (1977) Sensitivity of influenza A virus to amantadine. *J. Infect. Dis.* **136**: 301–302.

JACKSON, G. G., MULDOON, R. L. and AKERS, L. W. (1963) Serological evidence for prevention of influenzal infection in volunteers by an anti-influenzal drug adamantanamine hydrochloride. *Antimicrob. Agents. Chemother.* 703–707.

JAIN, M. K., YEN-MIN WU, N., MORGAN, T. K., BIGGS, M. S. and MURRAY, R. K. (1976) Phase transition in a lipid bilayer II. Influence of adamantane derivatives. *Chem. Phys. Lipids* 17: 71–78, North Holland.

JOHNSON, R. G., CARTY, S. E. and SCARPA, A. (1981) Accumulation of amantadine by isolated chromaffin granules. *Biochem. Pharmacol.* 30: 763–769.

KANELE, I., INDULEN, M., RYAZANTSEVA, G., DZEGUSE, D. and POLLS, J. (1972) Antiviral activity of 2-amino adamantane. *Izv. Akad. Nouk. Latv. SSR* 304: 42–47.

KATO, N. and EGGERS, H. J. (1969) Inhibition of uncoating of fowl plague virus by 1-adamantamine hydrochloride. *Virology* 37: 632–641.

KAWAKAMI, K. and ISHIHAMA, A. (1983) RNA polymerase of influenza virus. III isolation of RNA polymerase – RNA complexes from influenza virus PR8. *J. Biochem.* 93: 989–996.

KEENLYSIDE, R. A., SCHONBERGER, L. B., BREGMAN, D. J. and BOLYAI, J. Z. S. (1980) Fatal Guillain–Barré syndrome after the national influenza immunization program. *Neurology* 30: 929–933.

KENDAL, A. P., JOSEPH, J. M., KOBAYASHI, G., NELSON, D., REYES, C. R., ROSS, M. R., SARANDRIA, J. L., WHITE, R., WOODALL, D. F., NOBLE, G. R. and DOWDLE, W. R. (1979) Laboratory-based surveillance of influenza virus in the United States during the winter of 1977–78. I. Periods of prevalence of H1N1 and H3N2 influenza strains, their relative rates of isolation in different age groups and detection of antigenic variants. *Am. J. Epidemiology* 110: 449–461.

KILLEN, D. A., HATTORI, H and ZUKOSKI, C. F. (1969) Failure of amantadine hydrochloride to suppress canine renal homograft rejection. *Surgery*, 66: 550–554.

KITAMOTO, O. (1968) Therapeutic effectiveness of amantadine hydrochloride in influenza A2. Double blind studies. *Jap. J. Tuberc. Chest Dis.* 15: 17–26.

KITAMOTO, O. (1971) Therapeutic effectiveness of amantadine hydrochloride in naturally occurring Hong Kong influenza—double blind studies. *Jap. J. Tuberc. Chest. Dis.* 17: 1–7.

KITAMOTO, O. (1972) Therapeutic effectiveness of amantadine hydrochloride in naturally occurring Hong Kong influenza. *Jap. J. Tuberc. Chest. Dis.* 17: 1–7.

KNIGHT, V., MCCLUNG, H. W., WILSON, S. Z. *et al.* (1981) Ribavirin small-particle aerosol treatment of influenza. Lancet 2: 945–949.

KNIGHT, V., MCCLUNG, H. W., WILSON, S. Z., WATERS, B. K., QUARLES, J. M., CAMERON, R. W., GREGGS, S. E., ZERWAS, J. M. and COUCH, R. B. (1981) Ribavirin small particle aerosol treatment of influenza. *Lancet* i: 945–949.

KNIGHT, V., BLOOM, K., WILSON, Z. and WILSON, R. K. (1979) Amantadine aerosol in humans. *Antimicrob. Ag. Chem.* 16: 572–578.

KNIGHT, V., FEDSON, D., BALDINI, J., DOUGLAS, R. G. and COUCH, R. B. (1969) Amantadine therapy of epidemic influenza A2 Hong Kong. *Antimicrob. Agents Chemother.* 9: 370–371.

KRUG, R. M., PLOTCH, S. J., ULMANEN, I., HERZ, C. and BOULOY, M. (1981) The mechanism of initiation of influenza viral RNA transcription by capped RNA primers, In: *The Replication of Negative Strand Viruses*, BISHOP, DAVID, H. L., COMPANS, W. and RICHARD. (eds.). Elsevier. North Holland.

KYO, I., OKAMOTO, E. and KAITO, H. (1970) Effects of amantadine hydrochloride administered during pregnancy upon development of the foetus of rat and post natal growth. *Gendai no Rinsho* 4: 44–50.

LAEMMLI, U. K. (1970) Cleavage of structural proteins during the assembly of the head of bacteriophage T4. *Nature* 227: 680.

LAMAR, J. K., CALHOUN, F. J. and DARR, A. G. (1970) Effects of amantadine hydrochloride on cleavage and embryonic development in the rat and rabbit. Abstracts 9th meeting of *Society of Toxicology*.

LAMB, R. A. and CHOPPIN, P. W. (1976) Synthesis of influenza virus proteins in infected cells: translation of viral polypeptides including three P polypeptides, from RNA produced by primary transcription. *Virology* 74: 504–519.

LAMB, R. A., CHOPPIN, P. W., CHANOCK, R. M. and LAI, C. J. (1980) Mapping of the two overlapping genes for polypeptides NS1 and NS2 on RNA segment 8 of influenza virus genome. *Proc. Natn. Acad. Sci. USA* 77: 1857–1861.

LANG, G., NARAYAN, O. and ROUSE, B. T. (1970) Prevention of malignant avian influenza by 1-adamantanamine hydrochloride. *Archiv fur die gesamte virusforschung* 32: 171–184.

LAVROV, S. V., EREMKINA, E. I., ORLOVA, T. G., GALEGOV, G. A., SOLOVEV, V. D. and ZHDANOV, V. M. (1968) Combined inhibition of influenza virus reproduction in cell culture using interferon and amantadine. *Nature* 217: 856–857.

LAVROV, S. V., EREMKINA, E. I., ORLOVA, T. G., GALEGOV, G. A., SOLOVEV, V. D. and ZHDANOV, V. M. (1969) Synergism of interferon and amantadine in the inhibition of influenza virus reproduction in cell culture. *Vop. Virus.* 14: 427–431.

LENNETTE, E. H. (1981) Viral respiratory diseases: vaccines and antivirals. *Bull. WHO* 59: 305–324.

LIKAR, MIHA. (1970) Effectiveness of amantadine in protecting vaccinated volunteers from an attenuated strain of influenza A_2/Hong Kong virus. *Ann. N.Y. Acad. Sci.* 173: 108–112.

LUBECK, M. D., SCHULMAN, J. L. and PALESE, P. (1978) Susceptibility of influenza A viruses to amantadine is influenced by the gene coding for M protein. *J. Virol.* 28: 710–716.

LUNDAHL, K., SCHUT, J., SCHLATMANN, L. M. A., PAERELS, G. B. and PETERS, A. (1972) Synthesis and antiviral activities of adamantane Spiro compounds. 1. Adamantane and analogous spiro-3'-pyrrolidine. *J. Med. Chem.* 15: 129.

MCCAULEY, J. W. and MAHY, B. W. J. (1983) Structure and function of the influenza virus genome. *Biochem. J.* 211: 281–294.

MCCLUNG, H. W., KNIGHT, V., GILBERT, B. E., WILSON, S. Z., QUARLES, J. M., DIVINE (1983). Ribavirin aerosol treatment of influenza B virus infection. *JAMA* 249: 2671–2674.

McGAHEN, J. W. and HOFFMANN, C. E. (1968) Influenza infections of Mice. I. Curative activity of amantadine HCl. *Proc. Soc. exp. Biol. Med.* **129**: 678–681.

McGAHEN, J. W., NEUMAYER, E. M., GRUNERT, R. R. and HOFFMANN, C. E. (1970) Influenza infections of mice. II. Curative activity of α-methyl-l-adamantanemethylamine HCl (Rimantadine HCl), *Ann. N. Y. Sci.* **173**: 557–567.

McGEOCH, D., FELLNER, P. and NEWTON, C. (1976) The influenza virus genome consists of eight distinct RNA species. *Proc. Natn. Acad. Sci. USA* **73**: 3045.

MACIAG, W. J. and HOFFMANN, C. E. (1968) Production of antibody in amantadine hydrochloride-treated mice. *Virology* **35**: 622–624.

MAHY, B. W. J. and BARRY, R. D. (eds.) (1978) *Negative Strand Viruses and the Host Cell.* Academic Press, London.

MAIKOVSKIY, V. S., KANZANTSEV, A. P., STARSHOV, P. D., ZLYDNIKOV, D. M., ANTONOV, V. S., LEVITOV, T. A., ZHUK, L. N., STELMAKA, V. I. and RUMOVSKY, V. I. (1970) Preventive and therapeutic action of amantadine in acute respiratory diseases. *Vo.-med. Th. No.* 1, 17–20.

MARCHESI, V. T., TILLOCK, T. W., JACKSON, R. L., SEGREST, J. P. and SCOTT, R. E. (1972) *Proc. Natn. Acad. Sci. USA* **69**: 1445–1449.

MATE, J., SIMON, M. and JUVANEZ, I. (1971) Use of Viregyl (Amantadine HCl) in the treatment of epidemic influenza. *Ther. Hung.* **19**: 117–121.

MATE, J., SIMON, M., JUVANEZ, I., TAKATSY, G., HOLLOS, I. and FARKAS, E. (1970) Prophylactic use of amantadine during Hong Kong influenza epidemic. *Acta. Microbiol. Acad. Sci. Hung.* **17**: 285–296.

MAUGH, T. H. (1980) Editorial Panel urges wide use of antiviral drug. *Science* **206**: 1058–1060.

MILLET, VICTORIA, M., DREISBACH MELANIE and BRYSON YVONNE, J. (1982) Double-blind controlled study of central nervous system side effects of amantadine, rimantadine and chlorpheniramine. *Antimicrobial Agents and Chemotherapy* **21**: 1–4.

MONTO, A. S., GUNN, R. A., BANDYK, M. G. and KING, C. L. (1979) Prevention of Russian influenza by amantadine. *J. Am. Med. Ass.* **241**: 1003–1007.

MULDER, J. and HERS, J. F. (1972) *Influenza.* Wolters-Noordhorff Publishing, Gruningen.

MULDOON, R. L., STANLEY, E. D. and JACKSON, G. G. (1976) Use and withdrawal of amantadine chemoprophylaxis during epidemic influenza A. *Am. Rev. Resp. Dis.* **113**: 487.

NAFTA, I., TURCANU, A. G., BRAUN, I., COMPANETZ, W., SIMIONESCU, A., BIRI, E. and FLOREA, V. (1970) Administration of amantadine for the prevention of Hong Kong influenza. *Bull. WHO.* **42**: 423–427.

NAGATA, S., TAIRA, H., HALL, A., JOHNSRUD, L., STREVIL, M., ECSODI, J., BOLL, W., CANTELL, K. and WEISSMAN, C. (1980) Synthesis in *E. coli* of a polypeptide with human leukocyte interferon activity. *Nature* **284**: 316–320.

NEUMAYER, E. M., HAFF, R. F. and HOFFMANN, C. E. (1965) Antiviral activity of amantadine hydrochloride in tissue culture and *in ovo. Proc. Soc. Exp. Biol. Med.* **119**: 393–396.

NICKON, A., PANDIT, G. D. and WILLIAMS, R. O. (1967) Synthesis of noradamantane functionalized at C-2. *Tetrahed. Lett.* No. 30 2851–2854.

NORA, J. J., NORA, A. H. and WAY, G. L. (1975) Cardiovascular maldevelopment associated with maternal exposure to amantadine. *Lancet* **ii**: 607.

OBROSOVA-SEROVA, N. P., SLEPUSHKIN, A. N., KUPRYASHINA, L. M., VOLKOV, V. E., PUGAEVA, V. P., RYKHLETSKAYA, N. S., CHERNETSOV, V., SHTUNDERENKO, G. V. and GOLDENBURG, B. I. (1979) Investigation of the protective effect of rimantadine during an influenza A (H1N1) outbreak in December 1977. *Vop Virosol.* **4**: 353–357.

O'DONOGHUE, J. M., RAY, C. G., TERRY, D. W. and BEATY, H. N. (1973) Prevention of nosocomial influenza infection with amantadine A. *J. Epidemiol.* **97**: 276–282.

OHKUMA, S. and POOLE, B. (1978) Fluorescence probe measurement of the intralysosomal pH in living cells and the perturbation of pH by various agents. *Proc. Natn. Acad. Sci.* **75**: 3327–3331.

OKER-BLOM, N., HOVI, T., LEINIKKI, P., PALOSUO, T., PETTERSSON, R. and SUNI, J. (1970) Protection of man from natural infection with influenza A2 Hong Kong virus by amantadine: A controlled field trial. *Br. Med. J.* **3**: 676–678.

OXFORD, J. S. (1975a) Inhibition of the replication of influenza A and B viruses by a nucleoside analogue (Ribavirin). *J. gen. Virol.* **28**: 409–414.

OXFORD, J. S. (1977) In: *Chemoprophylaxis and Virus Infections of the Respiratory Tract*, Volume I. CRC Press, Cleveland.

OXFORD, J. S. (1981) Chemotherapy of influenza and herpes virus infections. *J. Roy. Coll. Phys. (Lond.)* **15**: 218–226.

OXFORD, J. S. and OBERG, B. (1984) *Prevention of Human Viral Disease: Antivirals and Vaccines.* Elsevier, North Holland (in press).

OXFORD, J. S. and PERRIN, D. D. (1977) Influenza RNA transcriptase inhibitors: Studies *in vitro* and *in vivo. Ann. N.Y. Acad. Sci.* **284**: 613–623.

OXFORD, J. S. and SCHILD, G. C. (1967) Inhibition of the growth of influenza and rubella viruses by amines and ammonium salts. *Br. J. Exp. Pathol.* **48**: 235–243.

OXFORD, J. S. and SCHILD, G. C. (1968) Immunofluorescent studies on the inhibition of influenza A and B antigens in mammalian cell cultures by amines. *J. gen. Virol.* **2**: 377–84.

OXFORD, J. S. and SCHILD, G. C. (1977) Inhibition of swine influenza virus A/New Jersey/76 (Hsw1N1) multiplication and polypeptide synthesis by amantadine. *FEMS Microbiol. Lett.* **1**: 223–226.

OXFORD, J. S., LOGAN, I. S. and POTTER, C. W. (1970) *In vivo* selection of an influenza A2 strain resistant to amantadine. *Nature* **226**: 82–83.

OXFORD, J. S., CORCORAN, T and SCHILD, G. C. (1981) Intratypic electrophoretic variation of structural and non-structural polypeptides of human influenza A viruses. *J. gen. Virol.*

OXFORD, J. S., CORCORAN, T. and SCHILD, G. C. (1980b) Naturally occurring *ts* influenza A viruses of the H1N1 and H3N2 antigenic subtypes. *J. Gen. Virology* **48**: 383–389.

PALESE, P. and SCHULMAN, J. L. (1976) Differences in RNA patterns of influenza A viruses. *J. Virol.* **17**: 876–884.

PATTERSON, S. and OXFORD, J. S. (1980) Pulse labelling and electron microscope studies of the inhibition of influenza A viruses by amantadine. In *Recent Development in Antiviral Chemotherapy*, COLLIER, L. and OXFORD, J. S. (Eds.). Academic Press, London.

PATTERSON, S., OXFORD, J. S. and DOURMASHKIN, R. R. (1979) Studies on the mechanism of influenza virus entry into cells. *J. gen. Virol.* **43**: 223–229.

PECKINPAUGH, R. O., ASKIN, F. B., PIERCE, W. E., EDWARDS, E. A., JOHNSON, D. P. and JACKSON, G. G. (1970) Field studies with amantadine: Acceptability and protection. *Ann. N.Y. Acad. Sci.* 173.

PERKINS, F. T. and REGAMEY, R. (1977) Editors International Symposium on Influenza Immunization. Developments in Biological Standard. **39**:

PERRIN, D. D. (1977) In: *Chemoprophylaxis and Virus Infections of the Respiratory Tract*, Volume II. OXFORD, J. S. (Ed). CRC Press, Cleveland.

PERRIN, D. D. and STUNZI, H. (1980) Viral chemotherapy: antiviral actions of metal ions and metal chelating agents. *Pharmac. Ther.* **12**: 255–297.

PORTER, A. G., BARBER, C., CAREY, N. H., HALLEWELL, R. A., HALLEWELL, R. A., THRELFALL, G. and EMTAGE, J. S. (1979) Complete nucleotide sequence of an influenza virus haemagglutinin gene from cloned DNA. *Nature* **282**: 471–477.

POTTER, C. W. and OXFORD, J. S. (1977) Animal models of influenza virus infection as applied to the investigation of antiviral compounds. In: *Chemoprophylaxis and Virus Infections of the Respiratory Tract*, Volume II. OXFORD, J. S. (ed.). CRC Press, Cleveland.

QUARLES, J. M., COUCH, R. B., CATE, T. R. and GOSWICK, C. B. (1981) Comparison of amantadine and rimantadine for prevention of type A (Russian) influenza. *Antiviral Res.* **1**: 149–155.

QUILLIGAN, J. J., HIRAYAMA, M. and BAERNSTEIN, H. D. (1966). The suppression of A2 influenza in children by the chemoprophylactic use of amantadine. *J. Paediat.* **69**: 572–5.

RABINOVICH, S. (1972) Rimantadine therapy of influenza A infection in mice. *Antimicrob. Ag. Chemother.* 408–411.

RICHARDSON, C. D., SCHEID, A. and CHOPPIN, P. W. (1980) Specific inhibition of Paramyxovirus and Myxovirus replication by oligopeptides with amino acid sequences similar to those at the *N*-termini of the F1 or HA2 viral polypeptides. *Virology* **105**: 205–222.

ROTT, R. (1979) Molecular basis of infectivity and pathogenicity of Myxovirus: a brief review. *Archiv. Virol.* **59**: 285–298.

SABIN, A. B. (1967) Amantadine hydrochloride: Analysis of data related to its proposed use for prevention of A2 influenza virus disease in human beings. *J. Am. Med. Ass.* **200**: 135.

SABIN, A. B. (1978) Amantadine and influenza: evaluation of conflicting reports. *J. Infect. Dis.* **1381**: 557–568.

SCHILD, G. C. (1979) Editor *Influenza. Br. Med. Bull.* **35**: 1–96.

SCHILD, G. C. (1977) Appendix. Influenza in man and animals: epidemiology, surveillance and immunoprophylaxis. In: *Chemoprophylaxis and Virus Infections of the Respiratory Tract*. OXFORD, J. S. (ed.). CRC Press, Cleveland, USA.

SCHILD, G. C. and SUTTON, R. N. P. (1965) Inhibition of influenza viruses *in vitro* and *in vivo* by L-adamantanamine hydrochloride. *Br. J. exp. Path.* **46**: 263–273.

SCHILD, G. C., OXFORD, J. S., DOWDLE, W. R., COLEMAN, M., PEREIRA, M. S. and CHAKRAVERTY, P. (1974) Antigenic variation in current influenza A viruses: evidence for a high frequency of antigenic drift for Hong Kong virus. *Bulletin WHO* **51**: 1–11.

SCHMIDT-RUPPIN, K. H. and PONCIONI, B. (1979) Effects of individual inhalation of aerosolised amantadine hydrochloride in mice infected with influenza virus A/Bethesda/10/63 (H3N2) and A/Hong Kong/1/68 (H3N2). *Drug. Res.* **29**: 652–659.

SCHOLTISSEK, C. and FAULKNER, G. P. (1979) Amantadine resistant and sensitive influenza A strains and recombinants *J. gen. Virol.* **44**: 807–815.

SCHULMAN, J. L. (1968) Effect of amantadine-HCl and rimantadine-HCl on transmission of influenza virus infection in mice. *Proc. Soc. Exp. Biol. Med.* **128**: 1173–1178.

SELBY, P. Editor (1976) *Influenza: Virus, Vaccines and Strategy*. Academic Press, London.

SIDWELL, R. W., HUFFMAN, J. H., KHARE, G. P., ALLEN, L. B., WITKOWSKI, J. T. and ROBINS, R. K. (1972) Broad spectrum antiviral activity of virazole; 1-β-D-ribofuranosyl-1,2,4-triazole-3-carboxamide. *Science* **177**: 705–706.

SIMPSON, R. W. and HIRST, G. K. (1968) Temperature-sensitive mutants of influenza A virus: isolation of mutants and preliminary observations in genetic recombination and complementation. *Virology* **35**: 41–49.

SKEHEL, J. J. (1972) Polypeptide synthesis in influenza virus infected cells. *Virology* **49**: 23–36.

SKEHEL, J. J., HAY, A. J. and ARMSTRONG, J. A. (1978) On the mechanism of inhibition of influenza virus replication by amantadine hydrochloride. *J. gen. Virology.* **38**: 97–110.

SMITH, J. W. G., FLETCHER, W. B. and WHERRY, P. J. (1976) Future prospects for the control of influenza by immunoprophylaxis and choice of groups for routine vaccination. *Post. Med. J.* **52**: 399.

SMITH, R. A. and KIRKPATRICK, W. (1980) In: *Recent Developments in Antiviral Chemotherapy*. COLLIER, L. and OXFORD, J. S. (eds.). Academic Press, London.

SMORODINTSEV, A. A., KARPUCHIN, G. I., ZLYDNIKOV, D. M., MALYSHEVA, A. M., SHVETSOVA, E. G., BUROV, S. A., CHRAMTSOVA, L. M., ROMANOV, Y. A., TAROS, L. YU., IVANNIKOV, Y. G. and NOVOSELOV, S. D. (1970a). The prospect of amantadine for prevention of influenza A₂ in humans (Effectiveness of amantadine during influenza A₂/Hong Kong epidemics in January–February, 1969 in Leningrad). *Ann. N.Y. Acad. Sci.* **173**: 44–61.

SMORODINTSEV, A. A., KARPUHIN, G. I., ZLYDNIKOV, D. M., MALYSEVA, SVECOVA, E. G., A. M., BUROV, S. A., HRAMCOVA, L. M., ROMANOVJU, A., TAROS, L. JU, IVANNIKOVJU, G. and NOVOSELOV, S. D. (1970b) The prophylactic effectiveness of amantadine hydrochloride in an epidemic of Hong Kong influenza in Leningrad in 1969. *Bull. WHO* **42**: 865–872.

SRIRAM, G., BEAN, W. J., HINSHAW, V. S. and WEBSTER, R. G. (1980) Genetic diversity among avian influenza viruses. *Virology* **105**: 592–599.

STUART-HARRIS, C. H. (1984) *Fifty Years of Influenza Research*. Academic Press, London (in press).

STUART-HARRIS, C. H. (1981) The epidemiology and prevention of influenza. *Am. Scient.* **69**: 166–172.

STUART-HARRIS, C. H. (1977) In: *Chemoprophylaxis of Virus Infections of the Respiratory Tract*, Volume I. OXFORD, J. S. (ed.). CRC Press, Cleveland.

STUART-HARRIS, C. H. and OXFORD, J. S. (1983) *Problems of Antiviral Therapy*. Academic Press, London.

STUART-HARRIS, C. H. and SCHILD, G. C. (1976) In: *Influenza, the Viruses and the Disease*. Edward Arnold, London (1976).

SWALLOW, D. L. (1978) Antiviral agents. *Prog. Drug Res.* **22**: 267–326.

TILLETT, H. E., SMITH, J. W. G., and CLIFFORD, R. E. (1980) Excess morbidity and mortality associated with influenza in England and Wales. *Lancet* **i**: 793–795.

TIMBERLAKE, W. H. and VANCE, M. A. (1978) Four years treatment of patients with Parkinsonism using amantadine alone or with Levodopa. *Ann. Neurol.* **3**: 119–128.

TOGO, Y., HORNICK, R. B. and DAWKINS, A. T. (1968) Studies on induced influenza in Man. 1. Double blind studies designed to assess prophylactic efficacy of amantadine hydrochloride against A2/Rockville/1/65 strain. *J. Am. Med. Ass.* **203**, 1089.

TOGO, Y., HORNICK, R. B., FELITTI, V. J., KAUFMAN, M. L., DAWKINS, A. T., KILPE, V. E. and CLAGHORN, J. L. (1970) Evaluation of therapeutic efficacy of amantadine in patients with naturally occurring A2 influenza. *J. Am. Med. Ass.* **211**: 1149–1156.

TONEW, E., GUMPERT, B. and ULBRICHT, H. (1974) Antiviral activity of 1-(p-(methyl-nitrosamino)-benzylidene amino)-adamantane on fowl plague virus in cell cultures. *Acta Virologica* **18**: 10–16.

TONEW, E., AUGSTEN, K., GUMPERT, B. and ULBRICHT, H. (1973) The antiviral activity of 1-(p-(methylnitrosamino)-benzylidenamino)-adamantane on the fowl plague virus in tissue cultures. II. *Acta Microbiologica Polonica* **5**: 221–223.

TUČKOVÁ, E., VONKA, V., ZÁVADOVÁ, H. and KUTINOVÁ, L. (1973) Sensitivity to 1-adamantanamine as a marker in genetic studies with influenza viruses. *J. Biol. Standard* **1**: 341–346.

TYRRELL, D. A. J., BYNOE, M. L. and HOORN, B. (1965) Studies on the antiviral activity of 1-adamantanamine HCl. *Br. J. Exp. Pathol.* **46**: 370–375.

TYRRELL, D. A. J. and SMITH, J. W. G. (1979) Vaccination against influenza A. *Br. Med. Bull.* **35**: 77–85.

VACZI, L., HANKOVSZKY, O. H., HIDEG, K. and HADHAZY, G. (1973) Antiviral effect of 1-aminoadamantane derivatives *in vitro. Acta microbiol. Acad. Sci. Hung.* **20**: 241–247.

VALE, J. A. and MACLEAN, K. S. (1977) Amantadine-induced heart-failure. *Lancet* **i**: 548.

VAN HES, R., SMIT, A., KRALT, T. and PETERS, A. (1972) Synthesis and antiviral activities of adamantane spiro compounds. 2. *J. Med. Chem.* **15**: 132–136.

VAN VORIS, L. P., BETTS, R. F., HAYDEN, F. G., CHRISTMAS, W. A. and DOUGLAS, G. (1981) Successful treatment of naturally occurring influenza A/USSR/77 (H1N1). *JAMA* **245**: 1128–1131.

VERNIER, V. G., HARMON, J. B., STUMP, J. M., LYNES, T. E., MARVEL, J. P. and SMITH, D. H. (1969) The toxicologic and pharmacologic properties of amantadine hydrochloride. *Toxicol. appl. pharmacol.* **15**: 642–665.

VOGT, B. R. and HOOVER, J. R. E. (1967) The synthesis of noradamantane. *Tetrahedron Letters* No. 30: 2841–2843.

WATSON, D. H. and HONESS, R. W. In: *Chemotherapy of Herpes simplex Virus Infections.* OXFORD, J. S., DRASÄR, F. A. and WILLIAMS, J. D. (eds.). Academic Press, London 1977.

WEBSTER, R. G. and LAVER, W. G. (1975) Antigenic variation of influenza viruses. In: *The Influenza Viruses and Influenza.* KILBOURNE, E. D. (ed.). Academic Press, New York.

WEBSTER, R. G., LAVER, W. G., AIR, G. M. and SCHILD, G. C. (1982) Molecular mechanisms of variation in influenza viruses. *Nature* **296**: 115–121.

WHITE, J., MATLIN, K. and HELENIUS, A. (1981) Cell fusion by Semliki Forest, influenza and vesicular stomatitis viruses. *Cell. Biol.* **89**: 674–679.

WILSON, I. A., SKEHEL, J. J. and WILEY, D. C. (1981) Structure of the haemagglutinin membrane glycoprotein of influenza virus at 3 Å resolution. *Nature* **289**: 366–373.

WILSON, S. Z., KNIGHT, V., WYDE, P. R., DRAKE, D. and COUCH, R. B. (1980) Amantadine and ribavirin aerosol treatment of influenza A and B infection in mice. *Antimicrob. Ag. Chemother.* **17**: 642–648.

WINGFIELD, W. L., POLLOCK, D. and GRUNERT, R. R. (1969) Therapeutic efficacy of amantadine HCl and rimantadine HCl in naturally occurring influenza A2 respiratory illness. *New Engl. J. Med.* **281**: 579–584.

YOUNG, J. F., DESSELBERGER, V. and PALESE, P. (1979) Evolution of human influenza A viruses in nature: sequential mutations in the genomes of new H1N1 isolates. *Cell* **18**: 73–83.

YOUNG, J. F. and PALESE, P. (1979) Evolution of human influenza A viruses in nature: Recombination contributes to genetic variation of H1N1 strains. *Proc. Natn. Acad. Sci.* **76**: 6547–6551.

YOUNKIN, S. W., BETTS, R. F., ROTH, F. K., DOUGLAS, R. G., Jr., (1983) Reduction in fever and symptoms in young adults with Influenza A/Brazil/78 H1N1 infection after treatment with aspirin or amantadine. *Antimicrob. Agents Chemother.*, **23**: 577–582.

ZLYDNIKOV, D. M., KUBAR, O. I., KOVALEVA, T. P. and KAMFORIN, L. E. (1981) Study of rimantadine in the USSR: a review of the literature. *Rev. Infect. Dis.* **3**: 408–421.

SUMMARY AND CONCLUSIONS

Almost two decades have passed since the initial discovery of the antiviral effect of the primary amine amantadine. During this period extensive clinical trials in more than 20,000 volunteers have established a prophylactic effect against influenza A viruses, approximately equivalent to that of inactivated influenza vaccines. Unexpectedly a mild therapeutic effect has been unequivocally demonstrated with both H3N2 and H1N1 viruses. Earlier fears that the new virus antigenic variants which constantly emerge and assume epidemiological significance would be less inhibited by amantadine have not been fulfilled. The majority of recent field viruses are as well inhibited *in vitro* and in the clinic as the first H2N2 viruses tested in the early 1960s.

Recently there has been more interest in finding ways of using the compound usefully on a large scale. This fresh approach has probably been stimulated by the continued absence of any more effective influenza inhibitors and also by the heightened interest in antiviral compounds in general, following the increasingly successful use in the clinic of a triumvirate of new anti-herpes compounds, acyclovir, phosphonoformate and bromovinyl deoxyuridine (reviewed by Collier and Oxford, 1980; Stuart-Harris and Oxford, 1983), and the increasingly large quantities of interferon which are becoming available as a result of the use of genetic engineering and large-scale tissue culture techniques. Unlike amantadine, the anti-herpes compounds have well-established modes of action at the molecular level. This has been an important omission by influenza research virologists, and is a result of a paucity of data and a poor understanding of early events following infection of the cell with the virus. Once the precise point of action is understood, the way may be open to the production of a whole new generation of molecules acting at this stage in the life-cycle. It is also of some importance to extend the antiviral action to include influenza B viruses which can cause mortality and large epidemics, although not so frequently or devastatingly as influenza A viruses. The earlier studies with other primary amines established quite clearly that certain of these compounds inhibit influenza B viruses as well as influenza A viruses.

The studies with amantadine have shown the difficulties of successfully using an anti-respiratory virus compound in the field. Nevertheless these problems should not be considered insurmountable and indeed may be less formidable than they seem to some. It is quite possible that amantadine used on a large scale and with some thought and planning may have a total degree of effectiveness in preventing spread of influenza A virus out of proportion to the apparent mild effect in small historical trials. As an example, we have the successful epidemiological intervention to prevent the spread of cerebro-spinal fever in army camps, which achieved unexpectedly successful results from simple recalculations of population density in barrack rooms. The basic epidemiology of influenza A virus is not understood, encompassing as it does possible genetic pools in animals and birds and then the emergence after the summer period of antigenic mutants to cause epidemics in the late autumn in the northern and southern hemispheres. Presumably a small change in habits of the population during the beginning of the winter months helps to trigger an epidemic (Hope-Simpson, 1979). Certainly, the demonstration of a reduction in virus titre in persons treated therapeutically with amantadine may be of marked epidemiological significance if a large proportion of the population at risk was using the compound and might even abort an outbreak. There is no reason why such large-scale trials could not now be initiated and may be encouraged by the recent WHO recommendations for the prophylactic use of rimantadine (100–200 mg per day for 4–6 weeks) and the therapeutic use of amantadine or rimantadine (200 mg per day for 3–5 days) (Galasso *et al.*, 1984).

CHAPTER 7

ANTIVIRAL ACTIONS OF METAL IONS AND METAL-CHELATING AGENTS

D. D. Perrin and H. Stünzi*

*Medical Chemistry Group, John Curtin School of Medical Research,
Australian National University, Canberra, Australia*

**Institut de Chimie, Université de Neuchâtel,
Avenue de Bellevaux 51, CH-2000 Neuchâtel, Switzerland*

CONTENTS

7.1. INTRODUCTION

The discovery of highly effective antibacterial agents such as the sulphonamides and antibiotics led to expectations of similar successes against diseases of viral origin. These hopes have not, in general, been fulfilled. Identification of antiviral drugs and elucidation of their mechanisms of action have lagged behind the results on antibacterial substances, largely because the cycle of virus production is intimately linked to that of the host cell, thereby narrowing the possible ways in which a virus can be selectively inhibited. To a large extent, viruses exploit the energy-supplying and synthetic systems of the host organism; the relatively few viral enzymes are similar to those of the host, so that it is difficult to find antiviral agents which do not simultaneously have toxic effects on the host cell. Nevertheless, if progress is to be made in antiviral chemotherapy, differences in chemical and biochemical properties of viruses and host cells must be found and exploited.

A distinction must be made between an antiviral agent and a tissue poison. Although many toxic substances, such as phenyl mercuric acetate, prevent virus reproduction they do so by killing the host cell. In the present context, an antiviral agent is understood to be a substance which inhibits viral multiplication, by whatever means, at concentrations that are not seriously damaging to the host cell.

In aiming at selective inhibition of virus multiplication, one approach would be to inactivate enzyme targets that are present in virus-infected cells but are absent from the normal host cell. A good example would be interaction with a virus-induced nucleic acid polymerase since this may differ biochemically and physically from the corresponding cellular polymerase. By comparison, competitive inhibition by substrates such as the nucleotide analogues or inhibition by binding to the DNA template (actinomycin, acridine dyes) may lack specificity.

One field which has been little explored is the contribution that might be made by the manipulation of metal ion equilibria. This is the subject of the present Review.

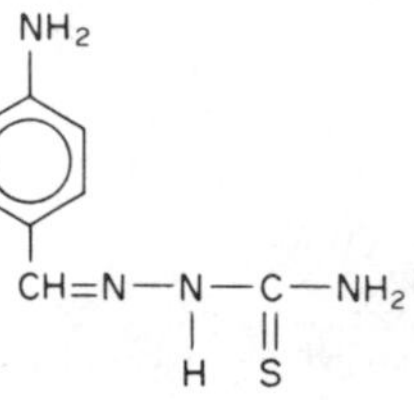

SCHEME I

The first synthetic agent to be shown to have antiviral activity was p-aminobenzaldehyde thiosemicarbazone (Scheme I) which reduced the severity of vaccinia infection of chick embryos and mice (Hamre et al., 1950). Similarly, the parent compound benzaldehyde thiosemicarbazone gave some protection to mice against intracerebral infection with vaccinia virus (Thompson et al., 1951). Extension to thiosemicarbazones of heterocyclic aldehydes such as nicotinaldehyde, isonicotinaldehyde, 2-thenylaldehyde, 3-thenylaldehyde and isatin followed (Thompson et al., 1953; Bauer, 1955; Bauer and Sadler, 1960; Bauer et al., 1963), leading to the discovery of the considerable antiviral activity of 1-methylisatin β-thiosemicarbazone (methisazone, Marboran) (Scheme II) and to its successful use as a prophylactic against smallpox (Bauer et al., 1963). It has also found clinical application in treating certain infective complications of smallpox vaccination (Bauer, 1965) and it is active against adenovirus (Bauer and Apostolov, 1966).

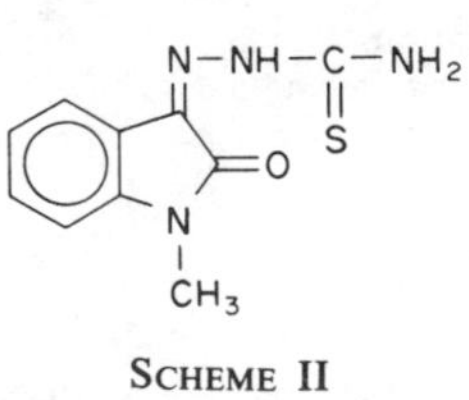

SCHEME II

Several thiosemicarbazones are known to owe their biological activity to chelation, i.e. metal ion binding (Crim and Petering, 1967; Agrawal et al., 1974). Chelation might thus be important for the mode of antiviral action of thiosemicarbazones.

Further support for a correlation between antiviral action and metal chelation comes from the observations that the anion of phosphonoacetic acid, also a chelating agent, inhibits herpes-type viruses (Shipkowitz *et al.*, 1973) and that antiviral activity has been reported for other chelating agents, including 8-hydroxyquinoline (Auld *et al.*, 1974), isonicotinic acid hydrazide (Levinson *et al.*, 1977b), sodium diethylenetriaminepentaacetic acid and 1,10-phenanthroline (Oxford and Perrin, 1974). In most cases, activity was tested in tissue cultures or in the absence of the viral envelope.

Biological reactions proceed by many successive steps and these are commonly studied *in vitro* by isolating the small number of enzymatic reactions making up one of these steps. If this group includes any metal—ion-mediated reaction, a chelating agent may act as an inhibitor. In a virus-infected cell there are many such steps, so that the same chelating agent may inhibit several enzymes; the likeliest inhibition *in vivo* is the step for which the lowest concentration of chelating agent is effective.

Conversely, the addition of more than traces of transition metal ions to test systems can also inhibit viral activity. Thus, added Cu^{2+} and Zn^{2+} (0.5 mM) inhibit the growth of foot-and-mouth disease virus in cell culture by interfering with the cleavage of large precursors of virus-specific protein and by preventing the formation of viral capsid protein (Polatnik and Bachrach, 1978). Zn^{2+} selectively inhibits herpes simplex virus type 1 DNA polymerase *in vitro* (Fridlender *et al.*, 1978a).

Because of the growing interest in bio-inorganic chemistry and the rapid increase in the knowledge of host—virus interactions, it is opportune to review the effects of metal ions and chelating agents on viral disease and the problems associated with the delivery of these possibly useful agents to their targets. Hopefully, this might suggest new or improved methods for the prophylaxis and chemotherapy of diseases of viral origin, especially those where vaccination is of only limited value.

7.2. METAL IONS IN BIOLOGICAL SYSTEMS

7.2.1. METAL IONS AND METALLOENZYMES

Besides alkaline and alkaline earth cations (Na^+, K^+, Mg^{2+}, Ca^{2+}), living organisms require trace amounts of many other metal ions (Underwood, 1977), especially the transition metal ions of copper, zinc, iron, manganese and cobalt which play vital roles in a very large number of biological processes (summarized by Ainscough and Brodie, 1976). Thus, a recent review (Vallee, 1976) lists more than eighty zinc-containing enzymes.

Whereas Na^+ and K^+ are present as "free" aquo ions, the transition metal ions are commonly bound to proteins and other metal-complexing species. The metalloenzymes are metal ion—protein complexes in which the metal ion is an integral part of the enzyme, usually situated at its active site. The metal ion may be tightly bound as the iron in haemoglobin (from which it cannot be removed except by destruction of the protein) or it may be easily exchangeable as in the zinc carboxypeptidases. The latter enzymes retain their activity when the zinc ion is replaced by a cobalt ion, but the apoenzyme (without the metal) is completely inactive (Coleman and Vallee, 1961). Metal-binding is more easily reversed in metal-activated enzymes, which are usually isolated as apoenzymes but require the presence of metal ions for their biological activity. (For example, neuraminidase needs Ca^{2+} as a cofactor.) Other metal—protein complexes, such as metallothioneins (Cherian and Goyer, 1978), function as a means of transportation for metal ions. In a less specific way, metal ions also stabilize the structures of proteins and nucleic acids.

The binding of a metal ion to a protein influences the structural arrangement and charge distribution of the atoms or groups surrounding the metal ion and affects their reactivity. Conversely, the reactivity of the metal ion is modified by the groups attached to it. Many of the copper and iron enzymes are involved in redox reactions whereas hydrolytic reactions and the formation of amide linkages are commonly catalysed by zinc enzymes. Often enzymes having similar properties contain the same metal ion, as illustrated by the zinc-containing nucleic acid polymerases listed in Table 1. Their synthesis requires dietary zinc, so that if the availability of the metal ion is decreased so, too, is the enzyme activity. For example, it has been observed that zinc-deficient suckling rats had decreased nuclear RNA polymerase activity (Terhune and Sandstead, 1972). Perhaps more importantly for our present purposes, the list includes a number of virus-induced enzymes, raising the possibility that they could be inhibited by the use of appropriate chelating agents. To understand how this and other metal ion manipulations might be achieved, it is desirable to outline briefly the salient aspects of metal ion binding by chelating agents.

TABLE 1. *Zinc-containing Polymerases and Related Enzymes*

Enzyme	Source	Reference
DNA-terminal nucleotidyl transferase	Calf thymus	Chang and Bollum, 1970
RNA polymerase	*Escherichia coli*	Scrutton et al., 1971
DNA polymerase	*E. coli*	Slater et al., 1971
DNA polymerase	Sea urchin	Slater et al., 1971
DNA polymerase	Chicken embryo	Stavrianopoulos et al., 1972
DNA polymerase I	*E. coli*	Springgate et al., 1973
DNA polymerases I, II and III	Sea urchin nuclei	Valenzuela et al., 1973
RNA polymerases I and II	Rat liver	Valenzuela et al., 1973
Reverse transcriptase	Rous sarcoma virus	Levinson et al., 1973
		Valenzuela et al., 1973
RNA polymerase	T7 phage	Coleman, 1974
RNA polymerase	Influenza virus	Oxford and Perrin, 1974
Reverse transcriptase	Avian myeloblastosis virus	Auld et al., 1974
		Poiesz et al., 1974
Reverse transcriptase	Murine leukaemia virus	Auld et al., 1975
Reverse transcriptase	Feline leukaemia virus	Auld et al., 1975
Reverse transcriptase	Woolly monkey type C virus	Auld et al., 1975
Reverse transcriptase	RD-114 RNA tumour virus	Auld et al., 1975
RNA polymerase II	*Euglena gracilis*	Falchuk et al., 1976
RNA polymerase I	Yeast	Auld et al., 1976
RNA polymerase II	Yeast	Lattke and Weser, 1976
RNA polymerase II	Wheat germ	Petranyi et al., 1977
RNA polymerase III	Yeast	Wandzilak and Benson, 1977.

7.2.2. SOME BASIC ASPECTS OF COMPLEX FORMATION

In water, Cu^{2+} exists as the pale-blue aquo ion, Cu^{2+}_{aq}, in which water molecules are coordinated to the metal ion. Addition of ammonia leads to an intense blue colour because some of the water molecules surrounding the metal ion are replaced by ammonia molecules, forming the complexes $Cu(NH_3)^{2+}_n$, where n varies from 1 to 5. A species that binds to a metal ion in this way is a ligand and the formation of a bond usually involves 'donation' (displacement) of electrons from the *donor atom* (in this case nitrogen) of the ligand towards the metal ion. Complex formation in solution involves the replacement of one kind of ligand (water molecule) by another.

Much the most important class of ligands is that which gives rise to *chelate* complexes in which the metal ion is attached to the ligand at two or more sites. If 5- or 6-membered rings are formed around the metal ion their metal complexes are much more stable than those of the monodentate ligands such as NH_3. (For a discussion of this 'chelate effect' see Anderegg, 1971.) With some sulphur ligands 4-membered chelate rings are also stable. Glycinate binds to copper ion through the NH_2 and the COO^- groups; it is a *bidentate* ligand. With excess glycinate ion the bis(glycinato) copper(II) complex (Scheme III) is formed. Perhaps the best known *multidentate* ligand is EDTA (ethylenediamine tetraacetate) with six donor atoms.

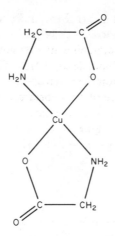

SCHEME III

7.2.3. STABILITY CONSTANTS

A metal ion, M, and ligand, L, may combine reversibly to form complexes ML_n:

$$M + L = ML$$
$$ML + L = ML_2$$
$$ML_{n-1} + L = ML_n$$

where the equilibrium concentrations of the different species depend on the total concentrations of M and L and the stabilities of the complexes. The latter are mathematically expressed by the stepwise formation constants K_n

$$K_1 = \frac{[ML]}{[M]\cdot[L]}, \quad K_2 = \frac{[ML_2]}{[ML]\cdot[L]}, \quad K_n = \frac{[ML_n]}{[ML_{n-1}]\cdot[L]}$$

or by the cumulative stability constants β_n:

$$M + nL = ML_n, \beta_n = \frac{[ML_n]}{[M]\cdot[L]^n} = K_1 \cdot K_2 \dots K_n$$

where the quantities in brackets are the molar concentrations.

Because stability constants cover a wide range of values they are usually expressed as log β. However, different constants may have different dimensions and a comparison of, say, a log K_1 value with a log β_2 value is meaningless.

Often, the situation is complicated by the formation of protonated complexes ML_nH_p, hydroxo complexes $ML_n(OH)_q$ and polynuclear complexes such as Cu_2 (histidinate)$_2$(OH)$_2$. In the presence of two or more different ligands, mixed complexes $ML'L''$ may be important. (For a detailed discussion of stability constants, see Anderegg, 1971.)

Extensive tables of stability constants are available (Sillén and Martell, 1964, 1971; Perrin, 1979), but care must be exercised in applying them to biological studies. In the above equations L signifies the form of the deprotonated ligand as in the complex: this may be a neutral molecule (ethylenediamine), a mono-anion (glycinate ion), a dianion (oxalate ion), etc. If, as is usually the case, the ligand can be protonated, so that there is competition between protons and metal ions for binding to the ligand, the extent of complex formation becomes pH-dependent. In comparing the effectiveness of different ligands as complexing agents *at a given pH* it is better to use 'apparent' or 'conditional' constants (Schwarzenbach and Flaschka, 1969; Ringbom, 1963) in which the free-ligand concentration is replaced by the total concentration of all ligand species, including protonated forms, that are not complexed with the metal ion.

Thus, a stability constant is not, in itself, an adequate indication of complexing ability at, say, physiological pH. The stability constant of Cu(2,2',2''-triaminotriethylamine) is very much larger (log K_1 = 19.3; Stünzi and Anderegg, 1976) than that of Cu-oxalate (log K_1 = 5.5; Ciavatta and Villafiorita, 1965) yet at pH 5 the latter is the more stable. Conditional constants are 5.2 and 5.5, respectively. At this pH, oxalate is present almost entirely as the dianion, which is the metal-complexing species, whereas the three strongly basic amino groups of 2,2',2''-triaminotriethylamine are 'blocked' by protonation so that the equilibrium concentration of the complex-forming species, the neutral amine, is very small. Stability constants are also dependent on temperature and ionic strength. For example, log K_1 for Cu (2,2',2''-triaminotriethylamine) changes from 19.3 in 1 M KNO$_3$ at 25° (Stünzi and Anderegg, 1976) to 18.5 in 0.15 M KNO$_3$ at 37° (Stünzi et al., 1979).

7.2.4. Factors Determining the Stability of Complexes

A convenient approach for describing the interaction of metal ions and ligands is the concept of 'hard and soft acids and bases' (HSAB), formulated by Pearson (1963, 1966). In metal complexes, the metal ions function as (Lewis) acids and the ligands as bases. A 'hard' metal ion forms chemical bonds which are electrovalent in character: its complexes are held together by electrostatic interaction between charges of opposite sign (positively charged metal ion and negatively charged ligand, or if the ligand is neutral, the negative side of the dipole). The higher the charge and the smaller the radius of the metal ion the stronger the resulting complexes. This is a good description of the bonding in, say, the fluoro complexes of Al^{3+}.

A 'soft' metal ion usually has a low charge, is of large atomic radius and forms chemical bonds of a covalent character with large, rather than small, donor atoms. An example is Ag^+ with iodide ion.

Similarly, 'hard' and 'soft' ligands can be distinguished on the basis of their size and polarizability. Fluoride ion is 'hard', Cl^-, Br^- and I^- are increasingly 'soft'. One useful classification of donor atoms in descending order of 'hardness' is oxygen > nitrogen > sulphur.

'Soft' metals form their strongest complexes with 'soft' ligands (for example, $RS^- > RNH_2 > HO^-$). 'Hard' metal ions form their strongest complexes with 'hard' ligands (for example, $RCOO^- > RNH_2 > RS^-$).

The transition metal ions are intermediate in properties, and an approximate classification for biologically important metal ions and donor atoms is given in Table 2. Among the divalent transition metal ions, the stability constants of complexes with most ligands follow the Irving–Williams series:

$$Mn < Fe < Co < Ni < Cu > Zn$$

and the differences are greatest for the 'softest' ligands. Copper(II) generally forms its more stable complexes with nitrogen than with oxygen-type ligands, and has the ability to displace a proton from peptide nitrogens to form chelate rings. Most of the transition metal ions are well suited to interact with oxygen and nitrogen atoms in proteins, nucleic acids and related molecules, whereas the 'soft' copper(I) tends to accumulate in tissues rich in lipids.

Stereochemical factors may favour coordination of a particular metal ion at a special binding site. Complexes are most stable when the cavity formed by a multidentate ligand accords with the size of the metal ion. Also, many metal ions (especially the 'soft' ones) have more or less rigid coordination geometries that have to be matched by the arrangement of the donor atoms of the ligands (e.g. Ag^+ usually forms linear complexes and binds to only two donor atoms).

These criteria may help to suggest whether a given ligand forms stable complexes with a given metal ion. But in order to find whether complexes are major species in a system comprising several metal ions and more than one kind of ligand it is necessary to know the relevant equilibrium constants and to process this information with a suitable computer programme. (For further general discussion of metal-complex formation, see Perrin, 1970, 1978.)

TABLE 2. *Some 'Hard' and 'Soft' Metal Ions and Ligands*

'Hard' Metal Ions
Na^+, Mg^{2+}, Ca^{2+}, Ba^{2+}, Al^{3+}, La^{3+}, Zr^{4+}, Mn^{2+}, Fe^{3+}, Ga^{3+}

Intermediate
Fe^{2+}, Co^{2+}, Ni^{2+}, Cu^{2+}, Zn^{2+}, Pb^{2+}, Bi^{3+}

'Soft'
Pt^{2+}, Cu^+, Ag^+, Au^+, Cd^{2+}, Hg^+, Hg^{2+}, Tl^+, Tl^{3+}

'Hard' Ligands
Binding through O^- as in RO^-, $RCOO^-$. Also F^-, Cl^-, NH_3

Intermediate
Binding through N, grading from RNH_2 to pyridine. Also Br^-, N_3^-

'Soft'
Binding through S as in R_2S, RS^-, $S_2O_3^{2-}$
Binding through P as in R_3P, $(RO)_3P$. Also I^-, CN^-

7.2.5. pM AND METAL ION BUFFERS

If a solution of a metal ion contains an excess of ligand, the concentration of the free metal ion is buffered (Perrin and Dempsey, 1974). Analogously to pH, pM can be defined as the negative logarithm of the free metal ion concentration:

$$pM = -\log [M_{aq}^{n+}]$$

However, in a given system the pM value is dependent not only on the metal ion, the ligand and their total concentrations but also on the pH value (because of the competition between hydrogen ion and metal ion, as described above). Thus at pH 7.3 in a solution 10^{-4} M in $CaCl_2$ and 10^{-3} M EDTA, the free calcium concentration is 2.8×10^{-9} M, corresponding to pCa = 8.55. At pH 8.3, pCa = 9.55. In Fig. 1, pM values of solutions of some representative metal ion–ligand pairs are given.

In a solution 0.003 M in ATP^{4-} and 0.001 M Cu^{2+} at pH 8, $CuATP^{2-}$ is formed almost quantitatively and pCu is approximately 6.2. If 0.003 M $EDTA^{4-}$ is added, pCu becomes approximately 17. This value combined with the stability constant K_1 for $CuATP^{2-}$ shows that virtually no $CuATP^{2-}$ is now present ($[CuATP] \approx 7.5 \times 10^{-14}$ M). Instead $CuEDTA^{2-}$ has become the predominant complex. This example illustrates a central problem in discussing the effect of chelating agents in biological systems. It is not sufficient to know that a metal ion and a ligand can form a complex: it is necessary that the resulting complex is at least as stable as other possible complexes that may be present. As biological systems contain much higher concentrations of ligands than of metal ions, the most effective complexing species will be the one which results in the greatest value of pM with the given total concentrations and pH. This approach can be seen as providing a partial answer to the question of whether the biological activity of a chelating agent could be due to its metal-binding properties.

7.2.6. ORGANISMS AS MULTI-METAL–MULTI-LIGAND SYSTEMS

Animal and plant tissues contain many different kinds and amounts of complex-forming species, such as amino acids, peptides, proteins, carboxylic acids and phosphates, together with small amounts of metal ions, so that each of the tissues of a living system can be likened to an arena in which these complexing species compete for the various kinds of metal ions that are present. The availability of extensive compilations of stability constants of metal complexes, pK values of organic ligands, and composition tables for biological systems, on the one hand, and electronic digital computers with large memories, on the other hand, has made it possible to simulate, semi-quantitatively, metal–ligand equilibria in biological

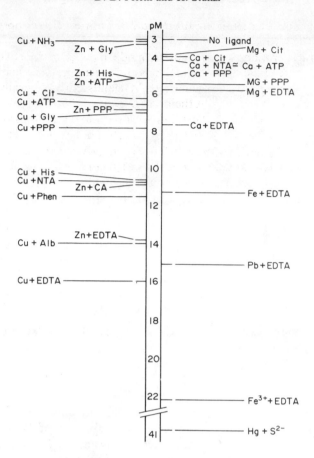

FIG. 1. Some representative metal ion buffers: pM of a solution of 0.001 M of a divalent metal ion in presence of 0.003 M of a ligand at pH 7.0

Alb	= serum albumin
ATP	= adenosine triphosphate
CA	= carbonic anhydrase
Cit	= citrate
EDTA	= ethylenediamine-tetraacetate
Gly	= glycinate
His	= histidinate
NTA	= nitrilotriacetate
Phen	= 1,10-phenanthroline
PPP	= tripolyphosphate

systems. Convenient computer programmes for this purpose include COMICS (Perrin and Sayce, 1967), HALTAFALL (Ingri et al., 1967), and EQUIL (I and Nancollas, 1972). Calculations using a theoretical blood plasma model with albumin, amino acids, citrate, lactate, phosphate and carbonate as ligands gave pCu = 15.5 and pZn = 8.8 (Agarwal and Perrin, 1976). These values are important as indicating concentrations likely to be near optimum for biological activity.

A significant departure from the normal levels may be deleterious to an organism: metal ions are toxic in excess, probably because the metal ion binds to inappropriate sites of biomolecules, possibly blocking active sites of enzymes or changing the conformation of a protein or a nucleic acid. If essential metals are present at too low concentrations, a metalloenzyme or a metal ion-activated enzyme may be deprived of its metal ion, leaving the inactive apoenzyme.

This biphasic character is illustrated by Menkes' kinky hair syndrome and Wilson's disease (hepatolenticular degeneration). In the first of these conditions, victims cannot absorb copper from the gut and die because of copper deficiency. In Wilson's disease, the level of exchangeable copper in the blood is too high and results in excessive storage of copper in the liver, kidney and brain. The latter condition can be controlled by appropriate chelation therapy (Walshe, 1969; Jones and Pratt, 1976).

The following considerations serve as a useful guide to the possibility of chelation therapy and to an understanding of the roles of metal ions and chelating agents in biological systems:

Most complexes formed by low molecular weight ligands and biologically important metal ions exist in dynamic equilibrium with their components. When a solution of a preformed metal complex is added to a biological medium the extent to which it dissociates is governed by the stability constant of the complex and the pM value of the system. Thus, the same result is obtained by adding ligand and metal ion separately, as a mixture or as a preformed complex. If the complex is not stable under the actual conditions the liberated ligand may exert its effects at a location different from the metal ion.

An extrapolation to *in vivo* conditions may be based on the stability constants of the complexes with the ligand in question. It is, however, necessary to take account of the multiple metal complex equilibria in the biological system and of the total concentrations of the components. Thus, computer blood plasma simulations show that most of the copper (99 per cent) and zinc (97 per cent) is bound to albumin. The major low-molecular weight complexes of copper and zinc are their histidinato complexes and the cysteinato complexes of zinc (Table 3). If the 'apparent' stability constants (see above) of complexes formed by a ligand with copper and zinc are smaller than those of the histidinato complexes of copper and the cysteinato complexes of zinc, the ligand is not likely to be competitive under biological conditions.

TABLE 3. *Conditional Stability Constants at pH 7.4 for Some Zinc Complexes and Distribution of Zinc Among Low Molecular Complexes in Blood Plasma Models*

Complex A	$\log \beta'_2$ $\log \beta_{1110'}$	% formed in blood plasma model		
		B	C	D
Zn(cys)$_2$	10.82	16	40	46
Zn(cys) (his)H$_{0.1}$	10.14	24	24	23
Zn(his) (s.a.a.)				10
Zn(his) (gly)	7.15			

(A) cys = cysteine, his = histidine, s.a.a. simple amino acids.
(B) (Hallman *et al.*, 1971): distribution among 17 amino acids.
(C) (Berthon *et al.*, 1978): Free zinc concentration estimated.
(D) (Stünzi and Perrin, 1979; Stünzi *et al.*, 1980): serum albumin as representative for metal binding proteins.

Many ligands form complexes with copper(II) that are more stable than those with zinc and other first-row transition metals. However, although the stability constant for $CuEDTA^{2-}$ is appreciably greater than for $ZnEDTA^{2-}$ or $CaEDTA^{2-}$, the copper(II) ion is bound so much more strongly by other ligands in blood plasma that administration of EDTA lowers zinc and calcium ion levels (raises pCa and pZn) more than it does pCu. This result emphasizes the importance of computer analysis of multi-metal–multi-ligand systems as models for equilibria in biological environments. As another example, calculations indicate that although polymeric species such as $Cu_2his_2(OH)_2$ may be important under laboratory conditions, they are usually negligible in a biological environment.

The presence of many ligands in a biological environment also leads to an extensive formation of mixed-ligand (ternary) complexes such as M(ligand A)-(ligand B) (Sigel, 1973; Perrin, 1977b, cf. Table 3). Often, especially where the ligands are of different types, such as oxalate dianion and ethylenediamine, the mixed complexes are more stable than expected on statistical grounds. This has been observed, especially, with Cu^{2+} (Sigel, 1975). The mixed-ligand complexes formed by copper(II), histidinate and another amino acid are about 6 times more stable than expected (Brookes and Pettit, 1977). Similarly, for Cu(histidinate)-(phosphonoacetate)$^{2-}$ the stability is enhanced by a factor of 16 (Stünzi and Perrin, 1979).

In the same way, metalloenzymes may form mixed-ligand complexes of the type apoenzyme–metal ion–substrate, thereby attaching the substrate to the active site of the enzyme. Addition of a ligand that binds more strongly than the substrate may result in the inhibition of the enzyme by the formation of a similar mixed complex in which this ligand replaces the substrate. Again a biphasic response is possible: yeast phosphoglucomutase, a zinc enzyme, is inhibited by EDTA, which forms a ternary complex; however, low concentrations of EDTA stimulated enzyme activity, probably by removing traces of undesirable metal ions (Hirose *et al.*, 1972).

Nucleic acids also bind metal ions, thereby possibly stabilizing the DNA double helix when metal ions are present in low concentrations or destabilizing it when metal ions are in high concentrations. This may bring about conformational changes, allowing interactions with polymerases, binding to histones and initiating cell differentiation or, conversely, neoplastic growth (Sissoëff *et al.*, 1976).

The distribution of metal ions and ligands is by no means uniform throughout an organism. There are barriers between organs, cells and subcellular organelles. These membranes are generally passively permeable for small neutral molecules. Charged species may also penetrate membranes but this often depends on their structure. Also, passage may be allowed only unidirectionally. Different cells and organelles achieve an active transport of selected molecules through their membranes against a concentration gradient. (Thus, the intracellular concentrations of Na^+ and Ca^{2+} are considerably smaller than those found extracellularly; for K^+ the reverse is true.)

7.3. HOST–VIRUS INTERACTION

7.3.1. THE CYCLE OF VIRUS REPLICATION

All viruses are obligate intracellular parasites (insofar as they can be considered as organisms) which divert the host cell's metabolism wholly or in part to the production of viral nucleic acid and protein. Because the viral nucleic acid may be either DNA or RNA, but never both, viruses are classified according to the type of nucleic acid they contain. Some common examples are given in Table 4. The ability of the genome of the virus to impress its control on the host cell is the major difference between bacterial and fungal diseases on the one hand and viral diseases on the other. At the same time the virion lacks the organelles required for energy generation so that it depends entirely on the cells of its host to provide its energy requirements. Unlike a bacterium or a fungus, a virion cannot multiply in a cell-free medium.

Although subject to individual variations, the cycle of host–virus interactions can be generalized as follows:

A virion existing outside the host cell becomes attached to its surface and penetrates the host cell. The protein coat surrounding the viral nucleic acid is removed and the viral nucleic acid takes over the control of nucleic acid and protein synthesis in the cell so that viral components are replicated. Virions are assembled from these new viral components in the cell. Finally, large numbers of newly formed virions are released from the host cell and they become dispersed. The cycle repeats itself and the viral infection spreads among a susceptible population if the disease is propagated.

To rationalize possibilities of virus control we first examine this cycle more closely:

(1) Free virions exist as discrete particles, each of which comprises a core of either DNA or RNA which may be singly or doubly stranded and which is surrounded by a protective capsid (shell) of protein. Over this may lie a lipoprotein envelope which is bounded by a lipid membrane. Enveloped viruses may contain enzymes and bear, on their surfaces, spikes which facilitate highly specific attachment to host cells. Thus the exterior of the influenza virion is studded with two sets of glycoprotein spikes, comprised of haemagglutinin and neuraminidase. The former are responsible for the adsorption of the virions to mucoprotein receptors on cells of the respiratory tract and red blood cells; the haemagglutinin binds to

TABLE 4. *Some Common Viruses Classified by Type of Nucleic Acid*

Major groups	Examples
DNA viruses (double-stranded DNA)	
Adenoviridae	
Herpetoviridae	Cytomegalo virus
	Epstein–Barr virus
	Herpes simplex virus
	Marek's disease virus
	Pseudorabies virus
	Varicella-zoster virus (chickenpox)
Papovaviridae	Papilloma viruses
Poxviridae	Vaccinia (cowpox) virus
	Variola (smallpox) virus
	Myxoma virus
Others	Hepatitis virus A and B
RNA viruses (single-strand RNA with positive (messenger) polarity)	
Picornaviridae	Enteroviruses: Coxsackie virus
	Echo virus
	Mengo virus
	Polio virus
	Rhinoviruses: Human rhinovirus
	Foot-and-mouth-
	disease virus
Retroviridae	Oncovirus, e.g. Rous sarcoma virus
	'Slow' viruses (maedi, kuru, visna)
Togaviridae	Rubella virus (German measles)
	Sindbis virus
	Tick-borne encephalitis virus
	Yellow fever virus
RNA viruses (single-strand RNA with negative (antimessenger) polarity	
Myxoviridae	Influenza virus
	Measles virus
	Mumps virus
	Parainfluenza virus
Rhabdoviridae	Rabies virus
	Vesicular stomatitis virus

sialic acid residues on the plasma membranes of the cells. This triggers the entry of the virion into the cell either by viropexis (pinacytosis) (Fazekas de St. Groth, 1948; Dourmashkin and Tyrrell, 1974), a phagocytic type of action, or by fusion of the viral lipid envelope with the plasma membrane. The functions of the neuraminidase are not yet clearly established. They may be to hydrolyse neuraminic acid present in the glycoproteins of mucus, and to facilitate passage through the mucus which lines the respiratory tract. Conversely, they may be concerned with the release of newly formed virions from cells. Inhibitors of neuraminidase would be expected to decrease the rate of penetration of influenza virus into the respiratory tract, slowing the spread of infection and hence favouring an enhancement of the natural defence mechanism of the host.

(2) Whereas most animal viruses probably penetrate the cell surface intact, most bacterial viruses leave their coats outside the cell. Penetration by the virion may be accompanied by partial degradation. Thus, cytoplasmic proteases and lipases disrupt the influenza virus envelope and liberate the viral transcriptase enzyme. The liberated viral nucleic acid is transported to the site of replication, which is the cytoplasm for pox viruses and myxoviruses. For herpes viruses, replication occurs in the nucleus. The genomes (or DNA copies of them) of herpes viruses and oncoviruses are incorporated into the host's chromosomes, where they remain latent. In response to stress the genes may be reactivated and produce a new outbreak of the disease: 'cold sore' (herpes simplex virus) is a familiar example. With oncoviruses there may be transformation of the cell into a malignant cell; *in vivo*, this may be one of the causes of some forms of cancer.

Depending on the virus, different pathways may be followed, the more common ones being as summarized in Fig. 2.

DNA viruses (double stranded DNA)[a] e.g. herpesvirus, poxvirus

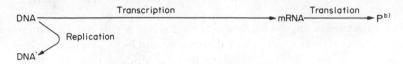

RNA viruses (single stranded RNA)[a]

Retroviruses (RNA with "message" polarity) e.g. Rous sarcoma virus, slow viruses

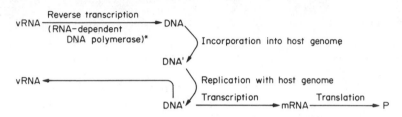

Viruses with "antimessage" RNA e.g. influenza virus

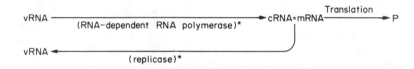

Viruses with "message" RNA e.g. rhinovirus

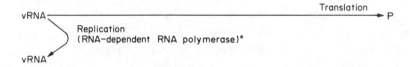

Fig. 2. Nucleic acids in reproduction of common viruses

* Types of enzymes not ordinarily used by healthy cells.
(a) Animal viruses with single-stranded DNA or double-stranded RNA are of minor importance.
(b) Proteins: early proteins are synthesized before replication of genome, late proteins are synthesized after replication of the genome.

(a) DNA viruses often employ the nucleus and enzymes of the host cell for the transcription of their double-stranded DNA into mRNA, except for the pox viruses which use their own transcriptase in the cytoplasm. The mRNA is then translated into virus-coded enzymes and other 'early' proteins which are synthesized on cellular ribosomes. Viral DNA is replicated and further ('late') mRNA is transcribed from progeny- and parental-DNA. These 'late' mRNA's are translated into structural proteins, enzymes and regulatory proteins.

DNA synthesis requires the availability of the appropriate deoxyribonucleotides. These occur at such low levels in animal cells that the reductive conversion of ribonucleotides to deoxyribonucleotides is believed to be a rate-controlling step in the biosynthesis of DNA. Thus a correlation was found between ribonucleotide reductase activity and growth rates of rat hepatomas (Elford et al., 1970).

(b) RNA tumour viruses (retroviruses, e.g. Rous sarcoma virus) contain single-stranded RNA which is translated by a viral enzyme, reverse transcriptase (RNA-dependent DNA polymerase), into an RNA–DNA hybrid which serves as a template for synthesizing double-stranded DNA (Temin, 1970). This DNA is integrated into cellular DNA prior to multiplication.

(c) Influenza virus contains a single-stranded RNA which has the 'antimessage' polarity ('negative strand') and cannot serve directly as mRNA. The parental vRNA molecule functions as a single-stranded template for the simultaneous transcription of several complementary cRNA strands by virus-dependent RNA polymerases and is translated on the cellular ribosomes. The complementary strand (cRNA) is mRNA (Pons, 1975).

(d) When single-stranded RNA is of the correct 'message' polarity in a virus it can serve both as mRNA and as a template for its own replication.

Multiplication of DNA and RNA viruses show many variations in detail. (For a fuller discussion of viral replication, see Fenner and White, 1976.)

(3) Many of the RNA viruses and some DNA viruses acquire their lipoprotein envelope by budding through cellular membrane which has been modified by incorporation of viral proteins. In the process of budding, the plasma membrane evaginates, becoming the envelope of a complete virion which is nipped off and released to its surroundings. Liberation of newly assembled influenza virions from the host cell appears to be facilitated by neuraminidase which removes neuraminic acid from the viral envelope and prevents aggregation of progeny virus on the cell surface (Palese *et al.*, 1974).

7.3.2. INTERFERENCE WITH THE VIRAL CYCLE

Examination of the different steps of the viral cycle may suggest ways of inhibiting viral activity and may also help interpret the observed antiviral activity of various compounds. Possibilities include the selective inhibition of viral multiplication by preventing the attachment of the virion to the plasma membrane, by preventing its penetration of the cell, or by interfering with the uncoating of the virion. Where viruses induce virus-specific enzymes their selective inhibition may be possible. Assembly and release of virus particles may also provide sites for application of antiviral chemotherapy.

For a substance to be considered as an antiviral agent it must be effective in treating a virus infection by inhibiting the multiplication of the virus. Unfortunately, there still remains at present a large mass of empirical information about antiviral agents without much indication of the mechanisms of their actions.

As can be seen from Table 5 most of the current antiviral agents act at sites within the host cell. The intimate relation between a virus and its host cell makes it difficult to develop a nontoxic agent which functions as a selective virus inhibitor within infected cells because both the virus and the host cell use similar substrate and enzyme systems for synthesis.

Nevertheless, some virion-associated and virus-induced enzymes differ appreciably from enzymes of host cells (Kit, 1979) and may be more sensitive to metal ions and chelating agents (cf. Section 7.4.3).

An ideal antiviral agent should specifically inhibit virus multiplication without affecting normal cell division. However, attempts to interfere biophysically or biochemically with viral activity often results in damage to the host cell. Many inhibitors of DNA synthesis bind to template DNA and are non-specific. Examples include actinomycin and anthracycline. Others, nucleoside analogues such as cytosine arabinoside, adenine arabinoside, trifluoro-thymidine and iododeoxyuridine, that affect the multiplication of DNA viruses also affect the replication of uninfected cells, are cytotoxic or even mutagenic and hence, in general, are unsuitable as antiviral drugs (Stalder, 1977). Thus the toxic effects of most antiviral agents arise from lack of specificity, due to the close dependence of viral replication on cell metabolism.

Far fewer substances are antiviral when tested *in vivo*. This is probably because of the added requirements that they must penetrate the host cell if they are to be active and they must at the same time not be metabolized rapidly. One means of overcoming this limitation is the use of liposomes as transport vehicles. Another is to attach lipid-soluble groups to an

TABLE 5. *Probable Modes of Action of Antiviral Agents*

Step in viral cycle	Agent
Attachment to cell	Immunoglobulins
Penetration of cell	Amantadine
Uncoating	Immunoglobulins
Eclipse of infectivity	
Synthesis of viral nucleic acid	Nucleoside analogues, e.g. cytosine arabinoside
(DNA)	α-(N)-heterocyclic thiosemicarbazones
	Phosphonoformic acid
	Phosphonoacetic acid
	Zinc ions
(RNA)	Rifamycin
	2-(α-Hydroxybenzyl)-benzimidazole
	Guanidine
	α-Amanitin
Synthesis of proteins:	
(i) transcription	Actinomycin D
	Isatin β-thiosemicarbazone
	Interferon
(ii) translation	Puromycin
	Interferon
(iii) post-translation	Isatin β-thiosemicarbazone
	Zinc ions
Assembly	Rifamycin
Release	

otherwise lipophobic or ionic species. Thus, by adding a long-chain alkylamido group to diethylenetriaminepentaacetic acid, the chelating agent was able to penetrate rats' livers to remove plutonium (Bulman, 1978).

To be infective, a virus must breach barriers such as skin or mucous membranes. Viral multiplication may be limited to the initial site, as in most respiratory infections, or it may spread to secondary sites via the blood stream, the lymphatic system or other possible routes. Also, the timing of antiviral therapy is important. Once replication and damage have become widespread and clinical symptoms are apparent there is often little advantage in a chemotherapeutic approach. This is particularly true when the symptoms are caused by the host's defence mechanisms and the peak of viral production has been passed.

7.4. APPLICATION OF METAL IONS AND CHELATING AGENTS IN VIRUS CONTROL

7.4.1. INHIBITION OF VIRAL ENZYMES

The viral cycle outlined in Fig. 2 indicates several points at which a virus might be susceptible to interference by chelating agents. One of the most promising areas is in the synthesis and functioning of nucleic acid polymerases. These enzymes are often virus-specific and especially the RNA-dependent RNA polymerases and the RNA-dependent DNA polymerases (reverse transcriptases) are not ordinarily utilized by healthy cells. This raises the possibility that substances may be found that inhibit selectively the viral polymerases within the host cell. In this context, many antiviral agents, even if they were not active *in vivo*, facilitated the study of molecular biology of viruses.

Transcriptase activity can be measured by incorporation of radioactively labelled ribonucleoside triphosphates in a suitable medium if the enzyme is liberated by disrupting the virion with a detergent. Maximum activity requires the presence of Mg^{2+} and/or Mn^{2+} as essential cofactors in the phosphoryl transferase reaction (Chow and Simpson, 1971; Skehel, 1971). These metal ions appear to be needed to facilitate the binding of the nucleoside triphosphate substrates to the polymerase whereas Zn^{2+} is involved in the interaction of nucleic acid with enzyme (Slater *et al.*, 1971). Reverse transcriptase activity is measured similarly by the uptake of tritium-labeled thymidine, added as its triphosphate, from an appropriate medium (Levinson et al., 1973).

From Table 1 it seems likely that most, if not all, nucleic acid polymerases are zinc enzymes. Typically, the removal of zinc from E. coli DNA polymerase by dialysis against 1,10-phenanthroline, a chelating ligand, led to loss of activity which was fully restored by addition of zinc to the apoenzyme (Springgate et al., 1973). Possibly the Zn^{2+} functions by coordinating the 3'-OH terminus or 'growing point'of the DNA (Springgate et al., 1973).

A common type of inhibition of zinc enzymes by chelating agents involves the formation of apoenzyme–zinc–ligand complexes from which the ligand can be removed by dialysis. The chelating agent would be a competitive inhibitor of the enzyme with respect to the substrate. Ternary complexes of this type have been suggested for yeast phosphogluco-mutase (Hirose et al., 1972) and carbonic anhydrase with chelating agents (Carpy, 1968).

1,10-Phenanthroline (Scheme IV, a) 8-hydroxyquinoline (Scheme V), and their deriva-tives, comprise two widely used types of bidentate ligands in which two donor atoms are held rigidly in positions suitable for chelation of a transition metal ion. Isomers such as the other six hydroxy quinolines and m-phenanthroline (1,7-phenanthroline) cannot form chelate complexes and lack antibacterial, antifungal and antiviral activity.

Examples where these chelating agents show antiviral effects include RNA-dependent DNA polymerase of Rous sarcoma virus which is inhibited by 8-hydroxyquinoline (Rohde et al., 1976) and the reverse transcriptase of avian myeloblastosis virus which is inhibited by 1,10-phenanthroline, 8-hydroxyquinoline and other chelating agents such as EDTA (Scheme VI) (or better, EGTA (Scheme VII); ethyleneglycol-bis(β-aminoethylether)-N,N,N',N'-tetraacetate) (Auld et al., 1974; Poiesz et al., 1974).

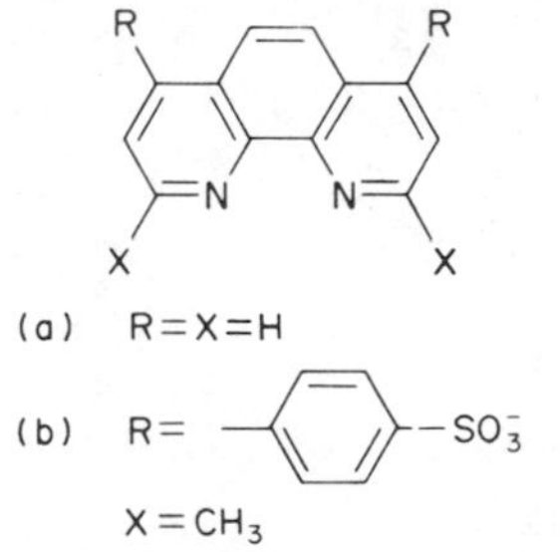

(a)   R=X=H

(b)   R= —⟨ ⟩— SO_3^-

X = CH_3

Scheme IV

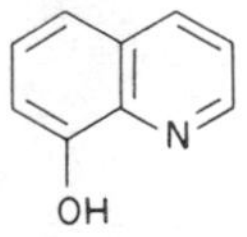

Scheme V

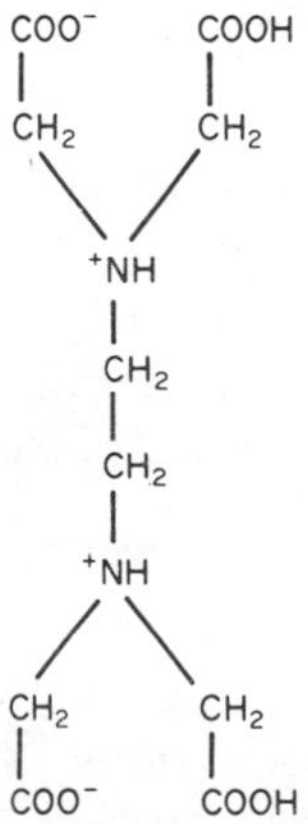

Scheme VI

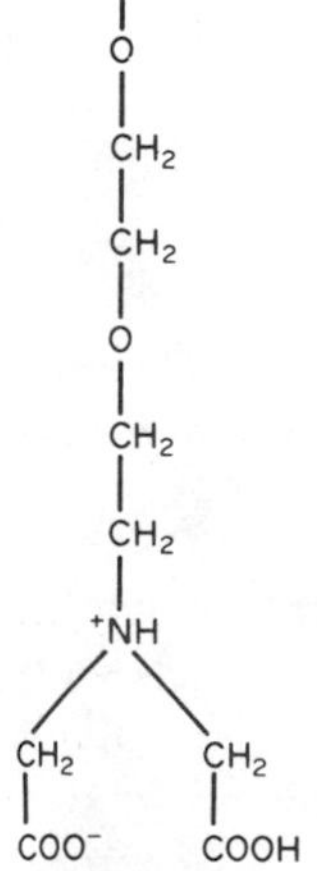

Scheme VII

Numerous polymerases and transferases have been inhibited using 1,10-phenanthroline (Chang and Bollum, 1970; Slater *et al.*, 1971; Stavrianopoulos *et al.*, 1972; Valenzuela *et al.*, 1973; Wandzilak and Benson, 1977). Similarly, bathocuproine disulphonate (Scheme IV, b) and selenocystamine inhibit DNA-dependent RNA polymerase of *E. coli* (Oxford, 1975). On the other hand, the terdentate ligand 5-amino-2-formylisoquinoline thiosemicarbazone did not inhibit four types of sea urchin nucleic acid polymerase (Venton *et al.*, 1977).

It seems probable that many polymerases contain at least one —SH group near the bound metal ion, so that the enzymes readily undergo oxidation during attempts to purify them. Addition of mercaptoethanol, by providing an alternative source of —SH groups, protects the enzymes unless it is added in such large excess that it complexes competitively with the enzyme-bound zinc. Complexation explains the effects of cystamine (Scheme VIII) and penicillamine (Scheme IX), which inhibit the particle-associated RNA-dependent RNA polymerase activity of influenza virus (Oxford and Perrin, 1974). The inhibition by selenocystamine (Scheme X) is reversed by addition of mercaptoethanol (Oxford, 1973) possibly due to reductive scission of the diselenide to selenol. This enzyme is also inhibited by the other chelating agents including selenocystine, heterocyclic thiosemicarbazones, aliphatic polyamines, bathophenanthroline and bathocuproine sulphonic acids, triethylenetetramine, diethylenetriamine, 2,2'-bipyridyl, dithizone, solochrome black, eriochrome blue, zincone, PAR and 8-hydroxyquinoline (Ho and Walters, 1970; Oxford and Perrin, 1974; Oxford, 1977). It is likely that in RNA-dependent RNA polymerase the zinc ion shows its usual octahedral stereochemistry and that three or four sites around the zinc are occupied by binding groups on the enzyme. (Two sites would not hold zinc strongly enough to withstand removal of the zinc by EDTA, while more than four sites occupied would leave too few for stable ternary complex formation. Three occupied sites and three free sites would favour terdentate ligands and explain why 2-acetylpyridine thiosemicarbazone is more effective than the bidentate 3- and 4-acetylpyridine thiosemicarbazones (Oxford, 1977).)

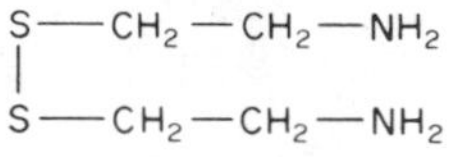

$$S\text{---}CH_2\text{---}CH_2\text{---}NH_2$$
$$|$$
$$S\text{---}CH_2\text{---}CH_2\text{---}NH_2$$

SCHEME VIII

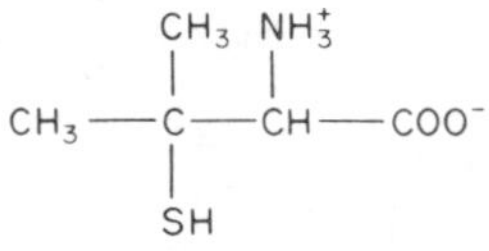

$$CH_3 \quad NH_3^+$$
$$| \qquad |$$
$$CH_3\text{---}C\text{---}CH\text{---}COO^-$$
$$|$$
$$SH$$

SCHEME IX

$$Se\text{---}CH_2\text{---}CH_2\text{---}NH_2$$
$$|$$
$$Se\text{---}CH_2\text{---}CH_2\text{---}NH_2$$

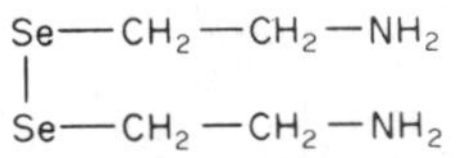

SCHEME X

Most reports implicate Zn^{2+} as a possible cofactor in many nucleotidyl transferase reactions but in complex multicomponent systems such as the polymerases using metal-nucleotide triphosphates as substrates it is difficult to establish unambiguously the role of any particular kind of metal ion. Chelating agents are selective but not specific for metal ions; for example, 1,10-phenanthroline forms stable complexes, with Zn^{2+}, Cu^{2+} and Fe^{2+}.

The T-even bacteriophages of *Escherichia coli* contain a zinc metalloenzyme on the phage baseplate and it is suggested (Kozloff and Lute, 1977) that zinc-chelating agents such as 1,10-phenanthroline and 8-hydroxyquinoline interfere with phage infection by binding to the zinc on the baseplate and bringing about conformational changes. If the zinc was removed from the plate it could be replaced, somewhat less efficiently, by Co^{2+}, Cd^{2+} or Ni^{2+}, but not by Fe^{2+}, Cu^{2+}, Mn^{2+} or Hg^{2+}.

In many cases, a transition metal ion other than zinc is involved in an enzymatic reaction. Thus, ribonucleoside diphosphate reductase is an iron(II) metalloenzyme (Moore *et al.*, 1970) which catalyses the reductive conversion of ribonucleotides to deoxyribonucleotides. α-(*N*)-Heterocyclic carboxaldehyde thiosemicarbazones such as 2-formylpyridine thiosemicarbazone (Scheme XI) inhibit tumour-derived and herpes virus-derived ribonucleoside diphosphate reductase (French *et al.*, 1974) and hence prevent the synthesis of viral DNA.

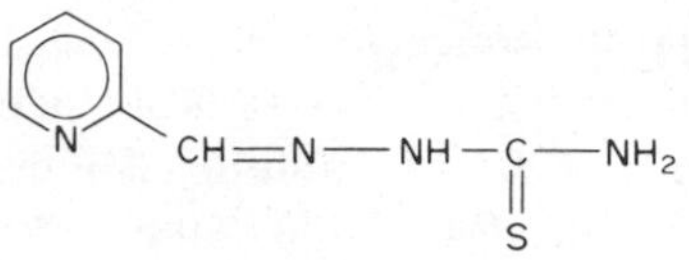

SCHEME XI

It is a matter of interest that there appear to be no known virus-specific enzymes containing copper.

Calcium ion is an essential cofactor of viral, bacterial and avian neuraminidases, so that all neuraminidases tested were inhibited to some extent by EDTA (Boschman and Jacobs, 1965). EDTA was effective against influenza viral neuraminidase at ligand concentrations around 10 mm. Activity could be restored by dialysis or by adding calcium ion (Boschman and Jacobs, 1965). Rafelson *et al.* (1963) found EDTA inhibited neuraminidase of Asian and PR 8 strain influenza viruses. Calcium ions are also required for the penetration by phage pL-1 genomes of the host cells of *Lactobacillus casei*. In the absence of calcium ion, growth of the host cells continues normally, and the phage remains adsorbed on their external surface (Watanabe and Takesue, 1972). Other phages are known which require calcium or magnesium ions for adsorption, for penetration or for multiplication of phage genomes.

The neuraminidase (*N*-acetylneuraminate glycohydrolase) activity of influenza virions may be important as a means of penetrating the mucus layer in the nasal passages to secure access to the underlying cells. Following replication of influenza virus in the upper respiratory tract, it facilitates the spread of infection by removing sialic acid from the surrounding mucus, thereby lowering the viscosity. This activity depends on the presence of calcium ion in the medium, the stimulating effect of Ca^{2+} being removed if the reaction mixture is made 3 mm in EDTA (Dimmock, 1971; Wilson and Rafelson, 1967). Similar behaviour has been shown by a mammalian neuraminidase (Warren and Spearing, 1960) and also by the purified neuraminidase from *Vibrio cholerae* (Rosenberg *et al.*, 1960). Conversely, inhibition by EDTA could be removed by dialysing or by adding Ca^{2+} or Mn^{2+}.

Inhibition of viral enzymes is achieved not only by ligands, but also by metal ions; reverse transcriptase of retroviruses is inhibited significantly by Ag^+, Co^{2+}, Zn^{2+}, Cd^{2+}, Ni^{2+} and Cu^{2+} (Levinson *et al.*, 1973) and DNA-dependent RNA polymerase of T7 bacteriophage is inhibited by Mn^{2+}, Co^{2+} and Cd^{2+} (Coleman, 1974). Inhibition by metal ions may be selective, for example among nucleotidyl transferases of a sea urchin, DNA polymerase α and the RNA polymerases II and III were inhibited by copper ion but DNA polymerase β was resistant (Venton *et al.*, 1977). The former three polymerases showed also varying degrees of sensitivity to Fe^{2+} and Cu^{2+} complexes but ferrous ion by itself was not inhibitory.

7.4.2. THIOSEMICARBAZONES

Bauer (1973) has reviewed antiviral chemotherapy, with particular reference to the thiosemicarbazones, up until 1970. The first antiviral agents (benzaldehyde thiosemicarbazone and derivatives) belonged to this class. Many thiosemicarbazones have been tested for activity against viruses, leading to the discovery of isatin β-thiosemicarbazone (Scheme XII) and its ring-*N* substituted derivatives which were highly active against viruses of the pox family and were successfully used in Man.

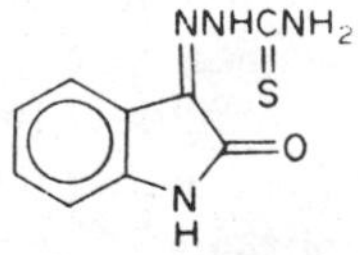

SCHEME XII

Methisazone (1-methyl isatin β-thiosemicarbazone), given orally, was used in a successful trial in Madras to prevent smallpox (variola) in persons at risk of infection following contact with cases of the disease (Bauer *et al.*, 1963). A similar trial of methisazone in the prophylaxis of contacts of alastrim was carried out in Sao Paulo (Ribeiro do Valle *et al.*, 1965). However, a therapeutic trial on patients already showing clinical signs failed to reveal any advantage of the treatment. Many cases of eczema vaccinatum (Turner *et al.*, 1962) and vaccinia gangrenosum (Bauer, 1965) responded to treatment with methisazone. Oral administration of methisazone gave rapid and complete recovery from vaccinial complications affecting skin and mucocutaneous junctions (McLean, 1977).

Similarly, M and B 7714 (3-methyl-4-bromo-5-formylisothiazole thiosemicarbazone (Scheme XIII) was effective against neurovaccinia and rabbitpox virus (Slack *et al.*, 1964) and also afforded significant protection against smallpox when administered prophylactically (Rao *et al.*, 1965).

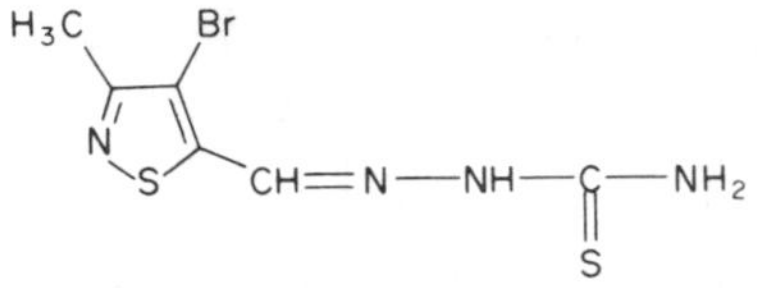

SCHEME XIII

These thiocarbazones have a broad spectrum of activity against DNA and RNA viruses (Bauer *et al.*, 1970) with structure activity relationships varying from one virus to another. However, the thiosemicarbazone sidechain is vital and replacement of the sulphur atom by NH or O abolishes activity completely (cf. Bauer, 1973).

Subsequently, two further classes of biologically active thiosemicarbazones came into use; namely the α-(*N*)-heterocyclic thiosemicarbazones of the general structure given in Scheme XIV, and bisthiosemicarbazone compounds. Both types were mainly studied as anticancer drugs but are active against viruses as well.

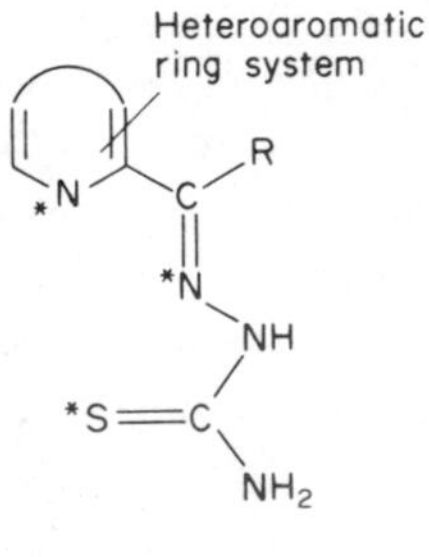

SCHEME XIV

The above examples by no means exhaust the biological activities of thiosemicarbazones. Besides their antiviral and antitumour activities, they have been found to be effective against protozoa and fungi, and also as pesticides. Considerable scope remains for designing further ligands of this class, modified so as to improve their water-solubility and to enhance their uptake in the body. A general criticism, however, is that they are highly toxic and there is little margin between therapeutic and toxic levels.

The metal binding of thiosemicarbazide and thiosemicarbazones was reviewed by Campbell (1975). The 1'-nitrogen* and sulphur* atoms are the donor atoms in their complexes (Scheme XV). Bidentate thiosemicarbazones, even in the deprotonated thiol form (Scheme XVI) are weak chelating agents. A study with p-sulphonatobenzaldehyde thiosemicarbazone (Stünzi, 1982) revealed that the complexes of only bidentate thiosemicarbazones are not stable enough to be of any importance under biological conditions. Furthermore, copper(II) is reduced by these ligands and copper(I) complexes are formed (Stünzi, 1981a).

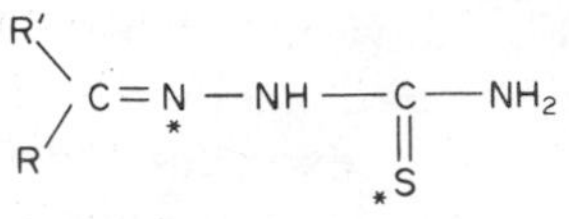

SCHEME XV 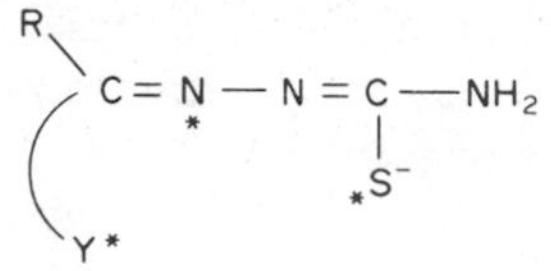   SCHEME XVI

The amide-type oxygen attached at position 2 of the pyrrolidine ring of isatin β-thiosemicarbazone is an example of a weak additional donor atom which further increases the stability of its metal complexes. The ring nitrogen of the α-(N)-heterocyclic thiosemicarbazones, on the other hand, is a strong donor, so that these compounds are powerful terdentate ligands and readily form two 5-membered chelate rings in their metal complexes.

Metal-binding ability is further enhanced in the bisthiosemicarbazones of aliphatic 1,2-diketones, which are tetradentate ligands.

7.4.2.1. Bis-thiosemicarbazones

Kethoxal bisthiosemicarbazone (H_2KTS, 3-ethoxy-2-oxobutyraldehyde bisthiosemicarbazone (Scheme XVII)) was active against vesicular stomatitis virus in chick embryo by inhibiting viral mRNA and protein synthesis (Levinson *et al.*, 1977a) but there was also marked inhibition of cellular DNA, RNA and protein synthesis. Methisazone and 2-formylpyridine thiosemicarbazone did not inhibit this virus.

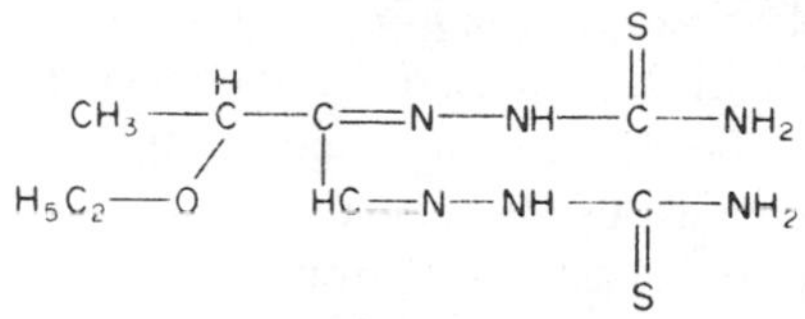

SCHEME XVII

Pyruvaldehyde and kethoxal bisthiosemicarbazones are carcinostatic, and dietary copper (or other metals to a lesser degree) enhances the anticancer activity of the parenterally administered drug (Cappuccino *et al.*, 1967). The copper chelate was found to be the active species for KTS (Crim and Petering, 1967), possibly as an oxidizing agent, interfering with the energy transport system (Petering, 1972). Warren *et al.* (1972) have shown that copper(II) complexes of 1,2-bisthiosemicarbazones readily undergo oxidation and reduction.

These 1,2-bisthiosemicarbazones form very stable complexes with metal ions. The conditional stability constant of the copper complex of KTS at pH 7.4 is reported to be $10^{18.4}$ (Petering, 1974) and the copper complexes of substituted kethoxal bisthiosemicarbazones do not dissociate appreciably in human plasma and mouse ascites fluid (Petering, 1974). The crystal structure of Cu(KTS) showed a planar coordination in which the copper is bound to two nitrogens and two (thiol) sulphur atoms (Taylor *et al.*, 1966). In the solid state two molecules of Cu(KTS) are joined by bonds between one S of one molecule to the fifth (axial) coordination site of the copper in the other molecule, suggesting that in solution a ligand might coordinate at this site on Cu(KTS).

We doubt the small reported value for the stability constant of the zinc-KTS complex because of the unsuitability of the spectrophotometric method used, based as it was on the assumption that only one complex was formed. Zinc ion does not itself absorb so that the observed spectroscopic differences are due to changes in the electronic structure of the ligand as in Scheme XV and Scheme XVI. The authors did not consider the possible formation of complexes with the neutral ligand.

The 1,2-bisthiosemicarbazones are linear ligands forming three chelate 5-rings when bound to a metal ion. With linear tetradentate ligands, expansion of the middle chelate ring by one CH_2-group often increases the stability of the copper complexes but decreases those with other bivalent first row transition metals including zinc, whereas expansion to a 7-membered ring generally drastically reduces the stability of metal complexes (e.g. Anderegg et al., 1975). If this were true as well for these sulphur ligands, a bisthiosemicarbazone of a 1,3-diketone could be even more active and more discriminating towards copper.

1,5-Bisthiosemicarbazones have been investigated as antitumour agents. Their metal-binding ability is substantially less than for 1,2-bisthiosemicarbazones. (In a comparable tetradentate system, increasing the inner chelate ring from six atoms to eight atoms, decreased the stability constant by seven logarithmic units (Bläuenstein, 1977).) Kessel and McElhinney (1975) showed, using an ^{30}S labelled drug and ^{64}Cu, that the metal chelate readily penetrated leukaemia L1210 cells, where the metal was tightly bound to ligands present in the cell. The drug then diffused from the cells to shuttle more metal ions inwards. Intracellular copper was several hundred times higher when the extracellular solution contained copper and a 1,5-bisthiosemicarbazone than when it was without such a ligand. This mechanism is unlikely to operate with 1,2- or 1,3-bisthiosemicarbazones because the metal complexes are probably too stable to be dissociated in this way. Tests with a series of homologous bisthiosemicarbazones could give more insight into the mode of action of these compounds, provided the stability constants are reliably determined.

7.4.2.2. α-(N)-Heterocyclic Thiosemicarbazones

The α-(N)-heterocyclic thiosemicarbazones comprise derivatives of 1-formylisoquinoline and 2-formylpyridine and other molecules of the structural type given in Scheme XIV. They exert antiviral and antineoplastic activity, inhibiting the growth of DNA viruses of the herpes family (Brockman et al., 1970), transplanted rodent neoplasma (French and Blanz, 1966) and lymphoma of dogs (Creasey et al., 1972). Their activity against vaccinia virus is suggested to be by a mechanism different from that of the isatin thiosemicarbazones and related substances (Katz et al., 1974). Appreciable antiviral activity against herpes virus types I and II is shown by derivatives of 2-acetylpyridine thiosemicarbazones in cell culture (Shipman et al., 1981). Thus, azacycloheptanyl-2-acetylpyridine thiosemicarbazone is active in vitro by suppressing RNA synthesis and, as a secondary effect, DNA synthesis. It is also inhibitory to E. coli, plasmodia and leishmanial promastigotes (Brown et al., 1981). 2-Formyl pyridine thiosemicarbazone, 1-formylisoquinoline thiosemicarbazone and diphenyl thiocarbazone inhibit Rous sarcoma virus intracellularly (Levinson et al., 1977b). Most of the biological studies of these thiosemicarbazones have concentrated on their antineoplastic activity, which has been reviewed elsewhere (Agrawal and Sartorelli, 1978). Their inhibition of RNA and protein synthesis is less sensitive than their effects on DNA.

However, although 5-hydroxy-2-formylpyridine thiosemicarbazone shows antineoplastic activity in animals, it is largely inactive in humans, possibly because of its relatively low inhibitory potency for the target enzyme (Moore et al., 1971) or because it is rapidly converted to its glucuronide conjugate and eliminated (Dé Conti et al., 1972). It also produces extensive gastrointestinal toxicity and has a relatively low therapeutic index.

One of the most successful antineoplastic agents of this group is 4-methyl-5-amino-1-formylisoquinoline thiosemicarbazone which is water-soluble and about 60 times more effective than 5-hydroxy-2-formylpyridine thiosemicarbazone as an inhibitor of ribonucleoside diphosphate reductase. The 4-methyl group decreases the ease of inactivation of the drug by biological acetylation of the 5-amino group (Agrawal et al., 1976b). Its antiviral activity has not been assessed.

The antiviral and antitumour activities of these thiosemicarbazones may have a common origin, the primary site of action being in the biosynthesis of DNA. The postulated metabolic lesion is the inhibition of the iron(II) enzyme ribonucleoside diphosphate reductase (Moore et al., 1970). This enzyme synthesizes the deoxyribonucleoside diphosphates, precursors of the deoxyribonucleoside triphosphates needed in the DNA synthesis.

These α-(N)-heterocyclic thiosemicarbazones have been postulated (French and

Freedlander, 1958) to act in biological systems as terdentate ligands for metal ions, in particular iron(II) (French and Blanz, 1966). Chelation through the ring nitrogen, the 1'-nitrogen and the sulphur atom gives complexes as shown in Scheme XVIII (Campbell, 1975). Supporting evidence for such structures comes from the synthesis of the iron, cobalt, nickel (Ablov and Belichuk, 1969) and copper(II) (Antholine *et al.*, 1976) complexes of 2-formylpyridine thiosemicarbazone and from the X-ray crystal structure determination (Mathew and Palenik, 1969) of bis(isoquinoline-1-carboxaldehyde thiosemicarbazonato) nickel(II) monohydrate which showed that the ligand was terdentate and present in the thiol form as in Scheme XVIII. Antonini *et al.* (1977) concluded from spectrometric studies that 2-formylpyridine and 1-formylisoquinoline thiosemicarbazones had predominantly the E (anti-) configuration as a ligand (see also, Brown and Agrawal, 1977).

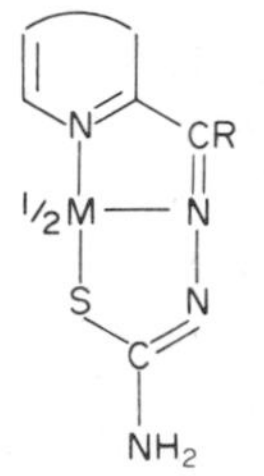

SCHEME XVIII

The inhibition of ribonucleoside diphosphate reductase may be the result of a ligand–Fe(II)–enzyme complex (Sartorelli *et al.*, 1971; Moore *et al.*, 1975). Enzyme studies have shown that α-(N)-heterocyclic thiosemicarbazones have some inhibitory activity, possibly by binding to the iron of the enzymes (Saryan *et al.*, 1979). Addition of ferric ions or the iron complexes of these ligands greatly enhanced the inhibitory response. This suggests that the iron complex was the actual inhibitor that interacts with the target enzyme (Saryan *et al.*, 1979; Agrawal *et al.*, 1974).

Inhibition of the formation of DNA in sarcoma 180 ascites cells was decreased considerably if an amino group was substituted for the sulphur atom of 1-formylisoquinoline thiosemicarbazone. Replacement of the sulphur by an oxygen atom eliminated activity. Similarly, the chelating ability and the extent to which DNA synthesis was inhibited by 5-hydroxy-2-formylpyridine thiosemicarbazone was greater than for the analogous seleno-semicarbazone, while the guanylhydrazone and semicarbazones were inactive, so that inhibition paralleled the iron-binding ability of these ligands (Michaud and Sartorelli, 1968). The α-N is essential for the antitumour activity of 6-formylpurine thiosemicarbazone: conversion to the N-oxide abolished this activity (Giner-Sorolla *et al.*, 1973).

By analogy with results for other ligands the Fe(II) complexes of these thiosemicarbazones would be expected to have stability constants similar to those of the zinc complexes. For the 1:2 Fe(II)-2-formylpyridine thiosemicarbazone complex the large value of $\log \beta_2' = 15.8$ at pH 7.4 has been reported (Antholine *et al.*, 1977b). $Fe(II)L_2$ and $Fe(III)L_{2+}$ were found to be very stable, kinetically inert and they did not dissociate in plasma. The ligand was able to remove Fe(III) from ferritin (Antholine *et al.*, 1977b). There is further evidence of the biological significance of the iron complexes of α-(N)-heterocyclic thiosemicarbazones: Administration of 5-hydroxy-2-formylpyridine thiosemicarbazone to patients with cancer led to a significant increase in excretion of iron, probably as the chelate (DéConti *et al.*, 1972; Krakoff *et al.*, 1974).

The stability constants of the copper and zinc complexes of 2-acetylpyridine thiosemicarbazone (= HL) have been determined conventionally, including the species $CuHL^{2+}$, CuL^+, CuLOH and $Cu(HL)L^+$ and $ZnHL^{2+}$, ZnL^+, ZnLOH, $Zn(HL)_2^{2+}$ and $Zn(HL)L^+$ (Agarwal and Perrin, 1976). The conditional stability constants $\log K_1'$ at pH = 7.4 are 13.1 for Cu^{2+} and 8.5 for Zn^{2+}. The former value agrees well with 13.4 found for 2-formylpyridine thiosemicarbazone (Antholine *et al.*, 1977a). However, Antholine *et al.*'s value for the zinc complexes (5.6) seems much too small and is probably due to the insensitivity of the spectrophotometric method and to the inclusion of only two complexes in their calculations.

Comparison with constants for amino acid complexes suggests that in biological systems the 1:1 copper–thiosemicarbazone complexes would be very little dissociated. The copper complex of 2-formylpyridine thiosemicarbazone survived in blood plasma, and it was found that also a mixed ligand complex, possibly with histidine, was formed (Antholine *et al.*, 1977b). This copper complex was found to be a catalyst for the oxidation of thiols by oxygen; the complex was thus cytotoxic for Ehrlich cells (Knight *et al.*, 1979).

The value of log K_1' for ZnL$^+$ is low, relative to copper(II) but this is partly offset by the higher concentration of zinc ion in biological systems. Comparison with other zinc complexes shows that the zinc complex of 2-acetylpyridine thiosemicarbazone is considerably more stable than, say, that of histidine (log $K_1' = 4.8$) or even albumin (log $K_1' = 7.6$, Agarwal and Perrin, 1976). And the tendency of zinc to form octahedral complexes could lead to significant contributions by the 1:2 complex ZnL$_2$ and by mixed ligand zinc complexes.

Calculation of metal–ion distributions in a computer model for blood plasma (Agarwal and Perrin, 1976) confirmed that 2-acetylpyridine thiosemicarbazone (active against influenza *in vitro* (Perrin, 1977)) is an effective chelating agent for zinc and copper under biological conditions. (Similar calculations have not yet been carried out for iron(II).) The inhibition *in vitro* of influenza virus RNA-dependent RNA polymerase (Oxford, 1977) may be due to complexation of the zinc ion of this enzyme.

The chelating agent 2-formyl-3-hydroxy-4,5-bis-(hydroxymethyl) pyridine thiosemicarbazone (Scheme XIX) was tested for its possible inhibitory effect on the zinc-requiring enzyme pyridoxal phosphokinase. However, its antineoplastic activity was associated with inhibition of DNA synthesis (Agrawal *et al.*, 1976a).

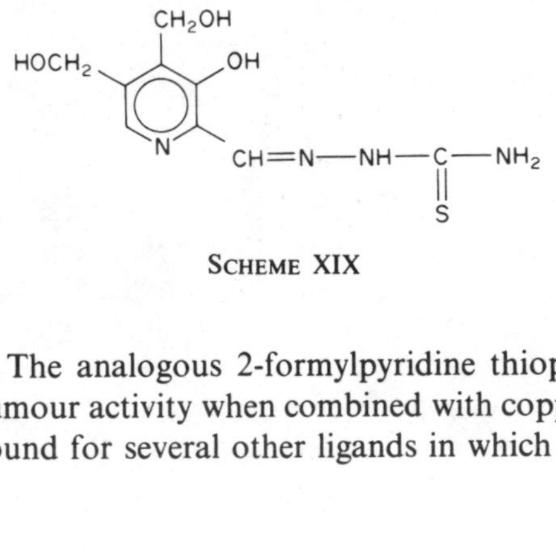

SCHEME XIX 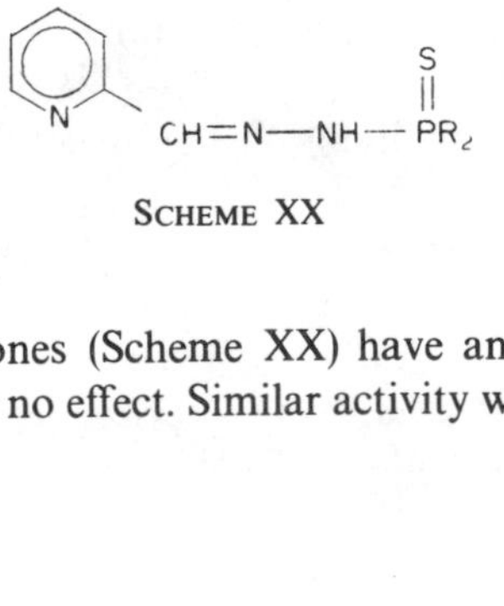   SCHEME XX

The analogous 2-formylpyridine thiophosphorus hydrazones (Scheme XX) have anti-tumour activity when combined with copper. Ferrous ion has no effect. Similar activity was found for several other ligands in which

$$
\begin{array}{c}
-\mathrm{PR_2} \\
\parallel \\
\mathrm{S}
\end{array}
$$

replaced the

$$
\begin{array}{c}
-\mathrm{C-NH_2} \\
\parallel \\
\mathrm{S}
\end{array}
$$

group (Cates *et al.*, 1976).

7.4.2.3. Isatin β-Thiosemicarbazone (IBT) and its Derivatives

7.4.2.3.1. *Effect on pox viruses.* Isatin β-thiosemicarbazone (Scheme XII) and its *N*-ethyl and *N*-methyl derivatives are efficient inhibitors of growth of pox viruses, comprising variola, alastrim, vaccinia, rabbitpox, monkeypox, ectromelia and cowpox. Rabbitpox virus that had become resistant to isatin β-thiosemicarbazone was also resistant to its *N*-methyl derivative (methisazone, 'marboran') and, to a lesser extent, to 4-bromo-3-methylisothiazole-5-carboxaldehyde thiosemicarbazone (Scheme XIII), indicating that these compounds have a common mode of action (Appleyard and Way, 1966). There was no cross-resistance with respect to *p*-fluorophenylalanine or 5-bromo-2′-deoxyuridine. The presence of isatin thiosemicarbazone does not impede the uptake of virus by the cells (Sheffield *et al.*, 1960). Hence the site of action is intracellular. Isatin β-thiosemicarbazone does not interfere with synthesis of viral DNA or other early stages of the viral cycle (Katz *et al.*, 1978). Its effects are produced late in the viral cycle and appear to lie in the assembly or maturation of viral components, so that the number of complete virus particles fails to increase (Easterbrook, 1962). Instead, immature virus particles appear in the cytoplasm (Katz *et al.*, 1973b). In the presence of isatin β-thiosemicarbazone the two main structural polypeptides of vaccinia virus are not formed, so that assembly of the viral cores is inhibited (Katz *et al.*, 1978). The precursor of one of the polypeptides (4a) is synthesized by the host cell but polypeptide 4a fails to cleave from it in the presence of isatin β-thiosemicarbazone (Katz *et al.*, 1973a). As a result of the failure of the viral DNA to combine with the necessary polypeptides it remains sensitive to destruction by nucleases (Katz *et al.*, 1978).

Earlier, Appleyard *et al.* (1965) had concluded that essentially the transcription (DNA-dependent RNA synthesis) was affected in the inhibition of rabbitpox virus by isatin thiosemicarbazone. Woodson and Joklik (1965) found the inhibition of vaccinia virus multiplication to be due to defective RNA synthesis: methisazone caused instability of the late messenger RNA of vaccinia virus so that the assembly of infective virus particles was prevented. Pennington (1977) concluded that isatin β-thiosemicarbazone inhibits growth in the pox viruses by interfering with the production of post-replicative viral proteins, resulting in premature cessation of synthesis of necessary proteins.

The mechanism by which viral polypeptides 4a and 4b are cleaved from their precursors is not known but a plausible speculation would be that a metal-activated enzyme, probably a peptidase, is involved in this step. Inhibition by isatin β-thiosemicarbazone was thought to be consistent with metal-chelating properties of thiosemicarbazones and with some of the effects of substitution. In particular, the sulphur atom in the sidechain was found to be essential for the antivaccinia activity of isatin β-thiosemicarbazones (Thompson *et al.*, 1953). Replacement of the sulphur by oxygen or an NH-group, which are both weak donors, abolished this activity (Sheffield *et al.*, 1960).

Tetradentate chelation of copper(II) by IBT as in Scheme XXI was reported by Barz and Fritz (1970). However, this complex had to be prepared at very low temperature to avoid reduction of copper(II) and formation of copper(I) complexes. These authors also suggested that in a neutral solution the zinc complexes contain the neutral ligand but gave no evidence for their proposed structures (cf. Campbell, 1975, p. 307). Contrarily, Hovorka and Holzbecher (1949) isolated a 1 : 2 zinc complex with the deprotonated ligand from an acetate buffered solution.

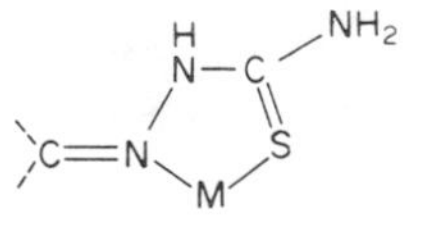

SCHEME XXI

The reactions of isatin β-thiosemicarbazones in aqueous solution have been investigated by Stünzi (1981, 1981a, 1982) with the water-soluble 5-sulphonatoisatin β-thiosemi-carbazone, SIBT (Scheme XXII). From pH-metric, kinetic and nuclear magnetic resonance (^{1}H and ^{13}C) studies it was concluded that this ligand is predominantly in the *Z* (*syn*) configuration (Scheme XXIIa). This agrees with a thorough study by Tomchin *et al.* (1974) for the non-sulphonated IBT. (Barz and Fritz (1970) postulated that the *E* (*anti*) isomer predominated.) In alkaline solutions, the ligand is deprotonated and isomerizes to the more stable *E* configuration (Scheme XXIIb). Only in this form is it possible that isatin β-thiosemicarbazones act as terdentate ligands as in Scheme XXI.

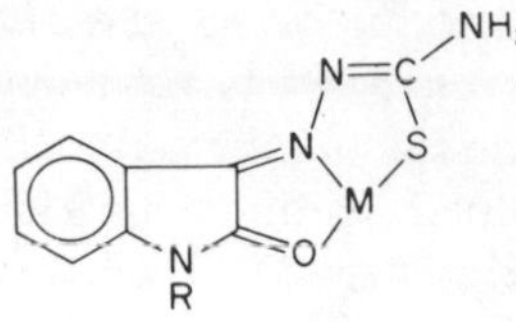

SCHEME XXII

In contrast to the speculations by Barz and Fritz (1970), at neutral pH zinc forms 1:2 complexes which contain the deprotonated ligand. The conditional stability constants at pH 7.4 for the zinc and iron(II) complexes of 5-sulphonatoisatin β-thiosemicarbazone and also its 1-methyl derivative are log $\beta'_1 = 4.5$ (Zn) and 3.6 (Fe) and log $\beta'_2 = 9.0$ (Zn) and 6.5 (Fe) (Stünzi, 1982). These values are comparable with those for the histidinato complexes, but log β_2' for $Zn(SIBT)_2^{3-}$ is much smaller than log β_2' for the bis-cysteinato zinc complex (10.8). The mixed ligand complex of zinc, SIBT and histidinate is less stable than statistically expected. The complexes of iron(III) are not stable enough to prevent extensive precipitation of ferric hydroxide.

Copper(II) is reduced by sulphonatoisatin β-thiosemicarbazones. With a moderate excess of ligand, the polymeric complex $Cu(I)_n L_n^{n-}$ (with $n > 6$) is a main species at physiological pH and total copper concentrations as low as 8 μM. With a very large excess of ligand monomeric 1:2 complexes $Cu(I)L_2^{3-}$ were formed (Stünzi, 1981a). As the sulphonate substituent is unlikely to affect the nature of the equilibria, similar reactions are likely with the non-sulphonated isatin β-thiosemicarbazone and its 1-methyl derivative, methisazone. The polymeric copper(I) complex would be uncharged and probably insoluble.

In contrast to many speculations, the complexes of isatin β-thiosemicarbazone are not very stable and are not expected to be important under biological situations. The stability of the complexes of bidentate thiosemicarbazones, such as benzaldehyde thiosemicarbazones, is considerably smaller (Stünzi, 1982); these complexes would not be formed *in vivo*.

Aromatic ring systems bearing the thiosemicarbazone sidechain, but lacking an additional donor atom to form a terdentate ligand (e.g. γ-thiochromanone-4-thiosemicarbazone) have antivaccinial activity (Katz *et al.*, 1974) and cross-resistance studies suggest that these have the same mode of action as isatin β-thiosemicarbazone, and this is different from that of the α-(*N*)-heterocyclic thiosemicarbazones (Katz *et al.*, 1974). Similarly, several *N*-substituted 2-chloro-3-formylindole thiosemicarbazones (Andreani *et al.*, 1975) were more active and the *N*-isopropyl derivative was comparable to methisazone in its action on vaccinia virus (Andreani *et al.*, 1977). These ligands are not expected to form more stable complexes than benzaldehyde thiosemicarbazones for which *in vivo* chelation can be excluded. The similar antivaccinia activity of isatin β-thiosemicarbazones is hence not the result of their modest chelating ability (Stünzi, 1982).

That steric effects are important in the activity of isatin β-thiosemicarbazone could explain the variations produced by substitution or by varying the structure of the molecule. Substitution in the 5-position of the benzene ring usually decreases or abolishes activity against vaccinia virus (Bauer and Sadler, 1960). A correlation has been suggested between the antiviral activity of these compounds and their lipophilicity (Bauer and Sadler, 1960; Andreani *et al.*, 1979).

7.4.2.3.2. *Effects on other viruses.* Isatin β-thiosemicarbazone and its derivatives also inhibit the growth *in vitro* of a wide range of both DNA and RNA viruses, but they exhibit different structure-activity relationships (Bauer *et al.*, 1970).

Like the pox viruses, adenoviruses are DNA-type, so that a similar structure-activity relationship to that of isatin β-thiosemicarbazones with vaccinia is found for methisazone with a number of adenoviruses in HeLa cells (Bauer and Apostolov, 1966). Unlike vaccinia virus, ectromelia virus is sensitive to the 4',4'-dimethyl derivative of isatin thiosemicarbazone

(Bauer and Sadler, 1961). Activity falls off if larger groups replace either or both of the methyl groups. On the other hand, isatin 3-(4',4'-dibutyl)thiosemicarbazone inhibits replication of polio virus in HeLa cells (Pearson and Zimmerman, 1969) and 1-methylisatin β-4',4'-diethyl-thiosemicarbazone inhibited Molony Leukaemia virus which is a RNA tumour virus (Sherman *et al.*, 1980). Methisazone decreases the reverse transcriptase activity and cytopathic effect of the RNA slow viruses which cause the diseases visna and maedi (Haase and Levinson, 1973). However, there is a serious problem in treating diseases caused by tumour viruses with these drugs. In mice infected with leukaemia virus, the leukaemia is enhanced by methisazone, probably because of a suppression of the immune system by this drug (Levy *et al.*, 1976).

Inserting an alkyl group on the sulphur atom to give isatin β-isothiosemicarbazones (Scheme XXIII) removes the complexing ability of the sulphur atom. These derivatives still inhibit Mungo virus RNA synthesis (Tonew and Tonew, 1974) and the corresponding RNA polymerase (Tonew *et al.*, 1974a, 1974b). Based on the preparation of copper and zinc complexes or salts it has been claimed (Heinisch and Tresselt, 1977) that this biological activity is due to complexation. However, they observed that the aqueous phase over the precipitated complex contained free ligand and metal ion but no complexes. Under the highly dilute *in vivo* conditions, complexation would therefore not be expected to be appreciable.

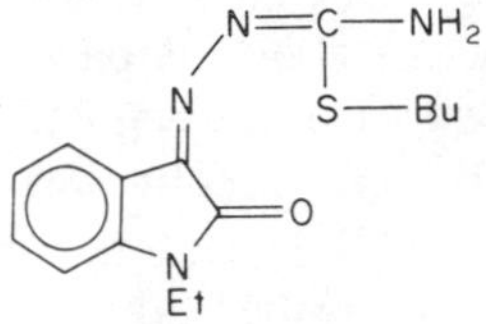

SCHEME XXIII

Thus it seems likely that substituted isatin β-thiosemicarbazones exert their antiviral effects at different points of the viral cycle, depending on the nature of the particular virus. Metal chelation is unlikely to be involved in the *in vivo* antiviral action of these compounds.

7.4.2.4. Contact Inhibition by Isatin-β-Thiosemicarbazones

Extracellular contact of retroviruses (Rous sarcoma, murine sarcoma or murine leukaemia virus) with isatin-β-thiosemicarbazones inactivates the malignant transforming ability of these viruses towards tissue cultures. At the same time there is inhibition of the viral reverse transcriptase (RNA-dependent DNA polymerase) and the viruses lose their ability to multiply in cells (Levinson *et al.*, 1971, 1973; Levy *et al.*, 1976).

Three other types of copper-binding ligands (8-hydroxyquinolines, 1,10-phenanthrolines and isonicotinic acid hydrazide) and their copper complexes also inactivate, on contact *in vitro*, the ability of these RNA tumour viruses to induce malignant transformation of chick embryo cells (Levinson *et al.*, 1977b, Valenzuela *et al.*, 1973).

Herpes simplex virus is sensitive to similar contact inhibition by isatin thiosemicarbazones in phosphate buffers but not in media (for example, Eagle's minimal essential medium) where proteins or free tryptophan or histidine apparently protects the virions (Levinson *et al.*, 1974). Contact inhibition of arenavirus was prevented by EDTA; it took place only in the presence of both methisazone and metal ions (Logan *et al.*, 1975). Many other viruses were subsequently found to be inhibited on contact with methisazone plus excess copper ion in a phosphate-buffered saline (Fox *et al.*, 1977) but not in media where other naturally occurring ligands were abundant. It is suggested that methisazone potentiated the inactivation of these viruses by divalent copper by serving as a scavenger and a vehicle to transport copper to the virus (Fox *et al.*, 1977). Similarly, methisazone, as its copper complex, but not as the free ligand, inhibits transfection by purified lambda phage DNA in *Escherichia coli* (Levinson and

Helling, 1976). Copper complexes of thiosemicarbazide inactivate lambda phage infectivity and transfection by lambda phage DNA. They also inhibit the activity of RNA-dependent DNA polymerase of Rous sarcoma virus (Pillai *et al.*, 1977).

On the other hand, methisazone has essentially the same activity as its copper chelate against Rous sarcoma virus, as measured by inhibition of the RNA-dependent DNA polymerase activity (Kaska *et al.*, 1978). This result is consistent with the effect being due to the *ligand* (methisazone) directly, or following dissociation of its copper complex, forming a complex with the enzyme, the copper ion presumably being bound elsewhere.

It has been conjectured, mainly on the basis of filter retention, centrifugation and gel filtration experiments that methisazone, copper(II) and nucleic acids (Mikelens *et al.*, 1976) or proteins (Rohde *et al.*, 1979) form ternary complexes in solution. This conclusion is doubtful because the experiments describe the co-precipitation of the copper methisazone complex (which is insoluble in water) onto poorly soluble nucleic acids. The copper complex is likely to be the polymeric copper(I) complex (Stünzi, 1981a) and not a copper(II) complex CuL^+ (Kaska *et al.*, 1978) which would have been quite soluble in water. When the copper methisazone complex was solubilized by larger concentrations of dimethyl sulphoxide, there was no evidence of interaction with nucleic acids. The coprecipitation was also prevented if EDTA, histidine and some other strong chelating agents were present. This effect is therefore unlikely to occur *in vivo*.

The *in vitro* contact inhibition as described above, however, may well be the result of the formation of the insoluble copper methisazone complex which would coprecipitate with the nucleic acids or proteins of the viruses. Such coprecipitation may also explain the inhibition of Rous Sarcoma Virus reverse transcriptase by interaction with the template DNA (Mikelens *et al.*, 1978; Levinson *et al.*, 1973). The interaction of copper(II), thiosemicarbazide and DNA (Pillai *et al.*, 1977) may, analogously, be due to the formation and coprecipitation of the insoluble copper(I) complex of the deprotonated thiosemicarbazide (Campbell, 1975).

7.4.3. PHOSPHONIC ACIDS

7.4.3.1. *Phosphonoacetic Acid*

Phosphonoacetic acid (PAA, Scheme XXIV) was shown to inhibit the replication of herpes simplex virus in mice and rabbits (Shipkowitz *et al.*, 1973) and in tissue cultures (Overby *et al.*, 1974). It blocks the replication of all herpes viruses so far examined, including herpes simplex viruses, cytomegalo virus (Huang, 1975), herpesvirus saimiri, Epstein—Barr virus (the causative agent of infectious mononucleosis), pseudorabies virus, equine abortion virus and Marek's disease virus (Hay *et al.*, 1977) by inhibiting a virus-induced DNA polymerase activity. It inhibited the production of Epstein—Barr virus capsid antigen and drastically decreased, but did not abolish, the synthesis of infectious virus particles (Rickinson and Epstein, 1978), so that PAA resistant mutants of Epstein—Barr virus could be selectively cultured. Subacute myeloopticoneuropathy virus (Nishiba and Inoue, 1978) and herpesvirus hominis (Kern *et al.*, 1977) have recently been found to be sensitive to PAA *in vitro* and *in vivo* (mice). It is also effective against varicella zoster (May *et al.*, 1977) and African swine fever virus (Moreno *et al.*, 1978) *in vitro*, and two pox viruses (vaccinia and Shope fibroma virus) in rabbits (Friedman-Kien *et al.*, 1976). It has been used in the treatment of warts (Clark, 1977). Other DNA viruses (such as simian virus-40 and human adenovirus-12) and RNA viruses (such as polio virus, rhinovirus or measles virus) were not inhibited (Overby *et al.*, 1977).

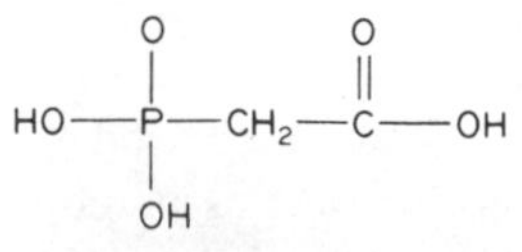

SCHEME XXIV

Using plaque reduction technique on cell cultures, PAA at the concentrations generally used (up to 200 μg/ml of the disodium salt) was not cytotoxic and non-mutagenic to uninfected cells in culture but it effectively blocked herpesvirus replication (Becker et al., 1976). At higher concentrations (200–1000 μg/ml) it is cytotoxic to normal or infected cells, inhibiting cell growth and cellular DNA synthesis (Huang, 1973, Nyormoi et al., 1976).

PAA seems to be of low topical and systemic toxicity in animals except in suckling mice (Nishiba and Inoue, 1978) and it was irritating when applied liberally in a 2–5 per cent cream-ointment to herpetic skin lesions on the genitalia of cebus monkeys (Palmer et al., 1977). This local irritancy and also the existence of PAA-resistant mutants (Newton, 1979) may limit its usefulness. Also, established infections do not always respond to treatment with PAA (Alenius and Öberg, 1978; Descamps et al., 1979). Nevertheless, in a comparison with four other antiviral drugs, PAA was the only compound with a good therapeutic activity for topical treatment of cutaneous herpesvirus infection in guinea pigs (Alenius and Öberg, 1978) and, with 1 per cent solution, skin irritation was seen only occasionally (see also Descamps et al., 1979).

PAA is often used topically, but when administered intraperitoneally it was also active against herpesvirus injected into the brains of hamsters (Overby et al., 1977).

The most valuable results have been obtained in the treatment of established herpetic keratitis and iritis in eyes of rabbits (Meyer et al., 1976; Gordon et al., 1977). Gerstein et al. (1975) applied PAA topically as a 5 per cent solution of the disodium salt and Meyer et al., (1976) used intravenous injection. No serious toxicity was encountered so that PAA was claimed to be suitable for trials in Man. It was also effective against herpetic keratitis resistant to iododeoxyuridine, the drug currently in use in Man (which was shown to be carcinogenic by Prusoff and Goz, 1973).

Treatment of the viruses or cells with PAA prior to infection had no effect on herpes simplex virus replication (Barahona et al., 1977). PAA did not inhibit absorption, penetration or release of the virus, nor the synthesis of RNA and 'early' proteins (Overby et al., 1974), but it affected the synthesis of DNA and the 'late' proteins (Honess and Watson, 1977) and was virostatic. PAA selectively binds to, and inhibits, the herpesvirus-induced DNA polymerase (Mao and Robishaw, 1975; Mao et al., 1975; Huang, 1975; Huang et al., 1976; Summers and Klein, 1976; Overby et al., 1977) at concentrations (around 1–2 μM) that do not significantly reduce cellular DNA synthesis. PAA did not prevent the formation of a DNA–enzyme complex, and inhibition was non-competitive with respect to the deoxyribonucleoside triphosphates. The mechanism of the phosphonoacetate inhibition of herpesvirus-induced DNA polymerase (from studies with Marek's disease virus and herpes virus of turkeys) is suggested to be by direct competition with pyrophosphate at a binding site on the DNA polymerase molecule (Leinbach et al., 1976). PAA acts as a competitive inhibitor by blocking the site that should accept pyrophosphate liberated in the formation of DNA from the deoxyribonucleoside triphosphates.

Several esters of PAA have been tested in an assay of herpesvirus-induced polymerase and orally in mice, but only the low molecular weight carboxyl esters of PAA were active (Herrin et al., 1977). Methylation of the CH_2-group decreased the activity. The dimethylated product (2-methyl-2-phosphonopropionate) and 2-aminophosphonoacetate were inactive against herpes virus of turkeys (Leinbach et al., 1976). Many similar compounds of the structure $X–CH_2–Y$ were also inactive, including methylene diphosphonate, malonate, sulphoacetate, aminomethyl phosphonate (Leinbach et al., 1976), and phosphonoacetaldehyde, phosphonoacetamide and longer chain analogues of PAA such as phosphonopropionate (Reno et al., 1978).

On the other hand, phosphonoformate is as effective as PAA in selectively inhibiting herpes virus-induced DNA polymerase (Helgestrand et al., 1978; Reno et al., 1978).

7.4.3.2. Phosphonoformic Acid

Phosphonoformate (PFA) also inhibits DNA polymerase of hepatitis B virus (Alenius et al., 1978) and vesicular stomatitis virus transcriptase (Chanda and Banerjee, 1980).

Influenza-virus RNA polymerase is inhibited by PFA (Helgestrand *et al.*, 1978) much more strongly than by PAA (Stridh *et al.*, 1979). This activity was enhanced in the presence of magnesium or manganese(II) ions. In cell culture, PFA has an antiviral effect on herpesvirus type 1 and 2, pseudorabies virus and infectious bovine rhinotrachitis virus (Helgestrand *et al.*, 1978) and also herpesvirus sylvilagus (Goodrich *et al.*, 1980). PFA inhibited the synthesis of Epstein–Barr virus capsid antigen at concentrations that were not toxic to cells but did not inhibit the synthesis of EBV nuclear antigen (Margalith *et al.*, 1980).

PFA is also effective against cutaneous herpes virus infections in the guinea pig but, unlike PAA, it is not locally skin-irritating (Alenius *et al.*, 1978; Alenius, 1980). A 2 per cent PFA topical cream showed marked therapeutic activity when applied on infected guinea-pig skin. It has also been similarly effective when tested on humans (Wallin *et al.*, 1980).

At concentrations up to 10 mM, phosphonoformate is not cytotoxic but is antiviral towards herpes virus. (A limitation to the use of phosphonoformate is its instability in acid solutions (Warren and Williams, 1971).) It primarily affected DNA synthesis and cell proliferation in cell cultures, but the inhibition was reversed if phosphonoformate was removed from the cells (Stenberg and Larsson, 1978). Phosphonoformate is also reported to inhibit DNA polymerase α of human cells (Sabourin *et al.*, 1978), but the viral DNA polymerase is 15–30 times more sensitive than the host DNA polymerase-α (Sabourin *et al.*, 1978; see also Modak *et al.*, 1980).

PAA-resistant mutants of herpes simplex virus induce a PAA-resistant DNA polymerase (Becker *et al.*, 1977; Hay and Subak-Sharpe, 1976; Honess and Watson, 1977; Purifoy and Powell, 1977). The presence of resistant variants in the viral population could lead to their accumulation, following repeated dosage of PAA, so that antiviral activity would be diminished. Intact nuclei were resistant to higher concentrations of PAA than the purified viral DNA polymerase, probably because the nuclear membrane prevented penetration of the drug (Fridlender *et al.*, 1978b).

PAA-resistant DNA polymerase is also resistant to PFA (Reno *et al.*, 1976, 1978) hence PAA and PFA apparently have the same mode of action (Kern *et al.*, 1978).

Phosphonoacetate (PAA^{3-}) is a bidentate ligand forming a chelate 6-ring with a metal ion (Scheme XXV). The stability constants of PAA with Mg^{2+}, Ca^{2+}, Cu^{2+} and Zn^{2+} have been determined (Stünzi and Perrin, 1979). Among similar ligands are malonate (with smaller stability constants) and methylenediphosphonate or pyrophosphate (with greater stability constants for the metal complexes).

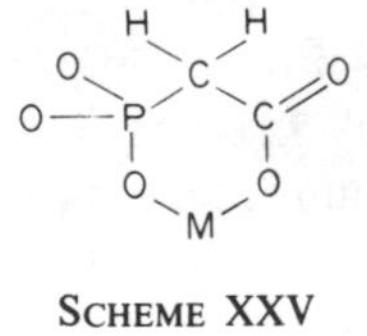

SCHEME XXV

A theoretical blood plasma model (based on that by Agarwal and Perrin, 1976), used to compute the extent of competition between PAA and other biomolecules for the complexation of metal ions, showed that PAA did not significantly affect the copper ion distribution. There was not a large reduction in the concentration of free zinc ion but zinc/PAA complexes were predominant among the low molecular weight zinc complexes. The free magnesium ion concentration was significantly reduced in this model. Hence it is reasonable to suggest that complex formation is involved in the inhibition of viral DNA polymerase by PAA as the DNA polymerases are zinc enzymes and need magnesium ion as a cofactor. Within the model, there is an appreciable amount of $CaPAA^-$ formed which could be connected with the retention of PAA in bones (Bopp *et al.*, 1977).

Like PAA, absorbed PFA can bind tightly, but reversibly, to the inorganic matrix of bone. No adverse effects of this binding have been noted, but the United States Food and Drug Administration have withdrawn PAA and PFA from clinical testing (Wallin *et al.*, 1980).

Phosphonoformate could bind to a metal ion in a similar manner to phosphonoacetate but forming a chelate 5-ring. From the experience with other ligands it seems reasonable to assume that the phosphonoformate complexes have stability constants similar to (or slightly larger than) the corresponding PAA complexes. On the other hand, phosphonopropionate is limited to formation of 7-membered rings and such complexes are known to have much lower stability constants. The antiviral activity of these three homologues is consistent with these expectations. The C-propyl and diethyl esters of PAA are also inhibitors although they are only weak ligands but it is not known whether the esters are catalytically hydrolysed by metal ions to give free PAA, under biological conditions (Margalith *et al.*, 1980).

A study has been made of PAA as a non-competitive inhibitor of sheep kidney pyruvate carboxylase with respect to MgATP (Ashman and Keach, 1975).

7.4.4. OTHER CHELATING AGENTS WITH ANTIVIRAL ACTIVITY

Because metal ions are involved in many enzymic reactions which are part of the virus cycle, any sufficiently strong chelating agent would be expected to exert antiviral activity. Many chelating agents have been used in *in vitro* studies on viral enzymes as discussed earlier in this Review. However, only those ligands that have shown activity against virions either *in vivo* or in tissue culture are included here.

The substances given below almost certainly form complexes in a biological environment but it is not known to what degree this is connected with their antiviral action.

7.4.4.1. β-Diketones

Aryl alkyl, aryloxy alkyl and aryl *bis*, β-diketones (Schemes XXVI–XXVIII) have antiviral activity against RNA and DNA viruses. (Diana *et al.*, 1977a, 1977b, 1978). The substituents in the phenyl rings contribute mainly to the lipophilicity of the molecules.

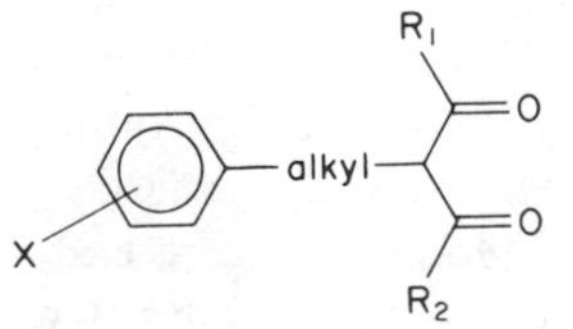

SCHEME XXVI

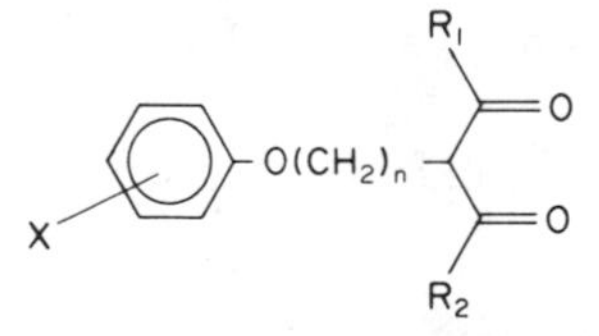

One of the most active has: X = 2–Cl, 4–OH

n = 6

$R_1 = R_2 = CH_3$

SCHEME XXVII

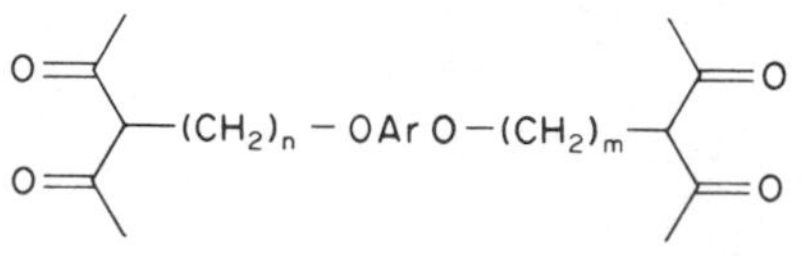

SCHEME XXVIII

Arildone, 4-(6-(2-chloro-4-methoxy)phenoxyl)-hexyl-3,5-heptane dione (Scheme XXVII) is a promising member of this series. It inhibits herpes simplex virus in tissue culture if it is added to the culture within 6 hr of infection (Kuhrt *et al.*, 1979). Arildone showed antiviral activity when tested *in vitro* against murine cytomegalovirus, herpes simplex virus 1 and 2, rhinoviruses, Semliki Forest virus, vesicular stomatitis virus and coxsackie virus A9 (Kim *et al.*, 1980). Results with polio virus suggest that uncoating of the virion is inhibited, preventing the virus-induced shutoff of host-cell protein synthesis (McSharry *et al.*, 1979).

Arildone is not virucidal and the inhibition can be removed by washing. It does not interfere significantly with the macromolecular synthesis in the host cells (Kuhrt *et al.*, 1979). Arildone (Pancic *et al.*, 1978) and other 3,5-heptanediones have been effective topically against herpesvirus infections in the rabbit eye, guinea-pig skin and mouse vagina.

These compounds (Schemes XXVI–XXVIII) are β-diketones and hence are derivatives of acetylacetone (pentane-2,4-dione) which is a well-known chelating agent. Because acetylacetonate has been shown to inhibit the iron enzyme peroxidase (Gemant, 1977), complexation of iron was suggested as the likely mode of action but an equally good case could be made out for other metal ions, especially copper. Thus, our computer-based blood plasma model shows that with published stability constants of Cu^{2+} and Zn^{2+} acetylacetonates (Gutnikov and Freiser, 1968) and estimates of the constants for mixed metal-(amino acid)-acetylacetonate complexes (based on known constants for ternary amino acid complexes with other two oxygen-type ligands) there would be a significant formation of copper acetylacetonate complexes (among the low molecular weight complexes) at ligand concentrations above 10^{-4} M.

Most of the antiviral testing of β-diketones has been done *in vitro*. Effects *in vivo* have been less dramatic probably because of limited penetrability of these agents into tissues. The use of vehicles to deliver these drugs more efficiently is under study. (Diana *et al.*, 1978a).

7.4.4.2. Flavonoids

Quercetin, morin and several other flavonoids were virucidal to the enveloped viruses, pseudorabies virus, parainfluenza virus and herpes simplex virus (Beladi *et al.*, 1977). Quercetin and morin had a prophylactic effect against rabies virus in mice (Cutting *et al.*, 1949, 1953) and they were also effective against Mengovirus-induced encephalitis in mice when administered orally (Veckenstedt *et al.*, 1978). Flavonoids also show activity against vesicular stomatitis virus when tested in cell culture (Wacker and Eilmes, 1978). Maximum inhibition was at $200\,\mu g$ flavonoid/ml, added 6–8 hr before viral infection.

Stability constant data for the metal complexes of these flavonoids are not available but their chelating group (Scheme XXIX) resembles that of Alizarin Red S (Scheme XXX) for complex formation through the carbonyl and deprotonated peri-hydroxyl group, so that comparable stability constants are expected. Alternatively, if the deprotonated 2-hydroxyl group binds to the metal ion, the flavonoids also resemble kojic acid (Scheme XXXI). At pH 7.4, the zinc complex of Alizarin Red S is 10 times as stable as the zinc histidine complex or the zinc kojate. The Alizarin Red S and kojic acid complexes of copper(II) are less stable than those of histidine. (Data from Sillén and Martell, 1964, 1971; Perrin, 1979.) Assuming comparable stability for the complexes of the flavonoids, complexation of zinc under biological conditions seems likely.

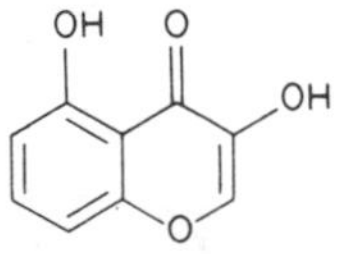

SCHEME XXIX

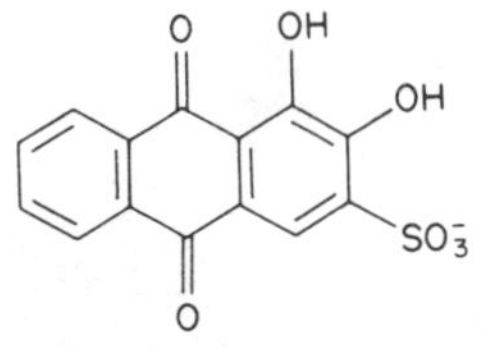

SCHEME XXX

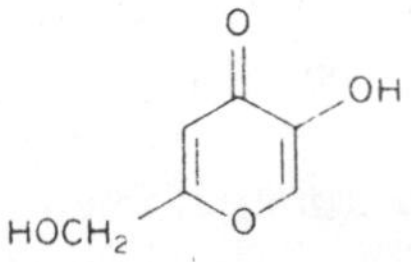

SCHEME XXXI

7.4.4.3. Selenocystine

Selenocystine (Scheme XXXII) was active against influenza virus PR8 in mice and Rous sarcoma virus in chicks by inhibiting selectively the viral RNA polymerase but not the DNA-dependent RNA polymerase (Ho *et al.*, 1967). Addition of 5 mM dithiothreitol may cleave the Se—Se bond in selenocystine, thereby reversing its inhibitory effect toward influenza RNA polymerase activity (Billard and Peets, 1974).

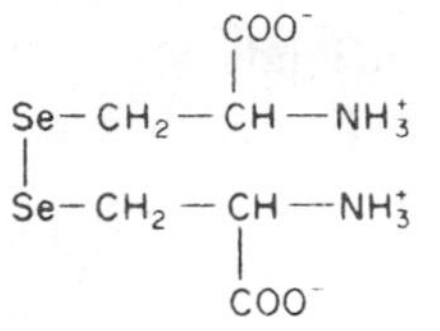

$$
\begin{array}{c}
\text{COO}^- \\
| \\
\text{Se—CH}_2\text{—CH—NH}_3^+ \\
| \\
\text{Se—CH}_2\text{—CH—NH}_3^+ \\
| \\
\text{COO}^-
\end{array}
$$

SCHEME XXXII

7.4.4.4. EDTA

EDTA (Scheme VI) inactivated purified tobacco rattle virus possibly due to removal of divalent metal ions from the virions, making the internal RNA accessible to attack by a ribonuclease present in the preparation (Robinson and Raschké, 1977). It is likely that EDTA lowers the intracellular free calcium ion concentration. Calcium ions bound to virions are removed, facilitating the separation of proteins from the nucleic acid (Brady *et al.*, 1977; Cohen *et al.*, 1979). This may trigger the uncoating process. If the virion is disassembled extracellularly the nucleic acid is accessible to attack by nucleases (Durham, 1977; Durham and Hendry, 1977). The ubiquitous nature of calcium makes it difficult to take advantage of calcium chelation for therapeutic purposes.

Calcium ion is also an essential cofactor for all neuraminidases, so that EDTA was effective against influenza virus neuraminidase (Rafelson *et al.*, 1963). We can speculate that application of EDTA solution by means of a nasal spray to people at risk might slow down the release and spread of the virus. This, in turn, would give more time for the host's immune system to become operative.

7.4.4.5. 8-Hydroxyquinoline

8-Hydroxyquinoline (Scheme V) and some of its derivatives inhibited the RNA-dependent DNA polymerase of avian myeloblastosis virus (Auld *et al.*, 1974) and of Rous sarcoma virus and abolished the ability of the latter virus to malignantly transform cells on contact (Levinson *et al.*, 1977b; Rohde *et al.*, 1976). The copper complex of 5-chloro-7-iodo-8-hydroxyquinoline is reported to coprecipitate with nucleic acid, but it is doubtful whether this is of any importance in the antiviral activity of the ligands. Treatment with 8-hydroxyquinoline had no effect on the resolution of herpetic keratitis in rabbits (Rohde *et al.*, 1976).

The antibacterial and antifungal activity of hydroxyquinoline in conjunction with the metal binding ability of this ligand are discussed by Albert (1973).

Rous sarcoma reverse transcriptase was also inhibited by 8-mercapto and 8-amino-quinoline and 8-hydroxyquinoline-5-sulphonate (Rohde *et al.*, 1976). The sulfonated ligand forms charged 1 : 2 metal complexes with stability constants similar to those of the parent compound and the increased solubility of the ligand and the complexes allows quantitative measurements in aqueous solution. The conditional stability constants at pH = 7.4, log K_1' and log K_2', of the copper and zinc complexes (Gutnikov and Freiser, 1968) are larger than those of the histidinato complexes by 3 and 2 logarithmic units, respectively. Hence complex formation in a biological environment can be considered certain. Compared with 8-hydroxyquinoline, the 8-mercaptoquinoline complexes with zinc ion are considerably more stable, and those with copper ion much less so (Gutnikov and Freiser, 1968). 8-Aminoquinoline is a much weaker ligand (Sillén and Martell, 1971). Quantitative studies of inhibition, taken in conjunction with differences in the measured metal binding selectivity and stabilities of the complexes, might provide more information about possible mechanisms of action and the involvement of metal ions.

7.4.4.6. 2-Mercapto-1-(β-4-pyridethyl)-benzimidazole

2-Mercapto-1-(β-4-pyridethyl)-benzimidazole inhibited the synthesis of a 'late' enzyme (RNA polymerase) of vaccinia virus (Nishigori and Nishimura, 1977) and the induction of herpes simplex DNA polymerase (Nishigori et al., 1978) in HeLa cells by disorganizing nucleolar structure.

The unsubstituted 2-mercaptobenzimidazole (Scheme XXXIII) was reported to form chelate (4-ring) complexes with Cu^{2+}, Al^{3+} and Fe^{3+} (Foye and Lo, 1972) and at pH 7.4 the 1:2 copper complex had a conditional stability constant of 10^{15} which is comparable with that of the 1:2 copper histidinate complex ($10^{14.3}$). Because of the magnitude of this constant, metal ion chelation may be involved in the biological action of 2-mercaptobenzimidazole derivatives. However, the formation of a copper(II) complex is doubtful in view of the reducing tendency of thiol compounds (cf. thiosemicarbazones).

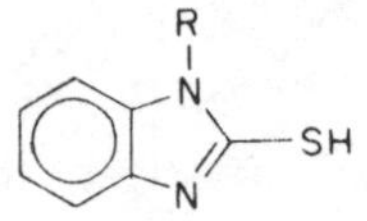

SCHEME XXXIII

7.4.4.7. Isoniazid

Isoniazid (pyridine-4-carboxylic acid hydrazide) (Scheme XXXIV) is a weak chelating agent. The conditional stability constants at pH 7.4 of the copper and zinc complexes with isoniazid (log K'_1 = 4.4 and 2.2) are considerably smaller than those of other ligands present in cells (compare ATP (6.0 and 5.2), or amino acids such as glycine (6.0 and 2.9) so that the isoniazid complexes are unlikely to survive inside a cell). In the presence of copper ion and isoniazid, the DNA polymerase and the malignantly transforming activity of Rous sarcoma virus were inhibited. It is suggested that an uncharged 1:2 metal–ligand complex enters cells or virions and on dissociation leads to toxicity due to the metal ion (Antony et al., 1978).

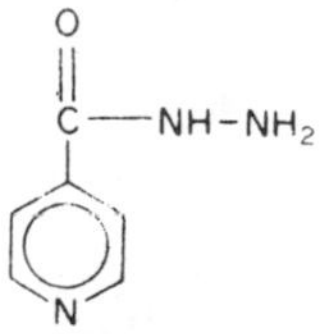

SCHEME XXXIV

7.4.5. ANTIVIRAL AGENTS WITH POSSIBLE CHELATING ABILITY

Other antiviral agents which are possible metal-chelating agents have been reported but it is not yet known whether the two properties are related. Often, the stability constants of the complexes have not been reported so that the extent of complex formation under physiological conditions can only be conjectured.

Flavonoid-type, metal-binding possibilities exist in the glycosidic anthracycline antibiotics such as daunomycin and adriamycin. They contain the chelating group given in Scheme XXXV and have been shown to have antitumour and antiviral activity. In vitro, they

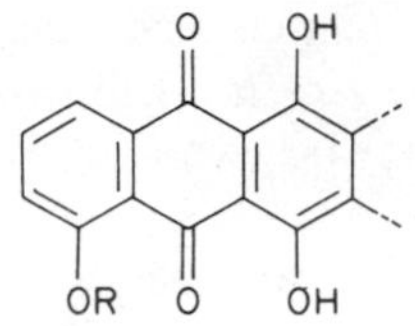

SCHEME XXXV

inhibit the DNA polymerase of Rous sarcoma virus (Apple *et al.*, 1971), Rauscher's leukaemia virus and avian myeloblastosis virus (Papas and Schafer, 1977) and there was a decrease in the number of sarcomas induced in chicks by Rous sarcoma virus (Apple *et al.*, 1972). The currently suggested mechanism of inhibition involves specific interaction with AT base pairs on the nucleic acid templates chosen (Sethi, 1977; Papas and Schafer, 1977).

Bleomycins, a family of glycopeptide antibiotics, have been isolated as their copper chelates. Copper-free bleomycins inhibit replication of vaccinia virus in HeLa cells and protect mice against vaccinia infection (Takeshita *et al.*, 1974; Takashita *et al.*, 1977). The significance of metal complexation in the biological activity of bleomycins has been reviewed (Umezawa and Takita, 1980). Bleomycin interacts with, and induces breaks in, DNA (Suzuki *et al.*, 1969). *In vitro*, the process requires iron and oxygen (Sausville *et al.*, 1976). Bleomycin also inhibits the synthesis of viral DNA (Takeshita *et al.*, 1977).

Modified rifamycin antibiotics (Scheme XXXVI) are potentially metal-chelating agents either through the peri phenolic OH groups or through the other phenolic OH and a nitrogen on the adjacent sidechain (R). Several of these compounds inhibit oncornavirus reverse transcriptase and also the morphological transformation of cell cultures with sarcoma-inducing oncornaviruses (Gurgo *et al.*, 1971).

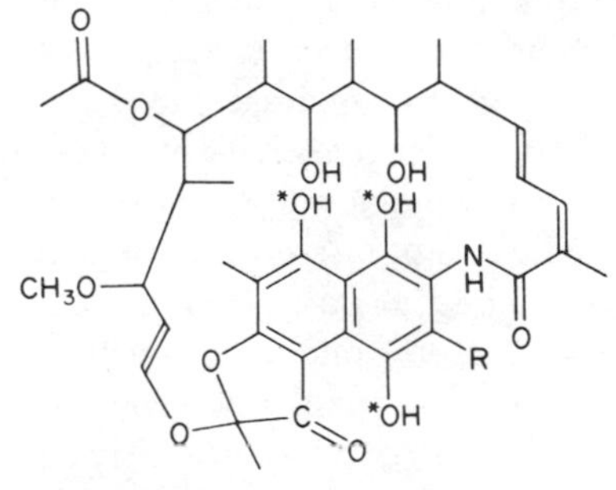

R = −CH=N−NR'R"
  −CH₂−NR'R"
  −NR'R"

SCHEME XXXVI

A potentially useful generalization seems to be that many antiherpes agents are bidentate ligands with two oxygens as metal-binding (donor) atoms. This is true for PAA, PFA and the β-diketones. This list can be extended by including the glyoxal derivative (Scheme XXXVII), 6-bromonaphthaquinone (Bonaphthon, Scheme XXXVIII) and the tetrazine (Scheme XXXIX) (Swallow, 1978), as well as humic acids and polyphenols (Klöcking *et al.*, 1978; Klöcking *et al.*, 1979).

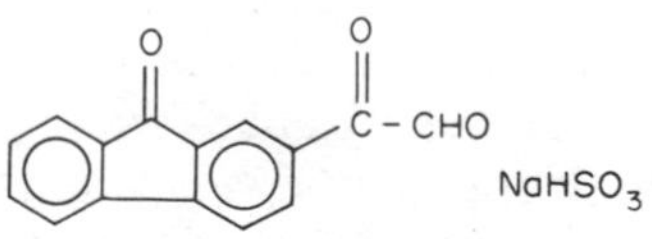

SCHEME XXXVII

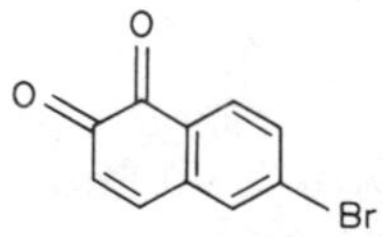

SCHEME XXXVIII

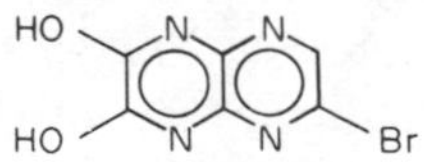

SCHEME XXXIX

Many other antiviral compounds (e.g. nucleoside analogues) may bind to metal ions to a limited extent in pure solutions. However, in a competitive ligand situation such as exists under physiological conditions they may be unable to compete for the low concentrations of metal ions.

1-Aminoadamantane (amantidine) is not a chelating agent and complex formation with copper or zinc ion in aqueous solution is negligible. Thus, any attempt to use its copper or zinc complexes, synthesized in non-aqueous solvents, in antiviral testing (Roos and Williams, 1977) results in immediate dissociation; observed effects are due to either the 1-aminoadamantane or the free metal ion.

7.4.6. METAL ION MANIPULATON

For optimal functioning of biological systems, free metal ion concentrations have to lie within controlled limits. Their levels are determined by the many complexing agents that are present in a biological environment. If the concentration of metal ions is too high, cellular reactions are inhibited by the metal binding to inappropriate sites of enzymes or to the substrate. Excess of a metal ion favours binary complex formation instead of the important ternary complexes substrate—metal—apoenzyme. If the concentrations are too low, deficiency symptoms are produced because metal ions are essential in very many cellular reactions. It is hazardous to seriously deplete free metal ion concentrations systemically in intact organisms. Where possible, antiviral chelation therapy aimed at depletion of metal ions should be local in its application and take advantage of cell barriers and tissue surfaces to limit the area involved. If the optimum pM range for a virus lies outside the normal pM range for the host cell there is scope for controlling the viral disease by administering appropriate chelating agents and metal ion buffers.

Excess zinc ions inhibit the replication of herpes simplex virus *in vitro* (Gordon *et al.*, 1975), a level of 0.2 mM zinc sulphate markedly inhibiting synthesis of herpes simplex virus DNA while not affecting cell DNA synthesis (Shlomai *et al.*, 1975). This is due to the selective inhibition of herpes simplex virus DNA polymerase: the α- and β-cellular DNA polymerases are resistant (Fridlender *et al.*, 1980a). The sensitivity of herpes simplex virus DNA synthesis to zinc ion may explain why 0.5 per cent zinc sulphate is effective in the treatment of herpes keratitis in man (de Roetth, 1963). It is of interest that an excess of zinc ion inhibits herpes virus and so does the zinc-chelating agent phosphonoacetate. This may be an example of how excess and deficiency of a metal ion might both lead to viral inhibition. As wound healing proceeds most rapidly when adequate zinc levels are maintained, use of a lipid-soluble zinc salt for the topical treatment of cutaneous herpetic lesions might be better than phosphonoacetate.

At 0.5 mM, zinc ions completely inhibit foot-and-mouth disease virus replication (Polatnick and Bachrach, 1978), the zinc apparently interfering with the proteolytic cleavage of the precursor of capsid proteins. Comparable concentrations interfered with the replication of some RNA viruses (rhino, picorna- and arboviruses), including human rhinovirus, encephalomyocarditis virus and poliovirus (Butterworth and Korant, 1974; Bracha and Schlesinger, 1976). It is suggested that zinc ions might be useful in blocking certain stages of replication of many kinds of bacteriophages and animal viruses, including RNA tumour viruses (Korant *et al.*, 1974). Although large picornaviral polypeptides are produced, their post-translational cleavage to capsid polypeptides is prevented in the presence of zinc ions (Korant *et al.*, 1974). Binding of zinc ions to these large polypeptides is suggested to prevent access of the protease which would cleave it (Butterworth *et al.*, 1976). On the other hand, depletion of zinc might abolish the activity of this protease which is probably a zinc enzyme. If so, this is another example of how excess and deficiency of a metal ion might lead to the same result.

Because many human rhinoviruses show marked inhibition of their plaque-forming ability on HeLa cells in the presence of 0.1 mM zinc chloride (Korant *et al.*, 1974), the possibility is suggested that aerosol therapy with dilute solutions of zinc ions might be useful in prevention of the common cold.

Treatment of Rous sarcoma virus with metal ions inhibited the activity of its RNA-dependent DNA polymerase and its cell transforming ability, whereas EDTA enhanced the polymerase activity, possibly by removing cations present as contaminants (Levinson *et al.*, 1973). Metal ion toxicity might well be involved in the *in vitro* inhibitions by metal complexes of antiviral drugs, if these complexes more easily penetrate virions. Thus, the activity of copper-isoniazid was suggested to result from the copper ion *per se* (Antony *et al.*, 1978) but to what extent this mechanism is important with the other antiviral drugs is not known.

Because of the toxicity of metal ions (Luckey and Venugopal, 1977) and the variability in their absorption from the gut, systemic administration of simple salts of heavy metals is not usually attempted for chemotherapy. Exceptions are the small amounts of ferrous and zinc salts which may be taken orally for the treatment of deficiencies. A controlled disturbance of mineral metabolism leading to antiviral activity is illustrated in the subcutaneous injection of copper(II) and rhodium salts into mice infected with neurovaccinia and ectromelia: therapeutic effects were observed (Bauer, 1958). Iridium and platinum chlorides also had some activity against neurovaccinia virus. On the other hand, a gold salt (aurothiomalate) potentiated Coxsackievirus infection in mice (Kabiri *et al.*, 1978).

Aquadichloro(2,6-diaminopyridine)palladium(II) was active against vaccinia virus *in vitro* by suppressing DNA synthesis (Tayim *et al.*, 1974). Inside a cell the chloride ligands are probably exchanged by water molecules whereas the organic ligand is unlikely to dissociate, so that the aquo ion exerts its effect as a modified Pd^{2+} ion. It might behave similarly to the antitumour, *cis*-diamino-dichloro-platinum(II) compounds which also bind to DNA and inhibit its proper functioning. (Cleare, 1974. This review also contains a summary of trials of metal ions in cancer therapy.)

There is scope for studying the uptake of zinc and other cations as their lipid-soluble salts. The iontophoretic method used to enhance penetration of anionic species, such as PAA, by applying an electric field (Hill *et al.*, 1977) could also be a means of administering metal ions locally without the risk of systemic toxicity.

7.4.7. SOME PHARMACOLOGICAL CONSIDERATIONS

Many chelating agents, active against viruses when tested *in vitro*, show little or no activity *in vivo*. This may be due to rapid degradation of the agent under biological conditions or to failure of the agent to reach the site of enzyme activity at a sufficient concentration. Thus the negatively charged $CaEDTA^{2-}$ complex and the $EDTA^{4-}$ anion, inhibitors of RNA-dependent RNA polymerase of influenza virus, cannot readily cross cell membranes to reach the cytoplasm of cells lining the respiratory tract, the target area of influenza. On the other hand they are rapidly excreted via the kidney. However, neutrality may not be a requirement for penetration: Caryen *et al.*, (1979) found that although a neutral ligand had a partition coefficient between 1-octanol and water of about 5, it was not readily absorbed by Ehrlich cells, whereas its copper complex (carrying a +1 charge) and two iron complexes were readily taken up.

Clinical administration of heterocyclic carboxaldehyde thiosemicarbazones, orally or parenterally, is of limited use because of their sparing solubility in water. To overcome this difficulty, many structural modifications have been made, such as the insertion of hydrophilic groups (amino and hydroxyl) into the molecules to improve solubility in water. Structure-activity considerations led to the design of 4-methyl-5-amino-1-formyl-isoquinoline thiosemicarbazone as an inhibitor of ribonucleoside diphosphate reductase (Agrawal *et al.*, 1977).

One way of enabling the penetration of cells may be by the use of liposomes, as described below, to carry the drug. An alternative approach might be to use a lipid-soluble pro-drug which could be metabolized in the target cells into the active form. Of considerable interest, but beyond the scope of this Review, is the vehicle or ointment to apply the antiviral agent and also the parameters of drug absorption and excretion. Untoward effects, such as local irritation, resulting from administration of simple metal salts could be minimized by using solutions of a moderately stable complex or, better still, a complex with a ligand that is rapidly metabolized (e.g. citrate).

Diets can be deficient in metal ions, especially zinc and this can modify the response of an organism to environmental stresses. Taking zinc deficiency as an example, wound healing proceeds more slowly in zinc-deficient animals and there is evidence that the immune response is also affected (Frost *et al.*, 1977). Another example of the importance of the diet is in the reported enhancement of the antitumour activity of pyruvaldehyde bisthiosemicar-bazone by dietary copper or other metal ions (Cappuccino *et al.*, 1967).

Most metal complexes exist in dynamic equilibrium with their components so that no distinction can ordinarily be made between appropriate mixtures of metal ion and ligand and a solution of a preformed complex. The extent and nature of complex formation in a biological medium is determined by the concentrations of the other ligands and metal ions that are also present and the pH of the solution. In an *in vitro* situation, pM may be much more easily affected and controlled than in a therapeutical application. Thus, contact inhibition of herpes simplex virus with methisazone was achieved in phosphate buffered saline but not in a medium containing many more potential ligands (Levinson *et al.*, 1974) possibly due to a larger *p*Cu value in the latter medium. Control of pH *in vivo* is much less easily achieved because pH and free metal ion concentrations (pM) are buffered in organisms. The total concentrations of metal ions in the body are also maintained within broad limits by a series of mechanisms which govern the absorption of metal ions from the digestive tract, the synthesis of chelating proteins such as thioneins (Cherian and Goyer, 1978), storage and excretion. There are also interactions between different metal ions which may facilitate or hinder their uptake, as well as self-regulating mechanisms where the amount of a metal ion taken up from the gut varies inversely with the level already present in the body. The overall result is that metal ion levels tend to be maintained within closely defined limits.

'Concentration quenching' (Albert, 1979) has been suggested as an explanation of why high concentrations of 8-hydroxyquinoline caused less inhibition of DNA synthesis by herpes simplex virus than was observed at lower concentrations (Rohde *et al.*, 1976). As originally observed, this is a phenomenon in which the antifungal and antibacterial action of 8-hydroxyquinoline depended on the formation of 1:1, metal:ligand complexes and the activity passed through a maximum with increasing concentration of the ligand in the presence of Fe(II) or Cu(II) because the free ligand and the fully formed complexes FeL_3 and CuL_2 were inactive.

One of the objectives in viral chemotherapy is that the treatment will slow down the rate of progression of a viral infection thereby giving the body's defence mechanisms time to operate so that the disease pursues only a mild course. Because the immune response mechanism involves metal–ion-mediated reactions, manipulation of free metal ion concentrations may impede the desired response.

7.5. LIPOSOMES: A POSSIBLE NEW TYPE OF DELIVERY AGENT

7.5.1. FORMATION

Liposomes (phospholipid vesicles) are particulate bodies consisting of aqueous dispersions of phospholipids in the form of little multi- or unilamellar lipid bilayers. They are non-toxic, biodegradable carriers formed by dispersing films of suitable phospholipids, or their mixtures, in aqueous solutions containing the solute it is desired to incorporate (Sessa and Weissmann, 1968). Alternatively, lipid-soluble substances can be accommodated in the lipid phase of liposomes. As prepared simply by shaking lipid films with aqueous solutions, liposomes comprise mainly concentric multiple bilayers around $1-10\,\mu m$ in diameter which incorporate water and solutes in compartments between the bimolecular lamellae (Bangham *et al.*, 1965). Sonication breaks up these multi-lamellar liposomes to give smaller monolamellar liposomes (down to about 25 nm). They can be separated from the external aqueous phase by gel filtration, by repeated centrifugation and washing, or by ultrafiltration under pressure.

By introducing an aqueous buffer into a mixture of phospholipid and organic solvent and then evaporating the organic solvent under reduced pressure, unilamellar and oligolamellar liposomes can be formed with much greater internal aqueous spaces. These liposomes also trap in a single step up to 30 times the amount of water-soluble material (drugs, proteins, nucleic acids) that is entrapped by the sonication technique (Szoka and Papahadjopoulos, 1978). This process makes more efficient use of the often valuable or rare materials dispersed in the aqueous phase, with entrapment of up to 65 per cent of the aqueous phase.

A range of membrane structures is possible for liposomes by varying the lipid composition. Charged lipids can be formed by incorporating bases such as stearylamine or anionic species such as dicetyl phosphate or phosphatidic acid, and this modifies their *in vivo* distribution.

Small molecules trapped in liposomes tend to leak through the lipid bilayers. This can be minimized by adding cholesterol (up to an equimolar amount) to the egg lecithin or by using dipalmitoyl lecithin (in which case the liposomes must be formed above 41°, the melting point of the lipid). If the solute is charged, permeation through the bilayer can be reduced by inclusion of similarly charged lipids in the bilayer. The use of charges in the bilayer has the advantage of increasing the volume of water in the liposomes. Amphiphilic compounds readily leak out of liposomes. Leakage can also occur because of interaction with serum components.

Externally, liposomes appear to be fat droplets and the body treats them as such, so that they may be taken into a cell by pinocytosis or they may be engulfed by phagocytes. Inside the cell the liposomes are broken down by lysosomal lipases and the contents of the liposomes are discharged.

7.5.2. APPLICATIONS

Administration of a drug encapsulated in a liposome may enable it to reach its target selectively and in a controlled fashion. Hence the trivial name of 'guided missile drugs'. The strategy behind their use has also been likened to that of the Trojan horse in Virgil's 'Aeneid'. Liposomes have great potential as a means of modifying cellular physiology and of improving chemotherapy. They have been applied successfully for the injection, into mice, of encapsulated DTPA which removed from liver a fraction of the metal plutonium that was not accessible to the usual DTPA therapy (Rahman *et al.*, 1973).

Rahman *et al.* (1974b) prepared liposomes containing the chelating agents EDTA and DTPA from a 3:1 mixture of phosphatidylcholine (egg lecithin) and cholesterol. Tissue retention of these liposomes was studied after intravenous injection of encapsulated [^{14}C]-EDTA (Rahman and Wright, 1975). Their results, given in Table 6, indicate that a high intracellular level of chelating agent can be maintained in liver, spleen and lung tissue.

Rahman and Wright (1975) observed that in the liver the liposomes were phagocytized by hepatocytes and Kupffer cells. After initial close contact of the liposome membrane with the exterior cell wall, the latter became invaginated to form a distinct vesicle surrounding the liposome. (Similar phagocytic vacuoles were found within cells of the reticuloendothelial system (Segal *et al.*, 1974) following intravenous injection of liposomes.) During the 24 hr following injection, large numbers of autophagic vacuoles and, sometimes, extensive areas of focal cytoplasmic degeneration were observed. (Similar lesions were seen in the kidney following intraperitoneal injection of CaEDTA (Schwartz *et al.*, 1970).) The morphology reverted to normal by 7 days post-injection.

Differences were observed in the distribution of EDTA-encapsulated liposomes prepared with different lipids and different surface charges following intravenous injection into mice. Uptake of EDTA by spleen and marrow was highest from negatively charged liposomes, by lungs from positively charged liposomes and by liver from neutral liposomes (Jonah *et al.*, 1975). The tendency of liposomes administered intravenously to be taken up predominantly by liver and spleen thereby decreasing the delivery to other organs is diminished if small liposomes (around 80 nanometers in diameter and prepared from larger liposomes by sonication) are used (Gregoriadis et al., 1977).

Initial experiments having demonstrated that liposomes can introduce agents into cells and alter their metabolism, the carriage of drugs by liposomes is seen as likely to improve drug-target contacts and hence their pharmacological effectiveness (Gregoriadis, 1977). Most of the work on liposomes as carriers of enzymes has been in enzyme replacement therapy of lysosomal storage diseases. A successful application (Belchetz et al., 1977) showed that this approach could circumvent problems such as immunogenicity of a foreign enzyme, its premature inactivation and its inability to reach and act in afflicted cells, but not all cases can be treated in this way (Tyrrell et al., 1976b).

TABLE 6. Distribution of $[^{14}C]$-EDTA as Percentage of Initial ^{14}C Following i.v. Injection of Liposomes Containing $CaNa_2EDTA$ into Mice

Tissue	$t = 0$	15 min	6 hr	1 day	3 days
Blood	100	8.5	1	0.5	0.8
Liver	0	39	41	24	9
Spleen	0	8	11	11	7
Lungs	0	26	10	7	4
Kidney	0	1	0.4	0.4	0.3

(Rahman et al., 1974b). When non-encapsulated EDTA was injected, less than 2 per cent remained in the body after 1 hr.

Closer to present considerations, liposomes have been proposed for use in cancer chemotherapy (Gregoriadis, 1973) and promising results have been reported in the use of liposomes containing cytotoxic agents to treat mice with ascites tumours (Neerunjun and Gregoriadis, 1974; Rahman et al., 1974a).

Clearly, in any application to the chemotherapy of virus infections, it is necessary for the liposome to deliver its drug to the site of action of the virus. This aspect has been little studied. Not only the surface charge and the size of a liposome affect its distribution in the body, but also alterations by blood components of its surface characteristic and properties. Also, anatomical barriers may exist between target cells and liposomes in the circulating blood.

Attempts have been made to administer liposomes intragastrically (Dupergolas and Gregoriadis, 1976/1977; Patel and Ryman, 1976) using semisynthetic phospholipids which are more resistant to pancreatic phospholipases. Liposomes have also been shown to cause delayed release of drugs when injected intramuscularly (Arakawa et al., 1975) and intraperitoneally (Rahman et al., 1974b).

The possibility of securing highly localized drug release from liposomes calls for caution in applying the technique; liposomes containing drugs may alter drug distribution in the body, leading to an unsuspected drug action or otherwise result in toxicity.

The tendency of liposomes to concentrate in particular tissues may be enhanced by enriching the liposomal surface with molecules (such as antibodies to tumours) which exhibit a specific affinity for target cells (Gregoriadis and Neerunjun, 1975).

Almeida et al. (1975) removed surface haemagglutin and neuraminidase projections from influenza viral envelopes, purified them and relocated them in the surfaces of unilamellar liposomes to give 'virosomes' which resembled the original virions. These may well potentiate immunological responses to viruses.

Liposomes may be used as adjuvants to vaccines. Immunity-stimulating substances or vaccines encapsulated in liposomes should be substantially more effective because liposomes tend to accumulate in lymph nodes, and hence are heavily exposed to macrophages.

Attempts, so far unsuccessful, have been made to inhibit influenza viral activity in ferrets by intranasal administration, post-infection, of liposomes containing the chelating agents CaEDTA and CaDTPA (Oxford and Perrin, 1977) with the aim of securing selective delivery of these agents to the interiors of cells of the respiratory tract so as to deplete local zinc concentrations and inhibit viral RNA replication. It seems likely that this approach would be improved if the liposomes were turned into virosomes as described above.

For a recent review of liposomes, see Tyrrell *et al.* (1976).

The liposomes concept can be broadened. Instead of phospholipid vesicles, use can be made of resealed erythrocyte 'ghosts' (made by rapid lysis of red cells (Ihler *et al.*, 1973) in a solution containing the substances to be entrapped, followed by bringing the cells to isoosmoticity and incubating at 37° for 15 min to 'reseal' them). These 'ghosts' can carry therapeutic agents and deliver them to the liver or the spleen. By modifying the 'ghost' surfaces, the vesicular carrier might acquire specificity for a particular target (Tyrrell and Ryman, 1976a).

7.6. ABBREVIATIONS

The following abbreviations are used:

ATP	Adenosine triphosphate
CYS	Cysteinate
DNA	Deoxyribonucleic acid
DTPA	Diethylenetriamine pentaacetate
EDTA	Ethylenediamine-N,N,N',N'-tetra-acetate
HEDTA	Hydroxyethylethylenediamine triacetate
his	Histidinate
IBT	Isatin-β-thiosemicarbazone
KTS	Kethoxal bisthiosemicarbazone
	(3-ethoxy-2-oxobutyraldehyde bisthiosemicarbazone)
L	General for ligand
M	General for metal ion
MIBT	Methisazone, 1-methylisatin β-thiosemicarbazone
mRNA	Messenger RNA
PAA	Phosphonoacetic acid
PFA	Phosphonoformic acid
pK	$-\log([X]\cdot(H)/[HX])$
RNA	Ribonucleic acid
SIBT	5-Sulfonatoisatin β-thiosemicarbazone
β_n	Cumulative stability constant: $[ML_n]/([M]\cdot[L]^n)$
β_n'	Conditional ("apparent") stability constant

7.7. REFERENCES

ABLOV, A. V. and BELICHUK, N. I. (1969) Complexes of iron(II), cobalt(II) and nickel with the thiosemicarbazone of 2-pyridine carboxaldehyde. *Zhur. Neorg. Khim.* **14**: 179–185.

AGARWAL, R. P. and PERRIN, D. D. (1976) Computer-based approach to chelation therapy: a theoretical study of some chelating agents for the selective removal of toxic metal ions from plasma. *Agents and Actions* **6**: 667–673.

AGRAWAL, K. C., BOOTH, B. A., MOORE, E. C. and SARTORELLI, A. C. (1974) Antitumor effects of transition metal chelates of 1-formylisoquinoline thiosemicarbazone. *Proc. Am. Ass. Cancer Res.* **15**: 73.

AGRAWAL, K. C., CLAYMAN, S. and SARTORELLI, A. C. (1976a) Synthesis of site-directed chelating agents—II. 2-Formyl-3-hydroxy-4,5-bis(hydroxymethyl)pyridine thiosemicarbazone. *J. Pharm. Sci.* **65**: 297–299.

AGRAWAL, K. C., LEE, M. H., BOOTH, B. A., MOORE, E. C. and SARTORELLI, A. C. (1974) Potential antitumor agents—II. Inhibitors of alkaline phosphatase, an enzyme involved in the resistance of neoplastic cells to 6-thiopurines. *J. Med. Chem.* **17**: 934–938.

AGRAWAL, K. C., MOONEY, P. D. and SARTORELLI, A. C. (1976b) Potential antitumour agents. 13.4-Methyl-5-amino-1-formylisoquinoline thiosemicarbazone *J. Med. Chem.* **19**: 970–975.

AGRAWAL, K. C. and SARTORELLI, A. C. (1978) The chemistry and biological activity of α-(N)-heterocyclic carboxaldehyde thiosemicarbazones. *Prog. in Med. Chem.* **15**: 321–356.

AGRAWAL, K. C., SCHENKMAN, J. B., DENK, H., MOONEY, P. D., MOORE, E. C., WODINSKY, I. and SARTORELLI, A. C. (1977) 4-Methyl-5-amino-1-formylisoquinoline thiosemicarbazone, a second-generation antineoplastic agent of the α-(N)-heterocyclic carboxaldehyde thiosemicarbazone series. *Cancer Res.* **37**: 1692–1696.

AINSCOUGH, F. W. and BRODIE, A. M. (1976) The role of metal ions in proteins and other biological molecules. *J. Chem. Educ.* **53**: 156–158.

ALBERT, A. (1979) *Selective Toxicity*, 6th edn. Chapman & Hall, London.

ALENIUS, S. (1980) Inhibition of herpes virus multiplication in guinea pig skin by antiviral compounds. *Arch. Virol.* **65**: 149–156.

ALENIUS, S., DINTER, Z. and ÖBERG, B. (1978) Therapeutic effect of trisodium phosphonoformate in cutaneous herpesvirus infection in guinea pigs. *Antimicrob. Ag. Chemother.* **14**: 408–413.

ALENIUS, S. and NORDLINDER, H. (1979) Effect of trisodium phosphonoformate in genital infection of female guinea pigs with herpes simplex virus type II. *Arch. Virol.* **60**: 197–206.

ALENIUS, S. and ÖBERG, B. (1978) Comparison of the therapeutic effect of five antiviral agents on cutaneous herpesvirus infection in guinea pigs. *Arch. Virol.* **58**: 277–288.

ALMEIDA, J. D., BRAND, C. M., EDWARDS, D. C. and HEATH, T. D. (1975) Formation of virosomes from influenza subunits and liposomes. *Lancet*, pp. 899–901.

ANDEREGG, G. (1971) *Multidentate Ligands. J. Coord. Chem.* **1**: 427–490 (ACS monograph, Ed. A. E. MARTELL, Van Nostrand Rheinhold Co.).

ANDEREGG, G., PODDER, N. G., BLÄUENSTEIN, P., HANGARTNER, M. and STÜNZI, H. (1975) Pyridine derivatives as complexing agents—X. Thermodynamics of complex formation of N,N'-bis(2-pyridylmethyl)-ethylene-diamine and of two higher homologues. *J. Coord. Chem.* **4**: 267–275.

ANDREANI, A., BONAZZI, D., CAVRINI, V., GATTI, R., GIOVANNINETTI, G., FRANCHI, L. and NANETTI, A. (1979) Ricerche su sostanze ad attività anti-virale, nota—VII. Attività e lipofilia di tiosemi-carbazoni di N-alchil-2-cloro-3-formylindoli. *Il Farmaco.* **32**: 703–712.

ANDREANI, A. C., CAVRINI, V., GIOVANNINETTI, G., MANNINI PALENZONA, A. and FRANCHI, L. (1975) Ricerche su sostanze ad attività antivirale, nota—II. Derivati di 2-cloro-3-formilindoli N-sostituti. *Il Farmaco*: **30**: 440–448.

ANTHOLINE, W. E., KNIGHT, J. M. and PETERING, D. H. (1976) Inhibition of tumour cell transplantability by iron and copper complexes of 5-substituted 2-formylpyridine thiosemicarbazone. *J. Med. Chem.* **19**: 339–341.

ANTHOLINE, W. E., KNIGHT, J. M. and PETERING, D. H. (1977a) Some properties of copper and zinc complexes of 2-formylpyridine thiosemicarbazone. *Inorg. Chem.* **16**: 569–574.

ANTHOLINE, W., KNIGHT, J., WHELAN, H. and PETERING, D. H. (1977b) Studies of the reaction of 2-formylpyridine thiosemicarbazone and its iron and copper complexes with biological systems. *Molec. Pharmac.* **13**: 89–98.

ANTONINI, L., CLAUDI, F., FRANCHETTI, P., GRIFANTINI, M. and MARTELLI, S. (1977) Elucidation of the structure of the antineoplastic agents, 2-formyl-pyridine and 1-formylisoquinoline thiosemicarbazones. *J. Med. Chem.* **20**: 447–449.

ANTONY, A., RAMAKRISHNAN, T., MIKELENS, P., JACKSON, J. and LEVINSON, W. (1978) Effect of isonicotinic acid hydrazide–copper complex on Rous sarcoma virus and its genome RNA. *Bioinorg. Chem.* **9**: 23–34.

APPLE, M. A. and HASKELL, L. M. (1971) Potent inhibition of sarcoma virus RNA-directed RNA–DNA duplex synthesis and arrest of ascites murine leukaemia and sarcoma *in vivo* by anthracyclines. *Physiol. Chem. Phys.* **3**: 307–312.

APPLE, M. A., OSOFSKY, L., LEVINSON, W., PAGANELLI, J. and WILDENRADT, E. (1972) Prevention of oncornavirus transformation *in vivo* and *in vitro* by anthracyclines and actinomycins. *Clin. Res.* **20**: 562.

APPLEYARD, G., HUME, V. B. M. and WESTWOOD, J. C. N. (1965) The effect of thiosemicarbazones on the growth of rabbitpox virus in tissue culture. *Ann. N.Y. Acad. Sci.* **130**: 92–104.

APPLEYARD, G. and WAY, H. J. (1966) Thiosemicarbazone-resistant rabbitpox virus. *Br. J. Exp. Path.* **47**: 144–151.

ARAKAWA, E., IMAI, Y., KOBAYISHI, H., OKUMURA, K. and SEZAKI, H. (1975) Application of drug-containing liposomes to the duration of the intramuscular absorption of water-soluble drugs in rats. *Chem. Pharmacol. Bull.* **23**: 2218–2222.

ASHMAN, L. K. and KEACH, D. B. (1975) Sheep kidney pyruvate carboxylase. Coupling of adenosine triphosphate hydrolysis and carbon dioxide fixation. *J. biol. Chem.* **250**: 14–21.

AULD, D. S., ATSUYA, I., CAMPINO, C. and VALENZUELA, P. (1976) Yeast RNA polymerase—I: a eucariotic zinc metalloenzyme. *Biochem. biophys. Res. Comm.* **69**: 548–554.

AULD, D. S., KAWAGUCHI, H., LIVINGSTON, D. and VALLEE, B. (1974) RNA-dependent DNA polymerase (reverse transcriptase) from avian myeloblastosis virus: a zinc metalloenzyme. *Proc. Nat. Acad. Sci. USA* **71**: 2091–2095.

AULD, D. S., KAWAGUCHI, H., LIVINGSTON, D. M. and VALLEE, B. L. (1975) Zinc reverse transcriptase from mammalian RNA type C viruses. *Biochem. biophys. Res. Comm.* **62**: 296–302.

BANGHAM, A. D., STANDISH, M. M. and WATKINS, J. C. (1965) Diffusion of univalent ions across the lamellae of swollen phospholipids. *J. Mol. Biol.* **13**: 238–252.

BARAHONA, H., DANIEL, M. D., BEKESI, J. G., FRASER, C. E. D., KING, N. W., HUNT, R. D., INGALLS, J. K. and JONES, T. C. (1977) *In vitro* suppression of herpesvirus saimiri replication by phosphonoacetic acid. *Proc. Soc. Exp. Biol. Med.* **154**: 431–434.

BARZ, P. and FRITZ, H. P. (1970) Spektroskopische Untersuchungen an Metallkomplexen des Antivirus-mittels Isatin-3-thiosemicarbazon. *Z. Naturforsch.* **25B**: 199–204.

BAUER, D. J. (1955) The antiviral and synergic action of isatin thiosemicarbazone and certain phenoxpyrimidines on vaccinia infection in mice. *Br. J. Exp. Path.* **36**: 105–114.

BAUER, D. J. (1958) The chemotherapeutic activity of compounds of copper, rhodium and certain other metals in mice infected with neurovaccinia and ectromelia virus. *Br. J. Exp. Path.* **39**: 480–489.

BAUER, D. J. (1965) Clinical experience with the antiviral drug Marboran (1-methylisatin 3-thiosemicarbazone). *Ann. N.Y. Acad. Sci.* **130**: 110–117.

BAUER, D. J. (1973) *Chemotherapy of Virus Diseases, Int. Encyl. Pharmacol. and Therapeutics*, Sec. 61, Vol. **1**, 1–114. Pergamon Press, Oxford.

BAUER, D. J. and APOSTOLOV, K. (1966) Adenovirus multiplication: inhibition by methisazone. *Science*, **154**: 796–797.

BAUER, D. J., APOSTOLOV, K. and SELWAY, J. W. T. (1970) Activity of methisazone against RNA viruses. *Ann. N.Y. Acad. Sci.* **173**: 314–319.

BAUER, D. J. and SADLER, P. W. (1960) The structure-activity relationship of the antiviral chemotherapeutic activity of isatin-β-thiosemicarbazone. *Br. J. Pharmac. Chemotherap.* **15**: 101–110.

BAUER, D. J., ST. VINCENT, L., KEMPE, C. H. and DOWNIE, A. W. (1963) Prophylactic treatment of smallpox contacts with *N*-methylisatin β-thiosemicarbazone (compound 33T57. Marboran). *Lancet* **2**: 494–496.

BECKER, Y., ASHER, COHEN, Y., WEINBERG-ZAHLERING, G. and SHLOMAI, J. (1977). Phosphonoacetic acid-resistant mutants of herpes simplex virus: effect of phosphonoacetic acid on virus replication and *in vitro* DNA synthesis in isolated nuclei. *Antimicrob. Agents Chemother.* **11**: 919–922.

BECKER, B. A., BOPP, B. A., BRUSICK, D. J. and LEHRER, S. B. (1976) Non-mutagenicity of phosphonoacetic acid (disodium salt) in *in vitro* tests and in rodents. *Fed. Proc.* **35**: 533.

BELADI, I., PUSZTAI, R., MUCSI, I., BAKAY, M. and GABOR, M. (1977) Activity of some flavonoids against viruses. *Ann. N.Y. Acad. Sci.* **284**: 358–364.

BELCHETZ, P. E., BRAIDMAN, I. P., CRAWLEY, J. C. W. and GREGORIADIS, G. (1977) Treatment of Gaucher's disease with liposome entrapped glucocerebroside: β-glucosidase. *Lancet* **2**: 116–117.

BERTHON, G., MAY, P. M. and WILLIAMS, D. R. (1978) Computer simulation of metal–ion equilibria in biofluids. Part II. *J. Chem. Soc., Dalton,* pp. 1433–1438.

BIKHAZI, A. B., AGHAZARIAN, S. M. and TAYIM, H. A. (1977) Degradation kinetics of a novel antimitogenic and antiviral palladium(II) coordination compound. *J. Pharm. Sci.* **66**: 1515–1520.

BILLARD, W. and PEETS, E. (1974) Sulfhydryl reactivity: mechanism of action of several antiviral compounds—selenocystine, 4-(2-propinyloxy)-β-nitrostyrene and acetylaranotin. *Antimicrob. Agents Chemother.* 19–24.

BLÄUENSTEIN, P. (1977) Über die Komplexbildung mit Tetraazaalkanen. Diss. no. 5921, E. T. H., Zürich.

BOPP, B. A., ESTEP, C. B. and ANDERSON, D. J. (1977) Disposition of disodium phosphonoacetate-^{14}C in rat, rabbit, dog and monkey. *Fed. Proc.* **36**: 939.

BOSCHMAN, T. A. C. and JACOBS, J. (1965) The influence of ethylenediaminetetraacetate on various neuraminidases. *Biochem. Z.* **342**: 532–541.

BRACHA, M. and SCHLESINGER, M. (1976) Inhibition of Sindbis virus replication by zinc ions. *Virology* **72**: 272–277.

BRADY, J. N., WINSTON, V. D. and CONSIGLI, R. A. (1977) Dissociation of polymer virus by the chelation of calcium ions found associated with purified virus. *J. Virol.* **23**: 717–724.

BROCKMAN, W., SIDWELL, R. W., ARNETT, G. and SHADDIX, S. (1970) Heterocyclic thiosemicarbazones: correlation between structure, inhibition of ribonucleotide reductase, and inhibition of DNA viruses. *Proc. Soc. Exp. Biol. Med.* **133**: 609–613.

BROOKES, G. and PETTIT, L. D. (1977) Complex formation and stereo-selectivity in the ternary systems Copper(II)-D/L-histidine-L-amino acid. *J. Chem. Soc. Dalton,* pp. 1918–1924.

BROWN, J. N. and AGRAWAL, K. C. (1977) Crystal and molecular structure of α-(N)-heterocyclic thiosemicarbazones—I. The structure of 2-formyl-4-phenyl pyridine thiosemicarbazone-dimethylformamide. *Acta Cryst.* **B33**: 980–984.

BROWN, R. E., STANCATO, F. A. and WOLFE, A. D. (1981) Preferential inhibition of ribonucleic acid synthesis by a new thiosemicarbazone possessing antibacterial and antiparasitic properties. *Antimicrob. Agents Chemother.* **19**: 234–237.

BULMAN, R. A. (1978) Chemistry of plutonium and the transuranics in the biosphere. *Structure and Bonding* **34**: 39–77.

BUTTERWORTH, B. E., GRUNERT, R. R., KORANT, B. D., LONBERG-HOLM, K. and YIN, F. H. (1976) Replication of rhinoviruses. *Arch. Virol.* **51**: 169–189.

BUTTERWORTH, B. E. and KORANT, B. D. (1974) Characterization of the large picornaviral polypeptides produced in the presence of zinc ion. *J. Virology* **14**: 282–291.

CAMPBELL, M. J. M. (1975) Transition metal complexes of thiosemicarbazide and thiosemicarbazones. *Coord. Chem. Rev.* **15**: 279–319.

CAPPUCCINO, J. G., BANKS, S., BROWN, G., GEORGE, M. and TARNOWSKY, G. S. (1967) The effect of copper and other metal ions on the antitumor activity of pyruvaldehyde bis-(thiosemicarbazone). *Cancer Res.* **27**: 968–973.

CARPY, S. (1968) Inhibition de l'anhydrase carbonique erythrocytaire bovine B par differents agents chelateurs á pH 7.4. *Biochim. Biophys. Acta* **151**: 245–59.

CATES, L. A., CHO, Y. M., SMITH, L. K., WILLIAMS, L. and LEMKE, T. L. (1976) Phosphorus-nitrogen compounds. 20. Thiophosphorus hydrazones. *J. Med. Chem.* **19**: 1133–1137.

CHANDA, P. K., and BANERJEE, A. K. (1980) Inhibition of vesicular stomatitis virus transcriptase *in vitro* by phosphonoformate and ara-ATP. *Virology* **107**: 962–966.

CHANG, L. M. S. and BOLLUM, F. J. (1970) Deoxynucleotide-polymerising enzymes of calf thymus gland—IV. Inhibition of terminal deoxynucleotidyl transferase by metal ligands. *Proc. Nat. Acad. Sci. USA* **65**: 1041–1048.

CHERIAN, M. G. and GOYER, R. A. (1978) Metallothioneins and their role in the metabolism and toxicity of metals. *Life Sci.* **23**: 1–10.

CHOW, N. and SIMPSON, R. W. (1971) RNA-dependent RNA polymerase activity associated with virions and subviral particles of myxoviruses. *Proc. Nat. Acad. Sci. USA* **68**: 752–756.

CIAVATTA, L. and VILLAFIORITA, M. (1965) Sui complexxi rame(II)-ossalato. Uno studio potenziometrico. *Gazzetta* **95**: 1247–1257.

CLARK, L. L. (1977) Wart treatment with phosphonoacetic acid or derivatives. U.S. Patent 4,016,264.

CLEARE, M. J. (1974) Transition metal complexes in cancer therapy. *Coord. Chem. Rev.* **12**: 349–405.

COHEN, J., LAPORTE, J., CHARPILIENNE, A. and SCHERRER, R. (1979) Activation of rotavirus RNA polymerase by calcium chelation. *Arch. Virol.* **60**: 177–186.

COLEMAN, J. E. (1974) The role of Zn(II) in transcription by T7 RNA polymerase. *Biochem. Biophys. Res. Comm.* **60**: 641–648.

COLEMAN, J. E. and VALLEE, B. L. (1961) Metallocarboxypeptidases: stability constants and enzymatic activities. *J. biol. Chem.* **236**: 2244–2249.

CREASEY, W. A., AGRAWAL, K. C., CAPIZZI, R. L., STINSON, K. K. and SARTORELLI, A. C. (1972) Studies of the antineoplastic activity and metabolism of α-(N)-heterocyclic carboxaldehyde thiosemicarbazones in dogs and mice. *Cancer Res.* **32**: 565–572.

CRIM, J. A. and PETERING, H. G. (1967) The antitumor activity of Cu(II)KTS, the copper(II) chelate of 3-ethoxy-2-oxobutyraldehyde bis(thiosemicarbazone). *Cancer Res.* **27**: 1278–1285.

CUTTING, W. C., DREISBACH, R. H. and NEFF, B. J. (1949) Antiviral chemotherapy—III. Flavones and related compounds. *Stanford Med. Bull.* **7(2)**: 137–138.

CUTTING, W. C., DREISBACH, R. H. and MATSUSHIMA, F. (1953) Antiviral chemotherapy—VI. Parenteral and other effects of flavonoids. *Stanford Med. Bull.* **11(4)**: 227–229.

DÉCONTI, R. C., TOFFNESS, B. R., AGRAWAL, R. C., TOMCHICK, R., MEAD, J. A. R., BERTINO, J. R., SARTORELLI, A. C. and CREASEY, W. A. (1972) Clinical and pharmacological studies with 5-hydroxy-2-formylpyridine thiosemicarbazone. *Cancer Res.* **32**: 1455–1462.

DE ROETTH, A. (1963) Treatment of herpetic keratitis. *Am. J. Ophthalmol.* **56**: 729–731.

DESCAMPS, J., DE CLERCQ, E., BARR, P. J., JONES, A. S., WALKER, R. T., TORRENCE, P. F. and SHUGAR, D. (1979) Relative potencies of different anti-herpes agents in the topical treatment of cutaneous herpes simplex virus infection of athymic nude mice. *Antimicrob. Agents Chemother.* **16**: 680–682.

DIANA, G. D., CARABATEAS, P. M., JOHNSON, R. E., WILLIAMS, G. L., PANCIC, F. and COLLINS, J. C. (1978a) Antiviral activity of some β-diketones—IV. Benzyl diketones. *In vitro* activity against both RNA and DNA viruses. *J. Med. Chem.* **21**: 689–694.

DIANA, G. D., CARABATEAS, P. M., SALVADOR, U. J., WILLIAMS, G. L., ZALAY, E. S., PANCIC, F., STEINBERG, B. A. and COLLINS, J. C. (1978b) Antiviral activity of some β-diketones—III. Aryl bis(β-diketones). *J. Med. Chem.* **21**: 689–692.

DIANA, G. D., SALVADOR, U. J., ZALAY, E. S., CARABATEAS, P. M., WILLIAMS, G. L., COLLINS, J. C. and PANCIC, F. (1977a) Antiviral activity of some β-diketones—II. Aryloxy alkyl diketones. *In vitro* activity against both RNA and DNA viruses. *J. Med. Chem.* **20**: 757–761.

DIANA, G. D., SALVADOR, U. J., ZALAY, E. S., JOHNSON, R. E., COLLINS, J. C., JOHNSON, D., HINSHAW, W. B., LORENZ, R. R., THIELKING, W. H. and PANCIC, F. (1977b) Antiviral activity of some β-diketones—I. Aryl alkyl diketones. *In vitro* activity against both RNA and DNA viruses. *J. Med. Chem.* **20**: 750–756.

DIMMOCK, N. J. (1971) Dependence of the activity of an influenza virus neuraminidase upon Ca^{2+}. *J. Gen. Virol.* **13**: 481–483.

DOURMASHKIN, R. R. and TYRRELL, D. A. J. (1974) Electron microscopic observations on the entry of influenza virus into susceptible cells. *J. Gen. Virol.* **24**: 129–141.

DUPERGOLAS, G. and GREGORIADIS, G. (1976) Hypoglycaemic effect of liposome-entrapped insulin administered intragastrically into rats. *Lancet* **2**: 824–827.

DUPERGOLAS, G. and GREGORIADIS, G. (1977) The effect of liposomal lipid composition on the fate and effect of liposome-entrapped insulin and tubocurarine. *Biochem. Soc. Trans.* **5**: 1383–1386.

DURHAM, A. C. (1977) Do viruses use calcium ions to shut off host cell functions? *Nature* **267**: 375–376.

DURHAM, A. C. and HENDRY, D. A. (1977) Cation binding by tobacco mosaic virus. *Virology* **77**: 510–519.

EASTERBROOK, K. B. (1962) Interference with the maturation of vaccinia virus by isatin β-thiosemicarbazone. *Virology* **17**: 245–251.

ELFORD, H. L., FREESE, M., PASSAMANI, E. and MORRIS, H. P. (1970) Ribonucleotide reductase and cell proliferation—I. Variations of ribonucleotide reductase activity with tumour growth rate in a series of rat hepatomas. *J. biol. Chem.* **245**: 5228–5233.

FALCHUK, K. H., MAZUS, B., ULPINO, K. and VALLEE, B. L. (1976) *Euglena gracilis* DNA dependent RNA polymerase—II. A zinc metalloenzyme. *Biochemistry* **15**: 4468–4475.

FAZEKAS DE ST. GROTH, S. (1948) Viropexis, the mechanism of virus infection. *Nature (London)* **162**: 294.

FELSENFELD, A. D., ABEE, C. R., GERONE, P. J., SOIKE, K. F. and WILLIAMS, S. R. (1978) Phosphonoacetic acid in the treatment of simian varicella. *Antimicrob. Agents Chemother.* **14**: 331–335.

FENNER, F. J. and WHITE, D. O. (1976) *Medical Virology*, 2nd edn. Academic Press, New York.

FOX, M. P., BOPP, L. H. and PFAU, C. J. (1977) Contact inactivation of RNA and DNA viruses by N-methylisatin beta-thiosemicarbazone and $CuSO_4$. *Ann. N.Y. Acad. Sci.* **238**: 533–543.

FOYE, W. O. and LO, J. R. (1972) Metal-binding abilities of antibacterial heterocyclic thiones. *J. Pharmaceut. Sci.* **61**: 1209–1212.

FRENCH, F. A. and BLANZ, E. J. (1966) The carcinostatic activity of thiosemicarbazones of formylheteroaromatic compounds—III. Primary correlation. *J. Med. Chem.* **9**: 585–589.

FRENCH, F. A., BLANZ, E. J., SHADDIX, S. C. and BROCKMAN, R. W. (1974) α-(N)-Formylheteroaromatic thiosemicarbazones. Inhibition of tumour-derived ribonucleoside diphosphate reductase and correlation with *in vivo* antitumour activity. *J. Med. Chem.* **17**: 172–181.

FRENCH, F. A. and FREEDLANDER, B. L. (1958) Carcinostatic action of polycarbonyl compounds and their derivatives—IV. Glyoxal bis(thiosemicarbazone) and derivatives. *Cancer Res.* **18**: 1290–1300.

FRIDLENDER, B., CHEJANOVSKY, N. and BECKER, Y. (1978a) Selective inhibition of herpes simplex virus type 1 DNA polymerase by zinc ions. *Virology* **84**: 551–554.

FRIDLENDER, B., CHEJANOVSKY, N. and BECKER, Y. (1978b) Deoxyribonucleic acid polymerase of wild-type and phosphonoacetic acid-resistant mutant of herpes simplex virus. *Antimicrob. Agents Chemother.* **13**: 124–127.

FRIEDMAN-KIEN, A. E., FONDAK, A. A. and KLEIN, R. J. (1976) Phosphonoacetic acid treatment of Shope fibroma and vaccinia virus skin infections in rabbits. *J. Invest. Dermatol.* **66**: 99–102.

FROST, P., CHEN, J. C., RABBANI, I., SMITH, J. and PRASAD, A. S. (1977) The effect of zinc deficiency on the immune response. *Prog. Clin. Biol. Res.* **14**: 143–153.

GEMANT, A. (1977) Inhibition of oxidation by peroxidase of human serum proteins. *Mol. Biol. Rep.* **3**: 283–287.

GERSTEIN, D. D., DAWSON, C. R. and OH, J. O. (1975) Phosphonoacetic acid treatment of experimental herpes simplex keratitis. *Antimicrob. Agents Chemother.* **7**: 285–288.

GINER-SOROLLA, A., McCRAVEY, M., LONGLEY-COOK, J. and BURCHENAL, J. H. (1973) Heterocyclic thiosemicarbazones and related derivatives. Synthesis and screening data. *J. Med. Chem.* **16**: 984–988.

GOODRICH, J. M., LEE, K. W. and HINZE, H. L. (1980) *In vitro* inhibition of herpesvirus sylvilagus by phosphonoacetic acid and phosphonoformate. *Arch. Virol.* **66**: 261–64.

GORDON, Y. J., ASHER, Y. and BECKER, Y. (1975) Irreversible inhibition of herpes simplex virus replication in BSC-1 cells by zinc ions. *Antimicrob. Agents Chemother.* **8**: 377–380.

GORDON, Y. J., LAHAV, M., PHOTIOU, S. and BECKER, Y. (1977) Effect of phosphonoacetic acid in the treatment of experimental herpes simplex keratitis. *Br. J. Ophthal.* **61**: 506–509.

GREGORIADIS, G. (1973) Drug entrapment in liposomes. *FEBS Lett.* **36**: 292–295.

GREGORIADIS, G. (1977) Targeting of drugs. *Nature (London)* **265**: 407–411.

GREGORIADIS, G. and NEERUNJUN, E. D. (1975) Homing of liposomes to target cells. *Biochem. Biophys. Res. Commun.* **65**: 537–544.

GREGORIADIS, G., NEERUNJUN, E. D. and HUNT, R. (1977) Fate of liposome associated agent injected into normal and tumour bearing rodents. Attempts to improve localisation in tumour tissues. *Life Sci.* **21**: 357–370.

GURGO, C., RAY, R. K., THIRY, L. and GREEN, M. (1971) Inhibitors of the RNA and DNA dependent polymerase activities of RNA tumour viruses. *Nature New Biol.* **229**: 111–114.

GUTNIKOV, G. and FREISER, H. (1968) Heats and entropies of formation of metal chelates of certain 8-quinolinols, quinoline-8-thiols and 2,4-pentanedione. *Anal. Chem.* **40**: 39–44.

HAASE, A. T. and LEVINSON, W. (1973) Inhibition of RNA slow viruses by thiosemicarbazones. *Biochem. biophys. Res. Comm.* **51**: 875–880.

HALLMAN, P. S., PERRIN, D. D. and WATT, A. E. (1971) The computed distribution of copper(II) and zinc(II) ions among seventeen amino acids present in human blood plasma. *Biochem. J.* **121**: 549–555.

HAMRE, D., BERSTEIN, J. and DONOVICK, R. (1950) Activity of *p*-aminobenzaldehyde 3-thiosemicarbazone in the chick embryo and in the mouse. *Proc. Soc. Exp. Biol. Med.* **73**: 275–278.

HARRIS, S. R. B. and BOYD, B. R. (1977) The activity of iododeoxyuridine, adenine arabinoside, cytosine arabinoside, ribavarin and phosphonoacetic acid against herpesvirus in the hairless mouse model. *J. Antimicrob. Chemother.* **3** (*Suppl. A*): 91–98.

HAY, J., BROWN, S. M., JAMIEŠON, A. T., RIXON, F. J., MOSS, H., DARGAN, D. A. and SUBAK-SHARPE, J. H. (1977) The effect of phosphonoacetic acid on herpes viruses. *J. Antimicrob. Chemother.* **3** (*Suppl. A*): 63–70.

HAY, J. and SUBAK-SHARPE, J. (1976) Mutants of herpes virus simplex virus type 1 and 2 that are resistant to phosphonoacetic acid induce altered DNA polymerase activities in infected cells. *J. Gen. Virol.* **31**: 145–148.

HEINISCH, L., and TRESSELT, D. (1977) Komplexbildung antiviraler Isatin-3-isothiosemicarbazone und -thio-carbonylhydrazone mit Uebergangsmetallen. *Pharmazie* **32**: 582–586.

HELGESTRAND, E. B., ERIKSSON, N. G., JOHANNSON, B., LANNERO, A., LARSSON, A., MISIORNY, J. O., NOREN, B., SJOBERG, K., STENBERG, G., STRIDH, S., ÖBERG, B., ALENIUS, S. and PHILIPSSON, L. (1978) Trisodium phosphonoformate, a new antiviral compound. *Science* **201**: 819–821.

HERRIN, T. R., FAIRGRIEVE, J. S., BOWER, R. R., SHIPKOWITZ, N. L. and MAO, J. C. H. (1977) Synthesis and anti-herpes simplex activity of analogues of phosphonoacetic acid. *J. Med. Chem.* **20**: 660–663.

HILL, J. M., GANGAROSA, L. P. and PARK, N. H. (1977) Iontophoretic application of antiviral chemotherapeutic agents. *Ann. N.Y. Acad. Sci.* **284**: 604–612.

HIROSE, M., SUGIMOTO, E. and CHIBA, H. (1972) Studies on crystalline yeast phosphoglucomutase: the presence of intrinsic zinc. *Biochim. biophys. Acta* **289**: 137–146.

HO, P. P. K. and WALTERS, C. P. (1970) Inhibitors of influenza-induced RNA polymerase. *Ann. N.Y. Acad. Sci.* **173**: 438–443.

HO, P. P. K., WALTERS, C. P., STREIGHTOFF, F., BAKER, L. A. and DELONG, D. C. (1967) *In vivo* activity of an inhibitor of influenza virus-induced ribonucleic acid polymerase. *Antimicrob. Agents Chemother.*, pp. 636–641.

HONESS, R. W. and WATSON, D. H. (1977) Herpes simplex virus resistance and sensitivity to phosphonoacetic acid. *J. Virol.* **21**: 584–600.

HOVORKA, V. and HOLZBECHER, Z. (1949) Sels métallique des β-thiosemicarbazones de l'isatine et ses dérivés. *Collect. Czech. Chem. Commun.* **14**: 248–262.

HUANG, E. S. (1975) Human cytomegalovirus—IV. Specific inhibition of virus-induced DNA polymerase activity and viral DNA replication by phosphonoacetic acid. *J. Virol.* **16**: 1560–1565.

HUANG, E. S., HUANG, C. H., HUONG, S. M. and SELGRADE, M. (1976) Preferential inhibition of herpes-group viruses by phosphonoacetic acid: effect on virus DNA synthesis and virus-induced DNA polymerase activity. *Yale J. biol. Med.* **49**: 93–98.

I, T. P. and NANCOLLAS, G. H. (1972) EQUIL—a general computational method for the calculation of solution equilibria. *Anal. Chem.* **44**: 1940–1950.

IHLER, G. M., GLEW, R. H. and SCHNURE, F. W. (1973) Enzyme loading of erythrocytes. *Proc. Nat. Acad. Sci. USA* **70**: 2662–2666.

INGRI, N., KAKOLOWICZ, W., SILLÉN, L. G. and WARNQVIST, B. (1967) Haltafall, a general programme for calculating the composition of equilibrium mixtures. *Talanta* **14**: 1261–1286.

JONAH, M. M., CERNY, E. A. and RAHMAN, Y. E. (1975) Tissue distribution of EDTA encapsulated within liposomes of varying surface properties. *Biochim. biophys. Acta* **401**: 336–348.

JONES, M. M. and PRATT, Th. H. (1976) Therapeutic chelating agents. *J. Chem. Educ.* **53**: 342–347.

KABIRI, M., BASIRI, E. and KADIVAR, D. (1978) Potentiation of Coxsackie virus B3 infection in adult mice pretreated with a gold salt. *J. Med. Virol.* **3**: 125–136.

KASKA, W. C., CARRANO, C., MICHALOWSKI, J., JACKSON, J. and LEVINSON, W. (1978) Inhibition of the RNA dependent DNA polymerase and the malignant transforming ability of Rous sarcoma virus by thiosemicarbazone-transition metal complexes. *Bioinorg. Chem.* **8**: 225–236.

KATZ, E., MARGALITH, E. and WINER, B. (1974) The effect of isatin β-thiosemicarbazone (IBT)-related compounds on IBT-resistant and on IBT-dependent mutants of vaccinia virus. *J. Gen. Virol.* **25**: 239–244.

KATZ, E., MARGALITH, E. and WINER, B. (1978) Formation of vaccinia virus DNA-protein complex in the presence of isatin β-thiosemicarbazone (IBT). *J. Gen. Virol.* **40**: 695–699.

KATZ, E., MARGALITH, E., WINER, B. and GOLDBLUM, N. (1973a) Synthesis of vaccinia virus polypeptides in the presence of isatin β-thiosemicarbazone. *Antimicrob. Agents and Chemother.* **4**: 42–48.

KATZ, E., MARGALITH, E., WINER, B. and LAZAR, A. (1973b) Characterization and mixed infection of three strains of vaccinia virus: wild type, IBT-resistant and IBT-dependent mutants. *J. Gen. Virol.* **21**: 469–475.

KERN, E. R., GLASGOW, L. A., OVERALL, J. C., RENO, J. M. and BOEZI, J. A. (1978) Treatment of experimental herpesvirus infections with phosphonoformate and some comparisons with phosphonoacetate. *Antimicrob. Agents Chemother.* **14**: 817–823.

KERN, E. R., RICHARDS, J. T. and OVERALL, J. C. (1977) Genital herpesvirus hominis infection in mice—II. Treatment with phosphonoacetic acid, adenine arabinoside and adenine arabinoside 5'-monophosphate. *J. Infect. Dis.* **135**: 557–567.

KESSEL, D. and MCELHINNEY, R. S. (1975) The role of metals in the antitumor action of 1,5-bisthiosemicarbazones. *Mol. Pharmacol.* **11**: 298–309.

KIM, K. S., SAPIENZA, V. J. and CARP, R. I. (1980) Antiviral activity of arildone on deoxyribonucleic acid and ribonucleic acid viruses. *Antimicrob. Agents Chemother.* **18**: 276–280.

KIT, S. (1979) Viral-associated and induced enzymes. *Pharmacol. Ther.* **4**: 501–585.

KLÖCKING, R., HELBIG, B., THIEL, K. D., BLUMÖHR, T., WURTZLER, P., SPRÖSSIG, M. and SCHILLER, F. (1979) Gewinnung, Charakterisierung und antivirale Aktivität von Phenolkörperpolymerisaten. Teil 2. Antivirale Aktivität von Phenolkörperpolymerisaten. *Pharmazie*, **34**: 293–294.

KLÖCKING, R., THIEL, K. D., WURTZLER, P., HELBIG, B. and DRABKE, P. (1978) Antivirale Aktivität von Phenolkörperpolymerisaten gegenüber Herpesvirus hominis. Teil 1. *Pharmazie*, **33**: 539.

KNIGHT, J. M., WHELAN, E. and PETERING, D. H. (1979) Electronic substituent effects upon properties of 5-substituted-2-formylpyridine thiosemicarbazones and their metal complexes. *J. Inorg. Biochem.* **11**: 327–338.

KORANT, B. D., KAUER, J. C. and BUTTERWORTH, B. E. (1974) Zinc ions inhibit replication of rhinoviruses. *Nature (London)* **248**: 588–590.

KOZLOFF, L. M. and LUTE, M. (1977) Zinc, an essential component of the baseplates of T-even bacteriophages. *J. biol. Chem.* **252**: 7715–7724.

KRAKOFF, I. M., ETCUBANAS, E., TAN, C., MAYER, K., BETHUNE, V. and BURCHENAL, J. H. (1974) Clinical trial of 5-hydroxypicolinaldehyde thiosemicarbazone (5HP; NSC 107392) with special reference to its iron-chelating properties. *Cancer Chemother. Rep.* **58**: 207–212.

KUHRT, M. F., FANCHER, M. J., JASTY, V., PANCIC, F. and CAME, P. E. (1979) Preliminary studies of the mode of action of arildone, a novel antiviral agent. *Antimicrob. Agents Chemother.* **15**: 813–819.

LATTKE, H. and WESER, U. (1976) Yeast RNA-polymerase B: A zinc protein. *FEBS Lett.* **65**: 288–292.

LEE, L. F., NAZERIAN, K., LEINBACH, S. S., RENO, J. M. and BOEZI, J. A. (1976) Effect of phosphonoacetate on Marek's disease virus replication. *J. Nat. Cancer Inst.* **56**: 823–827.

LEINBACH, S. S., RENO, J. M., LEE, L. F., ISBELL, A. F. and BOEZI, J. A. (1976) Mechanism of phosphonoacetate inhibition of herpesvirus-induced DNA polymerase. *Biochemistry* **15**: 426–430.

LEVINSON, W., COLEMAN, V., WOODSON, B., RABSON, A., LANIER, J., WITCHER, J. and DAWSON, C. (1974) Inactivation of herpes simplex virus by thiosemicarbazones and certain cations. *Antimicrob. Agents Chemother.* **5**: 398–402.

LEVINSON, W., FARAS, A., WOODSON, B., JACKSON, J. and BISHOP, J. M. (1973) Inhibition of RNA-dependent DNA polymerases of Rous sarcoma virus by thiosemicarbazones and several cations. *Proc. Nat. Acad. Sci., USA* **70**: 164–168.

LEVINSON, W. and HELLING, R. (1976) Inactivation of lambda phage infectivity and lambda deoxyribonucleic acid transfection by N-methyl-isatin-β-thiosemicarbazone–copper complexes. *Antimicrob. Agents Chemother.* **9**: 160–163.

LEVINSON, W., OPPERMAN, H. and JACKSON, J. (1977a) Inhibition of vesicular stomatitis virus by kethoxal bis-(thiosemicarbazone). *J. Gen. Virol.* **37**: 183–190.

LEVINSON, W., ROHDE, W., MIKELENS, P., JACKSON, J., ANTONY, A. and RAMAKRISHNAN, T. (1977b) Inactivation and inhibition of Rous sarcoma virus by copper-binding ligands: thiosemicarbazones, 8-hydroxy-quinolines, and isonicotinic acid hydrazide. *Ann. N.Y. Acad. Sci.* **284**: 525–532.

LEVINSON, W., WOODSON, B. and JACKSON, J. (1971) Inactivation of Rous Sarcoma virus on contact with N-ethyl isatin β-thiosemicarbazone. *Nature New Biology* **233**: 116–118.

LEVY, J., LEVY, S. B. and LEVINSON, W. (1976) Inactivation of murine RNA tumor viruses by isatin β-thiosemicarbazone, its derivatives and analogs. *Virology* **74**: 426–431.

LOGAN, J., FOX, P., MORGAN, J., MAKOHON, A. and PFAU, C. (1975) Arenavirus inactivation on contact with N-substituted isatin β-thiosemicarbazones and certain cations. *J. Gen. Virol.* **28**: 271–284.

LUCKEY, T. D. and VENUGOPAL, B. (1977) *Metal Toxicity in Mammals*, vol. 1. *Physiologic and Chemical Basis for Metal Toxicity*. Plenum Press, New York.

MCLEAN, D. M. (1977) Methisazone therapy in pediatric vaccinia complications. *Ann. N.Y. Acad. Sci.* **284**: 118–121.

MCSHARRY, J. J., CALIGUIRI, L. A. and EGGERS, H. J. (1979) Inhibition of uncoating of poliovirus by arildone, a new antiviral drug. *Virology* **97**: 307–315.

MAO, J. C. H. and ROBISHAW, E. E. (1975) Mode of inhibition of herpes simplex virus DNA polymerase by phosphonoacetate. *Biochemistry*, **14**: 5475–5479.

MAO, J. C. H., ROBISHAW, E. E. and OVERBY, L. R. (1975) Inhibition of DNA polymerase from herpes virus-infected WI-38 by phosphonoacetic acid. *J. Virol.* **15**: 1281–1285.

MARGALITH, M., MANOR, D., USIELI, V. and GOLDBLUM, N. (1980) Phosphonoformate inhibits synthesis of Esptein–Barr virus (EBV) capsid antigen and transformation of human cord blood lymphocytes by EBV. *Virology* **102**: 226–230.

MATHEW, M. and PALENIK, G. J. (1969) The crystal structure of bis(isoquinoline-1-carboxaldehyde thiosemicarbazonato) nickel(II) monohydrate. *J. Am. Chem. Soc.* **91**: 6310–6314.

MAY, C. D., MILLER, R. L. and RAPP, F. (1977) The effect of phosphonoacetic acid on the *in vitro* replication of varicella-zoster virus. *Intervirology* **8**: 83–91.

MEYER, R. F., VANELL, E. D. and KAUFMAN, H. E. (1976) Phosphonoacetic acid in the treatment of experimental ocular herpes simplex infections. *Antimicrob. Agents Chemother.* **9**: 308–311.

MICHAUD, R. L. and SARTORELLI, A. C. (1968) Antitumor and metal-coordinating activities of the thiosemicarbazone, semicarbazone and guanylhydrazine of 1-formyl-isoquinoline. *Abstr. Am. Chem. Soc. 155th Nat. Meet., San Francisco*, April. N-54.

MIKELENS, P. E., WOODSON, B. A. and LEVINSON, W. E. (1976) Association of nucleic acids with complexes of isatin β-thiosemicarbazone and copper. *Biochem. Pharm.* **25**: 821–827.

MIKELENS, P., WOODSON, B. and LEVINSON, W. (1978) Inhibition of *Escherichia coli* DNA polymerase I by association of the template with an *N*-methylisatin β-thiosemicarbazone-copper complex. *Bioinorg. Chem.* **9**: 469–478.

MODAK, M. J., SRIVASTAVA, A. and GILLERMAN, E. (1980) Observations on the phosphonoformic acid inhibition of RNA dependent DNA polymerase. *Biochem. Biophys. Res. Comm.* **96**: 931–938.

MOORE, E. C., AGRAWAL, K. C. and SARTORELLI, A. C. (1975) Ribonucleotide reductase substrate and metal interaction and inhibition by thiosemicarbazones. *Proc. Am. Ass. Cancer Res.* **16**: 160.

MOORE, E. C., BOOTH, B. A. and SARTORELLI, A. C. (1971) Inhibition of deoxyribonucleotide synthesis by pyridine carboxaldehyde thiosemicarbazones. *Cancer Res.* **31**: 235–238.

MOORE, E. C., ZEDECK, M. S., AGRAWAL, K. C. and SARTORELLI, A. C. (1970) Inhibition of ribonucleoside diphosphate reductase by 1-formylisoquinoline thiosemicarbazone and related compounds. *Biochemistry* **9**: 4492–4498.

MORENO, M. A., CARRASCOSA, A. L., ORTIN, J. and VINUELA, E. (1978) Inhibition of African swine fever (ASF) virus replication by phosphonoacetic acid. *J. Gen. Virol.* **93**: 253–258.

NEERUNJUN, E. D. and GREGORIADIS, G. (1974) Prolonged survival of tumor-bearing mice treated with liposome-entrapped actinomycin D. *Biochem. Soc. Trans.* **2**: 868–869.

NEWTON, A., (1979) Inhibition of the replication of herpes viruses by phosphonoacetate and related compounds. *Advan. Ophthal.* **38**: 267–75.

NISHIBA, Y. and INOUE, Y. K. (1978) Effects of phosphonoacetic acid on subacute myeloopticoneuropathy virus *in vitro* and *in vivo*. *J. Med. Virol.* **2**: 225–229.

NISHIGORI, H. and NISHIMURA, C. (1977) Failure of poxvirus replication in the presence of an inhibitor of nucleolar RNA synthesis. *Arch. Virol.* **53**: 163–166.

NISHIGORI, H., SATO, M. and NISHIMURA, C. (1978) Reversible inhibition of the induction of DNA polymerase of herpes simplex virus type 2 in HeLa cells. *Arch. Virol.* **58**: 335–340.

NYORMOI, O., THORLEY-LAWSON, D. A., ELKINGTON, J. and STROMINGER, J. L. (1976) Differential effect of phosphonoacetic acid on the expression of Epstein–Barr viral antigen and virus production. *Proc. Nat. Acad. Sci. USA* **73**: 1745–1748.

OVERBY, L. R., DUFF, R. G. and MAO, J. C. H. (1977) Antiviral potential of phosphonoacetic acid. *Ann. N.Y. Acad. Sci.* **284**: 310–320.

OVERBY, L. R., ROBISHAW, E. E., SCHLEICHER, J. B., RUETER, A., SHIPKOWITZ, N. L. and MAO, J. C. H. (1974) Phosphonoacetic acid: Inhibitor of herpes simplex virus. *Antimicrob. Agents and Chemother.* **6**: 360–365.

OXFORD, J. S. (1973) An inhibitor of the particle-associated RNA-dependent RNA polymerase of influenza A and B viruses. *J. Gen. Virol.* **18**: 11–19.

OXFORD, J. S. (1975) Specific inhibitors of influenza virus replication as potential chemoprophylactic agents. *J. Antimicrob. Chemother.* **1**: 7–23.

OXFORD, J. S. (1977) In *Chemoprophylaxis and Virus Infections of the Respiratory Tract*, Vol. 1, Ch. 5. J. S. OXFORD, (ed.). CRC Press, Ohio.

OXFORD, J. S. and PERRIN, D. D. (1974) Inhibition of the particle-associated RNA-dependent RNA polymerase activity of influenza viruses by chelating agents. *J. Gen. Virol.* **23**: 59–71.

OXFORD, J. S. and PERRIN, D. D. (1977) Influenza RNA transcriptase inhibitors. Studies *in vitro* and *in vivo*. *Ann. N.Y. Acad. Sci.* **284**: 613–623.

PALESE, P., TOBITA, K., UEDA, M. and COMPANS, R. W. (1974) Characterization of temperature sensitive influenza virus mutants defective in neuraminidase. *Virology* **61**: 397–410.

PALMER, A. E., LONDON, W. T. and SEVER, J. L. (1977) Disodium phosphonoacetate in cream base as possible topical treatment for skin lesions of herpes simplex virus in cebus monkeys. *Antimicrob. Agents Chemother.* **12**: 510–512.

PANCIC, F., STEINBERG, B., DIANA, G., GORMAN, W. and CAME, P., 17th Intersci. Conf. Antimicrob. Agents Chemother., New York, Oct. 12–14, 1977, Abstr. No. 239 (quoted in *Annual Reports in Med. Chem.*, 1978, p. 145).

PAPAS, T. S. and SCHAFER, M. P. (1977) The inhibition of Rauscher leukemia virus and avian myeloblastosis virus DNA polymerases by anthracycline compounds. *Ann. N.Y. Acad. Sci.* **284**: 566–575.

PATEL, H. M. and RYMAN, B. E. (1976) Oral administration of insulin by encapsulation within liposomes. *FEBS Lett.* **62**: 60–63.

PEARSON, R. G. (1963) Hard and soft acids and bases. *J. Am. Chem. Soc.* **85**: 3533–3539.

PEARSON, R. G. (1966) Acids and bases. *Science* **151**: 172–177.

PEARSON, G. D. and ZIMMERMAN, E. F. (1969) Inhibition of poliovirus replication by *N*-methylisatin-β-4′,4′-dibutylthiosemicarbazone. *Virology* **38**: 641–650.

PENNINGTON, T. H. (1977) Isatin-β-thiosemicarbazone causes premature cessation of vaccinia virus-induced late post-replicative polypeptide synthesis. *J. Gen. Virol.* **35**: 567–571.

PERRIN, D. D. (1970) *Masking and Demasking of Chemical Reactions*. Wiley, Interscience, New York.

PERRIN, D. D. (1977) In *Chemoprophylaxis and Virus Infections of the Respiratory Tract*, Vol. II, Ch. 8, J. S. OXFORD, (ed.). CRC Press, Cleveland, Ohio.

PERRIN, D. D. (1977) The formation and stability of mixed ligand complexes. *Analytical Chemistry, Essays in Memory of Anders Ringbom*, pp. 113–122. Pergamon Press, Oxford.

PERRIN, D. D. (1978) *Organic Complexing Reagents*. Robert E. Krieger Publ. Co., New York.

PERRIN, D. D. (1979) *Stability Constants—Suppl. 2 (Organic Ligands)*. Pergamon Press, Oxford.

PERRIN, D. D. and DEMPSEY, B. (1974) *Buffers for pH and Metal Ion Control*. Chapman & Hall, London.

PERRIN, D. D. and SAYCE, I. G. (1967) Computer calculation of equilibrium concentrations in mixtures of metal ions and complexing species. *Talanta*, **14**: 833–842.

PETERING, D. H. (1972) The reaction of 3-ethoxy-2-oxobutyraldehyde bis(thiosemicarbazonato) copper(II) with thiols. *Bioinorg. Chem.* **1**: 273–288.

PETERING, D. H. (1974) Concerning the role of zinc in the antitumor activity of 3-ethoxy-2-oxobutyraldehyde bis(thiosemicarbazonato) zinc(II) and related chelates. *Biochem. Pharmacol.* **23**: 567–576.

PETRANYI, P., JENDRISAK, J. J. and BURGESS, R. B. (1977) RNA polymerase II from wheat germ contains tightly bound zinc. *Biochem. Biophys. Res. Comm.* **74**: 1031–1038.

PILLAI, C. K. S., NANDI, U. S. and LEVINSON, W. (1977) Interaction of DNA with anti-cancer drugs: copper thiosemicarbazide system. *Bioinorg. Chem.* **7**: 151–157.

POIESZ, B. J., BATTULA, N. and LOEB, L. A. (1974) Zinc in reverse transcriptase. *Biochem. biophys. Res. Comm.* **56**: 959–964.

POLATNICK, J. and BACHRACH, H. L. (1978) Effect of zinc and other chemical agents on foot-and-mouth disease virus replication. *Antimicrob. Agents and Chemother.* **13**: 731–734.

PONS, N. W. (1975) Influenza virus messenger ribonucleoprotein. *Virology* **67**: 209–218.

PRUSOFF, W. H. and GOZ, B. (1973) Potential mechanisms of action of antiviral agents. *Fed. Proc.* **32**: 1679–1687.

PURIFOY, D. J. M. and POWELL, K. L. (1977) Herpes simplex virus DNA polymerase as the site of phosphonoacetate sensitivity: temperature sensitive mutants. *J. Virol.* **24**: 470–477.

RAFELSON, M. E., SCHNEIR, M. and WILSON, V. W. (1963) Studies on the neuraminidase of influenza virus—II. Additional properties of the enzymes from the Asian and PR 8 strains. *Arch. Biochem. Biophys.* **103**: 424–430.

RAHMAN, V. E., CERNY, E. A., TOLLAKSEN, S. L., WRIGHT, B. J., NANCE, S. L. and THOMSON, J. F. (1974a) Liposome-encapsulated actinomycin D: Potential in cancer chemotherapy. *Proc. Soc. Exp. Biol. Med.* **146**: 1173–1176.

RAHMAN, V. E., ROSENTHAL, M. W. and CERNY, E. A. (1973) Intracellular plutonium removal by liposome-encapsulated chelating agents. *Science (Wash., D.C.)* **180**: 300–302.

RAHMAN, V. E., ROSENTHAL, M. W., CERNY, E. A. and MORETTI, E. S. (1974b) Preparation and prolonged tissue retention of liposome-encapsulated chelating agents. *J. Lab. Clin. Med.* **83**: 640–646.

RAHMAN, V. E. and WRIGHT, B. J. (1975) Liposomes containing chelating agents. *J. Cell Biol.* **65**: 112–122.

RAO, A. R., McFADZEAN, J. A. and SQUIRES, S. (1965) The laboratory and clinical assessment of an isothiazole thiosemicarbazone (M and B 7714) against pox virus. *Ann. N.Y. Acad. Sci.* **130**: 118–127.

RENO, J. M., LEE, L. F. and BOEZI, J. A. (1978) Inhibition of herpesvirus replication and herpesvirus-induced deoxyribonucleic acid polymerase by phosphonoformate. *Antimicrob. Agents and Chemother.* **13**: 188–192.

RIBEIRO DO VALLE, L. A., RAPOSO DE MELO, P., DE SALLES GOMES, L. F. and MORATO PROENCA, L. (1965) Methisazone in prevention of variola minor among contacts. *Lancet* **2**: 976–978.

RICKINSON, A. B. and EPSTEIN, M. A. (1978) Sensitivity of the transforming and replicative functions of Epstein–Barr virus to inhibition by phosphonoacetate. *J. Gen. Virol.* **40**: 409–420.

RINGBOM, A. (1963) *Complexation in Analytical Chemistry.* Interscience, New York.

ROBINSON, D. J. and RASCHKÉ, J. H. (1977) Inactivation of tobacco rattle virus by EDTA, and the role of divalent metal ions in the stability of the virus. *J. Gen. Virol.* **34**: 547–550.

ROHDE, W., MIKELENS, P., JACKSON, J., BLACKMAN, J., WHITCHER, J. and LEVINSON, W. (1976) Hydroxyquinolines inhibit ribonucleic acid-dependent deoxyribonucleic acid polymerase and inactivate Rous sarcoma virus and herpes simplex virus. *Antimicrob. Agents Chemother.* **10**: 234–240.

ROHDE, W., SHAFER, R., IDRIS, J. and LEVINSON, W. (1979) Binding of *N*-methylisatin β-thiosemicarbazone–copper complexes to proteins and nucleic acids. *J. Inorg. Biochem.* **10**: 183–194.

ROOS, J. T. H. and WILLIAMS, D. R. (1977) Synthesis and evaluation of several compounds with potential antiviral activity. *J. Inorg. Nucl. Chem.* **39**: 1294–1297.

ROSENBERG, A., BENNIE, B. and CHARGAFF, E. (1960) Properties of purified sialidase and its action on brain mucolipid. *J. Am. Chem. Soc.* **82**: 4113–4114.

SABOURIN, C. C. K., RENO, J. M. and BOEZI, J. A. (1978) Inhibition of eucaryotic DNA polymerase by phosphonoacetate and phosphonoformate. *Arch. Biochem. Biophys.* **187**: 96–101.

SARTORELLI, A. C., AGRAWAL, K. C. and MOORE, E. C. (1971) Mechanism of inhibition of ribonucleoside diphosphate reductase by α-(*N*)-heterocyclic aldehyde thiosemicarbazones. *Biochem. Pharm.* **20**: 3119–3123.

SARYAN, L. A., ANKEL, E., KRISHNAMURTI, C., PETERING, D. H. and ELFORD, H. (1979) Comparative cytotoxic and biochemical effects of ligands and metal complexes of α-*N*-heterocyclic carboxaldehyde thiosemicarbazones. *J. Med. Chem.* **22**: 1218–1221.

SAUSVILLE, E. A., PEISACH, J. and HORWITZ, S. B. (1976) A role for ferrous ion and oxygen in the degradation of DNA by bleomycin. *Biochem. Biophys. Res. Comm.* **73**: 814–822.

SCHWARTZ, S. L., JOHNSON, C. B. and DOOLAN, P. D. (1970) Study of the mechanism of renal vacuologenesis induced in the rat by ethylenediaminetetraacetate. *Mol. Pharmacol.* **6**: 54–60.

SCHWARZENBACH, G. and FLASCHKA, H. (1969) *Complexometric Titrations*, 2nd edn. Methuen, London.

SCRUTTON, M. C., WU, C. W. and GOLDTHWAIT, D. A. (1971) The presence and possible role of zinc in RNA polymerase obtained from *Escherichia coli*. *Proc. Nat. Acad. Sci. USA* **68**: 2497–2501.

SEGAL, A. W., WILLS, E. J., RICHMOND, J. E., SLAVIN, G., BLACK, C. D. V. and GREGORIADIS, G. (1974) Morphological observations on the cellular and subcellular destination of intravenously administered liposomes. *Br. J. Exp. Pathol.* **55**: 320–327.

SESSA, G. and WEISSMANN, G. (1968) Phospholipid spherules (liposomes) as a model for biological membranes. *J. Lipid Res.* **9**: 310–318.

SETHI, V. S. (1977) Base specificity in the inhibition of oncornavirus reverse transcriptase and cellular nucleic acid polymerase by antitumor drugs. *Ann. N.Y. Acad. Sci.* **284**: 508–524.

SHEFFIELD, F. W., BAUER, J. D. and STEPHENSON, S. M. (1960) The protection of tissue cultures by isatin β-thiosemicarbazone from the cytopathic effects of certain pox viruses. *Br. J. Exp. Path.* **41**: 638–647.

SHERMAN, L., EDELSTEIN, F., SHTECHER, G., AVRAMOFF, M. and TEITZ, Y. (1980) Inhibition of Moloney leukaemia virus production by *N*-methylisatin β-4′,4′-diethylthiosemicarbazone. *J. Gen. Virol.* **46**: 195–203.

SHIPKOWITZ, N. L., BOWER, R. R., APPELL, R. N., NORDEEN, C. W., OVERBY, L. R., RODERICK, W. R., SCHLEICHER, J. B. and VON ESCH, A. M. (1973) Suppression of herpes simplex infection by phosphonoacetic acid. *Appl. Microbiol.* **27**: 264–267.

SHIPMAN, C., SMITH, S. H., DRACH, J. C. and KLAYMAN, D. L. (1981) Antiviral activity of 2-acetylpyridine thiosemicarbazones against herpes simplex virus. *Antimicrob. Agents Chemother.* **19**: 682–685.

SHLOMAI, J., ASHER, Y., GORDON, Y. J., OBSHEVSKY, U. and BECKER, Y. (1975) Effect of zinc ions on the synthesis of herpes simplex virus DNA in infected BSC-1 cells. *Virology* **66**: 330–335.

SIGEL, H. (1973) *Metal Ions in Biological Systems*, Vol. 2. *Mixed Ligand Complexes*. Marcel Dekker, New York.

SIGEL, H. (1975) Ternary Cu^{2+} complexes: stability, structure, and reactivity. *Angew. Chem.* **14**: 394–402.

SILLÉN, L. G. and MARTELL, A. E. (1971) *Stability constants of metal–ion complexes. Chem. Soc. (London), Suppl. 1, Spec. Publ. 25.*

SISSOËFF, I., GRISVARD, J. and GUILLÉ, E. (1976) Studies on metal ion–DNA interactions: Specific behaviour of reiterative DNA sequences, *Prog. Biophys. Mol. Biol.* **31**: 165–199.

SKEHEL, J. J. (1971) RNA-dependent RNA polymerase activity of the influenza virus. *Virology* **45**: 793–796.

SLACK, R., WOOLDRIDGE, K. R. H., MCFADZEAN, J. A. and SQUIRES, S. (1964) A new antiviral agent—4-bromo-3-methyl isothiazole-5-carboxaldehyde thiosemicarbazone, M and B 7714. *Nature (London)* **204**: 587.

SLATER, J. F., MILDVAN, A. S. and LOEB, L. A. (1971) Zinc in DNA polymerases. *Biochem. Biophys. Res. Comm.* **44**: 37–43.

SPRINGGATE, C. F., MILDVAN, A. S., ABRAMSON, R., ENGLE, J. L. and LOEB, L. A. (1973) *Escherichia coli* deoxyribonucleic acid polymerase—I, a zinc metalloenzyme. *J. biol. Chem.* **248**: 5987–5993.

STALDER, H. (1977) Antiviral therapy. *Yale J. Biol. Med.* **50**: 507–532.

STAVRIANOPOULUS, J. G., KARKAS, J. D. and CHARGAFF, E. (1972) DNA polymerases of chicken embryo: purification and properties. *Proc. Nat. Acad. Sci. USA* **69**: 1781–1785.

STENBERG, K. and LARSSON, A. (1978) Reversible effects on cellular metabolism and proliferation by trisodium phosphonoformate. *Antimicrob. Agents Chemother.* **16**: 727–729.

STRIDH, S., HELGESTRAND, E., LANNERO, B., MISIORNY, A., STENING, G. and OBERG, B. (1979) Effects of pyrophosphate analogues on influenza virus RNA polymerase and influenza virus multiplication. *Arch. Virol.* **61**: 245–250.

STÜNZI, H. (1981) Derivatives of isatin in aqueous solution. II. Z–E isomerism in isatin β-thiosemicarbazone. *Aust. J. Chem.* **34**: 373–381.

STÜNZI, H. (1981a) Copper complexation by isatin β-thiosemicarbazones in aqueous solution. *Aust. J. Chem.* **34**: 2549–2561.

STÜNZI, H. (1982) Can chelation be important in the antiviral activity of isatin β-thiosemicarbazones? *Aust. J. Chem.* **35**: 1145–1155.

STÜNZI, H. and ANDEREGG, G. (1976) Complex formation of copper(II) and nickel(II) with pyrrole ligands in aqueous solution. *Helv. Chim. Acta* **59**: 1621–1636.

STÜNZI, H., HARRIS, R. L. N., PERRIN, D. D. and TEITEI, T. (1980) Stability constants for metal complexation by isomers of mimosine and related compounds. *Aust. J. Chem.* **33**: 2207–2220.

STÜNZI, H. and PERRIN, D. D. (1979) Stability constants of metal complexes of phosphonoacetic acid. *J. Inorg. Biochem.* **10**: 309–316.

STÜNZI, H., PERRIN, D. D., TEITEI, T. and HARRIS, R. L. N. (1979) Stability constants of some metal complexes formed by mimosine and related compounds. *Aust. J. Chem.* **32**: 21–30.

SUMMERS, W. C. and KLEIN, G. (1976) Inhibition of EBV DNA synthesis and late gene expression by phosphonoacetic acid. *J. Virol.* **18**: 151–155.

SUZUKI, H., NAGAL, K., YAMAKI, H. and TANAKA, N. (1969) On the mechanism of action of bleomycin. Scission of DNA strands *in vitro* and *in vivo. J. Antibiol.* **22**: 446–448.

SWALLOW, D. L. (1978) Antiviral agents. *Prog. Drug. Res.* **22**: 267–326.

SZOKA, F. and PAPAHADJOPOULOS, D. (1978) Procedure for preparation of liposomes with large internal aqueous space and high capture by reverse-phase evaporation. *Proc. Nat. Acad. Sci. USA* **75**: 4194–4198.

TAKESHITA, M., HOROWITZ, S. B. and GROLLMAN, A. P. (1974) Bleomycin, an inhibitor of vaccinia virus replication. *Virology* **60**: 455–465.

TAKESHITA, M., HORWITZ, S. B. and GROLLMAN, A. P. (1977) Mechanism of the antiviral action of bleomycin. *Ann. N.Y. Acad. Sci.* **284**: 367–374.

TAYIM, H. A., MALAKIAN, A. H. and BIKHAZI, A. B. (1974) Synthesis and physicochemical, antimitogenic and antiviral properties of a novel palladium(II) coordination compound. *J. Pharm. Sci.* **63**: 1469–1471.

TAYLOR, M. R., GABE, E. R., GLUSKER, J. P., MINKIN, J. A. and PATTERSON, A. L. (1966) The crystal structures of compounds with antitumor activity. 2-Keto-3-ethoxybutyraldehyde bis(thiosemicarbazone) and its cupric complex. *J. Am. Chem. Soc.* **88**: 1845–1846.

TEMIN, H. M. (1970) Formation and activation of the provirus of RNA sarcoma viruses. In *Biology of Large Viruses*, p. 233. BARRY, R. D. and MAHY, B. W. J. (eds.). Academic Press, London.

TERHUNE, M. W. and SANDSTEAD, H. H. (1972) Decreased RNA polymerase activity in mammalian zinc deficiency. *Science* **177**: 68–69.

THOMPSON, R. L., MINTON, S. A., OFFICER, J. E. and HITCHINGS, G. H. (1953) Effect of heterocyclic and other thiosemicarbazones on vaccinia infection in the mouse. *J. Immunol.* **70**: 229–234.

THOMPSON, R. L., PRICE, M. L. and MINTON, S. A. (1951) Protection of mice against vaccinia virus by administration of benzaldehyde thiosemicarbazone. *Proc. Soc. Exp. Biol. Med.* **78**: 11–13.

TOMCHIN, A. B., IOFFE, I. S., KOL'TSOV, A. I. and LEPP, YU. K. (1974) Semicarbazones and thiosemicarbazones of the heterocyclic series. XXVII. Spectra and structures of isatin β-thiosemicarbazones. *Khim. Geterotsikl. Soedin.*, pp. 503–509.

TONEW, E., LOBER, G. and TONEW, M. (1974a) The influence of antiviral isatinisothiosemicarbazones on RNA-dependent RNA polymerase in mengovirus-infected FL cells. *Acta Virol.* **18**: 185–192.

TONEW, M., TONEW, E. and HEINISCH, L. (1974b) Antiviral thiosemicarbazones and related compounds—II. Antiviral action of substituted isatinisothiosemicarbazones. *Acta Virol.* **18**: 17–24.

302   D. D. Perrin and H. Stünzi

TURNER, W., BAUER, D. J. and NIMMO-SMITH, R. H. (1962) Eczema vaccinatum treated with *N*-methyl-isatin *β*-thiosemicarbazone. *Br. Med. J.* **1**: 1317–1319.

TYRRELL, D. A., HEATH, T. D., COLLEY, C. M. and RYMAN, B. E. (1976) New aspects of liposomes. *Biochim. biophys. Acta* **457**: 260–302.

TYRRELL, D. A. and RYMAN, B. E. (1976a) The entrapment of therapeutic agents in resealed erythrocyte ghosts and their fate *in vivo*. *Biochem. Soc. Trans.* **4**: 677–680.

TYRRELL, D. A., RYMAN, B. E., KEETON, B. R. and DUBOWITZ, V. (1976b) Use of liposomes in treating type II glycogenosis. *Br. Med. J.* **2**: 88.

UMEZAWA, H. and TAKITA, T. (1980) The bleomycins: antitumor copper-binding antibiotics. *Struct. Bonding.* **40**: 73–99.

UNDERWOOD, F. J. (1977) *Trace Elements in Human and Animal Nutrition*, 4th edition, Academic Press, New York.

VALENZUELA, P., MORRIS, R. W., FARAS, A., LEVINSON, W. and RUTTER, W. J. (1973) Are all nucleotidyl transferases metalloenzymes? *Biochem. Biophys. Res. Comm.* **53**: 1036–41.

VALLEE, B. L. (1976) Zinc biochemistry: a perspective. *Trends Biochem. Sci.* **1**: 88–91.

VECKENSTEDT, A., BELADI, I. and MUESI, I. (1978) Effect of treatment with certain flavonoids on mengovirus-induced encephalitis in mice. *Arch Virol.* **57**: 255–60.

VENTON, D. L., CHAN, C. K., PASSO, C., RACINE, F. M. and MORRIS, P. W. (1977) Inhibition of nucleotidyl transferase enzymes by metal ions in combination with 5-amino-1-formylisoquinoline thiosemicarbazone. *Biochem. Biophys. Res. Comm.* **78**: 547–53.

WALLIN, J., LENNESTEDT, J. O. and LYCKE, E. (1980) Therapeutic efficacy of trisodium phosphonoformate in treatment of recurrent herpes labialis. *Proc. Int. Conf. on Human Herpes Viruses, Atlanta, Georgia*, March.

WALSHE, J. M. (1969) Management of penicillamine nephropathy in Wilson's disease: A new chelating agent. *Lancet* **2**: 1401–1402.

WANDZILAK, T. M. and BENSON, R. W. (1977) Yeast RNA polymerase—III: a zinc metalloenzyme. *Biochem. Biophys. Res. Comm.* **76**: 247–252.

WARREN, L. E., HORNER, S. M. and HATFIELD, W. E. (1972) Chemistry of diketone bis(thiosemicarbazone) copper(II) complexes. *J. Am. Chem. Soc.* **94**: 6392–6396.

WARREN, L. and SPEARING, C. W. (1960) Mammalian sialidase (neuraminidase). *Biochem. Biophys. Res. Comm.* **3**: 489–492.

WARREN, S. and WILLIAMS, M. R. (1971) The acid-catalyzed decarboxylation of phosphonoformic acid. *J. Chem. Soc. B*: 618–621.

WATANABE, K. and TAKESUE, S. (1972) The requirement for calcium in infection with lactobacillus phage. *J. Gen. Virol.* **17**: 19–30.

WILSON, V. W. and RAFELSON, M. E. (1967) Studies on the neuraminidases of influenza virus. III. Stimulation of activity by bivalent cations. *Biochim. Biophys. Acta* **146**: 160–166.

WOODSON, B. and JOKLIK, W. K. (1965) The inhibition of vaccinia virus multiplication by isatin *β*-thiosemicarbazone. *Proc. Nat. Acad. Sci. USA* **54**: 946–953.

YAJIMA, Y., TANAKA, A. and NONOYAMA, M. (1975) Inhibition of productive replication of Epstein–Barr virus DNA by phosphonoacetic acid. *J. Virol.* **71**: 352–354.

CHAPTER 8

ARANUCLEOSIDES AND ARANUCLEOTIDES IN VIRAL CHEMOTHERAPY

Thomas W. North[1] and Seymour S. Cohen[2]

[1]Department of Biochemistry and Pharmacology, Tufts University Schools of Veterinary Medicine,
Medicine and Dental Medicine, Boston, MA 02111, USA
[2]Department of Pharmacological Sciences, State University of New York at Stony Brook,
Stony Brook, NY 11794, USA

CONTENTS

8.1. INTRODUCTION

Two toxic D-arabinosyl nucleosides, 1-β-D-arabinofuranosylcytosine (araC) and 9-β-D-arabinofuranosyladenine (araA), have been found to possess significant antiviral properties in experimental systems and in man. These two compounds, and particularly araA, have proven effective in the treatment of herpetic infections. Both have been used to treat herpetic eye infections (Kaufman and Maloney, 1963; Pavan-Langston et al., 1975) and araA has been approved for both topical and systemic use in treatment of human herpetic disorders. AraC has also proven effective in the treatment of certain leukemias (Livingston and Carter, 1968). After it was found to be effective in treatment of herpes simplex encephalitis (Whitley et al., 1977), a usually fatal disease, araA became the first antiviral agent approved for systemic treatment of herpes encephalitis in humans. AraA has also been found to be effective in treatment of herpes zoster infections in immunosuppressed patients (Whitley et al., 1976). It is the purpose of this review to analyze the antiviral properties of these and other aranucleosides in association with the known biochemical and pharmacological properties of these compounds. This approach is aimed not only at gaining an understanding of the antiviral activity of these analogs, but also at utilizing the biochemical information to maximize these properties. The compounds with which we will be concerned are shown in Fig. 1.

The first aranucleosides, spongothymidine (araT) and spongouridine (araU) were discovered in the sponge *Cryptotethya crypta* (Bergmann and Feeney, 1951). The

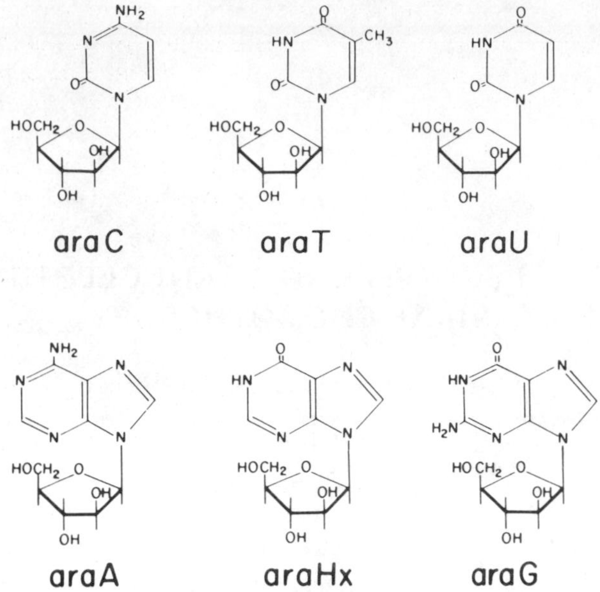

Fig. 1. Structures of the aranucleosides.

identification of these compounds as D-arabinosyl nucleosides (Bergmann and Burke, 1955) stimulated the synthesis of other aranucleosides. The most notable of these synthetic compounds are araC, first synthesized by Walwick *et al.* (1959), and araA, first synthesized by Lee *et al.* (1960). The corresponding nucleotides of these analogs were first synthesized by Cohen (see Cordeilhac and Cohen, 1964 and Cohen, 1966 for synthesis of araCMP, araCDP and araCTP; Cohen, 1966 and Furth and Cohen, 1967 for synthesis of araAMP, araADP and araATP). The availability of these nucleotides greatly facilitated studies of the metabolism of araC and araA. AraA was later found as an antibiotic produced by *Streptomyces antibioticus* (Parke, Davis and Co., 1967). The chemical properties of the D-arabinosyl nucleosides and early studies of their biological properties have been reviewed in some detail (Cohen, 1966; Suhadolnik, 1970). Recent reviews have also discussed the biochemistry and molecular biology of these compounds (Cohen, 1976; Cohen, 1977; Cass, 1978; Suhadolnik, 1979). This review will duplicate only those aspects covered in previous reviews that are necessary for an understanding of the antiviral properties of these compounds.

As we shall see, there are many similarities in the biochemical and pharmacological properties of araC and araA. Both are enzymatically deaminated to less toxic forms, and phosphorylation is necessary to convert both to active forms. Both are metabolized to the corresponding nucleoside-5'-triphosphates (araCTP and araATP) which are believed to be the active forms. These aranucleotides competitively inhibit mammalian DNA polymerases and are also incorporated into DNA. Their toxic effects are believed to involve one or both of these effects on DNA synthesis (reviewed in Cohen, 1976; Cohen, 1977).

As inhibitors of DNA synthesis, one might expect the aranucleosides to inhibit the replication of DNA viruses and those RNA viruses that require DNA synthesis via reverse transcriptase for replication. As we shall see, many DNA viruses and the RNA retroviruses are sensitive to aranucleosides, while most RNA viruses are not. Both araC and araA are also toxic to uninfected cells. Thus, their usefulness as antiviral agents depends upon their ability to inhibit virus replication at concentrations that do not produce adverse physiological effects.

Most studies of aranucleosides as antiviral agents, both in cell culture and in animal systems, have been upon herpesviruses. One reason for this is the demonstration by Kaufman that the infected eye (rabbit or human) is a great model system involving topical therapy with a built in control (the other eye) (see Kaufman and Maloney, 1963). A second reason is that a number of severe and often life-threatening diseases are produced by human herpesviruses. These include herpetic keratitis (a major cause of blindness) and herpes encephalitis both caused by herpes simplex virus (HSV), herpes zoster infections in immunosuppressed patients, and neonatal infections with cytomegalovirus and herpes simplex virus. For detailed information on these and other herpetic disorders see Kaplan (1973). The immunological approaches that have been so successful in treating some other viral diseases such as smallpox and polio have not yet been successfully applied to herpetic infections. This has stimulated much interest in chemotherapeutic approaches to deal with herpesviruses.

The first successful chemotherapy used against herpetic infections was with the thymidine analog 5-iodo-2'-deoxyuridine (IUdR). This compound was found to inhibit replication of herpes simplex virus in cell culture (Hermann, 1961) and was subsequently proven effective in treating herpetic keratitis in rabbits (Kaufman, 1962) and in man (Kaufman et al., 1962). In order to exert toxicity IUdR must be phosphorylated first to the monophosphate and then ultimately to the triphosphate which is incorporated into DNA (Eidinoff et al., 1959). The first step in this process, formation of 5-iodo-deoxyuridylate, is carried out by a virus-induced deoxypyrimidine kinase (which uses thymidine and deoxycytidine as well as a number of nucleoside analogs as substrates) (Kit et al., 1966; Jamieson and Subak-Sharpe, 1974). This enzyme also has dTMP kinase activity (Chen and Prusoff, 1978). Since corneal cells have low levels of thymidine kinase, IUdR is phosphorylated to a much greater extent in herpes-infected cells than in uninfected corneal cells. However, IUdR is toxic to those tissues that have an active thymidine kinase and its use has been nonsystemic and limited to herpetic eye infections.

Since the discovery of the antiherpes activity of IUdR a number of other compounds have been found to exhibit antiherpes properties. Those which have some specificity toward herpesviruses replication or that have met with success in treating herpetic infections are shown in Fig. 2. Most of these have made use of the virus-induced deoxypyrimidine kinase to convert nucleosides to toxic nucleotides. The recognition that this enzyme is significantly different than the host enzyme and has a wide substrate specificity has led to a search for compounds which are phosphorylated by this enzyme and not by host enzymes. Many compounds which are phosphorylated only by this virus-induced enzyme and which

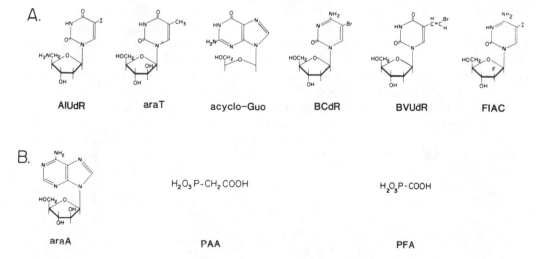

Fig. 2. Relatively specific inhibitors of herpes simplex virus multiplication. (A) Compounds whose antiviral activity requires phosphorylation by the herpes-induced deoxypyrimidine kinase: 5'-amino-5-iodo-deoxyuridine (AIUdR), araT, 9-(2-hydroxyethoxymethyl)-guanine (acyclo-Guo), 5-bromo-deoxycytidine (BCdR), (E)-5-(2-bromovinyl)-2'-deoxyuridine (BVUdR) and 2'-fluoro-2'-deoxy-5-iodo-araC (FIAC); (B) Compounds that do not utilize the herpes-induced deoxypyrimidine kinase: araA, phosphonoacetic acid (PAA) and phosphonoformic acid (PFA).

specifically inhibit replication of herpes simplex virus have been found. These include 5'-amino-5-iodo-deoxyuridine (Chen *et al.*, 1976), 9-(2-hydroxyethoxymethyl)guanine (Elion *et al.*, 1977), araT (Aswell *et al.*, 1977), 5-bromo-deoxycytidine (Dobersen and Greer, 1978), (*E*)-5-(2-bromovinyl)-2'-deoxyuridine (DeClercq *et al.*, 1979), and 2'-fluoro-2'deoxy-5-iodo-araC (Watanabe *et al.*, 1979), all of which are shown in Fig. 2. Although araC and IUdR can be phosphorylated by the herpes-induced enzyme, they are also phosphorylated by cellular enzymes and, therefore, do not show as much specificity as these other compounds.

In addition to deoxypyrimidine kinase there are a number of other enzymatic activities that increase or are changed following infection with herpes simplex virus. These include DNA polymerase (Keir *et al.*, 1966), DNase (Keir, 1968; Hoffmann and Cheng, 1978), deoxypyrimidine triphosphatase (Wohlrab and Francke, 1980), deoxycytidine deaminase (Chan, 1977), deoxycytidylate deaminase (Rolton and Keir, 1974), ribonucleotide reductase (Cohen, G., 1972) and uracil-DNA glycosylase (Caradonna and Cheng, 1981). The deoxypyrimidine kinase and DNA polymerase are known to be the products of viral genes; it has not yet been determined whether the other activities represent viral-encoded enzymes or viral modifications of host enzymes (reviewed by Kit, 1980). The dCMP deaminase appears not to be viral-encoded because this activity was not induced by HSV infection of a cell line devoid of this activity (Langelier *et al.*, 1978).

Each virus-induced or virus-modified host enzyme represents a potential target for viral chemotherapy. However, so far there are only three specific antiherpes compounds that do not utilize the viral deoxypyrimidine kinase. These are phosphonoacetic acid and phosphonoformic acid which selectively inhibit the herpes-induced DNA polymerase, and araA which, as will be discussed in detail in this review, is a relatively specific inhibitor of herpes DNA synthesis.

The relative specificity of an antiviral agent depends in part on the ability of the active form of the compound to inhibit processes in virus-infected cells to a greater extent than in uninfected cells, and also on the ability of the active form to be generated. Many of these compounds, including the aranucleosides, must be activated by phosphorylation and, since they can also be inactivated enzymatically, their relative metabolism in herpes-infected vs. uninfected cells helps determine specificity. Moreover, the phosphorylated derivatives must compete with a naturally occurring nucleotide (araATP and araCTP compete with dATP and dCTP, respectively) at their site of inhibition. Therefore, effects of viral infection and of the aranucleosides upon DNA precursor levels affect the antiviral activities of these compounds. All of these aspects must be considered in evaluating the antiviral activity of the aranucleosides.

Finally, certain biological properties must be considered in the evaluation of any antiviral agent. With the herpesviruses one must be concerned not only with the herpetic lesions but also with the latency and recurrences that often accompany these disorders. In addition some herpesviruses (e.g. HSV-2 and Epstein–Barr virus) have been implicated in human cancers (Rapp, 1974), and certain manipulations such as UV-irradiation allow herpesviruses to transform cultured cells (Duff and Rapp, 1971; Duff and Rapp, 1973). In life-threatening situations these factors are not of as great a concern as the survival of the patient. However, for widespread use of an antiviral agent under less threatening conditions these factors must certainly be considered.

8.2. AraC

Biological activity of araC was first demonstrated at the Upjohn Company by Evans *et al.* (1961) against mouse L1210 leukemia and then by Underwood (1962) who found it to be effective in treating herpes keratitis in rabbits. Shortly thereafter it was also found to be effective in treating human herpes keratitis (Kaufman and Maloney, 1963). The clinical use of araC in treating herpetic keratitis has been limited because it results in corneal toxicity (Kaufman *et al.*, 1964). These toxic effects include the appearance of small opacities in lower layers of the epithelium accompanied by pain and iritis. Occasionally araC treatment leads to corneal ulceration. All of these effects are reversed when araC treatment is stopped (Kaufman *et al.*, 1964).

The first demonstration that araC inhibits the replication of herpes simplex virus in cultured cells was by Buthala (1964). Both HSV type 1 and HSV type 2 are sensitive to inhibition by araC (Nutter and Rapp, 1973). Subsequent to these initial observations, the ability of araC to inhibit other viruses has been examined. Table 1 summarizes the results of these studies. AraC inhibits the replication of most DNA viruses. All of the herpesviruses examined are sensitive to araC. These include the human herpesviruses, herpes zoster and cytomegalovirus, as well as HSV. Vaccinia virus and SV40 are also inhibited by araC, while adenoviruses have been found to be either insensitive or slightly sensitive to araC. Table 1 also shows that most RNA viruses are insensitive to araC. The exceptions to this are the retroviruses whose replication requires DNA synthesis via reverse transcriptase, and the rhabdoviruses.

TABLE 1. *Antiviral Activity of araC*

Virus	Antiviral activity	References
A. DNA viruses		
Herpesviruses		
HSV-1	+	(Underwood, 1962)
HSV-2	+	(Fiala *et al.*, 1972)
Herpes zoster	+	(Rapp, 1964)
Cytomegalovirus	+	(Sidwell *et al.*, 1972)
Epstein–Barr virus	?	
Pseudorabies	+	(Buthala, 1964)
Herpes saimiri	+	(Adamson *et al.*, 1972)
Poxviruses		
Vaccinia	+	(Renis and Johnson, 1962)
Swinepox	+	(Buthala, 1964)
Fowlpox	+	(Buthala, 1964)
Fibroma	+	(Minocha and Maloney, 1970)
Papovaviruses		
SV40	+	(Butel and Rapp, 1965)
Adenoviruses	±	(Feldman and Rapp, 1966; Hermann, 1968)
B. RNA viruses		
Retoviruses		
Rous sarcoma	+	(Bader, 1965)
Murine sarcoma	+	(Hirschman, 1969)
Friend leukemia	+	(Yoshikura, 1968)
Rhabdoviruses		
Rabies	+	(Maes *et al.*, 1967)
Vesicular stomatitis virus	+	(Campbell *et al.*, 1968)
Picornaviruses	−	(Buthala, 1964)
Orthomyxoviruses	−	(Renis and Johnson, 1962)
Paramyxoviruses	−	(Buthala, 1964)
Reoviruses	−	(Campbell, *et al.*, 1968)

8.2.1. CELLULAR ASPECTS

Most of the studies on araC have been done in non-viral systems. AraC has proven useful in the treatment of certain leukemias (Livingston and Carter, 1968) and this has stimulated much work toward evaluating its mechanism of cellular toxicity. These studies have demonstrated that araC inhibits DNA synthesis and that the active form is a nucleotide, almost certainly araCTP (reviewed in Cohen, 1976).

That araC toxicity involves inhibition of DNA synthesis was first suggested by the finding that its toxicity was reversed by deoxycytidine but not by cytidine in mice (Evans *et al.*, 1961) and in cultured cells (Chu and Fischer, 1962). In addition it was found that araC could inhibit DNA synthesis in mouse L cells without much effect on RNA or protein synthesis (Chu and Fischer, 1962; Doering *et al.*, 1966). Moreover, several studies have shown that cells are killed by araC during the S-phase of the growth cycle (Kim *et al.*, 1968; Karon and Chirakawa, 1970). This is the period during which cellular DNA replication occurs.

It is well established that to exert toxicity araC must be phosphorylated to the corresponding nucleotide (Cohen, 1976). Deoxycytidine kinase is required for the first step in this process, namely formation of araCMP. Cells lacking this enzyme are not sensitive to killing by araC (Chu and Fischer, 1965). AraCDP and araCTP are formed by dCMP kinase and nucleoside diphosphokinase, respectively (Momparler, 1974). This sequence of reactions is shown in Fig. 3.

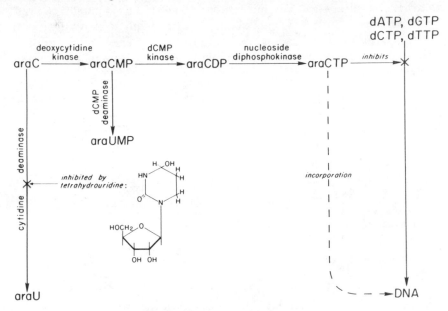

FIG. 3. Metabolism of araC by mammalian cells.

Following the discovery that deoxycytidine prevents the toxic effects of araC it was suggested that an araC nucleotide inhibited the production of dCDP by ribonucleotide reductase. The addition of deoxycytidine would thus eliminate the need for this metabolic pathway. However, neither araCDP nor araCTP inhibit mammalian ribonucleotide reductase at levels in which they are found in cells (Moore and Cohen, 1967). In addition, toxic levels of araC do not deplete any of the deoxyribonucleotide pools (Graham and Whitmore, 1970; Skoog and Nordenskjold, 1974). So the inhibition of DNA synthesis by araC is not due to an inhibition of ribonucleotide reductase.

AraCTP was synthesized by Cardeilhac and Cohen (1964) and was shown to have no inhibitory effect on *E. coli* DNA polymerase I. Thus, it was rather surprising to find that araCTP is a potent inhibitor of mammalian DNA polymerases (Furth and Cohen, 1968). This inhibition is competitive with respect to dCTP (Furth and Cohen, 1968). In addition, some araCTP is incorporated into DNA (Graham and Whitmore, 1970; Manteuil *et al.*, 1974). In studies of mammalian DNA polymerase *in vitro* the araCMP incorporated into DNA was found at terminal positions (Atkinson *et al.*, 1969; Momparler, 1972). These studies were performed in the absence of dCTP. However, studies in cell systems have demonstrated that araCMP in DNA is present mostly in internal positions (Graham and Whitmore, 1970; Manteuil *et al.*, 1974). Further demonstration that araCMP is incorporated into DNA in internucleotide linkage was provided by showing that it is incorporated into closed circular SV40 DNA (Manteuil *et al.*, 1974). Therefore araC is not a DNA chain terminator.

Fridland (1977) has provided evidence that araC inhibits the synthesis of new DNA chains to a greater extent than the elongation of pre-existing chains. In these studies, it was shown that araC blocks the incorporation of ³H-thymidine into low molecular weight DNA to a greater extent than its incorporation into high molecular weight DNA (Fridland, 1977; Bell and Fridland, 1980). Reichard *et al.* (1978) have provided evidence that the most sensitive target for inhibition of *E. coli* DNA replication by another cytidine nucleotide analog, 2′-deoxy-2′-azidocytidine triphosphate, is DNA primase. These studies suggest that inhibition of DNA synthesis and/or incorporation into DNA involve more than just the ability of araCTP to serve as a substrate for or an inhibitor of DNA polymerase. However, araCTP is not an effective inhibitor of DNA polymerase-β, the cellular enzyme thought to be responsible for DNA repair (Reinke *et al.*, 1978). It is possible that the high molecular weight DNA synthesized under the conditions described by Fridland is repair synthesis, since this would involve elongation of pre-existing DNA strands. Thus, care must be taken in interpreting these data until the nature of DNA made in the presence of araC is more fully characterized.

It is not known whether araC toxicity is due to the inhibition of DNA synthesis or the incorporation of the nucleotide into DNA. Kufe *et al.* (1980) have shown that araC incorporation into DNA correlates with the cytotoxicity of araC. Although these authors suggest that incorporation into DNA may be important, they have demonstrated only that both araC cytotoxicity and incorporation of araCMP into DNA are dependent upon araCTP concentration. The extent to which DNA synthesis was inhibited was not determined under these conditions. Moreover, as discussed below, the incorporation of araAMP into DNA does not correlate with its ability to inhibit virus replication. If the toxicity of araC is a result of araCMP incorporation into DNA, its mode of action appears to be different from that of araA. Nevertheless, Kufe and his colleagues have shown that the incorporation of araC into DNA is a useful parameter for measurement of effects of agents that modulate the activity of araC (Major *et al.*, 1981c). AraC treatment does cause chromosome breakage (Nichols and Heneen, 1964; Brewen, 1965) although it has not been established whether this is due to its incorporation into DNA. All of these biological effects are due to araCTP, and it appears that araCTP is the major, if not the sole toxic agent (Cohen, 1976; Cohen, 1977).

Phosphorylation to a toxic nucleotide is not the only metabolic fate of araC. Early studies by the Upjohn Company established that much of the araC administered to animals appears rapidly in the urine as araU. This is due to the action of cytidine deaminase as shown in Fig. 3. This enzyme is present in high levels in the liver, kidney and erythrocytes of humans (Ho and Frei, 1971). Because araU is less toxic and is rapidly excreted, this pathway decreases the therapeutic effectiveness of araC. The ability of some cancer patients to respond to araC treatment has been shown to be better in those with higher ratios of araC kinase to araC deaminase (Hart *et al.*, 1972).

This rapid inactivation of araC led to a search for inhibitors of cytidine deaminase. The result of this search was the discovery of tetrahydrouridine (THU), synthesized by Hanze (1960) (shown in Fig. 3), which is a potent inhibitor of this enzyme (Camiener, 1968). Cytidine deaminase is inhibited competitively by THU with a K_i of 1.3×10^{-7} M (Stoller *et al.*, 1975). Combined treatment with araC and THU results in higher levels of araCTP than treatment with araC alone (Chou *et al.*, 1975; Ho *et al.*, 1975). This is particularly true for acute myelogenous leukemia cells and chronic myelogenous leukemia cells, which have a high ratio of araC deaminase to araC kinase activities (Ho *et al.*, 1980).

The level of araCTP is, therefore, dependent upon the relative activities of kinase and deaminase activities. Moreover, the activity of araCTP is dependent upon the intracellular concentration of dCTP because araCTP must compete with this DNA precursor for inhibition of DNA polymerase or incorporation into DNA. As discussed above, deoxycytidine is able to prevent the cytotoxicity of araC. This is due to its ability to increase the level of dCTP. In addition, dCTP pools can be depleted by thymidine. This is due to an inhibition of CDP reduction by ribonucleotide reductase in the presence of high dTTP levels (Bjursell and Reichard, 1973). There have been several reports that thymidine potentiates the cytotoxicity of araC (Grant *et al.*, 1980; Kinahan *et al.*, 1981; Streifel and Howell, 1981). In addition, thymidine was shown to increase the antitumor activity of araC in rats and mice (Danhauser and Rustum, 1980; Kinahan *et al.*, 1981). Similarly, Harkrader *et al.* (1981) have shown that araC is potentiated by 2'-deoxyadenosine, 2'-deoxyguanosine, or thymidine, each of which leads to a decreased level of dCTP. From these data, it is apparent that the activity of araC is dependent upon the metabolism of naturally occurring nucleotides as well as by the metabolism to araCTP.

To summarize, araC must be phosphorylated to an active form, almost certainly araCTP, in order to exert its toxic effects. Toxicity to cells seems to be due mainly to inhibition of DNA synthesis or incorporation of araC into DNA (or both of these). And finally, the activity of araC can be greatly potentiated by preventing its inactivation with the inhibitor of cytidine deaminase THU, or by coadministration of a compound that leads to depletion of intracellular dCTP pools.

8.2.2. AraC and Herpesviruses

A number of investigations have been performed to analyze the effect of araC on replication of herpes simplex virus. Levitt and Becker (1967) found that 20 μg/ml of araC inhibited DNA synthesis immediately in either HSV type 1-infected or uninfected BSC monkey kidney cells. Similar results were obtained with FL human amnion cells (Levitt and Becker, 1967). When this treatment was performed at 6 hr post-infection or earlier, no progeny virus were formed. However, araC treatment after 6 hr allowed coating of the already formed viral DNA and the formation of infectious virus, although it did stop DNA synthesis immediately. Ben-Porat et al. (1968) studied the effect of araC addition at 3 hr post-infection on DNA synthesis and virus production in rabbit kidney cells infected with either HSV or pseudorabies virus. They found that araC inhibits DNA synthesis and virus production to the same extent. Both of these studies suggest that the antiviral effect of araC is due to its ability to inhibit viral DNA synthesis.

Although araC inhibits herpesvirus replication in cultured cells, no specific antiviral activity has been observed. Ben-Porat et al. (1968) reported that DNA synthesis in uninfected rabbit kidney cells was more sensitive to araC than DNA synthesis in those same cells infected with either HSV or pseudorabies virus. A concentration of araC (0.05 μg/ml) that inhibited cellular DNA synthesis by 50 per cent inhibited DNA synthesis in HSV-infected cells by only 15 per cent and had no effect on DNA synthesis in cells infected by pseudorabies virus. It has not been determined why araC fails to exhibit antiviral specificity whereas araA, which is similar to araC in most biochemical properties, exhibits a great deal of specificity toward herpesviruses.

The inhibition of HSV replication by araC also seems to be reversible, but not readily. O'Neill et al. (1972) found that both replication and cytopathology of HSV type 2 in human embryonic lung cultures was completely blocked by 10 μg/ml of araC. Following removal of araC from the cultures, HSV-2 reappeared and destroyed the cultures. However, there was a latent period of 5 to 6 days before infectious virus could be detected following araC removal. It was suggested that this system might be used to study latency of herpesviruses, although its relationship to latency in human herpesvirus infections has not been established. No studies of the effect of araC on herpesvirus latency in an animal system have been reported, although this matter is of great concern both in the treatment of herpes infections and in understanding the nature of latency.

Since, as discussed above, araC must first be phosphorylated to araCTP in order to exert its toxicity, the apparently decreased sensitivity of herpesviruses to araC may be due to lower araCTP levels. In pseudorabies virus-infected cells this seems to be the case. Ben-Porat et al. (1968) found only 20 to 25 per cent as much araC converted to acid-soluble phosphorylated derivatives in pseudorabies-infected as in uninfected rabbit kidney cells. The amount of araC incorporated into DNA was also only one-third as much in pseudorabies-infected as uninfected cells (Ben-Porat et al., 1968). However, Nutter and Rapp (1973) found that the amount of araC incorporated into DNA in HSV type-1 infected cells was decreased only slightly relative to uninfected cells, while it was considerably higher in HSV type-2 infected than in uninfected cells. The actual levels of araCTP that accumulate in HSV-infected cells have not been determined.

Herpes simplex virus types 1 and 2 both induce the synthesis of a new deoxypyrimidine kinase which is capable of phosphorylating both thymidine and deoxycytidine (Kit *et al.*, 1966; Jamieson *et al.*, 1974; Jamieson and Subak-Sharpe, 1974; Dobersen and Greer, 1978). This enzyme is also capable of phosphorylating araC (Kit *et al.*, 1966), although its K_m for araC is 10-fold higher than for deoxycytidine. Since the activity of deoxycytidine kinase increases several-fold following infection with HSV, one might expect higher intracellular levels of araCTP to accumulate in infected cells than in uninfected cells. This increase in deoxycytidine kinase does not appear after pseudorabies virus infection (Ben-Porat *et al.*, 1968). However, as discussed above, the toxicity of araC depends not only on phosphoryl-ation, but also to the extent that it is inactivated by deamination. The report that HSV induces the synthesis of a new deoxycytidine deaminase (Chan, 1977) is of particular importance in this consideration. Following infection of either BHK or LMTK⁻ cells with HSV the activity of this enzyme increased to 7- to 10-fold (Chan, 1977). However, this activity did not appear until 36 hr after infection with HSV, which is a much longer time than is necessary for induction of other viral enzymes. Moreover, this result has not been confirmed by others (Y.-C. Cheng, personal communication), and the level of deoxycytidine deaminase decreases after infection of HeLa cells by HSV (North, T. W. and Case, J., unpublished results). Thus, the possible existence of an HSV-induced deoxycytidine deaminase needs further scrutiny. Such an enzyme could reduce the sensitivity of HSV to araC.

The activity of dCMP deaminase has also been reported to increase after infection of cells with HSV and this activity is different from that of uninfected cells (Rolton and Keir, 1974). However, HSV cannot induce this activity in a cell line which lacks dCMP deaminase (Langelier *et al.*, 1978). Thus, it is not yet clear whether HSV produces a substantial alteration of araC metabolism through alteration of the activity of this enzyme. Increased deamination of araCMP to araUMP via dCMP deaminase could also be important in decreasing the araC sensitivity of HSV.

Some support for increased deaminase activity in HSV-infected cells has come from studies of deoxycytidine metabolism. Jamieson and Subak-Sharpe (1976) reported that exogenous deoxycytidine is poorly incorporated into DNA of HSV-infected cells, whereas it is readily incorporated into the DNA of uninfected cells. These investigators also showed that radioactively labeled deoxycytidine is converted to a nucleoside-monophosphate in HSV-infected cells. These results were confirmed by North and Mathews (1981), who also identified the nucleotide produced from labeled deoxycytidine as dUMP. These data suggest that the failure of HSV-infected cells to incorporate deoxycytidine is due to its deamination. Strong support for this was provided by the demonstration that tetrahydrouridine facilitates the incorporation of deoxycytidine into DNA as dCMP (North and Mathews, 1981). In the presence of THU the predominant nucleotide formed from exogenous deoxycytidine was dCTP.

In contrast to HSV-infected cells, uninfected cells are not impaired in their ability to incorporate exogenous deoxycytidine into DNA and this level of incorporation is only slightly increased by treatment with tetrahydrouridine (North and Mathews, 1981). From these data, it appears that deamination of deoxycytidine occurs to a much greater extent in HSV-infected cells than in uninfected cells. This is consistent with an increased role of either deoxycytidine deaminase or dCMP deaminase in HSV-infected cells.

In contrast to the potentiation by tetrahydrouridine of deoxycytidine incorporation into HSV DNA, tetrahydrouridine had little effect on the ability of araC to block HSV replication in HeLa cells (North and Mathews, 1981). Therefore, the enzyme(s) responsible for massive deamination of deoxycytidine in HSV-infected cells appear to be less important in araC metabolism. These results make it unlikely that the failure of araC to display antiviral specificity is due to its deamination. Although the deamination product (araU) displays some antiviral activity (DeClercq *et al.*, 1977), it is much less active than araC. The antiviral properties of araU will be discussed in a later section.

One hypothesis which has been proposed to explain the different antiviral specificities of araC and araA is that araCTP is less effective than araATP as an inhibitor of the HSV DNA polymerase. Although it was reported that araCTP does not inhibit the DNA polymerase induced by HSV (Muller et al., 1973), these results were not confirmed by others. Those experiments (of Muller et al.) were performed with a partially purified enzyme which was separated from the cellular DNA polymerases. This enzyme is almost certainly involved in HSV DNA synthesis since it is sensitive to inhibition with phosphonoacetic acid, a specific inhibitor of herpes DNA synthesis (Overby et al., 1974; Mao et al., 1975). In studies with a more highly purified preparation of the HSV-induced DNA polymerase, Reinke et al. (1978) have shown that this enzyme is inhibited by araCTP. Moreover, araCTP was more inhibitory to the HSV DNA polymerase than to cellular α-DNA polymerases; β-DNA polymerases were not sensitive to inhibition by araCTP (Reinke et al., 1978). Thus, the inability of araC to exhibit antiviral specificity is not due to a failure of araCTP to inhibit the HSV DNA polymerase.

Another potential site of inhibition of herpes DNA synthesis is ribonucleotide reductase. As mentioned above, the cellular ribonucleotide reductase is not inhibited by araCDP or araCTP. However, following infection with HSV a new ribonucleotide reductase appears which shows regulatory properties significantly different from the host enzyme (Cohen, G., 1972; Cohen, G. et al., 1974). For example, this enzyme is much less sensitive to inhibition by dTTP than the cellular enzyme (Cohen, G., 1972). This activity is also less sensitive to inhibition by dATP (Langelier et al., 1978) and has no requirement for ATP (Huszar and Bacchetti, 1981). At present it is not known whether this is a new virus-induced enzyme or a virus-modified host enzyme. The effects of araC nucleotides upon this enzyme have not been evaluated.

In summary, araC inhibits herpes DNA synthesis and is also incorporated into herpes DNA. DNA synthesis in herpes-infected cells is less sensitive to araC than DNA synthesis in uninfected cells. And finally the mechanism by which araC inhibits herpes DNA synthesis has not been fully elucidated.

8.2.3. Other Viruses

Replication of papovaviruses and poxviruses is also inhibited by araC (Table 1). Inhibition of these viruses also seems to be due to the ability of araC to inhibit viral DNA replication. AraC inhibits replication of SV40 DNA but does not block synthesis of early mRNA or production of T-antigen (Butel and Rapp, 1965; Rapp et al., 1965). Vaccinia virus DNA replication is also blocked by araC (Umeda and Heidelberger, 1969). AraC has been shown to be effective in treating vaccinial keratitis in rabbits (Underwood et al., 1964).

The only DNA viruses that appear insensitive to araC are the adenoviruses (Table 1). Although some reports that adenoviruses are sensitive to araC have appeared, the majority of the studies have found adenoviruses to be insensitive to araC. It has not been established whether this is due to araCTP-resistant viral DNA replication or to an alteration of araC metabolism in adenovirus-infected cells. Accordingly, these experiments should be repeated in the presence of tetrahydrouridine.

As expected, most RNA viruses are insensitive to araC (Table 1). However, the retroviruses, whose replication requires DNA synthesis via reverse transcriptase, are inhibited by araC. It has been shown that the RNA-dependent DNA polymerases (reverse transcriptases) of these viruses are inhibited by araCTP (Muller et al., 1972; Tuominen and Kenney, 1972; Schrecker et al., 1974). This inhibition is competitive with respect to dCTP. The ability of araCTP to inhibit this enzyme has been found to depend upon the template used. AraCTP is an effective inhibitor when an RNA template is used (Muller et al., 1972; Schrecker et al., 1974), but inhibits poorly with a DNA template (Tuominen and Kenney, 1972; Schrecker et al., 1974). Also the K_i values for inhibition of reverse transcriptase by araCTP vary considerably depending upon the RNA template used. Thus, it has not been established that the inhibition of oncornaviruses by araC is due to inhibition of reverse transcriptase by araCTP.

The only other RNA viruses inhibited by araC are the rhabdoviruses. Replication of both rabies virus and vesicular stomatis virus is inhibited by araC (Table 1). These viruses are not known to require DNA synthesis and are not sensitive to other inhibitors of DNA synthesis such as mitomycin C or fluorodeoxyuridine (Defendi and Wiktor, 1966). Evidence that araC is acting differently in inhibiting these viruses than the DNA viruses comes from the finding that this inhibition is reversed by either cytidine or deoxycytidine (Maes *et al.*, 1967). The inhibition of DNA viruses is reversed only by deoxycytidine. The mechanism by which araC inhibits rhabdoviruses has not been determined, although the extent to which rabies virus is inhibited by araC is dependent upon cell type, suggesting involvement of a cellular function (Campbell *et al.*, 1968). It has not been determined whether this cellular factor is cytidine deaminase. A possible mechanism for inhibition of rhabdovirus replication is inhibition of the virion-associated transcriptase by araCTP. As discussed in the next section, araATP is able to inhibit this transcriptase. Thus, the antiviral activity of aranucleosides may be due to inhibition of RNA synthesis in this case. Another possibility is based upon the work of Hawtrey *et al.* (1974) who showed that high concentrations of araC (10^{-3} M) inhibit both the activation of *N*-acetylneuraminic acid to CMP-sialic acid and the incorporation of glucosamine into membrane glycoproteins. AraC exposure also reduced the amount of sialic acid in glycoproteins of WI-38 cells (Myers-Robfogel and Spataro, 1980). Perhaps rhabdovirus replication requires the synthesis of a glycoprotein which is particularly sensitive to inhibition of araC. AraC has been tested against rabies virus infections in mice and was found to be ineffective (Harmon and Janis, 1976); however, these studies were done in the absence of THU.

8.3. AraA

In contrast to the rapid evaluation of araC as an antiviral agent, which took only 4 years from its synthesis in 1959 to its evaluation in human herpetic keratitis in 1963, the development of araA as an antiviral agent was much slower. AraA was synthesized in 1960 by Lee *et al.*, and found to be toxic to purine-requiring *E. coli* in 1962 by Hubert-Habart and

TABLE 2. *Antiviral Activity of araA*

Virus	Antiviral activity	References
A. DNA viruses		
Herpesviruses		
HSV-1	+	(Privat de Garilhe and De Rudder, 1964)
HSV-2	+	(Person *et al.*, 1970)
Herpes zoster	+	(Schabel, 1968; Miller *et al.*, 1968)
Cytomegalovirus	+	(Schabel, 1968; Miller *et al.*, 1968)
Epstein–Barr virus	+	(Benz *et al.*, 1978; Henderson *et al.*, 1979)
Pseudorabies	+	(Sidwell *et al.*, 1970)
Herpes saimiri	+	(Adamson *et al.*, 1972)
Herpes marmoset	+	(Schabel, 1968; Miller *et al.*, 1968)
Herpes simiae (B)	+	(Schabel, 1968; Miller *et al.*, 1968)
Poxviruses		
Vaccinia	+	(Privat de Garilhe and De Rudder, 1964)
Myxoma	+	(Sidwell *et al.*, 1970)
Papovaviruses		
Polyoma	±	(Freeman *et al.*, 1965)
Adenoviruses	±	(Schabel, 1968; Miller *et al.*, 1968)
B. RNA viruses		
Retroviruses		
Rous sarcoma	+	(Schabel, 1968; Miller *et al.*, 1968)
Murine leukemia	+	(Shannon *et al.*, 1974)
Rhabdoviruses		
Rabies	+	(Harmon and Janis, 1976)
Vesicular stomatitis virus	+	(Grant and Sabina, 1972)
Picornaviruses	−	(De Rudder and Privat de Garilhe, 1965)
Orthomyxoviruses	−	(Huffman *et al.*, 1973)
Paramyxoviruses	−	(De Rudder and Privat de Garilhe, 1965)
Reoviruses	−	(Shannon, 1977b)

Cohen. In 1966 it was shown that araA was toxic to mouse fibroblasts due to inhibition of DNA synthesis (Doering *et al.*, 1966). Privat de Garilhe and De Rudder demonstrated an anti-herpes activity of araA in 1964, but there was little additional work on this property of araA until 1968. Moreover, clinical evaluations of araA as an antiviral agent have begun only in the past few years (Pavan-Langston *et al.*, 1975). Between 1968 and the present much has been learned about the metabolism and mode of action of araA.

Privat de Garilhe and De Rudder (1964) found that araA inhibited the replication of both herpes simplex virus and vaccinia virus in cultured cells. Since then araA has been reported to inhibit replication of a broad spectrum of DNA viruses as well as some RNA viruses. The results of these studies are summarized in Table 2.

AraA has been particularly effective as an inhibitor of the replication of herpesviruses. All herpesviruses which have been examined are sensitive to this substance. These include all the known human herpesviruses: herpes simplex types 1 and 2, herpes zoster, cytomegalovirus, and Epstein–Barr virus. Of the other DNA viruses examined, poxvirus multiplication is inhibited by araA, while adenoviruses and papovaviruses are only slightly sensitive to araA (Table 2).

The spectrum of antiviral activity of araA toward RNA viruses is identical to that of araC. The retroviruses and rhabdoviruses are sensitive to araA while all other RNA viruses tested have been found insensitive.

As with araC, much of the information on the mechanism of araA toxicity and its metabolism has been derived from studies with uninfected cells. Like araC, araA must be phosphorylated to an active form; and it can also be inactivated by enzymatic deamination. Like araC, the primary, if not sole effect of araA is upon DNA synthesis. However, unlike araC a specific antiviral activity of araA has been established.

8.3.1. CELLULAR ASPECTS

AraA is cytotoxic to cultured mammalian cells only at relatively high levels (10^{-4} M or greater). This is 100-fold higher than the concentration of araC required to kill cultured cells. In addition, araA has a low solubility (2 mM in H_2O at room temperature). The low toxicity and low solubility seriously limited study of the efficacy of araA in early studies. Nonetheless, toxic levels of araA were shown to inhibit DNA synthesis but not RNA or protein synthesis in both bacterial (Hubart-Habart and Cohen, 1962) and mammalian cell systems (Doering *et al.*, 1966). AraA, like araC, also inhibits the synthesis of new DNA chains to a greater extent than the elongation of pre-existing chains (Bell and Fridland, 1980). As with araC, it was suggested that this may be due to an effect on initiation of DNA chains. However, in view of the low sensitivity of DNA polymerase-β to araATP, an alternative explanation is that DNA repair synthesis can occur in the presence of a level of araATP that blocks semi-conservative replication. The product of repair synthesis would be high-molecular weight DNA.

Like araC, araA must be phosphorylated to an active nucleotide (araATP) in order to exert its biological activity. This sequence of reactions is shown in Fig. 4. This process is believed to involve the enzymes adenosine kinase, adenylate kinase, and nucleoside diphosphokinase acting sequentially, although rigorous proof that these are the actual enzymes involved is lacking (Cohen, 1976). The first step in this sequence, conversion of araA to araAMP, may also be catalyzed by deoxycytidine kinase (Brockman *et al.*, 1980), an enzyme which seems to be solely responsible for phosphorylation of 2-fluoro-araA to the 5′-monophosphate (see below).

AraATP, like araCTP, is a potent inhibitor of mammalian DNA polymerase with a K_i of 1.3 μM (Furth and Cohen, 1967; Furth and Cohen, 1968). This inhibition is competitive with respect to dATP. In addition, araA is incorporated into DNA, and araAMP is found in internucleotide linkage within the DNA (Plunkett *et al.*, 1974; Plunkett and Cohen, 1975a). AraA treatment also produces chromosome breaks (Cohen, 1976). The lethality of araA to cultured cells is believed to involve either inhibition of DNA synthesis or incorporation of

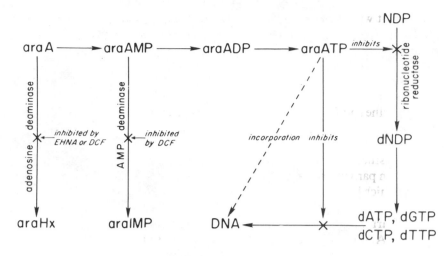

FIG. 4. Metabolism of araA by mammalian cells.

araAMP into DNA (or both). In support of this, cells resistant to araA have been obtained and these cells have a DNA polymerase that is resistant to araATP (LePage, 1978).

Unlike the araC nucleotides, araADP and araATP are significant inhibitors of ribonucleotide reductase, although less inhibitory than the naturally occurring dATP. Reduction of GDP by ribonucleotide reductase from rat tumor is inhibited 50 per cent by 30 μM araADP or araATP (Moore and Cohen, 1967). This concentration is higher than that required to inhibit DNA polymerase. However, concentrations of araATP in mouse fibroblasts have been shown to reach 200 μM (Plunkett et al., 1980) and under these conditions GDP reduction should be inhibited. Whether an effect on DNA precursor provision occurs in vivo, and whether such effects contribute to inhibition of DNA synthesis have not been determined. The cytotoxity of araATP has been recently reviewed (Cohen, 1976; Cohen, 1977).

In addition to metabolic activation via phosphorylation, araA is subject to inactivation via deamination. The enzyme responsible for this is adenosine deaminase, as shown in Fig. 4. This reaction produces 9-β-D-arabinofuranosylhypoxanthine (araHx) which is significantly less toxic than araA (Cohen, 1966). It is now well established that the low toxicity of araA results from high levels of adenosine deaminase present both within cells and in sera. Even when the serum enzyme is inactivated by heating (56°C for 20 hr), mouse fibroblasts contain sufficient activity to deaminate half of the araA supplied exogenously at 10^{-4} M within 4 hr (Plunkett and Cohen, 1975a).

This rapid inactivation of araA poses several problems to the investigator wishing to study its biochemical or pharmacological properties. First of all it is impossible to use a defined concentration of araA, since it rapidly changes during the experiment. Secondly, one cannot study only araA but must instead evaluate the effects of a mixture of araA and araHx. This mixture is also constantly changing its proportions. And finally, long-term experiments are difficult, if not impossible, due to this rapid elimination of araA.

Recently two very potent inhibitors of mammalian adenosine deaminase have been discovered. Their structures are shown in Fig. 5. The first of these was erythro-9-(2-hydroxy-3-nonyl)adenine (EHNA), synthesized by Schaeffer and Schwender (1974) and exploited by Plunkett and Cohen in 1975. EHNA is a competitive inhibitor of adenosine deaminase with a K_i of 10^{-8} M. The second, 2'-deoxycoformycin (DCF), was isolated from cultures of *Streptomyces antibioticus* by researchers at Parke, Davis & Company (Woo et al., 1974). Although originally thought to be an irreversible inhibitor it has more recently been shown to be a competitive inhibitor with a K_i of 10^{-11}–10^{-12} M (Agarwal et al., 1977). Another inhibitor of adenosine deaminase which has been studied less than EHNA and DCF is coformycin (Nakamura et al., 1974). This compound differs from DCF only in having a

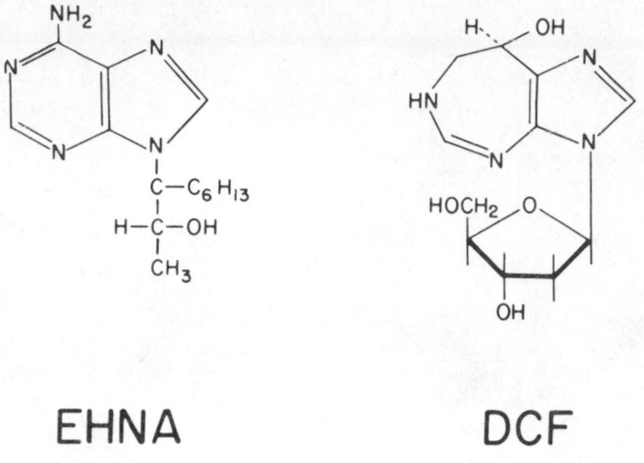

EHNA   DCF

Fig. 5. Inhibitors of adenosine deaminase. The two inhibitors are erythro-9-(2-hydroxy-3-nonyl)adenine (EHNA) and 2′-deoxycoformycin (DCF).

ribose rather than a deoxyribose sugar. Its activity toward adenosine deaminase is similar to that of DCF (Agarwal et al., 1977). Coformycin and DCF also inhibit AMP deaminase, while EHNA does not (Agarwal and Parks, 1977).

Both EHNA and DCF greatly increase the toxicity of araA and of another adenosine analog, cordycepin (3′-deoxyadenosine). This was demonstrated first with EHNA (Plunkett and Cohen, 1975b) and later with DCF (LePage et al., 1976; Johns and Adamson, 1976). Also, the activity of araA toward certain mouse tumors is greatly increased by simultaneous administration of EHNA (Plunkett and Cohen, 1975b). Both EHNA and DCF were shown to increase the plasma level and half-life of araA in mice (Suling et al., 1978; Plunkett et al., 1979a). Plunkett et al. (1979a; 1979b) showed that the combination of either inhibitor of adenosine deaminase with araA resulted in higher cellular concentrations of araATP and prolonged inhibition of cellular DNA synthetic capacity in comparison to araA alone. The ability of these inhibitors of adenosine deaminase to increase the antiviral activity of araA will be discussed below.

In addition to inhibition of DNA synthesis, araA also exerts some interesting effects on RNA metabolism. Although araA treatment has very little effect on RNA synthesis in cultured cells (Doering et al., 1966), and araATP does not inhibit cellular RNA polymerases (Furth and Cohen, 1968), araATP is a potent inhibitor of the chromatin-associated poly(A) polymerase (Rose and Jacob, 1978). This inhibition is competitive with respect to ATP, with a K_i of 4 μM. The poly(A) polymerase present in nuclear sap is also inhibited by araATP, but less effectively ($K_i = 60$ μM). It is not clear whether this contributes to the cytotoxicity produced by araA. AraA was shown to inhibit late gene expression by herpes simplex virus (Pedersen et al., 1981), but it was not determined whether this was due to a block of mRNA polyadenylation.

Although phosphorylation of araA is required to obtain biological activity, an interesting and possibly important effect is exerted by the nucleoside itself. Hershfield (1979) has shown that this nucleoside inhibits S-adenosylhomocysteine (SAH) hydrolase. Unlike adenosine, a product of SAH hydrolysis, araA does not simply reverse this reaction producing a buildup of SAH, but actually inhibits the enzyme. Both araA and 2′-deoxyadenosine are 'suicide inactivators' that bind tightly to the enzyme (Hershfield, 1979). Furthermore, Zimmerman et al. (1980) showed that araA treatment of lymphocytes leads to an elevated level of SAH. Treatment with araA (150 μM) + EHNA produced a 27-fold increase in intracellular SAH concentration. Since SAH is known to be a potent inhibitor of many SAM-dependent methylation reactions, including those of capping of mRNA, it may be asked if araA at high intracellular concentrations can inhibit synthesis of some RNA viruses.

8.3.2. ARAA AND HERPESVIRUSES

It is well established that multiplication of herpesviruses is more sensitive to inhibition by araA than the growth of cultured cells. The great potential that araA has shown for clinical treatment of herpetic disorders has stimulated a great deal of research into the antiviral properties of araA. Much of this work has been reviewed previously (Ch'ien *et al.*, 1973; Shannon, 1975a, Cohen, 1979). However, the recent discovery of inhibitors of adenosine deaminase has provided researchers with a tool to investigate the antiviral properties of araA under more controlled conditions. In this discussion, we shall discuss not only the antiviral activity of araA, but also the tremendous potentiation of this activity by simultaneous administration of an inhibitor of adenosine deaminase.

Following the initial report by Privat de Garilhe and De Rudder (1964) that araA inhibits the replication of herpes simplex virus, it was found that araA inhibits virus replication at concentrations that are not cytotoxic to uninfected cells. Miller *et al.* (1968) found that plaque formation by the HF strain of HSV in HEp-2 cells was completely blocked by 25 μg/ml of araA, while growth of uninfected HEp-2 cells was not completely arrested by 160 μg/ml of araA. Similar results were obtained for replication of HSV in KB cells (Miller *et al.*, 1968). Both Miller *et al.* (1968) and Schabel (1968) also found that araA had antiviral activity against herpes zoster and cytomegalovirus, as measured by inhibition of the cytopathic effects produced by these viruses in cell culture. The activity of araA against Epstein–Barr virus (EBV) was not examined until recently; araA was shown to selectively inhibit the replication of EBV-producing lymphocytes (Benz *et al.*, 1978) and the transformation of human leukocytes by EBV (Henderson *et al.*, 1979) (although these experiments were not performed in the presence of an inhibitor of adenosine deaminase).

In addition to the cell culture studies, araA has been tested against herpes infections in a number of animal systems. AraA had significant activity against experimental herpes keratitis and herpes skin lesions at concentrations that showed no toxicity to the host animal. These results are summarized in a recent review (Sloan, 1975).

A number of recent studies have shown that the deaminase inhibitors greatly increase both the toxicity and antiviral activity of araA. In the presence of low levels of DCF (which alone is neither cytotoxic toward cells nor inhibitory to virus replication) the anti-HSV activity of araA was increased about 20-fold as determined by the concentration necessary to inhibit plaque formation (Bryson *et al.*, 1974). Similar results were obtained with coformycin (Schwartz *et al.*, 1976). DCF also increases the ability of araA to inhibit plaque formation by herpes zoster (Bryson and Conner, 1976). We have found that low levels of EHNA (10^{-6} M) also increase the ability of araA to inhibit production of infectious virus in HSV-infected cells (Fig. 6). Surprisingly, we have also found that a higher level of EHNA (10^{-5} M) alone (in the absence of araA) significantly reduces HSV multiplication (North and Cohen, 1978). This observation will be discussed below.

The first study of the effect of araA on HSV DNA synthesis was reported by Shipman *et al.* (1976). In this study (done in the absence of an inhibitor of adenosine deaminase) herpes DNA synthesis was considerably more sensitive to araA than was cellular DNA synthesis. HSV DNA synthesis was inhibited by 75 per cent with a concentration of araA (3.2 μg/ml) that did not reduce cellular DNA synthesis. These experiments were later repeated in the presence of coformycin (Schwartz *et al.*, 1976). In these experiments it was demonstrated not only that the deaminase inhibitor potentiated the ability of araA to inhibit DNA synthesis, but also that the specificity toward inhibition of viral DNA synthesis remained under these conditions. EHNA also increases the ability of araA to inhibit DNA synthesis in HSV-infected HeLa cells (North, unpublished results).

The ability of an inhibitor of adenosine deaminase to increase the antiviral activity of araA in animal systems has also been reported. Sloan *et al.* (1977) of Parke, Davis & Co. have shown that an antiviral effect of araA toward HSV infections of mice is achieved at one-tenth the concentration of araA in the presence of DCF that is required in the absence of DCF. DCF has also been shown to increase the anti-HSV activity of araA in rabbit corneal infections (Falcon and Jones, 1977). Similarly, EHNA increases the activity of araA in systemic treatment of HSV infections in mice (Shannon *et al.*, 1980). These results are

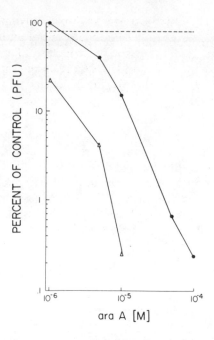

FIG. 6. Potentiation of the antiherpes activity of araA by EHNA. HeLa cells were infected with HSV (10 PFU/cell) in the presence (Δ) or absence (●) of 10^{-6} M EHNA and araA at the indicated concentrations. At 21 hr post-infection cells were disrupted and virus titers were determined by plaque assay.

promising in view of the fact that the most serious limitations to the systemic use of araA are its rapid deamination and its low solubility.

As mentioned above, there are two inhibitors of adenosine deaminase that are readily available to investigators, EHNA and DCF. Since both of these increase the antiherpes activity of araA (Bryson *et al.*, 1974; North and Cohen, 1978) the question arises as to which would be best for chemotherapeutic purposes. This must be determined in large part by toxicological studies which have not yet been completed. These toxicological studies will be of considerable interest because a deficiency of adenosine deaminase has been observed in some patients suffering from severe combined immunodeficiency disease (Meuwissen *et al.*, 1975). In the utilization of EHNA or DCF for viral chemotherapy it is imperative that they do not impair the host immune response for prolonged periods. Recent reports of deaths following DCF administration to humans (Sun, 1981) will probably exclude considerations of DCF.

Recent studies comparing the effects of EHNA and DCF in cultured cells also provide evidence that EHNA is better suited for chemotherapy than DCF. Lapi and Cohen (1977) have shown that the ability of EHNA to inhibit adenosine deaminase in cultured cells is readily reversible while DCF is not. In these experiments, cells were pretreated with one of the inhibitors and then extensively washed to remove the inhibitor. Following this treatment, the ability of the washed cells to detoxify the naturally occurring nucleoside deoxyadenosine was determined. The lethality of deoxyadenosine results from an increase in the level of dATP which is a strong inhibitor of ribonucleotide reductase. The toxicity exerted by deoxyadenosine is greatly increased in the presence of either EHNA or DCF. However, following removal of the deaminase inhibitor and extensive washing of cells, de-oxyadenosine was still toxic to cells pretreated with DCF but not to those pretreated with EHNA (Lapi and Cohen, 1977). These results are consistent with those of Agarwal *et al.* (1977) who showed that the adenosine deaminase-EHNA complex dissociates rapidly while the enzyme-DCF dissociation is very slow. For chemotherapeutic purposes it would seem more desirable to use the reversible inhibitor, particularly when the target of the drug is an enzyme whose long term inhibition may impair the immune response. The naturally occurring nucleoside deoxyadenosine is extremely toxic to lymphocytes in the presence of EHNA (Carson et al., 1977); this seems to be the result of an increased concentration of dATP, a known inhibitor of ribonucleotide reductase. Treatment of cells with deoxyadenosine (50 μM) in combination with EHNA (10 μM) elevated dATP levels more than 10-fold relative to controls, while levels of dGTP, dCTP and dTTP were greatly reduced by this treatment (Ullman et al., 1978). The combination of deoxyadenosine plus EHNA was also shown to reduce the activity of ribonucleotide reductase in HeLa cells (Lin and Elford, 1980). Moreover, erythrocytes from patients with severely-combined immunodeficiency disease and an absence of adenosine deaminase have elevated levels of dATP (A. Cohen et al., 1978; Coleman et al., 1978). These data suggest that prolonged exposure to an irreversible inhibitor of adenosine deaminase might be detrimental.

Another recent discovery that makes EHNA seem the more attractive of these two inhibitors is that EHNA alone (in the absence of araA) has significant antiviral activity in cultured cells (Fig. 7). In these experiments we found that 10^{-5} M EHNA inhibits production of HSV in infected HeLa cells by 75%. In parallel experiments it was shown that this concentration of EHNA had no toxic effects on uninfected HeLa cells (North and Cohen, 1978). This concentration of EHNA is also non-toxic to mouse fibroblasts (Plunkett and Cohen, 1975b; Lapi and Cohen, 1977). The ability of EHNA to inhibit HSV replication is not due to an inhibition of adenosine deaminase, since DCF does not show this antiviral effect (Sloan et al., 1977; Fig. 7). We have not determined the mechanism by which EHNA inhibits HSV replication, but we have shown that it specifically inhibits HSV DNA synthesis (North and Cohen, 1978). In these studies it was found that the extent to which HSV-specific DNA synthesis was inhibited correlated well with the extent that viral replication was inhibited. EHNA was not inhibitory to RNA or protein synthesis in HSV-infected cells and had no effect on macromolecular synthesis in uninfected HeLa cells. Therefore, EHNA seems to be a specific inhibitor of HSV DNA synthesis. Recently it has been shown that only one of the two enantiomers of EHNA inhibits adenosine deaminase (Frieden et al., 1980). The active form was subsequently shown to be the D-isomer (Baker et al., 1981; Bastian et al., 1981). The (+) 2S, 3R enantiomer of EHNA is 250-times as potent an inhibitor of adenosine deaminase as (−) 2R,3S EHNA. The two enantiomers of threo-9-(2-hydroxy-3-nonyl)adenine (THNA) are 40–60 times less active than (+) 2S, 3R EHNA (Bastian et al., 1981). It will be interesting to determine whether (+) 2S, 3R EHNA is also responsible for inhibition of HSV replication.

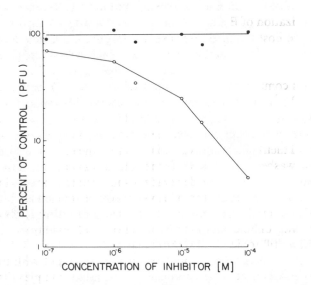

FIG. 7. Effect of inhibitors of adenosine deaminase on HSV multiplication. HeLa cells were infected with HSV (10 PFU/cell) in the presence of the indicated concentrations of DCF (●) or EHNA (○). At 21 hr post-infection cells were disrupted and virus titers were determined by plaque assay.

In animal systems EHNA has not proven effective when used alone against HSV infections. Shannon et al. (1980) determined that EHNA did not increase the mean survival time or decrease the morbidity of HSV infections in mice. However, this evaluation was made under condition of severe infection (mice were inoculated intraperitoneally with 6.4 LD_{50} of HSV) and it remains to be determined whether EHNA will exhibit antiviral activity following a milder challenge. In this same study it was shown that the combination of araA + EHNA was more effective than araA alone for treatment of HSV infections in mice.

Another inhibitor of adenosine deaminase, similar in structure to EHNA, (S)-9-(2,3-dihydroxypropyl)adenine (Schaeffer et al., 1965) also inhibits the replication of HSV and several other RNA and DNA viruses in cultured cells (DeClercq et al., 1978). Direct comparisons of the relative activities of these two compounds have not been made.

Direct comparisons of the relative toxicities of EHNA and DCF have not yet been published. However, preliminary studies indicate that EHNA is about one-tenth as toxic to mice as DCF (F. M. Schabel, Jr., personal communication). Long-term treatment of mice with DCF results in lung toxicity (Agarwal, 1980), kidney toxicity (Major et al., 1981a) and neurological toxicity (Major et al., 1981b). Toxicity of DCF has also been observed in phase I trials of DCF in humans (Poplack et al., 1981), and a recent report revealed that several patients have died after treatment with DCF (Sun, 1981). EHNA, on the other hand, seems to be relatively non-toxic to mice at dosages required to prevent deamination of araA (Shannon et al., 1980). However, an evaluation of the toxicity of EHNA in humans has not been carried out.

There have been several direct comparisons of the ability of these two compounds to inhibit adenosine deaminase in mice. Plunkett et al. (1979a) found that EHNA produces immediate inhibition of adenosine deaminase, while there is a lag of several hours before maximal inhibition by DCF is achieved. Furthermore, inhibition of adenosine deaminase by DCF is of much longer duration than inhibition by EHNA (Plunkett et al., 1979a). Both EHNA and DCF were shown to increase araA levels attained in plasma (Suling et al., 1978) and the peritoneal cavity (Plunkett et al., 1979a). Intracellular levels of araATP were elevated to about the same extent in the presence of either inhibitor (Plunkett et al., 1979a). Lambe and Nelson (1982) have also shown that EHNA produces a rapid and reversible inhibition of adenosine deaminase: a single oral dose inhibited adenosine deaminase for 4 hr. This suggests that administration of EHNA before araA might be the best way to potentiate the activity of araA. From these data it appears that EHNA displays the same desirable characteristics in vivo (at least in mice) that have been observed in cultured cells. If similar properties of EHNA and DCF are exerted in human, EHNA may well be the inhibitor of choice for use in combination chemotherapy with araA.

The mechanism of the specificity displayed by araA toward herpesviruses is of considerable importance since a knowledge of this mechanism might allow a more efficient use of araA in viral chemotherapy. The two most likely possibilities for this specificity are: (1) araA is metabolized to the active nucleotide araATP more efficiently in HSV-infected than in uninfected cells; or (2) that the site of inhibition of HSV replication is more sensitive to araATP than the site of inhibition in uninfected cells.

The metabolism of araA in uninfected and HSV-infected cells has not been compared in the presence of an adenosine deaminase inhibitor. Therefore, no information on the relative araATP levels in uninfected vs. HSV-infected cells is available. In the absence of a deaminase inhibitor Bennett et al. (1975) could detect no radioactively labeled araA converted to the corresponding nucleotides in either HSV-infected or uninfected HEp-2 cells. Since Plunkett and Cohen (1975a) found significant levels of araATP in uninfected mouse fibroblasts even in the absence of a deaminase inhibitor, it appears that the methods of Bennett et al. were not sufficiently sensitive to evaluate araATP levels.

As with araCTP, the activity of araATP may be modulated by the level of competing nucleotide, dATP. Levels of deoxyribonucleotides are known to change after infection of cells by HSV. However, there are conflicting reports as to whether dATP increases (Cheng et al., 1975) or decreases (Jamieson and Bjursell, 1976) after infection. Although these discrepancies may be partially explained by differences in cell and virus strains, problems with the techniques for assay of dNTPs have been encountered (North *et al.*, 1980). These problems have been eliminated (North *et al.*, 1980) and under such conditions dATP decreases after HSV-infection of HeLa cells to less than half the level in uninfected cells (North, unpublished results). Those studies were performed with the Miyama strain of HSV under conditions of infection described previously (North and Cohen, 1978). It remains to be determined whether dATP levels fall following infection under other conditions and with other cell types and virus strains. A decrease in dATP can clearly produce an increased ratio of araATP to dATP and this might account for some of the antiviral selectivity displayed by araA.

AraATP is known to inhibit mammalian DNA polymerases (Furth and Cohen, 1968) and its ability to inhibit DNA synthesis is most likely a result of this effect. This has prompted comparisons of the ability of araATP to inhibit the cellular and viral DNA polymerases. Conflicting results appeared from early studies of the specificity of araATP toward the herpes DNA polymerase. In studies of enzymes in crude extracts no specificity toward either viral or cellular DNA polymerases was found (Bennett *et al.*, 1975). However, using partially purified preparations, Muller *et al.* (1977b) found that the herpes-induced DNA polymerase was significantly more sensitive to araATP than either the α- or β-DNA polymerase of uninfected cells. These investigators reported that the HSV DNA polymerase was about 40-fold more sensitive to araATP than the cellular DNA polymerase-α. However, in studies of more highly purified enzymes Reinke *et al.* (1978) found that the HSV DNA polymerase is only slightly (at most four-fold) more sensitive to araATP than is DNA polymerase-α. These authors have cautioned that this effect may not be sufficient to account for all of the antiviral selectivity of araA.

The conflicting results of these studies comparing the ability of araATP to inhibit the HSV-induced and cellular DNA polymerases probably reflects the different state of purity of the enzymes in these investigations. Crude preparations may be expected to contain phosphatases and other enzymes which would affect determinations of the inhibition parameters. Likewise, certain of these contaminating enzymes might be enriched in one of the partially purified polymerase preparations. Therefore, it is essential to make these determinations with highly purified enzymes that lack interfering activities. Nevertheless, it is well established that HSV DNA synthesis is inhibited by araA to a greater extent than cellular DNA synthesis (Bennett *et al.*, 1975; Schwartz *et al.*, 1976). What has not been resolved is whether this specificity can be accounted for in part or in full by effects on DNA polymerase.

Another possible mechanism for the specificity toward herpesviruses displayed by araA has been suggested by Muller *et al.* (1977a) based upon studies of the incorporation of radioactively labeled araA into DNA. In these studies they confirmed the previous demonstration by Plunkett and Cohen (1975a) that araA is incorporated into cellular DNA in internucleotide linkage (Muller *et al.*, 1975). However, in HSV-infected cells most (90 per cent) of the radioactively labeled compound incorporated into HSV DNA was found at 3′-termini rather than in internucleotide linkage (Muller *et al.*, 1977a). Although it has been established that the radioactive material incorporated into cellular DNA was araA and not another metabolite (Plunkett and Cohen, 1975a; Muller *et al.*, 1975) this was not demonstrated with the material incorporated into HSV DNA (Muller *et al.*, 1977a). From these data it was suggested that araA was acting as a chain terminator in HSV DNA synthesis but not in cellular DNA synthesis.

In support of this model Muller *et al.* (1977a) reported that araA treatment of HSV-infected cells results in the accumulation of short DNA fragments which are not subsequently joined into long DNA chains. In addition, a large amount of single-stranded DNA was found to accumulate under these conditions. If it can be demonstrated that these short DNA fragments, and the single-stranded chains, are herpes DNA terminated with araAMP, it would argue strongly in favor of this model. These experiments of Muller *et al.* were done in the absence of an inhibitor of adenosine deaminase.

However, these results of Muller *et al.* have not been confirmed by others. Pelling *et al.* (1981) found that 92–96 per cent of the araAMP incorporated into HSV DNA was present in internucleotide linkage within the DNA. Moreover, they showed that commercial preparations of spleen phosphodiesterase (used to degrade DNA to 3'-nucleotides, giving rise to nucleosides from the 3'-termini) contain phosphatase activity which converts araAMP to araA. Muller *et al.* apparently took no precautions against this activity and this seems the best explanation for the discrepancy between their data and those of Pelling *et al.* (1981).

Pelling *et al.* (1981) also compared the amount of araAMP incorporated into viral DNA to that incorporated into cellular DNA following exposure to araA. With concentration of araA ranging from 0.1 to 3.2 μM, 2–4 times as much araAMP was incorporated into DNA of uninfected cells as was found in HSV DNA. These studies were done in the presence of the inhibitor of adenosine deaminase, deoxycoformycin. Under these conditions viral DNA synthesis is inhibited to a greater extent than is DNA synthesis in uninfected cells. Furthermore, Pelling *et al.* demonstrated that araAMP is found in internucleotide linkage within the DNA of virions that had been formed in the presence of araA, which rules out the possibility that araAMP-containing DNA cannot be packaged into virions. Thus, the antiviral specificity of araA cannot be explained solely by the selective incorporation of araAMP into viral DNA.

The lower level of incorporation of araAMP into HSV DNA relative to cellular DNA may be due to its removal by a 3'-exonuclease activity associated with the HSV DNA polymerase (Knopf, 1979). It has been shown that this exonuclease will remove 3'-terminal araAMP from DNA *in vitro* (Derse and Cheng, 1981). Further experiments will be necessary to determine whether this exonuclease or other DNA repair processes influence the amount of araAMP which is found within DNA.

Although early attempts to isolate HSV mutants resistant to araA failed (Klein, 1975; Shannon, 1977a), more recently such mutants have been obtained (Coen *et al.*, 1982). These mutants map in the locus for the HSV DNA polymerase, and the polymerase induced by these mutants is less sensitive to inhibition by araATP. These data confirm that the interaction of a nucleotide of araA (presumably araATP) with the herpes DNA polymerase produces the inhibition of viral multiplication.

In summary, studies in cultured cell systems have established that araA inhibits the replication of herpesviruses with a great deal of specificity relative to its effects on uninfected cells. This activity seems to be due to the ability of araA to inhibit herpes DNA synthesis specifically. The antiviral activity of araA is greatly increased by combining it with an inhibitor of adenosine deaminase. Under these conditions araA retains its specificity toward inhibition of herpesviruses. The specificity of araA toward herpesviruses and its potentiation by inhibitors of adenosine deaminase has also been demonstrated in animal systems. And finally the specific antiherpes activity of araA may result from (at least in part) its ability to inhibit the herpes DNA polymerase specifically, although this effect alone may not account for all of the antiviral specificity.

In addition to the antiviral activity displayed by araA, it has been encouraging that it exhibits low toxicity. Large doses of araA were tolerated well with little or no toxicity in mice, rats, rabbits and monkeys (Kurtz, 1975). Preliminary studies of araA in humans have also found it to be relatively non-toxic (Keeney, 1975). However, in the presence of an inhibitor of adenosine deaminase increased toxicity is expected. Nevertheless, a combination of araA + EHNA that displays antiviral activity in mice displays no toxicity in these mice (Shannon *et al.*, 1980).

Since herpesviruses have been implicated in cancer and since mutagenic agents increase the ability of HSV to transform cultured cells (Rapp, 1974), the ability of araA to act as a mutagen or a carcinogen must also be evaluated. It was reported that araA was negative in *Salmonella* tests of mutagenicity, although experimental details were not given (Kurtz *et al.*, 1977). In these studies it is likely that araA was extensively deaminated and that there was little accumulation of araATP, since apparently no steps were taken to inhibit the bacterial adenosine deaminase. It has also been reported that araA displays little or no teratogenicity (Adlard *et al.*, 1975; Fishaut *et al.*, 1975; Gasset and Akaboshi, 1976). However, these experiments were also done under conditions where deamination of araA was not prevented.

In contrast to these reports, Kurtz *et al.* (1977) found araA to be teratogenic to rabbits. It is apparent that further evaluation of the mutagenic and teratogenic potential of araA is needed.

8.3.3. OTHER VIRUSES

AraA inhibits most of the viruses that are inhibited by araC. The replication of vaccinia virus in cell culture is inhibited by araA (Privat de Garilhe and De Rudder, 1964). This inhibition is also relatively specific. Miller *et al.* (1968) found that replication of vaccinia virus is inhibited by concentrations of araA that are not cytotoxic to uninfected cells. In addition, araA has proven effective in the treatment of vaccinial keratitis in rabbits, vaccinial skin lesions in rabbits, and vaccinial encephalitis in mice (reviewed by Sloan, 1975). In cultured cells, the inhibition of vaccinia virus by araA is increased 40-fold by combining it with DCF (Conner *et al.*, 1974).

Results on the inhibition of other DNA viruses by araA are not conclusive. Adenoviruses and papovaviruses have been found either insensitive or slightly sensitive to araA (see Table 2). However, these studies were done in the absence of an inhibitor of adenosine deaminase and, therefore, need re-evaluation.

Replication of the retroviruses Rous sarcoma virus (Miller *et al.*, 1968; Schabel, 1968) and murine leukemia virus (Shannon *et al.*, 1974) is inhibited by araA. AraATP, like araCTP, also inhibits the viral reverse transcriptase (Shannon, 1975b). It has been reported that levels of adenosine deaminase are significantly reduced following transformation of chick embryo fibroblasts by Rous sarcoma virus (Chiang *et al.*, 1977). In these transformed cells, adenosine deaminase levels were decreased by 90 per cent. If this phenomenon is characteristic of transformation by all oncornaviruses, araA and other adenosine analogs should be particularly effective against these viruses.

The only other RNA viruses inhibited by araA are the rhabdoviruses. Like araC, araA inhibits the replication of both rabies virus (Harmon and Janis, 1976) and vesicular stomatitis virus (Grant and Sabina, 1972), although high concentrations of araA are required. Neither araA nor araC was found effective in treating mice infected with street-rabies virus (Harmon and Janis, 1976). However, deaminase inhibitors were not employed in these studies. The mechanism by which the aranucleosides inhibit replication of rhabdo-viruses in cultured cells has not been fully determined. It has recently been shown that high concentrations of araATP will inhibit the virion-associated RNA polymerase of vesicular stomatitis virus (Chanda and Banerjee, 1980). Perhaps when the significance of these effects has been clarified an effective treatment for rabies with araA or araC can be developed (in combination with an appropriate deaminase inhibitor).

As shown in Table 2 all other RNA viruses examined have been found insensitive to araA. But these studies too were all done in the absence of an inhibitor of adenosine deaminase and, therefore, should be repeated.

8.3.4. ARAAMP

Since the deamination of araA occurs at the nucleoside level a means of bypassing this step would be to provide the nucleotide, araAMP. AraAMP is the first product in the sequence of reactions which converts araA to the active form araATP (Fig. 4). AraAMP is also far more soluble than araA. Thus by supplying the compound at the nucleotide level the two problems of deamination and low solubility of araA could be solved. However, this approach depends on the ability of cells to utilize nucleotides without degradation to nucleosides, which would be subject to deamination.

AraAMP was first synthesized by Cohen (1966). In studies with nucleotides it was found that araAMP was more toxic to cultured fibroblasts than araA (Ortiz *et al.*, 1972). In these studies 2×10^{-4} M araAMP began to kill cells more slowly than araA. However, araA was rapidly deaminated and although some of the cells were killed, the survivors began growth at a normal rate. Thus, although araAMP exerted its toxicity more slowly at first it wasn't deaminated and, therefore, was able to exert toxicity over a much longer period. However, these studies did not distinguish between slow uptake of the intact nucleotide and slow cleavage to the nucleoside prior to uptake.

In subsequent studies using doubly-labeled (^{3}H, ^{32}P) araAMP it was demonstrated that araAMP enters cells without dephosphorylation (Plunkett et al., 1974). The rate of uptake of araAMP was found to be 3 to 5 per cent of the rate of araA uptake. Doubly-labeled araAMP was converted to araATP and incorporated into DNA in internucleotide linkage within the cell (Plunkett et al., 1974). In addition, almost all of the label was recovered in araAMP nucleotides, demonstrating that little deamination, dephosphorylation or reutilization of the free base was occurring (Plunkett et al., 1974; Cohen and Plunkett, 1975). The inhibitor of adenosine deaminase, EHNA, does not potentiate toxicity of araAMP (Plunkett and Cohen, 1975b).

3′,5′-Cyclic-araAMP (c-araAMP) was found to be as toxic as araAMP to L cells (Plunkett and Cohen, 1975b). This probably results from the ability of cells to convert c-araAMP to araAMP (Hughes and Kimball, 1972).

AraAMP has also been shown to exert biological activity in animals. AraAMP was as effective as araA in prolonging survival of mice with Ehrlich ascites carcinoma (Cohen and Plunkett, 1975). Similar results were obtained by Cass et al. (1979) in treatment of mouse L1210 leukemia with araAMP. In these studies, Cass et al. also found that the activity of araAMP is increased by combination with EHNA or DCF in contrast to the situation in cultured cells. These data suggest that a considerable amount of the araAMP administered to animals is converted to an intermediate which is sensitive to adenosine deaminase, presumably araA. Thus, in addition to its ability to penetrate intact into cells (albeit at a slow rate), araAMP may serve as a depot form of araA in animals.

AraAMP displays significant antiviral activity. Sidwell et al. (1973) found that araAMP inhibits the replication of HSV (both subtypes), cytomegalovirus, and vaccinia virus in cultured cells. In all cases inhibition of virus replication was achieved at approximately the same concentration of araAMP as was required for inhibition with araA. 3′,5′-Cyclic-araAMP had the same antiviral activity as araAMP (Sidwell et al., 1973).

AraAMP has also shown significant anti-HSV activity in animal studies. In these studies araAMP was shown to be successful in treatments of herpes simplex keratitis in rabbits (Kaufman and Varnell, 1976; Falcon and Jones, 1977). In mice araAMP was more effective than araA in systemic treatment of HSV-encephalitis (Kern et al., 1978). Because of its greater solubility higher concentrations of araAMP than araA may be used. Kaufman and Varnell (1976) found that increased levels of araAMP resulted in an increased therapeutic effect with no toxicity. In addition, Falcon and Jones (1977) found that araAMP was better at inhibiting the production of herpetic lesions in rabbit eyes than comparable levels of araA. Also Sloan (1975) reported that araAMP, given either subcutaneously or intravenously, significantly increased survival of mice with HSV-encephalitis.

In treatments of herpes simplex keratitis in rabbits, araAMP was more effective than a combination of araA and an inhibitor of adenosine deaminase (DCF) (Falcon and Jones, 1977). However, this involved topical application of the compounds. In systemic application the degradation of araAMP by phosphomonoesterase seems to occur (as discussed above). The product of this dephosphorylation, araA, is subject either to deamination or uptake by cells and rephosphorylation. Therefore, the combination of araAMP with an inhibitor of adenosine deaminase seems to merit clinical evaluation.

Of particular importance in comparison of araAMP with araA, and evaluation of the necessity for combination of araAMP with an inhibitor of adenosine deaminase, is the metabolism of araAMP in humans. It has been found that araAMP has a significant half-life in humans. In several patients more than half (and in all cases more than 25 per cent) of araAMP administered was retained for more than 24 hr (LePage et al., 1975). However, araAMP is not detected in plasma or urine following intravenous or intramuscular injection; the major metabolite found in those studies was araHx (Whitley et al., 1980). Once again these data suggest that the combination of araAMP with EHNA or DCF will be a potent antiviral treatment.

8.4. AraHx

9-β-D-Arabinofuranosylhypoxanthine (araHx), the product of adenosine deaminase attack upon araA, is known to be relatively non-toxic (Cohen, 1966). Nevertheless, a number of investigators have demonstrated an inhibition of the replication of herpes simplex virus (Conner et al., 1975; Shipman et al., 1976), herpes zoster (Bryson and Conner, 1976) and vaccinia virus (Conner et al., 1975) by araHx. However, this antiviral activity of araHx requires much higher concentrations than the concentrations of araA necessary to get the same activity. In the absence of inhibitors of adenosine deaminase, araA is about 10-fold more toxic than araHx (Shipman et al., 1976). When deamination of araA is prevented with a deaminase inhibitor, araA is 90 times more potent than araHx (Schwartz et al., 1976).

The mechanism by which araHx inhibits viral replication is not understood. AraHx selectively inhibits HSV DNA synthesis with a pattern similar to that of araA, but much higher levels of araHx are required (Schwartz et al., 1976). Because of these large dosages it is difficult to determine whether araHx or a metabolite of it is the toxic form. Possible ways in which araHx may be converted to araATP or araGTP have been suggested (Cohen, 1976). Experimental evidence has been provided which demonstrates that araIMP can be converted to araAMP by sequential action of the enzymes adenylosuccinate synthetase and adenylosuccinate lyase (Spector and Miller, 1976). Moreover, the antiviral activity of araHx is antagonized by deoxyadenosine (Smith et al., 1978). These data suggest that the low antiviral activity of araHx is due to its slow conversion to araATP.

AraHx displays some activity against herpes simplex keratitis of rabbits, but again it is much less effective than araA (Falcon and Jones, 1977). The 5'-monophosphate of araHx, araIMP, is also effective in treating rabbit herpetic keratitis, but is much less effective than araAMP (Sidwell et al., 1975; Kaufman and Varnell, 1976). Evaluation of these data will also require more information on araHx metabolism.

8.5. AraT

1-β-D-Arabinofuranosylthymine (araT, spongothymidine) was one of the original arabinosyl nucleosides isolated from the sponge Cryptotethya crypta (Bergmann and Feeney, 1951). AraT is relatively non-toxic to most cultured cells due to the inability of the cellular thymidine kinase to phosphorylate it to araTMP. However, araT is inhibitory to the replication of herpes simplex virus in cultured cells (Renis and Buthala 1965; De Rudder and Privat de Garilhe, 1965). It also shows some antiviral activity against herpes keratitis in rabbits (Underwood et al., 1964). This is due to the ability of the HSV-induced deoxypyrimidine kinase to phosphorylate araT (Aswell et al., 1977).

Gentry and Aswell (1975) have shown that 2×10^{-4} M araT completely inhibits replication of either HSV-1 or HSV-2 in BHK cells. This concentration of araT has no effect on growth of uninfected BHK cells. In addition, Aswell et al. (1977) have shown that araT is phosphorylated in HSV-infected but not in uninfected BHK cells; and DNA synthesis is inhibited by 2×10^{-4} M araT in infected but not uninfected cells. HSV mutants that lack viral deoxypyrimidine kinase activity are insensitive to araT (Aswell et al., 1977; Miller et al., 1977). These data convincingly demonstrate that phosphorylation of araT to a toxic nucleotide, presumably araTTP, occurs. It is supposed that araTTP inhibits DNA synthesis in a manner similar to araCTP and araATP. AraTTP is a competitive inhibitor of both the cellular DNA polymerase-α and the retroviral reverse transcriptase in a manner that is competitive with dTTP (Matsukage et al., 1978). It has not been determined whether araTTP is a selective inhibitor of herpesvirus DNA polymerases.

Miller et al. (1977) have also found that araT inhibits replication of and DNA synthesis by HSV in human embryo fibroblasts (HEF), but has no effect on growth of uninfected HEF cells. In addition, they found that herpes zoster was sensitive to araT while cytomegalovirus was not. These data are in agreement with other reports that cytomegalovirus does not induce an enzyme similar to the HSV deoxypyrimidine kinase (Zavada et al., 1976).

Interestingly, the replication of Epstein–Barr virus in P3HR-1 cells is inhibited by araT, whereas growth of P3HR-1 is not (Ooka and Calender, 1980; Yonemura *et al.*, 1981). It is not clear whether the phosphorylation of araT in Epstein-Barr virus-infected cells is performed by a viral-encoded thymidine kinase or a cellular enzyme that is induced after virus infection.

Although BHK and HEF cells are insensitive to araT, Miller *et al.* (1977) found that growth of CV-1 cells is inhibited by 50 μg/ml of araT. Thus it appears that some cells can phosphorylate araT. The effectiveness of araT in treating human herpes infections will depend upon whether human tissues phosphorylate it as well as herpes-infected cells. Aswell *et al.* (1977) have shown that araT has antiviral activity against equine herpesvirus infections of hamsters. However, in those studies in was found that araT was rapidly excreted in the urine and the antiviral activity required repeated injections at 4-hr intervals. More recently, araT was shown to be effective in treatment of HSV-encephalitis in mice (Machidda *et al.*, 1980). In these studies araT was effective when given twice daily by intraperitoneal injection, and exhibited some antiviral activity following a single large dose. Further pharmacological studies will be required in order to determine the appropriate dosage schedule for trials in humans.

8.6. AraG

9-β-D-Arabinofuranosylguanine (araG) was synthesized by Reist and Goodman (1964). AraG inhibits DNA synthesis in TA3 ascites cells and increases the survival of mice bearing TA3 cells; however, it is not nearly as effective as araA in these respects (Brink and LePage, 1964).

AraG inhibits the replication of herpes simplex virus and vaccinia virus in cultured cells (Elion *et al.*, 1975). AraG also has antiviral activity against HSV and vaccinia virus infections of rabbit eyes and against intracerebral infections of mice with these same viruses (Elion *et al.*, 1975). However, in these studies with mice the half-life of subcutaneously injected araG was only 45 min. Thus it is apparent that araG is either rapidly metabolized or poorly utilized by mice, despite the fact that it is readily phosphorylated by deoxynucleoside kinase (Elion *et al.*, 1975).

AraGMP, synthesized by Saneyoshi (Hokkaido University, Faculty of Pharmaceutical Sciences, Sapporo, Japan), also inhibits the replication of HSV. At 10^{-4} M araGMP, production of HSV in infected cells is inhibited by more than 99 per cent (North and Cohen, unpublished results). This level of araGMP inhibits growth of mouse fibroblasts, but is not lethal (Lapi and Cohen, unpublished results).

The metabolic fate of araG or araGMP has not been determined either in cultured cells or animals. These experiments have been discouraged in large measure by the difficulty in synthesizing the large quantities of appropriately labeled araG or araGMP to do the experiments. However, before these compounds can be evaluated as antiviral agents more should be known of their metabolism. Since the GC content of HSV DNA is approximately twice that of mammalian cells (Goodheart *et al.*, 1968; Kieff *et al.*, 1971), one might expect herpes simplex viruses to be particularly sensitive to deoxyguanosine analogs.

8.7. AraU

1-β-D-Arabinofuranosyluracil (araU, spongouridine), like araT, was one of the original arabinosyl nucleosides isolated from the sponge *Cryptotethya crypta* (Bergmann and Feeney, 1951). AraU was originally thought to be non-toxic to most cultured cells. As discussed above, the araU produced by enzymatic deamination of araC is rapidly excreted from humans. AraU can also be cleaved to free uracil (Tono and Cohen, 1962). More recently, Muller and Zahn (1979) have shown that araU inhibits growth of mammalian cells in culture. However, the concentration of araU required to achieve this effect was more than 100-times higher than the concentration of araC required to produce a similar effect. In mouse L5178Y cells araU was phosphorylated to araUMP, araUDP and araUTP. A small amount of araUMP was found in internucleotide linkage within DNA. Muller and Zahn determined that DNA from araU-treated cells contained 1 araUMP molecule per 45,500 dTMP molecules. AraUTP was also shown to inhibit cellular DNA polymerase-α and the reverse transcriptase of Rouse sarcoma virus, while it was less active against DNA polymerase-β and inactive against cellular RNA polymerases I, II and III. The inhibition of DNA polymerase was competitive with respect to both dUTP and dTTP. Interestingly, a strong synergism was achieved with the combination of araU and araC (Muller and Zahn, 1979).

In animal models araU was initially found to lack antiviral activity (Underwood *et al.*, 1964). However, in cell culture araU was shown to inhibit the replication of HSV, albeit at a 25-70-fold higher concentrations than required for inhibition by araT (DeClercq *et al.*, 1977). This antiviral activity was dependent upon the presence of the HSV-induced deoxypyrimidine kinase, suggesting that this enzyme is responsible for phosphorylation of araU to the corresponding 5′-monophosphate in HSV-infected cells.

The mechanism by which araU inhibits HSV replication has not been elucidated. The two most likely possibilities are: (1) conversion of araUMP to araTMP *via* thymidylate synthase, then subsequent conversion to araTTP and incorporation into DNA; or (2) conversion to araUTP and incorporation into DNA. Muller and Zahn (1979) have shown that the latter occurs in uninfected cells. AraUMP is a poor substrate of the bacteriophage T4-induced thymidylate synthase. It is converted to araTMP at only 2 per cent the rate at which dUMP is converted to dTMP (Cohen, 1960). The ability of araUMP to be incorporated into DNA of HSV-infected cells would depend upon the substrate specificities of uracil-DNA glycosylase and dUTP nucleotidylhydrolase. Both of these enzymes may be induced following infection of cells with HSV, and both are already present in uninfected cells (Caradonna and Cheng, 1981). Their abilities to act upon araUMP within DNA and upon araUTP have not been evaluated.

The low antiviral activity of araU combined with its rapid excretion make it unattractive as an antiviral agent. However, as will be discussed below, a number of 5-substituted derivatives of araU have excellent antiviral activity.

8.8. OTHER ARANUCLEOSIDES AND ARANUCLEOSIDE ANALOGS

As discussed above, one of the most serious limitations in the use of aranucleosides in chemotherapy is the detoxification of these compounds by cellular enzymes. One means of minimizing this problem is through utilization of another inhibitor that prevents this detoxification. Thus the activity of araA or araC is increased by using it in combination with an inhibitor of the deaminase which detoxifies it. However, another approach is to provide analogs of the aranucleoside that are not subject to inactivation by these enzymes yet still display biological activity. There are two different mechanisms by which this approach can work. The first is that the analog itself may be phosphorylated and that derivative exert biological activity similar to the parent nucleotide. And the second approach is that the analog be slowly converted back to the parent aranucleoside. Once this conversion has occurred the resulting aranucleoside would be subject to the same metabolic processes it normally faces. However, if the conversion of the analog to the respective aranucleoside is sufficiently slow, the analog can serve as a constant supply of aranucleoside and eliminate the problem of rapid depletion of the exogenous supply.

An excellent example of this latter type of compound is cyclocytidine (2,2′-anhydro-araC). This compound is not subject to deamination and is slowly converted to araC in humans. This slow conversion necessitates the use of high levels of cyclocytidine to continuously provide araC at effective levels. However, these high levels of cyclocytidine result in some toxic effects not seen with araC (Chawla *et al.*, 1974). Another analog, 2,2′-anhydro-5-fluoro-araC (AAFC), does not show these toxic effects (Schneyer and Galbraith, 1975). AAFC is hydrolyzed to 5-fluoro-araC which can also be deaminated to 5-fluoro-araU as

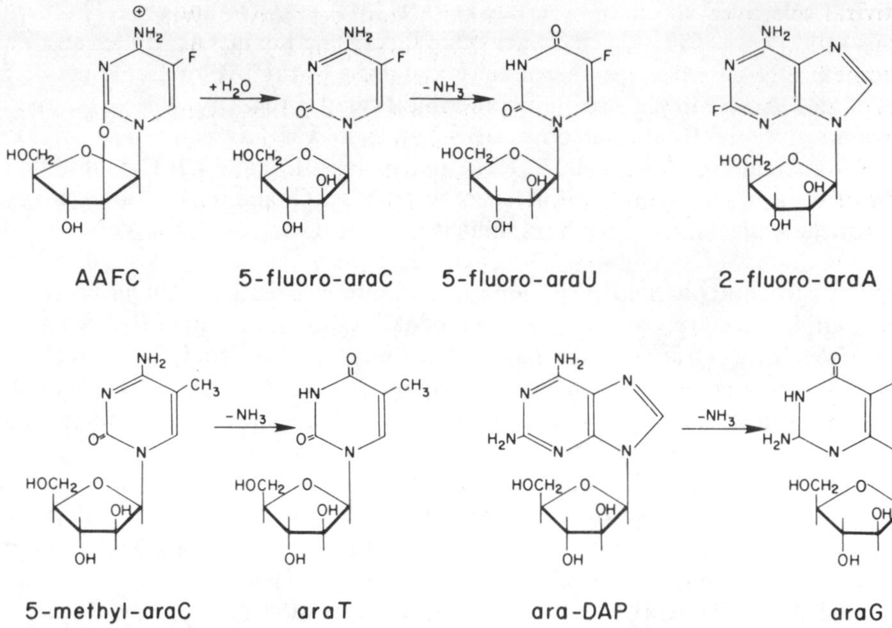

FIG. 8. Structure and metabolism of some aranucleosides and aranucleoside analogs.

shown in Fig. 8. 5-Fluoro-araC possesses many of the same inhibitory properties as araC (Fox *et al.*, 1966), and 5-fluoro-araUMP is an inhibitor of thymidylate synthetase (Cohen, 1961). Both of these compounds are active against leukemia cells (Burchenal *et al.*, 1975). The 5-halogenated derivatives of araC (5-fluoro-, 5-chloro-, 5-bromo- and 5-iodo-) all exhibit antiviral activity but are no more effective than araC (Fox *et al.*, 1966; Renis *et al.*, 1968; DeClercq and Torrence, 1978). Other compounds that may serve as a depot form of araC include 1-β-D-arabinofuranosyl-2-amino-1,4(2H)-4-iminopyrimidine (Khwaja *et al.*, 1979) and N^4-succinyl-araC (Oh-ishi *et al.*, 1981). Both of these compounds exhibit antitumor activity in mice that is equivalent or better than that of araC. The antiviral activities of these compounds have not been evaluated.

An interesting approach to avoid the deamination problem has been the development of lipophilic derivatives of araC nucleotides. Several araCDP-diacylglycerols have been made and shown to possess biological activity (MacCoss *et al.*, 1978; Turcotte *et al.*, 1980). Presumably these compounds are taken up by cells then converted to araCMP by CDP-diacylglycerol hydrolase. This would by-pass the need for phosphorylation of a nucleoside and the problems arising from deamination by cytidine deaminase. In addition to provision of araC nucleotides, the intact lipophilic-araCDP analogs may be responsible for some of their observed antitumor properties (Turcotte *et al.*, 1980).

Yet another araC analog which is resistant to deamination is 2′-azido-2′-deoxy-araC (Cheng *et al.*, 1981). This compound is converted to 2′-azido-2′-deoxy-araCTP which is an inhibitor of DNA polymerases. It is more effective than araC in treatment of some experimental leukemias; it inhibits replication of HSV but this requires a concentration 50-fold higher than a cytotoxic dose (Cheng *et al.*, 1981).

Another araC analog, 5-methyl-araC (Fig. 8), has been shown to possess antiviral properties. Aswell and Gentry (1977) found that this compound inhibits the replication of herpes simplex virus in cells that have high levels of deoxycytidine deaminase but not in cells that have low levels of this enzyme. From this they suggest that 5-methyl-araC is deaminated to araT (as shown in Fig. 8). Neither 5-methyl-araC nor araT is toxic to HEp-2 cells at concentrations that exert antiviral activity. Apparently the herpes-induced deoxycytidine deaminase reported by Chan (1977) does not utilize 5-methyl-araC as a substrate.

Several 5-substituted derivatives of araU have been synthesized and many of these have better antiviral selectivity than the corresponding araC derivatives. With most of these analogs the selectivity is due to selective phosphorylation by the herpes-encoded de-oxypyrimidine kinase (as with those compounds described in Fig. 2A). The 5-halogenated derivatives of araU have antiherpes activity (Underwood *et al.*, 1964; Renis *et al.*, 1968) and they exhibit more selectivity than the 5-halogenated derivatives of araC (DeClercq and Torrence, 1978). A number of 5-alkyl- and 5-alkenyl derivatives have also been made. The most active of these, 5-ethyl-araU, shows good antiviral selectivity but is less active than araT (Kulikowski *et al.*, 1979; Machida *et al.*, 1979). Of the 5-alkenyl derivatives, 5-bromo-vinyl-araU is about as active as 5-bromovinyldeoxyuridine, but others are less active than the corresponding deoxyuridine derivatives (Machida *et al.*, 1981).

Another aranucleoside which has antiviral activity is 2,6-diamino-9-β-D-arabinofuranosylpurine (ara-DAP) which is shown in Fig. 8. This compound inhibits replication of HSV (both subtypes) and vaccinia virus in cultured cells and is also active against infections of rabbit eyes and mouse brain by these viruses (Elion *et al.*, 1975). Ara-DAP is a poorer substrate for adenosine deaminase and adenosine kinase than araA (Elion *et al.*, 1975). The mechanism by which ara-DAP inhibits virus replication is not known but phosphorylation to ara-DAP nucleotides occurs. In animal studies ara-DAP was rapidly excreted but a significant portion was converted to araG. In fact, higher plasma levels of araG were obtained following treatment with ara-DAP than treatment with araG (Elion *et al.*, 1975).

A number of attempts have been made to obtain analogs of araA that are more soluble than araA and are not substrates for adenosine deaminase. One compound with these properties, araAMP, was discussed above. Another compound that is more soluble than araA and is resistant to adenosine deaminase is araA-5′-formate. In whole blood araA-5′ formate is rapidly converted to araA (Repta *et al.*, 1975). Since this conversion is complete within a few minutes araA-5′-formate does not serve as a depot form of araA. However, it does allow greater levels of araA to be achieved because of its greater solubility. The antiviral activities of araA and araA-5′-formate are equivalent at equimolar concentrations (Shannon, 1975a). Another araA analog that is resistant to adenosine deaminase is 2-fluoro-araA (shown in Fig. 8). This compound is phosophorylated to 2-fluoro-araATP, and is effective against L1210 leukemia (Brockman *et al.*, 1977). 2-Fluoro-araA was shown to inhibit cell growth as effectively as the combination of araA plus DCF; DCF did not increase the activity of 2-fluoro-araA (Plunkett *et al.*, 1980). Phosphorylation of 2-fluoro-araA to the corresponding monophosphate is catalyzed by deoxycytidine kinase and cells devoid of that enzyme are resistant to this analog (Brockman *et al.*, 1980; Dow *et al.*, 1980). Cells deficient in deoxycytidine kinase are not resistant to araA (Dow *et al.*, 1980). Recently it has been shown that there are two enzymes capable of phosphorylating deoxyadenosine, namely deoxycytidine kinase and adenosine kinase (Ullman *et al.*, 1981). These data suggest that araA can be phosphorylated by adenosine kinase. 2-Fluoro-araA inhibits DNA synthesis to a slightly greater extent than an equal concentration of araA (in the presence of DCF) (Plunkett *et al.*, 1980). The anti-herpes activity of 2-fluoro-araAMP is equivalent to the activity of araAMP (Shannon, 1980).

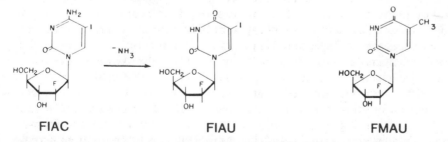

FIG. 9. Structures of 2′-fluoro-arabinosylpyrimidines which possess specific antiherpes activity. The compounds are 2′-fluoro-5-iodo-araC (FIAC), 2′-fluoro-5-iodo-araU (FIAU), and 2′-fluoro-5-methyl-araU (FMAU).

AraA-5'-valerate is an interesting analog of araA which is not subject to deamination, is more water-soluble than araA, and is more lipophilic than araA. Intracellularly, araA-5'-valerate is hydrolyzed to araA. Moreover, the parent compound (araA-5'-valerate) is an inhibitor of adenosine deaminase with a K_i of 11 μM (Lipper et al., 1978). Thus, this compound provides a depot form of araA and also protects the liberated drug from enzymatic deamination. Other analogs of araA that are resistant to adenosine deaminase include the α-anomer of araA and α-ara-8-azaadenine (Bennett et al., 1975), carbocyclic araA (Vince and Daluge, 1977) and arabinosyl-N^6-hydroxyadenine (Lopez and Giner-Sorolla, 1977). Preliminary studies have shown that all of these analogs have antiviral properties. Carbocyclic araA is as selective and as active as araA against HSV, vaccinia and Gross murine leukemia virus (Shannon, 1980).

Further studies will determine whether any of these other analogs will be of use in viral chemotherapy. Carbocyclic analogs of araG and araDAP have also been synthesized and only the latter is active against HSV (Lee and Vince, 1980).

Perhaps the most potent and selective antiherpes compounds yet developed are the 2'-fluoro-arabinosylpyrimidines synthesized by Watanabe et al. (1979). One of these compounds, 2'-fluoro-5-iodo-araC(FIAC), shown in Fig. 2, inhibits the replication of herpes simplex virus by > 90 per cent at a concentration below 0.01 μM. Little or no cytotoxicity was observed following treatment of human fibroblasts with 10 μM FIAC. In direct comparisons, FIAC was found to be 60 times more active than acycloguanosine against HSV-1 (Fox et al., 1981).

FIAC is deaminated to 2-fluoro-5-iodo-araU(FIAU) (Chou et al., 1981) which also exhibits potent and selective antiviral activity (Watanabe et al., 1979). This deamination may be prevented by combination with tetrahydrouridine (Chou et al., 1981). Following treatment of mice with FIAC, substantial levels of FIAU and of 2'-fluoro-5-methyl-araU (FMAU) were detected in urine (Chou et al., 1981). FMAU is more potent than FIAC in treatment of herpes infections in mice (Fox et al., 1981).

Fox et al. (1981) have also shown that the selectivity of FIAC is due to the ability of the herpes-induced deoxypyrimidine kinase to phosphorylate it to the corresponding nucleotide. Most uninfected cells fail to phosphorylate FIAC, although it does exhibit activity against some tumor cells. Viral mutants which fail to induce this kinase are also resistant to FIAC. Herpes DNA synthesis is inhibited by treatment of infected cells with FIAC. In addition the corresponding nucleotides of metabolites of FIAC (FIAU and FMAU) were found in DNA (Chou et al., 1981). DNA synthesis in uninfected cells was not inhibited at a concentration of FIAC 1000 times higher than that required to inhibit viral DNA synthesis by more than 90 per cent. Such promising results will certainly lead to further evaluation of these exciting aranucleoside analogs.

8.9. SUMMARY AND CONCLUSIONS

In this review the major goal has been to point out some aspects that must be considered in evaluating the aranucleosides as antiviral agents. We have seen that the active forms of these compounds are the aranucleotides and thus phosphorylation of the aranucleosides is essential for their biological activity. Likewise, most of these compounds are metabolized by cellular enzymes to an inactive form; araA and araC are enzymatically deaminated to araHx and araU, respectively, which are much less active. We have also seen that an inhibitor of the appropriate cellular deaminase will greatly increase the effectiveness of araA or araC. As another approach, the biological activity of these analogs is increased through utilization of derivatives that are not subject to deamination, such as araAMP. Thus an understanding of the metabolism of the aranucleosides has opened up the way for new chemotherapeutic approaches.

Of the aranucleosides studied, araA has shown the most promise as an antiviral agent, particularly in treating severe herpes infections in humans. In fact, araA has shown more promise in treating a wide range of herpes infections in animals and in clinical evaluations than any other compound tested to date, and is the only antiviral which has been approved for systemic treatment of herpetic disorders. In addition, this antiviral activity has been achieved with little or no toxic effects to the host. However, all of the clinical evaluations of araA were done under conditions where it was rapidly deaminated. It is apparent that these evaluations need to be done under the conditions that have been shown to increase effectiveness of araA. The combined use of araA and an inhibitor of adenosine deaminase or the use of araAMP may prove effective in treatment of herpes infections where araA alone has had little or no success, such as cytomegalovirus infections in humans (Ch'ien et al., 1974). However, increased toxicity may also be expected from such treatments.

AraC has proven too toxic for widespread use as an antiviral agent even though it has been used successfully to treat herpetic keratitis that has developed resistance to IUdR (Renis and Buthala, 1965). Treatment of human herpetic keratitis with araC has been limited due to its corneal toxicity. However, as pointed out above, very little is known about araC metabolism in virus-infected cells. Moreover, no antiviral selectivity is obtained with araC. Perhaps when this metabolism is understood effective ways to use araC as an antiviral agent can be devised.

The other aranucleosides have not been studied enough to determine how effective they would be in viral chemotherapy. One of those which shows some specificity toward herpes simplex virus is araT. It is phosphorylated by the HSV-induced deoxypyrimidine kinase and not by most cellular thymidine kinases. Therefore, it is converted to the active form, araTTP, only in HSV-infected cells. The mechanism by which araT exerts its antiviral effect is similar to that of many other nucleosides that are phosphorylated only by the HSV-induced enzyme (see Fig. 2).

Although these compounds that utilize the HSV-induced thymidine kinase might prove useful in certain situations, there are two problems that might limit their use. First of all they are not effective against other viruses that do not induce this deoxypyrimidine kinase. As discussed above, cytomegalovirus does not appear to induce such an enzyme. And secondly, HSV develops resistance to these compounds rather easily since the deoxypyrimidine kinase is not essential for its replication. This could seriously limit the use of these compounds in herpes infections subject to recurrences or in infections that require treatment for prolonged periods (such as in immunosuppressed patients).

So far the only specific antiherpes agents which have been found that do not utilize deoxypyrimidine kinase in this manner are araA, phosphonoacetic acid and phosphonoformic acid. HSV strains resistant to phosphonoacetic acid and phosphonoformic acid have been isolated (Klien, 1975; Honess and Watson, 1975). However, several attempts to obtain herpes mutants resistant to araA were unsuccessful (Klein, 1975; Shannon, 1977a). Under these conditions mutants resistant to phosphonoacetic acid and to 5-iododeoxyuridine were readily obtained. More recently, mutants resistant to araA have been obtained (Coen et al., 1982). However, it appears that these mutants arise less frequently than mutants resistant to most of the other antiherpes agents. Moreover, there have been no reports of viral resistance to araA developing during animal or clinical studies. The fact that herpesviruses develop resistance to araA slowly is a definite advantage for treating recurrent herpes infections.

AraA has proven effective in treating a number of life-threatening herpesvirus infections (Buchanan and Hess, 1980). Its approval for use in treatment of herpes simplex encephalitis is a case in point. Further studies on the mutagenicity, carcinogenicity and teratenogenicity of araA are necessary to determine the feasibility of more widespread use of araA in less threatening situations.

Other approaches to improve the effectiveness of araA in viral chemotherapy are now in progress and many new advances are to be expected in the next few years. New analogs that are metabolically stable and which exhibit improved antiviral properties are constantly being sought. In addition, improved means of administering these compounds are being explored. One possibility is the use of araA nucleotides entrapped within phospholipid vesicles. If such vesicles can be directed specifically to virus-infected cells they would confer another level of specificity and would also protect the entrapped compound from degradation by serum enzymes. Such specificity might be obtained by making vesicles whose surface contains antibodies to viral antigens expressed on infected cells. AraC entrapped within phospholipid vesicles was found effective against L1210 cells in culture (Mayhew *et al.*, 1976). AraC encapsulated within liposomes has also been used to selectively deliver this nucleoside to rat lungs (Julian and McCullough, 1980). Moreover, encapsulation within liposomes was shown to increase the efficacy of 5-iododeoxyuridine in treatment of herpetic keratitis in rabbits, presumably due to deeper penetration of the encapsulated drug (Smolin *et al.*, 1981). This exciting approach is just beginning. Another approach to increase the uptake of topically applied antivirals is iontophoresis. This has proven successful in increasing the activity of topically applied araAMP in mice (Park *et al.*, 1978).

Finally, it is hoped that these studies with aranucleosides will help toward the design of other antiviral agents that are even more specific than araA. Although araA inhibits viral DNA synthesis better than host DNA synthesis, the specificity is not absolute. What are desired are compounds that inhibit only a virus-induced enzyme and are directed against an enzyme that is essential for viral replication so that resistance does not easily develop. Herpesviruses have the genetic capacity for approximately 100 genes, many of which should determine essential virus-specific functions. Thus, a wealth of potential targets exists for the researcher willing to uncover them.

Acknowledgements—Thomas W. North is an Assistant Professor of Biochemistry and Pharmacology. Seymour S. Cohen is an American Cancer Society Professor of Pharmacological Sciences. The work reported here was supported in part by a grant from the National Institute of Allergy and Infectious Disease. We wish to thank Rachel Runfola for preparation of the manuscript.

REFERENCES

ADAMSON, R. H., ALBLASHI, D. V., ARMSTRONG, G. R., and ELLMORE, N. W. (1972) Effect of cytosine arabinoside, adenine arabinoside, tilorone, and rifamycin SV on multiplication of herpesvirus saimiri *in vitro*. *Antimicrob. Agents Chemother.* 1: 82–83.

ADLARD, B. P. F., DOBBING, J. and SANDS, J. (1975) A comparison of the effects of cytosine arabinoside and adenine arabinoside on some aspects of brain growth and development in the rat. *Br. J. Pharmacol.* 54: 33–39.

AGARWAL, R. P. (1980) Deoxycoformycin toxicity in mice after long-term treatment. *Cancer Chemother. Pharmac.* 5: 83–87.

AGARWAL, R. P. and PARKS, R. E. Jr. (1977) Potent inhibition of muscle AMP deaminase by the nucleoside antibiotics coformycin and deoxycoformycin. *Biochem. Pharmacol.* 26: 663–666.

AGARWAL, R. P., SPECTOR, T. and PARKS, R. E. Jr. (1977) Tight binding inhibitors—IV. Inhibition of adenosine deaminases by various inhibitors. *Biochem. Pharmacol.* 26: 359–367.

ASWELL, J. F., ALLEN, G. P., JAMIESON, A. T., CAMPBELL, D. E. and GENTRY, G. A. (1977) Antiviral activity of arabinosylthymine in herpesviral replication: mechanism of action *in vivo* and *in vitro*. *Antimicrob. Agents Chemother.* 12: 243–254.

ASWELL, J. F. and GENTRY, G. A. (1977) Cell-dependent antiherpesviral activity of 5-methylarabinosylcytosine, an intracellular araT donor. *Ann. N.Y. Acad. Sci.* 284: 342–350.

ATKINSON, M. R., DEUTSCHER, , M., KORNBERG, A., RUSSEL, A. F. and MOFFATT, J. G. (1969) Enzymatic synthesis of deoxyribonucleic acid. XXXIV. Termination of chain growth by a 2′,3′-dideoxyribonucleotide. *Biochemistry* 8: 4897–4904.

BADER, J. P. (1965) The requirement for DNA synthesis in the growth of Rous sarcoma and Rous-associated viruses. *Virology* 26: 253–261.

BAKER, D. C., HANVEY, J. C., HAWKINS, L. D. and MURPHY, J. (1981) Identification of the bioactive enantioner of erythro-9-(2-hydroxy-3-nonyl)adenine (EHNA), a semi-tight binding inhibitor of adenosine deaminase. *Biochem. Pharmacol.* 30: 1159–1160.

BASTIAN, G., BESSODES, M., PANZICA, R. P., ABUSHANAB, E., CHEN, S.-F, STOECKLER, J. D. and PARKS, R. E., Jr. (1981) Adenosine deaminase inhibitors. Conversion of a single chiral synthon into erythro- and threo-9-(2-hydroxy-3-nonyl)adenines. *J. Med. Chem.* 24: 1383–1385.

BELL, D. E. and FRIDLAND, A. (1980) Mode of action of 9-β-D-arabinofuranosyladenine and 1-β-D-arabinofuranosylcytosine on DNA synthesis in human lymphoblasts. *Biochem. Biophys. Acta* 606: 57–66.

BENNETT, L. L. Jr., SHANNON, W. M., ALLAN, P. W. and ARNETT, G. (1975) Studies on the biochemical basis for the antiviral activities of some nucleoside analogs. *Ann. N.Y. Acad. Sci.* 255: 342–358.

BEN-PORAT, T., BROWN, M. and KAPLAN, A. S. (1968) Effect of 1-β-D-arabinofuranosylcytosine on DNA synthesis. II. In rabbit kidney cells infected with herpes viruses. *Mol. Pharmacol.* 4: 139–146.

BENZ, W. C., SIEGEL, P. J. and BAER, J. (1978) Effects of adenine arabinoside on lymphocytes infected with Epstein–Barr virus. *J. Virol.* 27: 475–482.

BERGMANN, W. and BURKE, D. C. (1955) Contributions to the study of marine products. XXIX. Nucleosides of sponges III. Spongothymidine and spongouridine. *J. Org. Chem.* 20: 1501–1507.

BERGMANN, W. and FEENEY, R. (1951) Contributions to the study of marine products. XXXII. The nucleosides of sponges. *J. Org. Chem.* 16: 981–987.

BJURSELL, G. and REICHARD, P. (1973) Effects of thymidine on deoxyribonucleoside triphosphate pools and deoxyribonucleic acid synthesis in Chinese hamster ovary cells. *J. Biol. Chem.* **238**: 3904–3909.

BREWEN, J. G. (1965) The induction of chromatid lesions by cytosine arabinoside in post-DNA synthetic human leukocytes. *Cytogenetics* **4**: 28–36.

BRINK, J. J. and LePAGE, G. A. (1964) Metabolic effects of 9-D-arabinosylpurines in ascites tumor cells. *Cancer Res.* **24**: 312–318.

BROCKMAN, R. W., CHENG, Y.-C., SCHABEL, F. M., Jr. and MONTGOMERY, J. A. (1980) Metabolism and chemotherapeutic activity of 9-β-D-arabinofuronosyl-2-fluoroadenine against murine leukemia L1210 and evidence for its phosphorylation by deoxycytidine kinase. *Cancer Res.* **40**: 3610–3615.

BROCKMAN, R. W., SCHABEL, F. M., Jr. and MONTGOMERY, J. A. (1977) Biological activity of 9-β-D-arabinofuranosyl-2-fluoroadenine, a metabolically stable analog of 9-β-D-arabinofuranosyladenine. *Biochem. Pharmacol.* **26**: 2193–2196.

BRYSON, Y. J. and CONNER, J. D. (1976) *In vitro* susceptibility of varicella zoster virus to adenine arabinoside and hypoxanthine arabinoside. *Antimicrob. Agents Chemother.* **9**: 540–543.

BRYSON, Y., CONNER, J. D., SWEETMAN, L., CAREY, S., STUCKEY, M. A. and BUCHANAN, R. (1974) Determination of the plaque inhibitory activity of adenine arabinoside (9-β-D-arabinofuranosyladenine) for herpesviruses using an adenosine deaminase inhibitor. *Antimicrob. Agents Chemother.* **6**: 98–101.

BUCHANAN, R. A. and HESS, F. (1980) Vidarabine (Vira-A): Pharmacology and clinical experience. *Pharmac. Ther.* **8**: 143–171.

BURCHENAL, J. H., CURRIE, V. E., DOWLING, M. D., FOX, J. J. and KRAKOFF, I. H. (1975) Experimental and clinical studies on nucleoside analogs as antitumor agents. *Ann. N.Y. Acad. Sci.* **255**: 202–212.

BUTEL, J. S. and RAPP, F. (1965) The effect of arabinofuranosylcytosine on the growth cycle of simian virus 40. *Virology* **27**: 490–495.

BUTHALA, D. A. (1964) Cell culture studies on antiviral agents: 1. Action of cytosine arabinoside and some comparisons with 5-iodo-2'-deoxyuridine. *Proc. Soc. Exp. Biol. Med.* **115**: 69–77.

CAMIENER, G. W. (1968) Studies of the enzymatic deamination of aracytidine V. Inhibition *in vitro* and *in vivo* by tetrahydrouridine and other reduced pyrimidine nucleoside. *Biochem. Pharmacol.* **17**: 1981–1991.

CAMPBELL, J. B., MAES, R. F., WIKTOR, T. J. and KOPROWSKI, H. (1968) The inhibition of rabies virus by arabinosyl cytosine. Studies on the mechanism and specificity of action. *Virology* **34**: 701–708.

CARADONNA, S. J. and CHENG, Y-C. (1981) Induction of uracil-DNA glycosylase and dUTP nucleotidohydrolase activity in herpes simplex virus-infected human cells. *J. Biol. Chem.* **256**: 9834–9837.

CARDEILHAC, P. T. and COHEN, S. S. (1964) Some metabolic properties of nucleotides of 1-β-D-arabinofuranosylcytosine. *Cancer Res.* **24**: 1595–1603.

CARSON, D. A., KAYE, J. and SEEGMILLER, J. E. (1977) Lymphospecific toxicity in adenosine deaminase deficiency and purine nucleoside phosphorylase deficiency; possible role of nucleoside kinase(s). *Proc. Nat. Acad. Sci. USA* **74**: 5677–5681.

CASS, C. E. (1979) 9-β-D-arabinofuranosyladenine (araA). *Antibiotics* **5**: 85–109.

CASS, C. E., TAN, T. H. and SELNER, M. (1979) Antiproliferative effects of 9-β-D-arabinofuranosyladenine 5'-monophosphate and related compounds in combination with adenosine deaminase inhibitors against mouse leukemia L1210/C2 cells in culture. *Cancer Res.* **39**: 1563–1569.

CHAN, T. (1977) Induction of deoxycytidine deaminase activity in mammalian cell lines by infection with herpes simplex virus type 1. *Proc. Nat. Acad. Sci. USA* **74**: 1734–1738.

CHANDA, P. K. and BANERJEE, A. K. (1980) Inhibition of vesicular stomatitis virus transcriptase *in vitro* by phosphonoformate and ara-ATP. *Virology* **107**: 562–566.

CHAWLA, P. L., LOKICH, J. J., JAFFE, N. and FREI, E. (1974) Phase I study of cyclocytidine hydrochloride. *Proc. Am. Ass. Cancer Res. ASCO* **15**: 188.

CHEN, M. S. and PRUSOFF, W. H. (1978) Association of thymidylate kinase activity with pyrimidine deoxyribonucleoside kinase induced by herpes simplex virus. *J. Biol. Chem.* **253**: 1325–1327.

CHEN, M. S., WARD, D. C. and PRUSOFF, W. H. (1976) Specific herpes simplex virus-induced incorporation of 5-iodo-5'-amino-2',5'-dideoxyuridine into deoxyribonucleic acid. *J. Biol. Chem.* **251**: 4833–4838.

CHENG, Y-C, DERSE, D., TAN, R. S., DUTSCHMAN, G., BOBEK, M., SCHROEDER, A. and Block, A. (1981) Biological and biochemical effects of 2'-azido-2'deoxyarabinofuranosylcytosine on human tumor cells *in vitro*. *Cancer Res.* **41**: 3144–3149.

CHENG, Y.-C, GOZ, B. and PRUSOFF, W. H. (1975) Deoxyribonucleotide metabolism in herpes simplex virus infected HeLa cells. *Biochim. Biophys. Acta* **390**: 253–263.

CHIANG, P. K., CANTONI, G. L., RAY, D. A. and BADER, J. P. (1977) Reduced levels of adenosine deaminase in chick embryo fibroblasts transformed by Rous sarcoma virus. *Biochem. Biophys. Res. Commun.* **78**: 336–342.

CH'IEN, L. T., CANNON, N. J., WHITLEY, R. J., DIETHELM, A. G., DISMUKES, W. E., SCOTT, C. W., BUCHANAN, R. A. and ALFORD, C. A. Jr. (1974) Effect of adenine arabinoside on cytomegalovirus infections. *J. Infect. Dis.* **130**: 32–39.

CH'IEN, L. T., SCHABEL, F. M., Jr., and ALFORD, C. A., Jr. (1973). Arabinosyl nucleosides and nucleotides. In: *Selective Inhibitors of Viral Functions* p. 227–258, CARTER, W. A. (ed.). CRC Press, Cleveland, Ohio.

CHOU, T. C., CLARKSON, B. D. and PHILIPS, F. S. (1975) Metabolism of cytosine arabinoside (araC) *in vitro* by normal and leukemic blood and bone marrow. *Proc. Am. Ass. Cancer Res.* **35**: 225–236.

CHOU, T-C., FEINBERG, A., GRANT, A. J., VIDAL, P., REICHMAN, U., WATANABE, K. A., FOX, J. J. and PHILIPS, F. S. (1981) Pharmacological disposition and metabolic fate of 2'-fluoro-5-iodo-1-β-D-arabinofuranosylcytosine in mice and rats. *Cancer Res.* **41**: 3336–3342.

CHU, M. Y. and FISCHER, G. A. (1962) A proposed mechanism of action of 1-β-D-arabinofuranosylcytosine an inhibitor of the growth of leukemic cells. *Biochem. Pharmacol.* **11**: 425–430.

CHU, M. Y. and FISCHER, G. A. (1965) Comparative studies of leukemic cells sensitive and resistant to cytosine arabinoside. *Biochem. Pharmacol.* **14**: 333–341.

COEN, D. M., FURMAN, P. A., GELEP, P. T. and SCHAFFER, P. A. (1982) Mutations in the herpes simplex virus DNA polymerase gene can confer resistance to 9-β-D-arabinofuranosyladenine. *J. Virol.* **41**: 909–918.

COHEN, A., HIRCHHORN, R., HOROWITZ, S. D., RUBINSTEIN, A., PALMER, S. H., HONG, R. and MARTIN, D. W., Jr. (1978) Deoxyadenosine triphosphate as a potentially toxic metabolite in adenosine deaminase deficiency. *Proc. Nat. Acad. Sci. USA* **75**: 472–476.

COHEN, G. H. (1972) Ribonucleotide reductase activity of synchronized KB cells infected with herpes simplex virus. *J. Virol.* **9**: 408–418.

COHEN, G. H., FACTOR, M. N. and PONCE DE LEON, M. (1974) Inhibition of herpes simplex virus type 2 replication by thymidine. *J. Virol.* **14**: 20–25.

COHEN, S. S. (1961) Virus-induced acquisition of metabolic function. *Fed. Proc.* **20**: 641–649.

COHEN, S. S. (1966) Introduction to the biochemistry of D-arabinosyl nucleosides. *Prog. Nucleic Acid Res. Mol. Biol.* **5**: 1–88.

COHEN, S. S. (1976) The lethality of aranucleotides. *Medical Biol.* **54**: 299–326.

COHEN, S. S. (1977) The mechanisms of lethal action of arabinosyl cytosine (araC) and arabinosyl adenine (araA). *Cancer* **40**: 509–518.

COHEN, S. S. (1979) The mechanisms of inhibition of cellular and viral multiplication by aranucleosides and aranucleotides. In: *Nucleoside Analogues*, pp. 225–245. WALKER, R. T., DECLERCG, E. and ECKSTEIN, F. (eds.). Plenum Pub. Co., New York.

COHEN, S. S. and PLUNKETT, W. (1975) The utilization of nucleotides by animal cells. *Ann. N.Y. Acad. Sci.* **255**: 269–286.

COLEMAN, M. S., DONOFRIO, J., HUTTON, J. J., HAHN, L., DAOUD, A., LAMPKIN, B. and DYMINSKI, J. (1978) Identification and quantitation of deoxynucleotides in erythrocytes of a patient with adenosine deaminase deficiency and severe combined immunodeficiency. *J. Biol Chem.* **253**: 1619–1626.

CONNER, J. D., SWEETMAN, L., CAREY, S., STUCKEY, M. A. and BUCHANAN, R. (1974) Effect of adenosine deaminase upon the antiviral activity *in vitro* of adenine arabinoside for vaccinia virus. *Antimicrob. Agents Chemother.* **6**: 630–636.

CONNER, J. D., SWETMAN, L., CAREY, S., STUCKEY, M. A. and BUCHANAN, R. (1975) Susceptibility *in vitro* of several large DNA viruses to the antiviral activity of adenine arabinoside and its metabolite hypoxanthine arabinoside: relation to human pharmacology. In: *Adenine arabinoside: An Antiviral Agent*, pp. 177–196. PAVAN-LANGSTON, D., BUCHANAN, R. A. and ALFORD, C. A., Jr. (eds.). Raven Press, New York.

DANHAUSER, L. L. and RUSTUM, Y. M. (1980) Effect of thymidine on the toxicity, antitumor activity and metabolism of 1-β-D-arabinofuranosycytosine in rats bearing a chemically induced colon carcinoma. *Cancer Res.* **40**: 1274–1280.

DECLERCQ, E., DESCAMPS, J., DESOMER, P., BARR, P. J., JONES, A. S. and WALKER, R. T. (1979) (*E*)-5-(2-bromovinyl)-2′-deoxyuridine: a potent and selective antiherpes agent. *Proc. Nat. Acad. Sci. USA* **76**: 2947–2951.

DECLERCQ, E., DESCAMPS, J., DESOMER, P. and HOLY, A. (1978) (*S*)-9-(2,3-dihydroxypropyl)adenine: an aliphatic nucleoside analog with broad spectrum antiviral activity. *Science* **200**: 563–565.

DECLERCQ, E., KRAJEWSKA, E., DESCAMPS, J. and TORRENCE, P. F. (1977) Anti-herpes activity of deoxythymidine analogs: specific dependence on virus induced deoxythymidine kinase. *Mol. Pharmacol.* **13**: 980–984.

DECLERCQ, E. and TORRENCE, P. F. (1978) Nucleoside analogs with selective antiviral activity. *J. Carbohydrates. Nucleosides. Nucleotides* **5**: 187–224.

DEFENDI, V. and WIKTOR, T. J. (1966) Metabolic and autoradiographic studies of rabies virus-infected cells. *Int. Symp. Rabies, Talloires, 1965; Symp. Series, Immunobiol. Standard* **1**: 119–124. Karger, Basel.

DERSE, D. and CHENG, Y-C. (1981) Herpes simplex virus type I DNA polymerase. *J. Biol. Chem.* **256**: 8525–8530.

DE RUDDER, J. and PRIVAT DE GARILHE, M. (1965) Inhibitory effect of some nucleosides on the growth of various human viruses in tissue culture. *Antimicrob. Agents Chemother.* **5**: 578–583.

DOBERSEN, M. J. and GREER, S. (1978) Herpes simplex virus type 2 induced pyrimidine nucleoside kinase: enzymatic basis for the selective antiherpetic effect of 5-halogenated analogues of deoxycytidine. *Biochemistry* **17**: 920–928.

DOERING, A., KELLER, J. and COHEN, S. S. (1966) Some aspects of D-arabinosyl nucleosides on polymer synthesis in mouse fibroblasts. *Cancer Res.* **26**: 2444–2450.

DOW, L. W., BELL, D. E., POULAKOS, L. and FRIDLAND, A. (1980) Differences in metabolism and cytotoxicity between 9-β-D-arabinofuranosyladenine and 9-β-D-arabinofuranosyl-2-fluoroadenine in human leukemic lymphoblasts. *Cancer Res.* **40**: 1405–1410.

DUFF, R. and RAPP, F. (1971) Properties of hamster embryo fibroblasts transformed *in vitro* after exposure to ultraviolet-irradiated herpes simplex virus type 2. *J. Virol.* **8**: 469–477.

DUFF, R. and RAPP, F. (1973) Oncogenic transformation of hamster embryo cells after exposure to inactivated herpes simplex virus type 1. *J. Virol.* **12**: 209–217.

EIDINOFF, M. L., CHEONG, L. and RICH, M. A. (1959) Incorporation of unnatural pyrimidine bases into deoxyribonucleic acid of mammalian cells. *Science* **129**: 1550–1551.

ELION, G. B., FURMAN, P. A., FYFE, J. A., DEMIRANDA, P., BEAUCHAMP, L. and SCHAEFFER, H. J. (1977) Selectivity of action of an antiherpetic agent, 9-(2-hydroxyethoxymethyl)guanine. *Proc. Nat. Acad. Sci. USA* **74**: 5716–5720.

ELION, G. B., RIDEOUT, J. L., DEMIRANDA, P., COLLINS, P. and BAUER, D. J. (1975) Biological activities of some purine arabinosides. *Ann. N.Y. Acad. Sci.* **255**: 468–480.

EVANS, J. S., MUSSER, E. A., MENGEL, G. D., FORSBLAD, K. R. and HUNTER, J. H. (1961) Antitumor activity of 1-β-D-arabinofuranosylcytosine hydrochloride. *Proc. Soc. Exp. Biol. Med.* **106**: 350–353.

FALCON, M. G. and JONES, B. R. (1977) Antiviral activity in the rabbit cornea of adenine arabinoside, araA-5′-monophosphate, and hypoxanthine arabinoside; and interactions with adenosine deaminase inhibitor. *J. gen. Virol.* **36**: 199–202.

FELDMAN, L. A. and RAPP, F. (1966) Inhibition of adenovirus replication by 1-β-D-arabinofuranosylcytosine. *Proc. Soc. Exp. Biol. Med.* **122**: 243–247.

FIALA, M., CHOW, A. W. and GUZE, L. B. (1972) Susceptibility of herpesviruses to cytosine arabinoside:

standardization of susceptibility test procedure and relative resistance of herpes simplex type 2 strains. *Antimicrob. Agents Chemother.* **1**: 354–357.

FISHAUT, J. M., CONNOR, J. D. and LAMPERT, P. W. (1975) Comparative effects of arabinosyl nucleosides on the postnatal growth and development of the rat. In *Adenine Arabinoside: An Antiviral Agent*, pp. 159–170. PAVAN-LANGSTON, D., BUCHANAN, R. A. and ALFORD, C. A., Jr. (eds.). Raven Press, New York.

FOX, J. J., LOPEZ, C. and WATANABE, K. A. (1981) Potent antiviral activities and some chemistry of certain 2′-fluoro-arabinosylpyrimidine nucleosides. In: *Antiviral Chemotherapy: Design of Inhibitors of Viral Functions*, pp. 219–233. GAURI, K. K. (ed.). Academic Press, New York.

FOX, J. J., MILLER, N. and WEMPEN, I. (1966) Nucleosides. XXIV. 1-β-D-arabinofuranosyl-5-fluorocytosine and related arabinonucleosides. *J. Med. Chem.* **9**: 101–105.

FREEMAN, G., KUEHN, A. and SALTANIAN, I. (1965) Response of tumorogenic viruses and of cells to biologically active compounds. I. Method for determining response and application of methods. *Cancer Res.* **25**: 1609–1625.

FRIDLAND, A. (1977) Inhibition of deoxyribonucleic acid chain initiation: A new mode of action for 1-β-D-arabinofuranosylcytosine in human lymphoblasts. *Biochemistry* **16**: 5308–5312.

FRIEDEN, C., KURZ, L. C. and GILBERT, H. R. (1980) Adenosine deaminase and adenylate deaminase: comparative kinetic studies with transition state and ground state analogue inhibitors. *Biochemistry* **19**: 5303–5309.

FURTH, J. J. and COHEN, S. S. (1967) Inhibition of mammalian DNA polymerase by the 5′-triphosphate of 9-β-D-arabinofuranosyladenine. *Cancer Res.* **27**: 1528–1533.

FURTH, J. J. and COHEN, S. S. (1968) Inhibition of mammalian DNA polymerase by the 5′-triphosphate of 1-β-D-arabinofuranosylcytosine and the 5′-triphosphate of 9-β-D-arabinofuranosyladenine. *Cancer Res.* **28**: 2601–2607.

GASSET, A. R. and AKABOSHI, T. (1976) Teratogenicity of adenine arabinoside. *Investigative Opthalmol.* **15**: 556–557.

GENTRY, G. A. and ASWELL, J. F. (1975) Inhibition of herpes simplex virus replication by araT. *Virology* **65**: 294–296.

GOODHEART, C. R., PLUMMER, G. and WANER, J. L. (1968) Density differences of DNA of human herpes simplex viruses, types I & II. *Virology* **35**: 473–475.

GRAHAM, F. L. and WHITMORE, G. F. (1970) Studies in mouse L-cells on the incorporation of 1-β-D-arabinofuranosylcytosine into DNA and on inhibition of DNA polymerase by 1-β-D-arabino-furanosylcytosine-5′-triphosphate. *Cancer Res.* **30**: 2636–2644.

GRANT, J. A. and SABINA, L. R. (1972) Inhibition of vesicular stomatitis virus replication by 9-β-D-arabinofuranosyladenine. *Antimicrob. Agents Chemother.* **2**: 201–205.

GRANT, S., LEHMAN, C. and CADMAN, E. (1980) Enhancement of 1-β-D-arabinofuranosylcytosine accumulation within L1210 cells and increased cytotoxicity following thymidine exposure. *Cancer Res.* **40**: 1525–1531.

HANZE, A. R. (1960) Nucleic acids. IV. The catalytic reduction of pyrimidine nucleosides (human liver deaminase inhibitors). *J. Am. Chem. Soc.* **89**: 6720–6725.

HARKRADER, R. J., BORITZKI, T. J. and JACKSON, R. C. (1981) Potentiation of 1-β-D-arabinofuranosylcytosine in hepatoma cells by 2′-deoxyadenosine or 2′-deoxyguanosine. *Biochem. Pharmacol.* **30**: 1099–1104.

HARMON, M. W. and JANIS, B. (1976) Effects of cytosine arabinoside, adenine arabinoside, and 6-azauridine on rabies virus *in vitro* and *in vivo*. *J. Infect. Dis.* **133**: 7–13.

HART, J. S., HO, D. H., GEORGE, S. L., SALEM, P., GOTTLIEB, J. A. and FREI, E. (1972) Cytokinetic and molecular pharmacology studies of arabinosylcytosine in metastatic melanoma. *Cancer Res.* **32**: 2711–2716.

HAWTREY, A. O., SCOTT-BURDEN, T. and ROBERTSON, G. (1974) Inhibition of glycoprotein and glycolipid synthesis in hamster embryo cells by cytosine arabinoside and hydroxyurea. *Nature* **252**: 58–60.

HENDERSON, E. E., LONG, W. K. and RIBECKY, R. (1979) Effects of nucleoside analogs on Epstein–Barr virus-induced transformation of human umbilical cord leukocytes and Epstein–Barr virus expression in transformed cells. *Antimicrob. Agents. Chemother.* **15**: 101–110.

HERMANN, E. C. (1961) Plaque inhibition test for detection of specific inhibitors of DNA containing viruses. *Proc. Soc. Exp. Biol. Med.* **107**: 142–145.

HERMANN, E. C. (1968) Sensitivity of herpes simplex virus, vaccinia virus and adenoviruses to deoxyribonucleic acid inhibitors and thiosemicarbazones in plaque suppression test. *Appl. Microbiol.* **16**: 1151–1155.

HERSHFIELD, M. S. (1979) Apparent suicide inactivation of human lymphoblast S-adenosylhomocysteine hydrolase by 2′-deoxyadenosine and adenine arabinoside. *J. Biol. Chem.* **254**: 22–25.

HIRSCHMAN, S. F. (1969) Effect of cytosine arabinoside on the replication of the Maloney sarcoma virus in 3T3 cell cultures. *Proc. Am. Ass. Cancer Res.* **10**: 38.

HO, D. H. W., CARTER, C. J., BROWN, N. S., HESTER, J., McCREDIE, K., BENJAMIN, R. S., FREIREICH, E. J. and BODEY, G. P. (1980) Effects of tetrahydrouridine on the uptake and metabolism of 1-β-D-arabinofuranosylcytosine in human normal and leukemic cells. *Cancer Res.* **40**: 2441–2446.

HO, D. H. W., CARTER, C. K. and LOO, T. L. (1975) Effects of tetrahydrouridine (THU) on the uptake and metabolism of arabinosylcytosine (araC) by human acute myelogenous leukemia (AML). *Proc. Am. Ass. Cancer Res.* **16**: 57.

HO, D. H. W. and FREI, E. (1971) Clinical pharmacology of 1-β-D-arabinofuranosylcytosine. *Clin. Pharmacol. Ther.* **12**: 944–954.

HOFFMANN, P. J. and CHENG, Y.-C. (1978) The deoxyribonuclease induced after infection of KB cells by herpes simplex virus type 1 or type 2. *J. Biol. Chem.* **253**: 3557–3562.

HONESS, R. W. and WATSON, D. H. (1977) Herpes simplex virus resistance and sensitivity to phosphonoacetic acid. *J. Virol.* **21**: 584–600.

HUBERT-HABART, M. and COHEN, S. S. (1962) The toxicity of 9-β-D-arabinofuranosyladenine to purine-requiring *Escherichia coli*. *Biochem. Biophys. Acta* **59**: 468–471.

HUFFMAN, J. H., SIDWELL, R. W., KHARE, G. P., WITKOWSKI, J. T., ALLEN, L. B. and ROBBINS, R. K. (1973) *In vitro* effect of 1-β-D-ribofuranosyl,1,2,4,-triazole-3-carboxamide (Virazole, ICN 1229) on deoxyribonucleic acid and ribonucleic acid viruses. *Antimicrob. Agents Chemother*. **3**: 235–241.

HUGHES, R. G., Jr. and KIMBALL, A. P. (1972) Metabolic effects of cyclic-9-β-D-arabinofuranosyladenine 3',5'-monophosphate in L1210 cells. *Cancer Res*. **32**: 1791–1794.

HUSZAR, D. and BACCHETTI, S. (1981) Partial purification and characterization of the ribonucleotide reductase induced by herpes simplex virus infection of mammalian cells. *J. Virol*. **37**: 580–588.

JAMIESON, A. T. and BJURSELL, G. (1976) Deoxyribonucleoside triphosphate pools in herpes simplex type I infected cells. *J. gen. Virol*. **31**: 101–113.

JAMIESON, A. T., GENTRY, G. A. and SUBAK-SHARPE, J. H. (1974) Induction of both thymidine and deoxycytidine kinase activity by herpes viruses. *J. gen. Virol*. **24**: 465–480.

JAMIESON, A. T. and SUBAK-SHARPE, J. H. (1974) Biochemical studies on the herpes simplex virus-specified deoxypyrimidine kinase activity. *J. gen. Virol*. **24**: 481–492.

JAMIESON, A. T. and SUBAK-SHARPE, J. H. (1976) Herpes simplex virus specified deoxypyrimidine kinase and the uptake of exogenous nucleosides by infected cells. *J. gen. Virol*. **31**: 303–314.

JOHNS, D. G. and ADAMSON, R. H. (1976) Enhancement of the biological activity of cordycepin (3'-deoxyadenosine) by the adenosine deaminase inhibitor 2'-deoxycoformycin. *Biochem. Pharmacol*. **25**: 1441–1444.

JULAINO, R. L. and McCULLOUGH, H. N. (1980) Controlled delivery of an antitumor drug: localized action of liposome encapsulated cytosine arabinoside administered via the respiratory system. *J. Pharmacol. Expt. Ther*. **214**: 381–387.

KAPLAN, A. S. (ed.) (1973) *The Herpesviruses*. Academic Press, New York.

KARON, M. and CHIRAKAWA, S. (1970) The locus of action of 1-β-D-arabinofuranosylcytosine in the cell cycle. *Cancer Res*. **29**: 687–696.

KAUFMAN, H. E. (1962) Clinical cure of herpes simplex keratitis by 5-iodo-2'-deoxyuridine. *Proc. Soc. Exp. Biol. Med*. **109**: 251–252.

KAUFMAN, H. E., CAPELLA, J. A., MALONEY, E. D., ROBBINS, J. E., COOPER, G. M. and UOTILA, M. H. (1964) Corneal toxicity of cytosine arabinoside. *Arch. Ophthal*. **72**: 535–540.

KAUFMAN, H. E. and MALONEY, E. D. (1963) IDU and cytosine arabinoside in experimental keratitis. *Arch. Ophthal*. **69**: 626–629.

KAUFMAN, H. E., MARTOLA, E. L. and DOHLMAN, C. H. (1962) Use of 5-iodo-2'-deoxyuridine (IDU) in treatment of herpes simplex keratitis. *Arch. Ophthal*. **68**: 235–239.

KAUFMAN, H. E. and VARNELL, E. D. (1976) Effect of 9-β-D-arabinofuranosylhypoxanthine 5'-monophosphate on experimental herpes simplex keratitis. *Antimicrob. Agents. Chemother*. **10**: 885–888.

KEENEY, R. E. (1975) Human tolerance of adenine arabinoside. In: *Adenine Arabinoside: An Antiviral Agent*, pp. 265–273. PAVAN-LANGSTON, D., BUCHANAN, R. A. and ALFORD, C. A. Jr. (eds.). Raven Press, New York.

KERN, E. R., RICHARDS, J. T., OVERALL, J. C., Jr. and GLASGOW, L. A. (1978) Alteration of mortality and pathogenesis of three experimental herpesvirus hominis infections of mice with adenine arabinoside 5'-monophosphate, adenine arabinoside, and phosphonoacetic acid. *Antimicrob. Agents Chemother*. **13**: 53–60.

KEIR, H. M. (1968) Virus-induced enzymes in mammalian cells infected with DNA viruses. In: *The Molecular Virology of Viruses*, 18th Symposium of the Society for General Microbiology, Cambridge University Press, pp. 67–99.

KEIR, H. M., HAY, J., MORRISON, J. M., and SUBAK-SHARPE, J. H. (1966) Altered properties of deoxyribonucleic acid nucleotidyltransferase after infection of mammalian cells with herpes simplex virus. *Nature* **210**: 369–374.

KHWAJA, T. A., KIGWANA, L. J. and MIAN, A. M. (1979) Antileukemic activity of 1-β-D-arabinofuranosyl-2-amino-1,4(2H)-4-iminopyrimidine, a new depot form of 1-β-D-arabinofuranosylcytosine. *Cancer Res*. **39**: 3129–3133.

KIEFF, E. D., BACHENHEIMER, S. L. and ROIZMAN, B. (1971) Size, composition and structure of the deoxyribonucleic acid of herpes simplex virus subtypes 1 and 2. *J. Virol*. **8**: 125–132.

KIM, J. H., PEREZ, A. G. and DJORDJEVIC, B. (1968) Studies on unbalanced growth in synchronized HeLa cells. *Cancer Res*. **28**: 2443–2447.

KINAHAN, J. J., KOWAL, E. P. and GRINDEY, G. B. (1981) Biochemical and antitumor effects of the combination of thymidine and 1-β-D-arabinofuranosylcytosine against leukemia L1210. *Cancer Res*. **41**: 445–451.

KIT, S. (1980) Viral-associated and induced enzymes. *Pharmacol. Ther*. **4**: 501–585.

KIT, S., DeTORRES, R. A. and DUBBS, D. R. (1966) Arabinofuranosylcytosine-induced stimulation of thymidine kinase and deoxycytidylic deaminase activities of mammalian cultures. *Cancer Res*. **26**: 1859–1866.

KLEIN, R. J. (1975) Isolation of herpes simplex virus clones and drug resistant mutants in microcultures. *Arch. Virol*. **49**: 73–80.

KNOPF, K. W. (1979) Properties of herpes simplex virus DNA polymerase and characterization of its associated exonuclease activity. *Eur. J. Biochem*. **98**: 231–244.

KUFE, D. W., MAJOR, P. P., EGAN, E. M. and BEARDSLEY, G. P. (1980) Correlation of cytotoxicity with incorporation of araC into DNA. *J. Biol. Chem*. **255**: 8997–9000.

KULIKOWSKI, T., ZAWADZKI, Z., SHUGAR, S., DESCAMPS, J. and DeCLERCQ, E. (1979) Synthesis and antiviral activities of arabinofuranosyl-5-ethylpyrimidine nucleosides. Selective antiherpes activity of 1-(β-D-arabinofuranosyl)-5-ethyluracil. *J. Med. Chem*. **22**: 647–653.

KURTZ, S. M. (1975) Toxicology of adenine arabinoside. In: *Adenine Arabinoside: An Antiviral Agent*, pp. 145–157. PAVAN-LANGSTON, D., BUCHANAN, R. A. and AFORD, C. A. Jr. (eds.). Raven Press, New York.

KURTZ, S. M., FITZGERALD, J. E. and SCHARDEIN, J. L. (1977) Comparative animal toxicology of vidarabine and its 5'-monophosphate. *Ann. N.Y. Acad. Sci*. **284**: 6–8.

LAMBE, C. U. and NELSON, D. J. (1982) Pharmacokinetics of inhibition of adenosine deaminase by erythro-9-(2-hydroxy-3-nonyl)adenine in CBA mice. *Biochem. Pharmacol*. **31**: 535–539.

LANGELIER, Y., DECHAMPS, M. and BUTTIN, G. (1978) Analysis of dCMP deaminase and CDP reductase levels in hamster cells infected by herpes simplex virus. *J. Virol*. **26**: 547–553.

LAPI, L. and COHEN, S. S. (1977) Toxicities of adenosine and 2'-deoxyadenosine in L-cells treated with inhibitors of adenosine deaminase. *Biochem. Pharmacol*. **26**: 71–76.

LEE, H. and VINCE, R. (1980) Carbocyclic analogs of arabinosylpurine nucleosides. *J. Pharmaceut. Sci.* **69**: 1019–1021.

LEE, W. W., BENITEZ, A., GOODMAN, L. and BAKER, B. R. (1960) Potential anticancer agents. XL. Synthesis of the β-anomer of 9-(D-arabinofuranosyl)adenine. *J. Am. Chem. Soc.* **82**: 2648–2649.

LEPAGE, G. A. (1978) Resistance to 9-β-D-arabinofuranosyladenine in murine tumor cells. *Cancer Res.* **38**: 2314–2316.

LEPAGE, G. A., NAIK, S. R., KATAKKAR, S. B. and KHALIG, A. (1975) 9-β-D-arabinofuranosyladenine 5′-phosphate metabolism and excretion in humans. *Cancer Res.* **35**: 3036–3040.

LEPAGE, G. A., WORTH, L. S. and KIMBALL, A. P. (1976) Enhancement of the antitumor activity of arabinofuranosyladenine by 2′-deoxycoformycin. *Cancer Res.* **36**: 1481–1485.

LEVITT, J. and BECKER, Y. (1967) The effect of cytosine arabinoside on the replication of herpes simplex virus. *Virology*, **31**: 129–134.

LIN, A. L. and ELFORD, H. L. (1980) Adenosine deaminase impairment and ribonucleotide reductase activity and levels in HeLa cells. *J. Biol. Chem.* **255**: 8523–8528.

LIPPER, R. A., MACHKOVECH, S. M., DRACH, J. C. and HIGUCHI, W. I. (1978) Inhibition of drug metabolism by a prodrug: 9-β-D-arabinofuranosyladenine-5′-valerate as an inhibitor of adenosine deaminase. *Mol. Pharmac.* **14**: 366–369.

LIVINGSTON, R. B. and CARTER, S. K. (1968) Cytosine arabinoside (NSC-63878)-Clinical brochure. *Cancer Chemother. Rep.* **1**: 179–205.

LOPEZ, C. and GINER-SOROLLA, A. (1977) Arabinosyl-N[6]-hydroxyadenine: a new potent antivirus drug. *Ann. N.Y. Acad. Sci.* **284**: 351–357.

MACCOSS, M., RYU, E. K. and MATSUSHITA, T. (1978) The synthesis, characterization, and preliminary biological evaluation of 1-β-D-arabinofuranosylcytosine-5′-diphosphate-L-1,2-dipalmitin. *Biochem. Biophys. Res. Commun.* **85**: 714–723.

MACHIDA, H., ICHIKAWA, M., KUNINAKA, A., SANEYOSHI, M. and YOSHINO, H. (1980) Effect of treatment with 1-β-D-arabinofuranosylthymine of experimental encephalitis induced by herpes simplex virus in mice. *Antimicrob. Agents Chemother.* **17**: 109–114.

MACHIDA, H., SAKATA, S., KINNAKA, A., YOSHINO, H., NAKAYAMA, C. and SANEYOSHI, M. (1979) *In vitro* antiherpesviral activity of 5-alkyl derivatives of 1-β-D-arabinofuranosyluracil. *Antimicrob. Agent. Chemother.* **16**: 158–163.

MACHIDA, H., SAKATA, S., SHIBUYA, S., IKEDA, K., NAKAYAMA, C. and SANEYOSHI, M. (1981) Selective antiherpesviral activity of 5-substituted derivatives of 1-β-D-arabinofuranosyluracil. In: *Antiviral Chemotherapy: Design of Inhibitors of Viral Functions*, pp. 207–217. GAURI, K. K. (ed.). Academic Press, New York.

MAES, R. F., KAPLAN, M. W., WIKTOR, T. J., CAMPBELL, J. B. and KOPROWSKI, H. (1967) Inhibitory effect of a cytidine analog on growth of rabies virus. Comparative studies with other metabolic inhibitors. In: *The Molecular Biology of Viruses*, pp. 449–462. COLTER, J. S. and PARANCHYCH, W. (eds.). Academic Press, New York.

MAJOR, P. P., AGARWAL, R. P. and KUFE, D. W. (1981a) Clinical pharmacology of deoxycoformycin. *Blood* **58**: 91–96.

MAJOR, P. P., AGARWAL, R. P. and KUFE, D. W. (1981b) Deoxycoformycin: neurological toxicity. *Cancer Chemother. Pharmac.* **5**: 193–196.

MAJOR, P. P., SARGENT, L., EGAN, E. M. and KUFE, D. W. (1981c) Correlation of thymidine enhanced incorporation of ara-C into deoxyribonucleic acid with increased cell kill. *Biochem. Pharmacol.* **30**: 2221–2224.

MANTEUIL, S., KOPECKA, H., CURAUX, J., PRUNELL, A. and GIRARD, M. (1974) *In vivo* incorporation of cytosine arabinoside into simian virus 40 DNA. *J. Mol. Biol.* **90**: 751–756.

MAO, J. C.-H., ROBISHAW, E. E. and OVERBY, L. R. (1975) Inhibition of DNA polymerase from herpes simplex virus-infected Wi-38 cells by phosphonoacetic acid. *J. Virol.* **15**: 1281–1283.

MATSUKAGE, A., ONO, K., OHASHI, A., TAKAHASHI, T., NAKAYAMA, C. and SANEYOSHI, M. (1978) Inhibitory effect of 1-β-D-arabinofuranosylthymine 5′-triphosphate and 1-β-D-arabinofuranosylcytosine 5′-triphosphate on DNA polymerases from murine cells and oncornavirus. *Cancer Res.* **38**: 3076–3079.

MAYHEW, E., PAPAHADJOPOULOS, D., RUSTUM, Y. M. and DAVE, C. (1976) Inhibition of tumor cell growth *in vitro* and *in vivo* by 1-β-D-arabinofuranosylcytosine entrapped within phospholipid vesicles. *Cancer Res.* **36**: 4406–4411.

MEUWISSEN, H. J., PICKERING, R. J., POLLARA, B. P. and PORTER, I. H. (1975) *Combined Immunodeficiency Disease and Adenosine Deaminase Deficiency.* Academic Press, New York.

MILLER, F. A., DIXON, G. J., EHRLICH, J., SLOAN, B. J. and MCLEAN, I. W., Jr. (1968) Antiviral activity of 9-β-D-arabinofuranosyladenine. I. Cell culture studies. *Antimicrob. Agents Chemother.* 136–147.

MILLER, R. L., ILTIS, J. P. and RAPP, F. (1977) Differential effect of arabinofuranosylthymine on the replication of human herpesviruses. *J. Virol.* **23**: 679–684.

MINOCHA, H. C. and MALONEY, B. (1970) Inhibition of fibromal viral deoxyribonucleic acid synthesis by fluorodeoxyuridine and cytosine arabinoside. *Am. J. Vet. Res.* **31**: 1469–1475.

MOMPARLER, R. L. (1972) Kinetic and template studies with 1-β-D-arabinofuranosylcytosine 5′-triphosphate and mammalian deoxyribonucleic acid polymerase. *Mol. Pharmacol.* **8**: 362–370.

MOMPARLER, R. L. (1974) A model for the chemotherapy of acute leukemia with 1-β-D-arabinofuranosylcytosine. *Cancer Res.* **34**: 1775–1787.

MOORE, E. C. and COHEN, S. S. (1967) Effects of arabinonucleotides on ribonucleotide reduction by an enzyme system from rat tumor. *J. Biol. Chem.* **242**: 2116–2118.

MULLER, W. E. G., FALKE, D. and ZAHN, R. K. (1973) DNA dependent DNA polymerase pattern in noninfected and herpesvirus infected rabbit kidney cells. *Arch. ges. Virusforsch.* **42**: 278–284.

MULLER, W. E. G., ROHDE, H. J., BEYER, R., MAIDHOF, A., LACHMANN, M., TASCHNER, H. and ZAHN, R. K. (1975) Mode of action of 9-β-D-arabinofuranosyladenine on the synthesis of DNA, RNA and protein *in vivo* and *in vitro*. *Cancer Res.* **35**: 2160–2168.

MULLER, W. E. G., YAMAZAKI, Z., SOGTROP, H. H. and ZAHN, R. K. (1972) Action of 1-β-D-arabino-furanosylcytosine on mammalian tumor cells – 2. Inhibition of mammalian and oncogenic viral polymerases. *Eur. J. Cancer.* **8**: 421–428.

MULLER, W. E. G. and ZAHN, R. K. (1979) Metabolism of 1-β-D-arabinofuranosyluracil in mouse L5178Y cells. *Cancer Res.* **39**: 1102–1107.

MULLER, W. E. G., ZAHN, R. K., BEYER, R. and FALKE, D. (1977a) 9-β-D-arabinofuranosyladenine as a tool to study herpes simplex virus replication *in vitro. Virology.* **76**: 787–796.

MULLER, W. E. G., ZAHN, R. K., BITTLINGMAIER, K. and FALKE, D. (1977b) Inhibition of herpesvirus DNA synthesis by 9-β-D-arabinofuranosyladenine in cellular and cell-free systems. *Ann. N.Y. Acad. Sci.* **284**: 34–48.

MYERS-ROBFOGEL, M. W. and SPATARO, A. C. (1980) 1-β-D-arabinofuranosylcytosine nucleotide inhibition of sialic acid metabolism in WI-38 cells. *Cancer Res.* **40**: 1940–1943.

NAKAMURA, H., KOYAMA, G., IITAKA, Y., OHNO, M., YAGISAWA, N., KONDO, S., MEADA, K. and UMEZAWA, H. (1974) Structure of coformycin, an unusual nucleoside of microbial origin. *J. Am. Chem. Soc.* **96**: 4327–4328.

NICHOLS, W. W. and HENEEN, W. K. (1964) Chromosomal effects of arabinosylcytosine in a human diploid cell strain. *Hereditas* **52**: 402–410.

NORTH, T. W., BESTWICK, R. K. and MATHEWS, C. K. (1980) Detection of activities that interfere with the enzymatic assay of deoxynucleoside 5'-triphosphates. *J. Biol. Chem.* **255**: 6640–6645.

NORTH, T. W. and COHEN, S. S. (1978) Erythro-9-(2-hydroxy-3-nonyl)-adenine as a specific inhibitor of herpes simplex virus replication in the presence and absence of adenosine analogues. *Proc. Nat. Acad. Sci. USA* **75**: 4684–4688.

NORTH, T. W. and MATHEWS, C. K. (1981) Tetrahydrouridine specifically facilitates deoxycytidine incorporation into herpes simplex virus DNA. *J. Virol.* **37**: 987–993.

NUTTER, R. L. and RAPP, F. (1973) The effect of cytosine arabinoside on virus production in various cells infected with herpes simplex virus types 1 and 2. *Cancer Res.* **33**: 166–170.

OH-ISHI, J., KATAOKA, T., TSUKAGOSHI, S., SAKURAI, Y., SHIBUKAWA, M. and KOBAYASHI, H. (1981) Production of N⁴-succinyl-1-β-D-arabinofuranosylcytosine, a novel metabolite of N⁴-behanoyl-1-β-D-arabinofuranosyl-cytosine, in mice and its biological significance. *Cancer Res.* **41**: 2501–2506.

O'NEILL, F. J., GOLDBERG, R. J. and RAPP, F. (1972) Herpes simplex virus latency in cultured human cells following treatment with cytosine arabinoside. *J. gen. Virol.* **14**: 189–197.

OOKA, T. and CALENDAR, A. (1980) Effects of arabinofuranosylthymine on Epstein–Barr virus replication. *Virology* **104**: 219–223.

ORTIZ, P. J., MANDUKA, M. J. and COHEN, S. S. (1972) The lethality of some D-arabinosyl nucleotides to mouse fibroblasts. *Cancer Res.* **32**: 1512–1517.

OVERBY, L. R., ROBISHAW, E. E., SCHLEICHER, J. B., REUTER, A., SHIPKOWITZ, N. L. and MAO, J. C.-H. (1974) Inhibition of herpes simplex virus replication by phosphonoacetic acid. *Antimicrob. Agents Chemother.* **6**: 360–365.

PARK, N. H., GANGAROSA, L. P., KWON, B.-S. and HILL, J. M. (1978) Iontophoretic application of adenine arabinoside monophosphate to herpes simplex virus type 1-infected hairless mouse skin. *Antimicrob. Agents Chemother.* **14**: 605–608.

PARKE, DAVIS and CO. (1967) *Belgium Patent Number 671, 557.*

PAVAN-LANGSTON, D., BUCHANAN, R. A. and ALFORD, C. A., Jr. (1975) *Adenine Arabinoside: An Antiviral Agent.* Raven Press, New York.

PEDERSEN, M., TALLEY-BROWN, S. and MILLETTE, R. L. (1981) Gene expression of herpes virus. III. Effect of arabinosyladenine on viral polypeptide synthesis. *J. Virol.* **38**: 712–719.

PELLING, J. C., DRACH, J. C. and SHIPMAN, C., Jr. (1981) Internucleotide incorporation of arabinosyladenine into herpes simplex virus and mammalian cell DNA. *Virology* **109**: 323–335.

PERSON, D. A., SHERIDAN, P. J. and HERMANN, E. C. (1970) Sensitivity of types 1 and 2 herpes simplex virus to 5-iodo-2'-deoxyuridine and 9-β-D-arabinofuranosyladenine. *Infect. Immunity* **2**: 815–820.

PLUNKETT, W., ALEXANDER, L., CHUBB, S. and LOO, T. L. (1979a) Comparison of the toxicity of 2'-deoxycoformycin and erythro-9-(2-hydroxy-3-nonyl)adenine *in vivo. Biochem. Pharmac.* **28**: 201–206.

PLUNKETT, W., ALEXANDER, L., CHUBB, S. and LOO, T. L. (1979b) Biochemical basis of the increased activity of 9-β-D-arabinofuranosyladenine in the presence of inhibitors of adenosine deaminase. *Cancer Res.* **39**: 3655–3660.

PLUNKETT, W., CHUBB, S., ALEXANDER, L. and MONTGOMERY, J. A. (1980) Comparison of the toxicity and metabolism of 9-β-D-arabinofuranosyl-2-fluoroadenine and 9-β-D-arabinofuranosyladenine in human lym-phoblastoid cells. *Cancer Res.* **40**: 2349–2355.

PLUNKETT, W. and COHEN, S. S. (1975a) Metabolism of 9-β-D-arabinofuranosyladenine by mouse fibroblasts. *Cancer Res.* **35**: 415–422.

PLUNKETT, W. and COHEN, S. S. (1975b) Two approaches that increase the activity of analogs of adenine nucleosides in animal cells. *Cancer Res.* **35**: 1547–1554.

PLUNKETT, W. and COHEN, S. S. (1977) Increased toxicity of 9-β-D-arabinofuranosyladenine in the presence of an inhibitor of adenosine deaminase. *Ann. N.Y. Acad. Sci.* **284**: 91–102.

PLUNKETT, W., LAPI, L., ORTIZ, P. J. and COHEN, S. S. (1974) Penetration of mouse fibroblasts by the 5'-phosphate of 9-β-D-arabinofuranosyladenine and incorporation of the nucleotide into DNA. *Proc. Nat. Acad. Sci. USA* **71**: 73–77.

POPLACK, D. G., SALLAN, S. E., RIVERA, G., HOLCENBERG, J., MURPHY, S. B., BLATT, J., LIPTON, J. M., VENNER, P., GLAUBIGER, D. L., UNGERLEIDER, R. and JOHNS, D. (1981) Phase I study of 2'-deoxycoformycin in acute lymphoblastic leukemia. *Cancer Res.* **41**: 3343–3346.

PRIVAT DE GARILHE, M. and DE RUDDER, J. (1964) Effect de deux nucleosides de l'arabinose sur la multiplication des virus de l'herpes et de la vaccine en culture cellulaire. *CR Acad. Sci.* **259**: 2725–2728.

RAPP, F. (1964) Inhibition by metabolic analogues of plaque formation by herpes zoster and herpes simplex viruses. *J. Immunol.* **93**: 643–648.

RAPP, F. (1974) Herpesviruses and cancer. In: *Advances in Cancer Research* 19: 265–302. KLEIN, G., WEINHOUSE, S. and HADDOW, A. (eds.). Academic Press, New York.

RAPP, F., MELNICK, J. L. and KITAHARA, T. (1965) Tumor and virus antigens of simian virus 40: differential inhibition of synthesis by cytosine arabinoside. *Science* 147: 625–627.

REICHARD, P., ROWEN, L., ELIASSON, R., HOBBS, J. and ECKSTEIN, F. (1978) Inhibition of primase, the dnaG protein of *Escherichia coli* by 2′-deoxy-2′-azidocytidine triphosphate. *J. Biol. Chem.* 253: 7011–7016.

REINKE, C. M., DRACH, J. C., SHIPMAN, C., Jr. and WEISSBACH, A. (1978) Differential inhibition of mammalian DNA polymerases α, β, and herpes simplex virus-induced DNA polymerase by the 5′-triphosphates of arabinosyladenine and arabinosylcytosine. In: *Oncogenesis and Herpesviruses* III (Part 2) pp. 999–1005. DETHE, G., HENLE, W. and RAPP, F. (eds.). IARC, Lyon, France.

REIST, E. J. and GOODMAN, L. (1964) Synthesis of 9-β-D-arabinofuranosylguanine. *Biochemistry* 3: 15–18.

RENIS, H. E. and BUTHALA, D. A. (1965) Development of resistance to antiviral drugs. *Ann. N.Y. Acad. Sci.* 130: 345–354.

RENIS, H. E. and JOHNSON, H. G. (1962) Inhibition of plaque formation of vaccinia virus by cytosine arabinoside hydrochloride. *Bacterial. Proc.* 140.

RENIS, H. E., UNDERWOOD, G. E. and HUNTER, J. H. (1968) Antiviral properties of nucleosides structurally related to 1-β-D-arabinofuranosylcytosine. *Antimicrob. Agents Chemother.*, pp. 675–679.

REPTA, A. J., RAWSON, B. J., SHAFFER, R. D., SLOAN, K. B., BODOR, N. and HIGUCHI, T. (1975) Rational development of a prodrug of a cytotoxic nucleoside: Preparation and properties of arabinosyladenine 5′-formate. *J. Pharmacol. Sci.* 64: 392–396.

ROLTON, H. A. and KEIR, H. M. (1974) Deoxycytidylate deaminase. Evidence for a new enzyme in cells infected by the virus of herpes simplex. *Biochem. J.* 143: 403–409.

ROSE, K. M. and JACOB, S. T. (1978) Selective inhibition of RNA polyadenylation by araATP *in vitro*: a possible mechanism for antiviral action of araA. *Biochem. Biophys. Res. Commun.* 81: 1418–1424.

SCHABEL, F. M., Jr. (1968) The antiviral activity of 9-β-D-arabinofuranosyladenine (araA). *Chemotherapy* 13: 321–338.

SCHAEFFER, H. J. and SCHWENDER, D. F. (1974) Enzyme inhibitors. XXVI. Bridging hydrophobic and hydrophilic regions on adenosine deaminase with some 9-(2-hydroxy-3-alkyl)adenines. *J. Med. Chem.* 17: 6–8.

SCHAEFFER, H. J., VOGEL, D. and VINCE, R. (1965) Enzyme inhibitors VIII. Studies on the mode of binding of some 6-substituted 9-(hydroxyalkyl)-purines to adenosine deaminase. *J. Med. Chem.* 8: 502–506.

SCHNEYER, C. A. and GALBRAITH, W. M. (1975) Evaluation of sialogogic action of cyclocytidine (NSC-145668) and anhydro-ara-5-fluorocytidine (NSC-166641). *Cancer Chemother. Rep.* 59: 1019.

SCHRECKER, A. W., SMITH, R. G. and GALLO, R. C. (1974) Comparative inhibition of purified DNA polymerase from murine leukemia virus and human lymphocytes by 1-β-D-arabinofuranosylcytosine 5′-triphosphate. *Cancer Res.* 34: 286–292.

SCHWARTZ, P. M., SHIPMAN, C., Jr. and DRACH, J. C. (1976) Antiviral activity of arabinosyladenine and arabinosylhypoxanthine in herpes simplex virus-infected KB cells: selective inhibition of viral deoxyribonucleic acid synthesis in the presence of an adenosine deaminase inhibitor. *Antimicrob. Agents Chemother.* 10: 64–74.

SHANNON, W. M. (1975a) Adenine arabinoside: antiviral activity *in vitro*. In: *Adenine Arabinoside: An Antiviral Agent*, pp. 1–43. PAVAN-LANGSTON, D., BUCHANAN, R. A. and ALFORD, C. A., Jr. (eds.). Raven Press, New York.

SHANNON, W. M. (1975b) Inhibition of Rauscher murine leukemia virus replication and tumorigenesis by araA and inhibition of viral reverse transcriptase by ara-ATP. *Abstr. Am. Soc. Microbiol. Meet.* N.Y.

SHANNON, W. M. (moderator) (1977a) Discussion. *Ann. N.Y. Acad. Sci.* 284: 103–105.

SHANNON, W. M. (1977b) Introductory remarks on adenine arabinoside. *Ann. N.Y. Acad. Sci.* 284: 3–5.

SHANNON, W. M. (1980) Antiviral agents as adjuncts in cancer chemotherapy. *Pharmac. Ther.* 11: 263–390.

SHANNON, W. N., ARNETT, G., SCHABEL, F. M. Jr., NORTH, T. W. and COHEN, S. S. (1980) Erythro-9-(2-hydroxy-3-nonyl)adenine alone and in combination with 9-β-D-arabinofuranosyladenine in treatment of systemic herpesvirus infections in mice. *Antimicrob. Agents Chemother.* 18: 598–603.

SHANNON, W. M., WESTBROOK, L. and SCHABEL, F. M., Jr. (1974) Antiviral activity of 9-β-D-arabinofuranosyladenine (araA) against gross murine leukemia virus *in vitro* (37848). *Proc. Soc. Expt. Biol. Med.* 145: 542–545.

SHIPMAN, C. Jr., SMITH, S. H., CARLSON, R. H. and DRACH, J. C. (1976) Antiviral activity of arabinosyladenine and arabinosylhypoxantine in herpes simplex virus-infected KB cells: selective inhibition of viral deoxyribonucleic acid synthesis in synchronized suspension cultures. *Antimicrob. Agents Chemother.* 9: 120–127.

SIDWELL, R. W., ALLEN, L. B., HUFFMAN, J. H., KHWAJA, T. A., TOLMAN, R. L. and ROBBINS, R. K. (1973) Anti-DNA virus activity of the 5′-nucleotide and 3′,5′-cyclic nucleotide of 9-β-D-arabinofuranosyladenine. *Chemotherapy* 19: 325–340.

SIDWELL, R. W., ALLEN, L. B., HUFFMAN, J. H., REVANKAR, G. R., ROBBINS, R. K. and TOLMAN, R. L. (1975) Viral keratitis-inhibitory effect of 9-β-D-arabinofuranosylhypoxanthine 5′-monophosphate. *Antimicrob. Agents Chemother.* 8: 463–467.

SIDWELL, R. W., ARNETT, G. and SCHABEL, F. M., Jr. (1970) Effects of 9-β-D-arabinofuranosyladenine on myxoma and pseudorabies viruses. *Prog. Antimicrob. Anticancer Chemother.* 2: 44–48.

SIDWELL, R. W., ARNETT, G. and SCHABEL, F. (1972) *In vitro* effect of a variety of biologically active compounds on human cytomegalovirus. *Chemotherapy* 17: 259–282.

SKOOG, L. and NORDENSKJOLD, B. (1971) Effects of hydroxyurea and 1-β-D-arabinofuranosylcytosine on deoxyribonucleotide pools in mouse embryo cells. *Eur. J. Biochem.* 19: 81–89.

SLOAN, B. J. (1975) Adenine arabinoside: chemotherapy studies in animals. In: *Adenine Arabinoside: An Antiviral Agent*, pp. 45–94. PAVAN-LANGSTON, D., BUCHANAN, R. A. and ALFORD, C. A., Jr. (eds.). Raven Press, New York.

SLOAN, B. J., KIELTY, J. K. and MILLER, F. A. (1977) Effect of a novel adenosine deaminase inhibitor (Co-vidarabine, Co-V) upon the antiviral activity *in vitro* and *in vivo* of vidarabine (Vira-A) for DNA virus replication. *Ann. N.Y. Acad. Sci.* **284**: 60–80.

SMITH, S. H., SHIPMAN, C., Jr. and DRACH, J. C. (1978) Deoxyadenosine antagonism of the antiviral activity of 9-β-D-arabinofuranosyladenine and 9-β-D-arabinofuranosylhypoxanthine. *Cancer Res.* **38**: 1916–1921.

SMOLIN, G., OKUMOTO, M., FEILER, S. and CONDON, D. (1981) Idoxuridine-liposome therapy for herpes simplex keratites. *J. Ophthalmol.* **91**: 220–225.

SPECTOR, T. and MILLER, R. L. (1976) Mammalian adenylosuccinate synthetase: nucleotide monophosphate substrates and inhibitors. *Biochim. Biophys. Acta* **445**: 509–517.

STOLLER, R. G., DRAKE, J. C. and CHABNER, B. A. (1975) Purification and properties of human liver cytidine deaminase (CD). *Proc. Am. Ass. Cancer Res.* **16**: 88.

STREIFEL, J. A. and HOWELL, S. A. (1981) Synergistic interaction between 1-β-D-arabinofuranosylcytosine, thymidine, and hydroxyurea against human B cells and leukemia blasts *in vitro*. *Proc. Nat. Acad. Sci. USA* **78**: 5132–5136.

SUHADOLNIK, R. J. (1970) *Nucleoside Antibiotics.* John Wiley & Sons, Inc., New York.

SUHADOLNIK, R. J. (1979) *Nucleosides as Biological Probes.* John Wiley & Sons, New York.

SULING, W. J., RICE, L. S. and SHANNON, W. N. (1978) Effects of 2′-deoxycoformycin and erythro-9(-2-hydroxy-3-nonyl)adenine on plasma levels and urinary excretion of 9-β-D-arabinofuranosyladenine in mice. *Cancer Treat. Rep.* **62**: 369–373.

SUN, M. (1981) Cancer Institute's drug program reproved. *Science* **214**: 887–889.

TONO, H. and COHEN, S. S. (1962) The activity of nucleoside phosphorylase on 1-β-D-arabinofuranosyluracil within *Escherichia coli*. *J. Biol. Chem.* **237**: 1271–1282.

TOUMINEN, F. W. and KENNEY, F. T. (1972) Inhibition of RNA directed DNA polymerase from Rauscher leukemia virus by the 5′-triphosphate of cytosine arabinoside. *Biochem. Biophys. Res. Commun.* **48**: 1469–1475.

TURCOTTE, J. G., SRIVASTAVA, S. P., STEIM, J. M., CALABRESI, P., TIBBETTS, L. M. and CHU, M. Y. (1980) Cytotoxic liponucleotide analogs. II. Antitumor activity of CDP-diacylglycerol analogs containing the cytosine arabinoside moiety. *Biochim. Biophys. Acta* **619**: 619–631.

ULLMAN, B., GUDAS, L. J., COHEN, A. and MARTIN, D. W., Jr. (1978) Deoxyadenosine metabolism and cytotoxicity in cultured mouse T lymphoma cells: a model for immunodeficiency disease. *Cell* **14**: 365–375.

ULLMAN, B., LEVINSON, B. B., HERSHFIELD, M. S. and MARTIN, D. W., Jr. (1981) A biochemical genetic study of the role of specific nucleoside kinases in deoxyadenosine phosphorylation by cultural human cells. *J. Biol. Chem.* **256**: 848–852.

UMEDA, M. and HEIDELBERGER, C. (1969) Fluorinated pyrimidines. XXXI. Mechanism of inhibition of vaccinia virus replication in HeLa cells by pyrimidine nucleosides. *Proc. Soc. Exp. Biol. Med.* **130**: 24–29.

UNDERWOOD, G. E. (1962) Activity of 1-β-D-arabinofuranosylcytosine hydrochloride against herpes simplex keratitis. *Proc. Soc. Exp. Biol. Med.* **111**: 660–664.

UNDERWOOD, G. E., WISNER, C. A. and WEED, S. D. (1964) Cytosine arabinoside (CA) and other nucleosides in herpes virus infections. *Arch. Ophthal.* **72**: 505–512.

VINCE, R. and DALUGE, S. (1977) Carbocyclic arabinosyladenine, an adenosine deaminase resistant antiviral agent. *J. Med. Chem.* **20**: 612–613.

WALWICK, E. R., ROBERT, W. K. and DEKKER, C. A. (1959) Cyclisation during the phosphorylation of uridine and cytidine by polyphosphoric acid: a new route to the $O^2,2′$-cyclonucleosides. *Proc. Chem. Soc.* p. 84.

WATANABE, K. A., REICHMAN, U., HIROTA, K., LOPEZ, C. and FOX, J. J. (1979) Nucleosides. 110. Synthesis and antiherpes virus activity of some 2′-fluoro-2′-deoxyarabinofuranosyl-pyrimidine nucleosides. *J. Med. Chem.* **22**: 21–24.

WHITLEY, R. J., CH'IEN, L. T., DOLIN, R., GALASSO, G. J., ALFORD, C. A. Jr., editors, and the collaborative study group (1976) Adenine arabinoside therapy of herpes zoster in the immunosuppressed. *New Engl. J. Med.* **294**: 1193–1199.

WHITLEY, R. J., SOONG, S., DOLIN, R., GALASSO, G. J., CH'IEN, L. T., ALFORD, C. A., and the collaborative study group (1977) Adenine arabinoside therapy of biopsy-proved herpes simplex encephalitis. *New Engl. J. Med.* **297**: 289–294.

WHITLEY, R. T., TUCKER, B. C., KINKEL, A. W., BARTON, N. H., PASS, R. F., WHELCHEL, J. D., COBBS, C. G., DIETHELM, A. G. and BUCHANAN, R. A. (1980) Pharmacology, tolerance, and antiviral activity of vidarabine monophosphate in humans. *Antimicrob. Agents Chemother.* **18**: 709–715.

WOHLRAB, F. and FRANCKE, B. (1980) Deoxyribopyrimidine triphosphatase activity specific for herpes simplex virus type 1 infected cells. *Proc. Nat. Acad. Sci. USA* **77**: 1872–1876.

WOO, P. W. K., DION, H. W., LANGE, S. M., DAHL, L. F. and DURHAM, L. J. (1974) A novel adenosine and araA deaminase inhibitor (R)-3-(2′-deoxy-D-erythro-pentofuranosyl)-3,6,7,8-tetrahydro-imidazo[4,5,-d] [1,3]-diazepin-8-ol. *J. Hetercyclic Chem.* **11**: 641–643.

YONEMURA, K., SAIRERNJI, T. and HINUMA, Y. (1981) Inhibitory effect of 1-β-D-arabinofuranosylthymine on synthesis of Epstein–Barr virus. *Microbiol. Immunol.* **25**: 557–563.

YOSHIKURA, H. (1968) Requirement of cellular DNA synthesis for the growth of Friend leukemia virus. *Exp. Cell Res.* **52**: 445–450.

ZAVADA, V., ERBAN, V., REZACOVA, D. and VONKA, V. (1976) Thymidine kinase in cytomegalovirus infected cells. *Arch. Virol.* **52**: 333–339.

ZIMMERMAN, T. P., WOLBERG, G., DUNCAN, G. S. and ELION, G. B. (1980) Adenosine analogues as substrates and inhibitors of S-adenosylhomocysteine hydrolase in intact lymphocytes. *Biochemistry* **19**: 2252–2259.

CHAPTER 9

ANTIVIRAL IODINATED PYRIMIDINE DEOXYRIBONUCLEOSIDES: 5-IODO-2'-DEOXYURIDINE; 5-IODO-2'-DEOXYCYTIDINE; 5-IODO-5'-AMINO-2',5'-DIDEOXYURIDINE*

WILLIAM H. PRUSOFF, MING S. CHEN, PAUL H. FISCHER, TAI-SHUN LIN, WILLIAM R. MANCINI, MICHAEL J. OTTO, GEORGE T. SHIAU, RAYMOND F. SCHINAZI and JAMIESON WALKER

Department of Pharmacology, Yale University School of Medicine, New Haven, Connecticut, USA

CONTENTS

9.1. INTRODUCTION

Although iodinated pyrimidines were synthesized in the early part of this century by Johnson and Johns (1905–1906), the concept of their use as potential chemotherapeutic agents required almost a half century to be formulated. Thus Hitchings *et al.* (1945) initiated a systematic study of the biological activities of various purine and pyrimidine base analogs and found that analogs of thymine, in which the methyl moiety is replaced by a halogen such as 5-iodo-, 5-bromo- and 5-chlorouracil (Fig. 1), inhibited the reproduction of *Lactobacillus casei*. The chemical and physical relationships between these halogenated pyrimidines and thymine, which is a normal component of DNA, are such that these halogenated analogs readily replace thymine as a metabolic substrate and are incorporated into bacterial DNA in place of thymine (Weygand *et al.*, 1952; Dunn and Smith, 1954; Zamenhof and Griboff, 1954).

* The research emanating from our laboratories was supported by U.S. Public Health Service Grant CA05262 from the National Cancer Institute, and the Energy Research and Development Administration research contract AT (11-1)-2468.

VC–L

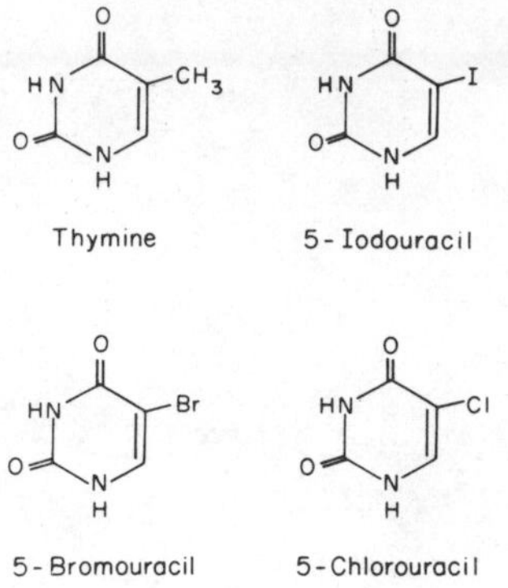

FIG. 1. Structure of thymine and related halogenated uracil analogs.

Examination of the periodic table of the elements shows that Group VIIA, the halogen group, is composed of the congeners—fluorine, chlorine, bromine, iodine and astatine. Some of the properties of the halogens are listed in Table 1 along with those of the methyl moiety of thymine for comparison. In this review we are concerned with the biological consequences that result from these new physicochemical forces when a member of the halogen group is introduced into the pyrimidine moiety of a deoxyribonucleoside (Table 2). This review will not include a discussion of fluorinated nucleosides since these have been well reviewed recently by Heidelberger (1975), but will be concerned primarily with nucleosides iodinated in the 5-position of the pyrimidine moiety. We will concentrate on three modifications of thymidine: (1) 5-iodo-2'-deoxyuridine (IdUrd) in which an iodine atom replaces the methyl group of the pyrimidine moiety of thymidine; (2) 5-iodo-2'-deoxycytidine (IdCyd) in which the oxygen on C4 of the pyrimidine moiety of IdUrd is replaced by an amino group; and (3) 5-iodo-5'-amino-2',5'-dideoxyuridine (AIdUrd; AIU) in which the 5'-hydroxyl of 5-iodo-2'-

TABLE 1. *Comparison of Some Characteristics of Group VIIA Congeners to the Methyl Group**

Halogen (CH$_3$)	Atomic number	Atomic weight (15)	Van der Waals radius (200 pm)	Covalent radius (pm)	Electronegativity	Single bond energy (C–X) (kcal/mole)
F	9	18.9984	135	64	4.0	107.0
Cl	17	35.453	180	99	3.0	66.5
Br	35	79.909	195	114	2.8	54.0
I	53	126.9044	215	135	2.4	45.5
At	85	210.0000				

*Pauling (1948); Pauling and Pauling (1975).

TABLE 2. *Some Properties of Thymidine and Various Halogenated Pyrimidine Deoxyribonucleosides*

R	Compound	pK_a^a	$\lambda_{max}^{H^+}$	$\varepsilon \times 10^{-3}$	$\lambda_{max}^{OH^-}$	$\varepsilon \times 10^{-3}$
CH$_3$	Thymidine	9.80	267	9.65	267	7.38
F	5-Fluoro-2'-deoxyuridine	7.80; 7.66[b]	271	9.17	271	7.3
Cl	5-Chloro-2'-deoxyuridine	7.90	279	9.16	276.5	6.5
Br	5-Bromo-2'-deoxyuridine	7.90; 8.1[c]	280	9.23	280	6.50
I	5-Iodo-2'-deoxyuridine	8.20; 8.25[d]	287	7.5	278	5.55
A$^+$	5-Astato-2'-deoxyuridine					

[a]Berens and Shugar (1963). [b]Wempen *et al.* (1961). [c]Lawly and Brookes (1962). [d]Prusoff (1963).

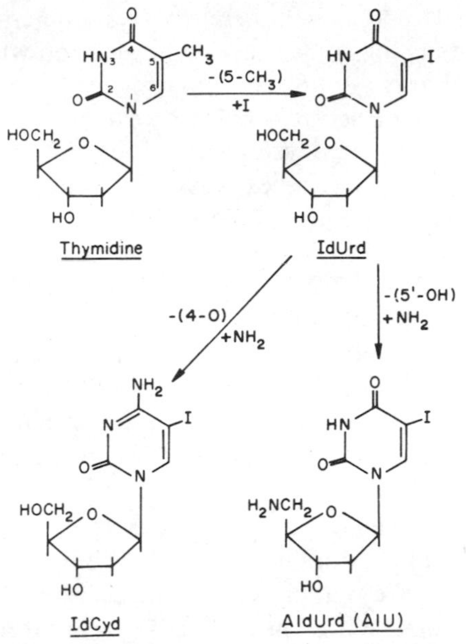

FIG. 2. Structural relationship between thymidine and three iodinated pyrimidine deoxyribo-nucleosides.

deoxyuridine is replaced by an amino group (Fig. 2). We shall concentrate on the halogenated *deoxyribo*nucleosides because one would not expect the free base, iodouracil, or its *ribo*nucleoside to be converted readily into the deoxyribonucleoside triphosphate, a form necessary for incorporation into DNA, since thymine (Plentle and Schoenheimer, 1944; Brown *et al.*, 1952; Holmes *et al.*, 1954; Reichard, 1955) and thymine ribonucleoside (Reichard, 1955) are very poor precursors of DNA-thymine in mammalian systems. Incorporation into DNA may be critical for expression of these halogenated analogs. Thus it is not surprising that Perkins *et al.* (1962) found that the ribonucleoside of 5-iodouracil had no antiviral activity in the therapy of experimental herpes simplex (a DNA virus) keratitis whereas the deoxyribonucleosides, 5-iodo-2′-deoxyuridine and 5-iodo-2′-deoxycytidine, were very efficacious. Nevertheless modest inhibition by 5-bromouracil of the replication of vaccinia virus in cell culture, and by 5-chlorouridine of the replication of Theiler's mouse encephalitis virus in mouse brain cultures was found by Thompson *et al.* (1949) and by Visser *et al.* (1952) respectively. A possible explanation for these latter findings is discussed later on.

An exciting recent development in the laboratories of Dr. K. Rössler and co-workers (1977) is the preparation of 5-astatodeoxyuridine (^{211}At) and a study of its distribution in normal and Sarcoma-180 bearing mice. Astatine is unique in the family of halogens in that it has no stable isotope.

Radioactive iodine-125 decays with release of Auger electrons (Feige and Gavron, 1975), and when [^{125}I]IdUrd is incorporated into DNA, double-strand breaks take place (Krisch and Sauri, 1975). Such action has been shown to be lethal to bacteriophage (Krisch and Sauri, 1975), bacteria (Krisch *et al.*, 1976), and mammalian cells (Bradley *et al.*, 1975; Burki *et al.*, 1973).

Robins and Taylor (1981) synthesized ^{123}I-labeled IdUrd for use as a semi-quantitative index of cell proliferation as well as an indicator of tumor response to treatment.

Bishop *et al.* (1981) and references cited therein describe the use of ^{125}I-labeled IdUrd as a marker of tumor cells; however replication is inhibited when the amount of radioactivity is in the range of 0.1–1.0 uCi per ml. They recommend that when labeling exponentially growing cells the concentration of ^{125}I-labeled IdUrd should not be in excess of 0.025 uCi per ml. Comparison of labeled thymidine and [^{125}I]-IdUrd as markers of cells have been made and reutilization of thymidine is more extensive than that of IdUrd (Webb *et al.*, 1980; Franko and Kallman, 1980; and references cited therein). This difference is presumably due to 5-halogenated deoxyuridylate being subject to dehalogenation when in a substrate complex with thymidylate kinase (Wataya *et al.*, 1977; Garrett *et al.*, 1979).

The structure of pyrimidine nucleosides has been extensively modified in the pyrimidine and pentose moieties in an attempt to develop biologically active compounds. A compilation of these compounds has been prepared recently by Schabel and Montgomery (1972), Prusoff *et al.* (1974), Langen (1975) and Prusoff and Ward (1976). Most of these modifications have been logical molecular manipulations from a synthetic point of view in that they represent isosteric replacement (Prusoff, 1955, 1959b; Beltz and Visser, 1955; Visser *et al.*, 1960; Chang and Welch, 1961; Lin and Prusoff, 1975, 1978a, b; Lin *et al.*, 1976a, b). Although the molecule has altered physicochemical properties, the hope is that it not only is transported readily into the cell but also is a good substrate for the appropriate enzyme, thereby enabling it to interact with a specific bioregulator (be it an enzyme with which it forms a complex or a macromolecule into which it is incorporated). The altered bioregulator can no longer perform its normal biological function.

Unfortunately our meager understanding of the physicochemical properties of a modified nucleoside is infinitely greater than our knowledge of the bioregulator. In the absence of such knowledge we hope that we are making intelligent decisions about the directions being pursued in our synthetic efforts. We acknowledge the fact that serendipity may have a very important input.

9.2. 5-IODO-2′-DEOXYURIDINE

9.2.1. Synthesis and Properties

The physicochemical and biological properties of IdUrd were reviewed in depth a few years ago by Langen (1975) and by Prusoff and Goz (1975) and more recently Goz (1978) has written a review on the effects of incorporation of halogenated deoxyribonucleosides into DNA of eukaryotic cells. This compound was first synthesized (Prusoff, 1959a; Fig. 3) as part of a program concerned with the development of anticancer drugs (Welch and Prusoff, 1960).

Analysis of the π-electron density of the uracil moiety of deoxyuridine indicates that the electron density is greater at C5 than at C6, making it more susceptible to electrophilic attack by the positive charged iodine during the synthesis of IdUrd (Bradshaw and Hutchinson, 1977).

In addition to the method of synthesis of IdUrd shown in Fig. 3, there are many other procedures for insertion of iodine into the pyrimidine moiety (references cited in Prusoff and Goz, 1975, and in Kochetkov and Budovskii, 1972).

9.2.2. Anticancer Activity

Prior to studies of the antiviral activity of IdUrd, investigations had been performed of its potential anticancer and radiation sensitizing properties. Jaffe and Prusoff (1960) found significant inhibition by IdUrd of the growth of Sarcoma-180, lymphoma-1210 and L5178Y without evidence of toxicity to the host mouse; however even at concentrations that produced severe toxicity to the mouse, and over 95 per cent inhibition of tumor growth, no 'cures' were obtained. An approach to augment the anticancer effect of IdUrd is based on the finding that halogenated uracil derivatives, when incorporated into DNA, sensitize bacteria (Greer, 1960; Greer and Zamenhof, 1957) and mammalian cells in culture (Djordjevic and Szybalski, 1960) to the lethal effects of UV and X-ray radiations. That IdUrd is incorporated into DNA of mammalian cells was documented by Prusoff (1959b), Mathias *et al.* (1959) and Eidinoff *et al.* (1959). In addition to an effect on the DNA polymer, iodinated substrate analogs, when bound to the active site of an enzyme, enhance the UV inactivation of these enzymes (Cysyk and Prusoff, 1972; Voytek *et al.*, 1972; Ku and Prusoff, 1974; Voytek, 1975;

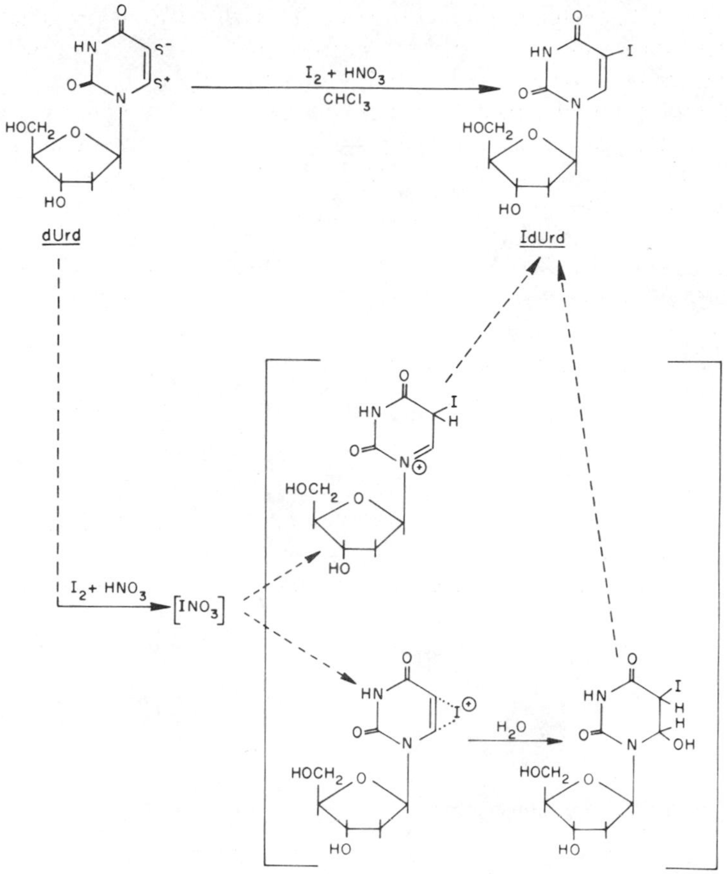

FIG. 3. Synthesis of 5-iodo-2'-deoxyuridine.

Chen *et al.*, 1976a; Chen and Prusoff, 1977), presumably by a radiation induced deiodination with formation of a uracil free radical (Rupp and Prusoff, 1964, 1965), which subsequently covalently interacts with the enzyme (Fig. 4). Although the *E. coli* thymidine kinase is readily sensitized to UV inactivation with IdUrd, the mammalian enzyme is considerably less susceptible.

The efficacy of IdUrd in patients with neoplastic disease was modest when used alone (Calabresi *et al.*, 1961; Papac *et al.*, 1962; Calabresi, 1963). However, when used in combination with X-ray, prolonged arrest of growth at the irradiated site was reported (Calabresi *et al.*, 1961). Nevertheless the use of IdUrd in combination with radiations for therapy of neoplasms in man remains to be exploited (see references in Prusoff and Goz, 1975).

9.2.3. ANTIVIRAL ACTIVITY

The primary importance of IdUrd today is the demonstration that nucleoside drugs not only have antiviral activity, but can be efficacious in an *established* virus infection. In contrast, most of the non-nucleoside antiviral agents such as interferon, adamantamine or *N*-methyl isatinthiosemicarbazide are most effective when administered prophylactically. This is of great importance during the initial stages of an epidemic or when one wishes to contain the outbreak of a contagious virus infection.

Thompson *et al.* (1949) documented a modest inhibition of vaccinia virus in cell culture by 5-bromouracil, as a consequence of the seminal studies of Hitchings and his co-workers

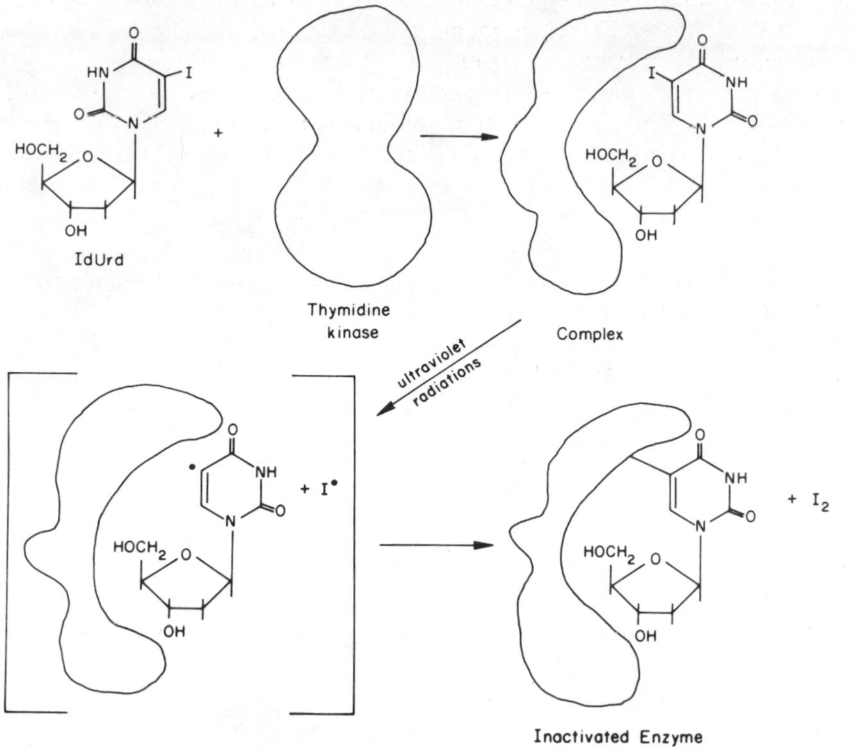

FIG. 4. Hypothetical mechanism of sensitization of thymidine kinase by IdUrd to the lethal effects of ultraviolet radiations.

(1945), who made a systematic study of the inhibitory potential of various purine and pyrimidine bases in bacteria. These findings stimulated a study by Visser *et al.* (1952), who demonstrated that certain *ribo*nucleoside analogs (5-chlorouridine, 5-hydroxyuridine, 5-aminouridine, etc.) inhibited the replication of Theiler's mouse encephalitis virus in mouse brain cultures. Soon after deoxyuridine became commercially available the halogenated deoxyribonucleosides were synthesized: 5-chloro-2′-deoxyuridine by Visser *et al.* (1960), 5-bromo-2′-deoxyuridine by Beltz and Visser (1955), and 5-iodo-2′-deoxyuridine by Prusoff (1959a). BrdUrd was found by Smith *et al.* (1960) to inhibit the replication of polyoma virus in mouse embryonic cells, and Herrmann (1961) found both BrdUrd and IdUrd to inhibit the replication of vaccinia and herpes simplex virus in cell culture.

IdUrd is primarily effective against DNA viruses (e.g. herpes simplex, pseudorabies, vaccinia, adenovirus, polyoma), but RNA-viruses are not affected with the exception of Columbia-SK (Force and Stewart, 1964a) and oncogenic RNA viruses such as Rous Sarcoma virus (Force and Stewart, 1964b). It is generally believed that replication of an RNA oncogenic virus involves a DNA intermediate which is formed from the viral RNA by the RNA-directed DNA polymerase (reverse transcriptase) present in the RNA oncogenic virion. This DNA is then integrated into the host cell DNA and can be transcribed into viral mRNA, which is then translated into viral polypeptides (Aaronson and Stephenson, 1976a, b). As we shall see later, incorporation of IdUrd into DNA is probably responsible for the inhibition of the replication of oncogenic RNA viruses as well as DNA viruses. The synthesis of DNA required for replication of Rous sarcoma virus occurs only during the early stages of the reproduction of this virus, and explains why IdUrd is inhibitory to this virus only when administered to cells at the time of infection.

The effectiveness of IdUrd against herpes keratitis in rabbits and in man was documented by Kaufman and his co-workers (1962a, b, c), soon after the report by Herrmann (1961) that IdUrd and BrdUrd, but not 5-bromouridine, inhibit the replication of herpes simplex virus *in vitro*. The animal experiments were confirmed by Perkins *et al.* (1962), who also provided evidence for the structural requirement of the pentose moiety of IdUrd since the corresponding 5-iodouracil*ribo*nucleoside (IUrd) was inactive. However, Maichuk *et al.* (1973) reported 5-bromouridine (BrUrd) not only inhibited the replication of herpes simplex virus, an effect which could be prevented by simultaneous use of uridine, but also that it was effective in therapy of herpes keratitis both in rabbits and in man. It had previously been established by Hanna (1966) that the free base, 5-iodouracil, neither prevented the replication of herpes simplex virus nor affected the synthesis of DNA. The reason for the efficacy of BrUrd in view of the lack of effectiveness of IUrd is unknown. However a recent finding in our laboratory indicated that 5-bromouracil at about 100-fold greater concentration than BrdUrd will exert an inhibitory effect on the replication of HSV-1 *in vitro*. Breitman *et al.* (1966), Gotto *et al.* (1969) and Cooper *et al.* (1972) found thymine and bromouracil incorporation into DNA can be enhanced markedly if a source of deoxyribose-1-phosphate is provided. Thus bromouracil *per se*, or derived from bromouridine by phosphorolysis, may be converted, albeit to a small extent, to the deoxyribonucleoside which is a potent antiviral agent.

The use of IdUrd in the therapy of herpes simplex infection of the corneal epithelium in man, a disease which is a major cause of blindness in the United States, has been unequivocally established and for this its use has been approved by the FDA. Juel-Jensen (1973, 1974) has reviewed the clinical utility of IdUrd and, in addition to therapy of herpes keratitis, beneficial results have been reported in the therapy of herpetic whitlow, genital herpes, cutaneous herpes, herpes zoster, vaccinia lesions and vaccinia whitlow when a concentrated solution of this drug in dimethylsulfoxide is used. The use of idoxuridine with or without dimethylsulfoxide in the topical therapy of varicella zoster or herpes genitalis is controversial (Juel-Jensen and MacCallum, 1972, 1974; MacCallum and Juel-Jensen, 1966; Dawber, 1974; Verbov, 1979; Wildenhoff *et al.*, 1979; Silvestri *et al.*, 1979). Kaufman (1980) has reviewed the use of various antimetabolites for clinical management of herpetic keratitis.

An approach under study to increase transport of IdUrd into areas of the skin infected with herpesvirus is the use of ionotophoresis (Gangarosa *et al.*, 1977; Hill *et al.*, 1977; Lekas, 1979).

Another approach to effect improved transport of drugs is to increase their lipophilicity. Therefore Chang and Welch (1961) first synthesized the 3',5'-diacetyl derivative of IdUrd. Preliminary data was obtained by Perkins *et al.* (1962) of the efficacy of this compound in the treatment of experimental HSV-1 keratitis. These findings were confirmed and extended by Hettinger *et al.* (1981) in a well-controlled statistical study.

Liposomes containing IdUrd have been used to treat experimental herpes keratitis in an attempt to increase the penetration of the drug into the cornea (Smolin *et al.*, 1981). They found the IdUrd-liposome preparation to be more effective than IdUrd alone in the therapy of epithelial and stromal herpes simplex virus keratitis in rabbits.

Although early reports indicated a beneficial effect from the use of IdUrd in the therapy of herpes encephalitis in man (references cited in Goz and Prusoff, 1970), most were not randomized double-blind experiments. A controlled study was performed in which *six* patients with proven herpes simplex virus encephalitis were treated, of which one who had received intraventricular as well as intravenous IdUrd survived (Boston Interhospital Virus Study Group and co-sponsor, 1975). The statistically inadequate number of patients involved is related to the decision to terminate the use of IdUrd because myelosuppression was 'unexpectedly' observed. Since this toxicity, as well as other toxicities that result from systemically administered IdUrd, have been well documented in the literature (Calabresi *et al.*, 1961), such toxicity should not have been unexpected. One of the two patients with proven herpes encephalitis who received intracerebral as well as intravenous IdUrd survived, although with severe neurological damage. Since the intraventricular dose (5 mg/kg) was only 10 per cent of that given systemically, one wonders whether a larger intraventricular dose would have been more beneficial. Lerner and Bailey (1972) found, during a slow infusion of IdUrd (4 mg/min) in patients with a suspected diagnosis of *Herpesvirus hominis* encephalitis, that the rate of inactivation or removal was very rapid. However, significant quantities of IdUrd (2.36 mM) were found in the cerebrospinal fluid of one patient soon after initiation of a fast rate of infusion of IdUrd (50 mg/min). They also reported that the minimal inhibitory concentration of IdUrd for fresh isolates of HSV-1 was about 18–70 μM.

Resistance to IdUrd by herpesvirus develops rapidly in cell culture (Buthala, 1964) and this is attributed to a decrease in the formation of herpesvirus encoded thymidine kinase (Dubbs and Kit, 1964; Lowry *et al.*, 1971). Hirano *et al.* (1979) isolated four strains of herpes simplex virus type-1 from two patients with recurrent herpes keratitis of which two were highly resistant to IdUrd in cell culture and the other two were susceptible to this drug. All four viruses induced thymidine kinase. Although the bases for resistance was not established, under consideration was a decreased affinity of IdUrd for thymidine kinase or of IdUTP for HSV–DNA polymerase. Resistant strains of HSV have been isolated from patients previously (Laibson *et al.*, 1963; Pavan-Langston *et al.*, 1972), however IdUrd resistance *in vivo* does not appear very easily (Nordenfelt and Nordenfelt, 1977) and clinically resistance may be due to pharmacokinetic problems. Thus Jawetz *et al.* (1970) found that of twelve strains of HSV isolated from 'clinically-IdUrd-resistant' patients, ten were equally sensitive to IdUrd and two had a 10–30-fold increase in resistance. Similar findings were made by Nordenfelt and Nordenfelt (1977).

It is clear there is a need for antiviral agents that are less toxic when given systemically. A logical question is whether one can obtain antiviral activity in the absence of toxicity. Before this question can be approached one should understand the biochemical basis for the antiviral activity of IdUrd as well as for its inhibition of uninfected cells. This has been discussed in great detail by Prusoff (1967), Goz and Prusoff (1970) and Prusoff and Goz (1975).

9.2.4. Metabolism and Biochemical Effects

Three major areas have been found where IdUrd or the appropriate phosphorylated derivative exert marked effects: (1) competitive inhibition of several enzymes concerned with the biosynthesis of DNA-thymine (thymidine kinase, thymidylate kinase and DNA polymerase); (2) allosteric or feedback inhibition by the triphosphate of IdUrd of the regulatory enzymes thymidine kinase, deoxycytidylate deaminase and ribonucleoside-diphosphate reductase; (3) alteration of gene expression subsequent to the incorporation of IdUrd into DNA (Fig. 5).

The two types of enzyme inhibition are competitive and readily reversible, whereas incorporation into DNA is not. Thus incorporation into DNA is believed to be responsible for toxicity as well as the antiviral effect of IdUrd. Incorporation of halogenated nucleosides (BrdUrd or IdUrd) into viral DNA has been found in vaccinia virus (Prusoff *et al.*, 1963;

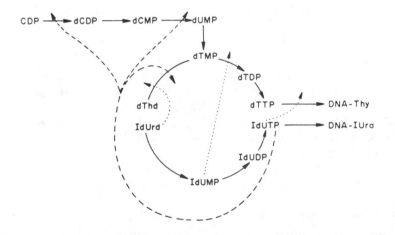

Fig. 5. Sites of inhibition by 5-iodo-2′-deoxyuridine and its phosphorylated derivatives.

Easterbrook and Davern, 1963), in pseudorabies (Kaplan *et al.*, 1965), in herpes simplex virus (Schiek and Schiek, 1969; Miyamoto *et al.*, 1969; Matsumura, 1973; Chen *et al.*, 1976b), in SV40 virus (Buettner and Werchau, 1973; Calothy *et al.*, 1973), in polyoma virus (Hirt, 1966), and in adenovirus (Wigand and Klein, 1974). Buettner and Werchau (1973) isolated infectious DNA from SV40 grown in the presence of IdUrd and showed a relationship between loss of infectivity and the extent of substitution of SV40 DNA-thymidine by IdUrd. Fischer *et al.* (1980) found a parallelism between the degree of incorporation of IdUrd into herpes simplex virus DNA and the inhibition of the replication of this virus. There was no evidence for either single- or double-stranded breaks even at about a 45 per cent substitution of DNA-thymidine by IdUrd.

Patch *et al.* (1981) investigated the effect of IdUrd-substituted SV40 on viral RNA transcription. Extensively substituted (18–35 per cent) SV-40 DNA decreased virus formation 100-fold, but induced 30–50 per cent more viral-specific RNA than control virus. However, lightly substituted (10–15 %) virions had only a slight effect on replication, but induced 5-fold more viral-specific RNA as well as longer viral m-RNA than control virions. Thus increased transcription is a consequence of incorporation of IdUrd into SV-40 DNA.

Lau *et al.* (1981) found that IdUrd increased the synthesis of EBV-RNA, and Davis *et al.* (1978) observed BrdUrd to amplify 40-fold virus specific RNA when retrovirus was activated in guinea-pig embryo cells.

Otto *et al.* (1982) studied the effect of IdUrd on the expression of herpes simplex virus induced proteins and found no effect on HSV-1 induced α proteins but β and γ proteins were markedly reduced. However, herpes simplex virus induced thymidine kinase is over-produced. The mechanism for this accumulation is unknown as yet. Second-generation IdUrd substituted virions exhibit altered protein synthetic patterns as analyzed by SDS-polyacrylamide gel electrophoresis.

Žemla (1974); Žemla and Petrik (1978) found polyoma virus in the presence of BrdUrd increased the activity of some enzymes involved in the synthesis of DNA. More recently Tarábek and Žemla (1980) and Žemla and Tarábek (1981) found BrdUrd to inhibit the synthesis of polyoma virus-specific RNA.

Commerford and Joel (1979) and Smellie and Parsons (1979) found that as much as 60 per cent of [^{3}H]-labeled IdUrd was incorporated into DNA as thymidine and such incorporation could be prevented by FdUrd. When a comparison was made by Gautschi *et al.* (1978) of the utilization of dTTP, BrdUTP and IdUTP for DNA synthesis by cells that were gently lysed, they found these compounds to be used with equal efficacy, whereas in the intact cell BrdUrd and dThd were used with equal efficacy but IdUrd less so.

The key question that remains is what is the lethal molecular event which is a consequence of such incorporation into viral DNA. Maass and Haas (1966) had previously found a marked decrease in the formation of virus specific SV40 antigens when the virus replicated in the presence of 280 μM IdUrd. However, analysis by Wigand and Klein (1974) of the capsid proteins derived from adenovirus grown in the presence of IdUrd, showed no difference in several physiological and immunological characteristics relative to control virions. Although Kan and Prusoff (1976) found no effect of IdUrd on the rate of synthesis of *early* proteins by adenovirus-2, the synthesis of *late* proteins was uniformly depressed. Whereas the early proteins are translated from mRNA transcribed off parental DNA, late proteins are derived from mRNA transcribed from progeny DNA which is synthesized in the presence of IdUrd. Similarly Pennington (1976) had found previously that, while BrdUrd did not affect the synthesis of most vaccinia virus polypeptides, a few post-replicative polypeptides were markedly inhibited. It would be ideal if one knew the specific biological role that an affected polypeptide has, since such a knowledge would accelerate and increase the sensitivity of analysis (Žemla, 1974; Žemla and Petrik, 1978; Žemla and Tarábek, 1981; Patch *et al.*, 1981, Otto *et al.*, 1982).

Specific biological effects of IdUrd and BrdUrd have been observed in other systems such as on embryonic development and expression of differentiated cell functions (Rutter *et al.*, 1973; Kreider *et al.*, 1974; Prusoff and Goz, 1975; Silagi, 1976; Wainwright and Wainwright, 1976; Bick, 1977; Biswas *et al.*, 1977; Hulanicka *et al.*, 1977; Murray and Russell, 1978;

Biquard and Aupoix, 1978; Garcia *et al.*, 1979; Lough, 1980; Ashman and Davidson, 1980; Scott, 1981; Kawamura and Hashimoto, 1981) as well as on the induction or repression of specific enzymes or proteins in mammalian cells (Stellwagen and Tomkins, 1971a, b; Koyama and Ono, 1971, 1972; Wrathall *et al.*, 1975; Gurr *et al.*, 1977; Bick and Soffer, 1976; Goz, 1974; Goz and Walker, 1976; Bulmer *et al.*, 1976; Coetzee and Gevers, 1977; O'Brien and Stellwagen, 1977; Evans and Bosmann, 1977; Miller *et al.*, 1977; Garcia *et al.*, 1981; Pawlowski *et al.*, 1981). These effects are probably a consequence of incorporation of these halogenated thymidine analogs into DNA.

Goz *et al.* (1980), however, found no correlation between the induction of alkaline phosphatase activity by IdUrd and its incorporation into DNA of HeLa cells. Whereas Goz and Walker (1978) found IdUrd and prednisolone can each induce alkaline phosphatase to a similar extent, Schneider and Falke (1980) found BrdUrd increased this enzyme in herpesvirus transformed hamster embryo cells about 10-fold whereas prednisolone had no effect. However, a 30-fold increase was observed by combination of these drugs by Schneider and Falke (1980).

Expression of *gene* activity may be controlled by the intermediate repetitive sequences in the DNA genome, and complex formation with these sequences by nonhistone proteins or hormones may be involved in the regulation of transcription. Initiation of gene transcription is believed to occur in pyrimidine-rich regions of the DNA (Jacob, 1966; Szybalski *et al.*, 1966; Taylor *et al.*, 1967; Shishido and Ikeda, 1970). Tracts of thymidine in DNA have been found and if specific genes have varying amounts of thymidine clusters and random incorporation of BrdUrd or IdUrd into DNA occurs, then those genes which are rich in thymidine tracts will have a greater probability for incorporation of those analogs and hence be specifically affected. Although a selective uptake of BrdUrd into specific regions of DNA was found by Strom and Dorfman (1976) and by Schwartz (1976, and references cited therein), Singer and co-workers (1977) found no such selectivity. Another possibility based on the studies of Stellwagen and Tomkins (1971a, b) supports a generalized effect on all mRNA transcription, with those proteins with a high turnover rate being primarily affected. A rapid decrease in enzyme activity is associated with a rapid turnover of the enzyme molecule as well as the specific mRNA (Barnett and Wicks, 1971; Steinberg *et al.*, 1975). However, Gurr *et al.* (1977) and Kasupski and Mukherjee (1977) found no simple relationship between turnover rates of a number of enzymes and the inhibition by BrdUrd of their synthesis, since the activity of enzymes with similar mRNA and protein half-lives were either decreased or increased by BrdUrd.

There is evidence for a greater binding affinity of substituted DNA to specific protein. In fact RNA polymerase is believed to bind selectively to pyrimidine-rich sequences (Jacob, 1966; Szybalski *et al.*, 1966; Taylor *et al.*, 1967; Shishido and Ikeda, 1970). Lin and Riggs (1972) found a ten-fold greater binding of the lac repressor to BrdUrd-substituted lac operator relative to unsubstituted lac operator. Goeddel *et al.* (1978) describe the synthesis of seventeen site-specific 5-bromouracil substituted *lac* operators and the dissociation kinetics for complexes formed between these operators and *lac* repressors. Matthes *et al.* (1977) incorporated BrdUrd extensively into rat liver after partial hepatectomy and found marked alterations in the histone-DNA binding. Thus a tighter binding of substituted DNA to chromosomal or regulatory proteins (Lapeyer and Bekhor, 1974; David *et al.*, 1974; Bick and Devine, 1977; Schwartz, 1977; Kallos *et al.*, 1978; Fasy *et al.*, 1980) could result in the inhibition of expression of differential cell functions (Gordon *et al.*, 1976; Lin *et al.*, 1976), and a tighter binding to RNA polymerase could affect not only the rate of RNA formation (Jones and Dove, 1972; Kotzin and Baker, 1972; Pawlowski, 1976), but also the relative amount of various RNAs normally transcribed (Kotzin and Baker, 1972; Grady and Campbell, 1974; Price, 1976; Palayoor, 1977; Lykkesfeldt, 1977) as well as the composition or properties of the transcripts (Hill *et al.*, 1974; Hill and Baserga, 1975). Kallos *et al.* (1979) incorporated equivalent molar amounts of CldUrd, BrdUrd and IdUrd into DNA and found an increased binding of estrogen receptor to DNA that was related to the specific halogen ($I > Br > Cl > CH_3$). Whether this increased binding is related to hydrophobicity, decreased electronegativity, base stacking, conformation differences, or destabilization of ordered water molecules enveloping the DNA have all been considered.

However, Simpson and Seale (1974) characterized chromatin extensively substituted with BrdUrd and found no difference from control chromatin in the composition of protein histones and nonhistones, as well as no difference in the ability of the proteins to be dissociated by sodium phosphate in 5 M urea. Thus, if differences in binding were present, they were not detected by the techniques used. Schwartz (1981) found the halogenated nucleoside triphosphates (BrdUTP and IdUTP) were utilized preferentially by eukaryotic DNA polymerase γ relative to dTTP, and this increased affinity was supported by an 8- to 20-fold lower K_m respectively relative to that of dTTP.

Circular dichroism studies have been performed to more clearly define the interaction between proteins and BrdUrd substituted DNA. Both an increase in positive ellipticity (Augenlicht et al., 1974; Simpson and Seale, 1974) and a change in the opposite direction (Lapeyer and Bekhor, 1974; Lin and Pagano, 1980) have been reported. These differences are believed by Nicolini and Baserga (1975) to be related to the extent of thymidine replacement by BrdUrd in the DNA.

There is very little difference sterically between thymidine and IdUrd since the size of the iodine atom as defined by its van der Waals' radius is 215 pm whereas that of the methyl group is 200 pm (Table 1). However, the electron configuration of the pyrimidine moiety is altered because the halogen may produce two different effects. The first of these results from the high electronegativity of the halogen atom, so that the electrons, by the inductive effect, are pulled away from the carbon atom to which it is attached (Fig. 6). The second effect is a consequence of the halogen atom having an unshared pair of electrons which can initiate a resonance effect in the pyrimidine ring by increasing the electron density of the ring. The inductive effect of the halogen is probably the dominant effect responsible for the labilization of the proton on the N3 position of IdUrd, which is readily measured by determination of the pK_a of thymidine (9.8) relative to that of IdUrd (8.2) (Fig. 7).

At physiological pH the proportion of the ionized or enolic form of IdUrd theoretically is greater than that of thymidine by a factor of over 30, and therefore it has been generally accepted that this is the basis for the increased ability of the halogenated analog relative to the thymidine moiety to base pair with guanine rather than adenine (Fig. 8). This explanation has been questioned. Thus, Sternglanz and Bugg (1975) postulate that the increase in stacking energy found in DNA substituted with halogenated bases may be primarily responsible for the mispairing, rather than ionization or enol-keto tautomerism. Furthermore, Shugar and his co-workers (Shugar et al., 1977; Kulikowski and Shugar, 1978) have found that the proportion of the two tautomers do not change appreciably when a halogen is inserted into the 5-position of a nucleoside, and hence factors other than tautomerism per se appear to be responsible for mispairing. No matter how errors in base pairing are produced, they may, during replication or transcription, have dramatic effects

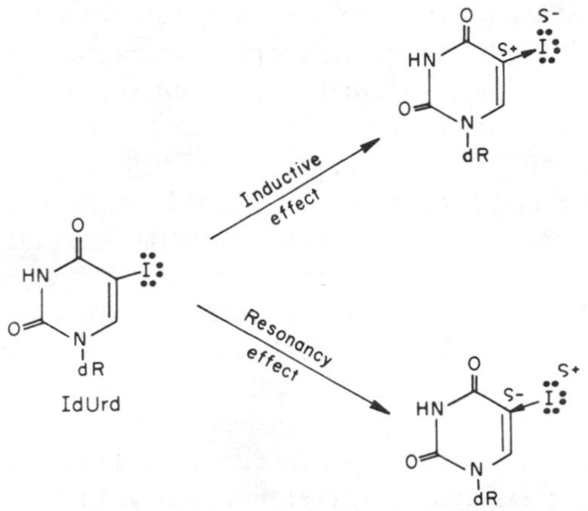

FIG. 6. Effect of iodine on the electron distribution of 5-iodo-2'-deoxyuridine.

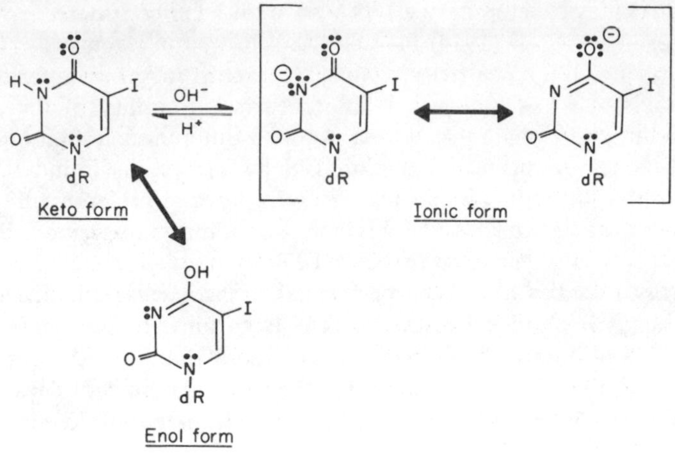

FIG. 7. Keto, enol and ionic forms of 5-iodo-2'-deoxyuridine.

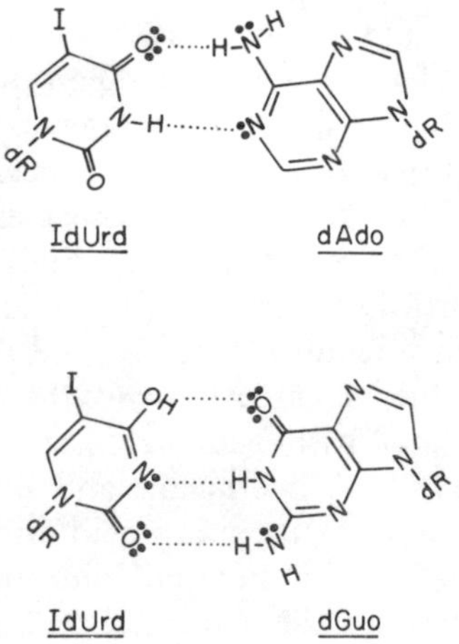

FIG. 8. The effect of the electronic form of IdUrd on its ability to base pair with purine moieties.

during translation of the mRNA derived from substituted DNA. These effects can also be manifest by the incorporation of an incorrect amino acid into a polypeptide, which would alter its properties so that it no longer might exert its catalytic activity or be utilized as a structural protein. Hopkins and Goodman (1980) support the primary determinant of mutagenesis by BrdUrd being base-pair errors due to analog mispairing as well as perturbation of deoxyribonucleotide triphosphate pools. Previous studies by Peterson *et al.* (1978) concluded that imbalances in precursor nucleotide pools may be involved not only in mutagenesis but also carcinogenesis and ageing. Kaufman and Davidson (1978) found a non-linear relationship between mutagenicity and the amount of BrdUrd in the DNA of mammalian cells. They suggested that more critical was the amount of BrdUrd in the medium. Davidson and Kaufman (1978) and Kaufman and Davidson (1979) found BrdUrd mutagenesis in mammalian cells to be suppressed by dCyd and to be stimulated by dThd as well as by purine deoxyribonucleosides, but the mechanism involved is not known. The dCyd effect was not due to an alteration in the distribution of BrdUrd in DNA (Reff and Davidson, 1979). Possible explanations suggested include induction of an 'error-prone' repair system, allosteric changes in DNA polymerase, an imbalance of dNTPs, and alteration of the cell membrane by an effect on nucleoside diphosphate sugars.

Pietrzykowska (1973) and Pietrzykowska and Krych (1977) invoked a role for DNA repair in mutagenesis effected by bromouracil. Recent studies by Krych *et al.* (1979) concerned the involvement of DNA-uracil *N*-glycosidase and endonuclease in the recognition and repair of DNA lesions that result from incorporation of BrdUrd into DNA (Arfellini *et al.*, 1977, 1978). The incorporation of IdUrd into DNA as dUrd has been established (Commerford and Joel, 1979; Smellie and Parsons, 1979).

An effect on transcription is supported by several studies: Jones and Dove (1972) found a seven-fold reduction in the synthesis of RNA in BrdUrd substituted bacteria and phage; Preisler *et al.* (1973) found BrdUrd decreased the amount of globin and of globin mRNA induced by dimethylsulfoxide in cultures of Friend leukemia cells; Hill *et al.* (1974) and Hill and Baserga (1975), working with a eukaryotic system, found that transcribed RNA from fibroblasts grown in the presence of BrdUrd had a marked increase in guanylate and a marked decrease in adenylate that was related to the extent of DNA-thymidine replacement by BrdUrd. On the other hand, Stambrook and Williamson (1974) analyzed functional 5-S RNA from ribosomes from cells grown in the presence of BrdUrd that allows a 50 per cent replacement of DNA-thymidine with bromouracil, and could not detect any errors in the nucleotide sequence. Colbert and Coleman (1977) in a study of transcription during inhibition of myogenesis in culture by BrdUrd found the rate of hybridization of RNA was significantly slower than that from untreated control cells.

Weintraub and co-workers (1972) studied the effect of BrdUrd incorporation into DNA of precursor erythroblasts and attributed the prevention of the formation of hemoglobin in progeny cells to an inhibitory effect on the initiation of new macromolecular synthesis. Once hemoglobin synthesis had been initiated, the cell was resistant to the effects of BrdUrd.

Faulty transcription can be manifested as an effect on translation. Several viruses grown in the presence of BrdUrd have been reported to synthesize abnormal proteins (Easterbrook and Davern, 1963; Kjellen, 1962; Vansanten, 1965). More recently, Kan and Prusoff (1976) and Pennington (1976) did find the synthesis of virus-induced specific proteins to be affected when virus replication occurred in the presence of IdUrd and BrdUrd respectively; and Gilbert *et al.* (1974) found BrdUrd in *Drosophila melanogaster* caused the disappearance of several proteins normally synthesized, as well as the appearance of an abnormal protein. In contrast Bick (1975) found no transcriptional errors in cell lines that had 60 or 100 per cent substitution of DNA-thymidine with BrdUrd, nor did Stambrook and Williamson (1974) find BrdUrd-induced transcriptional errors.

Another consequence of the presence of a halogen in the pyrimidine moiety was noted by Camerman and Trotter (1964) during X-ray diffraction analysis of crystalline IdUrd. They found an unusually short intermolecular distance of 2.96 A between the iodine atom and the carbonyl oxygen, whereas the calculated sum of their van der Waals radii is 3.55 A. They postulated that the ability of iodine to form charge transfer bonds may be responsible for the increased interchain attraction that could either prevent or delay the synthesis of virus DNA, or for that matter that of viral mRNA. A similar interaction between the halogenated uracil with an adjacent base in the same DNA strand may be responsible for the increase in stacking energy found by Sternglanz and Bugg (1975) in DNA substituted with halogenated uracil bases. The stacking energy is believed to be a consequence of electrostatic dipole-induced dipole forces (Plesiewicz *et al.*, 1976 and references cited therein).

Although the many biological effects of BrdUrd and IdUrd are generally attributed to incorporation into DNA, other possibilities have been entertained (Schubert and Jacob, 1970; Meuth and Green, 1974; Rogers *et al.*, 1975; Davidson and Kaufman, 1977). Schubert and Jacob (1970) found BrdUrd enhanced the induction of certain differentiated functions by neuroblastoma cells under conditions in which DNA biosynthesis was markedly inhibited by arabinosylcytosine (ara-C) or mitomycin. They attributed the phenomenon to a possible effect on the synthesis of carbohydrate moieties associated with the outer cellular membranes, such as glycoproteins and mucopolysaccharides, which could also be responsible for the increased affinity of the cells for the surface of the culture dish. Brown (1971) did indeed find BrdUrd to promote the synthesis of a cell surface glycopeptide which is characteristic of the differentiated state of a neuroblastoma cell.

Meuth and Green (1974) claim that many of the biological effects of BrdUrd may be due to a feedback inhibition by 5-bromo-2'-deoxyuridine triphosphate (BrdUTP) of ribonucleoside diphosphoreductase, thereby causing a deoxycytidineless state. Their interpretation was based on the observation that the lethal effect of BrdUrd on certain murine cells in culture could be prevented by deoxycytidine. Unfortunately no data were presented as to whether growth of these cells in low or moderate levels of BrdUrd was accompanied by any uptake into DNA. At the one concentration of BrdUrd (0.15 mM) investigated they found about a 40 per cent substitution of thymine residues by bromouracil. Thus it is difficult to attribute the toxicity of BrdUrd to a non-DNA effect, since deoxycytidine after phosphorylation, deamination and methylation forms deoxythymidylate which would be an effective competitive inhibitor of the utilization of the monophosphate of BrdUrd for DNA biosynthesis. Of relevance are the findings that ribonucleoside diphosphoreductase is induced by pseudorabies virus (Kaplan, 1964) and by both HSV-type 1 and -type 2 (Cohen, 1972; Cohen *et al.*, 1974), but that the enzyme is *not* inhibited significantly, unlike the host cell ribonucleoside diphosphoreductase, by thymidine triphosphate (Ponce de Leon *et al.*, 1977).

Rogers *et al.* (1975) were able to reverse the inhibition of myogenesis caused by BrdUrd with dThd, dCyd and dUrd without affecting its incorporation into DNA which amounted to not more than 1–2 per cent. This is a very low level of incorporation and one would have liked to be sure that the radioactivity incorporated into the DNA was indeed BrdUrd and not some radioactive impurity whose uptake is not affected by thymidine, deoxycytidine or deoxyuridine. Rogers *et al.* (1975) suggests the alternative explanation, mainly that a phosphorylated form of BrdUrd inhibits glycosyl-transferases of myoblasts so that specific glycoproteins or glycolipids responsible for the fusion of myoblasts into myotubules are not formed. However, Walther *et al.* (1974) found BrdUrd inhibited selectively the cytodifferentiation of embryonic rat pancreas under conditions in which there were no significant effects on the incorporation of precursors into phospholipid, sphingolipids, glycoproteins, sterols or free fatty acids and no evidence for the formation of BrdUrd-containing sugar nucleotides.

Deoxycytidine prevented the inhibition by BrdUrd of pigmentation and tumorigenicity in Syrian hamster melanoma cells, and this inhibition correlated with a decreased incorporation of the halogenated analog into DNA (Horn and Davidson, 1976). However, Davidson and Kaufman (1977), upon more detailed analysis, now claim that deoxycytidine did not reverse the suppression of pigmentation by changing the amount of BrdUrd in DNA. Concentrations of deoxycytidine (8 μM) which produced a maximal decrease in BrdUrd uptake into DNA had no significant effect on pigmentation suppression by BrdUrd. However, with massive doses of deoxycytidine (up to 1000 μM) although there was no further effect on BrdUrd incorporation into DNA, pigmentation inhibition did not occur. Since aminopterin prevented the deoxycytidine protection, conversion of deoxycytidine to thymidine is required for protection.

BrdUrd is known to affect the cell surface of cells, and nucleosides are co-factors in the synthesis of many cell surface components. Thus it is conceivable that deoxycytidine, as well as thymidine, may be exerting their anti-BrdUrd effect in this area. Furthermore, Fitzmaurice and Baker (1974) found that the effect of BrdUrd on the incorporation of RNA precursors (uridine) into sea urchin embryos that resulted in an altered composition from the control found previously by Kotzin and Baker (1972) may have been caused, not by an effect on DNA replication or transcription, but rather by an effect on transport into the cell. That BrdUrd can indeed exert an effect on transport processes is supported by the studies of Tsuboi and Baserga (1973), who found BrdUrd to inhibit the transport of deoxyglucose and cycloleucine into 3T6 fibroblasts.

Clearly much of our understanding of the specific biological and physical consequences that result from incorporation of BrdUrd or IdUrd into DNA is derived not only from non-viral systems, but much of the information is contradictory. Thus there is a great void in our knowledge of what is the penultimate event responsible for the antiviral effect of IdUrd.

Furthermore one cannot make the assumption that what is applicable to one species of virus is applicable to other viruses.

It should be noted that the basis of the antiviral activity of IdUrd is not one of specific attack on a unique virus function such as adsorption to a receptor on the cell wall, transport into the cell, uncoating of the virus, being a substrate for or inhibiting a virus specified enzyme, incorporation uniquely into viral DNA, etc. Rather its antiviral activity is based on a quantitative difference in the amount of thymidine kinase activity present in the virus infected, compared with the adjacent uninfected, cell. Thus certain viruses set the stage for their own demise by producing a marked increase in thymidine kinase activity which results in preferential accumulation of phosphorylated IdUrd for subsequent lethal incorporation into viral DNA, as well as an effect on viral DNA synthesis. Those virus strains that do not encode for thymidine kinase are completely resistant to IdUrd when grown in a host cell which is also incapable of producing thymidine kinase.

9.3. VIRUS ENHANCEMENT AND INDUCTION

9.3.1. ENHANCEMENT OF VIRUS REPLICATION BY IdUrd

A curious phenomenon is the enhancement of virus replication when cells are pretreated with IdUrd even though many, but not all, of these viruses are inhibited if the analog is present during the infective cycle. Munyon et al. (1964) exposed mouse embryo cells to IdUrd (10 µg/ml) for as long as 69 hr before infection with polyoma virus, and then transferred the cells to medium free of the drug. They found infectious polyoma virus was formed in normal, or even greater than normal, amounts. This concentration of IdUrd inhibited irreversibly the replication of mouse embryo cells and resulted in enlarged cells which may have permitted the formation of increased amounts of virus, since Dunnebacke and Reaume (1958) found that the yield of polio virus particles is directly related to the size of the host cell.

More recently the enhancement of virus replication by pretreatment of cells with IdUrd prior to infection has been confirmed and extended to other viruses such as human and murine cytomegalovirus, human adenovirus 7, rubella, vesicular stomatitis, Sindbis, mouse encephalitis, vaccinia, SV40 and mouse mammary tumor virus (St. Jeor and Rapp, 1973a, b; Paul et al., 1974; Plummer and Goodheart, 1974; Fine et al., 1974; Green and Baron, 1975; Jerkofsky and Rapp, 1975; Staal and Rowe, 1975; Suarez et al., 1976; Speers and Lehman, 1976; Suarez et al., 1977, 1980); however, replication of parvovirus is inhibited by IdUrd pretreatment of cells (Salo and Mayor, 1979). Incorporation of IdUrd into the host cell DNA appears to be necessary for this phenomenon (Staal and Rowe, 1975; Suarez et al., 1976). However, the molecular mechanism involved is yet to be elucidated. This enhancement phenomenon is not unique to IdUrd since mitomycin C (Lavialle et al., 1977) as well as cyclophosphamide (Ginsberg et al., 1977) markedly augment the replication of viruses in cell culture. These latter findings are compatible with a DNA effect being responsible for this phenomenon, although other factors may also be critically involved. These studies may add greatly to our knowledge of host cell factors involved in the mediation of viral replication.

9.3.2. VIRUS INDUCTION

It is well established that certain RNA-viruses and DNA-viruses are oncogenic (Aaronson and Stephenson, 1976a, b; Rapp and Reed, 1977; Klein and Smith, 1977). Thus C-type RNA viruses may cause leukemia, lymphomas and sarcomas in a number of vertebrates, and B-type RNA viruses are associated with mammary carcinomas. Among the oncogenic DNA viruses may be included members of pox viruses, papovavirus (polyoma virus and SV40), adenovirus (type 12) and herpes virus (Lucke's virus, Marek's disease virus, guinea pig herpes virus, irradiated herpes simplex virus, etc.). BrdUrd and IdUrd, when present in an appropriate concentration early during infection, inhibit the formation of oncogenic RNA-and DNA-viruses in cell culture (references cited in Prusoff and Goz, 1975). Studies of tumor induction by viruses in animals indicate that IdUrd will suppress the development of adenovirus type 12-induced tumors (Huebner *et al.*, 1963), and IdUrd as well as IdCyd will suppress the development of polyoma virus-induced tumors in newborn hamsters (Fischer *et al.*, 1965a, b).

A concern expressed by some, relative to the use of nucleosides such as IdUrd as antiviral agents, is related to the remarkable finding by Lowy *et al.* (1971) that exposure of growing cultures of cells from embryos of the high leukemic mouse strain AKR to non-inhibitory amounts of BrdUrd or IdUrd induces the formation of murine leukemia virus in as many as 0.5 per cent of the cells. There was no evidence of viral particles, antigens or RNA-directed DNA polymerase (reverse transcriptase) in these cells prior to such treatment. Similarly Aaronson *et al.* (1971) found BrdUrd-induced C-type virus in several clonal lines of virus-free BALB/3T3 cells, Weber *et al.* (1978) type A particles in rat hepatoma cells, and Klement *et al.* (1971) induced a murine sarcoma virus in rat cells transformed by this virus. Hirsch and Black (1974) have reviewed the various factors involved in the activation of mammalian leukemia viruses, and Aaronson and Stephenson (1976a) have written a general review on mammalian type-C RNA-viruses. The information for expression of endogenous C-type viruses is present within the DNA of such virus negative cells, and in some cases is activated spontaneously but at a higher rate by either exposure to BrdUrd, IdUrd or inhibitors of protein synthesis. By use of this technique, C-type viruses have been found in a number of mammalian species including avian, mice, rat, hamster, cat, pig and guinea pig. A concern has been raised by Manly *et al.* (1978) which indicates that biochemical measurement of C-type particle release by particle-bound DNA polymerase activity may be erroneous, since most of these particles have a different density from C-type particles.

BrdUrd increased in many, but not all, cases the rate of formation of a DNA virus, the SV40 virus, in SV 40-transformed cells (Dubbs *et al.*, 1967). There are many other examples of viral induction by halogenated deoxyribonucleosides, for example: Hsiung (1972), Klement *et al.* (1972), Rowe *et al.* (1972), Stewart *et al.* (1972a, b), and Hampar *et al.* (1972), Gerber (1972), Glaser and Rapp (1971), Lazar *et al.* (1975), Suarez *et al.* (1977), Carreno and Esparza (1977), Dunn and Nazerian (1977), Lasneret *et al.* (1981).

Incorporation of BrdUrd or IdUrd into DNA appears to be required for virus induction (Gerber, 1972; Fogel, 1972, 1973; Teich *et al.*, 1973) since induction can be prevented by arabinosylcytosine, a potent inhibitor of DNA biosynthesis, and by thymidine, which would compete with these analogs for incorporation into DNA. The molecular basis for the induction of virus by these halogenated analogs is not clear. Some of the physical and biochemical consequences that result from incorporation of these halogenated analogs into DNA have been discussed above.

Krych and Pietrzykowska (1979) found induction of λ prophage by 5-bromouracil may depend upon the formation of single-strand breaks in DNA, and strains of bacteria that can efficiently repair such bromouracil-induced lesions may have a low rate of prophage induction. Pietrzykowska *et al.* (1975) reported previously that the repair process can influence the lethal effects of bromouracil incorporation into DNA. Similarly Rydberg (1977) involved the repair mechanism in the mutagenesis of *E. Coli* caused by incorporation of bromouracil in DNA. However, studies by Witkin and Parisi (1974) and Hutchinson and Stein (1977) do not support the involvement of a repair process. Grippo *et al.* (1981) have reported the presence of a DNA glycosylase in extracts of chick embryo nuclei which catalyzes the removal of bromouracil from DNA.

Among the many possible simplistic explanations is an alteration in the binding of a protein which may be critical for regulation of the transcription of the viral genome present in the host cell DNA. Thus, as previously mentioned, the presence of BrdUrd in DNA has been shown to have a very marked effect on the binding of a repressor protein (Lin and Riggs, 1972), an effect on transcription that is manifest in a decrease in specific enzymes with high turnover (Stellwagen and Tomkins, 1971b). Whether protein inhibitors which induce C-type virions also function to affect the availability of a hypothetical regulatory protein remains to be established. Wu *et al.* (1972) found cordycepin (3'-deoxyadenosine), an inhibitor of messenger RNA synthesis, prevented induction by IdUrd of RNA oncogenic viruses. Thus transcription may be a critical event in virus induction. Yoshikura (1974) found caffeine also inhibits the induction of endogenous C-type viruses. Caffeine is an inhibitor of phosphodiesterase and of DNA repair, but the relationship between these effects and the prevention of virus induction is not clear. Chattopadhyay *et al.* (1979) found treatment of AKR murine cells with IdUrd not only activates endogenous murine leukemia virus, but also augments transcription of unique DNA by 60 per cent. Whether a causal relationship exists remains to be seen.

A major concern in the use of IdUrd clinically is whether viruses, if induced by halogenated nucleosides during therapy in man, will prove to be oncogenic. The mutagenic capabilities of halogenated uracil derivatives are well documented. Litman and Pardee (1956) found 5-iodouracil, 5-bromouracil and 5-chlorouracil were incorporated into the DNA of bacteriophage T4 and also were potent mutagens. Many investigators have found BrdUrd to be mutagenic to mammalian cells in culture (Huberman and Heidelberger, 1972; Chu *et al.*, 1972; Davidson and Bick, 1973; Stark and Littlefield, 1974; Peterson *et al.*, 1975; Aebersold, 1976). The deoxyribonucleoside of 5-bromouracil, BrdUrd, is a more potent mutagen than the free base (Freese, 1959; Litman and Pardee, 1960) a finding presumably related to their relative rates of conversion into the pool of BrdUMP. However, although carcinogens are generally considered to be mutagenic, all mutagens are not carcinogenic. Manak *et al.* (1981) found HSV-2 substituted with BrdUrd (11 per cent) and exposed to near ultraviolet radiations were inactivated but were capable of neoplastic transformation of Syrian hamster embryo cells.

Jones *et al.* (1976) found neither IdUrd nor BrdUrd induced oncogenic transformation of a murine cell line in culture even though endogenous oncornaviruses are indeed induced in this cell line (Rapp *et al.*, 1975). Furthermore, these halogenated nucleosides neither altered significantly the appearance of lung adenomas in strain A mice (Poirier *et al.*, 1975), nor in newborn Swiss mice (Poirier *et al.*, cited in Jones *et al.*, 1976). Thus Jones *et al.* (1976) concluded 'not all mutagens produce oncogenic transformation, nor does lack of mutagenicity . . . exclude . . . that a given agent is oncogenic'. The virus induced in a cell that was previously virus-free is generally xenotropic, meaning that the virus does not propagate infectiously in the host species of origin as do ecotropic or some amphotropic C-type viruses. This may explain why IdUrd can induce endogenous type-C RNA-viruses without resulting generally in carcinogenesis. Thus if these induced viruses were transferred to a foreign host cell, the infection, replication, and transformation to oncogenicity could occur.

Veselý and Čihák (1973) gave IdUrd to a strain of mice that has a high incidence of spontaneous leukemia and found an early induction of leukemia. Whereas untreated mice were all alive for 120 days, the IdUrd-treated mice had developed leukemia within 50 days and 67 per cent died with lymphoma by day 60. Stephenson *et al.* (1974) and Greenberger *et al.* (1975) used IdUrd to induce C-type viruses in mouse embryo cells in culture and demonstrated that these viruses were oncogenic in that they induced specific neoplasms in newborn mice.

A recent study of Yoshikura *et al.* (1977) was designed to determine whether a direct relationship exists between carcinogenicity of certain polycyclic hydrocarbons and their ability to increase the induction frequency of virus in IdUrd-pretreated cells as determined by the XC plaque assay (Rowe *et al.*, 1970). Whereas IdUrd or BrdUrd are excellent producers of C-type viruses, the potent carcinogens are poor inducers (Lowy *et al.*, 1971; Weiss *et al.*, 1971; Teich *et al.*, 1973). Although the carcinogens alone did not activate the virus, even when pretreated with microsomal enzymes, the enzyme-treated polycyclic hydrocarbons caused a five—ten-fold increase in the induction frequency in the IdUrd-pretreated cells (Yoshikura *et al.*, 1977). However, there was no parallelism between such enhancement and *in vivo* carcinogenicity (Yoshikura *et al.*, 1977). The mechanism involved is not clear.

In an attempt to clarify the relationship between virus induction and neoplasia, Hirsch and Black (1974) offered the hypothesis that '. . . both virus induction and neoplasia induction may be secondary to loss of cellular control mechanisms . . .'. Thus these investigators consider the activation of virus or cell transformation to be by-products of such an event which may be caused by viruses, chemicals, immunological reactions or irradiations. Thus, for example, endogenous, C-type RNA-virus (oncornavirus) may be induced by herpes simplex virus types 1 and 2 (references cited by Flugel *et al.*, 1977) either by UV-irradiated HSV-1 and 2, by superinfection with HSV-2 or after transformation of certain murine cells in culture by HSV-1 and 2.

9.4. 5-IODO-2′-DEOXYCYTIDINE (IdCyd)

9.4.1. Synthesis, Metabolism and Anticancer Activity

A compound was sought with similar biological properties to IdUrd, but with a lower rate of catabolism, a greater stability to heat and a greater solubility than IdUrd. This was achieved when 5-iodo-2′-deoxycytidine was synthesized by Chang and Welch (1961) as part of an anticancer program. A novel procedure has been recently described by Kobayashi *et al.* (1980) for the synthesis of the triacetyl derivative of IdCyd that involves the iodination of 5′-0-triacetyl-2′-deoxycytidine with silver trifluoroacetate and iodine. Studies were conducted with the comparable bromo-analog, 5-bromo-2′-deoxycytidine (BrdCyd) (Cramer *et al.*, 1961; Kriss *et al.*, 1962a, 1963).

With the advent of IdCyd, studies in cell culture and animals were initiated by Cramer *et al.* (1972) and by Kriss *et al.* (1962b). Cramer *et al.* (1962) found IdCyd to be less effective than IdUrd as an antineoplastic agent. Kriss *et al.* (1962b) found IdCyd was more stable than IdUrd in the rat to metabolic degradation, the main products being IdUrd and Iodouracil. Studies of radioactive IdCyd in the mouse indicated similar uptake into DNA and a similar pattern of distribution compared to IdUrd (Kriss *et al.*, 1962b).

Clinical and pharmacological studies with IdCyd were performed in man by Calabresi *et al.* (1963) and by Kriss *et al.* (1963). The manifestations of toxicity produced by IdCyd and IdUrd at comparable doses were identical, and included stomatitis, hair loss and hematopoietic depression. About 85 to 95 per cent of an intravenously injected IdCyd was deaminated, with subsequent cleavage of the formed IdUrd to 5-iodouracil, and deiodination of the latter to iodide (Calabresi *et al.*, 1963). However, these was a great variation in the rate of catabolism. Kriss *et al.* (1963) made similar observations in man. However, the rate of degradation of both BrdCyd and IdCyd is slower in the rat than in man, which they attributed to the fact that human serum possesses a deaminase not present in rat serum.

Thus the use of IdCyd as an anticancer agent in man proved to be disappointing in spite of the correct predictions by Welch (1961) that it would circumvent many of the undesirable properties of IdUrd. Two factors are responsible: (1) the presence in man of a very active deaminase for which IdCyd is a good substrate and (2) the rather low affinity (high K_m) of IdCyd for deoxycytidine kinase. Thus an inadequate amount of IdCyd is converted into the monophosphate, 5-iodo-2′-deoxycytidylate, a compound which is not susceptible to deamination by deoxycytidine deaminase. 5-Iodo-2′-deoxycytidylate, once formed, is subsequently deaminated by the enzyme deoxycytidylate deaminase to 5-iodo-2′-deoxyuridylate and further phosphorylated to the triphosphate derivative which is the necessary precursor for incorporation into DNA (Fig. 9). However, it is just this property of being a poor substrate for deoxycytidine kinase present in cells not infected with herpes simplex virus which afforded the opportunity of its being a good antiviral agent, as will be discussed below.

9.4.2. Antiviral Activity

IdCyd and BrdCyd, like IdUrd, markedly inhibit the replication of herpes simplex virus in cell culture (Herrmann, 1961; Renis, 1970; Renis and Buthala, 1965) and BrdCyd inhibits the replication of human cytomegalovirus (Jerkofsky *et al.*, 1980). IdCyd is as effective as IdUrd

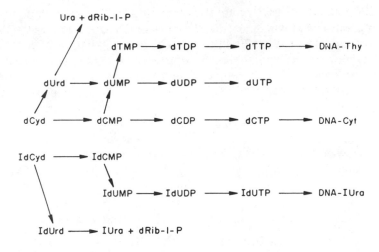

FIG. 9. Metabolic pathway of deoxycytidine and 5-iodo-2'-deoxycytidine.

in the therapy of experimental herpes keratitis in rabbits (Perkins *et al.*, 1962; Mendez *et al.*, 1971). Similarly Mendez and Martenet (1972) found IdCyd to be more effective than IdUrd in the therapy of deep stromal herpetic keratitis in the rabbit, based on clinical and histopathological evaluation. Furthermore, Martenet (1975) found IdCyd and 5-ethyl-2'-deoxyuridine to be equally effective in this condition. If applicable to man, the use of IdCyd would be of great importance since IdUrd is not efficacious in the therapy of deep herpetic keratitis. 5-Bromo-2'-deoxycytidine increased the survival rate of mice which had received an intracranial inoculation of herpes simplex virus type-1, provided that tetrahydrouridine, an inhibitor of deoxycytidine deaminase, was coadministered (Greer *et al.*, 1975). Again, if applicable to man, this would be of great value in therapy of herpes encephalitis, particularly since IdUrd is believed not to be efficacious.

A very important observation with significant clinical potential was made by Cooper (1973), who demonstrated that 5-bromodeoxycytidine is phosphorylated to 5-bromo-deoxycytidine-5'-phosphate (BrdCMP) in extracts of cells infected with herpes simplex virus, but not in extracts of uninfected cells. In uninfected cells BrdCyd is deaminated to BrdUrd, which is then phosphorylated to BrdUMP. The BrdCMP formed in the infected cells is deaminated to BrdUMP, phosphorylated to the diphosphate (BrdUDP) and subsequently to the triphosphate (BrdUTP). In the latter form it is a substrate for DNA polymerase and may be incorporated into DNA. Cooper (1973) suggested that advantage could be taken of the substrate specificity of BrdCyd for the virus-induced enzyme relative to the host-cell deoxycytidine kinase to allow selective chemotherapy of herpetic infections with BrdCyd or IdCyd. Thus BrdCyd and IdCyd were found to be poor substrates for the deoxycytidine kinase present in extracts of mouse and human lymphoid cells (Cooper and Greer, 1973b), and poor substrates for mammalian thymidine kinase (Bresnick and Thompson, 1965; Lee and Cheng, 1976). However, BrdCyd and IdCyd are twice as inhibitory as IdUrd of the phosphorylation of thymidine by mitochondrial pyrimidine deoxyribonucleoside kinase (Cheng, 1976; Lee and Cheng, 1976), and IdCyd is phosphorylated by this enzyme (Y. C. Cheng, personal communication). The K_m of mouse and of human cytosol deoxycytidine kinase for BrdCyd is about 200 times larger than the K_m for the normal substrate deoxycytidine. Once BrdCyd is phosphorylated to BrdCMP, it is a good substrate for deoxycytidylate deaminase (Maley, 1967). Thus, if IdCyd or BrdCyd were indeed not deaminated or phosphorylated in normal tissues, but were phosphorylated and then deaminated in the infected cells, then antiviral therapy would be achieved in the absence of toxicity.

The basis for the selective antiviral activity of IdCyd resides in the properties of the deoxycytidine kinase present in the herpes virus infected cell. It is well documented that infection of cells with herpes simplex virus results in the induction of a number of virally encoded enzymes including thymidine kinase (Kit and Dubbs, 1963; Klemperer *et al.*, 1967), deoxycytidine kinase (Hay *et al.*, 1970; Perera and Morrison, 1970) and DNA polymerase. Hay *et al.* (1970) provided evidence that a single protein was responsible for both thymidine and deoxycytidine kinase activities and that a single site may be involved (Jamieson and Subak-Sharpe, 1974; Leung *et al.*, 1975; Cheng, 1976). Thus this enzyme with dual activity has been termed a pyrimidine deoxyribonucleoside kinase. However, recent findings of Chen and Prusoff (1978) reveal that this enzyme also possesses deoxythymidylate kinase activity.

Dobersen *et al.* (1976) and Jerkofsky *et al.* (1977) have shown that the varicella zoster virus also induces an enzyme which, like that induced by herpes simplex virus, utilizes thymidine, deoxycytidine and 5-bromo-2'-deoxycytidine as good substrates (K_m for BrdCyd = 8.5 μM).

9.4.3. Effect of Tetrahydrouridine on Activity of BrdCyd

A major concern with the use of BrdCyd or IdCyd is that human tissues contain very potent cytidine deaminase activity (Camiener and Smith, 1965), which converts these analogs to BrdUrd and IdUrd respectively. Thus uninfected tissues would be exposed to the toxic effects of BrdUrd and IdUrd. An attempt to decrease toxicity by prevention of the deamination of BrdCyd or IdCyd takes advantage of the ability of tetrahydrouridine, a transition state analog (Cohen and Wolfenden, 1971), to inhibit the enzyme cytidine deaminase. Schildkraut *et al.* (1975) examined the toxicity of BrdCyd, IdCyd, BrdUrd and IdUrd in baby hamster kidney cells which do not have cytidine deaminase activity and showed that the halogenated deoxycytidine derivatives were significantly less toxic. All four analogs were equally toxic to HEp-2 cells which do contain high levels of cytidine deaminase; however, when tetrahydrouridine was included in the media, the halogenated deoxycytidine analogs were markedly less toxic.

Tetrahydrouridine is also active *in vivo* in the inhibition of cytidine deaminase in mice (Camiener, 1968; Neil *et al.*, 1970). Thus Cooper and Greer (1973a) decreased the utilization of BrdCyd for the biosynthesis of DNA by normal mouse tissues *in vivo* by the use of tetrahydrouridine, since it now could neither be deaminated to BrdUrd nor efficiently phosphorylated by cytosol deoxycytidine kinase; however, by prevention of the deamination process they increased the utilization of deoxycytidine for DNA biosynthesis. Tetrahydrouridine not only increased the efficacy of arabinosylcytosine (ara-C) as an antileukemic drug in mice (Neil *et al.*, 1970), but also the efficacy of BrdCyd in the therapy of experimental herpes encephalitis in mice (Greer *et al.*, 1975).

In order for tetrahydrouridine to be effective it must have a tissue distribution such that the infected cells maintain a concentration of at least 1 μg/g (Camiener, 1968; Chabner *et al.*, 1974; Wentworth and Wolfenden, 1975; El Dareer *et al.*, 1976). El Dareer *et al.*, (1976) prepared radioactive tetrahydrouridine and studied its distribution, metabolism and rate of excretion in various experimental animals who received an i.p. injection of 50 mg/kg. Within 3 hr the peak serum levels in mice (76 μg/ml) and rats (58 μg/ml) fell to less than 10 per cent of maximum with the kidneys of mice selectively accumulating the agent. Within 24 hr essentially all of the compound was excreted unchanged in the urine of mice, rats, dogs and monkeys. In mice 6 hr after injection, tissue levels of more than 1 μg/g tetrahydrouridine were present in kidney, liver, spleen, washed intestine and skeletal muscle. Tetrahydrouridine administered to dogs and rhesus monkeys is not toxic (Goldenthal *et al.*, 1974).

9.4.4. Use of IdCyd for Assay of Pyrimidinedeoxyribonucleoside Kinase Activity

Summers and Summers (1977) developed a simple, rapid, specific and very sensitive assay for herpes virus induced pyrimidine deoxyribonucleoside kinase which is based on the finding of Cooper (1973) that IdCyd is a substrate uniquely for the viral induced enzyme in the presence of tetrahydrouridine. As little as 0.0015 U of the viral induced enzyme can be detected which corresponds to about 10^{-4} of the normal *in vivo* level. Of concern, however, are the reports of Lee and Cheng (1976), and Cheng (1976), who found IdCyd not only interacted very effectively with human mitochondrial thymidine kinase, as well as HSV-1 and -2 induced enzyme, but also more importantly is a substrate for the mitochondrial thymidine kinase. In agreement with other investigators there is no interaction with human *cytosol* thymidine kinase. Therefore care should be exerted in using the phosphorylation of $[^{125}I]$-IdCyd as a specific test for the presence of herpes thymidine kinase, unless one excludes mitochondrial thymidine kinase activity as the responsible enzyme.

9.5. 5-IODO-5'-AMINO-2',5'-DIDEOXYURIDINE AND RELATED AMINO-DEOXYRIBONUCLEOSIDES

9.5.1. SYNTHESIS

Although 5-iodo-2'-deoxyuridine is a clinically effective antiviral nucleoside approved by the FDA for therapy of herpes simplex infection of the corneal epithelium in man, and is reported (Juel-Jensen and MacCallum, 1972), when a concentrated solution of IdUrd in dimethylsulfoxide is used, to be of value in therapy of other topical herpes virus infections, there is a need for agents for therapy of systemic virus infections. Many of the antiviral agents that are effective topically have limited value when used systemically. There are a number of reasons for this such as metabolic inactivation, problems of cell transport, teratogenicity, mutagenesis and general tissue toxicity. One is generally concerned about a drug which is either incorporated or interacts with cellular DNA. Thus the incorporation of 5-iodo-2'-deoxyuridine into the DNA of normal uninfected cells is most likely primarily responsible for the toxicity that has been found during either topical or systemic therapy. The antiviral nucleosides which are incorporated into DNA include 5-iodo-2'-deoxyuridine, 5-iodo-2'-deoxycytidine, 5-trifluoromethyl-2'-deoxyuridine, 5-ethyl-2'-deoxyuridine, 1-β-D-arabinofuranosylcytosine (ara-C), 9-β-D-arabinofuranosyladenine (ara-A), etc. Of course there is variation in the extent of toxicity produced by these antiviral agents, with ara-A being less toxic than IdUrd, and 5-ethyl-2'-deoxyuridine having the desirable feature of being non-mutagenic.

Our laboratory has been concerned with the synthesis of antiviral nucleosides which hopefully would have little or no toxicity to the host. Thus the design of a nucleoside that cannot be phosphorylated by normal uninfected cells would offer a significant therapeutic advantage. Langen and co-workers (1968, 1969, 1972) made a major conceptual contribution when they prepared analogs of thymidine that contained various halogens in the 5' position. These compounds are neither phosphorylated nor incorporated into DNA, but do preferentially inhibit thymidylate kinase. These findings formed the basis for our studies of the biological activity of nucleosides in which the 5'-hydroxyl moiety is replaced with an amino group. Baker *et al.* (1955) first indicated that amino sugar nucleosides possess biological activity in their report that the activity of puromycin against a mammary adenocarcinoma, and *Trypanosoma equiperdum* in mice, is due to the *in vivo* enzymic formation of N^6-dimethyl-3'-aminoadenosine.

The 3'-amino analog of thymidine (Fig. 10) was first synthesized by Horwitz *et al.* (1964) and by Miller and Fox (1964), and the 5'-amino analog of thymidine by Horwitz *et al.* (1962). However, their biological potential had not been extensively investigated. The 5'-amino analog of thymidine is a good competitive inhibitor of the phosphorylation of thymidine by Sarcoma-180 thymidine kinase (Neenan and Rohde, 1973; Cheng and Prusoff, 1974), and a modest inhibitor of thymidylate kinase (Cheng and Prusoff, 1973). The 3'-amino analog of thymidine is a modest inhibitor of Sarcoma-180 thymidine kinase (Cheng and Prusoff, 1974). The 3',5'-diamino-3',5'-dideoxythymidine was synthesized (Lin and Prusoff, 1978a) and its biological properties compared with that of the 3'- and the 5'-monoamino analogs of thymidine. Whereas the 3'-amino analog was markedly inhibitory to the replication of

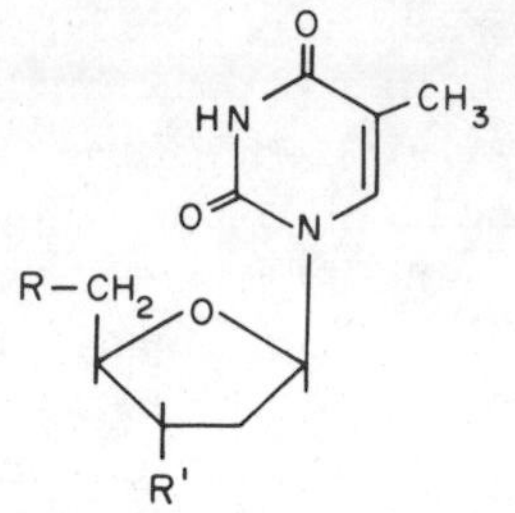

	R	R'
Thymidine	OH	OH
3'-amino-3'-deoxythymidine	OH	NH$_2$
5'-amino-5'-deoxythymidine	NH$_2$	OH
3',5'-diamino-3',5'-dideoxythymidine	NH$_2$	NH$_2$

Fig. 10. Structure of thymidine and several amino analogs of thymidine.

murine Sarcoma-180 and L1210 cells in cell culture, the 5'-amino and the 3',5'-diamino analogs of thymidine exerted little or no inhibition (Lin and Prusoff, 1978a).

Thus (1) the reports by Langen and Kowollik (1968) and (1969, 1972) referred to above; (2) the findings that the 5'-amino analog of thymidine is a potent inhibitor of thymidine kinase (Neenan and Rohde, 1973; Cheng and Prusoff, 1974), an enzyme with enhanced activity in many neoplastic and virus-infected cells, a modest inhibitor of thymidylate kinase, and yet was a poor inhibitor of mammalian cells; and (3) the finding that the 5'-amino analog of thymidine has significant antiviral activity (Lin *et al.*, 1976b), stimulated our interest in the antiviral potential of amino analogs in general.

The 3'-amino analog of thymidine is significantly less inhibitory than the 5'-amino analog of thymidine of the replication of herpes simplex virus *in vitro*, and the 3',5'-diamino analog of thymidine has no antiherpes virus activity at the concentrations evaluated (Lin and Prusoff, 1978a). The presence of an amino moiety in the 3'-position of thymidine decreases the antiviral activity relative to the 5'-amino analog, and the presence of an amino moiety in the 5'-position of the 3'-amino analog of thymidine abolishes its antineoplastic activity as well as its antiviral activity. Thus the 3',5'-diamino analog of thymidine appears to have acquired the undesirable qualities of both the 3'-amino- and the 5'-amino analogs of thymidine.

Based on the finding that the 5'-amino analog of thymidine has good antiviral activity, and 5-iodo-2'-deoxyuridine a potent antiviral agent, but poorly soluble and highly toxic, the 5'-amino analog of IdUrd was prepared. The hope was that, by substituting the 5'-hydroxy group of IdUrd with an amino moiety, not only would the solubility be increased by virtue of enhancement of polarity, but also, like Langen's compounds, such a structural modification would exert its biological activity, if any, without being incorporated into DNA.

The 5'-amino analog of 5-iodo-2'-deoxyuridine [5-iodo-5'-amino-2',5'-dideoxyuridine (AIU, AIdUrd)] was synthesized initially (Lin *et al.*, 1976b) by halogenation of the 5-mercuriacetate (Dale *et al.*, 1975) of 5'-amino-2',5'-dideoxyuridine, and later (Lin and Prusoff, 1978b) by reduction of the 5'-azido analog of 5-iodo-2'-deoxyuridine using the triphenylphosphine procedure (Mungall *et al.*, 1975) (Fig. 11). The latter procedure afforded the preparation of large amounts of the desired compound. Although the azido moiety is readily reduced by hydrogenation (Stout *et al.*, 1969), when applied to 5-iodo-5'-azido-2',5'-dideoxyuridine, the iodine in the 5-position of the pyrimidine moiety is also reduced with the formation of 5'-amino-2',5'-dideoxyuridine, whereas direct iodination of 2'-deoxyuridine occurs readily in the presence of aqueous nitric acid (Prusoff, 1959a), the presence of an amino group in the 5'-position prevents iodination by the more common iodination

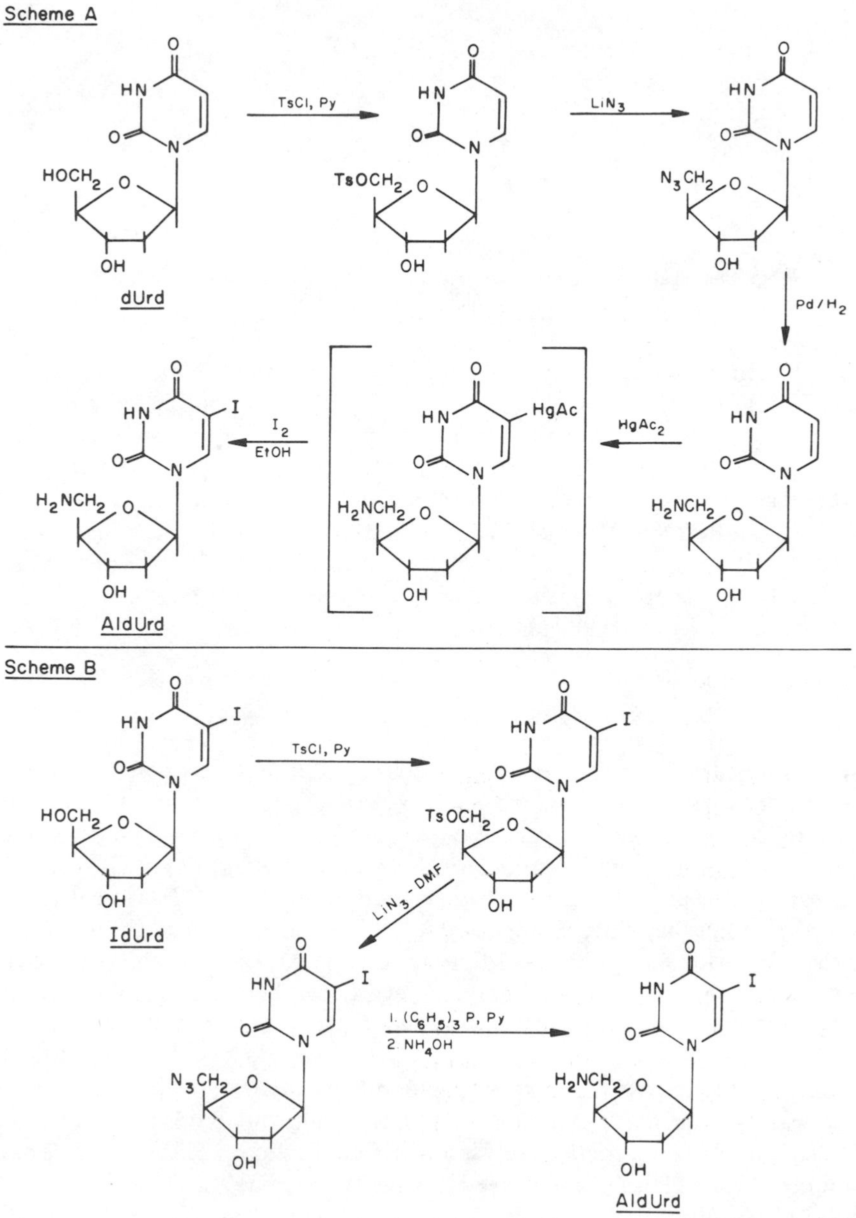

Scheme A

Scheme B

FIG. 11. Two procedures for the synthesis of 5-iodo-5'-amino-2',5'-deoxyuridine, Scheme A. Method of Lin *et al.* (1976b); Scheme B. Method of Lin and Prusoff (1978).

procedures (references cited in Prusoff and Goz, 1975). The amino group in the 5'-position may interact with the pyrimidine moiety, presumably at the 6-position, thereby decreasing the electron density on C5 (Fig. 12). Bradshaw and Hutchinson (1977) have discussed several mechanisms that may be involved in halogenation of pyrimidine nucleosides.

The structure and conformation of AIdUrd, both in the crystal as well as in solution, were examined by Birnbaum *et al.* (1979). The three-dimensional structure of 5-iodo-5'-amino-2',5'-dideoxyuridine, a potent inhibition of herpes simplex virus, was determined by x-ray crystallography. The crystals belong to the orthorhombic space group $P2_12_12_1$ and the cell dimensions are $a = 7.892(1)$, $b = 9.332(1)$, and $c = 15.749(2)$ A°. Intensity data were measured with a diffractometer and the structure was solved by the heavy-atom method. Least-squares refinement, which included hydrogen atoms, converged at $R = 0.047$. The structure is zwitterionic, with a protonated 5'-NH_2 group and a negative charge on N(3) in

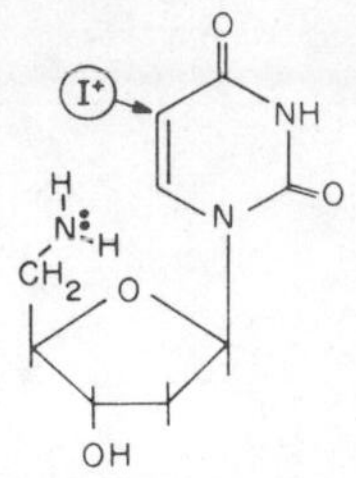

Fig. 12. Hypothetical attack by a positively charged iodine atom on the C-5 position of 5′-amino-2′,5′-dideoxyuridine.

the pyrimidine ring. The glycosyl bond is in the anticonformation (CN = 53.6°) and the exocyclic-$CH_2NH_3^+$ group is *gauche–trans*. The deoxyribose ring has the unusual $0(1')$ endo pucker. ^1H NMR spectroscopy was used to determine the conformation in solution. The spectra indicate an anticonformation about the glycosyl bond and equal contributions of the three staggered side-chain rotamers. The sugar ring may consist of a 36:64 equilibrium mixture of ^3E and ^2E conformers. It is pointed out, however, that the conventional interpretation may be inadequate, and that there may be a significant contribution of an $0(1')$ endo puckered ring. The relationship between the unusual structure of AIdUrd and its biological activity is yet to be elucidated.

9.5.2. ANTIVIRAL ACTIVITY

The initial studies by Cheng *et al.* (1975a, b) found AIdUrd to be a potent inhibitor of the replication of herpes simplex virus type 1 in Vero cells, a 400 μM concentration producing about a 3.5 log decrease in the number of plaque-forming units by the yield reduction assay. On a molar basis this analog is less potent than IdUrd, 5-trifluoromethyl-2′-deoxyuridine (F_3dThd), or ara-C but it possesses greater activity than ara-A. Of critical importance, however, is the finding that AIdUrd appeared totally devoid of cytotoxicity in sharp contrast to the extensive toxicity produced by IdUrd, F_3dThd and ara-C at comparable antiviral concentrations. Even ara-A, which is generally regarded as having a high therapeutic index, exerted significant toxicity at concentrations that produced less antiviral activity than AIdUrd.

A high degree of selectivity has now been achieved in experimental viral chemotherapy in both *in vitro* and *in vivo* models. A number of new agents, in addition to AIdUrd and 5′-amino-5′-deoxythymidine, can effectively inhibit the replication of HSV with little or no host cell toxicity, for example, 9-(2-hydroxyethoxymethyl)guanine, (acyclovir, ACV); E-5-(2-halovinyl)-2′-deoxyuridine (BrVdUrd, IVdUrd); arabinofuranosylthymine (ara-T); 1-(2-deoxy-2-fluoro-β-D-arabinosyl)-5-iodocytosine (FIAC), 5-propyl-2′-deoxyuridine; 5-methoxymethyl-2′-deoxyuridine and phosphonoformate (PFA). The basis for the high selectivity of these 'new generation' drugs is that their interactions with critical virally encoded enzymes are highly specific or preferential. They may have little or no interaction with the corresponding host-cell enzymes. In some cases, as with AIdUrd, the differences are essentially absolute and the activating reaction is catalyzed only by the virus enzyme (Chen and Prusoff, 1978). Thus, an important change in antiviral chemotherapy is that selectivity can now be based on qualitative as well as quantitative exploitation of viral associated enzymic activities.

Kit (1979), in an excellent review, discussed in detail the many enzymes which are known to be viral encoded. Certain viral-induced enzymes catalyze reactions which are unique to the virus-infected cell and are also necessary for viral replication and hence make excellent targets for selective viral chemotherapy: RNA transcriptase, RNA replicase, reverse transcriptase.

Another group of viral-induced enzymes catalyze reactions that normally occur in uninfected cells. Often these enzymes are sufficiently different from their host-cell counterparts that selective intervention may be possible – for example, HSV-induced thymidine kinase has proven susceptible to chemotherapeutic exploitation. The HSV-encoded DNA polymerase is also in this group of enzymes, and the selective antiherpes action of phosphonoformate is mediated through preferential inhibition of the viral polymerase (Mao and Robishaw, 1975). The high degree of selectivity of the unusual purine analog, acyclovir (acycloguanosine; ACG), also results from a preferential phosphorylation by the HSV-thymidine kinase followed subsequently after conversion to the triphosphate derivative to preferential interference of the HSV–DNA polymerase and/or incorporation into HSV–DNA as a chain terminator. Deoxycytidine deaminase, ribonucleoside diphosphate reductase and DNase activities as well as a recently described protein kinase (Blue and Stobbs, 1981) associated with HSV-infection provide other possible sites of intervention.

Variation has been found in the sensitivity of different strains of herpes simplex virus to IdUrd from two-fold to as much as 100-fold (de Lavergne *et al.*, 1965; Person *et al.*, 1970; Lowry *et al.*, 1971; Lerner and Bailey, 1972; Fiala *et al.*, 1974; Marks, 1974; Collins and Bauer, 1977). Similarly marked variation in sensitivity to AIdUrd and AIdCyd by fresh clinical isolates of HSV-1 and HSV-2 has been observed. The method of assay (plaque reduction or yield reduction) is also a major variable in the response of prototype HSV virus to these and other agents. Such variation in sensitivity to a drug has been attributed to the cell culture used, the virus strain, the passage history of the virus strains, size of inoculum, pH of media, composition of media, and method of assay. Collins and Bauer (1977) evaluated three *in vitro* methods (plaque inhibition, plaque reduction and yield reduction) for assay of the antiviral activity of IdUrd and several other compounds. They reported that the plaque inhibition method was *not* reliable, although convenient and rapid. Although the plaque reduction and the yield reduction methods were equally satisfactory, the plaque reduction method was claimed to be the most reliable method for *in vitro* assay of herpes virus. They found the plaque reduction method to be more sensitive for IdUrd; however, this method was either equally or less sensitive to ara-A than the yield reduction assay.

AIdUrd ($400\,\mu$M) was not cytotoxic to seventeen different cell lines in culture (Prusoff *et al.*, 1977), including murine, human and avian cells. At this concentration ($400\,\mu$M), or even at a considerably lower concentration, IdUrd, F_3dThd, ara-C and Ara-A are toxic. As indicated in the section devoted to 5-iodo-2′-deoxycytidine, this compound is quite toxic to those cells which have a deaminase and for which no precaution has been taken to inhibit deamination with an agent such as tetrahydrouridine.

Our laboratory in collaboration with Dr. Wilmer Summers have investigated the effect of AIdUrd on herpes simplex virus-transformed murine LMTK⁻ cells, as well as on the parental non-transformed strain, and have found that the virus-transformed cells, in contrast to the parental strain, are markedly sensitive to inhibition by this analog. Whereas the transformed cell lines in regular media were almost completely inhibited by 0.02–0.05 mM AIdUrd, the parental strain required concentrations of AIdUrd above 1 mM to produce significant inhibition. The molecular basis for the latter finding is based on the presence of the HSV-thymidine kinase genome in the HSV-transformed cell which, as discussed above, allows the formation of the virus-encoded enzyme required for phosphorylation of AIdUrd.

A very important finding relative to the potential use of AIdUrd in man was made by Capizzi (unpublished experiment) who found, under conditions in which 5-iodo-2′-deoxyuridine exerted a strong mutagenic effect on L5178Y cells in culture, that AIdUrd was totally devoid of such activity. The basis for the lack of mutagenicity for L5178Y cells (Capizzi and Prusoff, unpublished), the absence of cytotoxicity for the various cell lines evaluated (Prusoff *et al.*, 1977), as well as the marked cytotoxicity to the herpes simplex virus transformed, and the relative lack of toxicity to the parental cell line is related to the requirement of the herpes simplex virus-induced thymidine kinase for activation (phosphorylation) of AIdUrd. This is discussed in more detail below.

The immunosuppressive potential of AIdUrd and of 5′-amino-5′-deoxythymidine have been evaluated (Kan-Mitchell *et al.*, 1980; Bennett *et al.*, 1982) AIdUrd was found by Kan-Mitchell *et al.* (1980) to be a very mild immunosuppressive agent against either humoral or cell-mediated immunity, as compared to either IdUrd or ara-C. The inhibition produced by AIdUrd at the maximum feasible dose of 2 g/kg was significantly less than that observed with ara-C at 0.04 g/kg or that of IdUrd at 0.1 g/kg. Immunological function was analyzed by Bennett *et al.* (1982) in mice that received daily inoculations of 5'-amino-5'-deoxythymidine (1000 mg/kg/day, i.p.) or 5-iodo-2'-deoxyuridine (100 mg/kg/day, i.p.) following antigenic stimulation. 5'-Amino-5-'deoxythymidine did not suppress the development of: (1) delayed type hypersensitivity response to sheep red blood cells, (2) cell-mediated cytotoxicity response to allogeneic tumor cells, and (3) IgM and IgG antibody response to sheep red blood cells. In contrast 5-iodo-2'-deoxyuridine suppressed the development of all of these responses.

Toxicity studies of AIdUrd relative to IdUrd were performed in newborn and 8-day-old suckling mice and no detrimental effect on growth of tissues was produced by AIdUrd when administered intraperitoneally at doses up to 450 mg/kg for 5 days, with examination 20 days later (Albert *et al.*, 1979). In contrast, IdUrd significantly arrested neonatal growth when given at 125 and 250 mg/kg. Histopathological analysis of these teratological studies show no ocular, systemic neurological or renal abnormalities in the newborn mice treated with high doses of AIdUrd. However, cataracts, retinal dysplasia, cerebellar lesions, cortical lesions and general retardation of organ development were observed in the IdUrd-treated animals.

The apparent lack of toxicity both *in vitro* and *in vivo* encouraged an examination of the therapeutic effect of AIdUrd on experimental herpetic keratitis in rabbits (Albert *et al.*, 1976). Virus infections were established bilaterally in 40 animals using herpes simplex, type 1 (NIH strain 11124). Twenty-four hours after infection the rabbits were divided into five matched groups of eight and each group was treated, double blind, with topical drugs at 4-hr intervals for a total of 72 hr. The solutions instilled were: (1) saline; (2) IdUrd, 1 mg/ml; (3) AIdUrd, 1 mg/ml; (4) AIdUrd, 4 mg/ml; and (5) AIdUrd, 8 mg/ml. Each eye was examined daily for 12 days and graded independently by two ophthalmologists. Although IdUrd and AIdUrd (8 mg/ml) were effective therapeutically, IdUrd had a greater effect. A second similar but independent experiment gave essentially identical results.

Although AIdUrd is more soluble than 5-iodo-2'-deoxyuridine, its solubility at neutral pH is nevertheless limited to about 20 mg/ml. For this reason the efficacy of ointment preparations of IdUrd (0.5 per cent) and AIdUrd (10 and 30 per cent) against herpetic keratitis in rabbits were evaluated (Puliafito *et al.*, 1977). In agreement with earlier studies (Albert *et al.*, 1976) with aqueous preparations of these compounds, both ointment preparations of AIdUrd and of IdUrd (positive control) were found to be significantly effective therapeutically. Of particular importance is the finding that the ointment preparations of AIdUrd and IdUrd were *not* significantly different in their efficacy from each other.

The therapeutic efficacy of AIdUrd and acyclovir on oral infection in the mouse with HSV-2 was studied by Park *et al.* (1980). The earlier the treatment with these two drugs was initiated after infection, the better was the chemotherapeutic effect. A delay of 48 and 72 hr after infection showed no chemotherapeutic efficacy with AIdUrd and acyclovir respectively. Acyclovir was superior to AIdUrd as a topical agent for therapy of HSV-2.

Park *et al.* (1982) developed a novel oral model in mice for evaluation of drugs against HSV-1 infections. Early topical or systemic treatment with AIdUrd notably reduced the development of clinical lesions and the virus content in the inoculated lips; however, the establishment of latency was not prevented.

The corresponding analog of thymidine, 5'-amino-5'-deoxythymidine (5'-AdThd) is considerably more soluble than AIdUrd and like AIdUrd is specifically activated by HSV-thymidine kinase. Pavan-Langston *et al.* (1982) found 10 and 15 per cent AdThd eye drops were significantly better than placebo in therapy of herpetic keratouveitis in rabbits, and the slope of the therapeutic curve of 15 per cent AdThd was similar to that of IdUrd. Systemic administration of these drugs in the neonatal mouse model revealed no adverse effect *in vivo* or by histopathologic examination in AdThd or saline-treated animals but IdUrd was extremely toxic and teratogenic.

Sim *et al.* (1981) administered AIdUrd to HSV-1 infected mice at a dose of 1000 mg/kg for 5 days with no apparent toxicity or efficacy. However, higher doses were toxic. Of critical importance are our findings that AIdUrd was effective in the therapy of HSV-1 infection of the rabbit eye, whether given in aqueous or ointment preparation, and also that this occurred in the absence of any toxicity.

The next obvious question which is being approached is whether the efficacy of AIdUrd can be extended to other topical herpes simplex infections, and of even greater importance, whether systemic virus infections are susceptible to therapy with this agent. Before evaluation of an antiviral agent, or for that matter any drug, the pharmacokinetic properties should be determined. Such considerations are important for proper administration of an agent systemically.

Several of the more recently developed compounds such as acyclovir, BrVdUrd or FIAC are more potent and more effective antiviral agents. What the role is of AIdUrd or 5′-AdThd as antiviral agents, when used either alone or in combination with other drugs, is under active investigation.

Elucidation of the sites of inhibition, as well as its mechanism of action, is a major effort in our laboratories. Germane to such studies is the finding of selectivity in antiviral activity. Of the various DNA viruses examined (herpes simplex type 1, herpes simplex type 2, guinea pig herpes-like virus, guinea pig cytomegalovirus, human cytomegalovirus, vaccinia, SV40, adeno type 2, minute virus of mice) only type 1 and, to a lesser extent, type 2 strains of herpes simplex virus and guinea pig herpes-like virus are inhibited significantly (Prusoff *et al.*, 1977). More recently Iltis *et al.* (1979) evaluated the antiviral effect of AIdUrd against three isolates of varicella-zoster virus, and found that concentrations of 10 to 800 μM reduced the number of plaques produced by VZV-infected cells and cell-free VZV from approximately 30 to 95 per cent. Drug concentrations as high as 800 μM were not toxic to host cells (human diploid embryo fibroblast). Henderson *et al.* (1979) found AIdUrd to be a very potent inhibitor of the Epstein–Barr virus in cell culture. Among the RNA viruses AIdUrd also exhibits a high degree of selectivity, with murine leukemia viruses being sensitive to inhibition by AIdUrd, whereas Rous sarcoma virus, polio, sendai, influenza A, and measles viruses are resistant (Prusoff *et al.*, 1977).

9.5.3. Metabolism and Biochemical Effects

Thus the selectivity in antiviral action, the lack of mutagenicity in a mammalian cell line that is very susceptible to IdUrd induced mutagenicity, and the little or no host-cell toxicity support a virus-specific site of inhibition. The effect of AIdUrd on gross RNA, DNA and protein biosynthesis in herpes simplex virus-type 1 infected and uninfected Vero cells was investigated and no inhibition of incorporation of radioactive uridine into RNA, or of radioactive amino acids into protein, was found. However, there was significant inhibition of the incorporation into the DNA of ^{14}C-thymidine of infected cells. Upon infection of Vero cells with HSV-1 there is a significant increase in the pool size of all four nucleotides (dTTP, dCTP, dGTP, dATP), with a very marked increase in that of dTTP. When AIdUrd was included in the media during infection there was an additional very marked increase in the pool size of dCTP, dGTP and dATP. However, although there was a decrease in that of dTTP, the pool size of dTTP was still markedly greater than that of the mock infected control. The specific decrease in the pool size of dTTP may be a consequence of a decrease in the phosphorylation of dTMP or of dTDP, whether derived via the *de novo* or salvage pathways, by a phosphorylated derivative of AIdUrd which is functioning as an alternate substrate. The alternate substrate hypothesis is supported by the finding of the triphosphate derivative of AIdUrd in the infected cell. The marked increase in the pools of dATP, dGTP, dCTP and what may be a combination of dTTP plus the triphosphate of AIdUrd (AIdUTP) is compatible with the observed effect on the DNA biosynthetic pathway. Recently Otto *et al.* (1982) examined the effect of IdUrd, AIdUrd and 5-AdThd on the expression of HSV-1-induced proteins. Exposure of HSV-1-infected Vero cells to the nucleoside analogues 5-iodo-

5'-amino-2',5'-dideoxyuridine (AIdUrd), 5-iodo-2'-deoxyuridine (IdUrd) or 5'-amino-2',5'-dideoxythymidine (5'-AdThd) resulted in altered expression of HSV-1-induced proteins. Infected cell proteins (ICPs) synthesized in the presence of the nucleoside analogs were compared, by SDS polyacrylamide gel electrophoresis to ICPs from non-drug-treated cells and it was found that there was no effect on HSV-1-induced α proteins but β and γ proteins were reduced as much as 60 per cent. There were three exceptions; ICP 35 (MW 46K) and ICP 39 (MW 36K) were not reduced and ICP 36 (MW 42K) was increased during drug treatment. Progeny virions were isolated from drug-treated infected Vero cells and were compared to progeny isolated from control cells with respect to their polypeptide make-up and for their ability to induce HSV-1 proteins in non-drug-treated Vero cells. The progeny virus from drug-treated cells exhibited altered protein patterns on SDS-polyacrylamide gels with respect to control HSV-1. The progeny virions from AIdUrd or IdUrd but not from 5'-AdThd-treated cells were defective in their abilities to induce proteins upon subsequent infection of non-drug-treated Vero cells. Two new phosphoproteins were detected; one with an apparent molecular weight of 30 K was induced by progeny virus from AIdUrd-treated cells and another at approximately 69 K was induced by progeny virus from 5'-AdThd-treated cells.

The metabolism of AIdUrd was investigated by Chen *et al.* (1976b). 5-[^{125}I]Iodo-5'-amino-2',5'-dideoxyuridine, prepared by the procedure of Lin *et al.* (1976b), was incubated with various uninfected murine, simian, or human cells for up to 24 hr and essentially none of the nucleoside became cell associated. In contrast, upon infection of Vero cells with HSV-1, significant radiolabel was detected both in nucleotide pools and in DNA. The major acid-soluble metabolite was shown by enzyme and chromatographic analysis to be the triphosphate of AIdUrd. AIdUTP was synthesized (Chen *et al.*, 1976c) for comparison with the metabolically formed nucleoside triphosphate by a modification of the procedure of Letsinger *et al.* (1972). Neither iodide, iodouracil nor 5-iodo-2'-deoxyuridine were detected, and hence are not involved in the metabolism of AIdUrd under the incubation conditions used.

The DNA from HSV-1-infected Vero cells labelled with [^{125}I]AIdUrd was isolated by buoyant density centrifugation in CsCl, and subjected to digestion by pancreatic DNase I, spleen DNase II, micrococcal nuclease, spleen and venom phosphodiesterase, and alkaline phosphatase (Chen *et al.*, 1976a). AIdUrd is incorporated into both the host and viral DNA of the infected cells, and analysis of the digestion products clearly indicated that AIdUrd is incorporated internally into the DNA structure.

If incorporation of AIdUrd had been restricted to the 3'-terminus of the growing DNA chain, free AIdUrd should have been detected, (a) after acid hydrolysis of intact AIdUrd-labeled DNA since a phosphoramidate (P–N) bond is extremely acid labile, or (b) under acidic chromatographic conditions used to analyze the DNase II digestion products. Furthermore the 3'-OH group of AIdUrd was shown to be involved in a standard phosphodiester linkage since only after digestion of the DNase-treated AIdUrd-DNA with venom phosphodiesterase was free AIdUrd released.

The isolated AIdUrd-DNA exhibited a CsCl profile with a rather high background of ^{125}I throughout the gradient which was attributed to the lability of the phosphoramidate bond, causing extensive fragmentation during isolation and purification (Chen *et al.*, 1976a).

Fischer and coworkers (1979, 1980) investigated the relationship between the incorporation of AIdUrd and IdUrd into HSV-1 DNA, the effect on DNA structure and their antiviral activity. Isopycnic centrifugation in CsCl gradients was used to quantify the incorporation of 5-iodo-5'-amino-2',5'-dideoxyuridine and 5-iodo-2'-deoxyuridine into herpes simplex virus type I DNA. A parallelism between the degree of incorporation into viral DNA and the inhibition of herpes simplex virus type I replication was found for both thymidine analogs. A concentration of 5-iodo-5'-amino-2',5'-dideoxyuridine approximately 100 times greater than 5-iodo-2'-deoxyuridine was required to achieve similar levels of antiviral activity. However, the inhibitory effects of these compounds are similar when compared with respect to the per cent of substitution for thymidine in herpes simplex virus type I DNA. Damage to the viral DNA, as indicated by the presence of single- or double-stranded breaks was assessed by centrifugation in alkaline and neutral sucrose gradients. The incorporation of 5-iodo-5'-amino-2',5'-dideoxyuridine into herpes simplex virus type I DNA produced single and to a lesser extent, double-stranded breaks in a dose-dependent manner. 5-Iodo-2'-deoxyuridine did not, however, induce DNA breakage. These data indicate that the additional presence of a phosphoramidate bond in the DNA produced the extensive damage detected under these conditions, but that such damage is not required for antiviral activity. Even though the pH during isolation and purification of the AIdUrd-DNA was carefully maintained above neutrality to minimize cleavage of the phosphoramidate linkage in the DNA, there was some broadening of the DNA peak suggestive of DNA fragmentation. However, the extensive fragmentation found previously (Chen et al., 1976a) had been prevented. Under investigation are the chemical, physical and biological consequences of incorporation of AIdUrd into virus DNA.

A very important question that is basic to the unique antiviral effect of AIdUrd is why this compound is anabolized only in the herpes simplex virus-infected cell. Since the intracellular formation of AIdUTP, as well as its incorporation into DNA, has been clearly demonstrated (Chen et al., 1976a), it is logical to assume that AIdUrd had been phosphorylated to the mono- and diphosphate derivative before conversion to AIdUTP and subsequent incorporation into DNA.

It is well documented that infection of a cell with HSV-1 results in an increase in thymidine kinase and DNA polymerase activities. These virus-induced enzymes possess properties which distinguish them from the comparable enzymes present in uninfected host cells. Chen and Prusoff (1978) isolated HSV-1 induced thymidine kinase from infected murine LMTK$^-$ cells and purified the enzyme by the procedure of Cheng and Ostrander (1976) which involves an affinity column containing p-amino-phenylthymidine-3'-phosphate linked to CH-sepharose. A protein was isolated which has thymidylate kinase activity in addition to thymidine kinase and deoxycytidine kinase activities. The purified enzyme has a molecular weight of 85,000 daltons. The K_m for thymidine is 0.8 μM and for thymidylate 25 μM; the ratio of V_m for thymidylate kinase to thymidine kinase is 1.7. These two activities can not be separated by affinity column chromatography, glycerol density gradient centrifugation or isoelectric focusing. In contrast, the thymidine kinase derived from the uninfected host does *not* exhibit thymidylate kinase activity.

Kinetic studies of this enzyme were performed by Chen et al. (1979b). Chen and Prusoff (1979) investigated the phosphorylation of AIdUrd, and Chen et al. (1980) that of 5'-amino-5'-deoxythymidine, because of the inability to detect the monophosphoramidate when these compounds were incubated with whole cells. Herpes simplex virus type 1 (HSV-1) encoded thymidine kinase converts 5-iodo-5'-amino-2',5'-dideoxyuridine (AIdUrd), a highly specific anti-herpes agent, into the 5'-diphosphate (AIdUDP) derivative *in vitro*. AIdUDP was identified by its acid lability, sensitivity to alkaline phosphatase hydrolysis, chromatographic behavior, and ratio of double isotope (^{125}I, ^{32}P) labeling. ATP, but not AMP, is a phosphate donor, and the direct transfer of the β and γ phosphate of ATP as pyrophosphate to AIdUrd was ruled out. The presence of a phosphoramidate bond was supported by the acid lability of AIdUDP which has a half-life of ($t_{1/2}$) of 320 min at pH 3.0. At neutral pH, the hydrolysis products are AIdUrd and orthophosphate, with AIdUrd monophosphate being the probable hydrolytic intermediate at these pH values. However, at acidic pH, some pyrophosphate was detected in addition to AIdUrd and orthophosphate. AIdUrd competitively inhibited the phosphorylation of thymidine and deoxycytidine. *Escherichia coli* thymidine kinase, even though 100-fold higher in activity, was unable to phosphorylate AIdUrd under similar conditions.

Similarly the monophosphoramidate derivative of 5'-AdThd was not detected as a reaction product when radioactive 5'-AdThd was incubated with purified HSV-1 encoded pyrimidine deoxyribonucleoside kinase, but only the diphosphoramidate derivative (Chen et al., 1980). A purified mixture of non-viral kinase and thymidylate kinase derived from uninfected Vero cells was unable to phosphorylate 5'-AdThd. The rate of hydrolysis of 5'-AdThd diphosphate increased as the pH of the reaction mixture decreased, with a shoulder region appearing between pH 3 and 5. The rate of hydrolysis was markedly increased below pH 3. 5′-AdThd, but not the monophosphate derivative, was detected in the hydrolysis mixture. The hydrolysis of 5′-AdThd diphosphate below pH 3 also yielded some thymine in addition to 5′-AdThd.

Chen *et al.* (1979a) characterized the pyrimidine deoxyribonucleoside kinase present in cells transformed by HSV-1 as a multifunctional enzyme capable of phosphorylating thymidine and thymidylate. Pyrimidine deoxyribonucleoside kinase (thymidine kinase [TK]) was purified from two herpes simplex virus type 1 (HSV-1)-transformed TK-deficient mouse (LMTK⁻) cell lines and from LMTK⁻ cells infected with HSV-1 mutant viruses coding for variant TK enzymes. These preparations exhibited normal or variant virus-induced thymidylate kinase activities correlating with their relative TK activities. Neither virus-induced activity was detected in LMTK⁻ cells infected with an HSV-1 TK-deficient mutant. These results suggest that HSV-1 thymidylate kinase activity and TK activity are mediated by the same protein.

Thus the herpes simplex virus-induced enzyme may be characterized as a multifunctional protein (Cooper, 1973; Chen *et al.*, 1979) rather than a complex of three different polypeptides which can not be separated (Kirschner and Bisswanger, 1976). An advantage attributed to such a multifunctional protein is the increased efficiency of anabolism which results from having the product of the initial enzymic reaction in optimal juxtaposition for use as a substrate for the second reaction:

Reaction 1 thymidine ⟶ thymidine monophosphate
Reaction 2 thymidine monophosphate ⟶ thymidine diphosphate.

Although the monophosphate of AIdUrd is not found as a product of the reaction but rather that of the diphosphate of AIdUrd, this may be due to the instability of the monophosphate of AIdUrd, since similar incubation with thymidine does result in formation of thymidine monophosphate in the medium in addition to thymidine diphosphate.

Thus it has been demonstrated that AIdUrd and 5′-amino-5′-deoxythymidine are potentially clinically useful drugs. Although AIdUrd is less potent than the parent compound 5-iodo-2′-deoxyuridine, it, like 5′-AdThd, has the property of having little or no toxicity to cells in culture or to animals. This unique state of affairs is due directly to the requirement that activation of the drug is dependent on phosphorylation by the herpes simplex virus-induced thymidine kinase. Once phosphorylated, it can then be further phosphorylated and subsequently incorporated into viral as well as host cell DNA. Incorporation of this analog into the DNA of uninfected cells does *not* occur because AIdUrd is not a substrate for the thymidine kinase present in uninfected cells. This requirement for a viral specified enzyme for activation therefore prevents normal cells from utilizing AIdUrd or 5′-AdThd, hence the remarkable lack of toxicity of AIdUrd and 5′-AdThd for uninfected cells and animals (Fig. 13).

Based on the findings by Cheng and Prusoff (1974) that 5′-amino-5′-deoxythymidine is an inhibitor and not a substrate for cellular thymidine kinase whereas both are substrates for

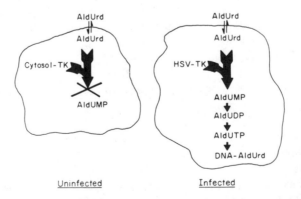

FIG. 13. Metabolic fate of AIdUrd in herpes simplex virus infected and uninfected cells.

HSV-thymidine kinase (Chen and Prusoff, 1979), Fischer *et al.* (1979) examined the potential therapeutic effect when 5′-AdThd was combined with IdUrd which is a substrate for both enzymes and highly toxic to uninfected cells. Fischer *et al.* (1979) showed that selective inhibition of IdUrd activation could be achieved with retention of antiviral activity by this combination. Thus, 5′-AdThd did prevent toxicity of IdUrd to uninfected Vero cells, but in HSV-infected cells the antiviral activity of the two agents in combination is enhanced. These findings if confirmed in animal systems, suggest that appropriate combinations may have clinical value in viral chemotherapy.

9.5.4. Prospectus

What can we do to take advantage of our serendipitous finding that AIdUrd appears to be a unique substrate for the herpes simplex virus induced enzyme? What are the unique features of the viral induced thymidine kinase required for utilization of AIdUrd as a substrate? Why is AIdUrd not a substrate for thymidine kinase present normally in uninfected mammalian cells? Is there a difference in the conformation, the hydrophobic, electronic or other physicochemical parameters of AIdUrd relative to thymidine which prevents AIdUrd from being a substrate for the mammalian enzyme, but allows it to be so for the herpes-induced enzyme? Does the herpes virus thymidine kinase direct the molecule of AIdUrd into the proper conformation for its phosphorylation, whereas the normal mammalian thymidine kinase can not do so? What is the amino acid sequence of the host cell and of the virus-induced thymidine kinases? What are the differences between virus and host-cell enzyme relative to the composition or configuration of the active site? Until we acquire such sophisticated physicochemical knowledge of the viral-induced and normal cellular thymidine kinase (cytosol and mitochondria), our best approach to obtain improved agents is chemical modification of the structure of AIdUrd in order to lower its K_m for the viral-induced enzyme while retaining its inability to be utilized as a substrate for the host cell enzyme.

It should be made clear that merely finding a compound which interacts with the herpes simplex virus induced thymidine kinase, but not that of human cytoplasmic or mitochondrial thymidine kinase, is not by itself adequate for identification of a potential antiherpetic agent. Inhibition of thymidine kinase alone should have little effect on the replication of a herpes virus, since herpes virus TK⁻ mutant can grow well in a TK⁻ host cell. The compound under study not only should be a good and unique substrate for the virus-induced thymidine kinase, but the product should also be capable of further phosphorylation up to the triphosphate so that inhibition of viral DNA synthesis or lethal incorporation into the virus DNA occurs.

In addition to being a unique substrate for a virus specified enzyme, modification of the structure of AIdUrd should produce compounds that retain its antiviral activity yet have, for example, increased solubility, increased lipophilicity and a broader spectrum of antiviral activity.

REFERENCES

AARONSON, S. A. and STEPHENSON, J. R. (1976a) Endogenous Type-C RNA viruses of mammalian cells. *Biochem. biophys. Acta* **458**: 323–354.

AARONSON, S. A. and STEPHENSON, J. R. (1976b) Viruses and the etiology of cancer. In: *Viral Infections*, pp. 251–291, DREW, W. L. (ed.). F. A. Davis, Philadelphia.

AARONSON, S. A., TODARO, G. T. and SCOLNICK, E. M. (1971) Induction of murine C-type viruses from clonal lines of virus-free BALB/T3 cells. *Science, N.Y.* **174**: 157–159.

AEBERSOLD, P. M. (1976) Mutagenic mechanism of 5-bromodeoxyuridine in chinese hamster cells. *Mutation Res.* **36**: 357–362.

ALBERT, D. M., PERCY, D. H., PULIAFITO, C. A., FRITSCH, E., LIN, T. S., WARD, D. C. and PRUSOFF, W. H. C. and PRUSOFF, W. D. (1976) Successful therapy of herpes hominis keratitis in rabbits by 5-Iodo-5′-amino-2′,5′-dideoxyuridine (AIU): A novel analog of Thymidine. *Invest. Opthal.* **15**: 470–478.

ALBERT, D. M., PERCY, D. H., PULIAFITO, C. A., FRITSCH, E., LIN, T. S., WARD, D. C. and PRUSOFF, W. H. (1979)

AIU: An antiherpetic drug with low neonatal toxicity in mice. *Adv. in Ophthalmol.* **38**: 89–98.

ARFELLINI, G., PRODI, G. and GRILLI, S. (1977) Removal of 5-bromo-2-deoxyuridine incorporated in DNA of regenerating rat liver. *Nature* **265**: 377–379.

ARFELLINI, G., PRODI, G. and GRILLI, S. (1978) Removal of 5-bromo-2-deoxyuridine incorporated in liver DNA of newborn and young adult rats. *Experientia* **34**: 185–186.

ASHMAN, C. R. and DAVIDSON, R. L. (1980) Inhibition of Friend erythroleukemic cell differentiation by bromodeoxyuridine: correlation with the amount of bromodeoxyuridine in DNA. *J. Cell. Physiol.* **102**: 45–50.

AUGENLICHT, T., NICOLINI, C. and BASERGA, R. (1974) Circular dichroism and thermal denaturation studies of chromatin from BrdU-treated mouse fibroblasts. *Biochem. biophys. Res. Commun.* **59**: 920–926.

BAKER, B. R., JOSEPH, J. P. and WILLIAMS, J. H. (1955) Puromycin. Synthetic studies. VII. Partial synthesis of amino acid analogs. *J. Am. chem. Soc.* **77**: 1–7.

BARASCH, J. M. and BRESSLER, R. S. (1977) The effect of 5-bromodeoxyuridine on the postnatal development of the rat testis. *J. Exper. Zool.* **200**: 1–8.

BARNETT, C. A. and WICKS, W. D. (1971) Regulation of PEP carboxykinase and tyrosine transaminase in hepatoma cell culture. *J. biol. Chem.* **246**: 7201–7206.

BELTZ, R. E. and VISSER, D. W. (1955) Growth inhibition of *Esherichia coli* by new thymidine analogs. *J. Am. chem. Soc.* **77**: 736–738.

BENNETT, J. A., SVOCOA, P. E., LIN, T. S. and PRUSOFF, W. H. (1982) Comparative effects of 5'-amino-5'-deoxythymidine, a new antiviral agent, and 5-iodo-2'-deoxyuridine on the immune response of mice. *Int. J. Immunopharmacol.* **4**: 557–566.

BERENS, K. and SHUGAR, D. (1963) Ultraviolet absorption spectra and structure of halogenated uracils and their glycosides. *Acta biochim. Pol.* **10**: 25–47.

BICK, M. D. (1975) Misincorporation of GTP during transcription of Poly dAT-dAT and poly ABU-dABU. *Nucleic Acid Res.* **2**: 1513–1523.

BICK, M. D. (1977) Bromodeoxyuridine inhibition of Friend leukemia cell induction. Mechanism of reversal by deoxycytidine. *Biochem. biophys. Acta* **476**: 279–286.

BICK, M. D. and DEVINE, E. A. (1977) Interaction of chromosomal proteins with BrdU substituted DNA as determined by chromatin DNA competition. *Nucleic Acid Res.* **4**: 3687–3700.

BICK, M. D. and SOFFER, M. (1976) Altered glucose-6-phosphate dehydrogenase in bromodeoxyuridine-substituted cells. *Nature, Lond.* **260**: 788–791.

BIQUARD, J.-M., AUPOIX, M. (1978) 5-Bromodeoxyuridine induces expression of a tumour-specific surface antigen on normal avian cells. *Nature* **272**: 284–286.

BIRNBAUM, I., LIN, T. S., SHIAU, G. T. and PRUSOFF, W. H. (1979) A novel Zwitterionic structure and an unusual sugar ring conformation in 5-iodo-5'-amino-2',5'-dideoxyuridine, an antiviral nucleoside. *J. Am. chem. Soc.* **101**: 3353–3358.

BISHOP, C. J., SHERIDAN, J. W. and DONALD, K. J. (1981) The effect of ^{125}I-5-iodo-2'-deoxyuridine labelling on murine tumour cells. *Br. J. Exp. Path.* **62**: 22–26.

BISWAS, D. K., LYONS, J. and TASHUIAN, A. H. JR (1977) Induction of prolactin synthesis in rat pituitary tumor cells by 5-bromodeoxyuridine. *Cell* **11**: 431–439.

BLUE, W. T. and STOBBS, P. G. (1981) Isolation of a protein kinase induced by herpes simplex virus type 1. *J. Virology* **38**: 383–388.

BOSTON INTERHOSPITAL VIRUS STUDY GROUP and the NIAID-SPONSORED COOPERATIVE ANTIVIRAL CLINICAL STUDY (1975) Failure of high dose 5-iodo-2'-deoxyuridine in the therapy of herpes simplex virus encephalitis. Evidence of unacceptable toxicity. *New Engl. J. Med.* **292**: 599–603.

BRADLEY, E. G., CHAN, P. S. and ADELSTEIN, S. J. (1975) The radiotoxicity of iodine-125 in mammalian cells. 1. Effects on the survival curve of radioiodine incorporated into DNA. *Radiat. Res.* **64**: 555–563.

BRADSHAW, T. K. and HUTCHINSON, D. W. (1977) 5-Substituted pyrimidine nucleosides and nucleotides. *Chem. Soc. Rev.* **6**: 43–62.

BREITMAN, T. R., PERRY, S. and COOPER, R. A. (1966) Pyrimidine metabolism in human leukocytes III. The utilization of thymine for DNA-Thymine synthesis by leukemic leukocytes. *Cancer Res.* **26**: 2282–2285.

BRESNICK, E. and THOMPSON, U. B. (1965) Properties of deoxythymidine kinase partially purified from animal tumors. *J. Biol. Chem.* **240**: 3967–3974.

BROWN, G. B., ROLL, P. M. and WEINFIELD, H. (1952) Biosynthesis of nucleic acids. In: *Phosphorous Metabolism*, pp. 384–486. MCELROY, W. D. and GLASS, B. (eds.). John Hopkins, Baltimore.

BROWN, J. C. (1971) Surface glycoprotein characteristic of the differentiated state of neuroblastomes C-1300 cells. *Expl Cell. Res.* **69**: 440–442.

BUETTNER, W. and WERCHAU, H. (1973) Incorporation of 5-iodo-2'-deoxyuridine (IUdR) into SV40 DNA. *Virology* **52**: 553–561.

BULMER, D., STOCCO, D. and MORROW, J. (1976) Bromodeoxyuridine induced variations in the level of alkaline phosphatase in several human heteroploid cell lines. *J. Cell. Physiol.* **87**: 357–365.

BURKI, N. H., ROOTS, H., FEINENDEGEN, L. E. and BOND, V. P. (1973) Inactivation of mammalian cells after disintegrations of ^{3}H or ^{125}I in cell DNA at $-196°C$. *Int. J. Radiat. Biol. Relat. Stud. Phys. Chem. Med.* **24**: 363–375.

BUTHALA, D. A. (1964) Cell culture studies on antiviral agents: Action of cytosine arabinoside and some comparison with 5-iodo-2-deoxyuridine. *Proc. Soc. Exp. Biol. (N.Y.)* **115**: 69–77.

CALABRESI, P., CARDOSO, S. C., FINCH, S. C., KLIGERMAN, M. M., VON ESSEN, C. F., CHU, M. Y. and WELCH, A. D. (1961) Initial clinical studies with 5-iodo-2'-deoxyuridine. *Cancer Res.* **21**: 550–559.

CALABRESI, P. (1963) Current status of clinical investigations with 6-azauridine, 5-iodo-2'-deoxyuridine, and related compounds. *Cancer Res.* **23**: 1260–1267.

CALABRESI, P., CREASEY, W. A., PRUSOFF, W. H. and WELCH, A. D. (1963) Clinical and pharmacological studies with 5-iodo-2'-deoxycytidine. *Cancer Res.* **23**: 583–592.

CALOTHY, C., HIRAI, K. and DEFENDI, V. (1973) 5-Bromodeoxyuridine incorporation into simian virus 40 deoxyribonucleic acid. Effects on simian virus 40 replication in monkey cells. *Virology* **55**: 329–338.

CAMERMAN, N. and TROTTER, J. (1964) 5-iodo-2'-deoxyuridine: relation of structure to its antiviral activity. *Science, N.Y.* **144**: 1348–1350.

CAMIENER, G. W. (1968) Studies of the enzymatic deamination of azacytidine—V. Inhibition *in vivo* by tetrahydrouridine and other reduced pyrimidine nucleosides. *Biochem. Pharmac.* **17**: 1981–1991.

CAMIENER, G. W. and SMITH, G. S. (1965) Studies of the enzymatic deamination of cytosine arabinoside—I. Enzyme distribution and species specificity. *Biochem. Pharmac.* **14**: 1405–1416.

CARRENO, G. and ESPARZA, J. (1977) Induction of Venezuelan equine encephalitis (Mucambo) virus by iododeoxyuridine in chronically infected 'cured' cultured mosquito cells. *Intervirology* **8**: 193–203.

CHABNER, B. A., JOHNS, D. G., COLEMAN, C. N., DRAKE, J. C. and EVANS, W. H. (1974) Purification and properties of cytidine deaminase from normal and leukemic granulocytes. *J. clin. Invest.* **53**: 922–931.

CHANG, P. K. and WELCH, A. D. (1961) Preparation of 5-iodo-2'-deoxycytidine. *Biochem. Pharmac.* **8**: 327–328.

CHATTOPADHYAY, S. K., JAY, G., LANDER, M. R. and LEVINE, A. S. (1979) Correlation of the induction of transcription of the AKR mouse genome by 5-iododeoxyuridine with the activation of an endogenous murine leukemia virus. *Cancer Res.* **39**: 1539–1546.

CHEN, M. S., CHANG, P. K. and PRUSOFF, W. H. (1976a) Photochemical studies and ultraviolet sensitization of *Escherichia coli* thymidylate kinase by various halogenated substrate analogs. *J. biol. Chem.* **251**: 6555–6561.

CHEN, M. S. and PRUSOFF, W. H. (1977) Kinetic and photochemical studies and alteration of ultraviolet sensitivity of *Escherichia coli* thymidine kinase by halogenated allosteric regulators and substrate analogues. *Biochemistry* **16**: 3310–3315.

CHEN, M. S. and PRUSOFF, W. H. (1978) Association of thymidylate kinase activity with pyrimidine deoxyribonucleoside kinase induced by herpes simplex virus. *J. biol. Chem.* **253**: 1325–1327.

CHEN, M. S., WARD, D. C. and PRUSOFF, W. H. (1976b) Specific herpes simplex virus-induced incorporation of 5-Iodo-5'-amino-2',5'-dideoxyuridine into deoxyribonucleic acid. *J. biol. Chem.* **251**: 4833–4838.

CHEN, M. S., WARD, D. C. and PRUSOFF, W. H. (1976b) Specific herpes simplex virus-induced incorporation of 5-Iodo-5'-amino-2'-dideoxyuridine into deoxyribonucleic acid. *J. biol. Chem.* **251**: 4833–4838.

CHEN, M. S., WARD, D. C. and PRUSOFF, W. H. (1976c) 5-Iodo-5'-amino-2',5'-dideoxyuridine-5'-*N*-triphosphate: Synthesis, chemical properties, and effect on *Escherichia coli* thymidine kinase. *J. biol. Chem.* **251**: 4839–4842.

CHEN, M. S. and PRUSOFF, W. H. (1978) Association of thymidylate kinase activity with pyrimidine deoxyribonucleoside kinase induced by herpes simplex virus. *J. Biol. Chem.* **253**: 1325–1327.

CHEN, M. S. and PRUSOFF, W. H. (1979) Phosphorylation of 5-iodo-5'-amino-2',5'-dideoxyuridine by herpes simplex virus type I encoded thymidine kinase. *J. Biol. Chem.* **254**: 10449–10452.

CHEN, M. S., SUMMERS, W. P., WALKER, J., SUMMERS, W. C. and PRUSOFF, W. H. (1979a) Characterization of pyrimidine deoxyribonucleoside kinase (thymidine kinase) and thymidylate kinase as a multifunctional enzyme in cells transformed by herpes simplex virus type 1 and cells infected with mutant strains of herpes simplex virus. *J. Virol.* **30**: 942–945.

CHEN, M. S., WALKER, J. and PRUSOFF, W. H. (1979b) Kinetic studies of herpes simplex virus type I encoded thymidine and thymidylate kinase, a multifunctional enzyme. *J. Biol. Chem.* **254**: 10747–10753.

CHEN, M. S., SHIAU, G. T. and PRUSOFF, W. H. (1980) 5'-Amino-5'-deoxythymidine, synthesis, specific phosphorylation by herpesvirus thymidine kinase and stability to pH of the enzymically formed diphosphate derivative. *Antimicrob. Agents and Chemother.* **18**: 433–436.

CHENG, Y. C. (1976) Deoxythymidine kinase induced in HeLa TK⁻ cells by herpes simplex virus type I and type II. *Biochem. biophys. Acta* **452**: 370–381.

CHENG, Y. C., GOZ, B., NEENAN, J. P., WARD, D. C. and PRUSOFF, W. H. (1975a) Selective inhibition of herpes simplex virus by 5'-amino-2',5'-dideoxy-5-Iodouridine. *J. Virol.* **15**: 1284–1285.

CHENG, Y. C., NEENAN, J. P., GOZ, B., WARD, D. C. and PRUSOFF, W. H. (1975b) Synthesis and biological activity of some novel analogs of thymidine. *Ann. N.Y. Acad. Sci.* **255**: 332–341.

CHENG, Y. C. and OSTRANDER, M. (1976) Deoxythymidine kinase induced in HeLa TK⁻ cells by herpes simplex virus type I and II. II Purification and characterization. *J. biol. Chem.* **251**: 2605–2610.

CHENG, Y. C. and PRUSOFF, W. H. (1973) Mouse ascites sarcoma 180 thymidylate kinase. General properties, kinetic analysis, and inhibition studies. *Biochemistry* **12**: 2612–2619.

CHENG, Y. C. and PRUSOFF, W. H. (1974) Mouse ascites sarcoma 180 deoxythymidine kinase. General properties and inhibition studies. *Biochemistry* **13**: 1179–1185.

CHU, E. H. Y., SUN, N. C. and CHANG, C. C. (1972) Induction of auxotrophic mutations by treatment of chinese hamster cells with 5-bromodeoxyuridine and black light. *Proc. natn. Acad. Sci. USA* **69**: 3459–3463.

COETZEE, G. A. and GEVERS, W. (1977) 5-Bromo-2'-deoxyuridine-stimulated calcium ion—or magnesium ion-dependent ecta—(adenosine triphosphatase) activity of cultured hamster cardiac cells. *Biochem. J.* **164**: 645–652.

COHEN, G. H. (1972) Ribonucleotide reductase activity of synchronized KB cells infected with herpes simplex virus. *J. Virol.* **9**: 408–418.

COHEN, G. H., FACTOR, M. N. and PONCE DE LEON, M. (1974) Inhibition of herpes simplex virus type 2 replication by thymidine. *J. Virol.* **14**: 20–25.

COHEN, R. M. and WOLFENDEN, R. (1971) Cytidine deaminase from *Escherichia coli*. Purification, properties, and inhibition by the potential transition state analog 3,4,5,6-tetrahydrouridine. *J. biol. Chem.* **246**: 7561–7565.

COLBERT, D. A. and COLEMAN, J. R. (1977) Transcriptional expression of non-repetitive DNA during normal and BUdR-mediated inhibition of myogenesis in culture. *Exp. Cell Res.* **109**: 31–42.

COLLINS, P. and BAUER, D. J. (1977) Relative potencies of anti-herpes compounds. *Ann. N.Y. Acad. Sci.* **284**: 49–59.

COMMERFORD, S. L. and JOEL, D. D. (1979) Iododeoxyuridine administered to mice is de-iodinated and incorporated into DNA primarily as thymidylate. *Biochem. Biophys. Res. Comm.* **86**: 112–118.

COOPER, G. M. (1973) Phosphorylation of 5-bromocleoxycytidine in cells infected with herpes simplex virus. *Proc. natn. Acad. Sci. USA* **70**: 3788–3792.

COOPER, G. M., DUNNING, W. F. and GREER, S. (1972) Role of catabolism in pyrimidine utilization for nucleic acid synthesis *in vivo*. *Cancer Res.* **32**: 390–397.

COOPER, G. M. and GREER, S. (1973a) The effect of inhibition of cytidine deaminase by tetrahydrouridine on the utilization of deoxycytidine and 5-bromodeoxycytidine for deoxyribonucleic acid synthesis. *Mol. Pharmac.* **9**: 698–703.

COOPER, G. M. and GREER, S. (1973b) Phosphorylation of 5-halogenated deoxycytidine analogues by deoxycytidine kinase. *Mol. Pharmac.* **9**: 704–710.

CRAMER, J. W., PRUSOFF, W. H. and WELCH, A. D. (1961) 5-Bromo-2'-deoxycytidine (BCDR)-II. Studies with murine neoplastic cells in culture and *in vitro. Biochem. Pharmac.* **8**: 331–335.

CRAMER, J. W., PRUSOFF, W. H., WELCH, A. D., SARTORELLI, A. C., DELAMORE, I. W., VON ESSEN, C. F. and CHANG, P. D. (1962) Studies on the biochemical pharmacology of 5-iodo-2'-deoxycytidine *in vitro* and *in vivo. Biochem. Pharmac.* **11**: 761–768.

CULLEN, B. R. and BICK, M. D. (1978) Bromodeoxyuridine induction of deoxycytidine deaminase activity in a hamster cell line. *Biochim. et Biophys. Acta* **517**: 158–168.

CYSYK, R. and PRUSOFF, W. H. (1972) Alteration of ultraviolet sensitivity of thymidine kinase by allosteric regulators, normal substrates, and a photoaffinity label, 5-iodo-2'-deoxyuridine, a metabolic analog of thymidine. *J. biol. Chem.* **247**: 2522–2532.

DALE, R. M. K., WARD, D. C., LIVINGSTON, D. C. and MARTIN, E. (1975) Conversion of covalently mercurated nucleic acids to tritiated and halogenated derivatives. *Nucleic Acid Res.* **2**: 915–930.

DAVID, J., GORDON, J. S. and RUTTER, W. J. (1974) Increased thermal stability of chromatin contained 5-bromodeoxyuridine-substituted DNA. *Proc. natn. Acad. Sci. USA* **71**: 2808–2812.

DAVIDSON, R. L. and BICK, M. D. (1973) Bromodeoxyuridine dependence—a new mutation in mammalian cells. *Proc. natn. Acad. Sci. USA* **70**: 138–142.

DAVIDSON, R. L. and KAUFMAN, E. R. (1977) Deoxycytidine reverses the suppression of pigmentation caused by 5-BrdUrd without changing the amount of 5 BrdUrd in DNA. *Cell* **12**: 923–929.

DAVIDSON, R. L. and KAUFMAN, E. R. (1978) Bromodeoxyuridine mutagenesis in mammalian cells is stimulated by thymidine and suppressed by deoxycytidine. *Nature* **276**: 722–723.

DAVIS, A. R., NAYAK, D. P. and LOFGREN, J. (1978) Induction of endogenous guinea pig retrovirus by 5-bromodeoxyuridine: amplification of virus-specific RNA. *J. Virol.* **26**: 603–614.

DAWBER, R. (1974) Idoxuridine in herpes zoster: Further evaluation of intermittent topical therapy. *Brit. Med. J.* **i**: 562–567.

DE LAVERGNE, E., OLIVE, D., GEORGES, J. C. and LE MOYNE, M. T. (1965) Action de la 5-iodo-2'-desoxyuridine (I.D.U.) sur quelque virus a A.D.N. en cultures cellulaires. *Revue Immunol.* **29**: 241–266.

DJORDJEVIC, B. and SZYBALSKI, W. (1960) Genetics of human cell lines. III. Incorporation of 5-bromo- and 5-iododeoxyuridine into the deoxyribonucleic acid of human cells and its effect on radiation sensitivity. *J. exp. Med.* **112**: 509–531.

DOBERSEN, M. J., JERKOFSKI, M. and GREER, S. (1976) Enzymatic studies on the basis for selective inhibition of herpes simplex virus and varicella zoster virus by 5-bromodeoxycytidine. *Fedn Proc.* **35**: 1689.

DOBERSEN, M. J., JERKOFSKY, M. and GREER, S. (1976) Enzymatic basis for the selective inhibition of varicella zoster virus by 5-halogenated analogues of deoxycytidine. *J. Virol.* **20**: 478–486.

DUBBS, D. R. and KIT, S. (1964) Mutant strains of herpes simplex deficient in thymidine kinase-inducing activity. *Virology* **22**: 493–502.

DUBBS, D. R., KIT, S., DE TORRES, R. A. and ANKEN, M. (1967) Virogenic properties of bromodeoxyuridine-sensitive and simian virus 40-transformed mouse kidney cells. *J. Virol.* **1**: 968–979.

DUNN, D. B. and SMITH, J. D. (1954) Incorporations of halogenated pyrimidines into the deoxyribonucleic acids of *Bacterium coli* and its bacteriophages. *Nature, Lond.* **174**: 305–306.

DUNN, K. and NAZERIAN, K. (1977) Induction of Marek's disease virus antigens by IdUrd in a chicken lymphoblastoid cell line. *J. Gen. Virol.* **34**: 413–419.

DUNNEBACKE, T. H. and REAUME, M. G. (1958) Correlation of the yield of poliovirus with the size of the isolated tissue cultured cells. *Virology* **6**: 8–13.

EASTERBROOK, K. B. and DAVERN, C. I. (1963) The effect of 5-bromodeoxyuridine on the multiplication of vaccinia virus. *Virology* **19**: 509–520.

EIDINOFF, M. L., CHEONG, L. and RICH, M. A. (1959) Incorporation of unnatural pyrimidine bases into deoxyribonucleic acid of mammalian cells. *Science, N.Y.* **129**: 1550–1551.

EL DAREER, S. M., WHITE, V., CHEN, F. P., MELLETT, L. B. and HILL, D. L. (1976) Distribution of tetrahydrouridine in experimental animals. *Cancer Treat. Rep.* **60**: 1627–1631.

EVANS, I. and BOSMANN, H. B. (1977) Bromodeoxyuridine (BUdR) treatment of melanoma cells decreases cellular proteolytic activity. *Exp. Cell Res.* **108**: 151–155.

FASY, T. M., CULLEN, B. R., LUK, D. and BICK, M. D. (1980) Studies on the enhanced interaction of halodeoxyuridine-substituted DNAs with H1 histones and other polypeptides. *J. biol. Chem.* **255**: 1380–1387.

FEIGE, Y. and GAVRON, A. (1975) Microdosimetry of auger electrons. In: *Radiation Research Proceedings of the Fifth International Congress of Radiation Research*, pp. 557–569. NYGAARD, O. E., ADLER, H. I. and SINCLAIR, W. K. (eds.).

FIALA, M., CHOW, A. W., MIYASAKI, R. and GUZI, L. B. (1974) Susceptibility of herpes viruses to three nucleoside analogues and their combinations and enhancement of the antiviral effect of acid pH. *J. Infect. Dis.* **129**: 82–85.

FINE, D. L., PLOWMAN, J. K., KELLY, S. P., ARTHUR, L. O. and HILLMAN, E. A. (1974) Enhanced production of mouse mammary tumor virus in dexamethasone-treated, 5-iododeoxyuridine-stimulated mammary tumor cell cultures. *J. Natn. Cancer Inst.* **52**: 1881–1886.

FISCHER, D. S., BLACK, F. F., CASSIDY, E. P. and WELCH, A. D. (1965a) Inhibition of the production of tumors by a polyoma virus. *Ann. N.Y. Acad. Sci.* **130**: 213–216.

FISCHER, D. S., BLACK, F. L. and WELCH, A. D. (1965b) Inhibition by nucleoside analogues of tumor formation by polyoma virus. *Nature, Lond.* **206**: 839–840.

FISCHER, P. H., CHEN, M. S. and PRUSOFF, W. H. (1979) A comparison of the effects of 5-iodo-5'-amino-2',5'-dideoxyuridine and 5-iodo-2'-deoxyuridine on the structure of herpes virus DNA. *Fedn. Proc.* **38**: 429.

FISCHER, P. H., LEE, J. J., CHEN, M. S., LIN, T. S. and PRUSOFF, W. H. (1979) Synergistic effect of 5-amino-5'-

deoxythymidine and 5-iodo-2'-deoxyuridine against herpes simplex virus infections *in vitro. Biochem. Pharmacol.* **28**: 3482–3486.

FISCHER, P. H., CHEN, M. S. and PRUSOFF, W. H. (1980) The incorporation of 5-iodo-5'-amino-2',5'-dideoxyuridine and 5-iodo-2'-deoxyuridine into herpes simplex virus DNA: A relationship to their antiviral activity and effects on DNA structure. *Biochim. Biophys. Acta* **606**: 236–245.

FITZMAURICE, L. C. and BAKER, R. F. (1974) Effect of 5-bromodeoxyuridine on incorporation of RNA precursors into sea urchin embryos. *J. cell. Physiol.* **83**: 259–261.

FLUGEL, R. M., DARAI, G., BRAUN, R. and MUNK, K. (1977) Activation of an endogenous C-Type RNA virus in rat embryo cells after transformation by herpes simplex virus types 1 and 2. *J. gen. Virol.* **36**: 365–369.

FOGEL, M. (1972) Induction of virus synthesis in polyoma-transformed cells by DNA antimetabolites and by irradiation after pretreatment with 5-bromodeoxyuridine. *Virology* **49**: 12–22.

FOGEL, M. (1973) Induction of polyoma virus by fluorescent (visible) light in polyoma-transformed cells pretreated with 5-bromodeoxyuridine. *Nature, New Biol.* **241**: 182–184.

FORCE, E. E. and STEWART, R. C. (1964a) Effect of 5-iodo-2'-deoxyuridine in the pathogenesis of Columbia—SK virus in mice. *J. Immunol.* **93**: 872–878.

FORCE, E. E. and STEWART, R. C. (1964b) Effect of 5-iodo-2'-deoxyuridine on multiplication of Rous sarcoma virus *in vitro. Proc. Soc. exp. Biol. Med.* **116**: 803–806.

FRANKO, A. J. and KALLMAN, R. F. (1980) Cell loss and influx of labeled host cells in three transplantable mouse tumors using [^{125}I]UdR release. *Cell Tissue Kinet.* **13**: 381–393.

FREESE, E. (1959) The specific mutagenic effect of base analogues on Phage T4. *J. molec. Biol.* **1**: 87–105.

GANGAROSA, L. P., PARK, N. H. and HILL, J. M. (1977) Iontophoretic assistance of 5-iodo-2'-deoxyuridine penetration into neonatal mouse skin and effects on DNA synthesis. *Proc. Soc. Exp. Biol. Med.* **154**: 439–443.

GARCIA, M., WESTLEY, B. and ROCHEFORT, H. (1981) 5-Bromodeoxyuridine specifically inhibits the synthesis of estrogen-induced proteins in MCF$_7$ cells. *Eur. J. Biochem.* **116**: 297–301.

GARCIA, R. I., WERNER, I. and SZABO, G. (1979) Effect of 5-bromo-2'-deoxyuridine on growth and differentiation of cultured embryonic retinal pigment cells. *In Vitro* **15**: 779–788.

GARRETT, C., WATAYA, Y. and SANTI, D. V. (1979) Catalysis of dehalogenation of 5-bromo- and 5-iodo-deoxyuridylate. *Biochemistry* **18**: 2798–2804.

GAUTSCHI, J. R., BURKHALTER, M. and BAUMANN, E. A. (1978) Comparative utilization of bromodeoxyuridine and iododeoxyuridine triphosphates for mammalian DNA replication *in vitro. Biochim. Biophys. Acta* **518**: 31–36.

GERBER, P. (1972) Activation of Epstein—Barr virus by 5-bromodeoxyuridine in 'virus-free' human cells. *Proc. natn. Acad. Sci. USA* **69**: 83–85.

GILBERT, E. F., PITOT, H. C., BRUYERE, H. J., JR and CHEUNG, A. L. (1974) Abnormal proteins in *Drosophila melanogaster* subsequent to 5-bromodeoxyuridine administration. *Comp. Biochem. Physiol.* **47B**: 229–232.

GINSBERG, A. H., MONTE, W. T. and JOHNSON, K. P. (1977) Effect of cyclophosphamide *in vitro* and on vaccinia virus replication in tissue culture. *J. Virol.* **21**: 227–283.

GLASER, R. and RAPP, F. (1971) Rescue of Epstein—Barr virus from somatic cell hybrids of Burkitts lymphoblastoid cells. *J. Virol.* **10**: 288–296.

GOEDDEL, D. V., YANSURA, D. G., WINSTON, C. and CARUTHERS, M. H. (1978) Studies on gene control regions. VII. Effect of 5-bromouracil-substituted lac operators on the lac operator—lac repressor interaction. *J. Mol. Biol.* **123**: 661–687.

GOLDENTHAL, E. I., COOKSON, K. M., GEIL, R. G. and WAZETER, F. X. (1974) Preclinical toxicologic evaluation of tetrahydrouridine (NSC-112907) in beagle dogs and rhesus monkeys. *Cancer Chemother. Rep. Part 3*, **5**: 15–16.

GORDON, J. S., BELL, G. I., MARTINSON, H. C. and RUTTLER, J. (1976) Selective interaction of 5-bromo-deoxyuridine substituted DNA with different chromosomal proteins. *Biochemistry* **15**: 4778–4786.

GOTTO, A. M., BELKHODE, M. L. and TOUSTER, O. (1969) Stimulatory effects of inosine and deoxyinosine on the incorporation of uracil-2-^{14}C, 5-fluorouracil-2-^{14}C and 5-bromouracil-2-^{14}C into nucleic acids of Ehrlich ascites tumor cells *in vitro. Cancer Res.* **29**: 807–811.

GOZ, B. (1974) An increase in deoxycytidine kinase (CD) activity in cells infected with herpes virus. *Proc. Am. Soc. Cancer Res.* **13**: 26.

GOZ, B. (1974) The induction of alkaline phosphatase activity in HeLa cells by 5-iodo-2'-deoxyuridine. *Cancer Res.* **34**: 2393–2398.

GOZ, B. (1978) The effects of incorporation of 5-halogenated deoxyuridines into the DNA of eukaryotic cells. *Pharmac. Rev.* **29**: 249–272.

GOZ, B. and PRUSOFF, W. H. (1970) Pharmacology of viruses. *Ann. Rev. Pharmac.* **10**: 143–170.

GOZ, B. and WALKER, K. P. (1976) The incorporation of 5-iodo-2'-deoxyuridine into the DNA of HeLa cells and the induction of alkaline phosphate activity. *Cancer Res.* **36**: 4480–4485.

GOZ, B., ORR, C. and WHARTON, W. (1980) Inhibition by deoxycytidine, cytidine, and β-cytosine arabinoside of the induction of alkaline phosphatase activity in HeLa cells. *J. Natl Cancer Inst.* **64**: 1355–1361.

GOZ, B. and WALKER, K. P. (1978) An immunological and biochemical analysis of alkaline phosphatase in HeLa cells exposed to 5-iodo-2'-deoxyuridine. *Biochem. Pharmacol.* **27**: 431–436.

GRADY, L. J. and CAMPBELL, W. P. (1974) The distribution of 5-bromodeoxyuridine in the DNA of polyoma-transformed mouse cells and some apparent effects on transcription. *Expl Cell. Res.* **87**: 127–131.

GREEN, J. A. and BARON, S. (1975) 5-Iododeoxyuridine potentiation of the replication *in vitro* of several unrelated RNA and DNA viruses. *Science, N.Y.* **190**: 1099–1101.

GREENBERGER, J. S., STEPHENSON, J. R., MOLONEY, W. C. and AARONSON, S. A. (1975) Different hematological diseases induced by type c viruses chemically activated from embryo cells of different mouse strains. *Cancer Res.* **35**: 245–252.

GREER, S. (1960) Studies on ultraviolet irradiation of *Escherichia coli* containing 5-bromouracil in its DNA. *J. gen. Microbiol.* **22**: 618–634.

GREER, S., SCHILDKRAUT, I., ZIMMERMAN, T. and KAUFMAN, H. (1975) 5-Halogenated analogs of deoxycytidine as selective inhibitors of the replication of herpes simplex viruses in cell culture and related studies of intracranial herpes simplex infections in mice. *Ann. N.Y. Acad. Sci.* **255**: 359–365.

GREER, S. and ZAMENHOF, S. (1957) Effect of 5-bromouracil in deoxyribonucleic acid of *E. coli* on sensitivity to ultraviolet radiation. *Am. chem. Soc.* Absts, papers 131st meeting: 3c.

GRIPPO, P., ORLANDO, P. and LOCOROTONDO (1981) 5-Bromouracil DNA glycosylase activity in differentiating muscle cells. *Cell Biol. Int. Repts.* **5**: 551.

GURR, J. A., BECKER, J. E. and POTTER, V. R. (1977) The diverse effects of 5-bromodeoxyuridine on enzyme activities in cultured H35 hepatoma cells. *J. Cell. Physiol.* **91**: 271–287.

HAMPAR, B., DERGE, J. G., MARTOS, L. M. and WALKER, J. L. (1972) Synthesis of Epstein–Barr virus after activation of the viral genome in a 'virus-negative' human lymphoblastoid cell (Ragi) made resistant to 5-bromodeoxyuridine. *Proc. natn. Acad. Sci. USA* **69**: 78–82.

HANNA, C. (1966) Effect of several analogs of idoxuridine on the uptake of tritium labeled thymidine in the rabbit cornea infected with herpes simplex. *Expl Eye Res.* **5**: 164–167.

HAY, J., PEREA, P. A. J., MORRISON, J. M., GENTRY, G. A. and SUBAK-SHARPE, J. H. (1970) Herpes virus-specified proteins. In: *Strategy of the Viral Genome*, pp. 355–376. WOLSTENHOLME, G. E. W., O'CONNOR, M. (eds.). Ciba Found. Symp. Churchill Livingstone, Edinburgh.

HEIDELBERGER, C. (1975) Fluorinated pyrimidines and their nucleosides. In: *Antineoplastic and Immunosuppressive Agents*, Vol. 2, pp. 193–231. SARTORELLI, A. C. and JOHNS, D. G. (eds.). Springer, Berlin.

HENDERSON, E. E., LONG, W. K. and RIBECK, R. (1979) Effects of nucleoside analogs on Epstein–Barr virus-induced transformation of human umbilical cord leukocytes and Epstein–Barr virus expressions in transformed cells. *Antimicrob. Agents Chemother.* **15**: 101–110.

HERRMANN, E. C. JR (1961) Plaque inhibition test for detection of specific inhibitors of DNA containing viruses. *Proc. Soc. exp. Biol.* **107**: 142–145.

HETTINGER, M. E., PAVAN-LANGSTON, D., PARK, N. H., ALBERT, D. M., DeCLERCQ, E. and LIN, T. S. (1981) Ac₂IDU, BVDU, and thymine arabinoside therapy in experimental herpes keratitis. *Arch. Ophthalmol.* **99**: 1618–1621.

HILL, B. T. and BASERGA, R. (1975) Effect of 5-bromodeoxyuridine on the transcriptional properties of the genome in W1-38 human diploid fibroblasts. *Chem. Biol. Interact.* **10**: 363–375.

HILL, B. T., TSUBUI, A. and BASERGA, R. (1974) Effect of 5-bromodeoxyuridine on chromatin transcription in confluent fibroblasts. *Proc. natn. Acad. Sci. USA* **71**: 455–459.

HILL, J. M., GANGAROSA, L. P. and PARK, N. H. (1977) Iontophoretic application of antiviral chemotherapeutic agents. *Ann. N.Y. Acad. Sci.* **284**: 604–612.

HIRANO, A., YUMURA, K., KURIMURA, T., KATSUMOTO, T., MORIYAMA, H. and MANABE, R. (1979) Analysis of herpes simplex virus isolated from patients with recurrent herpes keratitis exhibiting 'treatment-resistance' to 5-iodo-2'-deoxyuridine. *Acta Virol.* **23**: 226–230.

HIRSCH, M. S. and BLACK, P. H. (1974) Activation of mammalian leukemia viruses. *Adv. Virus Res.* **19**: 265–313.

HIRT, B. (1966) Evidence for semiconservative replication of circular polyoma DNA. *Proc. natn. Acad. Sci. USA* **55**: 997–1004.

HITCHINGS, G. H., FALCO, E. A. and SHERWOOD (1945) The effects of pyrimidines on the growth of *Lactobacillus casei*. *Science, N.Y.* **102**: 251–252.

HOLMES, W. L., PRUSOFF, W. H. and WELCH, A. D. (1954) Studies on metabolism of thymine-2-C¹⁴ by the rat. *J. biol. Chem.* **209**: 503–509.

HOPKINS, R. L. and GOODMAN, M. F. (1980) Deoxyribonucleotide pools, base pairing, and sequence configuration affecting bromodeoxyuridine- and 2-aminopurine-induced mutagenesis. *Proc. natl. Acad. Sci. USA* **77**: 1801–1805.

HORN, D. and DAVIDSON, R. L. (1976) Inhibition of biological effects of bromodeoxyuridine by deoxycytidine: correlation with decreased incorporation of bromodeoxyuridine into DNA. *Somatic cell Genetics* **2**: 469–481.

HORWITZ, J. P., CHUA, J. and NOEL, M. (1964) Nucleosides. V. The monomesylates of 1-(2'-deoxy-B-D-lyxofuranosyl) thymine. *J. org. Chem.* **29**: 2076–2079.

HORWITZ, J. P., TOMSON, A. J., URABANSKI, J. A. and CHUA, J. (1962) Nucleosides—I. 5'-Amino-5'deoxyuridine and 5'-amino-5'deoxythymidine. *J. org. Chem.* **27**: 3045–3048.

HSIUNG, G. D. (1972) Activation of guinea pig C-type virus in cultured spleen cells by 5-bromo-2'-deoxyuridine. *J. Natn. Cancer Inst.* **49**: 567–570.

HUBERMAN, E. and HEIDELBERGER, C. (1972) The mutagenicity to mammalian cells of pyrimidine nucleoside analogs. *Mutations Res.* **14**: 130–132.

HUEBNER, R. J., LANE, W. T., WELCH, A. D., CALABRESI, P., McCOLLUM, R. W. and PRUSOFF, W. H. (1963) Inhibition of 5-iododeoxyuridine of the oncogenic effects of adenovirus type 12 in hamsters. *Science, N.Y.* **142**: 488–490.

HULANICKA, B., BARRY, D. W. and GRIMLEY, P. M. (1977) Induction of tubuloreticular inclusions in human lymphoma cells (Raji line) related to S-phase treatment with halogenated pyrimidines. *Cancer Res.* **37**: 2105–2113.

HUTCHINSON, F. and STEIN, J. (1977) Mutagenesis of Lambda phage: 5-Bromouracil and hydroxylamine. *Molec. Gen. Genet.* **152**: 29–36.

ILTIS, J. P., LIN, T. S., PRUSOFF, W. H. and RAPP, F. (1979) Effect of 5-iodo-5'-amino-2',5'-dideoxyuridine on varicella-zoster virus *in vitro*. *Antimicrob. Agents Chemotherapy* **16**: 92–97.

JACOB, F. (1966) Genetics of the bacterial cell. *Science, N.Y.* **152**: 1470–1478.

JAFFE, J. J. and PRUSOFF, W. H. (1960) The effect of 5-iododeoxyuridine upon the growth of some transplantable rodent tumors. *Cancer Res.* **20**: 1383–1388.

JAMIESON, A. T. and SUBAK-SHARPE, J. H. (1974) Induction of both thymidine and deoxycytidine kinase activity of herpes virus. *J. gen. Virol.* **24**: 465–480.

JAWETZ, E., COLEMAN, V. R., DAWSON, C. K. and THYGESON, P. (1970) The dynamics of IUDR action in herpetic keratitis, and the emergence of IUDR resistance *in vitro*. *Ann. N.Y. Acad. Sci.* **173**: 282–289.

JERKOVSKY, M. A., DOBERSEN, M. J. and GREER, S. (1977) Selective inhibition of the replications of varicella-zoster virus by 5-halogenated analogs of deoxycytidine. *Ann. N.Y. Acad. Sci.* **284**: 389–395.

JERKOVSKY, M. and RAPP, F. (1975) Stimulation of adenovirus replication in simian cells in the absence of a helper virus by pretreatment of the cells with iododeoxyuridine. *J. Virol.* **15**: 253–258.

JERKOFSKY, M., DOBERSEN, M. J. and GREER, S. (1980) Inhibition of the replication of human cytomegalovirus by bromodeoxycytidine in the absence of detectable increases in bromodeoxycytidine kinase activity. *Intervirology* **14**: 233–238.

JOHNSON, T. B. and JOHNS, C. O. (1905–1906) Researchers on pyrimidines; some 5-iodo pyrimidine derivatives; 5-iodocytosine. *J. biol. Chem.* **1**: 305–318.

JONES, P. A., BENEDICT, W. F., BAKER, M. S., MONDAL, S., RAPP, U. and HEIDELBERGER, C. (1976) Oncogenic transformation of C3H/10T 1/2 clone 8 mouse embryo cells by halogenated pyrimidine nucleosides. *Cancer Res.* **36**: 101–107.

JONES, T. C. and DOVE, W. F. (1972) Photosensitization of transcription by bromodeoxyuridine substitution. *J. molec. Biol.* **64**: 409–416.

JUEL-JENSEN, B. E. (1973) Herpes simplex and zoster, *Br. med. J.* **1**: 406–410.

JUEL-JENSEN, B. E. (1974) Virus diseases. *Practitioner* **213**: 508–518.

JUEL-JENSEN, B. E. and MACCALLUM, F. D. (1972) In: *Herpes Simplex Varicella and Zoster*, pp. 1–194. J. B. Lippincott, Philadelphia.

JUEL-JENSEN, B. E. and MACCALLUM, F. P. (1974) Idoxuridine in herpes zoster. *Br. med. J.* **ii**: 41.

KALLOS, J., FASY, T. M., HOLLANDER, V. P. and BICK, M. D. (1978) Estrogen receptor has enhanced affinity for bromodeoxyuridine-substituted DNA. *Proc. natn. Acad. Sci. USA* **75**: 4896–4900.

KALLOS, J., FASY, T. M., HOLLANDER, V. P. and BICK, M. (1979) Estrogen receptor can distinguish among various halodeoxyuridine-substituted DNAs. *FEBS Letts.* **98**: 347–349.

KAN, J. and PRUSOFF, W. H. (1976) Effect of iododeoxyuridine (IdUrd) on adenovirus 2. *Fedn. Proc.* **35**: 624.

KAN-MITCHELL, J. and PRUSOFF, W. H. (1979) Studies on the effect of the 5-iodo-2′-deoxyuridine on the formation of adenovirus type 2 virions and the synthesis of virus induced polypeptides. *Biochem. Pharmacol.* 1819–1829.

KAN-MITCHELL, J., MITCHELL, M. S., LIN, T. S. and PRUSOFF, W. H. (1980) Comparative analysis of the immunosuppressive properties of two antiviral iodinated thymidine analogs, 5-iodo-2′-deoxyuridine and 5-iodo-5′-amino-2′,5′-dideoxyuridine. *Cancer Res.* **40**: 3491–3494.

KAPLAN, A. S. (1964) Studies on the replicating pool of viral DNA in cells infected with pseudorabies virus. *Virology* **24**: 19–25.

KAPLAN, A. S., BEN-PORAT, T. and KAMIYA, T. (1965) Incorporation of 5-bromodeoxyuridine and 5-iododeoxyuridine into viral DNA and its effect on the infective process. *Ann. N.Y. Acad. Sci.* **130**: 226–239.

KASUPSKI, G. J. and MUKHERJEE, B. B. (1977) Effects of controlled exposure of L cells to bromodeoxyuridine. II. Turnover rates and activity profiles during cell cycle of bromodeoxyuridine-sensitive and -resistant enzymes. *Expl Cell Res.* **108**: 393–401.

KAUFMAN, E. R. and DAVIDSON, R. L. (1978) Bromodeoxyuridine mutagenesis in mammalian cells: Mutagenesis is independent of the amount of bromouracil in DNA. *Proc. Natl. Acad. Sci. USA* **75**: 4982–4986.

KAUFMAN, E. R. and DAVIDSON, R. L. (1979). Bromodeoxyuridine mutagenesis in mammalian cells is stimulated by purine deoxyribonucleosides. *Somatic Cell Genetics* **5**: 653–663.

KAUFMAN, H. E. (1962a) Clinical cure of herpes simplex keratitis by 5-iodo-2′-deoxyuridine. *Proc. Soc. exp. Biol. Med.* **109**: 251–252.

KAUFMAN, H. E., MAROLA, E. and DOHLMAN, C. (1962b) Use of 5-iodo-2′-deoxyuridine (IDU) in treatment of herpes simplex keratitis. *Archs Opthal.* **68**: 235–239.

KAUFMAN, H. E., NESBURN, A. B. and MALONEY, D. E. (1962c) IDU therapy of herpes simplex. *Archs Opthal.* **67**: 583–591.

KAUFMAN, H. E. (1980) Anti-metabolites in the management of herpes simplex keratitis. *Metabolic & Pediatric Ophthal.* **4**: 175–177.

KAWAMURA, H. and HASHIMOTO, Y. (1981) Inhibitory effect of 5-halogenated deoxyuridines on *in vitro* keratinization of a transformed rat urinary bladder epithelial cell line. *Gann* **72**: 264–271.

KIRSCHNER, K. and BISSWANGER, H. (1976) Multifunctional proteins. *Ann. Rev. Biochem.* **47**: 143–166.

KIT, S. (1979) Viral-Associated and Induced Enzymes. Pharmac. Ther., **4**: 501–585.

KIT, S. and DUBBS, D. R. (1963) Acquisition of thymidine kinase activity by herpes simplex-infected mouse fibroblase cells. *Biochem. biophys. Res. Commun.* **11**: 55–59.

KJELLEN, L. (1962) Effect of 5-halogenated pyrimidines on cell proliferation and adenovirus multiplication. *Virology* **18**: 64–70.

KLEIN, P. A. and SMITH, R. T. (1977) The role of oncogenic viruses in neoplasia. *Ann. Rev. Med.* **28**: 311–327.

KLEMENT, V., NICOLSON, M. O., GILDEN, R. V., OROSZLAM, S., SARMA, P. S., RONGEY, R. W. and GARDNER, M. B. (1972) Rat C-type virus induced in rat sarcoma cells by 5-bromodeoxyuridine. *Nature, New Biol.* **238**: 234–237.

KLEMENT, V., NICOLSON, M. O. and HUEBNER, R. J. (1971) Rescue of the genome of focus forming virus from rat non-productive lines by 5-bromodeoxyuridine. *Nature, New Biol.* **234**: 12–14.

KLEMPERER, H., HAYNES, G., SHEDDEN, W. and WATSON, D. (1976) A virus-specific thymidine kinase in BKH21 cells infected with herpes simplex virus. *Virology* **31**: 120–128.

KOBAYASHI, Y., YAMAMOTO, K., ASAI, T., NAKANO, M. and KUMADAKI, I. (1980) Studies on organic fluorine compounds. Part 35. Trifluoromethylation of pyrimidine- and purine-nucleosides with trifluoromethyl-copper complex. *J. Chem. Soc. (Perkin)*, **1**: 2755–2761.

KOCHETKOV, N. K. and BUDOVSKII, E. I. (1972) In: *Organic Chemistry of Nucleic Acids*, p. 269. Plenum Press, London.

KOTZIN, B. L. and BAKER, R. F. (1972) Selective inhibition of genetic transcription in sea urchin embryos. Incorporation of 5-bromodeoxyuridine into low molecular weight nuclear DNA. *J. Cell Biol.* **55**: 74–81.

KOYAMA, G. and ONO, T. (1971) Induction of alkaline phosphatase by bromodeoxyuridine in a hybrid line between mouse and chinese hamster in culture. *Expl Cell Res.* **69**: 468–470.

KOYAMA, H. and ONO, T. (1972) Further studies on the induction of alkaline phosphatase by 5-bromodeoxyuridine in a hybrid line between mouse and chinese hamster in culture. *Biochim. biophys. Acta* **264**: 497–507.

KREIDER, J. W., MATHESON, D. W., BELTZ, B. and ROSENTHAL, M. (1974) Inhibition of melanogenesis with 5-bromodeoxyuridine treatment in a single period of DNA synthesis. *J. Natn. Cancer Inst.* **52**: 1537–1540.

KRISCH, R. E. and SAURI, C. J. (1975) Further studies of DNA damage and lethality from the decay at iodine-125 in bacteriophages. *Int. J. Radiat. Biol. Relat. Stud. Phys. Chem. Med.* **27**: 553–560.

KRISCH, R. E., KRASIN, F. and SAURI, C. J. (1976) DNA breakage, repair, and lethality after ^{125}I decay in Rec and Rec A strains of *Escherichia coli*. *Int. J. Radiat. Biol. Relat. Stud. Phys. Chem. Med.* **29**: 37–50.

KRISS, J. P., MARUYAMA, Y., TUNG, L. A., BOND, G. B. and RÉVÉSZ, L. (1963) Fate of 5-bromodeoxyuridine, 5-bromodeoxycytidine and 5-iododeoxycytidine in man. *Cancer Res.* **23**: 260–268.

KRISS, J. P., TUNG, L. A. and BONS, S. (1962a) Distribution and fate of bromodeoxyuridine and bromodeoxycytidine in the mouse and rat. *Cancer Res.* **22**: 254–265.

KRISS, J. P., TUNG, L. A. and BOND, S. (1962b) Fate of iododeoxycytidine in the mouse and rat. *Cancer Res.* **22**: 1257–1264.

KRYCH, M., PIETRZYKOWSKA, I., SZYSZKO, J. and SHUGAR, D. (1979) Genetic evidence for the nature, and excision repair, of DNA lesions resulting from incorporation of 5-bromouracil. *Molec. Gen. Genet.* **171**: 135–143.

KRYCH, M. and PIETRZYKOWSKA, I. (1979) BU-induction of prophage and its relation to repair processes. *Studia Biophysica, Berlin* **76**: 67–68.

KU, K. Y. and PRUSOFF, W. H. (1974) A comparative study of the effect of normal substrates and 5-iodo-2'-deoxyuridine triphosphate, a metabolic analog of thymidine triphosphate, on the inactivation of *Escherichia col)* deoxyribonucleic acid polymerase I and II by ultraviolet irradiation. *J. biol. Chem.* **249**: 1239–1246.

KULIKOWSKI, T. and SHUGAR, D. (1978) Methylation and tautomerism of 5-fluorocytocine nucleosides and their analogs. *Nucleic Acid Res.* Special Publication No. 4, 507–510.

LAIBSON, P. R., SERY, T, W. and LEOPOLD, I. H. (1963) The treatment of herpetic keratitis with 5-iodo-2-deoxyuridine (IDU). *Arch. Ophthal. (Chicago)* **70**: 52–58.

LANGEN, P. (1975) In: *Antimetabolites of Nucleic Acid Metabolism*, pp. 1–273. Gordon & Breach, New York.

LANGEN, P., ETZOLD, G. and KOWOLLIK, G. (1972) Inhibition of DNA synthesis and thymidylate kinase by halogeno derivatives of 2',5'-dideoxythymidine. *Acta biol. med. germ.* **28**: K5–10.

LANGEN, P. and KOWOLLIK, G. (1968) 5'-Deoxy-5'-fluorothymidine, a biochemical analogue of thymidine-5'-monophosphate selectively inhibiting DNA synthesis. *Eur. J. Biochem.* **6**: 344.

LANGEN, P., KOWOLLIK, G., SCHUTT, M. and ETZOLD, G. (1969) Thymidylate kinase as target enzyme for 5'-deoxythymidine and various 5'-deoxy-5'-halogeno pyrimidine nucleosides. *Acta. biol. med. germ.* **23**: K19.

LAPEYER, J. N. and BEKHOR, I. (1974) Effects of 5-bromo-2'-deoxyuridine and dimethylsulfoxide on properties and structure of chromatin. *J. molec. Biol.* **89**: 137–162.

LASNERET, J., CANIVET, M., BITTOUN, P. and PERIES, P. (1981) IdUr induction of a new type of retrovirus-like particle (E particle) in transformed fibroblastic mouse cells. *Ann. Virol. (Inst. Pasteur)* **132** E: 151–159.

LAU, R. Y., NONOYAMA, M. and KLEIN, G. (1981) Somatic cell hybrids between human lymphoma and human myeloid leukemia cells. *Virology* **110**: 259–269.

LAVIALLE, C., MORRIS, A. G., SUAREZ, H. G., ESTRADE, S., STEVENET, J. and CASSINGENA, R. (1977) Simian virus 40-chinese hamster kidney cell interactions. IV. Enhanced virus replication in infected cells upon treatment with mitomycin C. *J. gen. Virol.* **36**: 137–149.

LAWLY, P. D. and BROOKES, P. (1962) Ionization of DNA bases or base analogs as a possible explanation of mutagenesis, with special reference to 5-bromodeoxyuridine. *J. Molec. Biol.* **4**: 216–219.

LAZAR, A., SCHLESINGER, M., HOROWITZ, A. T. and HELLER, E. (1975) Induction of carcinogenic oncornavirus in C57 bl/6 mouse embryo cells by 5-iododeoxyuridine. *Nature, Lond.* **255**: 648–650.

LEE, L. S. and CHENG, Y. C. (1976) Human deoxythymidine kinase. II. Substrate specificity and kinetic behaviour of the cytoplasmic and mitochondrial isozymes derived from blast cells of acute myelocytic leukemia. *Biochemistry* **15**: 3686–3690.

LEKAS, M. D. (1979) Iontophoresis treatment. *Otolaryngol. Head Neck Surg.* **87**: 292–298.

LERNER, A. M. and BAILEY, E. J. (1972) Concentrations of idoxuridie in serum, urine, and cerebrospinal fluid of patients with suspected diagnoses of herpes virus hominis encephalitis. *J. clin. Invest.* **51**: 45–49.

LETSINGER, R. L., WILKES, J. S. and DUMAS, L. B. (1972) Enzymatic synthesis of polydeoxyribo-nucleotides possessing internucleotide phosphoramidate bonds. *J. Am. chem. Soc.* **94**: 292–293.

LEUNG, W., DUBBS, D. R., TRKULA, D. and KIT, S. (1975) Mitochondrial and herpes virus-specific deoxypyrimidine kinase. *J. Virol.* **16**: 486–497.

LIN, J. C. and PAGANO, J. S. (1980) Effect of 5-iodo-2'-deoxyuridine on physical properties and nonhistone chromosomal proteins of chromatin from Burkitt somatic cell hybrids. *Arch. Biochem. Biophys.* **200**: 567–574.

LIN, S. Y. and RIGGS, A. D. (1972) *Lac* operator analogues: bromodeoxyuridine substitution in the *lac* operator affects the rate of association of the *lac* repressor. *Proc. natn. Acad. Sci. USA* **69**: 2574–2576.

LIN, S. Y., LIN, D. and RIGGS, A. D. (1976) Histones bind more tightly to bromodeoxyuridine-substituted DNA than to normal DNA. *Nucleic Acid Res.* **3**: 2183–2191.

LIN, T-S., CHAI, C. and PRUSOFF, W. H. (1976a) Synthesis and biological activities of 5-trifluoromethyl-5'-azido-2',5'-dideoxyuridine and 5-trifluoromethyl-5'-amino-2',5'-dideoxyuridine. *J. med. Chem.* **19**: 915–918.

LIN, T-S., NEENAN, J. P., CHENG, Y. C., PRUSOFF, W. H. and WARD, D. C. (1976b) Synthesis and antiviral activity of 5 and 5'-substituted thymidine analogs. *J. med. Chem.* **19**: 495–498.

LIN, T-S. and PRUSOFF, W. H. (1975) Synthesis of 1-(5-azido-5-deoxy-B-D-arabinofuranosyl) cytosine and 1-(5-amino-5-deoxy-B-D-arabinofuranosyl) cytosine. *J. Carb. Nucleosides Nucleotides* **2**: 185–190.

LIN, T-S. and PRUSOFF, W. H. (1978b) A novel synthesis and biological activity of several 5-halo-5'-amino analogues of deoxyribopyrimidine nucleosides. *J. med. Chem.* **21**: 106–109.

LIN, T. S. and PRUSOFF, W. H. (1978a) Synthesis and biological activity of several amino analogues of thymidine. *J. med. Chem.* **21**: 109–112.

LITMAN, R. M. and PARDEE, A. B. (1956) Production of bacteriophage mutants by a disturbance of deoxyribonucleic acid metabolism. *Nature, Lond.* **178**: 529–531.

LITMAN, R. M. and PARDEE, A. B. (1960) The induction of mutants of bacteriophage T2 by 5-bromouracil. IV.

Kinetics of bromouracil-induced mutagenesis. *Biochim. biophys. Acta* **42**: 131–140.

LOUGH, J. (1980) Muscle specific traits display differential sensitivity to 5-bromo-2'-deoxyuridine. *Cell Differentiation* **9**: 247–260.

LOWY, D. R., ROWE, W. H., TEICH, N. and HARTLEY, J. W. (1971) Murine leukemia virus; high-frequency activation *in vitro* by 5-iododeoxyuridine and 5-bromodeoxyuridine. *Science, N.Y.* **174**: 155–156.

LOWRY, S. P., MELNICK, J. L. and RAWLS, W. G. (1971) Investigation of plaque formation in chick embryo cells as a biological marker for distinguishing herpes virus type 2 from type 1. *J. gen. Virol.* **10**: 1–9.

LOWRY, S. P., BRESNICK, E. and RAWLS, W. E. (1971) Differences in thymidine kinase-inducing ability of herpesvirus types 1 and 2. *Virology* **46**: 958–961.

LYKKESFELDT, A. E. and ANDERSEN, H. A. (1977) Preferential inhibition of rDNA transcription by 5-bromodeoxyuridine. *J. Cell Sci.* **25**: 95–102.

MAASS, G. and HAAS, R. (1966) Uber die bildung von virusspezifischem SV-40 Antigen in gengenwart von 5-Iod-2'-desoxyuridin. *Arch. ges. Virusforsch.* **18**: 253–256.

MACCALLUM, F. O. and JUEL-JENSEN, B. E. (1966) Herpes simplex virus skin infection in man treated with idoxuridine in dimethyl sulphoxide. Results of double blind controlled trial. *Br. med. J.* **ii**: 805–807.

MAICHUK, Y. F., POZDNYAKOV, V. L., GALEGOV, G. A. and BIKBULATOV, R. M. (1973) Antiviral activity of 5-bromouridine in an experiment and its therapeutic effectiveness in herpes virus infection of the eyes. *Vop. Virus.* **18**: 408–411.

MALEY, F. (1967) Deoxycytidylate deaminase. *Meth. Enzymol.* **12A**: 170–182.

MANAK, M. M., AURELIAN, L. and Ts'O, P. O. P. (1981) Focus formation and neoplastic transformation by herpes simplex virus type 2 inactivated intracellularly by 5-bromo-2'-deoxyuridine and near UV light. *J. Virol.* **40**: 289–300.

MANLY, K. F., GIVENS, J. F., TABER, R. L. and ZEIGEL, R. F. (1978) Characterization of virus-like particles released from the hamster cell line CHO-K1 after treatment with 5-bromodeoxyuridine. *J. Gen. Virol.* **39**: 505–517.

MAO, J. C. H. and ROBISHAW, E. E. (1975a) Mode of inhibition of herpes simplex virus DNA polymerase by phosphonacetate. *Biochemistry* **14**: 5475–5479.

MAO, J. C. H., ROBISHAW, E. E. and OVERBY, L. R. (1975b) Inhibition of DNA polymerase from herpes simplex virus-infected Wi-38 cells by phosphonacetic acid. *J. Virology* **15**: 1281–1283.

MARKS, M. I. (1974) Variables influencing the *in vitro* susceptibilities of herpes simplex viruses to antiviral drugs. *Antimicrob. Agents Chemother.* **6**: 34–38.

MARTENET, A. C. (1975) The treatment of experimental deep herpes simplex keratitis with ethyl-deoxy-uridine and iodo-deoxy-cytidine. *Ophthal. Res.* **7**: 170–180.

MATHIAS, A. P., FISCHER, G. A. and PRUSOFF, W. H. (1959) Inhibition of the growth of mouse leukemic cells in culture by 5-iododeoxyuridine. *Biochem. biophys. Acta* **36**: 560–561.

MATSUMURA, K., FUJIMOTO, M. and MITSUI, Y. (1973) Micro-autographic studies on incorporation of 5-iodo-2'-deoxyuridine into Herpes simplex virus. *Jap. J. Ophthal.* **17**: 125–132.

MATTHES, E., FENSKE, H., EICHORN, I., LANGEN, P. and LINDIGKERT, R. (1977) Altered histone–DNA interactions in rat liver chromatin containing 5-bromodeoxyuridine-substituted DNA. *Cell Differentiation* **6**: 241–251.

MENDEZ, M. S. and MARTENET, A. C. (1972) Activite de l'iodo-desoxy-cytidine (IDC) sur la keratite herpetique experimentale profone. *Annls Oculist* **205**: 199–206.

MENDEZ, M., MARTENET, A. C. and STEINBRUNNER, W. (1971) L'Iododesoxycytidine nouveau virostatique contre la keratite herpetique. *Annls Oculist* **204**: 1219–1228.

MEUTH, M. and GREEN, H. (1974) Induction of a deoxycytidineless state in cultured mammalian cells by bromodeoxyuridine. *Cell* **2**: 109–112.

MILLER, N. and FOX, J. J. (1964) Nucleosides XXI. Synthesis of some 3'-substituted 2',3'-dideoxyribonucleosides of thymine and 5-methylcytosine. *J. org. Chem.* **29**: 1772–1776.

MILLER, R. L., GLASER, R. and RAPP, F. (1977) Studies of an Epstein–Barr virus-induced DNA polymerase. *Virology* **76**: 494–502.

MIYAMOTO, H., MATSUMURA, K., NUNOMURA, H. and MITSUI, Y. (1969) The incorporation of IDU into viral DNA of herpes simplex virus. *Acta Soc. Ophthalmol. Japan* **73**: 1064–1070.

MUNGALL, W. S., GREENE, G. L., HEAVNER, G. A. and LETSINGER, R. (1975) Use of the azido group in the synthesis of 5'-terminal aminodeoxythymidine oligonucleotides. *J. org. Chem.* **40**: 1659–1662.

MUNYON, W. M., HUGHES, R., ANGERMANN, J., BERAZKY, E. and DMOCHOWSKI, L. (1964) Studies on the effect of 5-iododeoxyuridine and *p*-fluorophenylalanine on polyoma virus formation *in vitro*. *Cancer Res.* **24**: 1880–1886.

MURRAY, T. and RUSSELL, T. R. (1978) Effect of 5-bromodeoxyuridine on the induction of adenosine 3':5'-monophosphate phosphodiesterase in 3T3-L-fibroblasts. *Arch. Biochem. Biophys.* **190**: 705–711.

NEENAN, J. P. and ROHDE, W. (1973) Inhibition of thymidine kinase from Walker 256 carcinoma by thymidine analogs. *J. med. Chem.* **16**: 580–581.

NEIL, G. L., MOXLEY, T. E. and MANAK, R. D. (1970) Enhancement by tetrahydrouridine of 1-β-D-arabinofuranosyl cytosine (cytarabine) oral activity in L1210 leukemic mice. *Cancer Res.* **30**: 2166–2172.

NICOLINI, C. and BASERGA, R. (1975) Circular dichroism spectra and ethidium bromide binding of 5-deoxybromouridine-substituted chromatin. *Biochem. biophys. Res. Commun.* **64**: 189–195.

NORDENFELT, L. and NORDENFELT, E. (1977) Ocular herpes simplex infection, a clinical evaluation of virus isolation and studies on iodo-deoxyuridine resistance. *Acta Ophthalmologica* **55**: 919.

O'BRIEN, J. C. and STELLWAGEN, R. H. (1977) The effects of controlled substitution of 5-bromodeoxyuridine (BudR) for thymidine in hepatoma cell DNA. *Expl Cell. Res.* **107**: 119–125.

OTTO, M. J., LEE, J. J. and PRUSOFF, W. H. (1982) Effects of nucleoside analogues on the expression of herpes simplex type 1 induced proteins. *Antiviral Res.* **2**: 267–281.

PALAYOOR, T. (1977) Transcriptional effects of bromo-2'-deoxyuridine in post-implantation mouse embryos. *Experientia* **33**: 448–450.

PAPAC, R., JACOBS, E., WONG, F., COLLOM, A., SKOOG, W. and WOOD, D. A. (1962) Clinical evaluation of the pyrimidine nucleosides 5-fluoro-2'-deoxyuridine and 5-iodo-2'-deoxyuridine. *Cancer Chemother. Rep.* **20**: 143–146.

PARK, N. H., PAVAN-LANGSTON, D., HETTINGER, M. E., MCLEAN, S. L., ALBERT, D. M., LIN, T. S. and PRUSOFF, W. H. (1980) Topical therapeutic efficacy of 9-(2-hydroxyethoxymethyl)guanine and 5-iodo-5'-amino-2',5'-dideoxyuridine on oral HSV-2 infection in mice. *J. Infect. Diseases* **141**: 575–579.

PARK, N. H., PAVAN-LANGSTON, D., HETTINGER, M. E., GEARY, P. A., AUGUST, M. L., ALBERT, D. M., LIN, T. S. and PRUSOFF, W. H. (1982) Development of oral HSV-1 infection model in mice-evaluation of efficacy of 5'-amino-5-iodo-2',5'-dideoxyuridine. *Oral Surgery, Pathology and Oral Medicine* **53**: 256–262.

PATCH, C. T., CHATTOPADHYAY, S. K., HAUSER, J. and LEVINE, A. S. (1981) Regulation of viral transcription in cells infected with iododeoxyuridine-substituted simian virus 40 as a model for the activation by iododeoxyuridine of latent viral genomes. *Cancer Res.* **41**: 2421–2427.

PAUL, N. R., IWAKATU, S., RHODES, A. J. and LABZOFFSKY, N. A. (1974) Enhancing effect of halogenated pyrimidines (BUdR and IUdR) in the growth of rubella virus in BHK-21 cells. *Arch. ges. Virusforsch.* **44**: 144–146.

PAULING, L. (1948) In: *The Nature of the Chemical Bond*, p. 53, 2nd edn. Cornell University, Ithaca, N.Y.

PAULING, L. and PAULING, P. (1975) In: *Chemistry*, p. 204. W. H. Freeman, San Francisco.

PAVAN-LANGSTON, D. and DAHLMAN, C. H. (1972) A double-blind clinical study of adeninearabinoside therapy of viral keratoconjunctivitis. *Am. J. Ophthal.* **74**: 81–88.

PAVAN-LANGSTON, D., PARK, N. H., LASS, J., PAPALE, J., ALBERT, D. M., LIN, T. S., PRUSOFF, W. H. and PERCY, D. M. (1982) 5'-Amino-5'-deoxythymidine: Topical therapeutic efficacy in ocular herpes and systemic teratogenic and toxicity studies. *Proc. Soc. Exp. Biol. Med.* **170**: 1–7.

PAWLOWSKI, P. J., BRIERLEY, G. T. and LUKENS, L. N. (1981) Changes in the type II and type I collagen messenger RNA population during growth of chondrocytes in 5-bromo-2-deoxyuridine. *J. Biol. Chem.* **256**: 7695–7698.

PAWLOWSKI, P. J. (1976) Effect of 5-bromodeoxyuridine on the appearance of cytoplasmic poly-A containing RNA. *J. cell Physiol.* **89**: 19–27.

PENNINGTON, T. H. (1976) Effect of 5-bromodeoxyuridine on vaccinia virus-induced polypeptide synthesis: Selective inhibition of the synthesis of some post-replicative polypeptides. *J. Virol.* **18**: 1133.

PERERA, P. A. J. and MORRISON, J. M. (1970) Evidence for the induction of a new deoxycytidine kinase in cells infected with herpes virus. *Biochem. J.* **117**: 21P–22P.

PERKINS, E. S., WOOD, R. M., SEARS, M. L., PRUSOFF, W. H. and WELCH, A. D. (1962) Antiviral activities of several iodinated pyrimidine deoxyribonucleosides. *Nature, Lond.* **194**: 985–986.

PERSON, D. A., SHERIDAN, P. J. and HERRMANN, E. C. JR. (1970) Sensitivity of Types 1 and 2 herpes simplex virus to 5-iodo-2'-deoxyuridine and 9-β-D-arabinofuranosyladenine. *Infect. Immun.* **2**: 815–820.

PETERSON, A. R., PETERSON, H. and HEIDELBERGER, C. (1975) Reversion of the 8-azaguanine resistant phenotype of variant chinese hamster cells treated with alkylating agents and 5-bromo-2'-deoxyuridine. *Mutation Res.* **29**: 127–137.

PETERSON, A. R., LANDOLPH, J. R., PETERSON, H. and HEIDELBERGER, C. (1978) Mutagenesis of chinese hamster cells is facilitated by thymidine and deoxycytidine. *Nature* **276**: 508–510.

PIETRZYKOWSKA, I. (1973) On the mechanism of bromouracil-induced mutagenesis. *Mutation Res.* **19**: 1–9.

PIETRZYKOWSKA, I. and KRYCH, M. (1977) Lethal and mutagenic Bu-induced lesions in DNA and their repair. *Studia Biophysica, Berlin* **61**: 17–22.

PIETRZYKOWSKA, I., LEWANDOWSKY, K. and SHUGAR, D. (1975) Liquid-holding recovery of bromouracil-induced lesions in DNA of *Escherichia coli* CR-34 and its possible relation to dark-repair mechanisms. *Mutation Res.* **30**: 21–32.

PLENTLE, A. A. and SCHOENHEIMER, R. (1944) Studies of the metabolism of purines and pyrimidines by means of isotopic nitrogen. *J. biol. Chem.* **153**: 203–217.

PLESIEWICZ, E., STEPIEN, E., BOLEWSKA, K. and WIERZCHOWSKI, K. L. (1976) Stacking self-association of pyrimidine nucleosides and of cytosine: effects of methylation and thiolation. *Nucleic Acid Res.* **3**: 1295–1306.

PLUMMER, G. and GOODHEART, C. R. (1974) Growth of murine cytomegalovirus in a heterologous cell system and its enhancement by 5-iodo-2'-deoxyuridine. *Infect. Immun.* **10**: 251–256.

POIRIER, L. A., STONER, G. D. and SHIMKIN, M. D. (1975) Bioassay of alkyl halides and nucleotide base analogs by pulmonary tumor response in strain A mice. *Cancer Res.* **35**: 1411–1415.

PONCE DE LEON, M., EISENBERG, R. J. and COHEN, G. H. (1977) Ribonucleotide reductase from herpes simplex virus (types 1 and 2) infected and infected KB cells: Properties of the partially purified enzymes. *J. gen. Virol.* **36**: 163–173.

PREISLER, H. D., HOUSMAN, D., SCHER, W. and FRIEND, C. (1973) Effects of 5-bromo-2'-deoxyuridine on production of globin messenger RNA in dimethyl sulfoxide-stimulated Friend leukemic cells. *Proc. natn. Acad. Sci. USA* **70**: 2956–2959.

PRICE, P. M. (1976) The effect of 5-bromodeoxyuridine on messenger RNA production in cultured cells. *Biochim. biophys. Acta* **447**: 304–311.

PRUSOFF, W. H. (1955) Studies on the mechanism of action of 6 azathymine. 1. Biosynthesis of the deoxyribonucleoside. *J. biol. Chem.* **215**: 809–821.

PRUSOFF, W. H. (1959a) Synthesis and biological activities of iododeoxyuridine, an analog of thymidine. *Biochim. biophys. Acta* **32**: 295–296.

PRUSOFF, W. H. (1959b) Incorporation of iododeoxyuridine, an analog of thymidine into mammalian deoxyribonucleic acid. *Fedn. Proc.* **18**: 305.

PRUSOFF, W. H. (1963) A review of some aspects of 5-iododeoxyuridine and azauridine. *Cancer Res.* **23**: 1246–1259.

PRUSOFF, W. H. (1967) Recent advances in chemotherapy of virus diseases. *Pharmac. Rev.* **19**: 209–250.

PRUSOFF, W. H., BAKHLE, Y. S. and MCCAEA, J. F. (1963) Incorporation of 5-iodo-2'-deoxyuridine into the deoxyribonucleic acid of vaccinia virus. *Nature, Lond.* **199**: 1310–1311.

Prusoff, W. H., Cheng, Y. C. and Neenan, J. (1974) Present and future potential of nucleosides as antiviral agents. *Prog. Chemother.* **2**: 881–888.

Prusoff, W. H. and Goz, B. (1975) Halogenated pyrimidine deoxyribonucleosides. In: *Antineoplastic and Immunosuppressive Agents*, Vol. 2, pp. 272–347. Sartorelli, A. C. and Johns, D. G. (eds.). Springer, Berlin.

Prusoff, W. H. and Ward, D. C. (1976) Nucleoside analogs with antiviral activity. *Biochem. Pharmac.* **25**: 1233–1239.

Prusoff, W. H., Ward, D. C., Lin, T. S., Chen, M. S., Shaiu, G. T., Chai, C., Lentz, E., Capizzi, R., Idriss, J., Ruddle, N. H., Black, F. L., Kumari, H. L., Albert, D., Bhatt, P. N., Hsiung, G. D., Stricklands, S. and Cheng, Y. C. (1977) Recent studies on the antiviral and biochemical properties of 5-halo-5′-amino-deoxyribonucleosides. *Ann. N.Y. Acad. Sci. USA* **284**: 335–341.

Puliafito, C. A., Robinson, N. L., Albert, D. H., Pavan-Langston, D., Lin, T. S., Ward, D. C. and Prusoff, W. H. (1977) Therapy of experimental herpes simplex keratitis in rabbits with 5-iodo-5′-amino-2′,5′-dideoxyuridine. *Proc. Soc. exp. Biol. Med.* **156**: 92–96.

Rapp, F. and Reed, C. L. (1977) The viral etiology of cancer. A realistic approach. *Cancer* **40**: 419–429.

Rapp, U. R., Nowinski, R. C., Reznikoff, C. A. and Heidelberger, C. (1975) Endogenous oncornaviruses in chemically induced transformation. I. transformation independent of virus production. *Virology* **65**: 392–409.

Reff, M. E. and Davidson, R. L. (1979) Deoxycytidine reverses the suppression of pigmentation caused by 5-BrdUrd without changing the distribution of 5-BrdUrd in DNA. *J. Biol. Chem.* **254**: 6869–6872.

Reichard, P. (1955) Utilization of deoxyuridine and 5-methyluridine for the biosynthesis of thymine by the rat. *Acta Chem. Scand.* **9**: 1275–1285.

Renis, H. E. (1970) Comparison of cytotoxicity and antiviral activity of 1-β-D-arabinofuranosyl-5-iodocytosine with related compounds. *Cancer Res.* **30**: 189–194.

Renis, H. E. and Buthala, D. A. (1965) Development of resistance to antiviral drugs. *Ann. N.Y. Acad. Sci.* **130**: 343–354.

Robins, A. B. and Taylor, D. M. (1981) Iodine-123-iododeoxyuridine: A potential indicator of tumour response to treatment. *Int. J. Nuclear Med. Biol.* **8**: 53–63.

Rogers, J., Ng., S. K. C., Coulter, M. B. and Sanwal, B. D. (1975) Inhibition of myogenesis in a rat myoblast line by 5-bromodeoxyuridine. *Nature, Lond.* **256**: 438–440.

Rössler, K., Meyer, G. J. and Stocklin, G. (1977) Labelling and animal distribution studies of 5-astatouracil and 5-astatodeoxyuridine (211 AT). *J. Labelled Compounds Radiopharm.* **13**: 271.

Rowe, W. P., Lowy, D. R., Teich, N. and Hartly, J. W. (1972) Some implications of the activation of murine leukemia virus by halogenated pyrimidines. *Proc. natn. Acad. Sci. USA* **69**: 1033–1035.

Rowe, W. P., Pugh, W. E. and Hartley, J. W. (1970) Plaque assay technique for murine leukemia viruses. *Virology* **42**: 1136–1139.

Rupp, W. D. and Prusoff, W. H. (1964) Incorporation of 5-iodo-2′-deoxyuridine into bacteriophage T1 as related to ultraviolet sensitization of protection. *Nature, Lond.* **202**: 1288–1290.

Rupp, W. D. and Prusoff, W. H. (1965) Photochemistry of iodouracil. I. Photoproducts obtained in water. *Biochem. biophys. Res. Commun.* **18**: 45–151.

Rutter, W., Pictet, R. and Morris, P. (1973) Toward molecular mechanisms of developmental process. *Ann. Rev. Biochem.* **42**: 601–646.

Rydberg, B. (1977) Bromouracil mutagenesis in *Escherichia coli* evidence for involvement of mismatch repair. *Molec. Gen. Genet.* **152**: 19–28.

Salo, R. J. and Mayor, H. D. (1979) Inhibition of the replication of parvovirus X14 by 5-iodo-2; -deoxyuridine pre-treatment of cell cultures. *J. Gen. Virol.* **44**: 577–585.

Schabel, F. M. and Montgomery, J. A. (1972) Antiviral agents—purines and pyrimidines. In: *The Chemotherapy of Virus Diseases*, pp. 231–261. Bauer, D. J. (ed.). Pergamon Press, New York.

Schiek, W. and Schiek, E. (1969) Untersuchung uber infektiöses bromodesoxyuridinhaltiges Herpes virus hominis, Bestimmung der Dichte und der Sedimentationkonstanten in CsCl-H$_2$O Dichtergradienten. *Arch. ges. Virusforsch.* **28**: 229–238.

Schildkraut, I., Cooper, G. M. and Greer, S. (1975) Selective inhibition of the replication of herpes simplex virus by 5-halogenated analogues of deoxycytidine. *Molec. Pharmac.* **11**: 153–158.

Schneider, D. and Falke, D. (1980) Investigations on the mechanism of induction of the alkaline phosphatase by bromodesoxyuridine in herpes simplex virus transformed cells and the transport of uridine. *Z. Naturforsch.* **35**: 1036–1045.

Schubert, D. and Jacob, F. (1970) 5-Bromodeoxyuridine-induced differentiation of a neuroblastoma. *Proc. natn. Acad. Sci. USA* **67**: 247–254.

Schwartz, S. A. (1976) Enzymatic determination of nonrandom incorporation of 5-bromodeoxyuridine in rat DNA. *Biochemistry* **15**: 3097–3105.

Schwartz, S. A. (1977) Rat embryo nonhistone chromosomal proteins: Interaction *in vitro* with normal and bromodeoxyuridine-substituted DNA. *Biochemistry* **16**: 4101–4108.

Schwartz, S. A. (1981) Preferential utilization of bromodeoxyuridine and iododeoxyuridine triphosphates by DNA polymerase γ *in vitro*. *Biosci. Repts.* **1**: 387–398.

Scott, W. J. (1981) Pathogenesis of bromodeoxyuridine-induced polydactyly. *Teratology* **23**: 383–389.

Shishido, K. and Ikeda, Y. (1970) Preferential binding of RNA polymerase to the thymidylic acid-rich fragments obtained from bacteriophage FI DNA. *J. Biochem.* **68**: 881–884.

Shugar, D., Pietrzykowska, I. and Kulikowski, T. (1977) In: *Proc. 6th Oxford Int. Symp. on Genetic Expression*, pp. 141–156. Oxford University, Oxford. (Cited by Kulikowski and Shugar, 1978).

Silagi, S. (1976) Effects of 5-bromodeoxyuridine on tumorigenicity, immunogenecity, virus production, plasminogen activator, and melanogenesis of mouse melanoma cells. *Int. Rev. Cytol.* **45**: 65–111.

Silvestri, D. L., Corey, L., Winter, C., Remington, M. and Holmes, K. K. (1979) Controlled trial of topical idoxuridine in dimethyl sulfoxide for recurrent genital herpes. *Eleventh International Congress of Chemotherapy, Boston* (Abstract No. 970).

SIM, J. S., STEBBING, N. and CAREY, N. H. (1981) Studies on the antiviral activity of 5'-amino-2',5'-dideoxy-5-iodouridine (AIU) against herpes viruses *in vivo* and *in vitro*. *Antiviral Res.* 1: 393–404.

SIMPSON, R. T. and SEALE, R. L. (1974) Characterization of chromatin extensively substituted with 5-bromodeoxyuridine. *Biochemistry* 13: 4609–4616.

SINGER, J., STELLWEGEN, R. H., ROBERTS, J. and RIGGS, A. D. (1977) 5-Methylcytosine content of rat hepatoma DNA substituted with bromodeoxyuridine. *J. biol. Chem.* 252: 5509–5513.

SMELLIE, S. G. and PARSONS, P. G. (1979) Effects of thymidine analogues on murine and human cells. *Australian J. Exp. Biol. Med. Sci.* 57: 563–573.

SMITH, J. D., FREEMAN, G., VOGT, M. and DULBECCO, R. (1960) The nucleic acid of polyoma virus. *Virology* 12: 185–196.

SMOLIN, G., OKUMOTO, M., FEILER, S., and CONDON, D. (1981) Idoxuridine-liposome therapy for herpes simplex keratitis. *Am. J. Ophthalmol.* 91: 220–225.

SPEERS, W. C. and LEHMAN, J. M. (1976) Increased susceptibility of murine teratocarcinoma cells to simian virus 40 and polyoma virus following treatment with 5-bromodeoxyuridine. *J. Cell Physiol.* 88: 297–303.

STAAL, S. P. and ROWE, W. P. (1975) Enhancement of adenovirus in W1-38 and AGMK cells by pretreatment of cells with 5-iodo-2'-deoxyuridine. *Virology* 64: 517–519.

STAMBROOK, P. and WILLIAMSON, R. (1974) Error frequency in 5S RNA from cells grown in 5-bromodeoxyuridine. *Eur. J. Biochem.* 48: 297–302.

STARK, R. M. and LITTLEFIELD, J. W. (1974) Mutagenic effect of BUdR in diploid human fibroblasts. *Mutation Res.* 22: 281–286.

STEINBERG, R. A., LEVINSON, B. B. and TOMKINS, G. M. (1975) Kinetics of steroid induction and deinduction of tyrosine aminotransferase synthesis in cultural hepatoma cells. *Proc. natn. Acad. Sci. USA* 72: 2007–2011.

STELLWAGEN, R. H. and TOMKINS, G. M. (1971a) Preferential inhibition by 5-bromo-deoxyuridine of the synthesis of tyrosine aminotransferase in hepatoma cell cultures. *J. molec. Biol.* 56: 167–182.

STELLWAGEN, R. H. and TOMKINS, G. M. (1971b) Differential effect of 5-bromodeoxyuridine on the concentrations of specific enzymes in hepatoma cells in culture. *Proc. natn. Acad. Sci. USA* 68: 1147–1150.

STEPHENSON, J. R., GREENBERGER, J. S. and AARONSON, S. A. (1974) Oncogenicity of an endogenous C-type virus chemically activated from mouse cells in culture. *J. Virol.* 13: 237–240.

STERNGLANZ, H. and BUGG, C. E. (1975) Relationship between the mutagenic and base-stacking properties of halogenated uracil derivatives. The crystal structures of 5-chloro- and 5-bromouracil. *Biochim. biophys. Acta* 378: 1–11.

STEWART, S. E., KASNIC, G., JR., DRAYCOTT, C. and BEN, T. (1972a) Activation of viruses in human tumors by 5-iododeoxyuridine and dimethylsulfoxide. *Science, N.Y.* 175: 198–199.

STEWART, S. E., KASNIC, G., JR., DRAYCOTT, C., FELLER, W., GOLDIN, A., MITCHELL, E. and BEN, T. (1972b) Activation *in vitro* by 5-iododeoxyuridine, of a latent virus resembling C-type virus in a human sarcoma cell line. *J. Natn. Cancer Inst.* 48: 273–277.

ST. JEOR, S. and RAPP, F. (1973a) Cytomegalovirus replication in cells pretreated with 5-iodo-2'-deoxyuridine. *J. Virol.* 11: 986–997.

ST. JEOR, S. and RAPP, F. (1973b) Cytomegalovirus conversion of nonpermissive cells to a permissive state for virus replication. *Science, N.Y.* 181: 1060–1061.

STOUT, M. G., ROBINS, M. J., OLSEN, R. K. and ROBINS, R. D. (1969) Purine nucleosides XXV. The synthesis of certain derivatives of 5'-amino-5' deoxy- and 5'-amino-2',5'-dideoxy-β-D-ribofuranosylpurines as purine nucleotide analogs. *J. med. Chem.* 12: 658–662.

STROM, C. M. and DORFMAN, A. (1976) Distribution of 5-bromodeoxyuridine and thymidine in the DNA of developing chick cartilage. *Proc. natn. Acad. Sci. USA* 73: 1019–1023.

SUAREZ, H. G., LAVIALLE, C., STEVENET, J., ESTRADE, S., MORRIS, S. G. and CASSINGENA, R. (1977) Enhanced SV40 virus replication in fully permissive monkey kidney cells pre-treated with 5-iodo-2'-deoxyuridine (IdUrd). *J. Gen. Virol.* 37: 569–584.

SUAREZ, H. G., LAVIALLE, C. and CASSINGENA, R. (1980) Simian virus 40–Chinese hamster kidney cell interaction V. Cooperative effect of 5-iodo-2'-deoxyuridine and mitomycin C in the enhancement of virus replication in infected cells. *J. Virol.* 36: 295–297.

SUAREZ, H. G., LAVIALLE, CH., STEVENET, J., ESTRADE, S., MORRIS, A. G. and CASSINGENA, R. (1977) Enhanced SV40 replication for fully permissive monkey kidney cells pre-treated with 5-Iodo-2'-deoxyuridine (IdUrd). *J. gen. Virol.* 37: 569–584.

SUAREZ, H. G., MORRIS, A. G., LAVIALLE, CH. and CASSINGENA, R. (1976) Enhanced SV40-virus replication in chinese hamster kidney cells pretreated with 5-iodo-2'-deoxyuridine. *Archs Virol.* 50: 249–253.

SUMMERS, W. C. and SUMMERS, W. P. (1977) [^{125}I] deoxycytidine used in rapid, sensitive, and specific assay for herpes simplex virus type 1 thymidine kinase. *J. Virol.* 24: 314–318.

SZYBALSKI, W., KIBINSKI, H. and SHELDRICK, P. (1966) Pyrimidine clusters on the transcribing strand of DNA and their possible role in the initiation of RNA synthesis. *Cold Spring Harb. Symp. quant Biol.* 31: 123–127.

TARÁBEK, J. and ŽEMLA, J. (1980) Inhibition of polyoma virus-specific RNA formation by 5-bromo-2'-deoxyuridine. *Neoplasma* 27: 601–605.

TAYLOR, K., HRADECHA, Z. and SZYBALSKI, W. (1967) Asymmetric distribution of the transcribing regions on the complementary strands of coliphage λ DNA. *Proc. natn. Acad. Sci. USA* 57: 1618–1625.

TEICH, N., LOWY, D. R., HARTLEY, J. W. and ROWE, W. P. (1973) Studies of the mechanism of induction of infectious murine leukemia virus from AKR mouse embryo cell lines by 5-iododeoxyuridine and 5-bromodeoxyuridine. *Virology* 51: 163–173.

THOMPSON, R. L., WILKIN, M. L., HITCHINGS, G. H., ELION, G. B., FALCO, E. A. and RUSSEL, R. B. (1949) The effects of antagonists on the multiplication of vaccinia virus *in vitro*. *Science, N.Y.* 110: 454–455.

TSUBOI, A. and BASERGA, R. (1973) Effect of 5-bromo-2'-deoxyuridine on transport of deoxyglucose and cycloleucine in 3T6 fibroblasts. *Cancer Res.* 33: 1326–1330.

VANSANTEN, G. (1965) Phenotypic character of phase protein abnormalities induced by bromouracil. *Biochem. Pharmac.* 14: 215–222.

Verbov, J. (1979) Local idoxuridine treatment of herpes simplex and zoster. *J. Antimicrob. Chemother.* **5**: 126–128.

Veselý, J. and Cihák, A. (1973) High-frequency induction *in vivo* of mouse leukemia in AKR strain by 5-azacytidine and 5-iodo-2'-deoxyuridine. *Experientia* **29**: 1132–1133.

Visser, D. W., Frisch, D. M. and Huang, B. (1960) Synthesis of 5-chlorodeoxyuridine and a comparative study of 5-halodeoxyuridines in *E. coli*. *Biochem. Pharmac.* **5**: 157–164.

Visser, D. W., Lagerborg, D. L. and Pearson, H. E. (1952) Inhibition of mouse encephalomyelitis virus, *in vitro*, by certain nucleoprotein derivatives. *Proc. Soc. exp. Biol. Med.* **79**: 571–573.

Voytek, P. (1975) Purification of thymidine phosphorylase from *Escherichia coli* and its photo-inactivation in the presence of thymine, thymidine, and some halogenated analogs. *J. biol. Chem.* **250**: 3660–3665.

Voytek, P., Chang, P. K. and Prusoff, W. H. (1972) Kinetic and photochemical studies of 3-*N*-methyl-5-iodo-2'-deoxyuridine. *J. biol. Chem.* **247**: 567–572.

Wainwright, S. D. and Wainwright, L. R. (1976) Inhibition and stimulation by 5-bromodeoxyuridine of erythropoieses by chick blood island cells. *Experientia* **32**: 1473–1475.

Walther, B. T., Pictet, R. L., David, J. D. and Rutter, W. J. (1974) On the mechanism of 5-bromodeoxyuridine inhibition of exocrine pancreas differentiation. *J. biol. Chem.* **249**: 1953–1964.

Wataya, Y., Santi, D. V. and Hansch, C. (1977) Inhibition of *Lactobacillus casei* thymidylate synthetase by 5-substituted 2'-deoxyuridylates. Preliminary quantitative structure activity relationship. *J. med. Chem.* **20**: 1469–1473.

Webb, P., Chanana, A. D., Cronkite, E. P., Laissue, J. A. and Joel, D. D. (1980) Comparison of DNA renewal in germ-free and conventional mice using [^{125}I] iododeoxyuridine and [^{3}H]thymidine. *Cell Tissue Kinet.* **13**: 227–237.

Weber, H. W., Geddes, A. and Stellwagen, R. H. (1978) Induction of intracisternal type A particles by 5-bromo-2'-deoxyuridine in rat hepatoma cells: Brief communication. *J. Natl. Cancer Inst.* **60**: 919–923.

Weintraub, H., Campbell, G. and Holtzer, H. (1972) Identification of a developmental program using bromodeoxyuridine. *J. molec. Biol.* **70**: 337–350.

Weiss, R. A., Friis, R. R., Katz, E. and Vogt, P. K. (1971) Induction of avian tumor viruses in normal cells by physical and chemical carcinogens. *Virology* **46**: 920–938.

Welch, A. D. (1961) Some metabolic approaches to cancer chemotherapy. *Cancer Res.* **21**: 1475–1490.

Welch, A. D. and Prusoff, W. H. (1960) A synopsis of recent investigations of 5-iodo-2'-deoxyuridine. *Cancer Chemother. Rep.* **6**: 29–36.

Wempen, I., Duschinsky, R., Kaplan, L. and Fox, J. J. (1961) Thiation of nucleosides. IV. The synthesis of 5-fluoro-2'-deoxycytidine and related compounds. *J. Am. chem. Soc.* **83**: 4755–4766.

Wentworth, D. F. and Wolfenden, R. (1975) On the interaction of 3,4,5,6-tetrahydrouridine with human liver cytidine deaminase. *Biochemistry* **14**: 5099–5105.

Weygand, Von F., Wacker, A. and Dellweg, H. (1952) Stoffwechseluntersuchungen bei Mikroorganismen mit hilfe radioaktiver isotope II. *Z. Naturforsch.* **7B**: 18–25.

Wigand, R. and Klein, W. (1974) Properties of adenovirus substituted with iododeoxyuridine. *Arch. ges. Virusforsch.* **45**: 298–300.

Wildenhoff, K. E., Ipsen, J., Esmann, V., Ingemann-Jensen, J. and Poulsen, J. H. (1979) Treatment of herpes zoster with idoxuridine ointment, including a multivariate analysis of symptoms and signs. *Scand. J. Infect. Dis.* **11**: 1–9.

Witkin, E. M. and Parisi, E. C. (1974) Bromouracil mutagenesis: mispairins or misrepair? *Mutat. Res.* **75**: 407–409.

Wrathall, J. R., Newcomb, E. W., Balint, R., Zeitz, L. and Silagi, S. (1975) Suppression of melanoma cell tyrosinase activity and tumorigenicity after incorporation of bromouracil for one of two cell divisions. *J. cell Physiol.* **86**: 581–592.

Wu, A. M., Ting, R. C., Paran, M. and Gallo, R. C. (1972) Cordycepin inhibits induction of murine leukovirus production by 5-iodo-2'-deoxyuridine. *Proc. natn. Acad. Sci. USA* **69**: 3820–3824.

Yoshikura, H. (1974) Caffeine inhibits induction of endogenous C-type virus. *Nature, Lond.* **252**: 71.

Yoshikura, H., Zajdela, F., Perin, F., Perin-roussel, O., Jacquignon, P. and Latarjet, R. (1977) Enhancement of 5-iododeoxyuridine-induced endogenous C-type virus activation by polycyclic hydrocarbons. Apparent lack of parallels in between enhancement and carcinogenicity. *J. Natn. Cancer Inst.* **58**: 1035–1040.

Zamenhof, S. and Griboff, G. (1954) *E. coli* containing 5-bromouracil in its deoxyribonucleic acid. *Nature, Lond.* **174**: 307–308.

Žemla, J. (1974) Thymidine kinase induction in mouse embryo cells by polyoma virus. I. Effect of 5-bromo-2'-deoxyuridine. *Acta Virol.* **18**: 273–283.

Žemla, J. and Petrik, J. (1978) Effect of 5-bromo-2'-deoxyuridine on the *in vitro* DNA synthesizing activity of polyoma virus-infected cells. *Acta Virol.* **22**: 11–20.

Žemla, J. and Tarábek, J. (1981) Antiviral action of 5-bromo-2'-deoxyuridine and polyoma virus-specific RNA synthesis. *Antiviral Res.* **1**: 157–165.

CHAPTER 10

AZAPYRIMIDINE NUCLEOSIDES

Břetislav Rada and Jiří Doskočil*

Institute of Virology, Slovak Academy of Sciences, 817 03 Bratislava, Czechoslovakia;
* Institute of Molecular Genetics, Czechoslovak Academy of Sciences, 160 00
Prague, Czechoslovakia

CONTENTS

10.1. INTRODUCTION

The azapyrimidine analogs may be divided into two groups, substituted in position 6 or 5 of the pyrimidine ring, the most important members being 6-azauridine (z^6Urd) and 5-azacytidine (z^5Cyd), respectively.

6-Azauracil, i.e. 3,5-dioxo-2,3,4,5-tetrahydro-1,2,4-triazine, was first synthesized in 1947 by Seibert. Its potentialities as a metabolic inhibitor were discovered some 10 yr later by several groups who showed that it inhibited the growth of a number of microorganisms and several experimental tumours.

6-Azauridine was discovered in the course of studies on the mechanism of the antibacterial effect of 6-azauracil. In cultures of *Escherichia coli*, in the presence of sub-bacteriostatic concentrations of 6-azauracil, this analog disappeared gradually and a new compound accumulated, identified as z^6Urd (Škoda *et al.*, 1957a,b). Similarly z^6Urd was found as an intracellular anabolite in *Streptococcus faecalis*, cultivated in the presence of 6-azauracil (Handschumacher, 1957). The ribosylation of 6-azauracil in cultures of *Escherichia coli* was so efficient that this fermentation became the basis for industrial production of z^6Urd (Škoda and Šorm, 1958a). In addition, the analog has been prepared synthetically (Handschumacher, 1960a; Prystaš and Šorm, 1962; Cristescu, 1968).

As a consequence of the discoveries of the role of nucleic acids in viral replication, interest in the search for antiviral substances turned to analogs of pyrimidines, purines and nucleosides. Within 2 yr, 1960–1961, the antiviral activities of four nucleoside analogs, i.e. 5-fluorodeoxyuridine (Salzman, 1960), 6-azauridine (Rada *et al.*, 1960), 5-bromodeoxyuridine and 5-iododeoxyuridine (Herrmann, 1961) were demonstrated. The latter of these was used in practical chemotherapy. Simultaneously, with the detection of the antiviral effect of 6-azauridine, a new tissue culture method for studies of antiviral substances (agar-diffusion plaque-inhibition test) was developed (Rada *et al.*, 1960; Rada and Závada, 1962).

The first virus found sensitive to z^6Urd was vaccinia. This finding in 1960 represents one of the first lines of evidence that the synthesis of virus-specific RNA is a necessary step in the replication of DNA-containing animal viruses.

5-Azacytidine was synthesized by Pískala and Šorm (1964), in the course of systematic screening of potential anticancer nucleoside analogs. The same compound was later identified as a product of an actinomycete, *Streptoverticillium lakadanus*. Other compounds of the 5-azapyrimidine nucleoside series include 5-aza-2'-deoxycytidine, synthesized by Pliml and Šorm (1964). 5-Azauridine could not be prepared in crystalline form, being liable to dehydration; the resulting compound, 5',6-anhydro-6-hydroxy-5,6-dihydro-5-azauridine, generates 5-azauridine by hydrolysis when dissolved in aqueous medium (Piťhová *et al.*, 1965a,b) (Fig. 1).

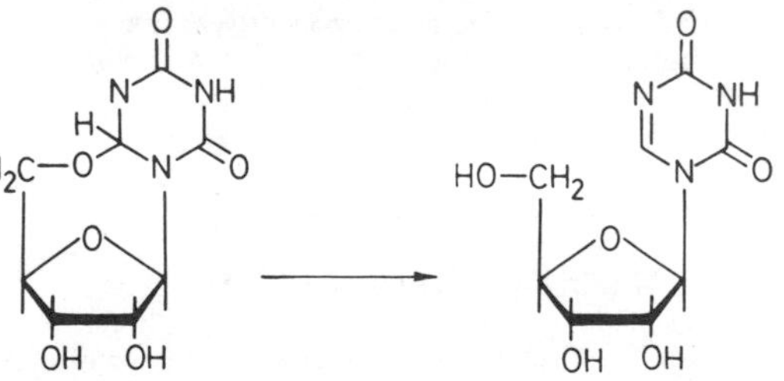

FIG. 1. Formation of 5-azauridine from 5',6-anhydro-6-hydroxy-5,6-dihydro-5-azauridine.

5-Azacytidine has been thoroughly investigated as an anticancer drug and has been covered in a review by Veselý and Čihák (1978), where a general survey on chemical reactivity and enzymatic conversion of 5-azapyrimidine nucleosides may also be found. In contrast to the field of oncology, only a few reports exist concerning the action of 5-azacytidine on the replication of animal viruses. A recent review on azapyrimidine nucleosides describes, in addition to mechanisms of action, their clinical application (Škoda, 1975).

10.2. 6-AZAURIDINE

10.2.1. CHEMISTRY OF 6-AZAURIDINE

z^6Urd (2-β-D-ribofuranosyl-*as*-triazine-3,5(2H, 4H) dione), MW 245.2, is a white, crystalline material, easily soluble in water (in excess of 1 g/ml). Aqueous solutions which are acid, are generally neutralized to physiological pH for biological use. Solutions of z^6Urd in the pH range 3–10 are stable to autoclaving and may be stored after sterilization. Since fermentation with *E. coli* effects conversion of the inexpensive 6-azauracil to the ribonucleoside in somewhat less than quantitative yield, it is important that the subsequent isolation procedures (charcoal absorption, ion-exchange chromatography and crystalliz-ation) remove as completely as possible all traces of unchanged 6-azauracil. Contamination of z^6Urd with as little as 1 per cent of 6-azauracil would be sufficient in many individuals to cause the appearance of central nervous system toxicity (Handschumacher *et al.*, 1962).

z^6Urd is ambivalent in its mimicry. It is sufficiently similar to uridine that its phosphorylation is catalyzed by uridine kinase. In the physiological pH range, ap-proximately 50 per cent of the triazine is unionized, a form which closely resembles uridine in its ionic and molecular configuration. Conversely, the active inhibitory form *in vivo* appears to be the ribonucleotide in which the negatively ionized triazine ring predominates in solutions above pH 7. The close ionic similarity between 6-azauridine 5′-phosphate and orotidylic acid, in which the carboxyl group is ionized in the physiological pH range, is apparent.

Crystallographic data reported by Schwalbe and Saenger (1973) demonstrate that z^6Urd crystallizes in the orthorhombic space group $P2_12_12_1$ with eight molecules per unit cell of dimensions $a = 20.230$, $b = 7.709$, $c = 12.863$ Å. The asymmetric unit contains two independent molecules of z^6Urd. Figure 2 shows bond distances between non-hydrogen atoms in these independent molecules A and B.

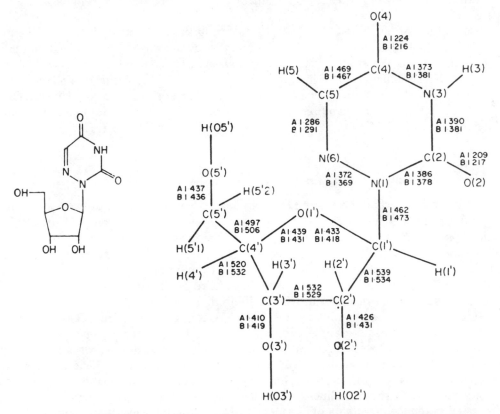

FIG. 2. Numbering convention with bond distances between non-hydrogen atoms in the molecule of 6-azauridine (estimated standard deviation 0.004Å). From Schwalbe and Saenger, 1973. Copyright © Academic Press Inc. (London) 1973. Reprinted with permission of the authors and publisher.

One of the most important parameters characterizing the conformation of a nucleoside is orientation around the glycosidic bond. It may be defined by the angle $C(2')-C(1')-N(1)-N(6)$ (Saenger and Scheit, 1970). This angle has a value of $-37.3°$ and $-42°$ in two independent molecules of z^6Urd, thus showing that, like uridine, z^6Urd has the *anti* conformation around this bond. Another characterization of the orientation of the sugar with respect to the base is the glycosyl torsion angle X_{CN}, defined according to Sundaralingam (1969), by the dihedral angle $O(1')-C(1')-N(1)-X(6)$. In studies of Singh and Hodgson (1974a) on 6-azacytidine, the unusual value of $+99.1°$ was found for this angle. Schwalbe and Saenger (1973) found that for z^6Urd this dihedral angle was $+81.3°$ in molecule A and $+76.3°$ in molecule B; however $+16.8°$ and $+23.8°$ were found in the two independent uridine molecules. Singh and Hodgson (1974b) noted that, except for formycin hydrobromide, all the 6-azapyrimidine and 8-azapurine nucleosides lie outside the conventional *syn* and *anti* ranges and are grouped together in a rather narrow range with an average X_{CN} of approximately $+100°$. It seems reasonable to conclude that the favored conformation describing the relative orientation of the base and the sugar in ribonucleosides with a nitrogen atom next to the glycosyl bond would have X_{CN} not far from $+100°$. This adoption of the '*high–anti*' conformation by both 6-azauridine and 6-azacytidine may be related to their biological effects.

Unlike uridine, z^6Urd exhibits a close approach of atom $N(6)$ to $C(2')$ of only 2.814 Å and 2.844 Å in the two independent molecules, compared with approximately 3.2 Å expected from the sum of the van der Waals' radii (Schwalbe and Saenger, 1973). Similar short intramolecular distances were also observed in 6-azacytidine (Singh and Hodgson, 1974a).

The ribose moieties in both molecules A and B take on the $C(3')$-endo envelope conformation (Schwalbe and Saenger, 1973), also observed in 6-azacytidine and cytidine (Singh and Hodgson, 1974a). The principal difference between the structures of z^6Urd and uridine is the conformation of the exocyclic $5'-CH_2OH$, which is *gauche-trans* in the former, a conformation only rarely observed for other $C(3')$-endo ribonucleosides in the crystalline state.

Calculations of Singh and Hodgson (1974a) using the complete neglect of differential overlap (CNDO/2) method on 6-azacytidine and z^6Urd have shown a net residual charge on $N(6)$ in both molecules of zero. There is probably very little coulombic interaction between $N(6)$ and $O(5')$ in either system, which explains why the barrier to rotation around the $C(4')-C(5')$ bond may be small. In uridine or cytidine, there is a positive attraction between $O(5')$ and $C(6)$ $H(6)$, which stabilizes the *gauche-gauche* conformation (Yathindra and Sundaralingam, 1973).

10.2.2. ANTIVIRAL SPECTRUM

z^6Urd inhibits several RNA and DNA viruses. Sixteen viruses out of twenty-six tested thus far are inhibited by z^6Urd (Table 1). The susceptible viruses are arranged in descending order of sensitivity to z^6Urd, dengue virus being the most sensitive, herpes virus showing borderline sensitivity. This order of sensitivity is approximate, since different viruses were studied in different cell systems, and the criteria of inhibition are not identical.

There are some differences in the sensitivity to z^6Urd of related viruses which are difficult to understand. Two viruses sensitive to inhibition by z^6Urd, dengue and Japanese encephalitis viruses, belong to the genus *Flavivirus*, formerly Arbovirus group B (Fenner, 1976); both are mosquito-borne viruses. Members of the genus *Alphavirus* (former Arbovirus group A), western equine encephalomyelitis virus, Sindbis virus and Semliki forest virus are insensitive to z^6Urd, whereas another alphavirus, Venezuelan equine encephalomyelitis virus, is sensitive. Similarly, in the genus *Influenzavirus*, fowl plague is sensitive to z^6Urd, whereas influenza viruses A, A1 and B1 are not. Smaller differences are expressed in the low sensitivity of cytomegalovirus, borderline sensitivity of human herpes virus, and complete resistance of five strains of porcine herpes (pseudo-rabies) virus. All three viruses are classified in the family *Herpetoviridae* and in one genus, *Herpesvirus*.

TABLE 1. *Antiviral Spectrum of 6-Azauridine*

Viruses inhibited	Viruses not inhibited
Dengue 2	Porcine herpes
Lymphocytic choriomeningitis	Influenza A, A1, B1
Reo 3	Newcastle disease*
Adeno 5	Vesicular stomatitis
Polyoma	Western equine encephalomyelitis
Measles	Sindbis
Turnip yellow mozaic	Semliki Forest
Fowl plague	Cardiovirus mengo
Venezuelan equine encephalomyelitis	
Rous sarcoma	
Vaccinia	
Enterovirus echo 7	
Japanese encephalitis	
Parainfluenza 3	
Cytomegalo	
Human herpes	

*Several strains have shown partial sensitivity.
Modified from Rada and Dragún, 1977.

Differences in sensitivity of related viruses are also observed with other antiviral substances, e.g. isatin 3-thio-semicarbazone, 2-(α-hydroxybenzyl)benzimidazole and guanidine (Bauer and Sheffield, 1959; Bauer, 1972).

10.2.2.1. *Dengue Virus*

Stollar *et al.* (1966) found that the multiplication of dengue virus was inhibited by z^6Urd at concentrations well below the cytotoxic range. The New Guinea B strain of dengue type 2 virus was grown in KB cells (cell line derived from human oral carcinoma). Under conditions of the one-step growth experiment, 5 μg/ml of z^6Urd inhibited virus yield by about 2 log units; 10 μg/ml caused inhibition by nearly 3 log units. The production of infectious virus, measured by plaque formation and virus hemagglutinin, was inhibited to the same extent by the analog. The dose-response curve is shown in Fig. 3. The inhibitory effect of 15 μg/ml of z^6Urd was fully reversible by 45 μg/ml of uridine when added during the first 6 hr post-infection.

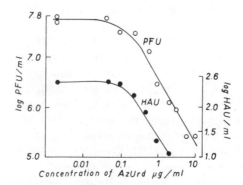

FIG. 3. Yield of plaque-forming units and hemagglutinin units of dengue virus as a function of concentration of 6-azauridine. Immediately after virus adsorption, z^6Urd was added to replicated cultures at the concentrations indicated. At 48 hr after infection, virus was harvested from each culture and assayed. From Stollar *et al.*, 1966. Copyright © Academic Press Inc. (London) 1966. Reprinted with permission of the authors and publisher.

10.2.2.2. Lymphocytic Choriomeningitis Virus

The inhibition of replication of lymphocytic choriomeningitis virus (strain Traub) by z^6Urd was studied in mouse L cells (Buck and Pfau, 1969). In the one-step growth experiments (multiplicity thirty mouse LD_{50} units per cell), virus replication was reduced about 80 per cent with the lowest concentration of analog tested (0.1 $\mu g/ml$). This inhibition increased to 98 per cent at 2.5 and 5 $\mu g/ml$ and 99 per cent at 10 $\mu g/ml$. A working concentration of 2.5 $\mu g/ml$ z^6Urd was used in further experiments because it inhibited the replication of the Traub strain by almost 2 log units, had no direct inactivating effect on the virus, elicited only slight inhibition of cell growth (10 per cent) and caused no cytotoxic effects over the 24-hr test period.

As the interval between infection and addition of the analog was increased, inhibition of virus replication progressively diminished. If z^6Urd was added either 2 or 4 hr after infection, the virus titers 24 hr after infection were 2 per cent of the controls not receiving z^6Urd. These titers increased to 56 per cent of the controls if z^6Urd was added at 6 hr after infection. There was no difference in titers between the controls and z^6Urd treated cultures if the analog was added after 8 hr post-infection. These data on the relation of the virus yield and the time of addition of z^6Urd can be taken to indicate that virus-specific RNA synthesis begins within 2 hr after infection, ends within 8 hr after infection, and precedes mature virion release by approximately 8 hr.

To test the assumption that z^6Urd was specifically blocking nucleic acid synthesis, experiments were carried out to determine if its inhibitory effect could be reversed by uridine. Three groups of cultures were infected with lymphocytic choriomeningitis virus; two of them received z^6Urd (2.5 $\mu g/ml$) after infection. To one of these groups with z^6Urd, uridine was added (final concentration 7.5 $\mu g/ml$) at 10 hr post-infection. At this time, in the presence of z^6Urd, there was virtually no increase over background infectivity in the tissue culture fluid, whereas the control cultures contained approximately forty times more virus than the inhibited cultures. An important finding was that, after uridine addition, peak titers were reached within 10 hr (from the 10–20 hr after infection), whereas a comparable rise in titer of the controls required the expected 16 hr. This shortened period for virus growth, not observed under normal conditions, may indicate that precursors necessary for viral reproduction, which are not dependent on genome replication, are formed within the cell in the presence of z^6Urd prior to uridine addition.

10.2.2.3. Reovirus

Reoviruses are an exception, since they contain double-stranded RNA. The Abney strain of reovirus type 3 was shown to be sensitive to z^6Urd (Rada and Shatkin, 1967). In one-step growth experiments (multiplicity 100 plague-forming units (PFU) per cell) in mouse L-929 cells, the formation of infectious virus was completely inhibited at a concentration of 50 $\mu g/ml$ or greater.

In reovirus-infected L cells which have been treated with 0.5 $\mu g/ml$ of actinomycin to suppress cellular RNA synthesis selectively, there is an increase in the rate of RNA synthesis beginning at about 6 hr after infection (Shatkin and Rada, 1967). It was shown that the newly formed RNA consists of virus-specific single-stranded RNA and double-stranded RNA. The effect of z^6Urd on the synthesis of these virus-specific RNAs was tested. z^6Urd (100 $\mu g/ml$), actinomycin (0.5 $\mu g/ml$) or both together were added to groups of infected and uninfected cultures. After 9.5 hr the cultures were exposed for one hour to ^{3}H-uridine and the specific activity of RNA determined. RNA synthesis in uninfected cells was reduced by 58 per cent, 86 per cent and 95 per cent in cells treated with 100 $\mu g/ml$ z^6Urd, 0.5 μg actinomycin/ml, or both together, respectively. In actinomycin-treated, virus-infected cells the RNA specific activity increased from 50 (actinomycin-treated uninfected cells) to 207 cpm/μg RNA; this 4-fold increase in rate of synthesis was due to virus-directed RNA formation. The increase did not occur in the presence of z^6Urd (57 cpm/μg), indicating that most virus-induced RNA synthesis is blocked by z^6Urd. However, the rate of RNA synthesis in infected cells treated with both drugs was 3-fold greater than in uninfected cells also treated with both drugs (57 cpm/μg vs 19 cpm/μg). The nature of the RNA which continues to be synthesized under these conditions remains to be determined (Rada and Shatkin, 1967).

10.2.2.4. Adenovirus

z^6Urd inhibits the multiplication of adenovirus type 5 in HeLa cell culture (Flanagan and Ginsberg, 1964). Dose response experiments (multiplicity 10 CC ID_{50} (cell culture median infective dose) per cell) showed that 100 μg/ml z^6Urd reduced virus multiplication so that the yield of virus at the end of the incubation period (30 hr) was equal to the amount present at the end of the adsorption period. By contrast addition of the base, 6-azauracil, in concentrations as high as 600 μg/ml, exerted no inhibitory effects on virus multiplication.

The sensitivity to z^6Urd of adenovirus types 1 and 4 was reported by Starcheus (Starcheus, 1965; Starcheus and Chernetsky, 1967). In HEp-2 (a cell line derived from human laryngeal carcinoma) cell monolayers, initiation of development of the virus cytopathic effect was delayed in the presence of z^6Urd by 2 days in both virus types. The intensity of the cytopathic effect was also decreased by the analog.

10.2.2.5. Polyoma Virus

The lytic cycle of polyoma virus was found to be sensitive to inhibition by z^6Urd (Gershon and Sachs, 1966). Two variants of polyoma virus, the large-plaque variant ILII and the small plaque SP2 variant, were studied using secondary cultures of mouse embryo cells. Under one-step growth conditions (multiplicity 100 PFU/cell) the virus yield of the ILII strain was reduced by 2 log units with 100 μg/ml of z^6Urd. Concentrations of 250 and 500 μg/ml resulted in maximum inhibition, i.e. virus titer at 40 hr post-infection was equivalent to that found at the end of the adsorption period.

The addition of 250 μg/ml of z^6Urd after the adsorption period resulted in 98–99 per cent inhibition of the synthesis of infectious DNA determined by plaque assay, and in complete inhibition of viral antigen synthesis determined by the fluorescent antibody technique. These results suggest that synthesis of RNA was required for the synthesis of viral DNA and viral antigen.

The mode of action of z^6Urd in the replication cycle of polyoma virus will be discussed further below (Section 10.2.5.4).

10.2.2.6. Measles Virus

z^6Urd inhibits the multiplication and cytopathic effect of measles virus (Leonard et al., 1971). Two strains, plaque-purified Edmonston strain in its 56–57th cell culture passage, and Woodfolk strain in its 7th passage, were examined in cultures of Vero cells (a continuous monkey cell line derived from African green monkey).

Incorporation of 100 μg/ml of z^6Urd into the agar overlay completely inhibited plaque development, 10 μg/ml of z^6Urd reduced plaque formation by approximately 2 log units, and 1 μg/ml had no effect. The analog also delayed plaque development.

In multiple-cycle experiments, suspension cultures were infected with measles virus at a multiplicity of approximately 0.01 (a low multiplicity more like that of natural infection). After either 1 or 18 hr of incubation, various concentrations of z^6Urd were added twice daily to cell cultures. The inhibitory effect was greater when z^6Urd was added 1 hr post-infection. In the case of the Edmonston strain, 100, 10 and 1 μg/ml of z^6Urd reduced the virus yield per total cell population by 4.3, 4.2 and 3.6 log units respectively, while the virus yield related to the number of infected cells (as determined by fluorescence antibody technique) was reduced by 2.8, 3.9 and 2.7 log units respectively. The same concentrations of z^6Urd also affected the replication of the Woodfolk strain, decreasing the virus yield per total cell population by

2.9–2.6 log units and the virus yield per infected cell by 3.7–2.2 log units. When the replication cycle was allowed to proceed for 18 hr before treatment, the inhibitory effect of z^6Urd was less marked. The decrease in the yield of the Edmonston strain on the basis of total cell population was 2.9, 2.3, 0.9 log units by 100, 10 and 1 μg/ml of z^6Urd respectively. The Woodfolk strain was not significantly affected by addition of the analog 18 hr post-infection. The interpretation was that the Woodfolk strain of measles virus synthesizes its RNA faster than does the Edmonston strain.

Subacute sclerosing panencephalitis (SSPE) is a rare, chronic and usually fatal inflammation of the brain which remained a disease of unknown aetiology until about 10 years ago. Since then histological, electronmicroscopic, serological and virological studies of the brain all indicate that measles virus is constantly present in neural and glial cells and the disease may be properly thought of as a chronic measles encephalitis. However, the precise nature of the association between virus and cell in this pathogenic state is not known, nor is it strictly certain, although generally assumed, that the virus has been present in brain cells since the attack of measles which has usually preceded the nervous condition by several years (Fraser and Martin, 1978).

Four viruses, wild measles (Woodfolk strain), attenuated measles (Edmonston strain), and JAC and LEC strains isolated from SSPE, were compared for their susceptibility to z^6Urd in culture of continuous cell line CV-1, derived from African green monkey kidney (ter Meulen et al., 1972).

Incorporation of 100 μg/ml of z^6Urd into the agar overlay completely inhibited plaque development of all four viruses. At a concentration of 10 μg/ml, plaque formation of the Woodfolk and Edmonston strains was reduced approximately 10-fold whereas the strains isolated from SSPE were completely inhibited. A concentration of 1 μg/ml had no effect on either strain of the standard measles virus, but resulted in a 10- to 100-fold plaque reduction of the strains isolated from SSPE. The analog also diminished the plaque size and delayed plaque development.

In multiple-cycle experiments, cells were infected in suspension at a multiplicity 0.01 PFU per cell. After either 1 or 18 hr of incubation various concentrations of z^6Urd were added twice daily to infected, as well as uninfected, cell cultures. When added 1 hr after infection, the strains isolated from SSPE were inhibited in the presence of 1 μg/ml by 3 log units and in the presence of 10 μg/ml completely. Under the same circumstances standard measles viruses could not be inhibited completely even by a concentration of 100 μg/ml. Addition of z^6Urd 18 hr after infection still substantially inhibited the replication of strains isolated from SSPE (3 log units). The two standard measles viruses were less affected by the analog at the later time.

The greater sensitivity of the strains isolated from SSPE to the action of z^6Urd serves as an additional characteristic distinguishing them from standard measles viruses. The present state of knowledge does not permit any specific predictions whether z^6Urd will be useful as a therapeutic agent in SSPE. It will be important to know whether some steps of the pathogenesis of SSPE occur outside the central nervous system, since z^6Urd does not pass the blood–brain barrier.

10.2.2.7. Turnip Yellow Mosaic Virus

Ralph and Wojcik (1976) studied the inhibition of turnip yellow mosaic virus by pyrimidine analogs. z^6Urd was used at concentration 100–200 μg/ml. In infected Chinese cabbage leaf discs the analog inhibited the synthesis of turnip yellow mosaic virus and increased the formation of empty virus protein shells. At the same molar concentrations, z^6Urd was more effective than 2-thiouracil and 6-azauracil.

10.2.2.8. Fowl Plague Virus

The action of z^6Urd on fowl plague virus in chick embryo cell cultures was investigated by Bukrinskaya and Asadullaev (1968). Under conditions of one-step growth (multiplicity 10 chick embryo ID_{50} per cell) the multiplication of the Baybridge strain of fowl plague virus was inhibited by more than 2 log units in the presence of 3 mg/ml of z^6Urd. Addition of the analog 2.5–3 hr post-infection still inhibited virus yield by 2 log units. But inhibition of hemagglutinin and complement fixing antigen formation was decreased on late addition of analog.

The Dobson strain was also found to be sensitive to z^6Urd. In the agar-diffusion test, z^6Urd suppressed plaque formation of this strain in an area of 48 mm in diameter in the absence of toxic effects (Rada, unpublished data).

10.2.2.9. Venezuelan Equine Encephalomyelitis Virus

z^6Urd at a concentration of 4 mg/ml completely inhibited the multiplication of Venezuelan equine encephalomyelitis virus in chick embryo cells (Kaverin and Emeliyanov, 1967). Further, the analog was used to study the course of the latent period of Venezuelan equine encephalomyelitis virus. Chick embryo cells were pretreated with 4 mg z^6Urd/ml for 2 hr. Then the cells were infected (multiplicity 100 PFU/cell) in the presence of z^6Urd. After adsorption the infected cells were washed and incubated again in the presence of the analog. Between 3–4 hr after infection z^6Urd was removed by careful washing, and medium without z^6Urd added. Subsequently at 30-min intervals, samples of the medium were taken for estimation of virus titer. The appearance of progeny·virus began 1–1.5 hr after the removal of the analog, whereas in nontreated control cultures progeny virus appeared 2.5–3 hr after infection. This indicates that the early stages of the latent period (before the onset of the synthesis of the bulk of virus RNA) occur in the presence of z^6Urd. The delay in appearance of progeny virus after removal of the analog coincides with virus RNA synthesis. It is suggested that there is no replication of Venezuelan equine encephalomyelitis virus RNA in the early stages of the latent period. If even limited early replication were necessary for the virus growth cycle then, after removal of z^6Urd up to the appearance of mature virions, the whole latent period of virus replication would be obliged to proceed.

10.2.2.10. Rous Sarcoma Virus

In studies using the agar-diffusion focus-inhibition technique, z^6Urd was found to inhibit focus formation by Rous sarcoma virus. The Prague strain of Rous sarcoma virus was grown in secondary chick embryo cells. The original method of Temin and Rubin (1958) was modified in that, instead of staining with neutral red, the cultures were fixed with Bouin's solution and subsequently stained with toluidine blue (Rada and Závada, 1962). A concentration of 200 mg/ml of z^6Urd used for the diffusion exerted complete inhibition of focus formation in dish cultures of 6 cm in diameter (Rada et al., 1964) (Fig. 4). This effect of z^6Urd was confirmed in in vivo experiments in chickens (see Section 10.2.6.1).

10.2.2.11. Vaccinia Virus

Vaccinia was the first virus found to be sensitive to z^6Urd. The analog inhibited plaque formation by the virus. Using the CL strain (derived from calf lymph) in chick embryo cells, the analog exerted an inhibitory zone of plaque formation of 62 mm in diameter. A high concentration of z^6Urd (500 mg/ml) was needed for the diffusion method. However, the absence of a toxic zone of damaged cells which do not take up neutral red documents a remarkably selective inhibition (Fig. 5).

The initial determination of selectivity was carried out in chorioallantoic membrane cultures, a technique developed by Tamm (1956) and used originally for the study of the antiviral effect of a large series of benzimidazole derivatives. The comparative semi-quantitative degree of macroscopic damage of the chorioallantoic membrane was exerted by a concentration of z^6Urd as high as 43 mg/ml; the comparative value of 75 per cent inhibition

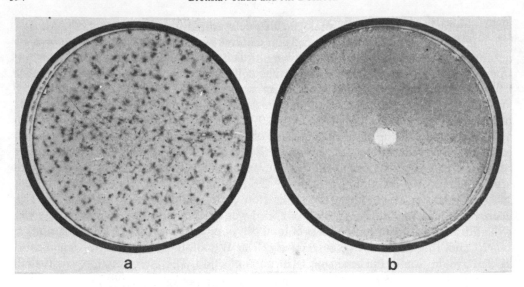

FIG. 4. Inhibitory effect of 6-azauridine on the formation of Rous sarcoma foci. (a) The culture of chick embryo cells was infected with about 400 focus-forming units of Rous sarcoma virus. Nine days after infection it was stained with toluidine blue. Control. (b) The culture of chick embryo cells was infected with the same dose of Rous sarcoma virus as in (a). After solidification of the agar overlay a glass well was mounted in the middle of the dish and 0.05 ml of z^6Urd solution, 200 mg/ml, was put into the well. Nine days after infection the cells were stained with toluidine blue. From Rada *et al.*, 1964.

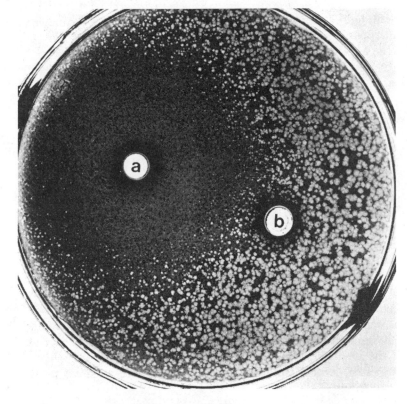

FIG. 5. Inhibitory effect of 6-azauridine on vaccinia virus. (a) z^6Urd—large zone of inhibition without zone toxicity. In the well 0.05 ml of z^6Urd solution, 500 mg/ml. (b) Benzimidazole—solution, 5 mg/ml. Monolayer of chick embryo cells was infected with 10^4 PFU of vaccinia virus. From Rada and Závada, 1962.

of virus multiplication was caused by 3 mg/ml of z^6Urd (99 per cent inhibition of virus multiplication by 10 mg/ml of z^6Urd). Thus the ratio toxic concentration/virus inhibitory concentration was 14 (Rada et al., 1960).

Further, the cytotoxic effect of the analog was studied in monolayers of chick embryo cells (Rada and Blaškovič, 1961). Concentrations of z^6Urd as high as 10 mg/ml caused minimal morphological changes (cytoplasmic granularity, cell rounding); even at 20 mg/ml, these changes were slight after 2 days exposure. In the presence of 5 mg/ml of z^6Urd the morphology of cells remained unchanged during a 6-day incubation period. In cultures with 10 and 5 mg/ml of z^6Urd the cell number was reduced in comparison with an untreated control. z^6Urd in chick embryo cultures exerted a cytostatic effect in the concentration range 2.5–10 mg/ml. Irreversible changes in cell multiplication were caused by 20 mg/ml of z^6Urd.

In experiments on the inhibition of virus cytopathic effect, tube cultures of chick embryo cells were inoculated with 50 CC ID_{50} of vaccinia virus and z^6Urd (1–5 mg/ml) was added immediately after infection. Infected untreated control cultures showed extensive cytopathic effect after 4 days incubation. In infected cultures containing 5 and 2.5 mg/ml of z^6Urd there were a few very small cytopathic foci. With 1 mg/ml z^6Urd the cytopathic foci were somewhat larger and more numerous. After 7 days post-infection a complete cytopathic effect developed in untreated control cultures. In cultures containing z^6Urd the cytopathic changes slightly increased but the great majority of the cells remained morphologically intact. The cytopathic foci did not spread. Thus, although the difference between the untreated group and the group of cultures with z^6Urd was very marked, at non-toxic concentrations, the analog was not able to completely inhibit the cytopathic effects of vaccinia virus.

One of the possible explanations of the small cytopathic foci in cultures treated with z^6Urd was the appearance of a mutant resistant to the analog. Several pyrimidine and puridine derivatives are mutagens. This possible resistance to z^6Urd was investigated. Virus material from cultures containing 5 mg/ml of z^6Urd in which the small cytopathic foci had developed was titered, and cultures without and with z^6Urd (5 mg/ml) were infected with 50 CC ID_{50} of this material. At the same time another two groups of cultures (with and without z^6Urd) were infected each with 50 CC ID_{50} of the original stock virus. No difference in sensitivity to z^6Urd between these two virus materials was found, i.e. development of complete cytopathic effect in both untreated groups, and development of small cytopathic foci in both groups of cultures containing the analog, were the same. It was assumed, therefore, that the development of the small cytopathic foci in cultures treated with z^6Urd was not caused by resistant mutants of vaccinia virus.

The cytotoxic effect of z^6Urd in HeLa cells (Rada and Blaškovič, 1966) was studied by means of the reduction of the single cell plating efficiency. However, this method yielded highly variable results. The inhibition of HeLa cell growth was then investigated by exposure of cell monolayers in tubes to several concentrations of the analog for 24 hr, i.e. for the same period as in the inhibition experiments. Subsequently the cell numbers in the cultures were estimated daily up to the 3rd day. z^6Urd caused irreversible damage of 20, 40 and 50 per cent to cells at concentrations of 0.1, 1 and 10 mg/ml, respectively. After removal of the analog, the cells multiplied at the same rate or slightly slower than those in untreated control cultures. Thus HeLa cells are sensitive to about ten times lower concentrations of z^6Urd than chick embryo cells.

In suspension cultures of HeLa cells the dose-response curve in one-step growth experiments showed that 1 mg/ml of z^6Urd exerted 99 per cent inhibition of the multiplication of the CL strain of vaccinia virus. The same sensitivity for another strain (strain not given) of vaccinia virus in HeLa cells was reported by Loh (1964). Further data are discussed below (Section 10.2.5).

10.2.2.12. Enterovirus Echo

z^6Urd was effective against echovirus type 7. Under one-step growth conditions in human embryo fibroblast cultures the analog (4 mg/ml) completely inhibited virus multiplication as measured by hemagglutinin production (Kaverin and Emeliyanov, 1967). Incubation of infected cells in the presence of z^6Urd resulted in a 45 min delay in the appearance of progeny virus after removal of the analog. This result is interpreted like those obtained with Venezuelan equine encephalomyelitis virus.

10.2.2.13. Japanese Encephalitis Virus and Hypr Virus

Several arboviruses have been examined for sensitivity to z^6Urd, with the aim of using this as a marker for classification within the arbovirus group (Grešíková and Rada, 1972). Chick embryo cell cultures were infected with a high dose, 10^6–10^7 mouse LD_{50} units of Japanese encephalitis virus (strain P3-Peking) or with Hypr (tick-borne encephalitis) virus. The antiviral activity was assessed from the degree of inhibition of the virus hemagglutination yield (at 48 hr post-infection). In control experiments, hemagglutinins of these viruses were exposed to z^6Urd (10 mg/ml) for 2 hr; the analog had no direct effect on the hemagglutinin activity.

The formation of Japanese encephalitis virus hemagglutinin was found to be sensitive to z^6Urd. The analog (10 mg/ml) completely inhibited virus hemagglutinin formation, whereas the titer of hemagglutinin in control cultures not treated with z^6Urd was 1280. The hemagglutinin formation of Hypr virus was less affected by the analog while that of Sindbis virus, and Western equine encephalomyelitis virus, was not inhibited by the analog.

10.2.2.14. Parainfluenza 3 Virus

z^6Urd at low concentrations, 125 μg/ml, inhibited multiplication of parainfluenza 3 virus (strain EA-106), with some inhibition of virus-induced giant cell formation in WISH cells (human amnion cell line). Concentrations up to 500 μg/ml did not exert any apparent damage to WISH cells as assessed from trypan blue staining. In the presence of 2 mg/ml of z^6Urd the virus-infected cultures were able to take up the vital stain (neutral red or Janus green) whereas in the absence of the analog they did not. These concentrations of z^6Urd strongly inhibited the cytopathogenicity of parainfluenza virus (Korbecki et al., 1968).

Another virus of this group, Newcastle disease virus, a thermostable mutant C of the strain Beaudette, was found to be partially sensitive to z^6Urd. In chick embryo cells the analog, at a concentration of 3.2 mg/ml, reduced multiplication by 90 per cent (Schäfer et al., 1967).

10.2.2.15. Cytomegalovirus

Cytomegalovirus causes cytomegalic inclusion disease, a serious infection among infants and a serious complication in intensive anticancer therapy and of organ and tissue transplantation. Chemotherapy would appear the most feasible approach to its control.

The effect of z^6Urd on cytomegalovirus was investigated by Demidova et al. (1969). The virus was grown in human embryo fibroblast cultures containing 250–750 μg/ml of z^6Urd. The analog exerted partial inhibition of virus cytopathic effect only when the cultures were pretreated with z^6Urd before infection and again supplemented with z^6Urd after infection. Despite this pretreatment, inhibition of the cytopathic effect was very low: the number of cytopathic foci was reduced from 30–73 in control cultures to 10–40 in cultures with 500 μg/ml of z^6Urd.

However, in studies by Sidwell et al. (1972), cytomegalovirus was found more sensitive to z^6Urd. Monolayers of WI-38 cells (a human diploid cell line) grown in tubes were infected with 32, 320 and 3200 CC ID_{50} of Casazza strain, i.e. conditions of a multiple-cycle experiment. z^6Urd (0.1–100 μg/ml) was added immediately after the virus and then at additional times in medium changes 2 and 4 days later. Antiviral activity was determined by inhibition of viral cytopathic effect. Thirty compounds out of 320 studied were considered markedly active against cytomegalovirus; z^6Urd was among those possessing virus ratings 1.0–1.2 (the virus rating method (Ehrlich *et al.*, 1965): a weighted measure of antiviral activity determined numerically by the degree of inhibition of viral cytopathic effect, concentration of compound, and cytotoxicity of compound. Virus rating > 1.0 represents definite antiviral activity, 0.5–0.9 moderate or questionable activity, and < 0.5 is considered insignificant). 6-Azauracil was not active (virus rating 0.3).

10.2.2.16. Human Herpes Virus

A low degree of sensitivity to z^6Urd in herpes viruses is dependent on the cell system and on the virus strain.

Kaufman and Maloney (1963) found no sensitivity to z^6Urd of herpes virus strain isolated from a patient with dentritic keratitis. They tested twenty pyrimidine, purine and nucleoside analogs in rabbit kidney cells infected with high virus doses. Only 5-chloro-, 5-bromo- and 5-iododeoxyuridine prevented the progression of cytopathic changes of herpes virus. z^6Urd at a concentration of 1 mg/ml did not inhibit.

On the other hand, Galegov *et al.* (1968a) found inhibition of more than 2 log units in the multiplication of the L-2 strain of herpes virus with 700 μg/ml of z^6Urd in human embryo cell cultures. In cultures pretreated with the analog for 1 hr before infection, inhibition of virus yield was higher than 3 log units. The analog was not able to inhibit the virus cytopathic effect completely, but it decreased and delayed the appearance of cytopathic changes.

Two giant cell-forming strains JES (fR variant) and L3-2S of herpes virus growing in rabbit kidney cells were employed by Falke and Rada (1970). Dose response experiments showed only a 1-log unit inhibition of virus yield with 10 mg/ml of z^6Urd. Assuming that starving of the cells could exhaust the pyrimidine pool, a procedure of cell starving (18 hr before infection in simple Hanks' solution) was included in the experiments. The virus yield in starved cells was inhibited by about 2 log units with 10 mg/ml of z^6Urd. Furthermore, a considerable reduction of giant cell formation in starved cells by z^6Urd treatment was observed.

10.2.2.17. Resistant Viruses

Multiplication of the following viruses was not affected by z^6Urd: porcine herpes (pseudorabies) virus—strains BUK, SPO 65/1, CVOS, SHO, RICE in chick embryo cells (Rada, unpublished data); influenza virus A—strain PR8 in surviving chorioallantoic membrane cultures (Rada *et al.*, 1960), influenza virus A1—strain Leningrad 3711/49 in surviving chorioallantoic membrane cultures and chick embryos (Sláviková and Rada, 1973); influenza virus B1—strain Košice 266-10/65 in surviving chorioallantoic membrane cultures and chick embryos (Sláviková and Rada, 1973); Newcastle disease virus—strain Hertfordshire in chick embryo cells (Rada *et al.*, 1960; Rada and Hanušovská, 1970); vesicular stomatitis virus—strain Indiana in chick embryo cells (Sláviková and Rada, 1973); western equine encephalomyelitis virus—strain WEE-15 in chick embryo cells (Rada and Hanušovská, 1970; Grešíková and Rada, 1972); Sindbis virus—strain AR-339 in chick embryo cells (Grešíková and Rada, 1972; Sláviková and Rada, 1973); Semliki Forest virus—prototype strain in chick embryo cells (Sláviková and Rada, 1973), cardiovirus Mengo in Novikoff rat hepatoma cell line N1S1-67 (Korbecki and Plagemann, 1969).

10.2.2.18. Rickettsiae and Chlamydiae

Brezina *et al.* (1962) investigated the effect of z^6Urd on the multiplication of *Coxiella burnetii*, *Rickettsia prowazekii* and *Rickettsia typhi (mooseri)*. Infection of chick embryos with high doses (10^5 ID$_{50}$ units) of Nine mile strain of *Coxiella burnetti* was significantly affected by a dose of 10 mg of z^6Urd per embryo; the analog caused a 2-day delay shift of 50 per cent mortality. With *Rickettsia prowazekii* (Breinl strain) the analog caused a shift of the 50 per cent mortality within the relative lethal phase, but the delay was not significant. Similarly, infection of mice with *Rickettsia typhi* (Mexico strain) was not significantly affected by 2.5 mg doses of z^6Urd administered s.c. at 8-hr intervals.

Inhibitory effect of z^6Urd on the growth of *Chlamydia psittaci (ornitosis agent)* was reported by Terskikh *et al.* (1968). The strain 15 of ornithosis agent was cultivated in A1-cells (human amnion cell line). The efficacy of the analog was assessed from inhibition of inclusion formation and infectivity (determined in mice or chick embryos). z^6Urd at 450 μg/ml added immediately after infection markedly inhibited the formation of cytoplasmic DNA inclusions. Addition of this dose 3 hr before infection caused complete inhibition of the growth of the ornithosis agent.

10.2.3. STRUCTURE—ACTIVITY RELATIONSHIPS

Structure–activity relationships of z^6Urd derivatives show that any modification in the pyrimidine ring or in the sugar moiety reduces or abolishes the antiviral activity.

Conversion of z^6Urd into its L-enantiometer L-z^6Urd resulted in a remarkable decrease of activity and selectivity. This analog (at the same concentration as z^6Urd) exerted a low inhibitory activity with vaccinia virus and moderate toxicity. Slight inhibitory effect was observed with Newcastle disease and western equine encephalomyelitis viruses (Rada, unpublished data). It is noteworthy that L-nucleosides can enter mammalian cells *in vivo* (Jurovčík *et al.*, 1971), whereas penetration of bacteria is not possible (Votruba *et al.*, 1971). The presence of toxic and inhibitory effects suggests penetration of the nucleoside into host cells.

6-Azacytidine did not inhibit plaque formation of vaccinia, Newcastle disease and western equine encephalomyelitis viruses. It did not cause any inhibition of the vaccinia virus cytopathic effect at nontoxic concentration (Rada, unpublished data). This analog was as effective in inhibition of cytomegalovirus (Casazza strain) as z^6Urd (Sidwell *et al.*, 1972). But in earlier *in vivo* studies with influenza and vaccinia viruses, 6-azacytidine was found to be ineffective (Sidwell *et al.*, 1968). It is possible that penetration of the analogs is the limiting factor in their biological activity. In noninfected tissues, such as liver or Ehrlich ascitic carcinoma, no essential difference was detected in the accumulation of 6-azacytidine 5′-phosphate or 6-azauridine 5′-phosphate. However, 6-azacytidine 5′-phosphate, compared with 6-azauridine 5′-phosphate, is about ten times less effective as an inhibitor of orotidylic acid decarboxylase (Handschumacher *et al.*, 1963). But the antitumour activities of z^6Urd and 6-azacytidine were similar (Šorm and Veselý, 1961).

5-Azacytidine (see Section 10.3) inhibited virus plaque formation with vaccinia (area diameter 45 mm), Newcastle disease (39 mm) and western equine encephalomyelitis (38 mm). In comparison, z^6Urd inhibited only vaccinia (62 mm) (Fig. 5). 5-Azacytidine was the most effective compound against Newcastle disease virus out of several hundreds of compounds tested. A minor toxic effect of 5-azacytidine, in diffusion test, was indicated by the appearance of a small toxic zone, in which after neutral red staining the cells were slighly orange and the cell monolayer density was reduced (Rada, unpublished data).

6-Azauridine 5′-phosphate did not inhibit vaccinia, Newcastle disease and western equine encephalomyelitis viruses. The penetration of nucleotides into mammalian cells is very limited. Some inhibitory or toxic effect might be due to the dephosphorylation product z^6Urd. It seems that, at least for several viruses, the *in vivo* conversion of z^6Urd to the nucleotide is the basis of selective inhibition.

6-Azauracil was ineffective in inhibition of the Casazza strain of cytomegalovirus, and in protection of mice infected with the PR8 strain of influenza A virus (Sidwell *et al.*, 1972). No activity was exhibited by 6-azauracil in plaque inhibition of vaccinia, Newcastle disease and western equine encephalomyelitis viruses (Rada, unpublished data). This base analog had moderate, but reproducible, activity against mouse neurovaccinia (IHD strain) infection (Sidwell *et al.*, 1968).

5-Azauracil does not show any inhibitory effect on plaque formation by vaccinia, Newcastle disease and western equine encephalomyelitis viruses. Nor does it inhibit the vaccinia virus cytopathic effect even at a concentration very close to the toxic one. 5-Azauracil and its derivatives were effective in inhibition of microorganisms and experimental tumours (Elion *et al.*, 1958; Šorm *et al.*, 1960; Škoda *et al.*, 1962).

The inhibitory effect of N-*methyl-*, *thio-*, and *methyl-mercaptoderivatives* of *6-azauracil* on vaccinia virus (Šmejkal *et al.*, 1962) was assessed from the degree of inhibition of cytopathic changes of the CL strain of vaccinia virus in monkey kidney cell cultures. The derivatives were tested at 100 μg/ml and the inhibitory effects were compared with that of z^6Urd. Out of twenty-two derivatives studied, eleven were ineffective, including one toxic derivative; four derivatives exhibited lower activity than z^6Urd; four derivatives exhibited the same activity as z^6Urd and three derivatives were more active than z^6Urd (Table 2).

TABLE 2. *Inhibitory Effect of* N-*Methyl-*,*Thio-*, *and Methylmercapto-Derivatives of 6-Azauracil on the Cytopathic Changes of Vaccinia Virus, in Comparison with 6-Azauridine*

Inhibitory effect	Derivatives of 6-azauracil
Ineffective	2-Thiouracil
	2-Thio-6-azauracil
	2-Thiothymine
	2-Methylmercapto-6-azathymine
	1-Methyl-2-methylmercapto-6-azauracil
	3-Methyl-2-methylmercapto-6-azathymine
	2-Thio-6-azauracil
	1-Methyl-4-thio-6-azauracil
	2,4-Dithio-6-azauracil
Toxic	1-Methyl-2,4-dithio-6-azauracil
Less effective than z^6Urd	2-Thio-6-azathymine
	1,3-Dimethyl-2-thio-6-azauracil
	2-Methylmercapto-6-azauracil
	1-Methyl-4-methylmercapto-6-azauracil
Effective similarly to z^6Urd	1-Methyl-2-thio-6-azauracil
	3-Methyl-2-thio-6-azauracil
	3-Methyl-4-thio-6-azauracil
	1,3-Dimethyl-4-thio-6-azauracil
More effective than z^6Urd	3-Methyl-2,4-dithio-6-azauracil
	3-Methyl-2-methylmercapto-4-thio-6-azauracil
	3,5-Dimethylmercapto-1,2,4-triazine

Monolayers of monkey kidney cells in tube cultures were infected with 10, 100 or 1000 CC ID_{50} of the CL strain of vaccinia virus. The analog was added immediately after virus infection.
From Šmejkal *et al.*, 1962.

3-Methyl-2,4-dithio-6-azauracil was the most effective derivative. Because it was toxic for monkey kidney cells at a concentration of 100 μg/ml, the effects of 10 μg/ml of this derivative were compared with the effects of 10 μg/ml of z^6Urd. 3-Methyl-2,4-dithio-6-azauracil was able to suppress almost completely virus cytopathic changes up to 48 hr post-infection when the cultures were infected with a virus dose of 10^3 CC ID_{50} or up to 24 hr when the virus infecting dose was 10^4 CC ID_{50}. Thereafter the development of virus cytopathic changes increased and peaked at 72–96 hr post-infection. The treatment with z^6Urd in parallel cultures caused a delay of the cytopathic effect which preceded by 12 hr the development of the cytopathic changes in cultures treated with 3-methyl-2,4-dithio-6-azauracil. Thus, this derivative is more effective at the lower concentration used and it is also more toxic than z^6Urd (it was necessary to use lower concentration for the inhibition). A comparison of both the toxic and virus-inhibitory concentrations of this derivative with those of z^6Urd would be necessary.

The delay of virus cytopathic changes caused by 3-methyl-2-methylmercapto-4-thio-6-azauracil and 3,5-dimethylmercapto-1,2,4-triazine was about 12–24 hr longer than that observed in cultures treated with z^6Urd. This delay was observed only in cultures infected with 10^2 and 10^3 CC ID_{50} of vaccinia virus but not in cultures infected with 10^4 CC ID_{50}.

3-Methylmercapto-4-thio-6-azauracil was reported to inhibit picorna virus multiplication (Zeitlenok *et al.*, 1965) at a concentration of 100 μg/ml, the highest not causing cell degeneration during 96 hr incubation. In monkey kidney cells under multiple-cycle experimental conditions this derivative inhibited the multiplication of the attenuated strain LSc 2ab of type 1 poliovirus by more than 3 log units and the virulent strain Mahoney by 1 log unit. In one-step growth experiments the derivative was unable to inhibit LSc strain multiplication by 2 log units. In pilot experiments enterovirus echo 7 was found to be inhibited by 3-methylmercapto-4-thio-6-azauracil.

6-Azathymidine (Sidwell *et al.*, 1972), in the concentration range 1–10 mg/ml, was found to inhibit markedly the cytopathic effect of the Casazza strain of cytomegalovirus in WI-38 cells, exhibiting a virus rating of 1.2–1.6.

10.2.4. ANTIVIRAL ACTIVITY OF 6-AZAURIDINE AND OTHER ANALOGS IN COMBINATION

Nine pyrimidine and purine analogs were studied for their single or combined inhibitory effect on the multiplication of adenovirus 9–15 (strain 5399, subgroup 11) in HeLa cell monolayer tube cultures (Wirjawan and Wigand, 1978). The criterion of inhibition was the total suppression of the formation of infectious virus. In combination experiments z^6Urd showed synergism in inhibition of adenovirus replication with all studied inhibitors (5-fluoro-2'-deoxyuridine, 5-iodo-2'-deoxyuridine, 1-β-D-arabinofuranosylcytosine, 9-β-D-arabinofuranosyladenine, 6-mercaptopurine, 6-thioguanine, amethopterin, hydroxyurea). The z^6Urd plus arabinofuranosyladenine or 5-fluoro-2'-deoxyuridine combination showed a high degree of synergism, i.e. reduction to 1/16 of the concentration of both inhibitors sufficient for complete inhibition of virus replication (in comparison with the concentration used for single inhibitor). Moreover, the z^6Urd plus arabinofuranosylcytosine combination was very effective, causing reduction to 1/128 of the arabinofuranosylcytosine concentration (Wirjawan and Wigand, 1978). However, in similar studies with vaccinia virus (strain IHD in Vero cell cultures), the z^6Urd combinations with the same substances showed indifference (Surjono and Wigand, 1981).

(S)-9-(2,3-Dihydroxypropyl)adenine ((S)-DHPA) is one of novel type nucleoside analogs in which the sugar moiety is substituted by an aliphatic chain resembling incomplete portion of sugar moiety. It was synthesized by Holý (1975). (S)-DHPA was shown to inhibit replication of several RNA and DNA viruses (De Clercq *et al.*, 1978; Sodja and Holý, 1980; Rada *et al.*, 1980). In agar-diffusion plaque-inhibition test (S)-DHPA alone exerted an inhibitory zone of 40–45 mm with vaccinia virus. However, the z^6Urd plus (S)-DHPA combination gave a very high degree of virus-inhibitory activity. This effect was demonstrated by an experimental arrangement in which z^6Urd (500 mg/ml) was diffusing from the center of the culture and (S)-DHPA was incorporated into the agar overlay at a subinhibitory concentration (100 μg/ml). In a separate control culture, (S)-DHPA alone at this concentration exerted a minute if any reduction of the plaque size of vaccinia virus. The z^6Urd plus (S)-DHPA combination exerted an inhibition of plaque formation of 135–140 mm in diameter thus exceeding the effect of cytosine arabinoside (Rada and Holý, 1980). In contrast to the marked effect found in the plaque-inhibition test, in one-step growth experiments in suspension cultures of HeLa cells the z^6Urd plus (S)-DHPA combination did not show any effect of synergism; additive inhibitory effect was found at lower concentration of both compounds. It remains to be established whether the synergic effect in plaque-inhibition test is based on pretreatment, since the plaque-inhibition test in contrast to one-step growth experiments also detects the compounds effective in the pretreatment only. Seventeen analogs related to DHPA modified at the base or at the aliphatic chain of DHPA were tested for the antiviral effect of their combination with z^6Urd. Several of these analogs caused enhancements of the inhibitory effect of z^6Urd but markedly lower than the enhancement caused by (S)-DHPA (Rada and Holý, 1980).

10.2.5. MODE OF ACTION OF 6-AZAURIDINE

10.2.5.1. 6-Azauridine 5'-Phosphate

In vivo z⁶Urd is not effective as such. It is converted by uridine kinase to 6-azauridine 5'-phosphate which is the actual inhibitor, inhibiting the enzyme orotidylic acid decarboxylase.

6-Azauridine 5'-phosphate was characterized by X-ray structure analysis and conformation energy computation in relation with functional mechanism by Saenger and co-workers (Saenger and Suck, 1973; Saenger *et al.*, 1979). 6-Azauridine 5'-phosphoric acid crystallizes as the trihydrate, space group $P2_12_12_1$ and cell constants $a = 20.615$, $b = 6.265$, $c = 11.881$ Å. The distances and bond angles within the 6-azauridine 5'-phosphoric acid molecules are comparable to those observed for z⁶Urd.

The conformation of 6-azauridine 5'-phosphoric acid about the glycosidic linkage is *anti* with the torsional angle $C(2')–C(1')–N(1)–N(6)$ $-33°$. The angle $N(6)–N(1)–C(1')–O(4')$ is $86.3°$.

The ribose moiety is in a twisted $C(2')$-exo, $C(3')$-endo (T_2^3) conformation. The orientation around the $C(4')–C(5')$ bond is not *gauche-gauche* as in all the ribonucleoside 5'-phosphates so far studied, but *gauche-trans* as in z⁶Urd, with torsional angles $O(1')–C(4')–C(5')$ $71°$, and $O(4')–C(4')–C(5')–O(5')$ $-172°$. Similarly, nuclear magnetic resonance studies (Hruska *et al.*, 1973) on solutions of 6-azauridine 5'-phosphate and z⁶Urd have shown that the presence of the 6-azauracil base has a destabilizing influence, relative to uracil, upon the *gauche-gauche* conformation around the $C(4')–C(5')$ bond. This destabilizing effect is more conspicuous for the monophosphate derivative. 6-Azauridine 5'-phosphate therefore retains its unusual solid state conformation in solution as well.

The change in molecular geometry of 6-azauridine 5'-phosphate caused by the change in conformation from *gauche-gauche* to *gauche-trans* is shown in Fig. 6. When uridine 5'-phosphate and 6-azauridine 5'-phosphate are superimposed so that the $C(1')$, $O(1')$, $C(4')$ atoms coincide, then the 5'-phosphate groups in both molecules are 4.25 Å apart. This difference is enough to produce different physical, chemical and biological properties for the two 5'-nucleotides.

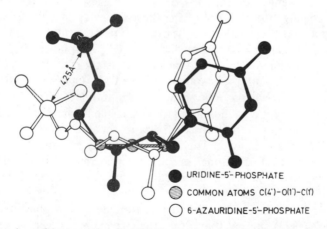

URIDINE-5'-PHOSPHATE

COMMON ATOMS C(4')–O(1')–C(1')

6-AZAURIDINE-5'-PHOSPHATE

FIG. 6. Comparison of the structures of uridine 5'-phosphate and of 6-azauridine 5'-phosphate. The two molecules were drawn from crystallographic atomic coordinates in such a way that the hatched atoms $C(4')–O(1')–C(1')$ are common to both. The sugar puckering modes, and the orientation of the $C(1')–N$ and $C(4')–C(5')$ bonds, are different. From Saenger and Suck, 1973. Copyright © Macmillan (Journals) Ltd, 1973. Reproduced with permission of the authors and publisher.

Conformational energy calculations of Saenger *et al.* (1979) indicate that 6-azauridine 5'-phosphate may adopt an extreme *anti* conformation not allowed for uridine 5'-phosphate and the same unusual *trans-gauche* conformation about the $C(4')–C(5')$ bond in orotidine 5'-phosphate. On this basis, the functioning of 6-azauridine 5'-phosphate as an inhibitor of orotidine 5'-phosphate decarboxylase can be explained as being due to its structural similarity to the substrate.

From calculations and experimental data, Saenger *et al.* (1979) suggest that orotidine 5′-phosphate, which is in the *syn* conformation, and *gauche-gauche*, is forced during decarboxylation to rotate the base moiety from *syn* towards *anti* and the exocyclic —CH₂—O-phosphate group to adopt the *gauche-gauche* conformation:

Substance	Ord-5′-P	U⁻rd-5′-P	Urd-5′-P
Conformation	*syn, trans-gauche*	*anti, trans-gauche*	*anti, gauche-gauche*

These conformational changes are shown in Fig. 7.

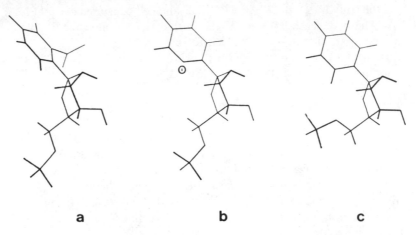

FIG. 7. Succession of conformation changes associated with the decarboxylation of orotidine 5′-phosphate to uridine 5′-phosphate. (a) Ord-5′-P (b) U⁻rd-5′-P (base rotation) (c) Urd-5′-P (—CH₂OP rotation). The three molecules are sketched in their lowest energy conformation. From Saenger *et al.*, 1979. Copyright © John Wiley and Sons Inc. 1979. Reproduced with permission of the authors and publisher.

A hypothesis on the mechanism of action of z⁶Urd based on the conformational structure was developed by Saenger *et al.* (1979). They suggest that orotidine 5′-phosphate decarboxylase recognizes the presence of the carboxyl group of orotidine 5′-phosphate on the one hand and its phosphate group on the other, so that the substrate binds to the enzyme simultaneously via its C(7) carboxyl group and its —CH₂—O-phosphate group. The oxygen atom was selected as that involved in binding and the distance O(5′)–O(7) determined. If the enzyme is able to bind the O(5′)–phosphate and the C(7)–O(7) groups 6.51 Å apart from each other, one should ask what atomic group of 6-azauridine 5′-phosphate could mimic the carboxyl group of orotidylic acid in binding to the enzyme. From distance determinations it appears that the carbonyl group C(2)=O(2) is a reasonable candidate for mimicking the carboxyl group of orotidylic acid. This hypothesis thus explains why 6-azauridine 5′-phosphate mimics, by conformational properties, a chemically unrelated substance like orotidine 5′-phosphate and is a competitive inhibitor of orotidine 5′-phosphate decarboxylase.

Concerning the conversion of z⁶Urd to 6-azauridine 5′-phosphate by uridine kinase, Saenger and Suck (1973) suggest that either the enzyme is not very specific, as both the substrate and reaction product exhibit an unusual *gauche-trans* conformation, or it forces the substrate z⁶Urd to assume a 'normal' *gauche-gauche* conformation like uridine during bonding at the active site.

10.2.5.2. *Studies in Uninfected Cells*

Inhibition of orotidylic acid decarboxylase by 6-azauridine 5′-phosphate. In cell-free extracts of *E. coli*, and in animal or tumour cells, z⁶Urd is phosphorylated to 6-azauridine 5′-phosphate (Škoda and Šorm, 1958b; Habermann and Šorm, 1958; Pasternak and Handschumacher, 1959). This conversion is carried out by uridine kinase and requires the presence of adenosine 5'-triphosphate. The affinity of the enzyme for z^6Urd is similar to that for uridine.

Studies in mouse liver and intestine, in L-5178-Y lymphoma, and in adenocarcinoma-755 *in vivo* yield data suggesting that the inhibition of orotidylic acid decarboxylase by 6-azauridine 5'-phosphate is the primary site of action responsible for the retardation of tumour growth when z^6Urd is administered. Incorporation of orotidylic acid into the nucleic acid of mouse tissues and mouse tumours *in vivo* is depressed by z^6Urd, whereas the incorporation of uridine is increased. Experimental mouse tumours, the growth of which has been inhibited by continued administration of z^6Urd, accumulate large amounts of orotidine. The metabolism of orotic acid by cell-free extracts from L-5178-Y tumours is inhibited by z^6Urd and its 5'-phosphate, leading to accumulation of orotidylic acid; however, uracil and uridine metabolism are unaffected by 6-azauracil or z^6Urd. Orotidine is not metabolized by such extracts, but orotidylic acid breaks down to orotidine in the presence of inhibitory concentrations of 6-azauridine 5'-phosphate (Pasternak and Handschumacher, 1959).

This unnatural ribonucleotide is a competitive inhibitor of orotidylic acid decarboxylase of yeast. Other phosphorylated derivatives of z^6Urd, 6-azauridine 2'- and 3'-phosphate, 6-azauridine 2',5'-diphosphate, 6-azauridine 3',5'-diphosphate, 6-azauridine 5'-diphosphate, 6-azauridine 5'-triphosphate and 6-azauracil or z^6Urd are noninhibitory (Handschumacher, 1960b).

Cultivation of human diploid cells in the presence of z^6Urd caused an augmentation of the levels of orotidylic acid phosphorylase and orotidylic acid decarboxylase (Pinsky and Krooth, 1967a,b). Metabolic conversions and site of action of z^6Urd are shown in Fig. 8.

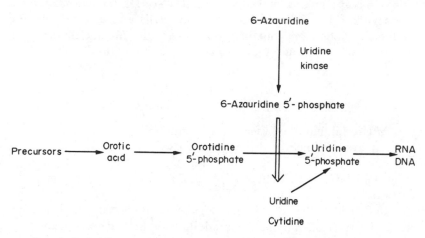

Fig. 8. Pyrimidine metabolic pathways with the site of action of 6-azauridine.

Generally, polyphosphates of z^6Urd have not been detected in biological systems. An interesting exception, the only one known, is *Trypanosoma equiperdum* (Rubin *et al.*, 1962). 6-Azauracil markedly suppresses the multiplication of *Trypanosoma equiperdum* and thus prolongs the survival time of mice infected with this parasitic organism. This protozoan converts the base analog, 6-azauracil, directly to the 5-ribonucleotide, i.e. 6-azauridylic acid, by condensation of the free base with 5-phosphoribosyl 1-pyrophosphate. Azauridylic acid in turn can be further phosphorylated to the di- and triphosphate derivatives. These reactions proceed, presumably, via the normal pathway used by the organism for incorporation of preformed uracil. Although z^6Urd can readily enter viable trypanosomes, the protozoan appears to lack significant capacity to phosphorylate this analog to azauridylic acid. Since the latter is the inhibitor of orotidylic acid decarboxylase, the capacity of trypanosomes to convert 6-azauracil, and not z^6Urd, to this derivative appears to account for the far greater potency of 6-azauracil in inhibiting the *de novo* synthesis of pyrimidines and suppressing the growth of this organism in mice. The extensive capacity of trypanosomes to convert 6-azauracil to 6-azauridylic acid, together with the limited capacity of mammalian cells to convert 6-azauracil by a totally different reaction sequence to the same ribonucleotide (via the intermediate formation of z^6Urd), points to the bichemical distinction between this protozoan and mammalian species.

Effects of 6-azauridine 5′-diphosphate and 6-azauridine 5′-triphosphate. 6-Azauridine 5′-diphosphate and 6-azauridine 5′-triphosphate, prepared by chemical synthesis, inhibit the biological synthesis of polynucleotides and ribonucleic acids. Škoda *et al.* (1959a,b) have shown that polynucleotide phosphorylase of *E. coli* does not catalyze the exchange of ^{32}P-orthophosphate with 6-azauridine 5′-diphosphate under conditions when this exchange is very marked with uridine 5′-diphosphate. Even low concentrations of 6-azauridine 5′-diphosphate inhibited the polynucleotide phosphorylase-catalyzed exchange of uridine 5′-diphosphate and adenosine 5′-diphosphate with ^{32}P-orthophosphate. 6-Azauridine 5′-monophosphate had no inhibitory effect whatever.

6-Azauridine 5′-triphosphate inhibits RNA polymerase of *E. coli* (Goldberg and Rabinowitz, 1963). 6-Azauridine 5′-di- and triphosphates probably play no significant role in the mechanism of action of z^6Urd in animal systems, since the inhibitory effects require relatively large concentrations of these nucleotides.

In contrast to 5-azacytidine and 5-halogeno substituted 2′-deoxyuridines, z^6Urd is not incorporated into nucleic acids of living cells. The finding of 6-azauridine 2′(3′)-phosphate (and 6-azacytidine 2′(3′)-phosphate) in the RNA of the brain cells after intracerebral injection of z^6Urd into cats is the only reported exception (Wells *et al.*, 1963).

Codon triplets containing 6-azapyrimidine nucleosides are inactive and unable to stimulate binding of aminoacyl-tRNA to ribosomes. Thus there is no risk of any potential incorporation of 6-azapyrimidine derivatives into RNA or DNA of organisms treated with z^6Urd or 6-azacytidine. Even if such incorporation (perhaps to a very limited extent) did occur, the codons and anticodons containing 6-azapyrimidine ribonucleotides would neither possess coding activity, nor would they cause errors in translation (Lisý *et al.*, 1968).

10.2.5.3. Reversal of the Virus Inhibitory Effect

Reversal of z^6Urd inhibition of vaccinia virus multiplication is possible by uridine or cytidine, but not by thymidine or deoxycytidine (Rada and Blaškovič, 1966). Figure 9 illustrates the effectiveness of uridine (strong effect), uracil (slight effect), and adenine (no effect), in reversal of the inhibitory effect of z^6Urd. Equimolar concentrations of uridine and cytidine reversed fully the inhibitory effect of z^6Urd (Table 3). However, a 3-fold higher concentration of thymidine than of z^6Urd, or an equimolar concentration of deoxycytidine, did not cause any reversal. Simultaneous addition of both deoxynucleotides was also ineffective.

A higher capacity of uridine and cytidine to reverse the inhibitory effect of z^6Urd on adenovirus replication was found (Flanagan and Ginsberg, 1964). z^6Urd (500 μg/ml) was added to cultures infected with adenovirus along with graded concentrations of uridine, cytidine or deoxycytidine. Uridine at a final concentration of 50 μg/ml completely reversed the inhibitory effect of z^6Urd. Cytidine, at a concentration of 250 μg/ml, permitted adenovirus multiplication equal to that in untreated infected cultures. Deoxycytidine, on the other hand, was without effect on the inhibition of virus multiplication produced by z^6Urd. Cytidine and uridine are interchangeable in replacing the deficit in pyrimidine precursors created by z^6Urd.

The inhibitory effect of 250 μg/ml of z^6Urd on polyoma virus yield could be completely overcome by addition of 50–250 μg/ml of uridine, but not deoxycytidine or thymidine. When infected cells were treated with 250 μg/ml of z^6Urd for 24 hr, followed by washing and replenishing with new medium containing 100 μg/ml of uridine, the virus yield at 40 hr was the same as that found in untreated cells at 40 hr post-infection. Hence the inhibitory effect of z^6Urd is not due to a nonspecific loss of ability of treated cells to produce virus (Gershon and Sachs, 1966).

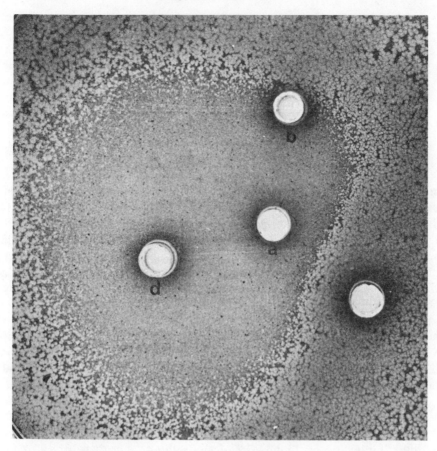

FIG. 9. Reversal of the inhibitory effect of 6-azauridine on vaccinia virus multiplication. Monolayers of chick embryo cells in dishes (15 cm diameter) were infected with 2×10^4 PFU of vaccinia virus. After solidification of the agar overlay, glass wells were mounted in the agar overlay and solutions were given into the wells: a—z^{6}Urd (4×10^{-1} M); b—uracil (10^{-1} M—not completely dissolved); c—uridine (10^{-1} M); d—adenine (10^{-1} M—not completely dissolved). The culture was stained 3 days after infection. From Rada and Blaškovič, 1966.

TABLE 3. *Reversal by Uridine and Thymidine of the Inhibitory Effect of 6-Azauridine on Vaccinia Virus Multiplication*

Molar concentration of		Virus titer	Molar concentration of		Virus titer
6-azauridine	uridine	(PFU/ml)	6-azauridine	thymidine	(PFU/ml)
0	0	1.7×10^6	0	0	1.2×10^6
4×10^{-3}	4×10^{-3}	1.3×10^6	4×10^{-3}	1.3×10^{-2}	7.9×10^3
4×10^{-3}	4×10^{-4}	5.8×10^5	4×10^{-3}	4×10^{-3}	1×10^4
4×10^{-3}	1.3×10^{-4}	2.3×10^5	4×10^{-3}	1.3×10^{-3}	9.5×10^3
4×10^{-3}	4×10^{-5}	1×10^5	4×10^{-3}	4×10^{-4}	7.9×10^3
4×10^{-3}	1.3×10^{-5}	3.7×10^4	4×10^{-3}	1.3×10^{-4}	8.4×10^3
4×10^{-3}	0	1.4×10^4	4×10^{-3}	0	1.5×10^4

Suspensions of HeLa cells were infected with 10 PFU/cell of vaccinia virus. After 1 hr adsorption the cultures were washed and the cells resuspended at a density of 2×10^5 cell per ml. z^{6}Urd, uridine or thymidine in concentration indicated were added thereafter. Virus titers were determined at 24 hr.
Modified from Rada and Blaškovič, 1966.

These results suggest that the site of action of z^{6}Urd in virus inhibition is the same as in uninfected cells and bacteria (discussed in previous section), i.e. inhibition of RNA synthesis by the block of orotidylic acid decarboxylase.

10.2.5.4. Kinetics of Formation of Viral Component Sensitive to Inhibition
by 6-Azauridine

Adenovirus. Studies on adenovirus infected cells were aimed at determining the relationship between time of analog addition and effect on virus multiplication to demonstrate the time at which virus specific RNA synthesis occurred in the sequence of biosynthetic events leading to production of infectious virions (Flanagan and Ginsberg, 1964). z^6Urd was added to virus-infected cultures at 1–2 hr intervals from 6 to 30 hr after infection. All cultures were harvested 30 hr after infection and infectivity titrations performed.

Additions of z^6Urd at a concentration of 490 μg/ml to cultures at any time up to 8 hr after infection resulted in complete suppression of adenovirus multiplication. After 8 hr the effect of z^6Urd on virus multiplication diminished rapidly. When the analog was added 16 hr or more after virus infection, no effect was noted on the virus titer. It can be inferred that the biosynthesis of RNA essential for adenovirus replication begins approximately 8 hr after infection, proceeds rapidly, and by 16 hr after infection sufficient RNA has been synthesized to permit maximal production of virus. These results were confirmed by studies in which the biosynthesis of virus-specific RNA was detected during the virus replication cycle by direct measurement of ^{32}P incorporation into RNA.

Similarly, formation of mRNAs of virus complement-fixing antigen and toxin, demonstrated with the aid of z^6Urd, was detected 30 hr after infection as complement-fixing antigen and toxin, respectively. The addition of the analog (490 μg/ml) to adenovirus-infected cultures at sequential time intervals resulted in a stepwise release of the inhibitory effect on the production of these proteins. The first appearance of complement-fixing antigen mRNA estimated in this way was found at 9 hr after infection, simultaneously with the initial formation of RNA determined for infectious virus. mRNA of adenovirus toxin was detected in cultures treated by z^6Urd 10 hr after infection. The analog effect decreased rapidly thereafter and addition of the inhibitor to infected cultures later than 16 hr after infection resulted in no reduction in the ultimate biosynthesis of virus antigen.

Vaccinia virus. The time-course of the z^6Urd-sensitive step in the vaccinia virus replicative cycle has been studied by addition of the analog to infected culture at various times after infection and determining the virus yield at the end of the replicative cycle (Rada and Blaškovič, 1966).

Figure 10 shows that formation of the component essential for virus replication is completely inhibited by z^6Urd up to 4 hr post-infection. Thereafter synthesis of this component becomes progressively resistant to the analog. The data on the reversal of the z^6Urd inhibitory effect (Section 10.2.5.3), in accord with studies on uninfected cells, indicate that the site of action of z^6Urd is inhibition of RNA synthesis. Figure 10 shows the kinetics of formation of the final species of RNA in the vaccinia virus replicative cycle. It precedes that of the appearance of infectious virus by 2 hr. Comparison with Fig. 11 shows that the synthesis of this late viral mRNA lasts 1 hr longer than the synthesis of viral DNA.

In parallel experiments the synthesis of viral DNA, as determined by 5-iododeoxyuridine inhibition, preceded the appearance of infectious virus by 3 hr (Fig. 11). Nearly the same curve was found with 5-fluorodeoxyuridine by Salzman *et al.* (1963).

These data on the kinetics of virus specific RNA synthesis, determined by z^6Urd inhibition, may be correlated with the detection of the synthesis of vaccinia virus mRNA (Salzman *et al.*, 1964; Becker and Joklik, 1964). Vaccinia virus mRNA formed in the cytoplasm of infected HeLa cells has a base composition similar to that of viral DNA and it hybridizes with viral DNA and not with HeLa cells DNA. It is first detectable 1–1.5 hr post-infection and is synthesized at a maximal rate about 4 hr post-infection (possibly 2–5-fold the rate of host cell mRNA synthesis in uninfected cells). After 4 hr post-infection the rate of synthesis of this virus mRNA declines, but is detectable even 9 hr post-infection.

Comparison of the curves obtained with z^6Urd and 5-iododeoxyuridine shows that the initial stages are different and that virus uncoating is inhibited by z^6Urd. The curve obtained with 5-iododeoxyuridine (Fig. 11) shows a low titer for addition at 2 hr post-infection. It is

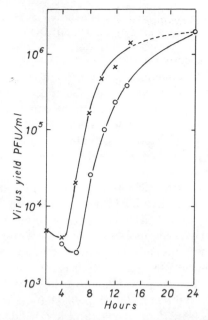

FIG. 10. The curve of formation of vaccinia virus messenger RNA, as determined by 6-azauridine inhibition and the curve of virus formation. Replicate cultures (2×10^5 HeLa cells per ml) infected with vaccinia virus (multiplicity 10) were established. The points of the virus growth curve (o——o) represent the virus titers determined in the untreated control cultures at the time indicated. The points of the viral mRNA curve (×——×) represent the virus yields obtained 24 hr after z^6Urd (1 mg/ml) was added at the time indicated by the position of the points. The yields of the virus, determined in this way, represent the relative quantity of viral mRNA formed before addition of the analog. From Rada and Blaškovič, 1966.

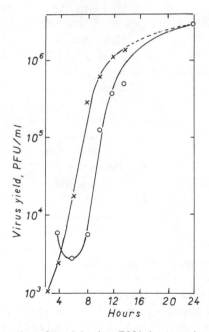

FIG. 11. The curve of formation of vaccinia virus DNA (×——×), as determined by 5-iododeoxyuridine inhibition, and the curve of virus formation (o——o). The experimental conditions were the same as in Fig. 10. 5-Iododeoxyuridine (10 μg/ml) was added at the time indicated by the points in the viral DNA curve. From Rada and Blaškovič, 1966.

possible to interpret this almost 1-log unit decrease of virus yield in such a way that, as the input virions undergo uncoating, they lose their infectivity; 5-iododeoxyuridine obviously is not inhibiting this process, but it prevents formation of new virus particles and thus unmasks the uncoating process. Since virus uncoating is undoubtedly not a synchronous process (similar to the appearance of new virions) it may be that a portion of input virions is still being uncoated at the time when new virions are already being synthesized. This seems to be the reason why the uncoating process is not fully expressed in the usual virus growth curve.

Comparison of the virus yield in the culture where 5-iododeoxyuridine (Fig. 11) was added 2 hr post-infection with that where this analog was added 4 hr post-infection shows that the eclipse period is about 2 hr shorter than that estimated in the usual way, i.e. new virions in fact are being synthesized at 4 hr post-infection. The virus titer in the culture with addition of 5-iododeoxyuridine at 2 hr post-infection indicates the lowest level of virus titer after uncoating. The remaining 3 log units of virus represent the input virions adsorbed but not uncoated.

On the other hand, the curve obtained with z^6Urd (Fig. 10) did not show a decrease in the amount of virus when the analog was added 2 hr post-infection, suggesting that the process of uncoating is inhibited by z^6Urd, in accord with findings of Joklik (1964a,b) on the molecular basis of uncoating of poxvirus DNA, which is a two-stage process. The first stage begins immediately after penetration of virus particles and is effected by enzymes present in the uninfected cell; the products of this stage are virus cores. Viral DNA within cores is not accessible to DNase. The second stage results in breakdown of the cores to release naked poxvirus DNA. This stage is inhibited by fluorophenylalanine and puromycin, inhibitors of protein synthesis, as well as by actinomycin D and u.v.-irradiation, inhibitors of mRNA synthesis. It was concluded that, for virus cores to be broken down, a protein must be synthesized after infection. This protein is synthesized only in response to infection with virus. It is postulated that viral coat protein released during the first stage of uncoating causes derepression of a portion of host cell DNA, permitting the synthesis, through the mediation of mRNA formation, of a protein which is instrumental in degrading virus cores and thus releasing viral DNA in the free state.

In summary, the time-course of the z^6Urd-sensitive step in the multiplication cycle of vaccinia virus indicates that this analog affects both the early (uncoating) as well as late events (synthesis of late m-RNA) in the latent period.

The above use of two different inhibitors, one inhibiting uncoating and the other viral nucleic acid synthesis, is a useful approach in the study of the virus uncoating process.

Polyoma virus. The necessity of RNA synthesis in the polyoma virus lytic cycle was proved by z^6Urd inhibition (Gershon and Sachs, 1966). To determine the kinetics of this RNA synthesis, 250 μg/ml of z^6Urd was added at different times to cultures of mouse embryo cells infected with polyoma virus. Virus yield was assayed at 40 hr post-infection. There was no detectable increase in the yield of new virus over background at the end of the adsorption period, when z^6Urd was added up to 6 hr post-infection. The RNA required for polyoma virus development started to be synthesized by about 7–8 hr post-infection, i.e. about 14 hr before new mature virions were first detected. After 20–24 hr post-infection no sensitivity to z^6Urd could be detected, showing that RNA essential for virion formation was synthesized up to about 24 hr.

In parallel experiments the synthesis of viral antigen was detected by the fluorescent antibody technique at 36 hr post-infection. Ninety-eight per cent inhibition of this synthesis was observed when z^6Urd was added 6 hr post-infection and a decrease in inhibition to 94 per cent and 89 per cent in two experiments, when z^6Urd was added 8 hr post-infection. These results indicate that RNA necessary for the synthesis of viral antigen was synthesized early during virus development.

Dengue virus. Similarly, the time course of viral RNA synthesis of dengue virus was determined by z^6Urd inhibition. The analog was added at various time intervals after infection to stop further RNA synthesis, and the virus yields at 21 hr were measured and plotted against the time of addition of the analog. Comparison with the control viral growth curve revealed that synthesis of an essential RNA began 6 hr post-infection and preceded release of mature virus by 6–7 hr, i.e. new mature virions appeared after 12 hr post-infection (Fig. 12). Parallel tests showed that hemagglutinin formation was similarly inhibited by z^6Urd (Stollar *et al.*, 1966).

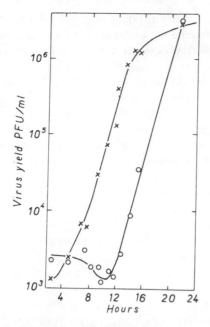

Fig. 12. The curve of formation of dengue virus RNA ($\times$——$\times$) as determined by 6-azauridine inhibition and the curve of virus formation ($\circ$——$\circ$). To the dengue virus infected KB cells z^6Urd (5 μg/ml) was added at the time indicated by the position of the points. Virus yields were determined 21 hr after infection. From Stollar et al., 1966. Copyright © Academic Press Inc. (New York) 1966. Reprinted with permission of the authors and publisher.

10.2.5.5. Role of Uridine Kinase in the Selectivity of the Antiviral Effect of 6-Azauridine

As discussed above (Section 10.2.5.2) z^6Urd exerts inhibitory effects as the nucleotide 6-azauridine 5'-monophosphate, formed intracellularly by uridine kinase. It was proposed (Škoda, 1963) that infection with some viruses, namely those sensitive to z^6Urd, led to an increase of intracellular uridine kinase activity, and an increased conversion of z^6Urd to its monophosphate, this being the basis of the selective antiviral action of z^6Urd.

Chick embryo cells infected with *Rous sarcoma virus* (strain Prague) exhibited a 5-fold increase in uridine kinase activity (Rada and Gregušová, 1964). Enzyme induction was observed in infected monolayers of chick embryo cells, as well as in tumours from the breast muscle of chicken. In studies of Gelbard et al. (1966), infection of the chorioallantoic membrane resulted in a 10-fold increase in uridine kinase activity in cell-free extracts prepared from the resulting tumour tissue. Enhancement of enzyme activity was evident 4 days after infection with appearance of the first pocks on the chorioallantoic membrane. Maximum activity was recorded 6 or 7 days after infection, when there was a confluent tumour on the chorioallantoic membrane. Uridine kinase activity was increased by infection with either the Bryan or Schmidt-Ruppin strain of Rous sarcoma virus.

To determine whether infection with Rous sarcoma virus resulted in a general increase in nucleoside kinase activities, several ribonucleosides and deoxyribonucleosides were tested as substrates for the corresponding nucleoside kinase. Besides uridine, only cytidine and z^6Urd were phosphorylated to a much greater extent in infected than in uninfected chorioallantoic membranes. The increase in phosphorylation of uridine in Rous sarcoma virus-induced tumours did not result from differential rates of catabolism of uridine or uridine 5'-phosphate, since the activities of uridine phosphorylase and uridine 5'-monophosphatase were similar in control and infected membranes.

A marked increase in rate and maximum phosphorylation (36-fold) of uridine was observed with cell-free extracts from chick chorioallantoic membrane tissue at 7 days post-infection with Fujinami virus, the morph^r strain. With this strain Dodge *et al.* (1970) confirmed the previous finding of Gelbard *et al.* (1966) that the increased phosphorylation of uridine (and uridine 5'-phosphate) obtained with cell-free extracts from infected tissues is indeed due to increased levels of uridine (and uridine 5'-phosphate) kinase and not a decreased activity of catabolic enzymes.

The studies on induction of uridine kinase by Rous sarcoma virus in cell culture were extended by Kára (1968), using a highly effective method of chick embryo cell infection, i.e. virus adsorption in cell suspension with subsequent cultivation in monolayers at 39°. Both the kinetics of enzyme induction and the rate of transformation of Rous sarcoma virus infected cells (strain Schmidt-Ruppin) were temperature dependent. Under these conditions more than 60 per cent of the cells were transformed into malignant Rous sarcoma cells within 72 hr post-infection. Uridine kinase activity was found to rise from 48 hr post-infection and to attain a 3-fold higher level than the uninfected culture after 72 hr. At 48 hr post-infection the activity of uridine kinase was significantly higher than in the control culture. At that time only a small number of the transformed cells was found in infected cultures. This indicates that expression of uridine kinase in infected cells precedes the morphological transformation. On incubating the infected cultures at 37° the increase in uridine kinase activity was retarded and was detectable 4 days post-infection.

The induction of uridine kinase was inhibited by puromycin, suggesting that the enhanced activity of the enzyme in infected chick embryo cultures was due to its increased *de novo* synthesis (Kára, 1968). Replication of Rous sarcoma virus in chick embryo cells was strongly inhibited by 5-iododeoxyuridine, when added at the time of infection. In the presence of this antimetabolite the induction of uridine kinase activity in Rous sarcoma virus infected cells was not blocked. Hence the increase in uridine kinase activity in Rous sarcoma virus infected cells is dependent on protein synthesis without being related to Rous sarcoma virus replication (Kára, 1968).

Under conditions of the one-step growth experiments the highly pathogenic Italian strain of *Newcastle disease virus* provoked a 2.5-fold increase of uridine kinase activity in chick embryo cells (Hammer *et al.*, 1976). By contrast the Roakin strain of Newcastle disease virus did not alter the activity of the enzyme (Consigli and Lerner, 1970).

Fowl plague virus (strain Rostock) and *Semliki forest virus* (strain Osterrieth) increased uridine kinase activity in chick embryo cells 2.2-fold and 1.5-fold respectively (Hammer *et al.*, 1976).

The CL strain of *vaccinia virus* derived from a calf lymph preparation, and passaged in chorioallantoic membrane of chick embryo, caused a 2-fold increase of uridine kinase activity in chorioallantoic membrane cultures (Rada and Gregušová, 1964). However, strain IHD of vaccinia virus did not induce activity in the mouse LM cell line (Kit *et al.*, 1964). Neither did mutants deficient in thymidine kinase activity (Dubbs and Kit, 1964). To explain this difference, the different properties of the strains have to be considered (compare herpes virus strains below) as well as the role of host cells. Compared with embryo cells, LM or HeLa cells contain about a 10-fold higher level of uridine kinase. Comparison of z^{6}Urd transport and uridine kinase activity in HeLa and chick embryo cells is illustrated in Fig. 13. It may be that virus multiplying in cells rich in uridine kinase does not induce this enzyme.

Dundaroff and Falke (1972) studied the activity of uridine kinase after infection of rabbit kidney cells with twenty-one strains of human *herpes virus* of serotype 1 or 2. The maximum uridine kinase activity was observed 12 hr post-infection. The late increase of enzyme activity cannot be easily explained, but cannot be attributed to a low multiplicity of infection. The herpes virus strains of type 1 isolated from non-genital herpetic lesions with high thymidine kinase activity induced more uridine kinase activity than the type 2 strains isolated from genital herpetic lesions. They enhanced uridine kinase by a factor of 1.5–2.5. The strains of serotype 2, the intermediate strain, and thymidine kinase deficient strain JES, did not affect uridine kinase levels in infected cells.

In pilot experiments Galegov *et al.* (1968b) observed an approximate 5-fold increase in activity of uridine kinase in bone marrow of chickens after infection with *avian myeloblastosis virus* (strain not given).

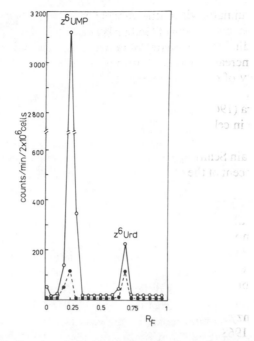

FIG. 13. Transport and metabolic conversion of 6-azauridine in HeLa and chick embryo cells. Suspension cultures (2×10^6 cells/ml) were supplemented with ^{14}C-6-azauridine (19 kBg/ml). After 1 hr incubation at 37° the cells were washed and the cell pellet was precipitated by trichloracetic acid. The respective supernatants were analyzed by paper chromatography in isopropanol-ammonium hydroxide-H_2O (7:1:2, v/v/v). ●---● chick embryo cells (Σ cpm 302); ○——○HeLa cells (Σ cpm 4003). In comparison with the amount of z^6Urd (19 kBg/ml $\sim 6 \times 10^5$ cpm/ml) added it can be seen that 0.05 per cent of z^6Urd was transported into chick embryo cells, whereas 0.7 per cent of z^6Urd was transported into HeLa cells. Out of the amount of z^6Urd which was transported into cells 48 per cent and 89 per cent were converted to monophosphate in chick embryo cells and HeLa cells, respectively (Rada and Dragún, unpublished data).

Enhancement of uridine kinase activity was also found in *T2 phage* infected *Escherichia coli* (Pravdina and Galegov, 1968). The enzyme activity was increased 10–15-fold at 8–15 min post-infection. Of special interest was the fact that the increase in uridine kinase activity after phage infection was not inhibited in the presence of chloramphenicol (200 μg/ml) suggesting that the increase of the enzyme activity is not dependent on protein synthesis *de novo*. Further experiments on the combined action of enzymatic extracts from T2 phage-infected and uninfected cells indicated the presence of an inhibitor of uridine kinase in uninfected bacteria. Thus in contrast to Rous sarcoma virus, the enhancement of enzyme activity by T2 phage infection may be due to blocking of an inhibitor of the enzyme in phage-infected cells. In spite of the high increase of uridine kinase activity upon T2 phage infection, the replication of the phage was not significantly inhibited by z^6Urd (Pravdina *et al.*, 1969).

Chick embryo cells infected with western equine encephalomyelitis, vesicular stomatitis and porcine herpes (pseudorabies) viruses, and mouse embryo cells infected with polyoma virus, did not enhance uridine kinase activity during the eclipse period of virus replication (Rada and Žemla, 1973).

Uridine kinase activities after virus infection are summarized in Table 4. Thus far eleven viruses (altogether twenty-nine strains) were tested for induction of uridine kinase activity. Five of these are sensitive to z^6Urd, five are not.

The data indicating a parallelism between increased activity of uridine kinase after virus infection and sensitivity to z^6Urd are as follows:

1. Rous sarcoma and fowl plague viruses are sensitive to z^6Urd and they enhance the activity of uridine kinase;
2. porcine herpes, vesicular stomatitis and western equine encephalomyelitis viruses are not sensitive to z^6Urd and do not change uridine kinase activity.

TABLE 4. *Induction of Uridine Kinase by Virus Infection*

Induction		No induction	
Virus (Strain)	Cells	Virus (Strain)	Cells
Rous sarcoma (Prague, Schmidt-Ruppin, Bryan, Fujinami-morf^r)	Chick embryo	Vaccinia (IHD) Human herpes type 2 (four strains) type intermediate (one strain)	Mouse fibroblast LM Rabbit kidney
Newcastle disease (Italian)	Chick embryo		
Fowl plague (Rostock)	Chick embryo	Porcine herpes (Such)	Chick embryo
Vaccinia (CL)	Chick embryo	Polyoma (SE)	Mouse embryo
Human herpes type 1 (nine strains)	Rabbit kidney	Newcastle disease (Roakin)	Chick embryo
		Vesicular stomatitis (Indiana)	Chick embryo
Semliki forest (Osterrieth)	Chick embryo	Western equine encephalomyelitis (WEE-15)	Chick embryo
Avian myeloblastosis	Chick bone marrow		

Modified from Rada and Dragúň, 1977.

The data for vaccinia and herpes viruses are inconclusive; these viruses show medium or low sensitivity to z^{6}Urd, some strains enhance activity of uridine kinase slightly while other strains are without effect. It is difficult to say whether, in the case of polyoma virus, the discrepancy between the high sensitivity to z^{6}Urd and the lack of uridine kinase induction is strain-specific. Only one strain of polyoma virus (strain SE) was investigated for induction of uridine kinase activity and did not influence the enzyme level. Two strains (1LII and SP2) studied by Gershon and Sachs (1966), and found highly sensitive to z^{6}Urd, were not investigated for induction of uridine kinase activity. The same holds for Semliki forest virus; the prototype strain was resistant to the analog, while the Osterrieth strain slightly increased enzyme activity.

In the following virus strains both z^{6}Urd sensitivity and uridine kinase activity induction were studied: Rous sarcoma virus—Prague strain, vaccinia virus—CL strain, vesicular stomatitis virus—Indiana strain, western equine encephalomyelitis virus—WEE-15 strain. Out of the herpes virus strains thus far tested for uridine kinase activity induction only strain JES, with low or zero induction of uridine kinase activity, was tested for sensitivity to z^{6}Urd. Its sensitivity was very slight.

The only strong argument against the hypothesis is the behavior of phage T2. The increase of uridine kinase activity after infection is very high, but the sensitivity to z^{6}Urd is low.

With z^{6}Urd as substrate in the uridine kinase assay, it was established that it has similar affinity for the enzyme as uridine (Sköld, 1960; Gelbard *et al.*, 1966). z^{6}Urd has two advantages over uridine: it is phosphorylated to monophosphate only; it is not cleaved by uridine phosphorylase.

10.2.6. STUDIES IN ANIMAL MODEL SYSTEMS AND CLINICAL APPLICATIONS

10.2.6.1. *Protective Effects in Animals*

z^{6}Urd has been found effective in the treatment of experimental dermal vaccinia virus infection in rabbits (Šmejkal and Šorm, 1962). Rabbits were inoculated with 10-fold dilutions of dermovaccinia intracutaneously. Half of the infected rabbits were treated with z^{6}Urd i.v. twice daily for 3 days, starting immediately after infection. The daily dose was 300 mg/kg. In untreated animals the skin lesions started as slight erythema 24 hr after infection and reached a maximum 3–4 days after infection as a pustule containing yellow purulent infiltrate surrounded by erythema.

In treated rabbits faint signs of erythema appeared after 3 days, but only in animals infected with the highest virus doses. Deeply red erythema did not occur in any treated rabbit. The pustules in these rabbits were pink, like the surrounding skin, and markedly smaller than in untreated controls. Treatment by z^{6}Urd was not accompanied by any serious side effects. At the end of the observation period (i.e. 14 days after infection) the treated rabbits showed a slight loss of hair and moderate skin necrosis at the site of z^6Urd administration. z^6Urd in these experiments displayed unequivocal inhibitory activity but did not inhibit vaccinia virus induced changes completely. Since there is difficulty in maintaining an adequate blood-level of z^6Urd, due to rapid renal excretion, it is possible that a more pronounced effect could be obtained if the daily dose of z^6Urd were divided in more than two doses.

In experimental therapy of herpes virus keratitis in rabbits (Galegov *et al.*, 1970), 2×10^4 mouse LD_{50} of keratotropic ELA strain of human herpes virus were inoculated on the scarified corneal epithelium of each eye of the rabbit. Drops of 0.75 per cent or 1 per cent solution of z^6Urd were administered to the eyes four times daily. In one experimental group the treatment was begun on appearance of the first symptoms (usually 3–4 days after infection) (Figs. 14a,b). Complete healing was observed 18–20 days after infection and was accompanied by opaque vascularized cicatrizing. Marked differences between the corneal epithelium of treated and untreated rabbit eyes were also found by histological examinations performed 10 days after treatment began.

In the other experimental group the treatment was begun 7 days after infection. z^6Urd was administered seven–eight times daily. Healing occurred 12–14 days after treatment began. In several cases small cicatrices of corneal epithelium persisted in place of the previous ulcers.

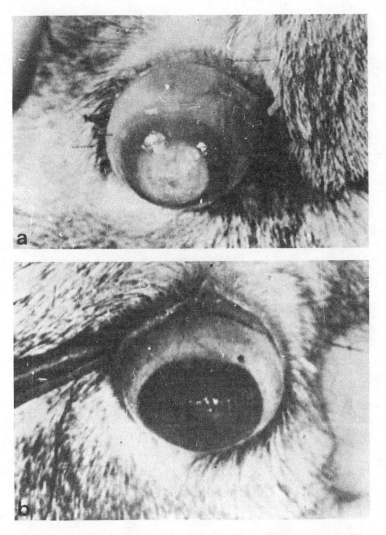

FIG. 14. Effect of 6-azauridine treatment on herpes keratitis in rabbit. (a) Untreated control eye. (b) The treatment, drops of 1 per cent solution of z^6Urd, was four times daily, starting with the first symptoms, 12 days after the beginning of treatment. From Galegov *et al.*, 1970.

In untreated eyes the experimental infection spread, forming marked interstitial keratitis which often resulted in large ulcers of the cornea. Application of drops of z^6Urd solution was shown to be effective. In toxicity tests, administration of the analog solution to the uninfected eyes of rabbits, and also to the eyes of experimentators, six–eight times daily for 7 days, did not cause any irritant effect. This suggests it is possible to apply z^6Urd in human therapy.

The relative efficacies of z^6Urd, adenine arabinoside and 5-iododeoxyuridine were evaluated in an experimental model system involving inoculation of the skin of hairless mice with herpes simplex virus (Klein *et al.*, 1974). The use of cutaneous herpes simplex infection in hairless mice offers the advantage of excellent reproducibility, high susceptibility to infection, and easy observation of the lesions on hairless skin and development of paralysis and death. For infection of mice, a dilution containing forty skin mean infective doses per ml of the S-type strain of herpes simplex virus ensured a maximal lesion score and a mortality rate greater than 50 per cent.

Adenine arabinoside and 5-iododeoxyuridine, when administered i.p. by several different dosage schedules, reduced the severity of cutaneous herpetic lesions and the incidence of paralysis and increased significantly the number of survivors. More rapid healing of lesions, and an increase in mean survival time, was also observed. A delay of 24–48 hr in initiation of treatment after infection was more effective than treatments started at the time of inoculation. Treatment with z^6Urd was totally ineffective with doses of 250 mg/kg daily for up to 10 days after inoculation. Although no toxic effect of the analog was demonstrable, there was significant reduction ($p < 0.05$) of the mean survival time of treated, infected animals as compared with that of the untreated infected control group. Klein *et al.* (1974) attributed this effect to the toxicity of the compound, which may influence the course of infection by diminishing the natural resistance of the treated mice.

z^6Urd was ineffective in protection of mice infected with IHD strain of vaccinia virus (Sidwell *et al.*, 1968). Mice were inoculated i.c. with ten or thirty-two LD_{50} of the virus and z^6Urd administered with one daily dose of 60–478 mg/kg/day. The data on the distribution of z^6Urd in the organism, as well as those on the maintenance of the blood level of the analog, could be related to these results (see Section 10.2.7.2).

Slight delay of 50 per cent survival of chicks infected with Rous sarcoma virus was observed after treatment with 6-azauracil (Jakubovič and Svoboda, 1960). However, if the daily dose of z^6Urd was increased to 90 mg, and divided into three doses per day, an inhibition of Rous sarcoma tumour growth was detected (Rada *et al.*, 1964). Experiments on the toxicity of the analog have shown that even a dose as high as 40 mg of z^6Urd per chick weighing 50 g, i.e. 800 mg/kg given three times daily (2.4 g/kg per day), was without any toxic effect and did not affect the weight increase of chicks (Fig. 15). In inhibition experiments the

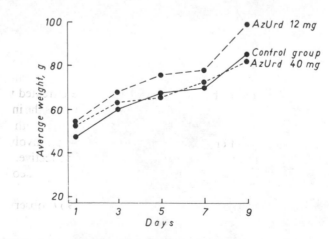

FIG. 15. Weight changes in chicks treated with 6-azauridine. Groups of four chicks were given z^6Urd (40 mg or 12 mg per chick weighing 50 g) three times daily. z^6Urd did not affect the weight increase of chicks for 9 days. From Rada *et al.*, 1964.

chicks were infected with 100 ID_{50} of the Prague strain of Rous sarcoma virus and treatment with 30 mg of z^6Urd s.c. at 8 hr intervals was begun on the day of virus inoculation. After 14 days the treated and untreated chicks were killed and the tumours removed and weighed (Fig. 16). At this time very small and rare metastases (mean diameter 0.5–2 mm) were found in the liver of a few chicks. z^6Urd at a dose of 30 mg per chick given three times a day (i.e. 1.8 g/kg per day) caused over 50 per cent inhibition of tumour growth as compared with the controls.

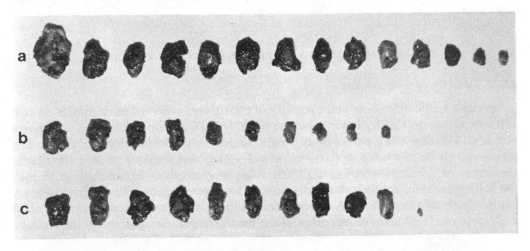

FIG. 16. Retardation of Rous sarcoma tumour growth by treatment with 6-azauridine. Groups of tumours removed from chicks infected with 100LD_{50} of Rous sarcoma virus. (a) Control group, not treated, 14 days after infection. (b) Group treated with z^6Urd (30 mg per chick) three times daily. (c) Group treated with z^6Urd (10 mg per chick) three times daily. From Rada *et al.*, 1964.

10.2.6.2. Clinical Applications

The first clinical application of z^6Urd was in patients with neoplastic disease. Calabresi (1965) examined the feasibility of suppressing infections by DNA-containing viruses in patients with advanced neoplastic disease receiving systemic therapy with antimetabolites of pyrimidine nucleosides. A 1:32 dilution of vaccinia virus (National Drug Co. vaccine) was applied directly to the skin of both arms. The vaccination sites were observed daily for evidence of vaccination 'takes'. z^6Urd administered every 8 hr i.v. to four patients in daily doses of 180–270 mg/kg was ineffective, as were 5-fluorodeoxyuridine, cytosine arabinoside or 5-azaorotic acid. Only 5-iododeoxyuridine (in doses ranging from 50 to 120 mg/kg daily) was able to suppress the primary vaccination reaction in eight out of eleven patients (Calabresi, 1965).

The usefulness of z^6Urd in the treatment of viral eye infections was shown in a study involving six patients (Myška *et al.*, 1967). Four had recurrent herpes simplex, one herpes zoster and one recurrent erosion of the cornea. All patients were treated with 6-azauridine triacetate orally for 3–21 days in total doses of 95–118 g. In five cases the infection was cured rapidly especially in the patients with dendritic ulcers combined with iridocyclitis. All patients selected for this study suffered from considerable stromal involvement for which other therapies, including topical 5-iododeoxyuridine, were ineffective. Although z^6Urd does not pass the blood-brain barrier, the drug penetrated into the aqueous humour of the rabbit eye easily.

In a trial carried out in Hyderabad, Jaffari and Hussain (1969) observed 140 smallpox patients for chemotherapeutic activity of z^6Urd. The unvaccinated smallpox patients admitted to the Fever Hospital in Hyderabad during 1967–1968 were randomized into drug-treated and placebo-treated groups. Only patients in the early stage of rash were included. No patient in the late stage of vesiculo-pustular eruption was taken for study. A daily dose of

100–200 mg/kg of z^6Urd, divided in two doses at an interval of 12 hr, was given as an intravenous drip for 3 days.

Jaffari and Hussain (1969) found 50 per cent reduction in mortality in drug-treated patients with ordinary smallpox over placebo-treated controls and increases in life span of drug-treated patients dying of hemorrhagic, flat or ordinary smallpox over placebo-treated control patients. The temperature responded well and this response was more appreciable in the pustular stage of the rash. The drug also exerted a favorable effect on focal eruption and the scabbing stage was reached early in patients under z^6Urd therapy. No toxic reactions were seen.

Since the disappearance of smallpox the chemotherapy of poxviruses lost its practical reason. The last known case of endemic smallpox in the world was reported from Somalia in October 1977. In December 1979, the World Health Organization concluded that the global eradication of smallpox had been achieved and the Organization formulated its policy for the post-eradication era. The Organization has recommended the cessation of smallpox vaccination. As part of the post-eradication 'insurance policy' to provide protection against presently unforeseen problems, the Organization is stockpiling enough vaccine to vaccinate 200 million persons and will ensure retention of vaccinia seed strains. In addition, many countries are developing their own national vaccine reserves (Ladnyi *et al.*, 1981). Also it is desirable, we suggest, to develop reserves of the drugs which were shown effective in the therapy and chemoprophylaxis of smallpox, i.e. z^6Urd and methisazone.

10.2.7. Pharmacology and other Biological Effects

10.2.7.1. Toxicity of 6-Azauridine

Species-specific differences in the toxicity of z^6Urd were observed in mammals. In mice and rats the acute toxicity is very low, the mean lethal doses (ID_{50}) after i.p. administration are 11.25 and 8.80 g per kg body weight, respectively. The toxicity of z^6Urd in dogs was found to be much higher (LD_{50} value = 3.4 g/kg) and similarly in cats (Handschumacher *et al.*, 1962; Novotný *et al.*, 1965). After repeated daily administration to mice, the following toxic manifestations developed: leukopenia, hemorrhagic diarrhoea and finally death of the animals. A linear relationship exists between the logarithm of the daily dose of z^6Urd and the logarithm of the mean lifespan. Small doses of the analog (50 mg/kg daily) cause a stimulation of lymphopoiesis in the spleen and the lymph nodes; whereas after higher dose progressive depressions of lymphopoieses, together with a proliferation of reticulum cells, were found. Daily administration of high doses for 17–32 days caused vacuolar degenerations, with necrosis and desquamation of the intestinal epithelium, fatty degeneration in the liver, as well as in the cortical tubuli of the kidney (Jiřička *et al.*, 1965). No significant pyrogenic reactions to solutions of z^6Urd were observed.

10.2.7.2. Absorption, Distribution and Excretion of z^6Urd

With two exceptions, the distribution of z^6Urd in the tissues, including neoplasms of mice, follows that of body water (Fig. 17). Unlike 6-azauracil, z^6Urd enters the cerebrospinal fluid to only a limited extent, while high concentrations, up to 3-fold higher than those in blood, are found in the kidney; this presumably reflects the rapid excretion of z^6Urd by this organ. Three hours after administration of ^{14}C-6-azauracil the highest activity was found in the kidney and blood; this analog penetrated the tumour tissue only slowly. However, ^{14}C-6-azauridine, 3 hr after administration, accumulated in the tumour tissue in much higher concentration than in other tissues; this nucleoside did not significantly accumulate in brain (Habermann and Šorm, 1958).

Intravenously administered z^6Urd (180 mg/kg) was without toxicity in man. Injected z^6Urd is rapidly excreted unchanged in the urine; 75 per cent of the dose is excreted within 4 hr and about 95 per cent within 8 hr. The level of the drug in the blood remained above

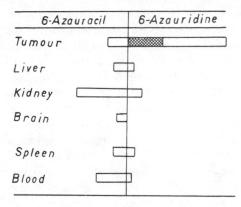

FIG. 17. Distribution of ^{14}C-6-azauracil and ^{14}C-6-azauridine in the tissues of mice with Ehrlich carcionoma. The relative radioactivity of 1 mg dry tissue at 3 hr after administration of ^{14}C-6-azauracil (on the left) and ^{14}C-6-azauridine (on the right). Conditions after 24 hr are shown by the hatched area. From Habermann and Šorm, 1958.

0.05 μmol/ml (1.2 mg/100 ml) for only 1 or 2 hr (Fig. 18). Orally administered z^{6}Urd was poorly absorbed and blood levels were detectable for only about 1 hr. The oral administration of this analog was accompanied by manifestations characteristic of central nervous system disturbance caused by 6-azauracil. About 80 per cent of the ingested z^{6}Urd was excreted primarily as 6-azauracil. This phenomenon is attributed to the cleavage of 6-azauracil from ingested z^{6}Urd by unidentified intestinal microflora; mammalian cells appear to have no enzyme capable of cleaving the ribose from z^{6}Urd. Previous clinical studies revealed that 6-azauracil invariably caused disturbances of the central nervous system. Thus it is not surprising that with oral doses of z^{6}Urd 180 mg/kg daily for 3 days, manifestation of central nervous system toxicity typical of that caused by 6-azauracil may be observed (Handschumacher et al., 1962).

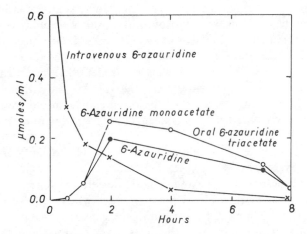

FIG. 18. Blood levels of 6-azauridine after equimolar dosage of 6-azauridine (intravenously) or 6-azauridine 2',3',5'-triacetate (orally). From Handschumacher et al., 1962. Copyright © National Institutes of Health, 1962. Reprinted with permission of the authors and publisher.

Neurotoxicity is also caused by z^{6}Urd, but to a much lesser extent than by 6-azauracil, because of the much lower penetration of the hematoencephalic barrier by the ribonucleoside. This naturally cannot exclude the appearance of neurotoxic side-effects when permeability of the hematoencephalic barrier is increased or when very large doses of z^{6}Urd are administered (Janku et al., 1965).

Synthetic 6-azauridine 2',3',5'-triacetate possesses advantages over z^{6}Urd in that it is orally effective and is not cleaved to 6-azauracil. Furthermore it produced more sustained blood levels of z^6Urd which is released during, or after, absorption from the intestine. Free z^6Urd appeared in the blood together with a smaller amount of 6-azauridine 5'-monoacetate (Fig. 18) (Handschumacher *et al.*, 1962).

The acute and chronic toxicity of 6-azauridine 2',3',5'-triacetate was studied and compared with the parent z^6Urd (Plevová *et al.*, 1970). In rats the LD_{50} (12 g/kg) corresponded in molar ratio to the values found for free z^6Urd; in mice the acetylated compound (LD_{50} = 7.8 g/kg) was more toxic than free z^6Urd. In chronic toxicity studies the symptoms found in rats were similar to those observed with z^6Urd (loss of weight, hemorrhagic diarrhoea); histopathologic findings in lymphadenic tissue were also alike. After repeated oral administration of 6-azauridine triacetate, a statistically significant lowering of red blood cell count was observed in rats and pigs given large doses. This erythrocytopenia was not observed after z^6Urd administration. In contrast to the high mortality and high incidence of hemorrhagic diarrhoea found in rats treated with 50 and 100 mg/kg of 6-azauridine triacetate three times per day, pigs survived similar treatment without any serious effects.

10.2.7.3. Suppression of the Immune Response by 6-Azauridine

The immunosuppressive activity of z^6Urd is not very strong. Complete inhibition of antibody formation in young rabbits was achieved only at very high doses of z^6Urd (5 g/kg of body weight). A significant inhibition could be obtained at a dose of 0.5 g/kg (Šterzl, 1961). Also in mice the ability of z^6Urd to suppress the primary immune response to the i.p. injection of sheep erythrocytes was weak. However, the combination with chloramphenicol exhibited potentiation of the weak immunosuppressive activity exerted by z^6Urd, while no such activity was demonstrated by chloramphenicol if administered alone (Fisher *et al.*, 1966).

Using the technique of localized hemolysis in agar gel, introduced by Jerne *et al.* (1963), z^6Urd was shown to have no effect on the number of these plaques upon *in vitro* incubation with suspensions of spleen cells taken from sheep-cell immunized mice. The analog was employed in the concentration range 0.5–50 mg/ml. Under similar conditions, actinomycin D, puromycin, 6-mercaptopurine and cytosine arabinoside were effective (Rose *et al.*, 1968).

Suppression of several cell-mediated immune responses in mice (transplantation reaction, graft-versus-host reactions and experimental autoimmune aspermatogenesis) by z^6Urd and 6-azauridine triacetate was studied by Nouza *et al.* (1970). In all of the reactions z^6Urd displayed a low to medium immunosuppressive activity, but only when limiting conditions of dose and timing were maintained. On the other hand, an enhancement of antibody synthesis *in vitro* was observed with low concentrations or short-term application of z^6Urd (Stejskalová *et al.*, 1970).

The effect of z^6Urd on interferon action was studied by Nichol and Tershak (1967). Chick embryo cell monolayers were exposed to interferon, z^6Urd (1 mg/ml) or interferon plus z^6Urd. After 2.5 hr exposure both the analog and interferon were removed and the cultures were infected with Sindbis virus (4 PFU per cell). The virus yields estimated after 17 hr of incubation showed that z^6Urd did not inhibit virus multiplication when present in the medium before infection, but it boosted the virus titer 4-fold in the presence of interferon. This result suggests that interferon action requires the synthesis of RNA and supports similar data obtained previously with actinomycin D.

10.2.7.4. The Effect of 6-Azauridine on Embryonic Development

The effect of z^6Urd on embryonic development was shown to depend on the period of gestation as well as on the dose. In rats the administration on days 1–6 was embryolethal or without any effect. Days 6–12 were the period of greatest embryonic susceptibility. Doses of 330 and 110 mg/kg caused 100 per cent resorption; 36 mg/kg caused embryolethality in 85 per cent, and 53.8 per cent of surviving fetuses had malformations. At a dose 12 mg/kg of the analog, 5.8 per cent of the fetuses were malformed, mostly with encephalocele and gastroschisis. Administered on days 12–18, a dose of 3 g/kg was 100 per cent embryolethal and 1 g/kg was 32.8 per cent embryolethal and all survivors had malformations of extremities. All fetuses from litters treated with z^6Urd showed growth retardation. After 330 mg/kg of z^6Urd, 65.2 per cent of fetuses survived without any visible damage (Gutová et al., 1971).

Similarly, the administration of z^6Urd into the yolk sack interfered with the development of the chick embryo. Doses of 5 and 10 mg of the analog increased the death of embryos and induced a striking incidence of malformation of a remarkably constant type frontal encephalocele, microcephalia and spastic paraplegia (Grafnetterová et al., 1966).

Furthermore, z^6Urd was used as an evoking agent in a study on the development of the syndrome of caudal regression (Jelínek et al., 1970) and in other morphogenetic studies.

The above data on the teratogenic effect of z^6Urd do not allow the use of large doses of z^6Urd in women during pregnancy, in spite of its low toxicity in adult humans. The use of this drug in women of child-bearing age should be undertaken only after weighing the possible risks to the fetus against benefit to the patient.

10.2.7.5. Other Effects

Clinical applications and miscellaneous biological effects of z^6Urd are summarized in reviews of Škoda (1975) and Elis and Rašková (1972).

Inhibitory action of z^6Urd in several experimental tumours including sarcoma 180, Ehrlich ascitic carcinoma, L-5178-Y lymphoma and others was described. In human infant leukemia z^6Urd produced complete remissions, in adults partial remissions were achieved. The analog did not affect solid tumours with the exception of some gynaecological tumours.

z^6Urd was shown to possess a therapeutic effect in the treatment of mycosis fungoides. Similarly, the usefulness of 6-azauridine triacetate was demonstrated in the treatment of psoriasis.

z^6Urd was shown not to be mutagenic (Rada and Závada, 1962).

10.3. 5-AZACYTIDINE

Chemical properties of 5-azapyrimidine nucleoside analogs and their mode of action in eukaryotic cells have been described by Veselý and Čihák (1978) in the section concerned with anti-tumour chemotherapy. Because of high toxicity 5-azacytidine has not been considered a prospective antiviral chemotherapeutic agent and only a few reports exist in the literature about this topic. The present review is concerned mainly with the effects of 5-azacytidine on the replication of bacteriophages. Some principles underlying the differential action of the drug on the replication of phage and the metabolism of its bacterial host could be found useful in devising new ways of administration of highly toxic drugs in order to direct their powerful inhibitory action selectively against virus replication.

10.3.1. CELLULAR UPTAKE OF NUCLEOSIDES

Bacterial and animal cells take up nucleosides by means of specific transport systems or permeases (Peterson and Koch, 1966; Doskočil, 1972; Plagemann and Richey, 1974; Mygind and Munch-Petersen, 1975). To enter the cell efficiently, a nucleoside analog must therefore possess a sufficiently high affinity for at least one of the nucleoside transport systems. The interaction of a nucleoside analog with the receptor site of the transport system thus represents the first controlling point on the metabolic pathway of the analog. Quite frequently mutants resistant to toxic nucleoside analogs arise by a loss or modification of a particular nucleoside transport system. Mutants of Escherichia coli resistant to 5-azacytidine were selected and classified according to the nature of the genetic defect. About one-half of these mutants was found to be pleiotropic, affecting the rate of uptake of 5-azacytidine and concurrently reducing the ability of the cells to take up many other purine or pyrimidine nucleosides and deoxynucleosides. All mutants of this class were resistant to showdomycin, indicating that both 5-azacytidine and showdomycin enter the cells by means of the same nucleoside-transport system. Mutants of the other class were not pleiotropic and were most probably deficient in uridine kinase (Doskočil, 1974).

Further analysis of the pleiotropic 5-azacytidine-resistant mutants has shown that they were deficient in a single nucleoside permease with high substrate affinity (K_m for cytidine uptake equal to 0.25 μM) and non-inducible (constitutive) character. Another nucleoside permease system with somewhat lower substrate affinity ($K_m = 7.1$ μM), and inducible with thymidine concurrently with the enzymes of the *deo* operon (Hammer-Jespersen *et al.*, 1971) was still operative in the mutants. The affinity of the inducible nucleoside permease system for 5-azacytidine, however, was at least 100 times less than that of the constitutive system of wild-type cells, so that the uptake rate of 5-azacytidine by non-induced mutant cells was not sufficient to cause any inhibitory effect. If, however, the inducible nucleoside-transporting sites of the mutant were augmented by induction with thymidine, resistant cells were converted to partially sensitive phenotype, in perfect agreement with the increased rate of uptake of labeled 5-azacytidine (Doskočil, 1974). These experiments underline the importance of nucleoside transport systems for determining the degree of sensitivity of different cell types to nucleoside analogues.

The broad range of specificity of nucleoside transport systems includes some 'gratuitous' inhibitors of transport, which are not metabolized by the cells but merely interact with receptor sites of permease systems. A large number of gratuitous transport inhibitors in *E. coli* has been described by Doskočil and Holý (1974). A typical representative is 2'-deoxy-2'-chlorouridine, a metabolically inert compound capable, however, of detoxicating 5-azacytidine or showdomycin by its mere presence in the medium. With a suitable ratio of concentrations of the toxic analog and the gratuitous transport competitor, it is possible to modulate the rate of uptake, and consequently the severity of inhibition. The use of transport inhibitors offers a distinct advantage over a simple decrease of the overall dose, because, due to very high substrate affinity of receptor sites, the uptake of a nucleoside analog is usually of zero kinetic order, even at very low concentrations. Hence by reducing the dose, we merely shorten the time of exposure but we cannot diminish the rate of uptake, by which the intracellular level of the analog and the intensity of inhibition are primarily determined. Although no data are available about the participation of nucleoside-transport systems in the uptake of 5-azapyrimidine nucleosides in mammalian cells, it may be expected, by analogy with other nucleoside analogs, that their transport is mediated by a permease and that suitable transport competitors could be found (Plagemann and Richey, 1974).

10.3.2. MODE OF ACTION OF 5-AZACYTIDINE AND 5-AZA-2'-DEOXYCYTIDINE IN *ESCHERICHIA COLI*

Growth of *E. coli* in the logarithmic phase is reversibly inhibited by 5-azacytidine. While the synthesis of RNA and DNA are primarily unaffected, protein synthesis is almost completely inhibited; the inhibition becomes apparent immediately after addition of the drug and is fully expressed 10 min later (Doskočil *et al.*, 1967). During the first few minutes of treatment the synthesis of a functional protein (β-galactosidase) still proceeds, apparently utilizing mRNA synthesized before addition of the drug (Pačes *et al.*, 1968a). After resuspending the cells in fresh medium, or upon addition of excess cytidine or uridine or of some gratuitous inhibitor of nucleoside transport, protein synthesis and growth recover in several minutes, reflecting the lifetime of faulty mRNA formed during the period of 5-azacytidine uptake. Complete reversibility of inhibition is observed if the cells are exposed to the drug for less than 30 min. After longer exposures the recovery takes longer and is incomplete, but no true bactericidal action has ever been observed.

Incorporation studies with 5-aza-4[^{14}C]-cytidine have shown that the analog is incorporated into all three classes of RNA, i.e. mRNA, tRNA and rRNA. Following a chase with excess non-radioactive cytidine, the label is retained within the cells and accumulates in stable forms of RNA, i.e. tRNA and rRNA. The sedimentation coefficients of the labeled RNA do not change upon subsequent incubation, indicating that no preferential degradation of 5-azacytidine-bearing RNA occurs. The ribosomes formed in the presence of 5-azacytidine, however, appear to be defective in initiation of translation (Pačes *et al.*, 1968b).

Labeled 5-azacytidine is incorporated into DNA. The incorporation lags slightly behind that into RNA initially, but a steady state is soon attained, when a constant fraction of 5-azacytidine taken-up is found in DNA. The overall extent of incorporation of 5-azacytidine into RNA and DNA is quite large; using a double-labeling technique it was found that the RNA formed during the period of exposure to 5-azacytidine may include up to 45 per cent replacement of cytidine by 5-azacytidine; in DNA the content of the analog was somewhat lower (Pačes *et al.*, 1968b); the analytically determined content of the analog in total RNA and DNA is, of course, much lower because a large excess of normal nucleic acids from the period prior to treatment is always present.

What derivative of 5-azacytidine is responsible for the non-functional state of mRNA? As pointed out by Veselý and Čihák (1978), 5-azacytidine undergoes cleavage of the *sym*-triazine ring, especially at alkaline pH. It was suggested that this reaction could take place even with the analog incorporated into RNA or DNA and attempts were made to explain the inhibitory and mutagenic effects of the drug by the ring-opening reaction (Piťhová *et al.*, 1965c). Furthermore most cells, bacterial and eukaryotic, contain cytidine deaminase (cytidine aminohydrolase, E.C. 3.5.4.5) converting 5-azacytidine into 5-azauridine (Čihák and Šorm, 1965); the latter may also be incorporated into RNA, but not into DNA, since methylation on the N_5 ring atom cannot take place so that no 5-azaanalog of thymidine is possible. We may presume that four forms of the base moiety of administered 5-azacytidine may actually occur in RNA: (1) intact 5-azacytosine; (2) its open-ring derivative *N*-amidinourea; (3) intact 5-azauracil; (4) its open-ring form, biuret.

To evaluate the effect of deamination on the inhibitory activity of 5-azacytidine, strains of *E. coli* deficient in cytidine deaminase (Karlström, 1970) were used. In these strains, inhibition of growth and total protein synthesis was weak, although the incorporation of the drug proceeded at a rate equal to about 60 per cent of that in wild-type strains (Doskočil and Šorm, 1970a,b). From this we conclude that complete inhibition of protein synthesis in wild-type (i.e. cytidine deaminase[+]) strains is due to incorporation of 5-azauridine into mRNA. This conclusion was confirmed by showing that 5′,6-anhydro-6-hydroxy-5,6-dihydro-5-azauridine, which generates 5-azauridine by hydrolysis, inhibits protein synthesis in cytidine deaminase-deficient strains to the same extent as does 5-azacytidine in wild-type strains of *E. coli* (Doskočil and Šorm, 1970a,b). If, however, the activity of a specific enzyme was followed, it was found that, even in cytidine deaminase-deficient strains, the synthesis of inducible β-galactosidase was suppressed much more than total protein synthesis. This is obviously due to miscoding caused by the presence of 5-azacytosine in mRNA.

5-Aza-2′-deoxycytidine was found to be non-inhibitory in cytidine deaminaseless strains, although in wild-type strains this compound inhibited protein synthesis as effectively as 5-azacytidine (Doskočil and Šorm, 1970c). We may conclude that deamination by cytidine deaminase is an obligatory step in the metabolism of 5-azadeoxycytidine in *E. coli*. This is understandable, since no kinase capable of phosphorylation of deoxynucleosides, except thymidine, has been detected in *E. coli* (Karlström, 1970). The conversion of 5-azadeoxycytidine to 5-azauracil in wild-type *E. coli* was confirmed by Čihák and Veselý (1977). On the other hand the ribonucleoside, 5-azacytidine, may be directly phosphorylated by uridine kinase (ATP : uridine/cytidine 5-phosphotransferase, E.C. 2.7.1.48) and this reaction accounts for its inhibitory activity in cytidine deaminase-deficient strains.

In order to determine the relative amounts of intact 5-azapyrimidines and the corresponding open-ring forms, RNA labeled *in vivo* with [^{14}C]-5-azacytidine was degraded by cold acid hydrolysis or enzymatically to nucleosides or nucleotides. In the hydrolysates of RNA from the cytidine deaminase-deficient bacteria the radioactive label was recovered as intact 5-azacytidine with a minor amount of *N*-amidino-*N*′-ribofuranosylurea. In the RNA from wild-type *E. coli* a third compound, 1-β-D-ribofuranosylbiuret, was detected, while no intact

5-azauridine could be found (Fig. 19). These results indicate that 5-azacytidine is present in the RNA mostly in intact form, while 5-azauridine, if present, is entirely converted to the open-ring form (Doskočil and Šorm, 1971b).

We may conclude that incorporation of 5-azauridine, followed by ring opening (i.e. depyrimidination) renders the mRNA non-translatable. On the other hand 5-azacytidine itself is not liable to rapid ring-opening when incorporated into RNA and permits translation with frequent miscodings.

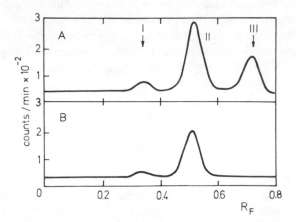

FIG. 19. Chromatographic analysis of cold acid hydrolysate of RNA labeled with 5-azacytidine. RNA was isolated from wild-type *E. coli* (A) or from strain OK 408 (Karlström, 1970) deficient in cytidine deaminase (B). RNA was hydrolysed with 1 N HCl at 45°C for 90 min. The hydrolysate was chromatographed in isopropanol–HCl–H$_2$O (170:41:39, v/v/v). Peak I, 5-azacytosine; peak II, 5-azacytidine-2'(3')-phosphate and *N*-amidino-*N*'-β-D-ribofuranosyl-urea-2'(3')-phosphate; peak III, 1-β-D-ribofuranosylbiuret-2'(3')-phosphate. From Doskočil and Šorm, 1971b.

10.3.3. DIFFERENTIAL INTERFERENCE OF 5-AZACYTIDINE WITH PHAGE f2 REPLICATION AND METABOLISM OF THE HOST

Inhibition of replication of the RNA phage f2 offers an example of a differential effect of 5-azacytidine on the synthesis of cellular and viral RNA.

Phage f2 is one of the simplest viruses known. The genomic single-stranded RNA molecule of about 1.21×10^6 daltons comprises three cistrons, i.e. maturation protein, coat protein and RNA-replicase genes. Phage RNA is synthesized by a specific RNA-replicase, a complex enzyme composed of one phage-coded subunit and three other subunits of host origin (Fedoroff, 1975). Unlike most RNA polymerases, the phage RNA-replicase holoenzyme is template-specific; apart from certain synthetic polynucleotides, phage plus (viral) or the complementary minus strands are exclusive templates. In infected cells the replication of phage starts as soon as the first molecules of phage-coded subunit of the replicase are formed by translation of the infecting viral RNA. The replication mechanism includes several unusual features. At first the replicase holoenzyme binds to the 3' end of the plus strand and synthesis from the 5' end of the complementary minus strand begins. According to the 'butterfly model' proposed by Robertson (1975) both the 3' end of the template and the 5' end of the nascent minus strand remain permanently attached to the enzyme, while the nascent RNA and the runoff template form single-stranded loops. When the synthesis of the minus-strand is finished, the enzyme switches over to the 3' end of the minus strand, where apparently a strong binding site for the enzyme is located. Now synthesis of a new plus strand starts, again with the 3' end of the template permanently attached to the enzyme. When the replication of the plus-strand is finished, no switchover of the replicase occurs, since the 3' end of the minus strand binds the enzyme more strongly than the 3' end of plus strand. Therefore the nascent plus strand is released and a new round of synthesis of plus strand begins on the same template. The proper functioning of this model depends on the presence of coat protein which, by forming a complex with a specific site on the plus strand, prevents the formation of excess RNA-replicase. If, however, no functional coat protein is present, e.g. if the infecting phage bears a non-polar suppressor-sensitive mutation in the coat protein gene, the replication of RNA takes an anomalous course. RNA-replicase is strongly over-produced and, in consequence of this, the phage-specific RNA has an atypical composition, consisting of nearly equal amounts of plus and minus strands which anneal to form double-stranded RNA (the so-called replicative form, or RF RNA).

If added immediately after infection, 5-azacytidine inhibits the synthesis of f2 phage completely. Neither phage-specific RNA nor proteins are formed with the exception of the RNA-replicase, the synthesis of which is directed by the infecting RNA. If, however, the inhibitor is added some 20 min after infection, enough viral particles, or RF RNA, is formed to permit determination of incorporated labeled 5-azacytidine. Deamination to 5-azauridine is mainly responsible for the inhibition of formation of new phage. If a cytidine deaminase-deficient host is used, a weak inhibitory effect is observed.

Double-stranded RF phage RNA was isolated from non-permissive bacteria infected with mutated phage f2 *sus* 11; labeled 5-azacytidine was added 20 min after infection. The RF RNA contained the same 5-azapyrimidine derivatives as host RNA, i.e. intact 5-azacytidine, N-amidino-N'-ribosylurea and ribosylbiuret. Therefore the f2 phage RNA replicase has no better discriminating power for 5-azacytidine than host RNA polymerase.

Differential incorporation of 5-azacytidine into host RNA, phage RF RNA and viral RNA was studied by double-labeling techniques, adding labeled 5-azacytidine and $^{32}P_i$ 20 min after infection. The relative amount of 5-azacytidine in RF RNA was slightly less than one-half the amount in host RNA concurrently synthesized. In the RNA of phage particles, however, the relative content of 5-azacytidine was as low as 7 per cent of the content in host RNA. It appears most likely that molecules with incorporated 5-azacytidine, or the open-ring form of 5-azauridine, cannot serve any more as templates for phage RNA replicase. Any utilizable template, whether plus or minus strands, must come from the period before addition of the drug, i.e. the first 20 min after infection. RF RNA would then always contain one analog-free strand, so that its total content of 5-azacytidine would be close to one-half of that in host RNA. The extremely low content of 5-azacytidine in viral RNA probably indicates that RNA molecules with high content of 5-azapyrimidines are incapable of encapsidation (Doskočil and Šorm, 1971a).

From this example we see that the mechanism of inhibition of RNA virus replication is entirely different from that responsible for growth inhibition of host cells; the susceptible target point is the two-stage synthesis of phage RNA, i.e. formation of minus-strand templates followed by synthesis of viral RNA on these templates. The template function of RNA is obviously more susceptible to the action of 5-azapyrimidines than that of DNA of host cells, which continues in the presence of the analog.

10.3.4. SPECIFIC INHIBITION OF SYNTHESIS OF T4 COLIPHAGE DNA BY 5-AZACYTIDINE

Cells of *E. coli* infected with T4 bacteriophage represent a system where 5-azacytidine exerts its full inhibitory effect on virus replication at internal pool levels completely harmless for host cells. Indeed, with T4 phage infection the response of the cells to 5-azacytidine is completely changed. Unlike inducible enzymes of the host cells, phage-induced early proteins are synthesized at normal rates in the presence of 5-azacytidine; synthesis of phage DNA is completely inhibited while in uninfected cells synthesis of chromosomal DNA proceeds unabated even for long periods of treatment (Doskočil and Šorm, 1967). These paradoxical findings were resolved by incorporation studies. First we found that upon phage infection the incorporation rate of 5-azacytidine drops instantaneously to less than 3 per cent of the rate before infection (Doskočil and Šorm, 1969). For comparison, incorporation of cytidine is decreased to 30–40 per cent of its preinfection rate. Further analysis of the phenomenon has shown that the dramatic decrease of incorporation of 5-azacytidine is due to inactivation of the constitutive nucleoside transport system which is mainly responsible for the uptake of 5-azacytidine (see above). Therefore the amount of 5-azacytidine taken up by the cells is far from sufficient to inhibit the synthesis of early phage-induced proteins. Nevertheless the synthesis of phage DNA *is* completely inhibited by the seemingly negligible amount of inhibitor taken up. Consequently phage DNA synthesis appears to be about two orders of magnitude more sensitive to the action of 5-azacytidine than protein synthesis in *E. coli*. Since the inhibition of DNA synthesis has been observed with T-even but not T-odd phages, it appears that the hydroxymethylation of deoxycytidylate, a key reaction in the synthesis of T-even phage DNA, is selectively inhibited by 5-azadeoxycytidylic acid present in the intracellular nucleotide pool.

Unlike the inhibition of host protein synthesis, suppression of T4 phage DNA replication is irreversible. This phenomenon becomes understandable from the kinetics of 5-azacytidine incorporation and elimination. As demonstrated above, 5-azacytidine migrates into stable forms of RNA and cannot be chased out of the cells. The bacteria with accumulated 5-azacytidine do not show any signs of inhibition. If these cells are infected with T4 phage, the presence of internal 5-azapyrimidine nucleotides in the intracellular nucleotide pools becomes apparent by inhibition of synthesis of phage DNA (Fig. 20). This 'antiphage state of the cells' persists for at least 1 hr after administration of the drug and may survive cell division. This condition is probably due to low stationary level of 5-azapyrimidine nucleotides in the internal nucleotide pool, which is due to limited turnover of tRNA; the level of this pool seems to be too low to inhibit protein synthesis, but sufficient to inhibit replication of phage DNA.

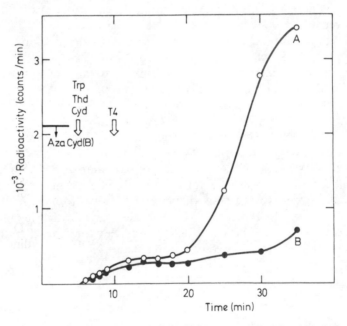

FIG. 20. Effect of pre-treatment with 5-azacytidine on incorporation of thymidine before and after infection with phage T4. One half of a bacterial culture (*E. coli* B) was treated with 5-azacytidine (20 μg/ml) for 4 min, rapidly filtered on a nitrocellulose membrane filter and resuspended in fresh medium containing cytidine (50 μg/ml), ³H-thymidine (0.5 μCi/ml, total conc. 2 μg/ml); the other half of the culture was processed in the same manner except that the treatment with 5-azacytidine was omitted. Five minutes later both cultures were infected with phage T4: *A*, untreated control (final yield of viable phage 2.55×10^{10} PFU/ml); *B*, culture pre-treated with 5-azacytidine (final yield 4.8×10^9 PFU/ml). From Doskočil and Šorm, 1969.

It will be noted that the inhibition of phage DNA synthesis is a function of 5-azacytidine itself while other inhibitory effects are caused mainly by 5-azauridine formed by deamination.

Phage T4 thus represents an example of a virus whose replication is sensitive to 5-azacytidine at concentrations far below those inhibitory for host cells. Of course, phage T4 is unique by its content of 5-hydroxymethyldeoxycytidylic acid which does not occur in the

DNA of animal viruses. The example shows, however, that selective inhibition of replication of viral DNA by very small doses of the inhibitor might be possible in special cases.

10.3.5. COMPARISON OF 5-AZACYTIDINE AND 6-AZAURIDINE

From the data compiled by Veselý and Čihák (1978) and those presented here, it follows that 5-azacytidine is recognized by a wide range of enzymes of pyrimidine nucleoside metabolism. Incorporation into RNA indicates that 5-azacytidine, or its phosphorylated derivatives, are substrates of uridine kinase, uridylate or cytidylate kinase and RNA-polymerase of E. coli, f2 phage and of mammalian cells. Furthermore the efficient incorporation into DNA implies that 5-azacytidine di- or tri-phosphates must be good substrates of cytidine di-(or tri-) phosphate 2′-oxidoreductase, and that 2′-deoxy-5-azacytidine triphosphate must be recognized by DNA-polymerase. Other enzymes recognizing 5-azapyrimidine nucleosides include cytidine aminohydrolase, uridine phosphorylase, UMP: pyrophosphate phosphoribosyltransferase, etc. Enzymes capable of discriminating 5-azapyrimidine analogs from normal nucleosides are exceptional, although the affinities for the former are usually lower. In E. coli 5-azacytidine is recognized by the constitutive nucleoside transport system, but not by the inducible system.

In contrast to 5-azacytidine, 6-azauridine fails to be recognized by most enzymes of pyrimidine nucleoside metabolism; in particular, it cannot be phosphorylated beyond the monophosphate level and thus cannot be incorporated into RNA or DNA. 6-Azauridine does not interact with nucleoside transport systems of E. coli and enters the cells by diffusion.

From the enzymological data we would assume that the conformation of 5-azapyrimidine nucleosides and nucleotides should be similar to corresponding derivatives of cytosine while 6-azapyrimidine should be dissimilar. Unfortunately few data concerning the conformation of 5-azapyrimidine nucleosides exist. Hruska et al. (1974) calculated the relative frequency of rotamers about $C_{4'}$—$C_{5'}$ bond from NMR data; the 5-azapyrimidines resemble cytidine and uridine by the predominance of the gauche-gauche conformer, while the opposite is true for 6-azauridine (cf. p. 388). Therefore 5-azacytidine resembles the normal nucleosides more closely than 6-azauridine, as predicted from enzymological data.

For obvious chemical reasons 5-azapyrimidine nucleosides cannot be substituted at N_5 of the sym. triazine ring, so that no analogs of thymidylic or 2′-deoxy-5-hydroxymethylcytidylic acids can be formed. The strong selective inhibition of T4 phage DNA synthesis indicates that 2′-deoxy-5-azacytidylic acid is a very strong inhibitor of deoxycytidylate hydroxymethyltransferase. Therefore it is noteworthy that 5-azapyrimidine nucleosides have apparently no effect on thymidylate synthetase, since the synthesis of DNA in E. coli is remarkably resistant to the action of both 5-azacytidine and 5-azauridine (Doskočil and Šorm, 1969).

10.3.6. ANTIVIRAL EFFECT OF 5-AZACYTIDINE

Several observations of interference with production of infectious viruses have been made in connection with the use of 5-azacytidine as a chemical mutagen. When applied as a liquid overlay to chick embryo cells infected with Venezuelan equine encephalomyelitis virus, 5-azacytidine (25 µg/ml) reduced virus production about 100-fold and greatly increased the frequency of large-plaque mutant of the virus (Halle, 1968). Toyoshima and Vogt (1969) used 5-azacytidine to obtain temperature-sensitive mutants of an avian sarcoma virus. Pringle (1970) compared the mutagenic efficiency of 5-azacytidine, 5-fluorouracil and ethylmethane sulfonate. In comparison with the high mutagenicity of 5-fluorouracil, 5-azacytidine had a relatively weak mutagenic, and much higher virostatic, effect when applied to baby hamster kidney cells infected with vesicular stomatitis virus; at about 50 µg/ml, 5-azacytidine reduced virus titer by five orders of magnitude while 5-fluorouracil under the same conditions caused reduction of virus titer by one log.

Antiviral activity of 5-azacytidine was evaluated by the agar-diffusion plaque-inhibition method (Rada, unpublished data), using vaccinia virus (CL strain), Newcastle disease virus (Hertfordshire strain) and western equine encephalomyelitis virus (strain WEE-15). 5-Azacytidine (20 $\mu g/ml$) caused large zones of plaque inhibition with all three viruses tested, while cytotoxicity as revealed by neutral red staining was not very strong. Of several hundred compounds tested, 5-azacytidine was the most effective against Newcastle disease virus, while 5-azauracil was without any effect.

By analogy with other mutagenic agents, 5-azacytidine was found to induce formation of infectious virus in a hamster cell line transformed with Schmitt-Ruppin strain of Rous sarcoma virus; the virus induced by 5-azacytidine deviated from the original transforming virus in host range and tumor-inducing ability, suggesting that a mutagenic effect might have taken place concurrently with induction (Altanerová, 1972; Altanerová and Altaner, 1972).

Extensive literature concerning antineoplasmic activity of 5-azacytidine, including neoplasias of viral aethiology, has been covered by Veselý and Čihák (1978). A recent study by von Hoff et al. (1976) reports on results for 200 patients with acute myelogenous leukemia, where 20 per cent complete and 16 per cent partial remissions were achieved by administration of 5-azacytidine (100–250 mg/m² body surface per day intravenously or by continuous infusion for five successive days). Most patients with remissions have previously been unsuccessfully treated with conventional antileukemic agents. Serious side-effects, however, were observed, of which hepatic coma was sometimes fatal, causing three deaths in a group of 745 patients treated with 5-azacytidine alone.

In an attempt to combine antineoplasmic and antiviral effectivity of 5-azacytidine and arabinosylcytosine, Beisler et al. (1977) synthesized 1-β-D-arabinofuranosyl-5-azacytosine. When tested on murine leukemia L 1210 system, the new drug was about as effective as 5-azacytidine. Antiviral activity of this compound has not yet been reported.

10.3.7. ACTIVATION OF GENES AND PROVIRUSES BY HYPOMETHYLATION

In the DNA of higher animals a small fraction of DNA-cytosine is methylated at the 5-carbon atom of pyrimidine ring. Methylation is a post-synthetic modification of DNA and is effected by DNA-methylase, with S-adenosyl methionine serving as the source of the methyl group. The distribution of 5-methylcytosine in the DNA is not random; most of it occurs in the sequence CpG (Doskočil and Šorm, 1962). Since CpG is a self-complementary sequence, fully methylated DNA would contain pairs of 5-methylcytosine residues, occurring at opposite sites of the double helix. The overall contents of 5-methylcytosine are not constant in a given species or individual, varying somewhat in the DNA of various tissues as compared with sperm DNA, where maximum degree of methylation is usually observed. In the DNA of differentiated tissues the lowered 5-methylcytosine contents are usually due to the presence of heavily undermethylated domains, alternating with fully methylated DNA (see Wigler, 1981, for a review). Amplified ribosomal DNA of amphibian embryos is non-methylated (Bird et al., 1981).

These data indicate the existence of a master pattern of methylation which is maintained in germline cells, while programmed omissions of methylation are introduced at specific sites of DNA in differentiating cells (Wigler, 1981). Any alteration of the master methylation pattern seems to be perpetuated in the course of subsequent cycles of DNA-replication. Wigler et al. (1981) prepared hypermethylated DNA by in vitro treatment of bihelical replication form of phage ØX 174 DNA with HpaII modification methylase. When introduced into mouse cells, this DNA has been observed to maintain its hypermethylated state for at least twenty-five generations, with infrequent losses of single methylation sites. Therefore it seems that animal cells contain a 'maintenance' methylase, which perpetuates any methylation pattern of DNA with relatively high degree of fidelity, provided it occurs in a self-complementary sequence. Rather than distinguishing any specific DNA sequence, the maintenance methylase recognizes the dissymmetry of methylation on opposite strands of the double helix of semiconservatively replicated DNA. Consequently, any accidental loss of a particular methyl group should cause a permanent hypomethylation at this site.

Clonally transmitted change in the methylation pattern appears to be a major tool in gene activation during cellular differentiation. In various differentiated cells, transcriptionally active chromatin is characterized by: (1) hypomethylation, (2) sensitivity to non-specific DNAases, e.g. micrococcal DNAase, (3) presence of sites hypersensitive to DNAase I (where DNAase I introduces a double cut at the same level of a double helix). From these alterations, hypomethylation appears to be the primary one, triggering the sequence of events ultimately leading to gene activation. Therefore DNA methylation plays a causative role in gene regulation during development and differentiation (Groudine et al., 1981; Compere and Palmiter, 1981; Christman et al., 1980).

For obvious chemical reasons 5-azacytidine cannot serve as acceptor of a methyl group in position 5. Therefore incorporation of 5-deoxyazacytidine into DNA instead of deoxycytidine must lead to the loss of methylation at this site, thus introducing a permanent hypomethylated site. Therefore, even a transient exposure of dividing cells to 5-azacytidine causes a random activation of genes, or groups of genes, causing a chaotic cellular differentiation. Examples of artificial differentiation provoked by 5-azacytidine have been observed (Constantinides et al., 1977; Constantinides et al., 1978; Taylor and Jones, 1979; Jones and Taylor, 1980). In a typical experiment, mouse 10T1/2 or 3T3 cells were exposed to 5-azacytidine (1–10 μg/ml) for 24 hr. The analog was then removed and cultivation was continued. Foci of differentiated cells (myoblasts, adipocytes or chondrocytes) appeared on the plates 2–4 weeks after the treatment (Taylor and Jones, 1979).

By inducing hypomethylation into proviral DNA, 5-azacytidine may activate endogenous retroviral genomes. As observed by Cohen (1980) and Struhlmann et al. (1981), hypomethylation of retroviral genomes is correlated with infectivity and expression in the animal. Groudine et al. (1981) were able to activate a silent locus of a retrovirus by treating chicken lymfocytes with 5-azacytidine for 24 hr; the activation was concurrent with hypomethylation in DNA as demonstrated by differential cleavage of proviral DNA sequences with restriction endonucleases MspI and HpaII; at the same time, acquisition of at least one DNAase I-hypersensitive site within the chromosomal domain of the provirus was detected. The effect of 5-azacytidine was found to be similar to that of other known inhibitors of methylation, i.e. ethionine, while the induction by other nucleoside analogs such as 5-bromo or 5-iododeoxyuridine appears to be due to a different mechanism.

Due to its proven ability to affect gene expression control via hypomethylation, 5-azacytidine has become a valuable tool of modern cytochemistry and virology; its therapeutic value is, however, severely limited by the risk of chaotic cell differentiation and retrovirus activation.

10.3.8. PERSPECTIVES

From the foregoing it follows that knowledge of antiviral activity of 5-azapyrimidine nucleosides is still incomplete, due to the fact that high toxicity of these compounds apparently prohibits their extensive use as chemotherapeutic agents. Symptoms of toxicity, however, may be relieved by continuous slow infusion (cf. Veselý and Čihák, 1978), and the overall efficiency may, in perspective, be modulated by simultaneous application of gratuitous inhibitors of transport, by analogy with bacterial systems (see Section 10.3.1). The effective utility of 5-azapyrimidine nucleosides for antiviral chemotherapy may then depend on the selectivity of antiviral action, i.e. whether an obligatory step of the virus replication cycle would be more sensitive than vital biochemical processes of host cells. Although the relevance of experiments with bacteriophages to animal viruses is limited, the results with T4 phage inhibition show that very large differences in the levels of sensitivity of host and phage may in fact exist; in this particular case, however, the selective antiphage effect was due to inhibition of synthesis of 2′-deoxy-5-hydroxymethylcytidylate, a specific precursor of phage DNA, which does not occur in the DNA of known animal viruses.

It appears that inactivation of RNA-template activity as observed with RNA-phage f2 may be the basis of a selective antiviral action. As shown above (see Section 10.3.3) the inactivation of an RNA template is a consequence of incorporation of 5-azauridine and may inhibit replication of all those RNA viruses dependent on two cycles of RNA synthesis by an RNA-directed RNA polymerase. Since no analogous RNA-directed RNA polymerase is vital for animal cells, the inhibition could be sufficiently selective. Replication of DNA viruses cannot be expected to be inhibitable by this mechanism, since template inactivation is due to incorporation of 5-azauridine, while 5-azacytidine itself is rather ineffective in this respect. From these considerations it appears that systematic investigation of the effect of 5-azapyrimidine nucleosides on the replication of RNA-viruses may prove useful.

Unfortunately, any potential benefit from antiviral or antitumour properties of 5-azapyrimidine nucleosides may turn out to be outweighed by the dangers of uncontrolled cellular differentiation and activation of proviruses.

10.4. 3-DEAZAURIDINE

3-Deazauridine (1-β-D-ribofuranosyl-2,4-(1H,3H)-pyridinedione) (Fig. 21), an analog of uridine, was synthesized by Robins and Currie (1968; Currie et al., 1970). This compound was shown to inhibit several bacteria and experimental tumours.

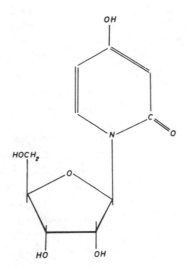

FIG. 21. The structure of 3-deazauridine.

3-Deazauridine was investigated for its effects on the replication of several RNA viruses (Shannon et al., 1972; Khare et al., 1972). Inhibition of virus-induced cytopathic effects was observed in cells infected with rhinovirus type 1A (strain 2060) and type 13 (strain 353), Coxsackie virus type A21 (strain Kuykendall) and influenza A0 virus (strain PR8/34). The extent of cytopathic changes in KB cells (a human nasopharyngeal carcinoma cell line) or in Madin—Darby canine cell line (in the case of influenza A0 virus) was determined statistically by the virus-rating procedure. The analog exhibited virus ratings of 1.4–2.0 and 1.3–1.7 for rhinovirus 1A and influenza A PR8, respectively. With influenza A2 virus (strain Aichi/2/68), B virus (strain Lee) and parainfluenza virus type 3 (Sendai strain) the hemagglutinin production by influenza A2 Sendai viruses was inhibited by about 90 per cent. 3-Deazacytidine, tested in parallel experiments, was more active than 3-deazauridine. The concentrations of the analogs employed in these studies were 10–1000 μg/ml. The virus dose per microculture panel well was 32–320 $CCID_{50}$. No inhibition of virus-induced cytopathic effect by 3-deazauridine or 3-deazacytidine was found in cells infected with the enteroviruses polio type 2 or echo type 12.

3-Deazauridine was evaluated for possible inhibitory activity against Gross murine leukemia virus (wild-type) in vitro by means of a u.v.-XC plaque-reduction assay procedure

(Shannon *et al.*, 1974). This method is based on the observation that when rat XC cells (a cell line originally derived from tumour cells induced in newborn Wistar albino rats by the Prague strain of Rous sarcoma virus) are placed in contact with mouse embryo cells infected with mouse leukemia virus, rapid and marked cytopathic effects consisting of cell fusion and syncytium formation occur. In multiple-cycle experiments 3-deazauridine inhibited significantly Gross leukemia virus replication in NIH strain Swiss mouse embryo cells and virus-induced plaque formation in rat XC cells at concentrations between 6.4 and 200 μg/ml. 3-Deazauridine was not obviously cytotoxic at concentrations which inhibited virus replication and plaque formation, nor was host cell protein synthesis affected by treatment of NIH-mouse cell cultures with the analog at these active concentrations. Although the analog had potent cytostatic properties, the synthesis of cellular DNA and RNA was partially inhibited by the compound at concentrations above 32 μg/ml and was not inhibited at all at concentrations of 10 μg/ml or below, i.e. analog levels at which virus inhibitory effects were still observed. While the analog displayed some selective inhibitory activity against the virus, the mechanism of action of 3-deazauridine against Gross leukemia virus appears to be primarily via its inhibitory effect on cell division *per se*, a process known to be required for RNA tumour virus replication. The combination 3-deazauridine plus polyadenylic acid was more effective in inhibiting Gross leukemia virus replication *in vitro* than either compound alone (Shannon, 1977). The combination of 6.4 μg 3-deazauridine/ml plus 3.2 μg poly(A)/ml yielded an 85 per cent inhibition of Gross leukemia virus replication, a response that would ordinarily require about 20 to 64 μg/ml of 3-deazauridine or about 10 μg/ml of poly(A) alone, i.e. about 3.2 to 10 times as much drug. The plotted isobole indicates a greater-than-additive (potentiating) effect for these two drugs in combination and probably reflects different mechanism of action.

3-Deazauridine failed to show any inhibitory activity on the development of Rauscher murine leukemia virus-induced splenomegaly *in vivo*, presumably because of its severe toxicity to mice (Shannon, 1977).

Studies on the metabolism of 3-deazauridine in microbial and tumour cells have shown that the analog is phosphorylated to form 3-deazauridine 5'-triphosphate, which is a potent, competitive inhibitor of cytidine triphosphate synthetase (McPortland *et al.*, 1974), but it is not incorporated into cellular RNA or DNA.

3-Deazauridine pharmacology was studied in twenty patients who received the analog by rapid or continuous infusion (Benvenuto *et al.*, 1979). The plasma clearance of 3-deazauridine after rapid (15 to 30 min) administration was biphasic, with an average terminal plasma half-life $t_{1/2}$ of 4.4 hr, an extrapolated volume of distribution of 0.57 liter/kg. After 5-day continuous infusion of 3-deazauridine, the plasma clearance was also biphasic with an average terminal $t_{1/2}$ of 21.3 hr and an extrapolated volume of distribution of 18.8 liter/kg. 2,4-Dihydroxypyridine, the aglycone of 3-deazauridine, was observed in plasma but not in urine of patients receiving the analog by rapid infusion. The urinary excretion of 3-deazauridine was low, only 7.8 per cent 24 hr after rapid infusion and 7.2 per cent up to 4 days after continuous infusion. This low urinary excretion of unchanged analog and the data from patients with hepatic and renal dysfunction suggest that hepatic clearance is the most important elimination pathway for 3-deazauridine. Tissue distribution of 3-deazauridine was determined from autopsy samples of two patients. Not only were high levels of 3-deazauridine in the tissues studied, but 3-deazauridine triphosphate, the active metabolite of 3-deazauridine, was present in brain, lung and liver.

REFERENCES

ALTANEROVÁ, V. (1972) Virus production induced by various chemical carcinogens in a virogenic hamster cell line transformed by Rous sarcoma virus. *J. natn. Cancer Inst.* **49**: 1375–1380.

ALTANEROVÁ, V. and ALTANER, C. (1972) Characterization of chicken sarcoma viruses induced with chemical carcinogens and mutagens in transformed hamster cells. *Neoplasma* **19**: 398–405.

BAUER, D. J. (1972) Thiosemicarbazones. In: *Chemotherapy of Virus Diseases*, Vol. 1 pp. 35–113, BAUER, D. J. (ed.). International Encyclopedia of Pharmacology and Therapeutics, Pergamon Press, Oxford.

BAUER, D. J. and SHEFFIELD, F. W. (1959) Antiviral chemotherapeutic activity of isatin β-thiosemicarbazone in mice infected with rabbitpox virus. *Nature* **184**: 149–167.

BECKER, A. and JOKLIK, W. K. (1964) Messenger RNA in cells infected with vaccinia virus. *Proc. natn. Acad. Sci. U.S.A.* **51**: 577–585.

BEISLER, J. A., ABBASI, M. I. and DRISCOLL, J. S. (1977) The synthesis and antitumor activity of arabinosyl-5-azacytosine. *Biochem. Pharmac.* **26**: 2469–2472.

BENVENUTO, J. A., HALL, S. W., FARQUHAR, D., STEWARD, D. J., BENJAMIN, R. S. and LOO, T. L. (1979) Pharmacokinetics and disposition of 3-deazauridine in humans. *Cancer Res.* **39**: 349–352.

BIRD, A., TAGGART, M. and MCLEOD, D. (1981) Loss of DNA methylation accompanies the onset of ribosomal gene activity in early development of *Xenopus laevis*. *Cell* **26**: 381–390.

BREZINA, R., KORDOVÁ, N. and LINK, F. (1962) The effect of 6-azauracil riboside on the multiplication of *Coxiella burneti, Rickettsia prowazeki* and *R. mooseri*. *Acta virol.* **6**: 266–270.

BUCK, L. L. and PFAU, CH. J. (1969) Inhibition of lymphocytic choriomeningitis virus replication by actinomycin D and 6-azauridine. *Virology* **37**: 698–701.

BUKRINSKAYA, A. G. and ASADULLAEV, T. A. (1968) Comparative effect of histon and 6-azauridine on myxovirus reproduction. *Vop. Virus.* **13**: 549–554 (in Russian).

CALABRESI, P. (1965) Clinical studies with systemic administration of antimetabolites of pyrimidine nucleosides in viral infections. *Ann. N.Y. Acad. Sci.* **130**: 198–208.

CHRISTMAN, J. K., WELCH, N., SCHOENBRUNN, B., SCHNEIDERMAN, N. and ACS, G. (1980) Hypomethylation of DNA during differentiation of Friend erythroleukemia cells. *J. Cell. Biol.* **86**: 366–370.

ČIHÁK, A. and ŠORM, F. (1965) Biochemical effects and metabolic transformations of 5-azacytidine in *Escherichia coli*. *Coll. Czech. Chem. Commun.* **30**: 2091–2102.

ČIHÁK, A. and VESELÝ, J. (1977) Transformation of 5-aza-2'-³H deoxycytidine in *Escherichia coli*. *FEBS Lett.* **78**: 244–246.

COHEN, J. C. (1980) Methylation of milk-borne and genetically transmitted mouse mammary tumor virus proviral DNA. *Cell* **19**: 653–662.

COMPERE, S. J. and PALMITER, R. D. (1981) DNA-methylation controls the inducibility of the mouse metallothionein-I gene in lymphoid cells. *Cell* **25**: 233–240.

CONSIGLI, R. A. and LERNER, M. P. (1970) Enzyme studies (phosphorylation) during Newcastle disease virus infection of chick embryo cells. *Can. J. Microbiol.* **16**: 635–638.

CONSTANTINIDES, P. G., JONES, P. A. and GEVERS, W. (1977) Functional striated muscle cells from non-myoblast precursors following 5-azacytidine treatment. *Nature* **267**: 364–366.

CONSTANTINIDES, P. G., TAYLOR, S. M. and JONES, P. A. (1978) Phenotypic conversion of cultured mouse embryo cells by azapyrimidine nucleosides. *Dev. Biol.* **66**: 57–71.

CRISTESCU, C. (1968) 6-Azauracil derivatives with potential cytostatic activity. VI. An improved synthesis of 2-β-D-ribofuranosyl-as-triazine-3,5(2H,4H) dione (6-azauridine). *Rev. Roum. Chim.* **12**: 365–369.

CURRIE, B. L., ROBINS, R. K. and ROBINS, M. J. (1970) The synthesis of 3-deazapyrimidine nucleosides related to uridine and cytidine and their derivatives. *J. heterocycl. chem.* **7**: 323–329.

DECLERCQ, E., DESCAMPS, J., SOMMER, P. and HOLÝ, A. (1978) (S)-9-(2,3-Dihydroxypropyl)adenine: an aliphatic nucleoside analog with broad-spectrum antiviral activity. *Science* **200**: 563–565.

DEMIDOVA, S. A., AZADOVA, N. B., MARTYNOVA, V. N., GALEGOV, G. A. and ZHDANOV, V. M. (1969) The injurious effect of 6-azauridine on the multiplication of cytomegalovirus in man. *Dokl. Akad. Nauk. SSSR* **186**: 709–710 (in Russian).

DODGE, W. H., MORSE, P. A. JR. and GENTRY, G. A. (1970) Rous sarcoma virus-induced changes in uridine and UMP metabolism in chick chorioallantoic membrane. *Biochim. biophys. Acta* **217**: 199–201.

DOSKOČIL, J. (1972) The components of the nucleoside-transporting system in *Escherichia coli*. *Biochim. biophys. Acta* **282**: 393–400.

DOSKOČIL, J. (1974) Inducible nucleoside permease in *Escherichia coli*. *Biochem. biophys. Res. Commun.* **56**: 997–1003.

DOSKOČIL, J. and HOLÝ, A. (1974) Inhibition of nucleoside binding sites by nucleoside analogs in *Escherichia coli*. *Nucleic Acids Res.* **1**: 491–502.

DOSKOČIL, J., PAČES, V. and ŠORM, F. (1967) Inhibition of protein synthesis by 5-azacytidine in *Escherichia coli*. *Biochim. biophys. Acta* **145**: 771–779.

DOSKOČIL, J. and ŠORM, F. (1962) Distribution of 5-methylcytosine in pyrimidine sequences of deoxyribonucleic acid. *Biochim. biophys. Acta* **55**: 953–959.

DOSKOČIL, J. and ŠORM, F. (1967) The action of 5-azacytidine on bacteria infected bacteriophage T4. *Biochim. biophys. Acta* **145**: 780–791.

DOSKOČIL, J. and ŠORM, F. (1969) Incorporation and phosphorylation of 5-azacytidine by normal and T4-phage-infected cells of *E. coli*. *Eur. J. Biochem.* **8**: 75–80.

DOSKOČIL, J. and ŠORM, F. (1970a) The inhibitory effects of 5-azacytidine and 5-azauridine in *Escherichia coli*. *Coll. Czech. Chem. Commun.* **35**: 1880–1891.

DOSKOČIL, J. and ŠORM, F. (1970b) The effects of 5-azacytidine and 5-azauridine on protein synthesis in *Escherichia coli*. *Biochem. biophys. Res. Commun.* **38**: 569–574.

DOSKOČIL, J. and ŠORM, F. (1970c) The mode of action of 5-aza-2'-deoxycytidine in *Escherichia coli*. *Eur. J. Biochem.* **13**: 180–187.

DOSKOČIL, J. and ŠORM, F. (1971a) Differential incorporation of 5-azapyrimidines into the RNA of phage f2 and of bacterial host. *Eur. J. Biochem.* **23**: 253–261.

DOSKOČIL, J. and ŠORM, F. (1971b) The determination of 5-azapyrimidines and their derivatives in bacterial RNA. *FEBS Lett.* **19**: 30–32.

DUBBS, D. R. and KIT, S. (1964) Isolation and properties of vaccinia mutants deficient in thymidine kinase-inducing activity. *Virology* **22**: 214–225.

DUNDAROFF, S. and FALKE, D. (1972) Thymidine-, uridine- and choline-kinase in rabbit kidney cells infected with Herpesvirus hominis, type I and II. *Arch. ges. Virusforsch.* **38**: 56–66.

EHRLICH, J., SLOAN, B. J., MILLER, F. A. and MACHAMER, H. E. (1965) Searching for anti-viral materials from microbial fermentations. *Ann. N.Y. Acad. Sci.* **130**: 5–16.

ELION, G. B., BIEBER, S., NATHAN, H. and HITCHINGS, G. J. (1958) Uracil antagonism and inhibition of mammary adenocarcinoma 755. *Cancer Res.* **18**: 802–817.

ELIS, J. and RAŠKOVÁ, H. (1972) New indications for 6-azauridine treatment in man. *Eur. J. clin. Pharm.* **4**: 77–81.

FALKE, D. and RADA, B. (1970) 6-Azauridine as an inhibitor of the synthesis of *Herpesvirus hominis*. *Acta virol.* **14**: 115–123.

FEDOROFF, N. (1975) Replicase of the phage f2. In: *RNA Phages*, pp. 235–258, ZINDER, N. D. (ed.). Cold Spring Harbor Laboratory.

FENNER, F. (1976) *Classification and Nomenclature of Viruses*, Second Report of the International Committee on Taxonomy of Viruses. Karger, Basel.

FISHER, D. S., CASSIDY, E. P. and WELCH, A. D. (1966) Immunosuppression by pyrimidine nucleoside analogs. *Biochem. Pharmac.* **15**: 1013–1022.

FLANAGAN, J. F. and GINSBERG, H. S. (1964) Role of ribonucleic acid biosynthesis in multiplication of type 5-adenovirus. *J. Bact.* **87**: 977–987.

FRASER, K. B. and MARTIN, S. J. (1978) *Measles Virus and its Biology*. Academic Press, New York. pp. 249.

GALEGOV, G. A., BIKBULATOVA, R. M., VANAG, K. A. and SHEN, R. M. (1968a) Inhibiting effect of 6-azauridine upon reproduction of *Herpes simplex* virus. *Vop. Virus.* **13**: 18–21 (in Russian).

GALEGOV, G. A., KUKHAR, E. E. and BIKBULATOV, R. M. (1970) Treatment of keratitis in rabbits due to *Herpes simplex* virus with 6-azauridine. *Vop. Virus.* **15**: 351–354 (in Russian).

GALEGOV, G. A., PRAVDINA, N. F., PARNES, A. and KARAPETYAN, D. K. (1968b) Synthesis of uridylic nucleosides and TMP in bone marrow of chicken infected with virus of avian myeloblastosis. *Biochimia* **33**: 338–342 (in Russian).

GELBARD, A. S., KIM, S. H. and EIDINOFF, L. M. (1966) Nucleoside kinase activities in tissues infected with Rous sarcoma virus. *Cancer Res.* **26**: 748–751.

GERSHON, D. and SACHS, L. (1966) The early synthesis of RNA in polyoma virus development. *Virology* **29**: 44–48.

GOLDBERG, I. H. and RABINOWITZ, M. (1963) Inhibition of RNA nucleotidyltransferase by 6-azauridine triphosphate. *Biochim. biophys. Acta* **72**: 116–119.

GRAFNETTEROVÁ, J., GROSSI, E., FUMAGALLI, R., MORGANTI, P. and GRAFNETTER, D. (1966) Effects of 6-azauridine on the developing chick embryo. *Neoplasma* **13**: 251–258.

GREŠÍKOVÁ, M. and RADA, B. (1972) Studies on arbovirus haemagglutinin: differential inhibition of haem-agglutinin formation by 6-azauridine and uridine kinase-containing cell-free extract. *Acta virol.* **16**: 239–243.

GROUDINE, M., EISENMAN, R. and WEINTRAUB, H. (1981) Chromatin structure of endogenous retroviral genes and activation by an inhibitor of DNA-methylation. *Nature* **292**: 311–317.

GUTOVÁ, M., ELIS, J. and RAŠKOVÁ, H. (1971) Teratogenic effect of 6-azauridine in rats. *Teratology* **4**: 287–294.

HABERMANN, V. and ŠORM, F. (1958) Mechanism of the cancerostatic action of 6-azauracil and its riboside. *Coll. Czech. Chem. Commun.* **23**: 2201–2206.

HALLE, S. (1968) 5-Azacytidine as a mutagen for arboviruses. *J. Virol.* **2**: 1228–1229.

HAMMER, G., SCHWARZ, R. T. and SCHOLTISSEK, C. (1976) Effect of infection with enveloped viruses on nucleoside metabolism. *Virology* **70**: 238–240.

HAMMER-JESPERSEN, K., MUNCH-PETERSEN, A., NYGAARD, P. and SCHWARTZ, M. (1971) Induction of enzymes involved in the catabolism of deoxyribonucleosides and ribonucleosides in *Escherichia coli* K12. *Eur. J. Biochem.* **19**: 533–538.

HANDSCHUMACHER, R. E. (1957) Studies of bacterial resistance to 6-azauracil and its riboside. *Biochim. biophys. Acta* **23**: 428–430.

HANDSCHUMACHER, R. E. (1960a) Azauracil ribonucleoside and ribonucleotide: isolation and chemical synthesis. *J. biol. Chem.* **235**: 764–768.

HANDSCHUMACHER, R. E. (1960b) Orotidylic acid decarboxylase: inhibition studies with azauridine 5′-phosphate. *J. biol. Chem.* **235**: 2917–2919.

HANDSCHUMACHER, R. E., CALABRESI, P., WELCH, A. D., BONO, V., FALLON, H. and FREI, E. (1962) Summary of current information on 6-azauridine. *Cancer Chemother. Rep.* **21**: 1–18.

HANDSCHUMACHER, R. E., ŠKODA, J. and ŠORM, F. (1963) Metabolic and biochemical effects of 6-azacytidine in mice with Ehrlich ascites carcinoma. *Coll. Czech. Chem. Commun.* **28**: 2983–2990.

HERRMANN, E. C. JR. (1961) Plaque inhibition test for detection of specific inhibitors of DNA containing viruses. *Proc. Soc. exp. Biol. Med.* **107**: 142–145.

HOLÝ, A. (1975) Aliphatic analogs of nucleosides, nucleotides and oligonucleotides. *Coll. Czech. Chem. Commun.* **40**: 187–214.

HRUSKA, F. E., WOOD, D. J., MYNOTT, R. J. and SARMA, R. H. (1973) ¹H NMR study of the conformation of the riboside phosphate moiety of 6-azauridine-5′-monophosphate—a nucleotide with an unusual conformation. *FEBS Lett.* **31**: 153–155.

HRUSKA, F. E., WOOD, D. J., McCAIG, T. N., SMITH, A. A. and HOLÝ, A. (1974) A nuclear magnetic resonance study of nucleoside conformation in solution. The effect of structure and confirmation of the magnetic nonequivalence of 5′-methylene hydrogens. *Can. J. chem.* **52**: 497–508.

JAFFARI, S. M. H. and HUSSAIN, A. (1969) 6-Azauridine in smallpox. *Indian J. Med. Res.* **57**: 809–814.

JAKUBOVIČ, A. and SVOBODA, J. (1960) The influence of 6-azauracil and 6-azauracil riboside on the growth of Rous sarcoma. *Neoplasma* **7**: 143–145.

JANKŮ, I., KRŠIAK, M., VOLICER, L., ČAPEK, R., SMETANA, R. and NOVOTNÝ, J. (1965) Studies on 6-azauridine and 6-azacytidine. II. The effects of 6-azauridine on the central nervous system. *Biochem. Pharmac.* **14**: 1525–1535.

JELÍNEK, R., RYCHTER, Z. and SEICHERT, V. (1970) Syndrome of caudal regression in the chick embryo. *Folia morphol.* **18**: 125–137.

JERNE, N. K., NORDIN, A. A. and HENRY, C. (1963) The agar plaque technique for recognizing antibody producing cells. In: *Cell Bound Antibodies*, pp. 109–125, AMOS, B. and KOPROWSKI, H. (eds). Wistar Institute Press, Philadelphia.

JIŘIČKA, Z., SMETANA, K., JANKŮ, I., ELIS, J. and NOVOTNY, J. (1965) Studies on 6-azauridine and 6-azacytidine. I. Toxicity studies of 6-azauridine and 6-azacytidine in mice. *Biochem. Pharmac.* **14**: 1517–1523.

JOKLIK, W. K. (1964a) The intracellular uncoating of poxvirus DNA. I. The fate of radioactively-labeled rabbitpox virus. *J. molec. Biol.* **8**: 263–276.

JOKLIK, W. K. (1964b) The intracellular uncoating of poxvirus DNA. The molecular basis of the uncoating process. *J. molec. Biol.* **8**: 277–288.

JONES, P. and TAYLOR, S. (1980) Cellular differentiation, cytidine analogs and DNA-methylation. *Cell* **20**: 85–93.

JUROVČÍK, M., HOLÝ, A. and ŠORM, F. (1971) Utilization of L-adenosine by mammalian tissues. *FEBS Lett.* **18**: 274–276.

KÁRA, J. (1968) Induction of deoxycytidylate deaminase and uridine kinase and activation of cellular DNA synthesis in the course of transformation of chicken embryo cells infected by Rous sarcoma virus *in vitro*. *Folia biol.* **14**: 249–265.

KARLSTRÖM, H. O. (1970) Inability of *E. coli* B to incorporate added deoxycytidine, deoxyadenosine and deoxyguanosine into DNA. *Eur. J. Biochem.* **17**: 68–71.

KAVERIN, N. V. and EMELIYANOV, B. A. (1967) The effect of 6-azauridine on the course of latent period in RNA viruses. *Vop. Virus.* **12**: 51–54 (in Russian).

KAUFMAN, H. E. and MALONEY, E. D. (1963) Therapeutic anti-viral activity in tissue culture. *Proc. Soc. exp. Biol. Med.* **112**: 4–7.

KHARE, G. P., SIDWELL, R. W., HUFFMAN, J. H., TOLMAN, R. L. and ROBINS, R. K. (1972) Inhibition of RNA virus replication *in vitro* by 3-deazacytidine and 3-deazauridine. *Proc. Soc. exp. Biol. Med.* **140**: 880–884.

KIT, S., VALLADARES, Y. and DUBBS, D. R. (1964) Effects of age of culture and vaccinia infection on uridine kinase activity of L-cells. *Expl. Cell. Res.* **34**: 257–265.

KLEIN, R. J., FRIEDMAN-KIEN, A. E. and BRADY, E. (1974) *Herpes simplex* virus skin infection in hairless mice: treatment with antiviral compounds. *Antimicrob. Ag. Chemother.* **5**: 318–322.

KORBECKI, M., LUCZAK, M. and KLIMOWICZ, Z. (1968) Influence of 6-azauridine on the multiplication of the parainfluenza 3 virus. *Bull. Acad. Polonaise Sci.* **16**: 539–543.

KORBECKI, M. and PLAGEMANN, P. G. W. (1969) Competitive inhibition of uridine incorporation by 6-azauridine in uninfected and mengovirus-infected Novikoff hepatoma cells. *Proc. Soc. exp. Biol. Med.* **132**: 587–595.

LADNYI, I. D., ARITA, I. and JEŽEK, Z. (1981) The global programme of smallpox eradication. *J. Hyg. Epidem. (Praha)* **25**: 217–232.

LEONARD, L. L., TER MEULEN, V. and FREEMAN, J. M. (1971) In vitro sensitivity of measles virus to 6-azauridine. *Proc. Soc. exp. Biol. Med.* **136**: 857–862.

LISÝ, V., ŠKODA, J., RYCHLÍK, I., SMRT, J., HOLÝ, A. and ŠORM, F. (1968) Changes in coding properties of poly- and oligonucleotides containing 6-azapyrimidine ribonucleosides. *Coll. Czech. Chem. Commun.* **33**: 4111–4119.

LOH, P. C. (1964) The role of RNA in the synthesis of vaccinia virus. *Proc. Soc. exp. Biol. Med.* **116**: 789–792.

McPORTLAND, R. P., WANG, M. C., BLOCK, A. and WEIFELD, H. (1974) Cytidine 5'-triphosphate synthetase as a target for inhibition by the antitumor agent 3-deazauridine. *Cancer Res.* **34**: 3107–3111.

MYGIND, B., and MUNCH-PETERSEN, A. (1975) Transport of pyrimidine nucleosides in cells of *Escherichia coli* K.12. *Eur. J. Biochem.* **59**: 365–372.

MYŠKA, V., ELIS, J., PLEVOVÁ, J. and RAŠKOVÁ, H. (1967) Azauridine in viral eye infections. *Lancet* i: 1230–1231.

NICHOL, F. R. and TERSHAK, D. R. (1967) Effects of 5-fluorouracil and 6-azauridine on interferon action. *J. Virol.* **1**: 450–451.

NOUZA, K., POKORNÁ, Z., SLAVÍK, M. and GOTTWALDOVÁ, A. (1970) The immunosuppressive effects of 6-azauridine. *Folia biol.* **16**: 188–195.

NOVOTNÝ, J., SMETANA, R. and RAŠKOVÁ, H. (1965) Studies on 6-azauridine and 6-azacytidine. III. The fate of 6-azacytidine in various animal species. *Biochem. Pharmac.* **14**: 1537–1544.

PAČES, V., DOSKOČIL, J. and ŠORM, F. (1968a) Incorporation of 5-azacytidine into nucleic acids of *Escherichia coli*. *Biochim. biophys. Acta* **161**: 352–360.

PAČES, V., DOSKOČIL, J. and ŠORM, F. (1968b) The effect of 5-azacytidine on the synthesis of ribosomes in *Escherichia coli*. *FEBS Lett.* **1**: 55–58.

PASTERNAK, C. A. and HANDSCHUMACHER, R. E. (1959) The biochemical activity of 6-azauridine: interference with pyrimidine metabolism in transplantable mouse tumors. *J. biol. Chem.* **234**: 2992–2997.

PETERSON, R. N. and KOCH, A. L. (1966) The relationship of adenosine and inosine transport in *Escherichia coli*. *Biochim. biophys. Acta* **126**: 129–145.

PINSKY, L. and KROOTH, R. S. (1967a) Studies on the control of pyrimidine biosynthesis in human diploid cell strains. I. Effect of 6-azauridine on cellular phenotype. *Proc. natn. Acad. Sci. U.S.A.* **57**: 925–932.

PINSKY, L. and KROOTH, R. S. (1967b) Studies on the control of pyrimidine biosynthesis in human diploid cell strains. II. Effects of 5-azaorotic acid, barbituric acid, and pyrimidine precursors on cellular phenotype. *Proc. natn. Acad. Sci. U.S.A.* **57**: 1267–1274.

PÍSKALA, A. and ŠORM, F. (1964) Synthesis of *l*-glycosyl derivatives of 5-azauracil and 5-azacytosine. *Coll. Czech. Chem. Commun.* **29**: 2060–2076.

PÍŤHOVÁ, P., PÍSKALA, A., PITHA, J. and ŠORM, F. (1965a) 5-Azauracil and its *N*-methyl derivatives. Formation and decomposition in aqueous solutions. *Coll. Czech. Chem. Commun.* **30**: 90–98.

PÍŤHOVÁ, P., PÍSKALA, A., PITHA, J. and ŠORM, F. (1965b) 5-Azacytidine and related compounds; study of structure, tautomerism and possibilities of pairing with purine derivatives. *Coll. Czech. Chem. Commun.* **30**: 1626–1634.

PÍŤHOVÁ, P., PÍSKALA, A., PITHA, J. and ŠORM, F. (1965c) Nucleic acid components and their analogues. LXVI. Hydrolysis of 5-azacytidine and its connection with biological activity. *Coll. Czech. Chem. Commun.* **30**: 2801–2811.

Plagemann, P. G. W. and Richey, D. P. (1974) Transport of nucleosides, nucleic acid bases, choline and glucose by animal cells in culture. *Biochim. biophys. Acta* **344**: 263–305.

Plevová, J., Jankŭ, J. and Šeda, M. (1970) Toxicity of 6-azauridine triacetate. *Toxic. appl. Pharmac.* **17**: 511–518.

Pliml, J. and Šorm, F. (1964) Synthesis of 2'-deoxy-D-ribofuranosyl-5-azacytosine. *Coll. Czech. Chem. Commun.* **29**: 2576–2578.

Pravdina, N. F. and Galegov, G. A. (1968) Increase of uridine kinase activity in *Escherichia coli* B following T2-phage infection or chloramphenicol treatment. *Biochim. biophys. Acta* **166**: 279–282.

Pravdina, N. F., Lysenko, A. M., Linevich, Yu. G. and Galegov, G. A. (1969) The action of 6-azauridine on reproduction of T2 phage. *Mikrobiologia* **38**: 295–298. (in Russian).

Pringle, C. R. (1970) Genetic characteristics of conditional lethal mutants of vesicular stomatitis virus induced by 5-fluorouracil, 5-azacytidine and ethyl methan sulfonate. *J. Virol.* **5**: 559–567.

Prystaš, M. and Šorm, F. (1962) Nucleic acid components and their analogues. XXII. Synthesis of 6-azauridine and 5-methyl-6-azauridine. *Coll. Czech. Chem. Commun.* **27**: 1578–1584.

Rada, B. and Blaškovič, D. (1961) Inhibition of vaccinia virus multiplication in vitro by 6-azauracil riboside. *Acta virol.* **5**: 308–316.

Rada, B. and Blaškovič, D. (1966) Some characteristics of the effects of 6-azauridine on vaccinia virus multiplication, in comparison with those of 5-iododeoxyuridine. *Acta virol.* **10**: 1–9.

Rada, B., Blaškovič, D., Šorm, F. and Škoda, J. (1960) The inhibitory effect of 6-azauracil riboside on the multiplication of vaccinia virus. *Experientia* **61**: 487–488.

Rada, B. and Dragúň, M. (1977) Antiviral action and selectivity of 6-azauridine. *Ann. N.Y. Acad. Sci.* **284**: 410–417.

Rada, B., Dragúň, M., Votruba, I. and Holý, A. (1980) Characteristics of the antiviral effect of 9-(S)-(2,3-dihydroxypropyl) adenine. *Acta virol.* **24**: 433–438.

Rada, B. and Gregušová, V. (1964) Increase of uridine kinase activity after infection of cell with vaccinia and Rous sarcoma viruses. *Biochem. biophys. Res. Commun.* **15**: 324–328.

Rada, B. and Hanušovská, T. (1970) Virus-inhibitory activity of 6-azauridine dependent on cell-free extracts containing uridine kinase. II. Quantitative aspects, efficacy of pretreatment. *Acta virol.* **14**: 435–444.

Rada, B. and Holý, A. (1980) Virus inhibitory effect of combination of 9-(S)-(2,3-dihydroxypropyl)adenine and 6-azauridine. *Chemotherapy* **26**: 184–190.

Rada, B. and Shatkin, A. J. (1967) The inhibitory effect of 6-azauridine on reovirus multiplication. *Acta virol.* **11**: 551–553.

Rada, B., Smidová, V. and Závada, J. (1964) The inhibitory effect of some antimetabolites and antibiotics on Rous sarcoma growth. *Neoplasma* **11**: 553–559.

Rada, B. and Závada, J. (1962) Screening-test for cytostatic and virostatic substances. *Neoplasma* **9**: 57–65.

Rada, B. and Žemla, J. (1973) Uridine kinase level in cells infected with western equine encephalomyelitis, vesicular stomatitis, pseudorabies and polyoma viruses. *Acta virol.* **17**: 111–115.

Ralph, R. K. and Wojcik, S. J. (1976) Inhibition of turnip yellow mosaic virus synthesis by pyrimidine analogues. *Biochim. biophys. Acta* **444**: 261–268.

Robertson, H. D. (1975) Functions of replicating RNA in cell infected by RNA bacteriophages. In: *RNA Phages*, pp. 113–145, Zinder, N. D. (ed.). Cold Spring Harbor Laboratory.

Robins, M. J. and Currie, B. L. (1968) The synthesis of 3-deazauridine [4-hydroxy-1-(β-D-ribopentofuranosyl)-2-pyridone]. *Chem. Commun.* **23**: 1547–1548.

Rose, N. R., Haber, J. A. and Calabresi, P. (1968) Immunosuppressive effects of selected metabolic inhibitors *in vivo* and *in vitro*. *Proc. Soc. exp. Biol. Med.* **128**: 1121–1128.

Rubin, R. J., Jaffe, J. J. and Handschumacher, R. E. (1962) Qualitative differences in the pyrimidine metabolism of Trypanosoma equiperdum and mammals as characterized by 6-azauracil and 6-azauridine. *Biochem. Pharmac.* **11**: 563–572.

Saenger, W. and Scheit, K. H. (1970) A pyrimidine nucleoside in the syn conformation: molecular and crystal structure of 4-thiouridine-hydrate. *J. molec. Biol.* **50**: 153–169.

Saenger, W. and Suck, D. (1973) 6-Azauridine-5'-phosphoric acid: unusual molecular structure and functional mechanism. *Nature* **242**: 610–612.

Saenger, W., Suck, D., Knappenberg, M. and Dirkx, J. (1979) Theoretical drug design. 6-Azauridine-5'-phosphate, its X-ray crystal structure, potential energy maps and mechanism of inhibition of orotidine-5'-phosphate decarboxylase. *Biopolymers.* **18**: 2015–2037.

Salzman, N. P. (1960) The rate of formation of vaccinia deoxyribonucleic acid and vaccinia virus. *Virology* **10**: 150–152.

Salzman, N. P., Shatkin, A. J. and Sebring, E. D. (1963) Viral protein and DNA synthesis in vaccinia virus-infected HeLa cell cultures. *Virology* **19**: 542–550.

Salzman, N. P., Shatkin, A. J. and Sebring, E. D. (1964) The synthesis of DNA-like RNA in the cytoplasm of HeLa cells infected with vaccinia virus. *J. molec. Biol.* **8**: 405–416.

Schäfer, W., Pister, L. and Schneider, R. (1967) Analyse des Vermehrungsmechanismus des Newcastle disease Virus (NDV) mit Hilfe verschiedener Inhibitoren. *Z. Naturforsch.* **22b**: 1319–1330.

Schwalbe, C. H. and Saenger, W. (1973) 6-Azauridine, a nucleoside with unusual ribose conformation. The molecular and crystal structure. *J. molec. Biol.* **75**: 129–143.

Shannon, W. H. (1977) Selective inhibition of RNA tumor virus replication *in vitro* and evaluation of candidate antiviral agents *in vivo*. *Ann. N.Y. Acad. Sci.* **284**: 472–507.

Shannon, W. M., Arnet, G. and Schabel, F. M. Jr. (1972) Deazauridine: inhibition of ribonucleic acid virus-induced cytopathogenic effect *in vitro*. *Antimicrob. Ag. Chemother.* **2**: 159–163.

Shannon, W. M., Brockman, R. W., Westbrook, L., Shaddix, S. and Schabel, F. M. Jr. (1974) Inhibition of Gross leukemia virus-induced plaque formation in XC cells by 3-deazauridine. *J. natn. Cancer. Inst.* **52**: 199–205.

Shatkin, A. J. and Rada, B. (1967) Reovirus-directed ribonucleic acid synthesis in infected L cells. *J. Virol.* **1**: 24–35.

SIDWELL, R. W., ARNETT, G. and SCHABEL, F. M. JR. (1972) *In vitro* effect of a variety of biologically active compounds on human cytomegalovirus. *Chemotherapy* **17**: 259–282.

SIDWELL, R. W., DIXON, G. J., SELLERS, S. M. and SCHABEL, F. M. JR. (1968) *In vitro* anti-viral properties of biologically active compounds. II. Studies with influenza and vaccinia viruses. *Appl. Microbiol.* **16**: 370–392.

SINGH, P. and HODGSON, D. J. (1974a) High-anti conformation in o-azanucleosides. The crystal and molecular structure of 6-azacytidine. *Biochemistry* **13**: 5445–5452.

SINGH, P. and HODGSON, D. J. (1974b) 8-Azaadenosine. Crystallographic evidence for a 'high-anti' conformation around a shortened glycosidic linkage. *J. Am. chem. Soc.* **96**: 5276–5278.

ŠKODA, J. (1963) Mechanism of action and application of azapyrimidines. In: *Progress in Nucleic Acid Research and Molecular Biology*, Vol. 2, pp. 197–210, DAVIDSON, J. M. and COHN, W. E. (eds.). Academic Press, New York.

ŠKODA, J. (1975) Azapyrimidine nucleosides. In: *Handbook of Experimental Pharmacology*. New series Vol. 38, pp. 348–372, SARTORELLI, A. C. and JOHNS, D. G. (eds.). Springer Verlag, Berlin.

ŠKODA, J., HESS, V. and ŠORM, F. (1957a) The biosynthesis of 6-azauracil riboside by *Escherichia coli* growing in the presence of 6-azauracil. *Experientia* **13**: 150–151.

ŠKODA, J., HESS, V. F. and ŠORM, F. (1957b) Production of 6-azauracil riboside by *Escherichia coli* growing in the presence of 6-azauracil. *Coll. Czech. Chem. Commun.* **22**: 1330–1333.

ŠKODA, J., KÁRA, J., ŠORMOVÁ, Z. and ŠORM, F. (1959a) Inhibition of *Escherichia coli* polynucleotide phosphorylase by 6-azauridine diphosphate. *Biochim. biophys. Acta* **32**: 579–580.

ŠKODA, J., KÁRA, J. and ŠORMOVÁ, Z. (1959b) Interaction of 6-azauridine-5′-diphosphate with *Escherichia coli* polynucleotide phosphorylase. *Coll. Czech. Chem. Commun.* **24**: 3783–3789.

ŠKODA, J., KÁRA, J., ČIHÁK, A. and ŠORM, F. (1962) Formation of the ribonucleoside of 5-azauracil by *Escherichia coli* and isolation of ribosyl biuret as the main decomposition product of 5-azauridine. *Coll. Czech. Chem. Commun.* **27**: 1692–1694.

ŠKODA, J. and ŠORM, F. (1958a) Czechoslovak patent No. 88063.

ŠKODA, J. and ŠORM, F. (1958b) Accumulation of nucleic acid metabolites in *Escherichia coli* exposed to the action of 6-azauracil. *Biochim. biophys. Acta* **28**: 659–660.

SKÖLD, O. (1960) Uridine kinase from Ehrlich tumor: purification and properties. *J. biol. Chem.* **235**: 3273–3279.

SLÁVIKOVÁ, K. and RADA, B. (1973) Inhibition of replication of some RNA viruses by 6-azauridine. *Rev. Roum. Virol.* **10**: 155–159.

ŠMEJKAL, F., GUT, J. and ŠORM, F. (1962) The effect of N-methyl, thio-, and methylmercaptoderivatives of 6-azauracil on vaccinia virus *in vitro*. *Acta virol.* **6**: 364–371.

ŠMEJKAL, F. and ŠORM, F. (1962) The effect of 6-azauracil riboside against vaccinia virus in rabbits. *Acta Virol.* **6**: 282.

SODJA, I. and HOLÝ, A. (1980) Effect of 9-(S)-(2,3-dihydroxypropyl) adenine on experimental rabies infection in laboratory mice. *Acta virol.* **24**: 317–324.

ŠORM, F., ŠKODA, J. and KÁRA, J. (1960) Antagonism between 5-azauracil and pyrimidine precursors of ribonucleic acid in *Escherichia coli*. *Experientia* **16**: 304–305.

ŠORM, F. and VESELÝ, J. (1961) Potentiation of cancerostatic effect of 6-azauridine and 6-azacytidine with 5-bis-(2-chloroethyl)-aminomethyluracil. *Experientia* **17**: 355.

STARCHEUS, A. P. (1965) Inhibition of type 1 adenovirus reproduction in tissue culture by azanucleosides. *Dopovidy Ukr. Acad. Sci.* **9**: 1219–1221 (in Ukrainian).

STARCHEUS, A. P. and CHERNETSKY, V. P. (1967) Effect of 6-azauridine, 6-azacytidine and 8-azaguanine on reproduction of IV type adenovirus in a tissue culture. *Mikrobiol. Zh. (Kiev)* **29**: 157–160 (in Ukrainian).

STEJSKALOVÁ, V., IVÁNYI, J. and KÁRA, J. (1970) Enhancement of antibody synthesis *in vitro* by 6-azauridine, uridine and actinomycin D. *Folia biol.* **16**: 250–258.

ŠTERZL, J. (1961) Effect of some metabolic inhibitors on antibody formation. *Nature* **189**: 1022–1023.

STOLLAR, V., STEVENS, T. M. and SCHLESINGER, R. W. (1966) Studies on the nature of dengue viruses. II. Characterization of viral RNA and effects of inhibitors of RNA synthesis. *Virology* **30**: 303–312.

STRUHLMANN, H., JÄHNER, D. and JAENISH, R. (1981) Infectivity and methylation of retroviral genomes is correlated with expression in the animal. *Cell* **26**: 221–232.

SUNDARALINGAM, M. (1969) Stereochemistry of nucleic acids and their constituents. IV. Allowed and preferred conformation of nucleosides, nucleotide mono-, di-, tri-, tetraphosphates, nucleic acids and polynucleotides. *Biopolymers* **7**: 821–860.

SURJONO, I. and WIGAND, R. (1981) Combined inhibition of vaccinia virus multiplication by inhibitors of DNA synthesis. *Chemotherapy* **27**: 179–187.

TAMM, I. (1956) Selective chemical inhibition of influenza B virus multiplication. *J. Bact.* **72**: 42–53.

TAYLOR, S. M. and JONES, P. A. (1979) Multiple new phenotypes induced in 10T$\frac{1}{2}$ and 3T3 cells treated with 5-azacytidine. *Cell* **17**: 771–779.

TEMIN, H. M. and RUBIN, H. (1958) Characteristics of an assay for Rous sarcoma virus and Rous sarcoma cells in tissue culture. *Virology* **6**: 669–688.

TER MEULEN, V., LEONARD, L. L., LENNETTE, E. H., KATZ, M. and KOPROWSKI, H. (1972) The effect of 6-azauridine upon subacute sclerosing panencephalitis virus in tissue cultures. *Proc. Soc. exp. Biol. Med.* **140**: 1111–1115.

TERSKIKH, I. I., GALEGOV, G. A., CHUTKOV, N. A. and BEKLESHOVA, A. IU. (1968) The inhibitory effect produced by 5-bromo-2′-deoxyuridine and 6-azauridine on the reproduction of the causative organism of ornithosis. *Dokl. Akad. Nauk. SSSR* **180**: 480–481 (in Russian).

TOYOSHIMA, K. and VOGT, P. K. (1969) Temperature sensitive mutants of an avian sarcoma virus. *Virology* **39**: 930–931.

VESELÝ, J. and ČIHÁK, A. (1978) 5-Azacytidine: Mechanism of action and biological effects in mammalian cells. *Pharmac. Ther.* A **2**: 813–840.

VON HOFF, D. D., SLAVIK, M. and MUGGIA, F. M. (1976) 5-Azacytidine. A new anticancer drug with effectiveness in acute myelogenous leukemia. *Ann. intern. Med.* **85**: 237–245.

VOTRUBA, I., HOLÝ, A. and ŠORM, F. (1971) L-Ribonucleosides do not penetrate bacterial cell walls. *FEBS Lett.* **19**: 136–138.

WELLS, W., GAINES, D. and KOENIG, H. (1963) Studies of pyrimidine nucleotide metabolism in the central nervous system. I. Metabolic effects and metabolism of 6-azauridine. *J. Neurochem.* **10**: 709–723.

WIGLER, H. M. (1981) The inheritance of methylation patterns in vertebrates. *Cell* **24**: 285–286.

WIGLER, H. M., LEVY, D. and PERUCHO, M. (1981) The somatic replication of DNA methylation. *Cell* **24**: 33–40.

WIRJAWAN, E. and WIGAND, R. (1978) Combined antiviral effect of DNA inhibitors on adenovirus multiplication. *Chemotherapy* **24**: 347–353.

YATHINDRA, N. and SUNDARALINGAM, M. (1973) Conformation studies on pyrimidine 5'-monophosphates and 3',5'-diphosphates. Effect of the phosphate groups on the backbone conformation of polynucleotides. *Biopolymers* **12**: 2261–2277.

ZEITLENOK, N. A., ROIHEL, V. M., PRYSTAŠ, M., GUT, J. and ŠORM, F. (1965) Effect of 3-methylmercapto-4-thio-6-azauracil on picorna virus multiplication. *Acta virol.* **9**: 60–64.

CHAPTER 11

ANTIVIRAL EFFECTS OF SINGLE-STRANDED POLYNUCLEOTIDES AND THEIR MODE OF ACTION

N. STEBBING

AMGen Inc., 1900 Oak Terrace Lane, Newbury Park, CA 91320, USA

CONTENTS

11.1. INTRODUCTION: THE CONCEPT OF STRATEGIC SEQUENCES

This review attempts to describe investigations on the antiviral effects of polynucleotides where the mechanism of action does not seem to depend primarily on the induction of interferon and updates an earlier review (Stebbing, 1979c). Induction of an antiviral material referred to as 'interferon' may be readily demonstrated with polynucleotide treatments of cells or animals, but a failure of stringent scientific logic (Popper, 1959) may well have led to an unwillingness by some to consider the possibility of other modes of action of polynucleotides. This review attempts to show that there are *a priori* reasons for asserting that polynucleotides, particularly single-stranded RNAs, should be capable of inhibiting replication of viruses, particularly those whose genome is single-stranded RNA. Some of the existing data concerning antiviral effects of polynucleotides can be interpreted in terms of such direct inhibitory effects on essential viral functions. A critical examination of the mechanisms of action of antiviral polynucleotides may thus lead to the development of clinically useful antiviral agents and, for this reason, this review is confined to the effects of polynucleotides mainly against animal viruses.

An additional complication in this review is the need to cover two distinct but related topics, namely polynucleotides which inhibit specific enzymes concerned with virus replication and polynucleotides which mimic parts of viral genomes. The former are identified by their effectiveness, using *in vitro* enzyme assays, while the latter require knowledge of nucleotide sequences within viral polynucleotides and, ideally, their role in virus replication.

Those nucleotide sequences within viral genomes which are directly involved in essential interactions with virus-coded or host cell-coded factors are here termed 'strategic sequences'. Analogs of such nucleotide sequences, if administered to infected cells, may inhibit virus replication by binding of factors that would otherwise interact with viral RNA. Early work on polynucleotide analogs of strategic regions in RNA 'phages and inhibitors of reverse transcriptases was reviewed by Pitha (1973). Any sequence in a viral genome may be considered as essential for virus replication. Within the limits of the present definition, however, strategic sequences are those where specific interactions occur between host or viral factors such that the presence of non-functional analogs of the sequence within an infected cell will be likely to have an effect on replication of the virus. Thus it seems likely that strategic sequences will occur mainly within *untranslated* regions of viral RNA. In this respect it is interesting to note that the untranslated sequences at the 3′ and 5′ ends of related RNA 'phages are more strictly conserved than the translated regions (see Min Jou and Fiers, 1976). The stringency of this conservation is indicated by a single nucleotide substitution in an untranslated region of Qβ RNA (G-> A, 16th nucleotide from the 3′ end) which causes loss of infectivity of the RNA, whereas other single nucleotide substitutions have little effect (Sabo *et al.*, 1977). It is therefore likely that strategic sequences in untranslated regions of viral genomes will generally show conservation, and analogs of these regions may prove effective even against viruses which show marked variability in the products of their translated regions, such as influenzas.

Presented and defined in this way, use of the concept of strategic sequences in developing an antiviral agent would appear to be open to logical criticism since, ultimately, a strategic sequence is recognized by the fact that analogs of it interfere with virus replication. However, if this problem is clearly recognized, no difficulties need arise. A similar problem arises in assessing the mechanism of action of any pharmacological agent. A number of properties of the agent may be investigated, e.g. *in vitro* effects on various factors recognized as contributing to the mechanism under study, but these effects may not be the ones which actually operate *in vivo*. In the case of a single-stranded polynucleotide, which is antiviral and which mimics a sequence within a viral genome, it may be supposed that the polynucleotide is antiviral *because* it mimics a viral RNA sequence. However, this hypothesis should be subjected to separate further investigation. Nevertheless, the concept of strategic sequences provides a relatively unexplored approach for finding antiviral agents which could in principle be applied to any virus disease. The remainder of this introduction is concerned with the background that leads to the concepts of both strategic sequence analogs and specific inhibitors of enzymes, particularly polymerases, involved in virus replication.

Studies on inhibition by polynucleotides of viral polymerases associated with replication of animal viruses have their origin in earlier analyses of the replication of bacteriophages, particularly Qβ. Haruna and Spiegelman (1966) demonstrated that synthetic homopolynucleotides inhibit *in vitro* replication of Qβ RNA by the Qβ replicase. In this case only one replicase molecule binds per Qβ genome (August *et al.*, 1968) and poly(U) and poly(A) strongly inhibit *in vitro* initiation but not elongation of the polymerization reaction whereas poly(C) and poly(G) show no effect (Haruna and Spiegelman, 1966). Inhibition is less marked if the enzyme is mixed with the inhibiting polynucleotide prior to addition of the template RNA. These results strongly suggest that there is one specific binding site in Qβ RNA to which the replicase binds and that single-stranded RNAs can interfere with this binding. In contrast, non-viral polymerases do not appear to show such specific binding to polynucleotide templates (Englund et al., 1968). The polynucleotides inhibiting the Qβ replicase were thought to mimic the actual initiation site (Haruna and Spiegelman, 1966) but, whatever the mechanism of action, in vitro examination of potential inhibitors of enzymes essential for, and specific to, virus replication ought to provide a means of devising and testing modifications of promising inhibitors.

The work with Qβ replicase also yielded another novel means of devising polynucleotide inhibitors of an essential viral activity. By serially selecting, in vitro, fast replicating products of the Qβ replicase, beginning with its natural template, molecules with only 13 per cent of the original length were obtained and these replicated about 15 times faster than the original template (Mills et al., 1967). Presumably polynucleotides containing nucleotide sequences essential for replication, and obviously including the enzyme recognition site, had been generated. However, there are no obvious sequence homologies between the binding sites found in Qβ and small RNA variants produced by these means (Mills et al., 1977). Recognition most likely depends on particular secondary and tertiary structures in the RNA. In contrast, initiation of RNA synthesis does appear to depend on specific sequences, particularly the presence of cytidines at the 3' terminus (Mills et al., 1977).

Replication of animal viruses, particularly those with small RNA genomes, is dependent on direct interactions between the viral genome or RNA products of the genome. Examples of such interactions can be most readily recognized for the small RNA viruses in which the genome is single-stranded and acts as messenger RNA. In these cases, where the RNA alone is infectious, the infecting viral genome must first act as messenger RNA. Viral RNA synthesis can only commence when translation of the mRNA produces an RNA-dependent RNA polymerase (replicase). This enzyme is likely to be, in part at least, coded for by the viral genome and to bind to, or initiate, replication at a specific nucleotide sequence, as occurs in the replication of Qβ. The nucleotide sequences in the ribosome binding site of the viral RNA, or other nucleotide sequences affecting binding to ribosomes, may also be unique to viral messengers and provide for particularly avid binding to polynucleotides. Later in the virus replicative cycle, assembly of virus particles is also likely to involve specific regions of the viral RNA sequence. The importance of such interactions between viral nucleotide sequences and proteins for virus replication is seen to be enhanced when one considers the very small number of viral genomes and translation products that exist, particularly in the early stages of virus replication, in an environment (the host cell) which is replete with other proteins and nucleic acids. These arguments apply with equal force to nucleotide sequences in DNA virus genomes and their mRNA products, but at present there is less relevant information for DNA viruses.

Biological generation of antiviral polynucleotides, as achieved for Qβ 'phage using a viral replicase, has not yet proved feasible even for the smaller animal RNA viruses and a primer-dependent replicase was obtained only with some difficulty (Flanegan and Baltimore, 1977). However, the RNAs in defective interfering (DI) particles do seem to provide examples of biologically generated polynucleotides which may be antiviral by virtue of being analogs of strategic sequences in the standard viral RNAs. Antiviral effects have been observed with DI particles from a range of viruses (Huang and Baltimore, 1977) but whether or not DI particles are generated may depend on the mode of RNA replication (Huang, 1977). In some cases antiviral activity of DI particles may largely be due to interferon induction, but it can occur independently of interferon production (Huang and Baltimore, 1977), even in vivo (see Dimmock and Kennedy, 1978). The antiviral activity of DI particles appears to occur intracellularly and not at the cell surface, probably at the level of RNA replication (Huang and Baltimore, 1977). Moreover, their effect is moderately specific in that less antiviral activity is observed against closely related viruses and no activity occurs against unrelated viruses (Huang and Baltimore, 1977) as would be expected if the effect depends on particular nucleotide sequences in RNAs. The terminal homologies within viral RNA and other particular complementary nucleotide sequences which cause strong intramolecular annealing ('snap-back' RNA) may be important for recognition by polymerases, and their presence in DI RNA could allow DI RNA to compete more effectively for polymerase than the standard RNA (Huang, 1977). The nucleotide sequences in RNA from DI particles responsible for interference have not been determined, hence this interesting and promising means of producing strategic sequence analogs will not be considered further in this review.

Up to the present antiviral effects of single-stranded polynucleotides, known or suspected of mimicking parts of viral RNAs, have been largely considered for only the small RNA viruses, while our knowledge of the effects of polynucleotides on known viral factors is principally that with the reverse transcriptase enzyme of the RNA tumor viruses.

11.2. CANDIDATE STRATEGIC SEQUENCES IN ANIMAL VIRUS GENOMES

Not enough comparative work has as yet been done on the nucleotide sequences of animal virus genomes to determine with any certainty which sequences are peculiar to viral polynucleotides, and what their functions might be in the replicative cycle of viruses. However, determination of viral genome sequences is progressing extremely rapidly and the complete structure of the genome is now known for SV40 (Fiers *et al.*, 1978), BK virus (Seif *et al.*, 1979; Yang and Wu, 1979), Polyoma virus (Soeda *et al.*, 1980; Deininger *et al.*, 1980), Hepatitis virus (Galibert *et al.*, 1979), Polio virus (Kitamura *et al.*, 1981; Racaniello and Baltimore, 1981) and Moloney murine leukemia virus (Sutcliffe *et al.*, 1980) and major portions of other viral genomes have also been determined. The nucleotide sequences known at present, and their possible functional significance, have been reviewed for the picorna-viruses (Fellner, 1979). Although sequencing of DNA virus genomes is progressing rapidly, candidate strategic sequences have proved more difficult to identify in these viruses on the basis of sequence information alone. The extent to which mechanisms of antiviral effects of particular polynucleotides are explicable in terms of mimicking sequences in viral RNA or inhibiting viral polymerases are discussed in context in Section 11.3 and 11.4 below and alternative mechanisms of action are considered in Section 11.5.

11.2.1. FACTORS INVOLVED IN THE ANTIVIRAL ACTIVITY OF STRATEGIC SEQUENCE ANALOGS

Analogs of strategic sequences may be positive analogs, i.e. mimic a sequence present, for example, in the virion RNA of a single-stranded RNA virus, or a negative analog, i.e. complementary to such a sequence. In the latter case the analog will be a positive analog of a sequence present in the polynucleotide complementary to the virion RNA, which must be produced at some step during replication of the genome. For a + strand RNA virus, i.e. one where the virion RNA acts as messenger RNA, a polynucleotide which is complementary to a part of the virion RNA could act as a positive analog of a viral mRNA function or a negative analog of − strand functions.

Of course, an analog of a strategic sequence need not be an exact copy of the sequence present in viral RNA. It may, for example, incorporate features designed to increase its binding to proteins, or include modified bases which increase its ability to hybridize to the complementary sequence. In addition it may include specific modifications to increase the antiviral efficacy of the analog, for example by substituents which increase its cellular uptake. Since natural RNAs which have messenger activity or act as templates for polymerases show considerable secondary structure, it may be argued that negative analogs, which anneal to parts of these RNAs, would be readily displaced and prove ineffective as inhibitors. However, such effects have been demonstrated, *in vitro*, where messenger activity is inhibited in the presence of cDNA (Hastie and Held, 1978; Paterson *et al.*, 1977) or complementary RNA (Inglis *et al.*, 1977), in the latter case the messengers being those of influenza virus. The best example to date of an antiviral polynucleotide acting as a positive analog of a virion RNA sequence is tRNA (see Section 11.3.2.1), if only because the complementary sequence is unlikely to have any biological significance. A good example of an antiviral polynucleotide acting as a negative analog (complementary) to a viral RNA sequence is a DNA sequence complementary to a nucleotide tract occurring near the 3' and 5' ends of RSV, and in this case there appears to be an effect on virus production (Zamecnik and Stephenson, 1978) as well as *in vitro* effects (Stephenson and Zamecnik, 1978).

To claim that a particular antiviral polynucleotide is an analog of a sequence within a viral genome requires some knowledge of the structure of the viral genome. That the antiviral effect, in cell cultures or *in vivo*, arises because the analog is a mimic of a sequence within the viral RNA is more difficult to ascertain, although negative analogs annealed to viral RNA might be isolated from infected cells. In the case of positive analogs some knowledge of the factors which interact with the analog and their role in virus replication would seem to be important. Since replication of single-stranded polynucleotides occurs via intermediate complementary polynucleotides it is possible that positive or negative analogs of a particular viral nucleotide sequence may have effects by both mechanisms.

An antiviral polynucleotide which mimics some part of a viral genome may be effective partly or completely for reasons unrelated to its structural similarity to a sequence in the viral genome. It should be noted that ribonucleic acids generally inhibit the activity of nucleic acid polymerases and may therefore suppress, in a non-specific manner, the replication of viral RNAs by affecting viral polymerases. A DNA-dependent RNA polymerase of yeast (RNA polymerase β or 2) transcribes polypyrimidines, especially polydeoxycytidylic acid, most efficiently and this reaction is inhibited by poly(I), poly(G) and poly(U) but not by poly(C) (Dezelee *et al.*, 1974). This effect is not observed with poly(G) if it is complexed to poly(C), indicating that the effect is due to single-stranded polymers. Investigations of the inhibitory effects of polynucleotides on the reverse transcriptase of RNA tumor viruses are now quite extensive (see Section 11.4). Although some polynucleotides inhibit host and viral polymerases, others seem to be more inhibitory for the viral polymerase and these are of interest in the present context even though the polynucleotides may not be mimics of viral nucleotide sequences. The polymerases of other viruses are not as well characterized as the reverse transcriptases, but examination of the effects of polynucleotides on isolated viral polymerases is likely to become as extensive as reverse transcriptase studies.

11.2.2. HOMOPOLYNUCLEOTIDE TRACTS

T_1 RNase digestion of several picornavirus RNAs has revealed the presence of a single poly(C) tract per viral RNA molecule between 70 and 200 nucleotides in length (Porter *et al.*, 1974; Brown *et al.*, 1974). Homopolymer tracts of this length are really quite remarkable and their conservation in particular sub-groups of the picornaviruses indicates some significant function. Curiously, a poly(C) tract does not occur in all groups of picornaviruses and this indicates that its function may be fulfilled in some groups by cytidine-rich tracts that cannot be detected by T_1 RNase-resistance because they are interrupted by G residues or the function of the cytidine-rich tract is not basic to the mode of replication of the picornaviruses. The poly(C) tract found in the cardiovirus and FMD virus groups appears to be single-stranded, at least in the case of EMC virus, since it can be converted to a poly(U) tract by bisulphite treatment under conditions which only affect single-stranded poly(C) (Goodchild *et al.*, 1975), and because in the native state, EMC virus RNA acts as a template for cDNA synthesis using oligo(dG) as a primer (Emtage *et al.*, 1976).

The poly(C) tract in EMC virus RNA appears to be located near the 5' terminus, since only alkaline digestion products close to the size of the complete genome are retained by both poly(U) and poly(I)-cellulose columns (Chumakov and Agol, 1976). A similar location of the poly(C) tract was deduced from competitive hybridization of oligo(dT) and oligo(dG) primed cDNAs to EMC virus RNA and this method located the poly(C) tract approximately 500 nucleotides from the 5'-terminus (Emtage *et al.*, 1976). The poly(C) tract of FMD virus has also been located in a similar position close to the 5' terminus of the viral RNA (Harris and Brown, 1976; Rowlands *et al.*, 1978). The single-stranded nature of the poly(C) tract in picornaviruses, and its location near one end of the genome, indicate that it is in an untranslated region (see also discussion of Fellner, 1979) and poly(C) is therefore an analog of this region which could inhibit some function necessary for virus replication. Antiviral studies based on this observation are considered in Section 11.3.1, below.

The function of the poly(C) tract in picornaviruses remains obscure. However, if it acts as a recognition site for a protein (see Fellner, 1979) its length indicates that it could bind several proteins. The poly(C) tract of an FMD virus strain attenuated by serial passage of a virulent strain is shortened from about 170 to 100 nucleotides by deletion (Harris and Brown, 1977), suggesting that virulence may be associated with length of the poly(C) tract. However, further analyses of other FMD virus strains of known virulence are necessary to confirm this interesting observation since other nucleotide differences between the two strains so far examined could account for the differences in virulence. Since picornavirus infections generally induce significant amounts of circulating interferon in animals, it is also possible that the poly(C) tract evolved to limit the antiviral effect of induced interferon and a decrease in length of the poly(C) tract could thus result in attenuation *in vivo*.

Those +strand RNA viruses examined to date also have a 3'-terminal poly(A) tract similar to cellular mRNAs, while such tracts appear to be absent in −strand RNA viruses. The function of the poly(A) tracts in viral RNAs is unknown but it may not be the same as the poly(A) tract of cellular mRNAs (for discussion see Fellner, 1979). While the poly(A) tract of cellular mRNAs is added post-transcriptionally, in the case of polio virus and Sindbis virus, at least, it appears to be transcribed since a poly(U) tract has been found in the −strand (Yogo and Wimmer, 1973; Frey and Strauss, 1978) and this tract is located at the 5' terminus of the −strand in polio virus (Yogo *et al.*, 1974). Partial removal of the poly(A) tract of polio virus causes a decrease in infectivity of the RNA but the progeny virus contains a poly(A) tract of normal size, indicating that it can be regenerated (Spector and Baltimore, 1974). The infectivity of EMC virus RNA purified from virions has also been found to be dependent on the length of the poly(A) tract (Hruby and Roberts, 1976). The infectivity of Sindbis virus RNA which does not bind to oligo(dT)-cellulose, and therefore essentially lacks a poly(A) tract, is also very much lower than that of polyadenylated Sindbis RNA (Frey and Strauss, 1978). Whatever the function of these viral poly(A) tracts, poly(A) has not been found to be antiviral *in vivo* against picorna- or togaviruses while poly(C) is so active (see Section 11.3.1).

11.2.3. HETEROPOLYNUCLEOTIDE TRACTS

11.2.3.1. *Viral mRNA Ribosome Binding Sites*

The ribosome binding sites of viral mRNAs are obvious candidate strategic sequences. However, it is noteworthy that although all bacterial mRNA initiation sequences examined show similarities (Steitz and Jakes, 1975), only minor similarities are apparent in the initiation sequences determined so far for EMC virus, reovirus and VSV mRNAs and SV40 mRNA (Smith, 1975; Kozak, 1977; Rose, 1977, 1978; Van de Voorde *et al.*, 1976; see also Kozak and Shatkin, 1978; Barelle and Brownlee, 1978). The absence of common sequences also occurs for non-viral initiation sites of eukaryotic mRNAs (Barelle and Brownlee, 1978). Nucleotide sequences protected by the 40S ribosome subunit include the 5' terminal cap structure (m^7GpppN), absent in the picornaviruses (Shatkin, 1976), so that the only sequence common to viral mRNA initiation sites seems to be the AUG initiator codon (Kozak and Shatkin, 1978; Barelle and Brownlee, 1978). This is somewhat surprising since an intact cap structure appears to be essential for translation of capped mRNAs (Shatkin, 1976). Although the 5'-terminal cap is generally protected against nuclease digestion in the presence of ribosomes, in the case of the reovirus mRNAs partial digestion products of the mRNAs which retain the cap, but not the AUG initiator codon, do not associate stably with ribosomes, indicating that the cap is not essential for initiation of protein synthesis and may play a quantitative role in initiation (Kozak and Shatkin, 1978).

There is evidence that, in eukaryotic cells, control of protein synthesis can occur at the level of translation and this makes it likely that some viral mRNAs which possess specific nucleotide sequences could act as particularly efficient messengers. There is evidence that EMC virus and VSV mRNAs out-compete cellular mRNAs (Lawrence and Thach, 1974; Nuss et al., 1975). Differential affinity of mRNAs for ribosomes has been attributed to specific internal nucleotide sequences which have varying affinity for the eukaryotic initiation factor which forms a complex with Met-tRNA and GTP (eIF-2) (Kaempfer et al., 1978b). This initiation factor appears to bind to mRNAs with high affinity (Kaempfer et al., 1978a) and this reaction is inhibited by cap analogs. Surprisingly a non-capped picornavirus RNA (Mengo) is also inhibited if the concentration of cap analogs is increased about fifty-fold (Kaempfer et al., 1978b). It has therefore been suggested that initiation of protein synthesis involves binding of eIF-2 to a specific sequence in mRNAs and the 5'-terminal cap, but that with the picornaviruses the internal sequence has such a high affinity for eIF-2 that a cap is superfluous for these mRNAs. Clearly the nucleotide sequence in picornavirus RNAs which binds to eIF-2 is a candidate strategic sequence and could provide a means for specifically inhibiting picornavirus replication. The internal site that binds to eIF-2 has not been identified for any mRNA, but may well include the AUG initiator codon, since the binding studies of Kozak and Shatkin (1978) employed unwashed ribosomes which must have included eIF-2.

In contrast, another group has found evidence for production of initiation factors specific for polio virus mRNA after infection, so that *in vivo* viral mRNA selection may not depend entirely on a particular nucleotide sequence (Helentjaris and Ehrenfeld, 1978).

A nucleotide sequence near the 3' end of 16S ribosomal RNA appears to be capable of binding to a sequence within the ribosome binding sites of several RNA 'phage messengers, first considered to be of significance by Shine and Dalgarno (1974). Such base pairings do actually occur during initiation of protein synthesis in bacteria, and it is possible that these interactions determine the relative efficiency of initiation of different (host or viral) cistrons (Steitz and Jakes, 1975). All bacterial messenger RNA initiation sequences examined show some similarities and complementarity to the Shine and Dalgarno (1974) sequence at the 3' end of 16S ribosomal RNA (Steitz and Jakes, 1975). A purine-rich sequence (AGGAGGCG) at the 3' end of 18S ribosomal RNA is highly conserved in eukaryotes and shows complementarity to 5'-terminal non-coding regions of some mRNAs (Hagenbuchle et al., 1978) and there is evidence that viral mRNAs anneal to this site in 18S ribosomal RNA (see Sections 11.2.3.4 and 11.2.3.5). The 3' terminus of 18S ribosomal RNA shows strong similarities to that of 16S ribosomal RNA of E. coli but the Shine and Dalgarno (1974) sequence is absent (Hagenbuchle et al., 1978). Different tetranucleotide sequences in mRNAs, some outside the 80S ribosome-protected region, show complementarity to parts of the purine-rich sequence in 18S ribosomal RNA (Hagenbuchle et al., 1978) and this explains why the possibility of such interactions was not observed previously. Other RNA–RNA interactions which occur in protein synthesis, are the codon–anticodon interactions, and the interactions between 5S RNA and the TψCG region of tRNAs, whereby tRNAs are aligned on the ribosome (Erdmann et al., 1973; Richter et al., 1973). Antiviral effects of modified or unmodified RNA extracts of cells could well involve RNA–RNA interactions of this type.

11.2.3.2. TRANSFER RNA-LIKE STRUCTURES

Salomon and Littauer (1974) first reported the presence, in an animal virus RNA, of a tRNA-like structure which was an integral part of the RNA. Mengo virus was shown to be aminoacylatable with histidine but this was accompanied by fragmentation of the viral RNA (Salomon and Littauer, 1974). The fragments were larger than tRNA, indicating that the aminoacylation was not due to a contaminating tRNA. Lindley and Stebbing (1976) observed aminoacylation of EMC virus RNA with serine and periodate oxidation of the RNA did not prevent the reaction, indicating that the effect was not due to contaminating tRNAs and that the tRNA-like structure could not be at the 3' terminus of the viral RNA. In this case the synthetases used were contaminated with nucleases and nucleotidyl transferase, which could be important for cleaving out a tRNA-like structure and allowing it to assume an aminoacylatable form. The extent of aminoacylation with these animal virus RNAs was low: for Mengo virus it was 0.18 mol histidine per mol viral RNA, and for EMC not more than 0.08 mol serine per mol viral RNA. Other picornaviruses have been found not to be aminoacylatable, viz. polio and FMD viruses (Oberg and Philipson, 1972; Chatterjee *et al.*, 1976), but this could be due to the synthetases used being free of other enzymes necessary to demonstrate aminoacylation.

The location of the tRNA-like structures within EMC and Mengo virus RNAs is unknown. In the case of EMC virus RNA it would not appear to be within the 129 nucleotides adjacent to the 3′ terminal poly(A) tract, in which very little secondary structure is possible (Porter *et al.*, 1978). Although the nucleotide sequence of the tRNA-like structure in TMV shows some similarities to tRNA[his], notably a common sequence of sixteen nucleotides, there are considerable differences (Guilley, *et al.*, 1975). Further sequence analysis of animal virus RNAs may reveal tRNA-like structures, but development of the present observations is more likely to come from studies of binding between viral RNAs and proteins which recognize tRNAs.

Plant viruses have generally been shown to have aminoacylatable structures at or near their 3′ termini and the particular amino acid which can be esterified to the viral RNA shows constancy within the taxonomic grouping of these viruses. Some functional differences between aminoacylated and non-aminoacylated viral RNAs have been considered for the plant viruses. Litvak *et al.* (1973) suggested that this difference could be a means of differentiating + and − strand replication and promoting translation of viral mRNA by formation of a complex with elongation factors. Although plant virus RNAs can donate amino acids in protein synthesis, this activity is low (Chen and Hall, 1973; Haenni *et al.*, 1973) and Lindley and Stebbing (1976) suggested that even in plant viruses aminoacylation *per se* plays no functional role in virus replication: the tRNA-like structure serves primarily as a strategic sequence which interacts with proteins, such as elongation factors, in processes essential for virus replication.

The presence of sequences annealing to tRNAs involved in replication of the RNA tumor viruses are considered in Section 11.2.3.4. Clover-leaf structures have been found in the two non-coding regions of the polyoma virus genome (Soeda *et al.*, 1980). One, in the non-coding early region (nucleotides 715–799), may regulate splicing events which allow production of mRNAs for the three early proteins. In the late region there is also a clover-leaf structure (nucleotides 5231 to 5160) but in neither case is it known whether transcription occurs and no low molecular weight RNA products have been associated with virus replication. The function of these structures in virus replication remains obscure.

11.2.3.3. The 3′ and 5′ Ends of RNA Viruses

The possible roles of the 5′-terminal cap (m⁷GpppN), and the 3′-terminal poly(A) tract when present, have been considered in Sections 11.2.3.1. and 11.2.2, respectively. Although the relatedness of the translated regions of different picornaviruses is not great, there is considerable conservation of sequences in untranslated regions particularly the 5′-terminal sequence adjacent to the terminal VPg protein (Hewlett and Florkiewicz, 1980). This sequence does not show any complementarity to known 3′ sequences and therefore is unlikely to function as a replicase recognition sequence. Very little secondary structure seems possible in the 3′-terminal region of EMC virus and it has been suggested that this could allow easy access for the viral replicase during initiation of replication (Porter *et al.*, 1978). However, in the FMD viruses there is the possibility of strong secondary structure close to the 3′-terminal poly(A) (Fellner, 1979). Interestingly, in the five FMD viruses which have been examined, a sequence of eleven nucleotides within the 3′-terminal twenty nucleotides next to the poly(A) is conserved, and this could well serve some function essential for replication of FMD viruses (see Fellner, 1979).

It is curious that, close to the 3′-terminal poly(A) tract of EMC virus RNA, there are ten nonsense triplets blocking all three reading frames, suggesting that prevention of read-through to the poly(A) tract is of some importance. However, in the FMD and cardio-viruses there are fewer such nonsense triplets (Fellner, 1979). The sequence 5'-AAUAA-3' occurs close to the poly(A) tract in EMC virus RNA, and the same sequence occurs in a similar location in the 3'-terminal untranslated region of polyadenylated eukaryotic mRNAs, suggesting that the sequence may be a signal involved in polyadenylation (Porter *et al.*, 1978). However, polio virus lacks this sequence (Fellner, 1979) but seems capable of being polyadenylated since partially de-polyadenylated polio virus RNA produces virus particles with a normal size poly(A) tract (Spector and Baltimore, 1974).

Transcription of the genome of RNA tumor viruses occurs by means of the viral reverse transcriptase from the tRNA primer near the 5' terminus, and formation of complete genome transcripts appears to involve a sequence reiterated at the 5' end and immediately adjacent to the 3' terminal poly(A) tract (Haseltine *et al.*, 1977b; Collett and Faras, 1978). The ends of RNA tumor viruses in general contain repeated sequences of 300–1200 nucleotides, the long terminal repeats (LTRs) (Shank *et al.*, 1978). These tracts may serve to circularize the genome during synthesis of the provirus (Collett and Faras, 1978). Isolation and cloning of DNA from cells recently infected with an RNA tumor virus indicates incorporation of viral genomes with LTRs at each end (Shoemaker *et al.*, 1980). The insertion mechanism appears to be analogous to that of transposable elements in bacteria which involves repeated terminal sequences (insertion sequences). However, integrated RNA tumor virus genomes are not known to transpose although multiple integration sites are possible. Similar sequences have been detected in the DNA of several species including man and in general these sequences are most similar between viruses and their normal hosts (Kominami *et al.*, 1980). Thus LTRs appear to play a role in integration of the virus but may also enhance expression of viral genes (Levinson *et al.*, 1982).

Complementary DNA transcripts can be formed from EMC virus RNA using oligo(dG) priming on the poly(C) tract near the 5' end (Emtage *et al.*, 1976), implying that a reiterated sequence may be present in this picornavirus RNA. Moreover, it has been proposed that circular structures are formed during replication of picornaviruses (Brown and Martin, 1965). To date the only sequence data for the 5' end of a picornavirus concern the 5' terminal ten nucleotides of polio virus and this sequence is not repeated in the 156 nucleotides adjacent to the 3' terminal poly(A) tract. Thus, in the case of the picornaviruses, circularization may not involve reiteration of a nucleotide sequence, but other factors. For example, the 5'-terminal, covalently linked, protein detected on the virion RNA of polio, FMD and EMC viruses (Flanegan *et al.*, 1977; Sanger *et al.*, 1977; Hruby and Roberts, 1978) may serve to form circular structures. Although this protein is present on picornavirus RNAs which lack the 5'-terminal cap structure m^{7}GpppN, the protein cannot fulfill the same function as a cap (see Section 11.2.3.1) since polio virus RNA isolated from polysomes lacks the protein (Flanegan *et al.*, 1977). It has been suggested that the terminal protein of picornaviruses initiates transcription of the genome (Nomoto *et al.*, 1977) in the same manner as the terminal protein of adenovirus (Rekosh *et al.*, 1977; see also Section 11.2.3.5).

Current data on the 3' termini of influenza virus RNAs, and the process of transcription in this virus, strongly indicate that all eight influenza virus RNAs have the same initial sequence which is important for replication of the viral RNAs. *In vitro* synthesis of the influenza mRNA strands from the virion RNAs occurs by means of a virion-associated transcriptase which requires the presence of primer mono-, di- or trinucleoside phosphates (McGeoch and Kitron, 1975; Plotch and Krug, 1977). The most effective of the sixteen possible dinucleoside monophosphate primers is ApG and in this case apparently full-length genome transcripts can be obtained *in vitro*; these contain poly(A) tracts as found *in vivo* during virus replication (Plotch and Krug, 1977). The trinucleoside diphosphate ApGpC also acts as a primer (Plotch and Krug, 1977). Since the primers appear in the transcript, and the virion RNA species all have a 3'-terminal U (Lewandowski *et al.*, 1971), it is most likely that the 5' terminus of all eight genome transcripts of influenza virus commence with the sequence (5') ApGpC and that transcription is initiated at such sites. Formation of complete RNA transcripts *in vitro* is dependent on addition of a primer and thus modified primers should specifically interfere with initiation of influenza virus RNA replication (see Section 11.3.2).

The sequences at the 5′-termini of several influenza A viral RNAs have been determined directly; this work confirms the start sequence ApGpC and shows that the first twelve nucleotides are identical in all the viral RNA transcripts examined (Skehel and Hay, 1978). Moreover, the first thirteen nucleotides at the 5′ ends of the virion RNAs of A and B strain influenzas are identical and there are marked similarities up to the 23rd nucleotide (Skehel and Hay, 1978). These studies show that the 3′ and 5′ ends of virus RNAs or the cRNAs are extensively complementary and these structures may be important for virus replication, e.g. by acting as replicase and transcriptase recognition sequences (Skehel and Hay, 1978).

Other examples of terminal sequences that are constant in the several genome segments of a virus are a sequence of eleven nucleotides at the 5′ end of two VSV mRNAs (Rose, 1977) and the 5′-terminal tetranucleotides of six of the reovirus mRNAs (Kozak, 1977). In the case of VSV the leader RNA contains repetitive and palindromic sequences with a polypurine sequence at its 3′ terminus (Colonno and Banerjee, 1978). The polypurine sequence may be involved in base pairing with the pyrimidine-rich sequence near the initiation AUG codon or act as a recognition site for the cleavage enzyme involved in processing VSV mRNAs (Colonno and Banerjee, 1978).

Although each genome segment of the influenza viruses appears to code for a single polypeptide, the smallest RNA segment codes for two proteins. The coding regions are overlapping and involve different reading frames (Porter *et al.*, 1980). If internal initiation of transcription is the mechanism that generates a second mRNA one might expect a recognition sequence similar to that at the 3′ end of all eight influenza RNA segments. There are two internal sequences resembling that of the 3′ end but also a more extensive homology between a sequence close to the 3′ end (Porter *et al.*, 1980). However, this region is not conserved near the 3′ end of any other influenza virus RNA segment and is therefore unlikely to be part of a general transcriptase binding sequence.

11.2.3.4. Sequences in RNA Tumor Virus Genomes

Replication of the RNA tumor viruses occurs by synthesis of a complementary DNA strand with specific host cell tRNAs acting as primers at around 100 nucleotides from the 5′ end of the genome. Complete covalently linked double-stranded DNA copies of the genome are formed and integrated into the host cell genome. For the murine viruses the initiator tRNA is a tRNApro and for the avian viruses, tRNAtrp. In the case of AMV, reverse transcriptase is known to interact with tRNAs (Panet *et al.*, 1975; Haseltine *et al.*, 1977a) and tRNAs have been shown to inhibit the reverse transcriptase (Cavalieri and Yamaura, 1975; Haseltine *et al.*, 1977a; Yamaura and Cavalieri, 1978). These inhibitory effects may in part be due to their mimicking the initiation complex and the results are considered further in Section 11.4.1.2. The initiator tRNAs are annealed, in virus particles, to the viral RNA by about sixteen nucleotides at the 3′ ends of the tRNAs.

Analogs of the tRNA sequences which anneal to the viral RNA could act as competitive inhibitors of viral functions by hybridizing to new viral RNAs in place of the initiator tRNA. But such mimics would not be expected to inhibit all RNA tumor viruses since different tRNAs are used as initiators in different groups of RNA tumor viruses. However, the initial DNA sequence synthesized from the initiator tRNA of RSV and MLV (Moloney) are very similar: AATGAAGC and AATGAAAGA, respectively (Haseltine *et al.*, 1976), and in AMV the initial sequence is identical to that found in RSV (Eiden *et al.*, 1975) so that mimics of this sequence may prove antiviral against a wide range of RNA tumor viruses.

In MLV (Moloney), immediately after the initial nonomer just described, the DNA synthesized from the initiator tRNA continues with a sequence of five cytidines and a C_6 sequence occurs at over ninety nucleotides. These two cytidine sequences appear to occur only once in the first 1000 nucleotides synthesized from the initiator tRNA of MLV (Moloney), indicating that they could be strategic for this virus (Haseltine *et al.*, 1976; see also Section 11.4.2.1). However, these cytidine sequences do not occur in the first 1000 nucleotides synthesized from the initiator tRNA of RSV (Haseltine *et al.*, 1976).

In vitro synthesis of DNA from the initiator tRNAs of tumor viruses tends to stop at around 100 nucleotides (strong-stop DNA) and sequence analysis of this DNA from RSV and the sequence adjacent to the poly(A) tract at the 3′ end of the viral RNA has shown that an identical sequence of twenty-one nucleotides occurs at both the 3′ and 5′ ends of the viral RNA (Haseltine *et al.*, 1977b; Schwartz *et al.*, 1977). This reiterated sequence of twenty-one nucleotides could allow synthesis of cDNA to jump to the 3′ end of the same or another viral RNA and thus allow synthesis of the entire genome and circularization of the provirus DNA prior to its integration into the host cell genome (Haseltine *et al.*, 1977b). A similar reiterated sequence has been found to occur in the same locations in AMV RNA (Stoll *et al.*, 1977). Such terminally reiterated sequences are clear candidate strategic sequences and specific antiviral effects of mimics of part of this sequence have already been observed (Zamecnik and Stephenson, 1978; Stephenson and Zamecnik, 1978; see also Section 11.4.1.4.).

The strong-stop DNA sequence of RSV also contains several possible protein synthesis initiator triplets, one of which (AUG commencing at eighty-three nucleotides from the 5′ end) is not in phase with a terminator triplet and is close to a sequence of seven nucleotides (commencing at nucleotide 63 from the 5′ end) which is complementary to the 3′ end of chicken fibroblast 18S ribosomal RNA and could therefore act in the same way as the Shine and Dalgarno (1974) sequence in prokaryotic mRNAs (Haseltine *et al.*, 1977b). The proximity of this possible protein synthesis initiator site to the tRNA which initiates replication of the genome could mean that the initiator tRNA interferes with ribosome attachment and thus controls translation (Haseltine *et al.*, 1977b). The strong-stop DNA of RSV, together with its complementary strand, also contains a palindromic sequence (between nucleotides 64 and 116 from the 5′ end of the genome) which could allow the two 35S viral RNAs in each virion to anneal together by more than thirty bases near their 5′ ends (Haseltine *et al.*, 1977b). Clearly there are several sequences within the strong-stop DNA which could fulfill important roles at various stages in virus replication and further elucidation of their significance is likely to indicate additional antiviral polynucleotides.

11.2.3.5. Sequences in DNA Viruses

Nucleotide sequence analyses of DNA viruses is progressing rapidly. In the case of SV40 the entire sequence of 5224 base pairs is now known, and of this at least 15.2 per cent is not used for coding proteins (Fiers *et al.*, 1978). The organization of the genome of this small virus is remarkable for its efficiency, for it shows that different proteins can be initiated at the same position but terminate at different points and the same sequences may be used for different proteins by utilizing different reading frames. A number of distinctive features are apparent in the untranslated regions of the DNA (see Section 11.2.3.2), which very likely are strategic for virus replication, but as yet there have been no related antiviral studies.

In adenovirus 2 there is an inverted terminal repetition of about 140 bases (Roberts *et al.*, 1974; Wu *et al.*, 1977) and a protein which binds to the ends of adenovirus DNA has been identified (Rekosh *et al.*, 1977). The inverted terminal repetitions in adenovirus permit formation of single-stranded circular DNA. The length of the inverted terminal repetitions correlates with oncogenicity (Shinagawa and Padmanabhan, 1980). The inverted terminal repetitions are bounded by a conserved hexanucleotide and a 14-nucleotide sequence is present in all the inverted terminal repetition sequences of adenovirus serotypes studied to date (Shinagawa and Padmanabhan, 1980). SV40 also contains a terminally repeated sequence involving 72 base pairs and in this case the sequence is known to enhance expression of viral (Levinson *et al.*, 1982) and other genes (Banerji *et al.*, 1981). The symmetrical distribution of restriction enzyme cleavage sites at the ends of vaccinia virus and rabbit pox virus DNAs also indicates the presence of identical sequences of inverse polarity at the ends of these viral DNAs which, in the case of vaccinia virus, are considerably longer than those of adenovirus and rabbit pox virus (Wittek *et al.*, 1978). The inverted terminal repeats of vaccinia virus are about 10,000 base pairs in length and contain transcribed and non-transcribed regions (Wittek *et al.*, 1980). Repeated sequences of inverse polarity have also been described for human papilloma virus DNA (Gissmann and Zurhausen, 1977). The herpes viruses have extensive regions of reiterated and palindromic sequences which, in some cases, gives rise to four genome isomers differing in the relative orientation of two major unique nucleotide segments, and the reiterated sequences show considerable conservation (see Honess and Watson, 1977). The terminally repeated sequences of these viruses may be related to transcription since in the case of adenovirus 2 the terminal protein seems to act as an initiator of transcription (Rekosh et al., 1977).

It is very likely that herpes viruses contain sequences which control expression of their structural genes since there is extensive evidence for patterns of coordinate control of protein synthesis during replication (Honess and Roizman, 1975). However, the nature of the control elements in the viral genome, in terms of nucleotide sequences, is unknown.

All the late mRNAs of adenovirus 2 have a common 150–200 nucleotide leader sequence at their 5′ ends which is coded for by three genome segments remote from the map positions of the mRNAs (Chow et al., 1977). Proteins of SV40 are also derived from discontinuous sequences in the genome (Fiers et al., 1978). Whether the splicing regions of viral mRNAs and their leader sequences have distinctive features conferring selective advantage for their translation is presently unknown. The 5′ non-coding part of the hexon mRNA of adenovirus 2 has been estimated at 235 nucleotides and between the leader sequence and the initiation codon there are thirty-nine nucleotides containing three sequences of four nucleotides complementary to the purine-rich sequence at the 3′ end of 18S ribosomal RNA (Akusjarvi and Pettersson, 1979). The presence of three sequences complementary to the 18S ribosomal sequence could serve to increase translation of the viral mRNA compared with other mRNAs. It is to be expected that splicing of mRNA sequences occur between looped-out sections of RNA and a hair-pin structure is possible at the leader junction in adenovirus 2 hexon mRNA (Akusjarvi and Pettersson, 1979).

11.3. INHIBITION OF LYTiC VIRUSES BY SINGLE-STRANDED RNAs

11.3.1. HOMOPOLYNUCLEOTIDES

Poly(C) or poly(I) administered to mice protects them against lethal infections of EMC virus and SFV and these treatments do not cause production of detectable circulating interferon (Stebbing et al., 1976a). Poly(A) and poly(U) were found to have no antiviral effects in these systems (Stebbing et al., 1976a). Sequential treatments with poly(I) and poly(C) also caused significant protection against EMC virus and SFV, using a treatment regime which did not cause production of interferon (4 hr between polynucleotide treatments) (Stebbing and Grantham, 1976). Various modified forms of poly(C) which have decreased stacking interactions also show antiviral activity against EMC virus and other picornaviruses of the cardiovirus and FMD virus groups (Stebbing et al., 1977c). One modified form of poly(C), a copolymer composed largely of 5-hydroxycytidylic acid residues, has been found not to anneal to poly(I) (Stebbing et al., 1977d) and treatment of mice with mixtures of this copolymer and poly(I) produced significant potentiation of the antiviral effects of these polynucleotides, again without evidence of interferon production (Stebbing et al., 1977d). These antiviral effects are consequent on the polymeric nature of the compounds since the nucleosides and nucleotides alone are without activity (Stebbing and Grantham, 1976; Stebbing et al., 1976a) and if the polynucleotides are too short (below about 4S) the antiviral activity is decreased or lost (Stebbing et al., 1977e). Moreover, antiviral activity seems to be dependent on single-strandedness because annealing of poly(C) or poly(I) to the complementary polydeoxyribonucleotides results in loss of antiviral activity (Stebbing, 1981).

In addition to the absence of detectable circulating interferon, there is evidence against induction of interferon as the mode of action of these single-stranded polynucleotide treatments. The optimum time of treatment is around 6 hr before infection, not 24 hr before infection or earlier, as is the case for polynucleotides that induce interferon (Stebbing and

Grantham, 1976; Stebbing *et al.*, 1977d) and the hyporeactivation response of mice to interferon production by poly(I).poly(C), by repeated prior administration of an interferon inducing polynucleotide, does not occur with the various treatment regimes with single-stranded polynucleotides (Stebbing and Grantham, 1976; Stebbing *et al.*, 1976a). Moreover, the single-stranded polynucleotide treatments give only short-lived protection and doses of the single-stranded polynucleotides conferring the same degree of protection as poly(I).poly(C) show no detectable levels of interferon (Stebbing *et al.*, 1976a; Stebbing and Grantham, 1976). Additional evidence against an interferon-mediated mechanism of action comes from a study of protective effects against an interferon-sensitive mutant of Mengo virus (Stebbing, 1979a). The single-stranded polynucleotide treatments were equally effective against the wild-type and interferon-sensitive strains of virus whereas poly(I).poly(C) was more effective against the mutant than the wild-type virus. The toxicity of the single-stranded polynucleotide treatments is also lower than that of double-stranded polynucleotides (see Section 11.6). The relation of the sequential poly(I), poly(C) treatment of mice to earlier work in tissue culture systems is discussed in Section 11.5.1.3.

Antiviral effects of the single-stranded polynucleotides considered here could be due to mechanisms other than interferon induction or mimicking the poly(C) tracts of the viruses, and some additional factors are considered in Section 11.5. However, certain possibilities were considered and dismissed, as follows: the antiviral effects are not simply due to some local effect at the site where the materials were administered, as occurs with polycarboxylates in the peritoneal cavity (Billiau *et al.*, 1971) since the effects occur when the routes of treatment and infection are different (Stebbing and Grantham, 1976; Stebbing *et al.*, 1976a, 1977d). Serum obtained from mice after treatment with the single-stranded polynucleotides did not confer protection to other mice, indicating the absence of protective factors in addition to interferon (Stebbing and Grantham, 1976; Stebbing *et al.*, 1976a, 1977d). The possibility that the single-stranded polynucleotides merely 'prime' subsequent interferon production by infection itself or poly(I).poly(C) was also examined, with negative results (Stebbing *et al.*, 1976b). Stimulation by single-stranded polynucleotides of immune responses capable of protecting mice do not appear to occur and protection by these polynucleotides occurs even in immunosuppressed mice (Stebbing *et al.*, 1976b, 1977d). It seemed possible that the single-stranded polynucleotide treatments might simply limit the pathological lesions leading to death of mice infected with a lethal virus. This possibility can be dismissed because antiviral effects are also observed against avirulent Semliki Forest virus infection of mice and avirulent infection of rats with EMC virus (Stebbing and Lindley, 1980). However, macrophages are required for the polynucleotides to be antiviral and this is discussed in Section 11.5.3.

The *in vivo* mode of action of these single-stranded polynucleotides remains obscure but protection has been observed with these single-stranded polynucleotides against infection of mice by SFV (Stebbing and Grantham, 1976; Stebbing *et al.*, 1976a) and there is no evidence, from T_1 RNase digests, that the RNA of this virus possesses a poly(C) tract (Brown *et al.*, 1974; Wengler and Wengler, 1976). Antiviral effects have also been observed with these single-stranded polynucleotides against a human influenza A virus infection of hamsters and ferrets (Round and Stebbing, 1981) and none of the genome segments of influenza viruses appear to possess a poly(C) tract (McGeoch *et al.*, 1976). However, it remains possible that there is a short oligo(C) tract in these viruses which is strategic for their replication or that there is a C-rich tract broken by G residues.

Identification of polynucleotides which inhibit replication of viruses may also be achieved directly in cases where some stages of virus replication can be carried out *in vitro*. Various polyribonucleotides such as poly(A), poly(I) and poly(U) significantly inhibit the virus transcriptase activity of detergent-disrupted influenza viruses (Smith *et al.*, 1980). The most effective polynucleotides against a range of influenza viruses are poly(U) and particularly a thiolated derivative poly(4-thiouridylic acid) and a copolymer of cytidine and 4-thiouridine residues, $poly(C,S^4U_{10})$. The sugar phosphate backbone appears to be necessary for inhibition by polynucleotides because vinyl analogs of poly(U) and poly(A) have little or no effect on transcriptase activity (Smith *et al.*, 1980) and polydeoxyribonucleotides are less effective than the corresponding polyribonucleotides (Weck et al., 1981). These inhibitory effects appear to require single-strandedness because annealing of poly(A) to poly(U) or poly(C) to poly(I) cause a marked decrease in inhibitory activity. Inhibition only occurs when the polynucleotides are added before in vitro transcriptase activity is initiated. Inhibition occurs with a range of influenza A strains and also a B strain and occurs at concentrations as low as 10^{-8} M (Smith et al., 1980). Antiviral effects have also been observed against influenza virus infections of hamsters and ferrets with poly(C,S^4U_{10}) and these effects do not occur with double-stranded polynucleotides including poly(C,S^4U_{10}) annealed to poly(A) (Round and Stebbing, 1981). The in vitro transcriptase activity of disrupted influenza virions is primed by the dinucleotide ApG and various analogs of this primer have been found to inhibit transcriptase activity (Weck et al., 1981). A deoxytetranucleotide dp(AG)$_2$ is the most active compound identified so far but the concentration causing 50 per cent inhibition is high (140 μg/ml). By examining inhibitory activity in magnesium or manganese buffers and the effects before and after initiation of transcriptase activity it is clear that dp(AG)$_2$ inhibits initiation, as predicted for an analog of the in vitro primer (Weck et al., 1981).

11.3.2. HETEROPOLYNUCLEOTIDES

Isaacs (1961) first proposed that an antiviral substance was released by virus-infected cells and that this material, termed 'interferon', was induced by the viral RNA because it was heterologous to the RNAs of the host cells and that this represented a means of excluding foreign RNAs. These ideas seemed to be confirmed by the observation that heterologous, but not homologous, RNAs caused appearance in tissue culture medium of an antiviral material (Rotem et al., 1963). The source of RNA used in this study was unspecified but presumably was a total cellular RNA extract consisting mainly of single-stranded material. Isaacs et al. (1963) obtained similar results. For example, these authors found that chick liver ribosomal RNA extracts were not effective in chick cells unless deaminated with nitrous acid and that the medium collected from cells treated overnight reduced plaque formation of vaccinia and chikungunya virus ten-fold, at most. This effect now seems to be small, since polynucleotide concentrations of up to 500 μg/ml were used, but this could be accounted for by the fact that most of the RNA used was single-stranded. The difficulty with this rationalization is that other single-stranded RNAs (from EMC virus and TYMV virus) showed no interferon production (Isaacs et al., 1963). Another report (Kohlhage and Falke, 1964) seemed to confirm these results: rabbit kidney RNA caused production of an interferon-like substance in HeLa cells but not in rabbit kidney cells. Much later work in the same vein (Befort et al., 1974) indicated that methylated, but not unmethylated, chick embryo RNA protected chick embryo cells against Sindbis virus infection. T$_1$ RNase fragments of this material (40 to 90 nucleotides in length) proved even more antiviral. These authors demonstrated that on fractionation of cells treated with the RNAs, in labeled form, most of the RNA was found in the ribosome and membrane fractions which they believed showed that the RNAs were taken up into these sub-cellular regions by the cells. The possibility of interferon production is mooted by the authors but their results are not related to the then known features of interferon induction.

Jensen et al. (1963) considered that their results supported those of Isaacs et al. (1963) but they differ in important features. Firstly, unlike Isaacs et al. (1963), they found that DNA was as effective as RNA in inducing interferon. Secondly, insignificant interferon was detected in cell culture supernatants until at least 10 days after addition of the polynucleotides. Rather high concentrations of material were used in this study and the authors note that interferon did not accumulate 'until after the cultured cells were in a rather poor state of nutrition'. One suspects that the cause of interferon production in these experiments was due to nucleic acids released by damage of cells rather than the added polynucleotides, particularly since various mononucleotides produced the same effects. There is, however, no reason to doubt that the material assayed was interferon since it was stable at pH 2.0 and susceptible to trypsin digestion.

Fukada *et al.* (1968) reported detailed and careful studies on the effect of various single-stranded RNAs in an interference assay in chick embryo cells. Protamine sulphate was added with the RNAs and serum was not used with the polynucleotides since without these precautions interference effects were greatly reduced. Cellular resistance was tested against Sindbis, VSV and NDV. MS2 phage RNA showed activity which was increased when it was degraded and chick embryo ribosomal RNA, ineffective when intact, was highly effective after digestion with T_1 RNase (but not pancreatic RNase). The authors note as follows: 'Apparently, not all oligonucleotides produced by T_1 RNase digestion are active, since *E. coli* and yeast RNAs, inactive as such, remained entirely inactive after the digestion, mild or extensive. This, combined with the finding that oligonucleotide mixtures produced from 'phage RNA by pancreatic RNase are only weakly effective, makes it appear evident that certain structural specificity is required for an oligonucleotide to be an effective inducer of interference.' These effects were produced with polynucleotide concentrations of 10–500 μg/ml and comparable effects were achieved with only 0.01–0.1 μg/ml of poly(I).poly(C), indicating that the assays were not inherently insensitive. However, little or no interferon production was found in cells treated with the various natural heteropolynucleotides. In view of the direct antiviral effects of poly(I) and poly(C) against EMC virus, discussed in Section 11.3.1, it is worth noting that in the studies of Fukada *et al.* (1968) poly(A), poly(U), polyC and poly(I) all showed no activity in their interference assay.

When we turn to antiviral studies with polynucleotides in animals, some work reported before formulation of the interferon hypothesis now seems particularly interesting. O'Dell *et al.* (1953) examined the antiviral activity of yeast RNA and sperm DNA against intradermal (foot-pad) infection of mice with MM virus. These experiments seem quite sensitive since the virus dose used caused paralysis or death in approximately 90 per cent of control mice and the number of mice per group was never less than thirty. With high doses of the polynucleotides (200 mg/kg), daily intraperitoneal treatments for 4, 6 or 12 days immediately prior to infection protected up to half of the mice. The DNA proved as effective as RNA in this study, so that it seems unlikely that interferon induction contributed significantly to the effect. Merely local effects, limiting passage of the virus from the site of inoculation, as occurs for example with polycarboxylates (Billiau *et al.*, 1971), are also not involved since the routes of treatment and infection were different. No antiviral effects were obtained when the polynucleotides were administered orally. Takano *et al.* (1965) examined the antiviral activity of the same polynucleotides against EMC and influenza virus infections of mice. Intranasal treatments of 3 mg on each of 1–4 days immediately before infection, 1–4 treatments per day, reduced susceptibility to intranasal infection, but not infections by other routes. The antiviral effect was proportional to the dose of polynucleotide administered and inversely proportional to the virus dose. Protection lasted for several days but was not observed with intranasal treatments against EMC when the virus was inoculated by the intraperitoneal or intracranial routes, indicating that the polynucleotides do not act solely by interacting with cells of the nasal passages. Interferon induction does not seem to be the explanation of these observations since DNA was as effective as RNA and the effects were only obtained when the infections and treatments were by the intranasal route. However, a protein material does seem to be involved in the effects since lung extracts of treated mice interfered with growth of vaccinia virus in chick embryo cultures and this antiviral activity was destroyed by trypsin treatment. But for this observation, one might suspect that the intranasal polynucleotide treatments merely inhibited nasal excretion of virus despite the observation that intranasal treatments with 5 per cent hydrolysed gelatin did not show antiviral activity.

All these studies demonstrate that RNAs, particularly single-stranded RNAs, may have antiviral effects without inducing interferon, or in addition to interferon induction. During this period a series of studies with a range of natural and synthetic materials showed that double-stranded, but not single-stranded, RNAs could induce interferon (Lampson *et al.*, 1967; Tytell *et al.*, 1967; Field *et al.*, 1967). These findings have been repeatedly confirmed, although interferon induction by synthetic single-stranded polynucleotides may now have been demonstrated (see Section 11.5.1.3). However, these studies have tended to obscure non-interferon mediated mechanisms of action for RNAs. Moreover, it should be borne in mind that when interferon induction is put forward as an explanation for antiviral effects of polynucleotides, the proposal really requires quantitative assessment of its contribution to the observed antiviral effect, if additional mechanisms of action are not to be overlooked.

11.3.2.1. Transfer RNA

Unfractionated transfer RNAs from bacteria protect mice against lethal infections of several picornaviruses and SFV (Stebbing et al., 1977a,c). The effect is relatively short-lived and the optimum response time appears to be around 6 hr before infection (Stebbing et al., 1977a). The effect is abolished on nuclease treatment of the tRNAs, and several of the rare nucleosides that occur in tRNAs show no antiviral activity, indicating that the effect is due to essentially intact tRNAs (Stebbing et al., 1977a). Transfer RNAs from eukaryotic sources are generally less active (Stebbing et al., 1977a) unless they are chemically modified (Stebbing et al., 1977b), and not all species of tRNA from antiviral batches of bacterial tRNA show activity (Stebbing et al., 1977a). No interferon is detectable in mice after treatment with tRNA, and tRNA does not 'hypo-reactivate' the protection conferred by poly(I).poly(C), implying that the tRNA does not act by producing even small undetectable amounts of interferon (Stebbing et al., 1977a).

In addition to the absence of interferon in mice treated with tRNA, the molecular size and low T_m of the polynucleotide indicate that it is unlikely to act as an interferon inducer. The antiviral effect of tRNA is not simply due to some local effect at the site where the material is administered since antiviral effects occur when the routes of treatment and infection are different (Stebbing et al., 1977a,c). Moreover, tRNA does not seem to 'prime' interferon production by subsequent treatment with a polynucleotide interferon inducer since there is no increase in antiviral activity of poly(I).poly(C) by prior treatment with tRNA; on the contrary, a decrease can occur (Stebbing et al., 1977c). Stimulation of immune responses to EMC virus does not seem to occur with tRNA treatments and protection occurs even in immunosuppressed mice (Stebbing et al., 1977a), but macrophages are necessary for in vivo activity and this point is discussed in Section 11.5.3.

Although a number of possible modes of action of tRNA have been eliminated, its in vivo activities contributing to the antiviral effect remain obscure. Treatment of mice with exogenous tRNA could cause infidelity in translation of EMC virus RNA since this is known to occur in vitro using tRNA from malignant cells (Sharma and Kuchino, 1977), and the tRNAs from this source are known to differ quantitatively and qualitatively from those of normal cells (Kuchino and Borek, 1976). Administration of tRNA to infected mice could also cause a reversal of host-cell shut-off and thus block viral protein synthesis in the manner in which modified tRNAs cause cessation of E. coli protein synthesis after 'phage infection (Kano-Sueoka and Sueoka, 1969). In the case of the E. coli RNA polymerase it is known that tRNAs bind to the core enzyme with a long residence time and a dissociation constant less than 1 nM (Spassky et al., 1979). There is little binding to the holoenzyme and binding results in loss of the sigma factor and tight binding to the core. Although the physiological function of such binding is unclear it is likely to occur in vivo because of the high concentration of RNA polymerase and tRNA in E. coli. Thus tRNAs may modulate transcription in as yet undefined ways and this may also occur in eukaryotic cells and affect replication of viruses. Furthermore, clover-leaf structures in viral genomes may have functional roles in virus replication (see Section 11.2.3.2).

11.4. INHIBITION OF REVERSE TRANSCRIPTASES BY SINGLE-STRANDED RNAs

11.4.1. ENZYME AND CELL CULTURE STUDIES

Several studies of polynucleotide inhibitors of reverse transcriptase have combined in vitro and cell culture effects so these aspects have not been segregated here, but the validity of interpreting results from cell studies in terms of *in vitro* effects is examined. Possibilities for treatment of human tumors based on reverse transcriptase inhibition are complex because of the uncertainty of involvement of RNA tumor viruses with human neoplasms. Only if recruitment of cells is essential for tumor development would reverse transcriptase inhibition be significant, as discussed elsewhere (Stebbing, 1979c).

11.4.1.1. Synthetic polynucleotides

Several studies have shown that single-stranded polynucleotides inhibit reverse transcription using purified reverse transcriptase preparations from various RNA tumor viruses. The first study demonstrated that MLV (Rauscher) reverse transcriptase was inhibited by homopolyribonucleotides, particularly poly(U) (Tuominen and Kenney, 1971). Purified DNA polymerase from mouse embryo cells was unaffected. Subsequent studies have shown that viral reverse transcriptases are generally inhibited by single-stranded polynucleotides, different polynucleotides showing different degrees of inhibition with various viral enzymes; but the effects are not specific to reverse transcriptases since some non-viral polymerases are also inhibited (Abrell *et al.*, 1972; Srivastava, 1975; Arya *et al.*, 1976a).

One factor complicating comparison of the various studies is the use of different primer/template complexes and enzymes of differing degrees of purity. The number of studies on inhibition of reverse transcriptase using purified enzyme free of natural primer/template are rather limited (Tuominen and Kenney, 1971; Abrell *et al.*, 1972; Mikke *et al.*, 1976). Detergent-disrupted virus preparations have been used and a series of papers by Arya *et al.* (1976a,b) indicate that in this system, using added synthetic primer/templates, purine polyribonucleotides are more active than pyrimidine-containing ones (Arya *et al.*, 1976b). De Clercq *et al.* (1974, 1975a,b) examined the inhibitory effect of a range of modified polynucleotides using the natural complex of viral template and enzyme obtained by simply treating purified virus with detergents. Their assays therefore determine effects on reverse transcriptase still associated with the natural primer/template. In this system poly(I) showed no inhibition whereas poly(2-azainosinic acid) (De Clercq *et al.*, 1977) and poly(2-methylthioinosinic acid) (De Clercq *et al.*, 1975a) were effective. Copolymers of inosinic acid and 2-methylthioinosinic acid showed intermediate effects, depending on the ratio of the two residues (De Clercq *et al.*, 1975a). The lack of any inhibition with poly(I) is in conflict with the observation of Arya *et al.* (1974) whose assay utilized an exogenous primer/template, unless poly(I) affects utilization of exogeneous, but not the natural endogenous, primer/template. Consequently it is difficult to explain why derivatives of poly(I) should be active in the assay utilizing the natural template. With the azo derivative of poly(I) the azo group seems important since this substitution on poly(A) renders the polynucleotide active in the same assay (De Clercq *et al.*, 1977). The effect of poly(U) and poly(C) and their 2′-azo derivatives have also been examined, in the assay lacking added primer/template, against the reverse transcriptases of a range of murine leukemia and sarcoma viruses (De Clercq *et al.*, 1975b). Poly(C) was without activity but poly(U) and the 2′-azo derivates of both poly(C) and poly(U) were active.

The assays of De Clercq *et al.* (1975a,b), using detergent-disrupted virus as a source of enzyme and primer/template complex, also included a carboxypolymethylene (Carbopol) since this material was found to increase the sensitivity of the assays by increasing the rate of DNA synthesis (De Clercq and Claes, 1973). Carbopol does not seem to have the same effect as detergent treatment of virus particles since increased DNA synthesis with Carbopol is observed even at optimum detergent concentrations (De Clercq and Claes, 1973). However, the effect of polynucleotide inhibitors of reverse transcriptase does not appear to be simply a reversal of the stimulatory effect of Carbopol: the 2′-azo derivative of poly(U) inhibited MLV (Moloney) reverse transcriptase to the same extent in reaction mixtures with and without Carbopol (De Clercq *et al.*, 1975b). Other studies have also utilized disrupted virions with the natural primer/template, but with addition of synthetic primer/templates (Arya *et al.*, 1974, 1975; Erickson and Grosch, 1974). Although it has been observed that in this system 'there is negligible incorporation of precursors catalysed by the endogenous murine leukemia virus template' (Arya et al., 1975), it is quite possible that the presence of the natural primer/template affects inhibition by polynucleotides when synthetic primer/templates are utilized. In fact, kinetic parameters of purified AMV reverse transcriptase have been found to be different from those of the disrupted virus using synthetic primer/templates (Erickson and Grosch, 1974).

Introduction of ε-adenosine into poly(A) by chloroacetaldehyde treatment prevents annealing to oligo (dT) and this modified polymer inhibits transcription of poly(A) primed with oligo(dT) using purified AMV reverse transcriptase (Chirikjian and Papas, 1974). Using the natural primer/template (AMV 70s RNA with primer tRNA attached) ε-adenosine containing poly(A) inhibited polymerization to a greater extent than poly(A). In these cases inhibition could be by competition for the template-recognition sites of the enzyme, as originally suggested by Tuominen and Kenney (1971). However, with the natural primer/template plus oligo(dT), DNA synthesis was stimulated but neither poly(A) nor the ε-adenosine containing poly(A) caused inhibition of polymerization. The authors imply that poly(A) and the modified form compete with the poly(A) tract of the viral RNA but that this does not occur when transcription is also occurring from this tract due to addition of oligo(dT). If true, one would predict that transcription from the natural primer (tRNA[phe]) would be stimulated on removal of the 3'-terminal poly(A) tract which, by implication, would then have some role in viral RNA transcription.

Although poly(U) is a more potent inhibitor of MLV reverse transcriptase in vitro than poly(A), the latter polynucleotide inhibits virus production in cell culture more effectively (Tennant et al., 1972, 1973). The 2'-O-methyl derivative of poly(A) is more effective in vivo, perhaps because it is more nuclease resistant (Tennant et al., 1973) and similar observations have been made for 2'-azo derivatives of poly(U) and poly(C) (De Clercq et al., 1975b). Substitutions of active polynucleotides which increase their nuclease resistance does not always increase their inhibition of virus replication. Various substitutions are likely to affect different activities contributing towards antiviral activity in vivo. Thus single-stranded polynucleotides have been shown to inhibit uptake of RNA tumor viruses. This occurs with poly(A) and poly(2'-O-methyl A) at higher concentrations (100 μg/ml) than those necessary for inhibition of replication (10 μg/ml) and some specificity seems to be involved since uptake of Sindbis virus is not affected (Tennant et al., 1973). Studies with several polynucleotides have shown that their relative potency in vitro against reverse transcriptase is the same as the relative effect on virus replication in vivo, implying that the prime effect on replication is via an effect on reverse transcriptase activity (Arya et al., 1975, 1976b). In view of the differences in nucleases between the two systems, the effects on virus uptake and the fact that the in vitro assays involved addition of a synthetic primer/template, these correlative observations are surprising and should be interpreted with caution.

The majority of studies concerning polynucleotide effects on reverse transcriptase activity have examined single-stranded polynucleotides without considering the possibility that double-stranded polynucleotides may have similar or different effects. The role of strandedness of polynucleotide inhibitors of reverse transcriptase was first considered by Erickson and Grosch (1974) who noted that the inhibitory effect of poly(2'-fluoro-2'-deoxy U) was greatly decreased when complexed with poly(A). De Clercq et al. (1975) noted a similar effect on the activity of the 2'-azo derivative of poly(U) against MLV (Moloney) reverse transcriptase when the polymer was complexed with poly(A). It has been noted that, since polynucleotides which tend to form multi-stranded complexes show the most pronounced inhibitory effects on MLV reverse transcriptase, their activity could reside in multistranded forms of these polynucleotides (Arya et al., 1976b). Although the strandedness of some polynucleotides in solution cannot be readily controlled, this is possible with the double- and triple-stranded structures formed between poly(A) and poly(U), which have been shown to inhibit synthesis of MLV in cell cultures much less than the single-stranded components (Arya and Chawda, 1977).

The role of polynucleotide chain-length in inhibiting reverse transcriptases has only been examined for poly(U) with the AMV enzyme. In this case inhibition of enzyme activity decreased sharply as the polynucleotide length decreased below 200 residues and below twenty residues no inhibition was observed (Erickson *et al.*, 1973). The length of fully effective poly(U) fragments in this system is not very different from polynucleotide lengths bound by other polymerases (see Erickson *et al.*, 1973). In view of the differences in inhibitory effects observed with various polynucleotides against different enzymes, further investigations on the role of chain-length would seem of value.

11.4.1.2. Natural Heteropolynucleotides

Studies on inhibition of reverse transcriptases by natural heteropolynucleotides are at present very limited. The differences between the inhibitory activity of various synthetic polynucleotides against different reverse transcriptases indicates that some specificity is involved and this could be due to recognition of particular nucleotide sequences by the enzymes. Nucleotide sequences in tRNAs are particularly interesting since the natural primers for reverse transcriptases are tRNAs and studies with fragments of RNA tumor virus genomes could be most informative since enzyme-recognition sites may be different from polymerization-initiation sites. Earlier related work on inhibition of other template specific polymerases was considered in Section 11.1.

The natural primer for reverse transcription of AMV RNA is a tRNA[trp] (Harada *et al.*, 1975) and analyses by gel filtration have shown that tRNA[trp] binds specifically to the purified enzyme and other tRNAs do not (Panet *et al.*, 1975). However, sucrose density gradient studies have shown that up to four molecules of *E. coli* tRNA[phe] can bind per enzyme molecule, that tRNA[met] binds less efficiently, and a mixed population of *E. coli* tRNAs also binds (Cavalieri and Yamaura, 1975). The mixed tRNA population was not found to bind to native AMV RNA. Various tRNA preparations were reported by Cavalieri and Yamaura (1975) to inhibit transcription of AMV RNA by the native reverse transcriptase using the natural primer and, in view of their interaction studies, this was attributed to direct interaction with the enzyme. The activity of an oligomeric form of this reverse transcriptase arising at low ionic strengths was not inhibited by the tRNAs so that, although oligomerization masked these binding sites, recognition of the natural initiation site was unaffected and enzyme activity not inhibited by the presence of tRNAs. It would seem particularly interesting to know whether the tRNA[phe] binding site, which is distinct from the primer binding site, also interacts with the various synthetic polynucleotide inhibitors of this reverse transcriptase or whether additional sites are involved.

11.4.1.3. Mode of Action of Polynucleotide Inhibitors of Reverse Transcriptases

In the first report of inhibition of reverse transcriptase by single-stranded poly-ribonucleotides (Tuominen and Kenney, 1971), it was noted that these polynucleotides do not act as templates for the enzyme and that inhibition showed classical reversible competitive kinetics, indicating that the inhibitors bind to the same site as the template. Arya *et al.* (1975) reported non-competitive inhibition of MLV (Moloney) reverse transcriptase by several polynucleotides. Curiously poly(A) and 2'-*O*-alkyl derivatives showed classical competitive inhibition of this reverse transcriptase with poly(A).oligo(dT) as the primer/template but non-competitive effects with poly(C).oligo(dG), and poly(I) also showed non-competitive inhibition with the former primer/template (Arya *et al.*, 1974). Erickson and Grosch (1974) found that the kinetics of inhibition of AMV reverse transcriptase by poly(2'-fluoro-2'-deoxy U) was clearly non-competitive, whereas poly(U) showed competitive kinetics in the same system. They noted that the assays measure polymerization, not enzyme binding, so that an avidly binding polynucleotide such as poly(2'-fluoro-2'-deoxy U), by rendering the reaction essentially irreversible, could inhibit polymerization in a non-competitive manner with the deoxynucleoside triphosphates as the true substrates. It is clear that reverse transcriptase assays involve so many components that they cannot be satisfactorily analysed by existing kinetic models and classical competitive inhibition data cannot be taken as evidence that the inhibitor competes with the template binding site of the enzyme.

On balance the evidence suggests that single-stranded RNAs which inhibit reverse transcriptases actually bind to the enzymes. Erickson and Grosch (1974) observed that the k_i for inhibition of AMV reverse transcriptase by poly(U) can be reduced about four-fold if the enzyme is pre-incubated with the inhibitor before addition of the template. Chandra and Bardos (1972) observed a similar effect with partially thiolated poly(C) on the reverse transcriptase of Friend leukemia virus, and ultracentrifugation studies with this copolymer have been claimed to show direct interaction with the enzyme (Chandra et al., 1975). However, these observations, like the kinetic analyses, do not mean that the inhibitor necessarily acts by binding to the template recognition sites of the enzymes. The observations that double-stranded polynucleotides do not act as inhibitors of reverse transcriptases argue against this notion since reverse transcription only occurs when template polynucleotides also have primers annealed to them. It is of course possible that enzyme recognition sites are single-stranded and remote from the primer sites with the latter merely determining the site at which already attached enzymes can commence polymerization. It has been suggested (Arya et al., 1974, 1975) that existing data is consistent with the notion of a template binding site which has sub-sites with different affinities for different polynucleotide inhibitors, as appears to be the case for different templates on E. coli DNA polymerase 1 (Marcus et al., 1974b). Binding sites on reverse transcriptases for polynucleotides remote from the template recognition site might be expected to cause allosteric effects but there is at present no data to support this notion.

A factor complicating interpretation of certain studies is the possibility of interactions between the potential inhibitor and the primer/template. Inability of polynucleotides to base pair with synthetic primers or templates is in some instances associated with increased inhibition of reverse transcriptase (Chirikjian and Papas, 1974; De Clercq et al., 1975a; Mikke et al., 1976). The most interesting of these cases seems to be poly (2′-O-ethyl C) which anneals readily to poly(I) but not to poly(dI). Even annealed to poly(I), poly(2′-O-ethyl C) does not act as a template for AMV reverse transcriptase so that the 2′-O-ethyl substitution must affect polymerization with the enzyme. Poly(2′-O-ethyl C) inhibits poly(A).oligo(dT) directed reverse transcription with the AMV enzyme. However, using poly(C).poly(dI) as template/primer (to avoid annealing of the inhibitor to the complex) no detectable inhibition of reverse transcriptase activity was found (Mikke et al., 1976). This was attributed to a high affinity of the reverse transcriptase for poly(C), and so a lower affinity for poly(A) could explain why the 2′-O-alkyl derivatives of poly(A) do act as inhibitors of reverse transcriptase when poly(A).oligo(dT) is used as the primer/template (Arya et al., 1974).

Indirect evidence that single-stranded polynucleotides which inhibit reverse transcriptase in vitro have effects on RNA tumor virus infected cells in culture by acting on the enzyme, comes from observations on effects of the polynucleotides on functions not dependent on reverse transcriptase. Infection and transformation of cells in culture by RNA tumor viruses are dependent on reverse transcriptase activity and are inhibited by single-stranded polynucleotides but production of virus particles from cells known to harbor leukemia viruses (De Clercq et al., 1975b), including those induced by iododeoxyuridine in AKR mouse embryo cells (Tennant et al., 1973), are not affected and these effects are not dependent on reverse transcriptase. In addition, it should be noted that the 2′-O-methyl derivative of poly(A) is a very potent inhibitor of the Moloney leukemia and sarcoma virus reverse transcriptases but, when added to cells after infection, is only effective within the first 4 hr, indicating an effect on some early virus function such as reverse transcriptase (Tennant et al., 1973). Evidence that inhibition of RNA tumor virus production in cell cultures occurs by effects on reverse transcriptase, rather than interferon production, is provided by the observation that single-stranded preparations of poly(A) and poly(U) are more effective inhibitors of murine leukemia virus production than the multistranded complexes of these two polynucleotides (Arya and Chawda, 1977).

A note of warning should be recorded with respect to observations indicating that polynucleotide inhibitors of reverse transcriptase do not affect virus production from cells harboring RNA tumor viruses. Poly(2′-azido U) has only been shown not to affect production of viruses from murine cells harboring leukemia and sarcoma viruses by monitoring ^{3}H-labeled virus production (De Clercq et al., 1975b), and Tennant et al. (1973) only showed that poly(A) and its 2'-alkyl derivatives did not affect virus specific cellular fluorescence. It is important to know whether production of released virus was affected in the latter study, and in both studies it would be interesting to know whether infectivity of released virus is affected, in view of the decreased in vivo infectivity of MLV incubated with poly(A) and its 2'-O-alkyl derivatives (Arya et al., 1975).

It remains unclear to what extent inhibition of RNA tumor virus production in cell cultures by single-stranded polynucleotides can be attributed to effects on reverse transcriptase. This question really requires some quantitative assessments of this effect and other factors influencing virus production which may be influenced by polynucleotides, such as uptake of the viruses by cells (Tennant et al., 1973). In addition to inhibition of reverse transcriptase, poly(C) could inhibit virus replication by mimicking the cytidine-rich regions found in the virion RNA of mammalian oncornaviruses (Pang and Phillips, 1975). These regions could even be concerned with the functioning of reverse transcriptase since the only synthetic template specific for viral reverse transcriptases is poly(C) (Goodman and Spiegelman, 1971; Roberts et al., 1972). The affinity of AMV reverse transcriptase for poly(C) has been used for affinity column purification of the enzymes (Marcus et al., 1974a) indicating that the cytidine-rich regions may be enzyme binding sites. Moreover, poly(C) containing templates are utilized better than poly(A) containing templates by several different reverse transcriptases (Spiegelman et al., 1970) and this has been shown in the case of MLV (Moloney) reverse transcriptase to be due to higher affinity for poly(C) containing primer/template complexes (Arya et al., 1974; Mikke et al., 1976).

In attempting to relate in vitro and cell culture studies, it is perhaps worth noting that the affinity of reverse transcriptase for RNAs is high both for the natural templates and the inhibitors, so that reverse transcriptase molecules free of polynucleotides must be rare in vivo. Polynucleotide inhibition of reverse transcriptase activity seems to act on initiation rather than polymerization (Erickson and Grosch, 1974) and newly synthesized viral DNA in cells seems to be circular (Guntaka et al., 1975) possibly because the viral RNA is circularized (Collett and Faras, 1978). Thus, inhibition by polynucleotides of reverse transcription in cells could be much less effective than with purified or semi-purified enzyme preparations since reinitiation events may be rare. Moreover, in one case it is clear that a polynucleotide (poly(I)) does not inhibit MLV (Moloney) reverse transcriptase using the natural primer/template (De Clercq et al., 1975a) although the polynucleotide does inhibit this enzyme when a synthetic primer/template (poly(A).oligo(dT)) is added to the assay system (Arya et al., 1974). It is possible that polynucleotide inhibitors of reverse transcriptases can bind to the template recognition sites or other remote sites. It is likely that polynucleotides which show effective in vitro inhibition of reverse transcriptase will not be effective in vivo unless they affect polymerization rather than initiation, i.e. enzyme sites remote from the template recognition site.

The electroneutral polyvinyl analog, poly(1-vinyluracil) like poly(U), inhibits MLV (Moloney) reverse transcriptase using poly(A).oligo(dT) as primer/template while poly(9-vinyladenine) does not (Pitha et al., 1973). However, both these polyvinyl analogs inhibit production of MLV in mouse embryo cells but have no effect on replication of Sindbis or VSV (Pitha et al., 1973). These vinyl analogs have been shown to inhibit all three classes of DNA polymerase from mouse cells only when they base-pair with the template and inhibition seems to occur by blocking elongation without displacement of the enzyme from its template (Pitha and Wilson, 1976). Such a mechanism of inhibition is unlike that of polynucleotide inhibitors and is consistent with the notion that the polyvinyl analogs may be recognized as primers by reverse transcriptase but that they cannot be extended by addition of nucleotides. On this basis a differential effect of the polyvinyl analogs against MLV production, compared with Sindbis and VSV is curious. If the 3'-terminal poly(A) tract of MLV is the site at which poly(1-vinyluracil) acts, then why does this analog not affect replication of Sindbis, which also has terminal poly(A)? One would anticipate tracts of oligo(U) in MLV RNA at which poly (9-vinyladenine) acts and that such tracts are absent from the virion RNA of the lytic viruses.

11.4.1.4. A Strategic Sequence Analog Inhibitor of RSV

Antiviral effects have been investigated with a tridecamer oligodeoxynucleotide which is complementary to thirteen of the twenty-one nucleotide sequence reiterated at the 3' and 5' ends of RSV (Zamecnik and Stephenson, 1978; Stephenson and Zamecnik, 1978; see also Section 11.2.3.3). The tridecamer, and the same tridecamer with the terminal hydroxyl moieties blocked, both delay and suppress release of virus from RSV-infected chick embryo cells, as monitored by reverse transcriptase activity in the medium and this effect is more pronounced as the dose of virus is decreased. The oligomers were used at a concentration of 10 μg/ml (2 μM) from the time of infection but the inhibitory effect, of higher concentrations at least, was reversed if the tridecamer was removed on changing the medium at 96 hr. Addition of the tridecamer to cell cultures which are already visibly transformed also cause suppression of reverse transcriptase in the medium. The greater efficacy of the blocked tridecamer, in these studies, was attributed to a possible increased resistance to nucleolytic breakdown (Zamecnik and Stephenson, 1978) but an alternative would be that the blocked tridecamer would not be displaced so readily during virus replication.

In vitro, the tridecamer primes cDNA synthesis with both RSV and AMV, but this is 7 times less efficient with AMV (Stephenson and Zamecnik, 1978). When the viral RNAs are translated in the wheat germ cell-free system, a molar ratio of as little as two tridecamers per 35S RSV RNA causes a 27 per cent inhibition of RSV and 10 per cent inhibition of AMV protein synthesis without any effect on the synthesis of rabbit globin or brome mosaic virus RNAs (Stephenson and Zamecnik, 1978). The extent of inhibition is dependent on the concentration of the tridecamer and the inhibitory effect is greater for RSV than AMV presumably because the tridecamer is not completely complementary to the terminal sequence in AMV RNA. At higher concentrations of tridecamer the inhibition of protein synthesis exceeds 85 per cent for RSV, although at these concentrations there was appreciable inhibition of globin and brome mosaic virus RNAs. At these higher concentrations, other oligodeoxynucleotides of similar size showed no inhibition of protein synthesis and the effect of the tridecamer on globin mRNA could be due to partial complementarity (Stephenson and Zamecnik, 1978).

The apparent antiviral effects in tissue-culture of the tridecamer have been attributed to its annealing to the viral RNA and thereby inhibiting translation and possibly other functions, the one most favored being circularization of the provirus DNA prior to integration into the host cell genome (Zamecnik and Stephenson, 1978). However, the data presented by Zamecnik and Stephenson (1978) do not allow any conclusion to be drawn on inhibition of transformation after circularization of the provirus DNA since an effect, like that on virus shedding, might be manifested by a delay in the time of transformation and the studies did not include time course effects on transformation. The conclusion favored by Zamecnik and Stephenson (1978) is further complicated by the absence of information concerning the effect of oligonucleotides annealing to any other sequence within the genome. It is possible that a tridecamer complementary to any thirteen nucleotides would produce the same effects.

11.4.2. STUDIES IN ANIMALS

11.4.2.1. Effects of Inhibitors of Reverse Transcriptase on RNA Tumor Virus Infected Animals

To date only a few of the polynucleotides that have been found to inhibit reverse transcriptase *in vitro* and in cell cultures have been tested for activity in RNA tumor virus infected animals and the results are not easily interpreted.

Tennant *et al.* (1974) found that 10 μg of the 2'-O-methyl derivative of poly(A) suppresses sarcoma formation and death of new-born mice challenged with the Moloney sarcoma-leukemia virus complex. At 1 hr before infection this effect was observed with 10^3 focus-forming units of virus and, at 4 hr before infection, against 10^4 units of the virus. Deaths seemed to occur primarily as a result of the leukemia component of the inoculated viruses.

Although the polynucleotide used is a particularly effective inhibitor of murine leukemia and sarcoma viruses in tissue cultures (Tennant *et al.*, 1972, 1973), its primary effect in new-born mice could be due to stimulation of immune responses to the virus since precipitating antibody levels to the virus were increased. However, this immunomodulatory effect occurred even in uninfected mice treated with the polynucleotide and could be due to stimulation of antibodies to endogenous RNA tumor viruses which cross-react with the experimentally inoculated viruses (Tennant *et al.*, 1974). Since development of antibodies to the endogenous virus occurs normally, the results may simply reflect a stimulation of immune responses before immune competence had developed. Such effects are difficult to relate to treatments of adult, competent animals which may be infected with viruses immunologically unrelated to endogenous viruses, particularly since the deaths in the mice infected as new-borns did not occur until 50–200 or more days after infection (Tennant *et al.*, 1974).

As with the 2'-*O*-methyl derivative of poly(A), the 2-methylthio derivative of poly(I) also inhibited reverse transcriptase and cell transformation by Moloney leukemia and sarcoma viruses, but did not inhibit sarcoma development or death of new-born mice treated 4 hr before infection, possibly because this polynucleotide does not have immunostimulatory properties (De Clercq *et al.*, 1975a).

Arya *et al.* (1975) observed that if polyadenylic acids are incubated at 37°C for 30 min with Friend MLV, the number of foci per spleen formed after 9 days in 8-week-old DBA/2 male mice was decreased. The most effective compound was poly(2'-*O*-ethyl A), followed by poly (2'-*O*-methyl A), and poly(A) was the least effective although it inhibited focus formation by about 60 per cent when incubated with the virus at a concentration of 3.4 μg/ml. Such a concentration of poly(2'-*O*-ethyl A) inhibited focus formation by 94 per cent. The degree of inhibition on focus formation was dose-dependent. The authors comment that the mode of action of these polynucleotides on focus formation is uncertain and that immune responses may be involved. However, they note that the relative inhibition by the different polynucleotides is the same as their relative effects on reverse transcription *in vitro*, and virus synthesis in cell cultures. These studies, since they are concerned with adult, rather than suckling, mice, may be more relevant to natural infections but they need to be extended to treatments of animals rather than the virus before it is administered.

It should be noted that although uptake of MLV (Moloney) is inhibited in tissue culture by poly(A) and its 2'-*O*-methyl derivative only at concentrations higher than those which affect virus replication (Tennant *et al.*, 1973), the principal effect of such polynucleotides in mice could be due to effects on cellular uptake of the viruses. The effects on immune responses of mice to RNA tumor viruses as a result of single-stranded polynucleotide treatments may arise from effects on uptake of the viruses by immunoresponsive cells such that enhanced antiviral effects are achieved.

Stebbing (1977) examined the effect on time of death from spontaneous leukemia of female AKR mice treated intraperitoneally once weekly from the tenth week of life with poly(C), poly(I) or both these polynucleotides given 4 hr apart. Poly(C) alone was without any effect, but doses of 400 μg/mouse/week of poly(I) caused significant prolongation of life and a greater effect occurred with weekly treatments of 100 or 400 μg/mouse/week of poly(I) followed 4 hr later by 100 or 400 μg/mouse of poly(C). These treatments prolonged life by 46 days or more and did not stimulate interferon production. The effectiveness of these treatments appear greater, on a weight basis, than those achieved after repeated treatments of AKR mice with the known interferon inducer, poly(A).poly(U) (Drake *et al.*, 1974). Poly(C) and poly(I) have been shown not to act as immunostimulators (Schmidtke and Johnson, 1971) but unfortunately the susceptibility of the reverse transcriptase of AKR leukemia virus to inhibition by poly(I) and poly(C) has not been examined. The antileukemia effects observed with poly(C) and poly(I) treatments (Stebbing, 1977) could be by direct effects on replication of the virus by inhibition of reverse transcriptase or perhaps by mimicking the cytidine-rich regions detected in virion RNA of mammalian oncornaviruses (Pang and Phillips, 1975) and their complements in the negative strand RNA. In the case of MLV (Moloney) there appears to be two unique cytidine sequences in the first 1000 nucleotides synthesized from the natural initiator tRNA (Haseltine *et al.*, 1976). Antitumor effects of polynucleotides could arise by adjuvant effects but immunostimulation would seem of dubious significance in AKR leukemia since an antibody response to the putative causative agent (Gross virus) occurs normally (Oldstone *et al.*, 1972) and onset of leukemia does not seem to depend on immunological factors (Gershwin *et al.*, 1976). It is possible, as argued elsewhere (Stebbing, 1977), that antitumor effects in intact animals of repeatedly administered double-stranded polynucleotides could be due primarily to effects on reverse transcriptase.

The adverse effect of repeated poly(A) treatments on development of leukemia in AKR mice (Stebbing, 1977) is curious since poly(A) itself inhibits the reverse transcriptase and cellular uptake of a murine leukemia virus (Tennant *et al.*, 1972, 1973). The 2'-*O*-methyl derivative of poly(A) was also found to enhance MLV (Rauscher)-induced splenomegaly in new-born mice (Tennant *et al.*, 1974). It is possible that these effects are in part due to aggravation of infection attributable to an immune response to the polynucleotides themselves since this is known to occur, particularly with poly(A) when it is conjugated with a protein (Braun and Nakano, 1967).

Poly(9-vinyladenine) and poly(1-vinyluracil) both inhibit MLV reverse transcriptase (Pitha *et al.*, 1973; Tennant *et al.*, 1974; Arya *et al.*, 1975) and suppress virus replication in cultured cells and mice (Noronha-Blob *et al.*, 1977; Vengris *et al.*, 1978). Immune responses were not involved in these mouse studies, but the polymers had no effect when given once: repeated, daily treatments were necessary. There was no evidence of interferon induction or effects against a transplantable tumor in these treatments of adult mice, indicating that polymeric inhibitors of reverse transcriptase can be effective *in vivo* by virtue of effects observed *in vitro* (Vengris *et al.*, 1978). Nevertheless results with polynucleotides and polyvinyl analogs suggest that single-stranded polymers may influence several processes in mice, some of which may be adverse. Moreover, the fact that the same polynucleotide shows protective effects against one RNA tumor virus and adverse effects with another, in mice (Tennant *et al.*, 1974) indicates that the effects are dependent on the particular viruses involved. The function of the poly(A) tracts in the virion RNA of AKR leukemia virus (Ihle *et al.*, 1974) and other oncornaviruses (Lai and Duesberg, 1972) is unclear but effects of poly(A) *in vivo* may be related to the role of the poly(A) tracts in virus replication.

11.4.2.2. Polynucleotide Effects on Tumors in Animals

Several studies have been made of the antitumor effects of double-stranded poly-nucleotides with evidence that this activity is not entirely due to induction of interferon. However, the possibility that similar antitumor effects may arise with single-stranded polynucleotides was not examined in these studies. Nevertheless there are a few studies of antitumor effects of single-stranded polynucleotides, including a study in man. Esposito (1969) reported the effect of treating ten pleural mesothelioma patients with 1 g hog's liver RNA daily for 10 days. The treatments were commenced after washing out the pleural cavity and all treatments were directly into the pleural cavity. Two patients relapsed within 3 months of remission but in eight cases all symptoms disappeared. The cause of this antitumor effect is obscure but would seem to warrant further investigation.

Geddes-Dwyer and Cameron (1976) treated cell suspensions from a ^{32}P-induced osteosarcoma of DA rats with 500 μg/ml tRNA overnight and then inoculated the cells subcutaneously into syngeneic rats. Treatment with rat embryo or normal mesenchymal tissue tRNA reduced the tumor weight at 22 days by 76 per cent and 60 per cent, respectively, while tRNA from the tumor cells increased tumor weight slightly. The authors suggest that non-neoplastic cells in the tumor cell suspensions could be involved but their notion that antitumor effects of total RNA extracts is primarily due to tRNA remains unconfirmed since there were no appropriate controls. Moreover, the results are difficult to assess since tumor weights were determined after only 22 days and no absolute weights were recorded, only relative changes. Similar studies, with purified tRNAs, have been carried out in mice by Stern and Schreiber (1977) except that these authors treated the animals rather than the tumor cells. C57 B1 mice treated 3 times/week before and after inoculation of syngeneic methyl-cholanthrene-induced tumors showed decreased incidence and weight of tumors with yeast tRNA treatments but rat liver and syngeneic mouse liver tRNAs had no effect. Mice which failed to develop tumors as a result of treatment with yeast tRNA succumbed to re-inoculation with 5×10^5 but not 5×10^4 tumor cells. This effect is difficult to interpret since no data are given for the effect of these cell doses in untreated animals. No effects were observed with yeast tRNA treatments of C_3H mice inoculated with a similar syngeneic tumor. Stern and Schreiber suggest that these results may be due to interaction of tRNA with macrophages and the effectiveness of the treatments in C57 B1 mice but not C_3H mice is attributed to differences in reticuloendothelial and immune responses.

Clearly the development of single-stranded polynucleotides for treatment of RNA tumor virus infections requires much more extensive and better designed *in vivo* experiments for the *in vitro* work to be meaningful, in view of other factors which may influence *in vivo* activity.

In comparison with the limited studies on antitumor effects of single-stranded poly-nucleotides, there is a large but conflicting literature on antitumor effects of double-stranded polynucleotides (Drake *et al.*, 1974; Lacour *et al.*, 1975; see references in Gresser *et al.*, 1978). Whether interferon induction by double-stranded polynucleotides can account for their antitumor activity was examined by Gresser *et al.* (1978) by simultaneous administration of anti-interferon serum. The results indicate that interferon production could quantitatively account for antitumor effects. However, it is likely that the tumor cells themselves produce interferon which partially slows or limits tumor development(Trinchieri *et al.*, 1978) so that administration of anti-interferon serum would be deleterious for this reason alone, but appropriate controls for this effect were not included in the study of Gresser *et al.* (1978).

11.5. ALTERNATIVE MECHANISMS OF ACTION OF ANTIVIRAL AND ANTITUMOR POLYNUCLEOTIDES

11.5.1. The Interferon Hypothesis

Strategic sequences within viral RNA may involve contiguous or non-contiguous regions which form double-stranded structures or loops. It is also possible that double-stranded polynucleotides may inhibit the activity of various factors necessary to complete virus replication. In other words, there is no necessity for antiviral polynucleotides acting in the ways considered in this review to be single-stranded. However, the possibility that double-stranded polynucleotides have antiviral effects by means other than interferon induction has only rarely been considered. Careful examination of the data and analysis of features of the interferon hypothesis as generally conceived, indicates that double-stranded polynucleotides may in fact have direct antiviral activities by other means. Antiviral effects of treatments of intact animals with single-stranded polynucleotides have also generally been interpreted in terms of interferon induction although many of these antiviral effects may be due to other mechanisms, as discussed in Section 11.3. This section is concerned with the relation of the interferon hypothesis to antiviral effects of polynucleotides and in so far as effects of single-stranded polynucleotides are concerned, only those effects attributed by authors to interferon induction are analysed. Firstly, however, the interferon hypothesis itself must be considered.

The interferon hypothesis for explaining antiviral effects of RNAs has now become quite elaborate, but its main features may be concisely stated as follows. In general double-stranded polyribonucleotides cause the *de novo* synthesis of a protein (interferon) which is secreted by cells and which is capable of protecting other cells against virus infection. Secreted interferons are generally stable at pH2, and generally show species specificity for the cells or animals which they can protect. Cellular RNA and protein synthesis are required for exogenously added interferon to protect cells and another protein (the antiviral protein) is therefore postulated as the agent directly causing protection of cells, with interferon itself acting as a de-repressor for synthesis of the antiviral protein. The observation that metabolic inhibitors, added after interferon induction in cells, cause greater amounts of interferon to be synthesized is generally interpreted to mean that the messenger RNA for interferon is degraded rather rapidly by another agent whose synthesis can be inhibited, thereby prolonging the life of interferon messenger RNA.

As described so far, the only limiting feature of this scheme as a hypothesis is the liberal use of the qualification 'generally'. It is true that several proteins satisfy the definition of interferon and the properties of these vary, e.g. molecular weight, stability to pH2, and the types of cells in which they are formed. However, the leeway provided for by these observations should not be too readily used as precedents for explaining new experimental data, since opportunities for testing the interferon hypothesis seem in practice to have been ignored. The most serious criticism of the data invoked to support the hypothesis is that in many studies, measurement of antiviral activity has involved assays of interference, rather than of interferon.

A further important feature of interferon induction is the phenomenon of hyporeactivity: repeated treatments with interferon inducers may cause measurable levels of released interferon to decrease without a decrease in protection, yet the protection is still ascribed to interferon. Indeed, undetected interferon has rather readily been put forward as an explanation of antiviral effects associated with polynucleotides. In whole animals, tissue rather than circulating levels of interferon are considered important. This view has rarely been tested experimentally. It should also be noted that while the interferon hypothesis allows for indirect effects, since it requires RNA and protein synthesis, indirect antiviral effects where they are observed, should not be taken as evidence that they involve the interferon mechanism.

The purpose of presenting the interferon hypothesis in this rather critical fashion is primarily aimed at overcoming the present readiness to interpret almost any antiviral effect mediated by polynucleotides in terms of interferon, with little regard for other possible mechanisms. Future work may well show that some of the phenomena considered in this review are rightly interpreted on the basis of interferon. However, the lack of alternative hypotheses does generally limit definitive experimentation (Popper, 1959) and has, in the issues under review, produced consensus views not based on critical considerations of the experimental data on crucial points.

11.5.1.1. Evidence that Interference Assays Measure Interferon

It must be said that interference assays are quite inappropriate for analysing the mode of action of antiviral substances suspected of inducing interferon and their use disregards the important conceptual advance made by Isaacs and Lindenmann (1957). Some justifications for interpreting interference effects on the basis of interferon production have been made and these seem ultimately to rely on observations that interferon inducers need only interact briefly with cells to induce interferon (Friedman, 1967) and that interferon can induce the antiviral state after only a short period in contact with cells (Dianzani and Baron, 1977).

Antiviral effects in cells in the absence of detectable interferon have been reported for normal cells (Henderson and Taylor, 1961) and even for cells resistant to interferon (Mayer, 1962; Stancek, 1965). These effects have been attributed to interferon (Baron, 1973) on the basis that undetectably small amounts of interferon can induce protection of cells (Buckler *et al.*, 1966; Youngner *et al.*, 1966; Friedman, 1967; Goldsby, 1967). The development of resistance to infection in cells before appearance of extracellular interferon has also been interpreted on the basis of the interferon hypothesis and formation of 'messenger RNA for antiviral substance' has been offered as an explanation for this phenomenon (Baron, 1973) even though the nature of the antiviral substance has only been postulated to be protein on the basis of studies with antimetabolites. The messenger RNA in question is therefore an even more remote abstraction. Although metabolic inhibitors do prevent development of the antiviral state by interferon (Buckler *et al.*, 1968) the interpretation of interference phenomena on the basis of these features of interferon induction demonstrate a profound confusion of the observations with the hypotheses which they are supposed to formulate and test. It suggests that many authors believe that a hypothesis can be proved by experiments in which the results can be interpreted in accord with the hypothesis. The continued adoption of this fallacious position (Popper, 1959) has greatly hampered our understanding of the mechanism of action of interferon and its inducers, and other antiviral substances.

11.5.1.2. Hyporeactivity

Interferon formation by cells and animals in response to inducers generally decreases with each successive treatment and this phenomenon is generally termed 'hyporeactivity', and lasts for several days (Ho, 1973). A number of explanations for this phenomenon have been put forward based on the possibility that interferon inhibits its own synthesis; that an inhibitory factor is also induced, or that in animals inducers are not rapidly cleared (see Ho, 1973). Cells and animals in the hyporeactive state remain resistant to infection. It should be noted that analysis of the mechanism involved in maintaining this antiviral state depends on interference assays: the resistance of treated cells or animals has, of necessity, to be tested directly. Consequently whether interferon, even undetectable interferon (!), is involved cannot be tested (see Section 11.5.1.1). Repeated treatments with an inducer during the hyporeactive stage do not confer significant additional protection so that from a therapeutic point of view, it would be most important to overcome this problem in some way since repeated treatments are likely to be necessary for significant effects after infection.

11.5.1.3. Synthetic Single-stranded Polynucleotides that Appear to Induce Interferon

Single-stranded polynucleotides have not generally been found to induce interferon, or do so only poorly, and then only when they are highly structured or used under conditions which cause formation of multi-stranded structures (De Clercq and Merigan, 1969; Colby, 1971). Baron et al. (1969) reported that poly(I) and poly(C) could induce interferon in several cell lines and in rabbits to about 10 per cent of the levels found with poly(I).poly(C). Some care was taken in this study to exclude the possibility of contaminating double-stranded RNA in the preparations of single-stranded RNAs but poly(I) and poly(C) from different sources and different solutions varied considerably in their ability to induce interferon. An extension of this work (Billiau et al., 1969) was concerned with the possibility that these variations in interferon induction by poly(I) and poly(C) arose from varying nucleases present in the assays. To protect polynucleotides against degradation and facilitate their uptake by cells, various polybasic materials were added in the assays. Billiau et al. (1969) found that cellular resistance to VSV increased to twenty-fold with poly(I).poly(C) on addition of polybasic materials, with similar effects on the activity of poly(I) and poly(C) so that some single-stranded RNA preparations which showed no activity alone, conferred significant protection. Unfortunately, these results, interpreted by the authors in terms of interferon, relied on an interference assay which means that their interpretation must be treated with caution. Only in the case of combined treatments with poly(I).poly(C) and polybasic materials were the media assayed for interferon-like activity, and as expected in this case the results support the notion that the increased antiviral activity was due to interferon.

Marked increase in antiviral activity of the synthetic alternating copolymer riboadenylic-ribouridylic acid has been reported if the phosphates are substituted by thiophosphate groups (De Clercq et al., 1969). In human skin fibroblasts VSV plaque formation was reduced to an equivalent extent by as little as 10,000-fold less of the thiophosphate-substituted copolymer in an interference assay, although on assaying the medium from treated cells for interferon, there was a difference of only 200-fold. Using equal weights the thiophosphate copolymer proved equivalent to poly(I).poly(C) in terms of interferon induction, although the thiophosphate copolymer induced greater cellular resistance to virus infection. It is therefore possible that some of the antiviral activity of the thiophosphate polymer is due to non-interferon mediated mechanisms. Curiously, in mice the thiophosphate copolymer stimulated about ten-fold lower amounts of interferon than poly(I).poly(C) but in rabbits about forty-fold more interferon was induced, compared with the unsubstituted copolymer. Unfortunately the resistance of animals to virus infection following treatments with these various polynucleotides was not examined.

Sequential poly(I), poly(C) treatments of a variety of cell lines have been shown to protect the cells against virus infections (De Clercq and De Somer, 1971, 1972; De Clercq et al., 1973). A range of time intervals between the two treatments produced this effect but generally the poly(I) treatment had to precede the poly(C) treatment. However, production of interferon, rather than interference, was demonstrated by direct assay in only one case: poly(I) treatment for 1 hr followed by poly(C) treatment for 1 hr in primary rabbit kidney cells (De Clercq and De Somer 1972; De Clercq et al., 1973). In this case the production of interferon extended over a longer period than with poly(I).poly(C) and the order of the poly(I) and poly(C) treatments was not crucial for induction (De Clercq et al., 1973). The formation of interferon in this case would therefore seem unusual and an explanation for the phenomena in other treatment regimes and cell lines based on interferon is presumptuous. Sequential treatment of primary chick embryo fibroblasts with poly(I) and poly(C), in a regime identical to one used by De Clercq and De Somer (1971), was found to cause no inhibition of poxvirus replication although poly(I).poly(C) in comparable amounts caused marked inhibition (Hiller et al., 1973).

Sequential treatment of mice with single-stranded polynucleotides produces no detectable interferon except when poly(I) is followed within 10 min by poly(C) (De Clercq and De Somer, 1971). With longer intervals between the treatments no interferon was detected in mice (De Clercq and De Somer, 1971; Stebbing and Grantham, 1976) but when the susceptibility of the mice to infection was examined they were found to be partially protected (Stebbing and Grantham, 1976). Curiously the order of treatments necessary for antiviral activity in mice was found to be the same as that necessary in most of the tissue culture studies of De Clercq and De Somer (1972). However, in addition to the absence of detectable interferon a number of features of the protection in mice are inconsistent with an interferon-mediated mechanism: in particular sequential treatments with non-base pairing poly-nucleotides also conferred protection (Stebbing and Grantham, 1976). The notions that antiviral effects of sequential poly(I).poly(C) treatments are due to interferon induction and that poly(I) is more important than poly(C) for interferon induction due to cellular receptors for poly(I), have been criticized elsewhere (Stebbing et al., 1977e).

More recently, Thang et al. (1977) reported that some preparations of poly(I) can induce interferon. No reference was made by these authors to the earlier work of Baron et al. (1969), but Thang et al. (1977) also reported that some preparations of poly(I) can reproducibly induce up to one-third of the amount of interferon induced by poly(I).poly(C). Interferon-inducing batches of poly(I) behave like poly(I).poly(C) in primed and superinduced protocols but their interferon inducing capacity varies considerably from one cell system to another and were much less active in vivo than would be expected from in vitro assays (De Clercq et al., 1978). The inducer preparations of poly(I) were indistinguishable from other poly(I) preparations by X-ray diffraction but were distinguishable by their interaction with antipoly(I) antibodies, suggesting that some conformational feature is important for interferon induction by inducer preparations of poly(I). Pitha and Pitha (1974) found that conjugation, with DEAE-dextran or poly-D-lysine, of poly(I) (from Miles Laboratories) caused the polynucleotide to become antiviral and to inducer interferon when applied to primary human fibroblasts or mouse L-cells. Possibly these aggregates induced poly(I) to assume the same conformation as the inducer poly(I) preparations of Thang et al. (1977). This work seems to show quite convincingly that some conformation, of poly(I) at least, can act as an efficient interferon inducer but it remains generally unclear to what extent earlier studies can be explained on the basis of inducer-type batches of poly(I). The poly(I) used by Stebbing et al. (1976) and Stebbing and Grantham (1976) was material from P-L Biochemicals of the same type as that which was found not to induce interferon by Thang et al. (1977). A highly structured form of poly(I) seems unlikely to provide an explanation of the observations of Thang *et al.* (1977) and the significant features of inducer preparations of poly(I) remain unclear.

11.5.1.4. *Direct Antiviral Effects of Double-stranded Polynucleotides not Explicable by Interferon*

Kjeldsberg and Flikke (1971) demonstrated that low concentrations of poly(I).poly(C) inhibited polio virus RNA synthesis in L-cells when they were treated with actinomycin D at the same time as the polynucleotide treatment. Since DNA-dependent RNA synthesis was inhibited by this treatment the authors concluded that interferon was not produced and they suggested some direct effect on virus replication, such as inhibition of the virus coded RNA polymerase. Subsequently Vilcek and Varacalli (1971) showed that actinomycin D greatly reduced interferon production in rabbit kidney cells up to $1\frac{1}{2}$ hr after adding poly(I).poly(C) and that at 1 hr and $1\frac{1}{2}$ hr after poly(I).poly(C) treatment, inhibition of interferon production was progressively decreased. They also showed that actinomycin D added 1 hr after poly(I).poly(C) completely suppressed the inhibitory effect of poly(I).poly(C) on VSV multiplication, and this effect of actinomycin D was still pronounced $1\frac{1}{2}$ hr after poly(I).poly(C) treatment. These observations were considered to be consistent with the notion that interferon mRNA synthesis was virtually complete $1\frac{1}{2}$ hr after addition of poly(I).poly(C) and that protection by interferon is indirect with a time delay between addition of inducer and development of the antiviral state. The observations of Kjeldsberg and Flikke are not contradicted by these results, but Vilcek and Varacalli criticized the suggestion of Kjeldsberg and Flikke, that a direct effect of poly(I).poly(C) on virus replication is involved in these observations, on the grounds of the time delay just noted. Vilcek and Varacalli (1971) ignore that a direct effect on virus replication may also involve a time delay in appearance of the effect and that their proposal that 'it has to be assumed that cellular resistance produced by such low poly(I).poly(C) concentrations is mediated by endogenous cellular interferon, that becomes undetectable once released into the culture medium' is unwarranted. The nature of these antiviral effects in the presence of actinomycin D remains unclear and the possibility of differences between the cells or viruses used by the two groups has not been explored.

Curiously, direct inhibitory effects of poly(I), poly(C) and poly(I).poly(C) have been observed against the virion transcriptase of VSV (Hiller *et al.*, 1973). At concentrations of $82.5\,\mu$g/ml all three polynucleotide preparations produced comparable levels of inhibition but at lower concentrations poly(C) was less effective than the other polynucleotides and no effect was observed in similar assays on the virion transcriptase of poxvirus using poly(I).poly(C).

It is clear that mice and rabbits with antibodies to poly(I).poly(C) fail to produce interferon when injected with poly(I).poly(C) (Steinberg *et al.*, 1971; Dianzani *et al.*, 1972). Mice immunized with a natural double-stranded RNA from a fungal source also show little or no interferon production on subsequent treatment with the RNA (Naysmith *et al.*, 1974). However, mice immunized in this way were as fully protected against EMC virus infection by a subsequent single dose of the double-stranded RNA, as were normal mice (Naysmith *et al.*, 1974). Although this observation may be explained by asserting that the level of circulating interferon in mice is merely material in excess of that required in tissues for protection, it is also possible that other mechanisms are involved. Naysmith *et al.* (1974) suggest that a direct effect on cells of the reticuloendothelial system may be involved and that this effect, unlike interferon induction, is unaffected by antibodies.

Recently Gresser *et al.* (1978) examined whether the antiviral activity of poly(I).poly(C) against EMC virus infection of mice could be accounted for by interferon induction by using antimouse-interferon serum raised in sheep. This study indicated that the antiviral activity of poly(I).poly(C) was destroyed with simultaneous administration of the anti-interferon serum. However, mice treated with anti-interferon serum, without simultaneous poly(I).poly(C) treatment, died earlier than control mice and with extensive replication of virus in visceral organs (Gresser et al., 1976). This earlier study was interpreted to mean that EMC virus infection induces sufficient interferon to alter the course of disease but the results also imply that poly(I).poly(C)-induced interferon may be insufficient to overcome infection if virus induced interferon is also eliminated. Thus, it remains possible that poly(I).poly(C) has antiviral effects in addition to interferon induction.

11.5.2. KNOWN EFFECTS OF POLYNUCLEOTIDES

The interferon-inducing activity of polynucleotides and their direct inhibitory effects on virus replication by affecting viral polymerases or mimicking strategic sequences have already been considered and in this section other effects of polynucleotides which may contribute or affect their antiviral and antitumor activities are considered. The diverse effects of synthetic and naturally produced double-stranded RNAs on the in vitro and in vivo course of virus infections were considered earlier by Carter and De Clercq (1974). Here, their review is updated and extended to single-stranded polynucleotides and antitumor effects. However, it is not possible to discuss in depth the known effects of polynucleotides on relevant activities since in very few cases have quantitative assessment been made of the individual effects. There can be no doubt that assessment of the effects of polynucleotides on a range of activities in vivo is now most important for a clear understanding of the in vivo mode of action of polynucleotides and the future development of clinically useful antiviral or antitumor polynucleotides.

Several potential antiviral and antitumor activities of polynucleotides are only apparent from in vivo studies because they influence particular reactions dependent on cells not present in tissue cultures. Several interferon inducers, including double-stranded polynucleotides, cause increased ingestion of IgG-coated erythrocytes in mice by macrophages (Hamburg et al., 1978). Several interferon inducers are known also to increase natural killer-cell activity (Gidlund et al., 1978; Herberman et al., 1978). Double-stranded polynucleotides are also known to stimulate immune responses (Braun and Nakano, 1967; Schmidtke and Johnson, 1971) but this does not seem to occur with single-stranded polynucleotides (Braun and Nakano, 1967; Schmidtke and Johnson, 1971) unless they are complexed with a protein such as methylated serum albumin (Braun and Nakano, 1967). The adjuvant effects of double-stranded RNA appear to be dependent on the times of administration relative to antigen and treatment 24 hr prior to antigen can cause a suppressed response (Cunnington and Naysmith, 1975). The contribution of adjuvanticity and interferon induction has been shown to vary with the dose of the double-stranded polynucleotide, poly(I).poly(C) (Stebbing et al., 1980). Thus quantitation of interferon-mediated effects are really very difficult. In addition double-stranded RNA is involved at various stages of the biochemical events leading to the antiviral state (Baglioni, 1979) and direct induction of interferon alone may not be the only stage at which an interferon inducing double-stranded polynucleotide is involved. The double-stranded complex poly(I).poly(C) has also been shown to have adjuvant-like effects on graft-vs-host activities in mice, which could in part account for the antitumor activities of this polynucleotide (Cantor et al., 1970). Poly(I).poly(C) also stimulated a graft-vs-host reaction in rats but only with donor cells differing at a major histocompatibility locus (Kreider and Cecalupo, 1975). Single-stranded polynucleotides, particularly poly(I) and some derivatives, stimulate the alternative pathway of complement mediated cell lysis (Yachin, 1963; De Clercq et al., 1975a) and this effect has been shown to occur in vivo in the case of rats (Yachin and Rosenblum, 1964). To be effective against lytic viruses, which can cause effects, even death, within a few days, immune responses, cellular or humoral, would have to be rapid. Nevertheless there is evidence for such rapid immune responses as the basis for the difference between virulent and avirulent strains of viruses (Bradish et al., 1975).

It is possible that polynucleotides may have indirect antiviral effects in vivo by limiting pathological sequelae of virus infection. In this regard it is interesting to note that treatment of dogs with calf-liver transfer RNA limits lipopolysaccharide-induced shock and this may be due to stabilization of lysosomes (Okude *et al.*, 1969). Breakdown products of polynucleotides may also affect potential antiviral activities *in vivo* and it may be noted that nucleosides and nucleotides are known to stimulate macrophage pinocytosis (Cohn and Parks, 1967).

A number of effects of polynucleotides have been studied *in vitro* but the extent to which they are affected *in vivo*, after treatment of animals or cells in culture, remains generally unclear. Polynucleotides have been found to inhibit DNA-dependent RNA polymerases to varying extents (Dezelee *et al.*, 1974; Sasaki *et al.*, 1974) and poly(I) has been shown to release DNA template restriction of isolated nuclei and soluble chromatin using *E. coli* DNA polymerase (Brown and Coffey, 1972). This effect is dependent on the size of poly(I). Below about 4S poly(I) becomes inactive and when complexed with poly(C) or methylated in the N-7 position activity is also lost. Poly(C) is without activity and comparisons of assays using nuclei and isolated chromatin indicate that the specificity of this phenomenon is not dependent on differences in transport of the polymers across the nuclear membrane (Brown and Coffey, 1972). Thermal denaturation profiles have confirmed that nucleohistone complexes are destabilized by several polyanions and that the effect depends on the presence of secondary structure: ribosomal RNA is also active in this assay while poly(C) shows only a small effect (Ansevin *et al.*, 1975).

Low concentrations of double-stranded RNAs, but not single-stranded RNA or DNA, inhibit protein synthesis in cell-free systems (Hunter *et al.*, 1975) and this appears to be due to activation of a protein kinase which modifies eIF-2 causing inhibition of protein synthesis (Farrell *et al.*, 1977; Levin and London, 1978). In the presence of ATP and cytoplasmic extracts double-stranded RNA causes production of a trinucleotide containing 2′–5′ linkages of adenylic acid and this compound inhibits protein synthesis *in vitro* (Kerr and Brown, 1978). This trinucleotide is produced by extracts of normal cells, although more appears to be made using interferon-treated cells and there is evidence that the trinucleotide activates a nuclease which degrades mRNA and thereby inhibits protein synthesis (Baglioni *et al.*, 1978). This mode of action has been proposed as the ultimate molecular mechanism of interferon-mediated antiviral effects (Baglioni *et al.*, 1978) but the mechanism would also allow other agents, such as polynucleotides, to activate the nuclease and have antiviral effects without the necessity of producing interferon. A number of other related activities of double-stranded RNAs have been reported to affect viral RNA activities using cell extracts from interferon-treated cells (see Lewis *et al.*, 1978) and these activities could also be affected by potential therapeutic RNA treatments.

For antiviral polynucleotides which induce interferon, in addition to acting primarily by direct inhibition of a viral polymerase or mimicking a strategic sequence, the consequence of interferon production should be considered. In addition to antiviral and antitumor activities, interferons are known to affect many activities *in vivo* (see articles in Stewart, 1977).

11.5.3. Antiviral and Antitumor Agents and Host Defense Mechanisms

A most important activity of polynucleotides *in vivo* may be their effect on natural host-defense mechanisms, in particular the extent to which polynucleotide treatments augment favorable reactions and limit adverse ones. The known effects of polynucleotides affecting such defense mechanisms are considered in Section 11.5.2, and here are considered only those natural defense mechanisms which may occur independently of polynucleotide effects or are not presently known to be affected by polynucleotides.

There is clear evidence that macrophages mediate natural defense mechanisms against viral infections and macrophages have been considered the most important factor limiting infections of several different types of virus (Mims, 1964; Hirsch *et al.*, 1970; Zisman *et al.*, 1971; Allison, 1974; Virelizier and Allison, 1976; Lindenmann *et al.*, 1978). In rodents, at least, the natural macrophage-mediated antiviral and antitumor activities seem to be genetically determined (Virelizier and Allison, 1976; Lindenmann *et al.*, 1978; Miller and

Feldman, 1976) and may only be manifest in adult animals (Hirsch *et al.*, 1970; Allison, 1974). Cytotoxic T-cells from mice immunized by a particular virus are also known to kill specific cells in culture infected with the same virus, but this occurs only if both cell types share at least part of the major histocompatibility region (Doherty *et al.*, 1976). This phenomenon also occurs with the influenza viruses and in this case it has been shown that the antigenic determinants of the virus do not affect cytotoxic T-cell activity even where distinct humoral antibodies can be produced against different viruses (Zweerink *et al.*, 1977).

The data demonstrating the involvement of macrophages and cytotoxic T-cells in natural defense against virus infections and tumor development raise the possibility that no antiviral or antitumor therapy will be effective *in vivo* unless these cellular activities are preserved during treatment. The nature of the necessary macrophage activity remains unclear. Agents known to stimulate pinocytosis by macrophages or release enzymes from macrophage do not cause similar antiviral effects to polynucleotides whose antiviral effects are known to depend on macrophages (Stebbing *et al.*, 1977c). The possibility that macrophages simply accumulate virus and become the first cells to be infected has been ruled out in the case of antiviral studies of EMC-virus-infected mice, since the virus does not replicate in these cells in mice which can be protected by the polynucleotides (Stebbing *et al.*, 1978). However, there is now *in vitro* data to suggest that the antitumor activity of activated macrophages is due to release of arginase by these cells (Currie, 1978). Reversal of secondary effects resulting from viral infection or tumor development may also be most important for antiviral and antitumor effects to be manifest and macrophages are known to reverse immunosuppression arising from leukemia virus infection of mice (Bendinelli *et al.*, 1975). Macrophages from regressing Moloney sarcomas are known to be more cytotoxic than those recovered from mice with progressing sarcomas (Russell and McIntosh, 1977) and this may be related to activation of the macrophages. Humoral factors have also been implicated in progression of tumors and subsequent regression in animals which recover (Ting *et al.*, 1977).

The antiviral activity of single-stranded polynucleotides which do not induce interferon and are ineffective in tissue culture has been shown to depend on the presence of macrophages *in vivo* (Stebbing *et al.*, 1976b, 1977a,c). More surprisingly, the antiviral effect of interferon, which is effective in tissue culture, has also been shown to depend on the presence of macrophages *in vivo* (Stebbing *et al.*, 1978). Whether the macrophage-mediated antiviral and antitumor effects are stimulated by polynucleotides, interferon or other antiviral and antitumor agents has been discussed previously (Stebbing, 1977; Stebbing *et al.*, 1977c, 1978) but remains unresolved. If the natural macrophage activities act independently of therapeutic agents then it must be concluded that the natural defense mechanisms and the therapy are independently inadequate but jointly can produce antiviral or antitumor effects. In such situations it is clear that any potential therapeutic agents should be designed so as not to interfere with the natural mechanisms and should preferably stimulate them.

11.6. CONCLUSIONS

Progress in sequencing viral genomes has become rapid and should lead to determination of the function of virus specific sequences. Where comparative data exist the untranslated regions of the genomes of related viruses appear to be more conserved than translated regions. Thus strategic sequence analogs of specific untranslated regions could be effective against viruses whose antigenic determinants vary frequently. Elucidation of the functions of particular regions of viral genomes is now likely to be the limiting step in developing strategic sequence analogs. In addition the uptake, metabolism and other indirect effects of viral specific sequences and their analogs will require elucidation in order to assess specific antiviral effects of such materials.

The studies of the middle and late 1960s, which demonstrated that interferon induction was a property of double- rather than single-stranded polynucleotides, were associated with development of sensitive assay methods particularly using rabbit kidney cells for human interferons. One must therefore suspect that although these assays are extremely sensitive, they may not be of particular relevance to analyses of the mode of action of polynucleotides in other systems, particularly whole animals. That a polynucleotide may, or may not, induce interferon in an exquisitely sensitive assay system is ultimately of little use when analysing the mode of action of the polynucleotide in another system. It has been suggested that very sensitive interferon and other biological assays may be used to determine the structure of polynucleotides (De Clercq *et al.*, 1974, 1975c). While one cannot dispute such a claim, it does seem regrettable that assay methods designed to elucidate the mode of action of antiviral polynucleotides have not been more appropriately applied for their original purpose.

Interpretation of antiviral activities of polynucleotides in terms of interferon induction is further complicated by the absence of a quantitative *correspondence* between the antiviral activity of double-stranded polynucleotides and the amount of interferon that they induce. The interpretations of the correlations that have been observed between structural features of double-stranded polynucleotides, such as T_m and their antiviral activity on the one hand, and their ability to induce interferon on the other, have not taken into account the other possible antiviral effects here described which are all simply absorbed in the proportionality constants involved. Furthermore, the structural features of polynucleotides and their antiviral activities do not all correlate (see De Clercq, 1974), so that the conclusion that the antiviral activity is due solely to the ability to induce interferon is somewhat dubious. Moreover, preparations of poly(I).poly(C) contain free single-stranded ends whose role in the overall antiviral effect has not been elucidated. Poly(I).poly(C) has been shown to exist partly in an open state involving long runs of separated base pairs that re-anneal surprisingly slowly (Teitelbaum and Englander, 1975). Furthermore, at cell surfaces the component polynucleotides of poly(I).poly(C) appear to separate and they are then accumulated in different amounts (Schell, 1971). Thus the formation of a double-stranded complex between poly(C) and poly(I), while producing a moeity that induces interferon, could also allow activities attributable to the component homopolynucleotides. With further studies employing anti-interferon antibodies it should be possible to determine to what extent the antiviral activity of a polynucleotide can be accounted for by induction of interferon. At the present time there is evidence that the antiviral activity, even of good double-stranded interferon inducers, is in part attributable to other mechanisms (see Section 11.5).

Whether polynucleotides which mimic parts of the viral genome have antiviral effects because they specifically interfere with virus replication is still unclear. However, the limited studies to date suggest that this is a promising approach to development of antiviral agents. The extensive work on polynucleotide inhibitors of reverse transcriptase has demonstrated the feasibility of devising polynucleotides which inhibit viral polymerases. This work has also highlighted current problems with this approach to therapy, in particular whether agents that mainly affect initiation rather than polymerization will be effective and generally the need for establishing correlations between *in vitro* enzyme effects and *in vivo* effects. The studies on polynucleotides which inhibit the transcriptase activity of disrupted influenza virus particles have clearly demonstrated that single-stranded polynucleotides can have potent effects on virus replication and these studies have been extended to infected animals (Round and Stebbing, 1981). This work has also allowed examination of the relation between effects *in vitro* and studies in animals. Oligonucleotide inhibitors of *in vitro* initiation of the influenza virus transcriptase have also been detected and these are analogs of the *in vitro* primer, ApG. Clearly further studies are required to understand the mode of action of these polynucleotides *in vivo* and define problems that may be common to developing polynucleotides as effective antiviral agents. Limited cellular uptake of polynucleotides is an obvious problem but may be less significant after administration to intact animals than predicted from cell culture studies (Stebbing, 1979b).

Although polynucleotides which mimic strategic sequences in viral RNA or their complements have been discussed in this review, it is possible that peptides of specific amino acid sequence could be effective. Tripeptides containing aromatic residues show strong electrostatic interactions, including stacking, with bases of polynucleotides, and these interactions occur principally with single-stranded polynucleotides (Brun *et al.*, 1975). The indole ring is the same size as a purine and many proteins may make use of their aromatic acids to bind selectively to single-stranded regions of nucleic acids (Toulme and Helene, 1977). This notion is strengthened by the finding that tryptophan residues in gene 32 protein of T4 phage are involved in its binding to denatured DNA (Helene *et al.*, 1976).

Acknowledgement—The reader and I are indebted to Jeanne Arch for her patience and skill in typing the manuscript.

REFERENCES

ABRELL, J. W., SMITH, R. G., ROBERTS, M. S. and GALLO, R. C. (1972) DNA polymerases from RNA tumor viruses and human cells; inhibition by polyuridylic acid. *Science, N.Y.* **177**: 1111–1114.

AKUSJARVI, G. and PETTERSSON, U. (1979) Nucleotide sequence at the junction between the coding region of the adenovirus 2 hexon messenger RNA and its leader sequence. *Proc. natn. Acad. Sci. USA* **75**: 5822–5826.

ALLISON, A. C. (1974) On the role of mononuclear phagocytes in immunity against viruses. *Prog. Med. Virol.* **18**: 15–31.

ANSEVIN, A. T., MACDONALD, K. K., SMITH, C. E. and HNILICA, L. S. (1975) Mechanics of chromatin-template activation. Physical evidence for destabilization of nucleoproteins by polyanions. *J. biol. Chem.* **250**: 281–289.

ARYA, S. K. and CHAWDA, R. (1977) Polyribonucleotide inhibition of murine leukemia virus replication: effect of strandedness. *Molec. Pharmac.* **13**: 374–377.

ARYA, S. K., CARTER, W. A., ALDERFER, J. L. and TS'O, P. O. P. (1974) Inhibition of RNA directed DNA polymerase of murine leukemia virus by 2'-*O*-alkylated polyadenylic acids. *Biochem. biophys. Res. Commun.* **59**: 608–615.

ARYA, S. K., CARTER, W. A., ALDERFER, J. L. and TS'O, P. O. P. (1975) Inhibition of ribonucleic acid-directed deoxyribonucleic acid polymerase of murine leukemia virus by polyribunucleotides and their 2'*O*-methylated derivatives. *Molec. Pharmac.* **11**: 421–426.

ARYA, S. K., CARTER, W. A., ALDERFER, J. L. and TS'O, P. O. P. (1976a) Inhibition of synthesis of murine leukemia virus in cultured cells by polyribonucleotides and their 2'-*O*-alkyl derivates. *Molec. Pharmac.* **12**: 234–241.

ARYA, S. K., HELSER, T. L., CARTER, W. A. and TS'O, P. O. P. (1976b) Polyxanthylic and polyguanylic acid inhibition of murine leukemia virus activities. *Molec. Pharmac.* **12**: 844–853.

AUGUST, J. T., BANERJEE, A. K., EOYANG, L., DE FERNANDEZ, M. F. T., HORI, K., KUO, C. H., RENSING, U. and SHAPIRO, L. (1968) Synthesis of bacteriophage Qβ RNA. *Cold Spring Harbor Symp. Quant. Biol.* **33**: 73–81.

BAGLIONI, C. (1979) Interferon-induced enzymatic activities and their role in the antiviral state. *Cell* **17**: 255–264.

BAGLIONI, C., MINKS, M. A. and MARONEY, P. A. (1978) Interferon action may be mediated by activation of a nuclease by pppA2'p5'A2'p5'A. *Nature, Lond.* **273**: 684–687.

BANERJI, J., RUSCONI, S. and SCHAFFNER, W. (1981) Expression of a β-globin gene is enhanced by remote SV40 DNA sequences. *Cell* **27**: 299–308.

BARELLE, F. E. and BROWNLEE, G. G. (1978) AUG is the only recognisable signal sequence in the 5' non-coding regions of eukaryotic mRNA. *Nature, Lond.* **274**: 84–87.

BARON, S. (1973) The defensive and biological roles of the interferon system. In: *Interferons and Interferon Inducers*, pp. 267–293. FINTER, N. B. (ed.). North-Holland, Amsterdam and London.

BARON, S., BOGOMOLOVA, N. N., BILLIAU, A., LEVY, H. B., BUCKLER, C. E., STERN, R. and NAYLOR, R. (1969) Induction of interferon by preparations of synthetic single-stranded RNA. *Proc. natn. Acad. Sci. USA.* **64**: 67–74.

BEFORT, N., BECK, G., EBEL, J. P. and LOUISOT, P. (1974) Inhibition of viral multiplication by homologous methylated ribonucleic acids. IV. Subcellular localisation after uptake into fibroblasts and relation between antiviral activity and chain length. *Chem. Biol. Interactions* **9**: 181–185.

BENDINELLI, M., KAPLAN, G. S. and FRIEDMAN, H. (1975) Reversal of leukemia virus-induced immunosuppression *in vitro* by peritoneal macrophages. *J. natn. Cancer Inst.* **55**: 1425–1432.

BILLIAU, A., BUCKLER, C. E., DIANZANI, F., UHLENDORF, C. and BARON, S. (1969) Induction of the interferon mechanism by single-stranded RNA: Potentiation by polybasic substances. *Proc. Soc. exp. Biol. Med.* **132**: 790–796.

BILLIAU, A., MUYEMBE, J. J. and DE SOMER, P. (1971) Mechanism of antiviral activity *in vivo* of polycarboxylates which induce interferon production. *Nature, New Biol.* **232**: 183–186.

BRADISH, C. J., ALLNER, K. and FITZGEORGE, R. (1975) Immunomodification and expression of virulence in mice by defined strains of Semliki Forest virus: the effects of Myocrisin and 1-asparaginase. *J. gen. Virol.* **28**: 239–250.

BRAUN, W. and NAKANO, M. (1967) Antibody formation: Stimulation by polyadenylic and polycytidylic acids. *Science, N.Y.* **157**: 819–821.

BROWN, D. G. and COFFEY, D. S. (1972) Effects of polyinosinic acid and polycytidylic acid on the deoxyribonucleic acid template activity of isolated nuclei and soluble chromatin from rat liver. *J. biol. Chem.* **247**: 7674–7683.

BROWN, F. and MARTIN, S. J. (1965) A new model for virus ribonucleic acid replication. *Nature, Lond.* **208**: 861–863.

BROWN, F., NEWMAN, J., STOTT, J., PORTER, A., FRISBY, D., NEWTON, C., CAREY, N. and FELLNER, P. (1974) Poly(C) in animal viral RNAs. *Nature, Lond.* **251**: 342–344.

BRUN, F., TOULME, J-J. and HELENE, C. (1975) Interactions of aromatic residues of proteins with nucleic acids. Fluorescence studies of the binding of oligopeptides containing tryptophan and tyrosine residues to polynucleotides. *Biochemistry* **14**: 558–563.

BUCKLER, C. E., BARON, S. and LEVY, H. B. (1966) Interferon: lack of detectable uptake by cells. *Science, N.Y.* **152**: 80–82.

BUCKLER, C. E., WONG, K. T. and BARON, S. (1968) Induction of the interferon system by various inducers. *Proc. Soc. exp. Biol. Med* **127**: 1258–1262.

CANTOR, H., ASOFSKY, P. and LEVY, H. B. (1970) The effect of polyinosinic-polycytidylic acid upon graft-vs-host activity in balb/c mice. *J. Immun.* **104**: 1035–1038.

CARTER, W. A. and DE CLERCQ, E. (1974) Viral infection and host defense. *Science, N.Y.* **186**: 1172–1178.

CAVALIERI, L. F. and YAMAURA, I. (1975) *E. coli* tRNAs as inhibitors of viral reverse transcription *in vitro*. *Nucleic acid Res.* **2**: 2315–2328.

CHANDRA, P. and BARDOS, T. J. (1972) Inhibition of DNA polymerases from RNA tumor viruses by novel template analogues: partially thiolated polycytidylic acid. *Res. Commun. Chem. Path. Pharmac.* **4**: 615–619.

CHANDRA, P., EBENER, V. and GOTZ, A. (1975) Inhibition of oncorna-viral DNA polymerases by 5-mercapto polycytidylic acid: mode of action. *FEBS Lett.* **53**: 10–14.

CHATTERJEE, N. K., BACKRACH, H. L. and POLANTNICK, J. (1976) Foot-and-mouth disease virus RNA: presence of 3′ terminal polyriboadenylic acid and absence of amino acid binding ability. *Virology* **69**: 369–377.

CHEN, J. M. and HALL, T. C. (1973) Comparison of tyrosyl transfer ribonucleic acid and brome mosaic virus tyrosyl ribonucleic acid as amino acid donors in protein synthesis. *Biochemistry* **12**: 4570–4573.

CHIRIKJIAN, J. G. and PAPAS, T. S. (1974) Inhibition of AMV DNA polymerase by poly A containing -adenosine residues. *Biochem. biophys. Res. Commun.* **59**: 489–495.

CHOW, L. T., GELINAS, R., BROKER, T. and ROBERTS, R. J. (1977) An amazing sequence arrangement at the 5′ ends of adenovirus 2 messenger RNA. *Cell* **12**: 1–8.

CHUMAKOV, K. M. and AGOL, V. T. (1976) Poly(C) sequence is located near the 5′ end of encephalomyocarditis virus RNA. *Biochem. biophys. Res. Commun.* **71**: 551–557.

COHN, Z. A. and PARKS, E. (1967) The regulation of pinocytosis in mouse macrophages III. The induction of vesicle formation by nucleosides and nucleotides. *J. exp. Med.* **125**: 457–466.

COLBY, C. (1971) The induction of interferon by natural and synthetic polynucleotides. *Prog. Nucleic Acid Res. Molec. Biol.* **11**: 1–32.

COLLETT, M. S. and FARAS, A. J. (1978) Avian retrovirus RNA-directed DNA synthesis: transcription at the 5′ terminus of the viral genome and the functional role of the viral terminal redundancy. *Virology* **86**: 297–311.

COLONNO, R. J. and BANERJEE, A. K. (1978) Complete nucleotide sequence of the leader RNA synthesized *in vitro* by vesicular stomatitis virus. *Cell* **15**: 93–101.

CUNNINGTON, P. G. and NAYSMITH, J. D. (1975) Naturally occurring double-stranded RNA and immune responses. I. effects on plaque-forming cells and antibody formation. *Immunology* **28**: 451–468.

CURRIE, G. A. (1978) Activated macrophages kill tumour cells by releasing arginase. *Nature, Lond.* **273**: 758–759.

DE CLERCQ, E. (1974) Synthetic interferon inducers. *Topics Curr. Chem.* **52**: 173–208.

DE CLERCQ, E. and CLAES, P. J. (1973) A more sensitive assay system for the detection of RNA-dependent DNA polymerase in oncogenic RNA viruses. *Biochim. biophys. Acta* **331**: 328–332.

DE CLERCQ, E. and MERIGAN, T. C. (1969) Requirement of a stable secondary structure for the antiviral activity of polynucleotides. *Nature, Lond.* **222**: 1148–1152.

DE CLERCQ, E. and DE SOMER, P. (1971) Antiviral activity of polyribocytidylic acid in cells primed with polyriboinosinic acid. *Science, N.Y.* **173**: 260–262.

DE CLERCQ, E. and DE SOMER, P. (1972) Mechanism of the antiviral activity resulting from sequential administration of complementary homopolyribonucleotides to cell cultures. *J. Virol.* **9**: 721–731.

DE CLERCQ, E., BILLIAU, A., HATTORI, M. and IKEHARA, M. (1975a) Inhibition of oncornavirus functions by poly(2-methylthioninosinic acid). *Nucleic Acid Res.* **2**: 2305–2313.

DE CLERCQ, E., BILLIAU, A., HOBBS, J., TORRENCE, P. F. and WITKOP, B. (1975b) Inhibition of oncornavirus functions by 2′-azido polynucleotides. *Proc. natn. Acad. Sci. USA* **72**: 284–288.

DE CLERCQ, E., ECKSTEIN, F. and MERIGAN, T. C. (1969) Interferon induction increased through chemical modification of a synthetic polyribonucleotide. *Science, N.Y.* **165**: 1137–1139.

DE CLERCQ, E., HUANG, G-F., TORRENCE, P. F., FUKUI, T., KAKIUCHI, N. and IKEHARA, M. (1977) Biologic activities of poly(2-azaadenylic acid) and poly(2-azainosinic acid). *Nucleic Acid Res.* **4**: 3643–3653.

DE CLERCQ, E., STEWARD, W. E. and DE SOMER, P. (1973) Poly(rI) more important than poly(rC) in the interferon induction process by poly(rI).poly(rC). *Virology* **54**: 278–282.

DE CLERCQ, E., STOLLER, B. D. and THANG, M. N. (1978) Interferon inducing activity of polyinosinic acid. *J. gen. Virol.* **40**: 203–212.

DE CLERCQ, E., TORRENCE, P. F., HOBBS, J., JANIK, B., DE SOMER, P. and WITKOP, B. (1975c) Anti-complement activity of polynucleotides. *Biochem. biophys. Res. Commun.* **67**: 255–263.

DE CLERCQ, E., TORRENCE, P. F., WITKOP, B., STEWART, W. E. and DE SOMER, P. (1974) Interferon induction: tool for establishing interactions among homopolyribonucleotides. *Science, N.Y.* **186**: 835–837.

DEININGER, P. L., ESTY, A., LAPORTE, P., HSU, H. and FRIEDMANN, T. (1980) The nucleotide sequence and restriction enzyme sites of the polyoma genome. *Nucleic Acid Res.* **8**: 855–860.

DEZELEE, S., SENTENAC, A. and FROMAGEOT, P. (1974) Role of deoxyribonucleic acid-ribonucleic acid hybrids in eukaryotes. *J. biol. Chem.* **249**: 5978–5983.

DIANZANI, F. and BARON, S. (1977) The continued presence of interferon is not required for activation of cells by interferon. *Proc. Soc. exp. Biol. Med.* **155**: 562–566.

DIANZANI, F., FORNI, G., PONZI, A. N., PUGLIASE, A. and CAVALLO, G. (1972) Decreased interferon response to polyinosinic-polycytidylic acid in rabbits immunised against the inducer. *Proc. Soc. exp. Biol. Med.* **139**: 93–95.

DIMMOCK, N. J. and KENNEDY, S. I. T. (1978) Prevention of death in Semliki Forest virus-infected mice by administration of defective-interfering Semliki Forest virus. *J. gen. Virol.* **39**: 231–242.

DOHERTY, P. C., BLANDEN, R. V. and ZINKERNAGEL, R. M. (1976) Specificity of virus-immune effector T cells for H-2K or H-2D compatible interactions: implications for H-antigen diversity. *Transplantation Rev.* **29**: 89–124.

DRAKE, W. P., CIMINO, E. F., MARDINEY, M. R. and SUTHERLAND, J. C. (1974) Prophylactic therapy of spontaneous leukemia in AKR mice by polyadenylic-polyuridylic acid. *J. natn. Cancer Inst.* **52**: 941–944.

EIDEN, J. J., BOLOGNESI, D. P., LANGLOIS, A. J. and NICHOLS, J. L. (1975) The initial nucleotide sequence of DNA transcribed from avian myeloblastosis virus 70S RNA by RNA-dependent DNA polymerase. *Virology* **65**: 163–172.

EMTAGE, J. S., CAREY, N. H. and STEBBING, N. (1976) Structural features of encephalomyocarditis virus RNA from analysis of reverse transcription products. *Eur. J. Biochem.* **69**: 69–78.

ENGLUND, P. T., DEUTSCHER, M. P., JOVIN, T. M., KELLEY, R. B., COZZARELLI, N. R. and KORNBERG, A. (1968) Structural and functional properties of *Escherichia coli* DNA polymerase. *Cold Spring Harbor Symp. Quant. Biol.* **33**: 1–9.

ERDMANN, V. A., SPRINZL, M. and PONGS, O. (1973) The involvement of 5S RNA in the binding of tRNA to ribosomes. *Biochem. biophys. Res. Commun.* **54**: 942–948.

ERICKSON, R. J. and GROSCH, J. C. (1974) The inhibition of avian myeloblastosis virus deoxyribonucleic acid polymerase by synthetic polynucleotides. *Biochemistry* **13**: 1987–1993.

ERICKSON, R. J., JANIK, B. and SOMMER, R. G. (1973) The inhibition of the avian myeloblastosis virus DNA polymerase by poly(U) fractions of varying chain length. *Biochem. biophys. Res. Commun.* **52**: 1475–1482.

ESPOSITO, S. (1969) RNA therapy for pleural mesothelioma. *Lancet* **2**: 1203–1204.

FARRELL, P. J., BALKOW, K., HUNT, T. and JACKSON, R. J. (1977) Phosphorylation of initiation factor eIF-2 and the control of reticulocyte protein synthesis. *Cell* **11**: 187–200.

FELLNER, P. (1979) General organisation and structure of the picornavirus genome. In: *The Molecular Biology of Picornavirus*, pp. 25–47. PEREZ-BERCOFF (ed.). Plenum Press.

FIELD, A. K., TYTELL, A. A., LAMPSON, G. P. and HILLEMAN, M. R. (1967) Inducers of interferon and host resistance. II. Multistranded synthetic polynucleotide complexes. *Proc. natn. Acad. Sci. USA* **58**: 1004–1011.

FIERS, W., CONTRERAS, R., HAEGEMAN, G., ROGIERS, R., VAN DE VOORDE, A., VAN HEUVERSWYN, H., VAN HERREWEGHE, J., VOLCKAERT, G. and YSEBAERT, M. (1978) Complete nucleotide sequence of SV40 DNA. *Nature, Lond.* **273**: 113–120.

FLANEGAN, J. B. and BALTIMORE, D. (1977) Poliovirus-specific primer-dependent RNA polymerase able to copy poly(A). *Proc. natn. Acad. Sci. USA* **74**: 3677–3680.

FLANEGAN, J. B., PETTERSSON, R. F., ANBROS, V., HEWLETT, M. J. and BALTIMORE, D. (1977) Covalent linkage of a protein to a defined nucleotide sequence at the 5′ terminus of virion and replicative intermediate RNAs of poliovirus. *Proc. natn. Acad. Sci. USA* **74**: 961–965.

FREY, T. K. and STRAUSS, J. H. (1978) Replication of Sindbis virus VI. poly(A) and poly(U) in virus-specific RNA species. *Virology* **86**: 494–506.

FRIEDMAN, R. M. (1967) Interferon binding: the first step in establishment of antiviral activity. *Science, N.Y.* **156**: 1960–1961.

FUKADA, T., KAWADE, Y., UJIHARA, M., SHIN, C. and SHIMA, T. (1968) Interference with virus infection induced by RNA in chick embryo cells. *Jap. J. Microbiol.* **12**: 329–341.

GALIBERT, F., MANDART, E., FITOUSSI, F., TIOLLAIS, P. and CHARNAY, P. (1979) Nucleotide sequence of the Hepatitis B virus genome subtype *ayw* cloned in *Escherichia coli*. *Nature* **281**: 646–650.

GEDDES-DWYER, V. and CAMERON, D. A. (1976) Influence of exogenous tRNA on growth of transplantable ^{32}P-induced osteosarcomata. *Br. J. Cancer* **33**: 600–605.

GERSHWIN, R. J., GERSHWIN, E., STEINBERG, A. D., AHMED, A. and OCHIAI, T. (1976) Relationship between age and thymic function on the development of leukemia in AKR mice. *Proc. Soc. exp. Biol. Med.* **152**: 403–407.

GIDLUND, M., ORN, A., WIGZELL, H., SENIK, A. and GRESSOR, I. (1978) Enhanced NK cell activity in mice injected with interferon and interferon inducers. *Nature, Lond.* **273**: 759–761.

GISSMANN, L. and ZURHAUSEN, H. (1977) Inverted repetitive sequences in human papilloma virus 1(HPA-1)-DNA. *Virology* **83**: 271–276.

GOLDSBY, R. A. (1967) The implications of the temperature-independent binding and the temperature-dependent action of interferon. *Experientia* **23**: 1073–1075.

GOODCHILD, J., FELLNER, P. and PORTER, A. G. (1975) The determination of secondary structure in the poly(C) tract of encephalomyocarditis virus RNA with sodium bisulphite. *Nucleic Acid Res.* **2**: 887–895.

GOODMAN, N. C. and SPIEGELMAN, S. (1971) Distinguishing reverse transcriptase of an RNA tumor virus from other known DNA polymerases. *Proc. natn. Acad. Sci. USA* **68**: 2203–2206.

GRESSER, I., TOVEY, M. G., BANDU, M-T., MAURY, C. and BROUTY-BOYE, D. (1976) Role of interferon in the pathogenesis of virus diseases in mice as demonstrated by the use of anti-interferon serum. 1. Rapid evolution of encephalomyocarditis virus infection. *J. exp. Med.* **144**: 1305–1315.

GRESSER, I., MAURY, C., BANDU, M-T., TOVEY, M. and MAUNOURY, M-T. (1978) Role of endogenous interferon in the anti-tumor effect of poly I:C and statolon as demonstrated by the use of anti-mouse interferon serum. *Int. J. Cancer* **21**: 72–77.

GUILLEY, H., JONARD, G. and HIRTH, L. (1975) Sequence of 71 nucleotides at the 3′ end of tobacco mosaic virus RNA. *Proc. natn. Acad. Sci. USA* **72**: 864–868.

GUNTAKA, R. V., MAHY, B. W., BISHOP, J. M. and VARMUS, H. W. (1975) Ethidium bromide inhibits appearance of closed circular viral DNA and integration of virus-specific DNA in duck cells infected by avian sarcoma virus. *Nature, Lond.* **253**: 507–511.

HAENNI, A. L., PROCHIANTZ, A., BERNARD, O. and CHAPEVILLE, F. (1973) TYMV valyl-RNA as an amino acid donor in protein biosynthesis. *Nature, New Biol.* **241**: 166–168.

HAGENBUCHLE, O., SANTER, M., ARGETSINGER-STEITZ, J. and MANS, R. J. (1978) Conservation of the primary structure at the 3′ end of 18S rRNA from eucaryotic cells. *Cell* **13**: 551–563.

HAMBURG, S. I., MANEJIAS, R. E. and RABINOVITCH, M. (1978) Macrophage activation. Increased ingestion of IgG-coated erythrocytes after administration of interferon inducers to mice. *J. exp. Med.* **147**: 593–598.

HARADA, F., SAWYER, R. C. and DAHLBERG, J. E. (1975) A primer ribonucleic acid for initiation of *in vitro* Rous sarcoma virus deoxyribonucleic acid synthesis. *J. biol. Chem.* **250**: 3487–3497.

HARRIS, T. J. R. and BROWN, F. (1976) The location of the poly(C) tract in the RNA of foot-and-mouth disease virus. *J. gen. Virol.* **33**: 493–501.

HARRIS, T. J. R. and BROWN, F. (1977) Biochemical analysis of a virulent and an avirulent strain of foot-and-mouth disease virus. *J. gen. Virol.* **34**: 87–105.

HARUNA, I. and SPIEGELMAN, S. (1966) Selective interference with viral RNA formation *in vitro* by specific inhibition of synthetic polyribonucleotides. *Proc. natn. Acad. Sci. USA* **56**: 1333–1338.

HASELTINE, W. A., KLEID, D. G., PANET, A., ROTHENBERG, E. and BALTIMORE, D. (1976) Ordered transcription of RNA tumor virus genomes. *J. molec. Biol.* **106**: 109–131.

HASELTINE, W. A., PANET, A., SMOLER, D., BALTIMORE, D., PETERS, G., HARRADA, F. and DAHLBERG, J. E. (1977a) Interaction of tryptophan tRNA and avian myeloblastosis virus reverse transcriptase: further characterization of the binding reaction. *Biochemistry* **16**: 3625–3632.

HASELTINE, W. A., MAXAM, A. M. and GILBERT, W. (1977b) Rous sarcoma virus genome is terminally redundant: the 5′ sequence. *Proc. natn. Acad. Sci. USA* **74**: 989–993.

HASTIE, N. D. and HELD, W. A. (1978) Analysis of mRNA populations by cDNA. mRNA hybrid-mediated inhibition of cell-free protein synthesis. *Proc. natn. Acad. Sci. USA* **75**: 1217–1221.

HELENE, C., TOULME, F., CHARLIER, M. and YANIV, M. (1976) Photosensitized splitting of thymine dimers in DNA by gene 32 protein from phage T4. *Biochem. biophys. Res. Commun.* **71**: 91–98.

HELENTJARIS, T. and EHRENFELD, E. (1978) Control of protein synthesis in extracts from poliovirus infected cells. I. mRNA discrimination by crude initiation factors. *J. Virol.* **26**: 510–521.

HENDERSON, J. R. and TAYLOR, R. M. (1961) Studies on mechanisms of arthropod-borne virus interference in tissue culture. *Virology* **13**: 477–484.

HERBERMAN, R. B., DJEU, J. V., ORTALDO, J. R., HOLDEN, H. T., WEST, W. H. and BONNARD, G. D. (1978) Role of interferon in augmentation of natural and antibody-dependent cell-mediated cytotoxicity. *Cancer Treat. Rep.* **62**: 1893–1896.

HEWLETT, M. J. and FLORKIEWICZ, R. Z. (1980) Sequence of picornavirus RNAs containing a radioiodinated 5′-linked peptide reveals a conserved 5′ sequence. *Proc. natn. Acad. Sci. USA* **77**: 303–307.

HILLER, G., JUNGWIRTH, C., BODO, G. and SCHULTZE, B. (1973) Biological activity of poly rI: poly rC; Effect on poxvirus-specific functions. *Virology* **52**: 22–29.

HIRSCH, M. S., ZISMAN, B. and ALLISON, A. C. (1970) Macrophages and age-dependent resistance to Herpes simplex virus in mice. *J. Immun.* **104**: 1160–1165.

HO, M. (1973) Factors influencing interferon production. In: *Interferons and Interferon Inducers*, pp. 73–105. FINTER, N. B. (ed.). North-Holland, Amsterdam and London.

HONESS, R. W. and ROIZMAN, B. (1975) Regulation of herpes virus macromolecular synthesis: sequential transition of polypeptide synthesis requires functional viral polypeptides. *Proc. natn. Acad. Sci. USA* **72**: 1276–1280.

HONESS, R. W. and WATSON, D. M. (1977) Unity and diversity in the herpes viruses. *J. gen. Virol.* **37**: 15–37.

HRUBY, D. E. and ROBERTS, R. K. (1976) Encephalomyocarditis virus RNA: variations in polyadenylic acid content and biological activity. *J. Virol.* **19**: 325–330.

HRUBY, D. E. and ROBERTS, R. K. (1978) Encephalomyocarditis RNA. III. Presence of a genome associated protein. *J. Virol.* **25**: 413–415.

HUANG, A. S. (1977) Viral pathogenesis and molecular biology. *Bact. Rev.* **41**: 811–821.

HUANG, A. S. and BALTIMORE, D. (1977) Defective interfering animal viruses. In: *Comprehensive Virology*, Vol. 10, pp. 73–116. FRAENKEL-CONRAT, H. and WAGNER, R. R. (eds.). Plenum Publishing, New York.

HUNTER, T., HUNT, T., JACKSON, R. J. and ROBERTSON, H. D. (1975) The characteristics of inhibition of protein synthesis by double-stranded ribonucleic acid in reticulocyte lysates. *J. biol. Chem.* **250**: 409–417.

IHLE, J. N., LEE, K. and KENNEY, F. T. (1974) Fractionation of 34S ribonucleic acid subunits from oncornaviruses on polyuridylate-sepharose columns. *J. biol. Chem.* **249**: 38–42.

INGLIS, S. C., McGEOCH, D. J. and MAHY, B. W. J. (1977) Polypeptides specified by the influenza virus genome. 2. Assignment of protein coding functions to individual genome segments by *in vitro* translation. *Virology* **78**: 522–536.

ISAACS, A. (1961) Mechanisms of virus infections. *Nature, Lond.* **192**: 1247.

ISAACS, A. and LINDENMANN, J. (1957) Virus interference. I. The interferon. *Proc. R. Soc. Lond.* B **147**: 258–267.

ISAACS, A., COX, R. A. and ROTEM, Z. (1963) Foreign nucleic acids as the stimulus to make interferon. *Lancet* **2**: 113–116.

JENSEN, K. E., NEAL, A. C., OWENS, R. E. and WARREN, J. (1963) Interferon responses of chick embryo fibroblasts to nucleic acids and related compounds. *Nature, Lond.* **200**: 433–434.

KAEMPFER, R., HOLLANDER, R., ABRAMS, W. and ISRAELI, R. (1978a) Specific binding of messenger RNA and methionyl-tRNA$_f^{Met}$ by the same initiation factor for eukaryotic protein synthesis. *Proc. natn. Acad. Sci. USA* **75**: 209–213.

KAEMPFER, R., ROSEN, H. and ISRAELI, R. (1978b) Translational control: recognition of the methylated 5′ end and an internal sequence in eukaryotic mRNA by the initiation factor that binds methionyl-tRNA$_f^{Met}$. *Proc. natn. Acad. Sci. USA* **75**: 650–654.

KANO-SUEOKA, T. and SUEOKA, N. (1969) Leucine tRNA and cessation of *Escherichia coli* protein synthesis upon phage T_2 infection. *Proc. natn. Acad. Sci. USA* **62**: 1229–1236.

KERR, I. M. and BROWN, R. E. (1978) pppA2′p5′A2′p5′A: an inhibitor of protein synthesis synthesized with an enzyme fraction from interferon-treated cells. *Proc. natn. Acad. Sci. USA* **75**: 256–260.

KITAMURA, N., SEMLER, B. L., ROTHBERG, P. C., LARSEN, G. R., ADLER, C. J., DORNER, E. A. (1981) Primary structure, gene organization and polypeptide expression of poliovirus RNA. *Nature* **291**: 547–553.

KJELDSBERG, E. and FLIKKE, M. (1971) Anti-viral activity of polyinosinic-polycytidylic acid in the absence of cell-controlled RNA synthesis. *J. gen. Virol.* **10**: 147–154.

KOHLHAGE, H. and FALKE, D. (1964) Vermehrungshemmung des Herpes-simplex-virus durch Ribonukleinsauren. *Arch. ges. Virusforsch.* **14**: 404–409.

KOMINAMI, R., TOMITA, Y., CONNORS, E. C. and HATANAKA, M. (1980) Conserved sequence related to the 3′-terminal region of retrovirus RNAs in normal cellular DNAs. *J. Virol.* **34**: 684–692.

KOZAK, M. (1977) Nucleotide sequences of 5′ terminal ribosome-protected initiation regions from two reovirus messages. *Nature, Lond.* **269**: 390–394.

KOZAK, M. and SHATKIN, A. J. (1978) Identification of features in 5′ terminal fragments from reovirus mRNA which are important for ribosome binding. *Cell* **13**: 201–212.

KREIDER, J. W. and CECALUPO, A. J. (1975) Stimulation of rat graft-versus-host reactions by polyinosinic-polycytidylic acid. *Transplantation* **19**: 470–474.

KUCHINO, Y. and BOREK, E. (1976) Changes in transfer RNAs in human malignant trophoblastic cells (BeWo) line. *Cancer Res.* **36**: 2932–2936.

LACOUR, F., DELAGE, G. and CHIANALE, C. (1975) Reduced incidence of spontaneous mammary tumors in C3H/He mice after treatment with polyadenylate.polyuridylate. *Science, N.Y.* **287**: 256–257.

LAI, M. M. C. and DUESBERG, P. H. (1972) Adenylic acid-rich sequences in RNAs of Rous sarcoma virus and Rauscher mouse leukemia virus. *Nature, Lond.* **235**: 383–386.

LAMPSON, G. P., TYTELL, A. A., FIELD, A. K., NEMES, M. M. and HILLEMAN, M. R. (1967) Inducers of interferon and host resistance. 1. Double stranded RNA from extracts of *Penicillium funiculosum. Proc. natn. Acad. Sci. USA* **58**: 782–791.

LAWRENCE, C. and THACH, R. (1974) Encephalomyocarditis virus infection of mouse plasmacytoma cells. I. inhibition of cellular protein synthesis. *J. Virol.* **14**: 598–610.

LEVIN, D. and LONDON, I. M. (1978) Regulation of protein synthesis: activation by double-stranded RNA of a protein kinase that phosphorylates eukaryotic initiation factor 2. *Proc. natn. Acad. Sci. USA* **75**: 1121–1125.

LEVINSON, B., KHOURY, G., VANDE WOUDE, G. and GRUSS, P. (1982) Activation of SV40 genome by 72 base pair tandem repeats of Moloney sarcoma virus. *Nature, Lond.* **295**: 568–572.

LEWANDOWSKI, L. J., CONTENT, J. and LEPPLA, S. H. (1971) Characterisation of the subunit structure of the ribonucleic acid genome of influenza virus. *J. Virol.* **8**: 701–707.

LEWIS, J. A., FALCOFF, E. and FALCOFF, R. (1978) Dual action of double-stranded RNA in inhibiting protein synthesis in extracts of interferon-treated mouse L cells. *Eur. J. Biochem.* **86**: 497–509.

LINDENMANN, J., DEUEL, E., FANCONI, S. and HALLER, O. (1978) Inborn resistance of mice to myxoviruses: macrophages express phenotypes *in vitro. J. exp. Med.* **147**: 531–540.

LINDLEY, I. J. D. and STEBBING, N. (1976) Aminoacylation of encephalomyocarditis virus RNA. *J. gen. Virol.* **34**: 177–181.

LITVAK, S., TARRAGO, A., TARRAGO-LITVAK, L. and ALLENDE, J. E. (1973) Elongation factor–viral genome interaction dependent on the aminoacylation of TYMV and TMV RNAs. *Nature, New Biol.* **241**: 88–90.

McGEOCH, D. and KITRON, N. (1975) Influenza virion RNA-dependent RNA polymerase: stimulation by guanosine and related compounds. *J. Virol.* **15**: 686–695.

McGEOCH, D., FELLNER, P. and NEWTON, C. (1976) Influenza virus genome consists of eight distinct RNA species. *Proc. natn. Acad. Sci. USA* **73**: 3045–3049.

MARCUS, S. L., MODAK, M. J. and CAVALIERI, L. F. (1974a) Purification of avian myelobastosis virus DNA polymerase by affinity chromatography on polycytidylate-agarose. *J. Virol.* **14**: 853–859.

MARCUS, S. L., MODAK, M. J. and CAVALIERI, L. F. (1974b) Evidence for template-specific sites in DNA polymerases. *Biochem. biophys. Res. Commun.* **56**: 516–521.

MAYER, V. (1962) Interactions of mammalian cells with tick-borne encephalitis virus. II. Persisting infection of cells. *Acta Virol.* **6**: 317–326.

MIKKE, R., KJELANOWSKA, M., SHUGAR, D. and ZMUDZKA, B. (1976) Poly 2′-O-ethylcytidylate, an inhibitor and poor template for AMV reverse transcriptase. *Nucleic Acid Res.* **3**: 1603–1611.

MILLER, G. A. and FELDMAN, J. D. (1976) Genetic role of rat macrophage cytotoxicity against tumor. *Int. J. Cancer* **18**: 168–175.

MILLS, D. R., PETERSON, R. L. and SPIEGELMAN, S. (1967) An extracellular Darwinian experiment with a self-duplicating nucleic acid molecule. *Proc. natn. Acad. Sci. USA* **58**: 217–224.

MILLS, D. R., NISHIHARA, T., DOBKIN, C., KRAMER, F. R., COLE, P. E. and SPIEGELMAN, S. (1977) The role of template structure in the recognition mechanism of Qβ replicase. In: *Nucleic Acid-Protein Recognition*, pp. 533–547. CRC Press, Cleveland, Ohio.

MIMS, C. A. (1964) Aspects of the pathogenesis of viral diseases. *Bact. Rev.* **28**: 30–71.

MIN JOU, W. and FIERS, W. (1976) Studies on the bacteriophage MS2 XXXIII. Comparison of the nucleotide sequences in related bacteriophage RNAs. *J. molec. Biol.* **106**: 1047–1060.

NAYSMITH, J. D., SHARPE, T. J. and PLANTEROSE, D. N. (1974) The anti-virus activity of double-stranded RNA in the presence of antibody to double-stranded RNA. *Eur. J. Immun.* **4**: 629–632.

NOMOTO, A., DETJEN, B., POZZATTI, R. and WIMMER, E. (1977) The location of the polio genome protein in viral RNAs and its implication for RNA synthesis. *Nature, Lond.* **268**: 208–213.

NORONHA-BLOB, L., VENGRIS, V. E., PITHA, P. M. and PITHA, J. (1977) Uptake and fate of water-soluble, nondegradable polymers with anti-viral activity in cells and animals. *J. med. Chem.* **20**: 356–359.

NUSS, D., OPPERMANN, H. and KOCH, G. (1975) Selective blockage of inhibition of host protein synthesis in RNA-virus-infected cells. *Proc. natn. Acad. Sci. USA* **72**: 1258–1262.

OBERG, B. and PHILIPSON, L. (1972) Binding of histidine to tobacco mosaic virus RNA. *Biochem. biophys. Res. Commun.* **48**: 927–932.

O'DELL, T. B., WRIGHT, H. N. and BIETER, R. N. (1953) Chemotherapeutic activity of nucleic acids and high protein diets against the infection caused by the MM virus in mice. *J. Pharmac.* **107**: 232–240.

OKUDE, S., TOLLEY, W. B., STUYVESANT, V. W., SMITH, L. L. and HINSHAW, D. B. (1969) Intracellular enzyme behaviour following soluble ribonucleic acid treatment of endotoxic shock in the dog. *Surgical Forum* **20**: 20–22.

OLDSTONE, M. B., AOKI, T. and DIXON, F. J. (1972) The antibody response of mice to murine leukemia virus in spontaneous infection: absence of classical immunological tolerance. *Proc. natn. Acad. Sci. USA* **69**: 134–138.

PANET, A., HASELTINE, W., BALTIMORE, D., PETERS, G., HARADA, F. and DAHLBERG, J. (1975) Specific binding of tryptophan transfer RNA to avian myeloblastosis virus RNA dependent DNA polymerase (reverse transcriptase). *Proc. natn. Acad. Sci. USA* **72**: 2535–2539.

PANG, R. H. L. and PHILLIPS, L. A. (1975) Nucleotide sequences in the RNA of mammalian leukemia and sarcoma viruses. *Biochem. biophys. Res. Commun.* **67**: 508–517.

PATERSON, B. M., ROBERTS, B. F. and KUFF, E. L. (1977) Structural gene identification and mapping by DNA. mRNA hybrid-arrested cell-free translation. *Proc. natn. Acad. Sci. USA* **74**: 4370–4374.

PITHA, P. M. (1973) Analogues of viral genomes. In: *Selective Inhibitors of Viral Functions*, pp. 349–360. CARTER, W. A. (ed.). CRC Press, Cleveland, Ohio.

PITHA, P. M. and PITHA, J. (1974) Interferon induction by single-stranded polynucleotides modified with poly bases. *J. gen. Virol.* **24**: 385–390.

PITHA, J. and WILSON, S. H. (1976) Template specific inhibitor of mammalian DNA polymerases. *Nucleic Acid Res.* **3**: 825–834.

PITHA, P. M., TEICH, N. M., LOWY, D. R. and PITHA, J. (1973) Inhibition of murine leukemia virus replication by poly(vinyluracil) and poly(vinyladenine). *Proc. natn. Acad. Sci. USA* **70**: 1204–1208.

PLOTCH, S. J. and KRUG, R. M. (1977) Influenza virion transcriptase: synthesis *in vitro* of large, polyadenylic acid-containing complementary RNA. *J. Virol.* **21**: 24–34.

POPPER, K. R. (1959) *The Logic of Scientific Discovery.* Hutchinson, London.

PORTER, A., CAREY, N. and FELLNER, P. (1974) Presence of a large poly(rC) tract within the RNA of encephalomyocarditis virus. *Nature, Lond.* **248**: 675–678.

PORTER, A. G., MERREGAERT, J., EMMELO, J. V. and FIERS, W. (1978) Sequence of 129 nucleotides at the 3' terminus of EMC virus RNA. *Eur. J. Biochem.* **87**: 551–561.

PORTER, A. G., SMITH, J. C. and EMTAGE, J. S. (1980) Nucleotide sequence of influenza virus RNA segment 8 indicates that coding regions for NS_1 and NS_2 proteins overlap. *Proc. natn. Acad. Sci. USA* **77**: 5074–5078.

RACANIELLO, V. R. and BALTIMORE, D. (1981) Molecular cloning of poliovirus cDNA and determination of the complete nucleotide sequence of the viral genome. *Proc. natn. Acad. Sci. USA* **78**: 4887–4891.

REKOSH, D. M. K., RUSSELL, W. C. and BELLET, A. J. D. (1977) Identification of a protein linked to the ends of adenovirus DNA. *Cell* **11**: 283–295.

RICHTER, D., ERDMANN, V. A. and SPRINZL, M. (1973) Specific recognition of GTUC loop (loop IV) of tRNA by 50S ribosomal subunits from *E. coli. Nature, New Biol.* **246**: 132–135.

ROBERTS, M. S., SMITH, R. G., GALLO, R. C., SARIN, P. S. and ABRELL, J. W. (1972) Viral and cellular DNA polymerase: Comparison of activities with synthetic and natural RNA templates. *Science, N.Y.* **176**: 798–800.

ROBERTS, R., ARRAND, J. R. and KEDER, W. (1974) The length of the terminal repetition in adenovirus 2 DNA. *Proc. natn. Acad. Sci. USA* **71**: 3829–3833.

ROSE, J. K. (1977) Nucleotide sequences of ribosome recognition sites in messenger RNAs of vesicular stomatitis virus. *Proc. natn. Acad. Sci. USA* **74**: 3672–3676.

ROSE, J. K. (1978) Complete sequences of the ribosome recognition sites in vesicular stomatitis virus mRNAs: recognition by the 40S and 80S complexes. *Cell* **14**: 345–353.

ROTEM, Z., COX, R. A. and ISAACS, A. (1963) Inhibition of virus multiplication by foreign nucleic acid. *Nature, Lond.* **197**: 564–566.

ROUND, E. and STEBBING, N. (1981) Antiviral effects of single-stranded polynucleotide inhibitors of the influenza virion-associated transcriptase against influenza virus infection of hamsters and ferrets. *Antiviral Res.* **1**: 237–248.

ROWLANDS, D. J., HARRIS, T. J. R. and BROWN, F. (1978) A more precise location of the poly(C) tract in foot-and-mouth disease virus RNA. *J. Virol.* **26**: 335–343.

RUSSELL, S. W. and MCINTOSH, A. T. (1977) Macrophages isolated from regressing Moloney sarcomas are more cytotoxic than those recovered from progressing sarcomas. *Nature, Lond.* **268**: 69–71.

SABO, D. L., DOMINGO, E., BANDLE, E. F., FLAVELL, R. A. and WEISSMAN, C. (1977) A guanosine to adenosine transition in the 3' terminal extracistronic region of bacteriophage Qβ RNA leading to loss of infectivity. *J. molec. Biol.* **112**: 235–252.

SALOMON, R. and LITTAUER, U. Z. (1974) Enzymatic acylation of histidine to mengo virus RNA. *Nature, Lond.* **249**: 32–34.

SANGER, D. V., ROWLANDS, D. J., HARRIS, T. J. R. and BROWN, F. (1977) Protein covalently linked to foot-and-mouth disease virus RNA. *Nature, Lond.* **268**: 648–650.

SASAKI, R., GOTO, H., ARIMA, K. and SASAKI, Y. (1974) Effect of polyribonucleotides on eukaryotic DNA-dependent RNA polymerases. *Biochim. biophys. Acta* **366**: 435–442.

SCHELL, P. L. (1971) Uptake of polynucleotides by intact mammalian cells. VIII. Synthetic homoribopolynucleotides. *Biochim. biophys. Acta* **240**: 472–484.

SCHMIDTKE, J. R. and JOHNSON, A. G. (1971) Regulation of the immune system by synthetic polynucleotides. I. Characteristics of adjuvant action on antibody synthesis. *J. Immun.* **106**: 1191–1200.

SCHWARTZ, D. E., ZAMECNIK, P. C. and WEITH, H. L. (1977) Rous sarcoma virus genome is terminally redundant: the 3' sequence. *Proc. natn. Acad. Sci. USA* **74**: 994–998.

SEIF, I., KHOURY, G. and DHAR, R. (1979) The genome of human papovavirus BKV. *Cell* **18**: 963–977.

SHANK, P. R., HUGHES, S. H., KUNG, H., MAJORS, J. E., QUINTRELL, N., GUNTAKA, R. U., BISHOP, J. M. and VARMUS, H. E. (1978) Mapping unintegrated avian sarcoma virus DNA: Termini of linear DNA bear 300 nucleotides present once or twice in two species of DNA. *Cell* **15**: 1383–1395.

SHARMA, O. K. and KUCHINO, Y. (1977) Infidelity of translation of encephalomyocarditis viral RNA with tRNA from human malignant trophoblastic cells. *Biochem. biophys. Res. Commun.* **78**: 591–595.

SHATKIN, A. J. (1976) Capping of eukaryotic mRNAs. *Cell* **9**: 645–653.

SHINAGAWA, M. and PADMANABHAN, R. (1980) Comparative sequence analysis of the inverted terminal repetitions from different adenoviruses. *Proc. natn. Acad. Sci. USA* **77**: 3831–3835.

SHINE, J. and DALGARNO, L. (1974) The 3'-terminal sequence of *Escherichia coli* 16S ribosomal RNA: complementarity to nonsense triplets and ribosome binding sites. *Proc. natn. Acad. Sci. USA* **71**: 1342–1346.

SHOEMAKER, C., GOFF, S., GILBOA, E., PASKIND, M., MITRA, S. W. and BALTIMORE, D. (1980) Structure of a closed circular Moloney murine leukemia virus DNA molecule containing an inverted segment: implications for retrovirus integration. *Proc. natn. Acad. Sci. USA* **77**: 3932–3936.

SKEHEL, J. J. and HAY, A. J. (1978) Nucleotide sequences at the 5' termini of influenza virus RNAs and their transcripts. *Nucleic Acid Res.* **5**: 1207–1219.

SMITH, A. E. (1975) Control of translation of animal virus messenger RNA. In: *Control Processes in Virus Multiplication*, pp. 183–224. BURKE, D. C. and RUSSELL, W. C. (eds.). Cambridge University Press, Cambridge, England.

SMITH, J. C., RAPER, R. H., BELL, L. D., STEBBING, N. and MCGEOCH, D. (1980) Inhibition of influenza virion transcriptases by polynucleotides. *Virol.* **103**: 245–249.

SOEDA, E., ARRAND, J. R., SMOLAR, N., WALSH, J. E. and GRIFFIN, B. E. (1980) Coding potential and regulatory signals of the polyoma virus genome. *Nature* **283**: 445–453.

SPASSKY, A., BUSBY, S. J. W., DANCHIN, A. and BUC, H. (1979) On the binding of tRNA to *Escherichia coli* RNA polymerase. *Eur. J. Biochem.* **99**: 187–201.

SPECTOR, D. H. and BALTIMORE, D. (1974) Requirement of 3′ terminal poly(adenylic acid) for the infectivity of poliovirus RNA. *Proc. natn. Acad. Sci. USA* **71**: 2983–2987.

SPIEGELMAN, S., BURNY, A., DAS, M. R., KEYDAR, J., SCHLOM, J., TRAVNICEK, M. and WATSON, K. (1970) Synthetic DNA-RNA Hybrids and RNA-RNA Duplexes as Templates of the Polymerases of the Oncogenic RNA Viruses. *Nature Lond.* **228**: 430–432.

SRIVASTAVA, B. I. S. (1975) Modified nucleotide polymers as inhibitors of DNA polymerases. *Biochim. biophys. Acta* **414**: 126–132.

STANCEK, D. (1965) Interferon production by and recovery of persistently infected L cells after treatment with immune serum. *Acta virol.* **9**: 275–279.

STEBBING, N. (1977) Effects of treatments with single-stranded polynucleotides on spontaneous AKR mouse leukaemia. *Leukemia Res.* **1**: 323–331.

STEBBING, N. (1979a) Protection of mice against infection with wild-type Mengo virus and an interferon sensitive mutant (IS-1) by polynucleotides and interferons. *J. gen. Virol.* **44**: 255–260.

STEBBING, N. (1979b) Cellular uptake and *in vivo* fate of polynucleotides. *Cell Biol. Int. Rep.* **3**: 485–502.

STEBBING, N. (1979c) The design of antiviral agents based on strategic sequences in viral RNA and antiviral effects of single stranded polynucleotides. *Pharmac. Ther.* A **6**: 291–332.

STEBBING, N. (1981) Studies on the mode of action of single-stranded polynucleotides which are antiviral against encephalomyocarditis virus infection of mice. *Arch. Virol.* **68**: 291–295.

STEBBING, N. and GRANTHAM, C. A. (1976) Anti-viral activity against encephalomyocarditis virus and Semliki Forest virus and acute toxicity of polyI and polyC administered sequentially to mice. *Arch. Virol.* **51**: 199–215.

STEBBING, N., GRANTHAM, C. A. and CAREY, N. H. (1976a) Anti-viral activity of single-stranded homopolynucleotides against encephalomyocarditis virus and Semliki Forest virus in adult mice without interferon induction. *J. gen. Virol.* **30**: 21–39.

STEBBING, N., GRANTHAM, C. A. and KAMINSKI, F. (1976b) Investigaton of the anti-viral mechanism of poly I and poly C against encephalomyocarditis virus infection in the absence of interferon induction in mice. *J. gen. Virol.* **32**: 25–35.

STEBBING, N., GRANTHAM, C. A., KAMINSKI, F. and LINDLEY, I. J. D. (1977a) Protection of mice against encephalomyocarditis virus infection by preparations of transfer RNA. *J. gen. Virol.* **34**: 73–85.

STEBBING, N., LINDLEY, I. J. D. and GRANTHAM, C. A. (1977b) Protection of mice against encephalomyocarditis virus infection by chemically modified transfer RNAs. *J. gen. Virol.* **36**: 351–355.

STEBBING, N., GRANTHAM, C. A., LINDLEY, I. J. D., EATON, M. A. W. and CAREY, N. H. (1977c) *In vivo* anti-viral activity of polynucleotide mimics of strategic regions in viral RNA. *Ann. N.Y. Acad. Sci.* **284**: 682–696.

STEBBING, N., LINDLEY, I. J. D. and EATON, M. A. W. (1977d) The direct antiviral activity of single-stranded polyribonucleotides. I. Potentiation of activity by mixtures of polymers which do not anneal. *Proc. R. Soc. Lond.* B **198**: 411–428.

STEBBING, N., LINDLEY, I. J. D. and EATON, M. A. W. (1977e) The direct antiviral activity of single-stranded polyribonucleotides. II. The effect of molecular size and the involvement of cellular receptors. *Proc. R. Soc. Lond.* B **198**: 429–437.

STEBBING, N., DAWSON, K. M. and LINDLEY, I. J. D. (1978) Requirement for macrophages for interferon to be effective against encephalomyocarditis virus infection of mice. *Infect. Immun.* **19**: 5–11.

STEBBING, N. and LINDLEY, I. J. D. (1980) Antiviral effects of single-stranded polynucleotides against avirulent Semliki Forest virus infection of mice and avirulent infection of rats with encephalomyocarditis virus. *Arch. Virol.* **64**: 57–66.

STEBBING, N., LINDLEY, I. J. D. and DAWSON, K. M. (1980) Variations in the contribution of induced interferon and adjuvanticity to the antiviral effect of different poly(I) and poly(C) formulations in mice infected with encephalomyocarditis virus. *Infect. Immun.* **29**: 960–965.

STEINBERG, A. D., BARON, S., UHLENDORF, C. and TATAL, N. (1971) Depression of the interferon response to polyinosinic.polycytidylic acid by specific antibody. *Proc. Soc. exp. Biol. Med.* **137**: 558.

STEITZ, J. A. and JAKES, K. (1975) How ribosomes select initiator regions in mRNA: Base pair formation between the 3′ terminus of 16S rRNA and the mRNA during initiation of protein synthesis in *Escherichia coli*. *Proc. natn. Acad. Sci. USA* **72**: 4734–4738.

STEPHENSON, M. L. and ZAMECNIK, P. C. (1978) Inhibition of Rous sarcoma viral RNA translation by a specific oligodeoxyribonucleotide. *Proc. natn. Acad. Sci. USA* **75**: 285–288.

STERN, K. and SCHREIBER, R. (1977) Inhibition of transplanted mouse tumors by heterologous transfer RNA. *Experientia* **33**: 508–509.

STEWART, W. E. (ed.) (1977) *Interferons and their Actions.* CRC Press, Cleveland, Ohio.

STOLL, E., BILLETER, M. A., PALMENBERG, A. and WEISSMANN, C. (1977) Avian myeloblastosis virus RNA is terminally redundant: implications for the mechanism of retrovirus replication. *Cell* **12**: 57–72.

SUTCLIFFE, J. G., SHINNICK, T. M., VERMA, I. M. and LERNER, R. A. (1980) Nucleotide sequence of Moloney leukemia virus. *Proc. natn. Acad. Sci. USA* **77**: 3302–3306.

TAKANO, K., WARREN, J., JENSEN, K. E. and NEAL, A. L. (1965) Nucleic acid-induced resistance to viral infection. *J. Bact.* **90**: 1542–1547.

TEITELBAUM, H. and ENGLANDER, S. W. (1975) Open states in native polynucleotides. II. Hydrogen-exchange study of cytosine-containing double helices. *J. molec. Biol.* **92**: 79–92.

TENNANT, R. W., KENNEY, F. T. and TUOMINEN, F. W. (1972) Inhibition of leukaemia virus replication by polyadenylic acid. *Nature, New Biol.* **238**: 51–53.

TENNANT, R. W., FARRELLY, J. G., IHLE, J. N., PAL, B. C., KENNEY, F. T. and BROWN, A. (1973) Effects of polyadenylic acids on functions of murine RNA tumor viruses. *J. Virol.* **12**: 1216–1225.

TENNANT, R. W., HANNA, M. G. and FARRELLY, J. G. (1974) Effects of poly(2′-O-methyl-adenylic acid) on susceptibility and autogenous immunity to RNA tumor virus oncogenesis *in vivo. Proc. natn. Acad. Sci. USA* **71**: 3167–3171.

THANG, M. N., BACHNER, L., DE CLERCQ, E. and STOLLAR, B. D. (1977) A continuous high molecular weight base-paired structure is not an absolute requirement for a potential polynucleotide inducer of interferon. *FEBS Lett.* **76**: 159–165.

TING, C. C., TSAI, S. C. and ROGERS, M. J. (1977) Host control of tumor growth. *Science, N.Y.* **197**: 571–573.

TOULME, J-J. and HELENE, C. (1977) Specific recognition of single-stranded nucleic acids. Interaction of tryptophan-containing peptides with native, denatured, and ultraviolet-irradiated DNA. *J. biol. Chem.* **252**: 244–249.

TRINCHIERI, G., SANTOLI, D., DEE, R. R. and KNOWLES, B. B. (1978) Anti-viral activity induced by culturing lymphocytes with tumor derived or virus-transformed cells. Identification of the anti-viral activity as interferon and characterization of the human effector lymphocyte subpopulation. *J. exp. Med.* **147**: 1299–1313.

TUOMINEN, T. W. and KENNEY, F. T. (1971) Inhibition of the DNA polymerase of Rauscher leukemia virus by single-stranded polynucleotides. *Proc. natn. Acad. Sci. USA* **68**: 2198–2202.

TYTELL, A. A., LAMPSON, G. P., FIELD, A. K. and HILLEMAN, M. R. (1967) Inducers of interferon and host resistance. III. Double stranded RNA from reovirus type 3 virions (Reo 3-RNA). *Proc. natn. Acad. Sci. USA* **58**: 1719–1721.

VAN DE VOORDE, A., CONTRERAS, R., ROGIERS, R. and FIERS, W. (1976) The initiation region of the SV40 VP$_1$ gene. *Cell* **9**: 117–120.

VENGRIS, V. E., PITHA, P. M., SENSENBRENNER, L. L. and PITHA, J. (1978) Polymeric drugs: direct compared with indirect inhibition of leukemia virus replication in mice. *Molec. Pharmac.* **14**: 271–277.

VILCEK, J. and VARACALLI, F. (1971) Sequential suppression by actinomycin D of interferon production and cellular resistance induced by poly I:C. *J. gen. Virol.* **13**: 185–187.

VIRELIZIER, J-L. and ALLISON, A. C. (1976) Correlation of persistent mouse hepatitis virus (MHV-3) infection with its effect on mouse macrophage cultures. *Archs Virol.* **50**: 279–285.

WECK, P. K., JACKSON, M., STEBBING, N. and RAPER, R. (1981) Studies on the action of nucleic acid inhibitors of the influenza virion transcriptase. In: *The Replication of Negative Strand Viruses*, pp. 325–332. BISHOP, D. H. L. and COMPANS, R. W. (eds.). Cambridge University Press.

WENGLER, G. and WENGLER, G. (1976) Localization of the 26-S RNA sequence on the viral genome type 42-S RNA isolated from SFV-infected cells. *Virology* **73**: 190–199.

WITTEK, R., MENNA, A., MULLER, H. K., SCHUMPERLI, D., BOSELY, P. G. and WYLER, R. (1978) Inverted terminal repeats in rabbit poxvirus and vaccinia virus DNA. *J. Virol.* **28**: 171–181.

WITTEK, R., COOPER, J. A., BARBOSA, E. and MOSS, B. (1980) Expression of the vaccinia virus genome: analysis and mapping of mRNAs encoded within the inverted terminal repetition. *Cell* **21**: 487–493.

WU, M., ROBERTS, and DAVIDSON, N. (1977) Structure of inverted terminal repetitions of adenovirus 2 DNA. *J. Virol.* **21**: 766–777.

YACHIN, S. (1963) Biologic properties of polynucleotides. I. the anti-complementary activity of polynucleotides. *J. clin. Invest.* **42**: 1947–1955.

YACHIN, S. and ROSENBLUM, D. (1964) Biologic properties of polynucleotides. IV. Studies on the mechanism of complement inhibition by polyinosinic acid together with observations on the *in vivo* effect of polyinosinic acid in complement activity. *J. clin. Invest.* **43**: 1175–1184.

YAMAURA, I. and CAVALIERI, L. F. (1978) Inhibition of reverse transcription of 70S and 35S avian myeloblastosis RNAs by non-primer tRNAs. *J. Virol.* **27**: 300–306.

YANG, R. C. A. and WU, R. (1979) BK virus DNA: Complete nucleotide sequence of a human tumor virus. *Science* **206**: 456–462.

YOGO, Y. and WIMMER, E. (1973) Poly(A) and poly(U) in polio-virus double-stranded RNA. *Nature, New Biol.* **242**: 171–174.

YOGO, Y., TENG, M. H. and WIMMER, E. (1974) Poly(U) in polio-virus minus RNA is 5′-terminal. *Biochem. biophys. Res. Commun.* **61**: 1101–1109.

YOUNGNER, J. S., TAUBE, S. E. and STINEBRING, W. R. (1966) Inhibition of viral replication by interferons with different molecular weights. *Proc. Soc. exp. Biol. Med.* **123**: 795–797.

ZAMECNIK, P. C. and STEPHENSON, M. L. (1978) Inhibition of Rous sarcoma virus replication and cell transformation by a specific oligodeoxynucleotide. *Proc. natn. Acad. Sci. USA* **75**: 280–284.

ZISMAN, B., WEELOCK, E. F. and ALLISON, A. C. (1971) Role of macrophages and antibody in resistance of mice against yellow fever virus. *J. Immun.* **107**: 236–243.

ZWEERINK, H. J., COURTNEIDGE, S. A., SKEHEL, J. J., CRUMPTON, M. J. and ASKONAS, B. A. (1977) Cytotoxic T cells kill influenza virus infected cells but do not distinguish between serologically distinct type A viruses. *Nature, Lond.* **267**: 354–356.

CHAPTER 12

CRITICAL REVIEW AND RISK EVALUATION OF PHOTODYNAMIC THERAPY FOR HERPES SIMPLEX

LARRY E. BOCKSTAHLER*[1], THOMAS P. COOHILL[2], KIKI B. HELLMAN[1], C. DAVID LYTLE[1] and JOAN E. ROBERTS[3]

[1] Bureau of Radiological Health, Food and Drug Administration, Rockville, Maryland 20857, USA
[2] Biophysics Program, Western Kentucky University, Bowling Green, Kentucky 42101, USA
[3] Fordham University, Lincoln Center Campus, New York City, New York 10023, USA

CONTENTS

* The authors contributed equally to this review and are therefore listed in alphabetical order.

12.1. INTRODUCTION

Herpes simplex virus, a common human virus, causes primary and recurrent infections of the skin and mucous membranes. Herpetic infections occur primarily in the oral and genital regions, in the eye, and in the brain (encephalitis). Genital infection with herpes simplex virus is considered a prevalent venereal disease. A recent analysis by the Centers for Disease Control (CDC), U.S. Public Health Service, suggests that an epidemic of genital herpes infection is presently occurring in the United States (CDC Report, 1982). Furthermore, the virus has been implicated in human cancer. Except for corneal herpes, therapy has been relatively unsuccessful in achieving rapid healing of oral and genital infections or in preventing symptomatic recurrences. A procedure involving photodynamic inactivation was developed in 1973 for treating both oral and genital forms of herpes simplex (Felber *et al.*, 1973). This treatment, termed the dye-light procedure, consists of applying a photosensitizing vital dye such as neutral red (3-amino-7-dimethylamino-2-methylphenazine hydrochloride) or proflavine (3,6-diaminoacridine) to herpetic lesions and then exposing them to radiation from visible incandescent or fluorescent lamps. Loss of virus infectivity presumably results through photodynamic inactivation. The procedure has been tested in several clinical trials. Earlier trials appeared to be successful; however, later, more detailed trials demonstrated the procedure to be ineffective. The procedure is also criticized by some investigators as being potentially carcinogenic and therefore clinically hazardous.

The purpose of this review is to provide a critical analysis of photodynamic therapy for herpes simplex. It updates an earlier report (Bockstahler *et al.*, 1979), presents basic principles of photodynamic action which provide a basis for the therapeutic treatment and for potential risks, describes medical aspects of herpes simplex, and discusses the current status of clinical photodynamic therapy for herpes simplex virus infections.

12.2. NEED FOR EFFECTIVE THERAPY: MEDICAL ASPECTS OF HERPETIC INFECTIONS

12.2.1. HERPESVIRUSES: ASSOCIATION WITH CARCINOGENESIS

Herpesviruses are large (150–200 nm diameter) intranuclear replicating animal viruses containing a genome of double-stranded DNA (deoxyribonucleic acid) and a glycoprotein envelope. The structures of these viruses and the molecular biology of their replication in host cells have been documented (Tooze, 1973; Fenner and White, 1970). Virus replication in a cell permissive for productive infection results in cell lysis and release of infectious virus from cells *in vitro* and *in vivo*. Incomplete or abortive infections, resulting in lack of infectious virus production, can occur in certain cells. In this case, results suggest that the virus can establish a stable association with the host cell genome by integration, similar to that of simian virus 40 (SV40) DNA and polyoma virus DNA in their host cells (Tooze, 1973).

Tumors in many animal species have been etiologically associated with herpesviruses. Marek's disease virus of chickens (Churchill and Biggs, 1967; Nazerian *et al.*, 1968), guinea-pig herpesvirus (Hsiung and Kaplow, 1969) and herpesvirus saimiri of monkeys (Melendez *et al.*, 1968; Wolfe *et al.*, 1971) have been established as etiologic agents of the tumors produced. In man, Epstein–Barr virus (EBV) has been associated with malignant lymphoreticular proliferative disease (e.g. Burkitt's lymphoma) and nasopharyngeal carcinoma (Tooze, 1973; Epstein *et al.*, 1964). Accumulated evidence also suggests an association between herpes simplex virus type 2 (HSV-2) and human cervical carcinoma (Nahmias *et al.*, 1970b; Melnick and Adam, 1978; Rotkin, 1973).

12.2.2. HERPES SIMPLEX VIRUS: PATHOGENIC PROPERTIES

Herpesvirus hominis, or herpes simplex virus (HSV), causes lesions of the skin and mucous membranes and is one of the most ancient parasites of man (Lennette and Magoffin, 1973). The original isolation of herpesvirus from a case of human herpes keratitis by corneal inoculation of the rabbit (Scott and Tokumaru, 1965) made laboratory research with the virus feasible, both in animal and cell culture systems.

Although several antigenic variants have been described, there are two major subtypes of human HSV, types 1 and 2 (HSV-1, HSV-2). These subtypes can be distinguished both antigenically (Dowdle et al., 1967) and biologically (Nahmias et al., 1968). They also differ with respect to their biochemical and epidemiological aspects (Josey et al., 1968). HSV-1 has been isolated primarily from the oral cavity, eye, skin vesicles above the waist, and brain (encephalitis) (Josey et al., 1968). The majority of human HSV infections are due to HSV-1 (Lennette and Magoffin, 1973). Herpes simplex virus recovered from the genitalia is predominantly type 2. In addition to venereal infection in the primary host, the virus is responsible for herpetic neonatal infections which are acquired by the infant at birth in passage through the genital tract of the mother (Nahmias et al., 1971).

In vitro and in vivo laboratory studies, clinical observations, and epidemiological data have all contributed to our present understanding of the behavior of HSV as an etiological agent of disease. Primary (initial) infections occur in the absence of circulating antibody and may be manifested either as a subclinical, inapparent infection or as one of several forms of the clinical disease, such as gingivostomatitis (mouth and gums become covered with vesicles which rupture to become ulcers), keratoconjunctivitis (ulcers of the cornea), and vulvovaginitis (Fenner and White, 1970). In all instances a humoral antibody response is produced upon initial infection. The infected individual subsequently becomes an asymptomatic carrier of the virus subject to recurrent manifestations any time later in life (Lennette and Magoffin, 1973).

Localized disease is typical of recurrent herpetic infection (Chang, 1971). Recurrent vesicular lesions tend to occur on the same part of the body of any given individual (Fenner and White, 1970). The oral form of recurrent herpetic infection is known variously as herpes simplex, herpes labialis, herpes facialis, or herpes febrilis, the corneal form as recurrent keratoconjunctivitis, and the genital form as herpes genitalis. An occasional serious complication of herpetic infection is encephalitis, which may result from recurrent as well as primary infection with HSV-1 (Scott and Tokumaru, 1965; Blank and Rake, 1955; Leider et al., 1965). Protection against recurrent infection is apparently not provided by circulating humoral antibody. Deficiencies in the cellular immune response (Park et al., 1967; Nahmias et al., 1969), as well as certain systemic factors which produce minor aberrations in cellular immunity (e.g. allergic reactions, menstruation, certain emotional stresses, or fever), may permit recurrence of infection with HSV-1 (Scott, 1957; Thygeson et al., 1953; Blank and Brody, 1950). In addition, local factors such as surgery involving the trigeminal nerve (Carton and Kilbourne, 1952; Carton, 1953; Kibrick and Gooding, 1965), excessive exposure to sunlight or cold wind, as well as inadvertent or deliberate exposure to artificially produced ultraviolet (UV) radiation (L. F. Mills, personal communication) can precipitate episodes of recurrent disease. It is not clear whether a common mechanism exists for virus reactivation in recurrent infection.

These observations, and studies showing intermittent release of virus in the absence of clinical disease (Douglas and Couch, 1970), support the notion that recurrent disease stems from activation of latent virus. It is believed that HSV-1 remains in a latent state in the body, apparently in the nerve sheath and sensory ganglia (Paine, 1964; Bastian et al., 1972; Baringer and Swoveland, 1973). Thus, the fact that high levels of humoral antibody do not protect individuals from recurrent attacks of HSV infections is consistent with the notion that latent intracellular virus is inaccessible to circulating antibody (Lennette and Magoffin, 1973).

12.2.3. Herpes Simplex Virus: Associated with Human Carcinoma

Although HSV-1 and HSV-2 normally destroy the cells they infect (Roizman et al., 1972; Nahmias et al., 1970b), studies have implicated these viruses in human carcinoma. Associations have been reported between HSV-1 and carcinoma of the lip (Sabin and Tarro, 1973). Numerous studies have related HSV-2 with human genital carcinoma. While HSV-2 has been most often associated with cervical carcinoma (Blank and Rake, 1955; Sabin and Tarro, 1973; Naib *et al.*, 1966; Rawls *et al.*, 1968, 1969; Aurelian *et al.*, 1970; Melnick and Rawls, 1970; Sprecher-Goldberger *et al.*, 1970; Adam *et al.*, 1972), a study has implicated this virus in Bowen's disease, a rare form of intraepidermal squamous cell carcinoma (Berger and Papa, 1977). Epidemiological studies suggest that cervical carcinoma may be fundamentally a venereal disease of herpesvirus etiology (Aitken-Swan and Baird, 1966; Pereyra, 1971; Terris *et al.*, 1967; Kessler, 1976, 1977).

The association between HSV-2 and human carcinoma is based on viral and seroepidemiological studies (Nahmias *et al.*, 1970b; Rawls *et al.*, 1969). Studies have confirmed the correlation between the presence of HSV-2 antibodies and cervical carcinoma (Christenson and Espmark, 1977; Thiry *et al.*, 1974; Heise *et al.*, 1979). Titers of HSV-2 neutralizing antibody are related to the evolution of precancerous and cancerous cervical lesions (Christenson and Espmark, 1977; Kawana and Yoshino, 1980). Long-term follow-up studies have confirmed that women with cervical carcinoma have higher titers of HSV-2 neutralizing antibody (Christenson and Espmark, 1977). In addition, an absence of low levels of neutralizing or cytotoxic HSV-2 antibodies may be prognostically unfavorable (Christenson and Espmark, 1977; Thiry *et al.*, 1974). Studies have also shown that, in addition to humoral immunity, women with invasive cervical carcinoma possess enhanced cellular immunity to HSV-2 as demonstrated by *in vitro* studies of lymphocyte reactivity (Smith *et al.*, 1977, 1979). The presence of viral antigens in exfoliated cells from patients with cervical dysplasias and carcinomas also suggests an association between HSV-2 and carcinoma (Royston and Aurelian, 1970; Aurelian *et al.*, 1977; Smith *et al.*, 1980; Smith *et al.*, 1981). Studies with mice have shown that both HSV-1 and HSV-2 persist for prolonged periods in vaginal and uterine tissue of vaginally inoculated mice (Walz *et al.*, 1977). The authors suggest that prolonged presence of virus in normal uterine tissue may also increase the likelihood of malignant cellular transformation (Walz *et al.*, 1977). The ability of HSV-2 to produce tumors in experimental animals such as hamsters (Nahmias *et al.*, 1970a) and mice (Nahmias *et al.*, 1970b), and to transform normal hamster cells into malignant cells *in vitro* (Duff and Rapp, 1971, 1973) testifies to its potential oncogenicity. Herpes simplex virus, rendered defective by either UV-irradiation (Hampar *et al.*, 1976; Hampar and Hatanaka, 1977; Brewer and Hellman, 1980b) or proflavine and visible light (Brewer and Hellman, 1980a), has been shown to induce endogenous type C RNA tumor virus from mouse cell systems. This suggests another possible mechanism by which HSV may be associated with malignancy.

Detection of HSV-2 virus DNA fragments (Frenkel *et al.*, 1972) and virus-specific RNA (McDougall *et al.*, 1979, 1980) in human cervical tumor cells is consistent with the hypothesis that the tumor could have arisen from a viral infection. Although some herpesviruses have been shown to be oncogenic in animals, absolute proof that HSV causes cancer in humans has not yet been established. However, evidence associating cervical carcinoma with HSV-2, together with the widespread occurrence of herpes simplex viral infections, including venereal disease attributed to HSV-2, leads to the need for effective therapy.

12.2.4. ALTERNATIVE THERAPY FOR HERPETIC INFECTIONS

There has been no single, generally effective treatment for herpetic lesions of the skin and mucous membranes or method of preventing recurrences of lesions. Infections of the cornea, due to HSV-1, is one of the very few viral infections amenable to specific chemotherapy. Inhibitors of DNA synthesis, such as the halogenated pyrimidines 5-iodo-2′-deoxyuridine (IUdR or idoxuridine) or 5-trifluoromethyl-2′-deoxyuridine, halt corneal infection provided the treatment is commenced early (Fenner and White, 1970). These drugs, however, have no discernible effect on other herpetic infections.

Some success in the treatment of HSV infections of the lip and eye has been obtained with the synthetic polynucleotide poly I:C (polyriboinosinic acid: polycytidylic acid), an inducer of interferon. Clinical trials, however, have shown that this drug can be toxic for man when administered systemically (Fenner and White, 1970).

Other therapeutic approaches include cryotherapy (liquid nitrogen), superficial x-ray therapy to the involved area, smallpox vaccination, use of aspirin to keep body temperature depressed (especially for so-called 'premenstrual herpes') and application of ether (Fenner and White, 1970). Therapy for HSV-2 infections includes use of cold Burrow's solution, corticosteroid creams, hot boric acid soaks and idoxuridine liquifilm (Friedrich, 1973). Different antibiotic ointments have been used in treating discomfort produced from secondary bacterial or mycotic infections. Many of the procedures mentioned above provide only symptomatic relief.

Antiviral chemotherapy (Alford and Whitley, 1976) includes the use of arabinosyladenosine (ara A), arabinosylcytosine (ara C), and acyclic guanosine (acyclovir, recently approved by the Food and Drug Administration, USA) which may have more general applicability. Experimental evidence indicates that arabinosylthymine (ara T) may also be effective against HSV infections (Gentry et al., 1977).

Some success has been achieved with the immunologic approach to treatment through the use of specific antigen therapy (Nasemann, 1970; Schneider and Rohde, 1972; Nasemann and Schaeg, 1973). Antigens to HSV-1 and HSV-2, available in Europe and Mexico, have been used successfully for certain patients. The use of leukocyte interferon is currently being evaluated in clinical studies both in the United States and Europe. Studies have shown that live and formalin-inactivated HSV-2 vaccine significantly protects experimentally infected animals against primary, but not recurrent infections (Scriba, 1977). Moreover, virus-free preparations containing virus-coded antigens, such as plasma membrane vesicles isolated from herpesvirus-infected cells, have been effective in protecting monkeys against infections with herpesvirus saimiri (Pearson and Scott, 1977). The applicability of this immunization technique to treatment of other herpetic infections, such as HSV-1 and HSV-2, has been considered.

12.3. BASIS FOR PHOTODYNAMIC THERAPY

This section describes fundamental principles of photodynamic action which provide a basis for antiviral photodynamic therapy and for potential long-term adverse effects. Early *in vitro* studies on photodynamic inactivation of viruses, which led to development of the dye-light therapeutic procedure, are discussed.

In clinical dye-light therapy some uninfected cells surrounding the herpetic lesions are likely to absorb dye and also be subjected to photodynamic action. The fact that photosensitizing dyes plus light can photoinactivate normal cellular DNA and other cellular components is frequently understated in medical literature concerned with dye-light therapy. The impression is generally given that the dyes find their way exclusively to herpesvirus DNA and that only this molecule is photo-inactivated. Since the viral DNA is not the sole target, and since basic information from studies on photodynamic inactivation of normal cells and their components is essential for risk evaluation, such material has been included in this section.

12.3.1. PHOTODYNAMIC INACTIVATION

Photosensitized oxidation is a reaction in which a sensitizer that has been excited by light causes a substrate to be oxidized by molecular oxygen. The substrate may be a simple organic molecule (unsaturated or aromatic compound) or it may be a macromolecule (DNA, RNA, protein, lipid, carbohydrate), isolated or part of a living system. The sensitizer may be endogenous or exogenous to the system. It is usually a tricyclic (consisting of three fused aromatic rings), heterocyclic compound. The structures of several photodynamic sensitizer (dye) molecules are shown in Fig. 1. The excitation wavelengths are dependent upon the absorption spectrum of the sensitizers and may be in the near-UV or visible range. In general, the action spectrum for the photodynamic oxidation of a substrate mimics the absorption spectrum of the particular sensitizer being used rather than that of the substrate (Smith and

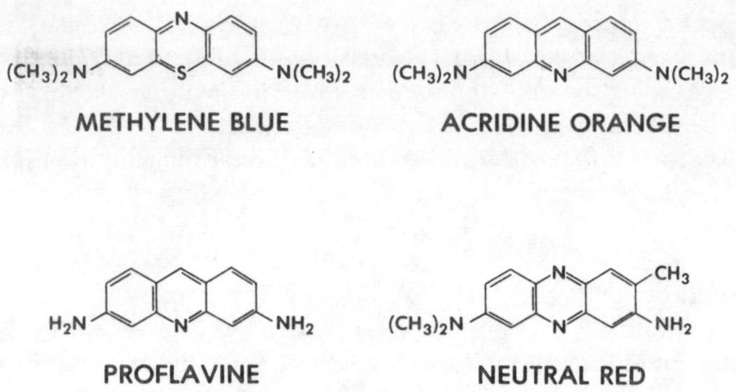

FIG. 1. Structures of selected photodynamic dyes.

Hanawalt, 1969). Oxygen concentrations as low as 10^{-5} M are sufficient for photooxidation to occur.

The damaging or killing of a biological system by photooxidation is known as 'photodynamic inactivation', 'photodynamic action', or the 'photodynamic effect'.

The rate of sensitized photooxidation of simple organic molecules is dependent on (1) light intensity, (2) substrate concentration, (3) sensitizer concentration, (4) oxygen concentration and (5) pH. Photooxidation of macromolecules involves all of the above and these additional parameters: (1) accessibility of photooxidizable groups and (2) the degree of binding of sensitizer to the macromolecule.

Consideration of photodynamic inactivation of cells requires all of the above parameters as well as these additional points: (1) inhibition of photooxidation by molecules naturally occurring within the cells (sugars, ascorbic acid, ions), (2) the ability of the sensitizer to penetrate the cell and associate with cell components and (3) the nature of the numerous potential sites of damage (membrane, DNA, RNA, ribosomes, enzymes) where the photodynamic action might be enhanced or repaired.

The fundamental molecular mechanism by which photooxidation of a substrate molecule may occur is as follows:

(1) Certain wavelengths of light radiation (dependent upon the absorption spectrum of the sensitizer) are absorbed by the sensitizer (dye) molecules, which are promoted from the ground state to an excited singlet state, most commonly the first excited singlet state.

(2) Here, through an intersystem crossing, the excited singlet state goes to a longer-lived triplet state. Most photosensitizations proceed via the triplet states of the sensitizers (Oster *et al.*, 1959).

(3) From the triplet state of the sensitizer there are two major mechanisms which eventually lead to the oxidation of the substrate molecule:

   (a) photoredox reaction of the triplet sensitizer in which a hydrogen atom or an electron is transferred to or from the sensitizer, from or to the substrate with the production of free radicals; these react rapidly with oxygen to oxidize the substrate (type I mechanism) (Schenck *et al.*, 1963);

   (b) energy transfer from the excited triplet state sensitizer to ground state (triplet) molecular oxygen to form excited singlet oxygen, which in turn oxidizes the substrate (type II mechanism) (Kautsky, 1937; Foote, 1968).

The efficiency of reaction and its mechanism is determined by several considerations: (1) the nature of the sensitizer, i.e. its ability to undergo photoredox reactions or to produce singlet oxygen, (2) the nature of the substrate, (3) concentration of reacting molecules: high sensitizer, and low substrate and oxygen concentration favors type I; the reverse favors type II, and (4) association of sensitizer to substrate: substrate-sensitizer binding favors type I.

In complex systems photooxidation can occur by either type I or type II mechanism, or both, concurrently.

Distinctions between type I and type II mechanisms can be made by chemical methods and in simple systems by kinetic methods. For further details on mechanisms of photodynamic inactivation of cells, cellular components and isolated macromolecules, see reviews by Spikes and Livingston (1969), Foote (1968), Grossweiner (1969), Bourdon and Schnuriger (1967), McLaren and Shugar (1964) and Blum (1964).

12.3.2. PHOTOOXIDATION OF ISOLATED CELLULAR MACROMOLECULES

12.3.2.1. Amino Acids, Peptides and Proteins

Although most amino acids are resistant to photooxidation, the following have been shown to be affected: histidine, tryptophan, tyrosine, methionine and cysteine are rapidly photooxidized, while cystine, serine and phenylalanine are photooxidized comparatively slowly (Blum, 1964; Spikes and Livingston, 1969; McLaren and Shugar, 1964; Spikes and MacKnight, 1971; Spikes, 1975; Matheson et al., 1975; Matheson and Lee, 1979; Rizzuto and Spikes, 1977). The sensitizing efficiency is dependent upon the nature of the sensitizer (Cauzzo et al., 1977) and the pH (Sysak et al., 1977).

Photodynamic changes in proteins are primarily the result of the photooxidation of their amino acid residues. Histidine and tryptophan are the most efficiently photooxidized residues (Spikes and Straight, 1967; Fowlks, 1959). The macromolecular changes observed are generally due to cross-linking and side chain modifications rather than to peptide bond rupture (Spikes and Ghiron, 1964; Girotti et al., 1979). The extent of photooxidation is influenced by the reaction conditions as well as the accessibility of the photooxidizable amino acid residues, i.e. the more accessible the amino acid residue, the more readily photooxidized is the protein (Ray and Koshland, 1962; Grossweiner, 1976).

The biological and chemical damage in photoinactivation of proteins is influenced by the dye used as sensitizer. Trypsin, for example, loses biological activity when sensitized by flavine (acriflavine hydrochloride), but not with other dyes (Ghiron and Spikes, 1965a; Ghiron and Spikes, 1965b). Methylene blue (methylthionine chloride) sensitizes the destruction of histidine and tryptophan in ribonuclease T_2, while riboflavine [vitamin B_2: 7,8-dimethyl-10-(D-ribo-2,3,4,5-tetrahydroxypentyl) isoalloxazine] sensitization results in only histidine destruction (Yamagata et al., 1962).

The photooxidation of specific amino acid residues disrupts not only the function of the macromolecule at specific sites, but also can result in changes in secondary and tertiary structures. Physical studies (e.g. viscosity, optical rotatory dispersion, sedimentation properties, surface tension, digestibility) indicate gross changes in conformation, and possible cross-linking, of proteins (Spikes and Livingston, 1969).

Macromolecules whose biological activity depends on higher-order structure lose that activity when the above changes occur. Some examples are loss of toxicity in bacterial toxins, loss of catalytic activity of enzymes and loss of hormonal action for peptide hormones (Spikes, 1968, 1975).

12.3.2.2. Purines, Pyrimidines and Nucleic Acids

Guanine derivatives are the most sensitive nucleic acid components toward photooxidation with the majority of sensitizer dyes (Waskell et al., 1966; Simon and VanVunakis, 1962; Sussenbach and Berneds, 1965; Lochmann et al., 1965a; Lober and Kittler, 1977). However, with methylene blue as sensitizer, there is also a slight effect on uracil, thymine and thymidylic acid (Simon and Van Vunakis, 1962; Simon et al., 1965; Sastry and Gordon, 1966). Eosine (4′, 5′-dibromo-2′,7′-dinitrofluorescein disodium salt) photooxidizes uracil (Spikes, 1977) and riboflavine photooxidizes adenine derivatives (Uehara et al., 1964).

Many photosensitizing dyes including methylene blue, neutral red and proflavine bind to DNA (Bellin and Grossman, 1965). These 'hetero-tricyclic' dyes consist of three coplanar fused aromatic rings (see Fig. 1) and therefore are capable of being inserted into the space between neighboring base pairs in the DNA helix (intercalation) (Lerman, 1961) or inserted between neighboring bases of the same strand in RNA (Pritchard *et al.*, 1966). In addition, there can be external weak binding by electrostatic attraction of the dye molecules to the outside of the polymer nucleotide (Nagata *et al.*, 1966; Georghiou, 1977). Photodynamic treatment of both DNA and RNA results primarily in the destruction of guanine residues (Simon and VanVunakis, 1962; Sussenbach and Berneds, 1965; Wacker *et al.*, 1964; Lochmann *et al.*, 1965b; Piette *et al.*, 1981; Gutter *et al.*, 1977c) with some destruction of thymine also noted (Simon and VanVunakis, 1962). These chemical modifications of base residues result in configurational changes and strand scissions (Boye and Moan, 1980; Piette *et al.*, 1979). There is a viscosity decrease for both DNA (Freifelder *et al.*, 1961) and RNA (Koffler and Markert, 1951) indicating polymerization. In addition, a decrease in sedimentation coefficient (Berg *et al.*, 1972; Jacob *et al.*, 1973; Triebel *et al.*, 1978) and melting temperature (T_m) occurs for DNA; this indicates single-strand breaks in both strands and possibly double-strand breaks in the DNA (Freifelder *et al.*, 1961), or initial single-strand breaks followed eventually by double-strand scission (Bellin and Yankus, 1966). The choice of sensitizer influences these effects; methylene blue and riboflavine are efficient, while thioflavine and proflavine are ineffective (Bellin and Yankus, 1966).

Changes in T_m for photooxidized DNA have been correlated with the content of guanine (G) plus cytosine (C) (Bellin and Grossman, 1965). Also, the ability of various dyes to photodegrade DNA can be approximately correlated with their ability to inactivate bacterial transforming DNA, to sensitize photopolymerizations and to photooxidize *p*-toluenediamine (Bellin and Grossman, 1965).

Photodynamic treatment of DNA leads to inhibition of enzymatic degradation by deoxyribonuclease and phosphodiesterase (Lochmann *et al.*, 1965a; Piette *et al.*, 1981). Photodynamically inactivated polymers containing guanine can neither be digested by ribonuclease T_1 (which is specific for guanine residues) nor can they act as specific messengers in the amino acid incorporation system (Simon *et al.*, 1965).

Physical and chemical changes in DNA and RNA from photodynamic effects result in considerable loss of biological activity of these macromolecules. For example, bacterial transforming activity of DNA can be destroyed after treatment with various dyes and light (Bellin and Oster, 1960). In addition, the biological activity of other nucleotide cell components is effected by photodynamic inactivation. A loss of acceptor activity of transfer-RNA can occur (Amagasa and Ito, 1970). A reduction in messenger activity of poly rU:rG (polyribouridylic acid: polyriboguanylic acid) has been demonstrated, while messengers without guanine residues remain active (Wacker *et al.*, 1964; Chandra and Wacker, 1966). A decrease in infectivity is noted with phage DNA (Calberg-Bacq *et al.*, 1977; Piette *et al.*, 1978). Loss of template activity of irradiated DNA may also occur (Kuratomi and Kobayashi, 1976).

12.3.2.3. *Lipids and Liposomes*

Cholesterol as well as methyl oleate, linoleate, linolenate and arachidonate have been photooxidized (Kopecky and Reich, 1965; Wilson, 1966). The products of this photooxidation are 3-β-hydroxy-5α-hydroperoxy-Δ6-cholestene, plus $^1O_2$ for cholesterol (Lamola *et al.*, 1973) and hydroperoxides with the allylic groups present in the unsaturated lipids (Rawls and Van Santen, 1970).

Photodynamic damage to liposomes may proceed by singlet oxygen mechanism, or may go via the production of free radicals (Anderson and Krinsky, 1973; Anderson *et al.*, 1974; Muller-Runkel and Grossweiner, 1981; Copeland *et al.*, 1976). The same is true of photodynamic membrane damage in cells (Lamola *et al.*, 1973; Rawls and Van Santen, 1970; Anderson and Krinsky, 1973; Anderson *et al.*, 1974).

12.3.3. PHOTODYNAMIC INACTIVATION OF CELLS AND CELLULAR COMPONENTS

The extent of photodynamic inactivation by a particular dye during *in vivo* cellular studies is influenced by factors in addition to those encountered in the aforementioned *in vitro* systems: (1) the extent to which the dye penetrates the cell membrane will determine the type of phototoxic damage; methylene blue, neutral red and proflavine are known to efficiently penetrate the cell membrane (Lochmann and Micheler, 1973; Ito, 1980); (2) the dyes usually bind to cell components to produce a phototoxic effect (however, this binding of the dye itself (dark effect) can impair the functioning of the cell (Webb and Kubitschek, 1963; Zampieri and Greenberg, 1965; Ball and Roper, 1966; Lerman, 1964; Lochmann and Micheler, 1973)); (3) previously irradiated photosensitizers added to cells in the dark can in some cases produce cytotoxic effects (Ledoux-Lebard, 1902; Menke, 1935; Bolande and Wurz, 1963); and finally, (4) some dyes are irreversibly reduced by mechanisms in the cell system and undergo chemical modification such that they can no longer act as photosensitizers (Jacob, 1974).

Photodynamic inactivation in cells can produce several sites of damage and impair the functioning of the cell in many ways (Ito, 1978). Therefore, the primary effect on a particular cell system is not always clear. The following sections outline major sites of damage and other biological effects due to photooxidation of cells that have been reported to date.

12.3.3.1. Nucleus

Evidence exists for both single- and double-strand breaks and changes in sedimentation pattern for DNA from photooxidized bacteria (Jacob, 1971; Jacob et al., 1973) and bacteriophage (Freifelder and Uretz, 1966; Simon and Van Vunakis, 1962; Piette et al., 1979). These observed physical and chemical changes are similar to those noted in the isolated DNA experiments (Section 12.3.2.2). In addition, possible DNA-protein cross-links have been noted for photooxidized Escherichia coli (E. coli) cells (Smith, 1962). Guanine is the base primarily damaged in these systems (Simon and Van Vunakis, 1962); however, thymine and cytosine also react to a lesser extent (Simon and Van Vunakis, 1962; Wacker et al., 1964).

In the case of human (HeLa) (Speck, et al., 1973), NHIK-3025 cells (Moan et al., 1980), normal skin fibroblasts and fibroblasts from patients with Xeroderma pigmentosum (Regan and Setlow, 1977), there is a reduction in the molecular weight of the DNA isolated after photooxidation. There is evidence of single-strand breaks which are repaired within 2 hr for both fibroblast cell lines (Regan and Setlow, 1977). Excision repair is possibly stimulated in human cells by photodynamic treatment (Trosko and Isoun, 1971). Modifications of guanosine in HeLa cells photooxidized with riboflavine (Speck et al., 1973), and thymine and cytosine in HeLa cells photooxidized with proflavine, have been reported (Roberts, 1981b). After photodynamic treatment, gene conversion has been noted with Saccharomyces cerevisae (Ito and Kobayashi, 1975, 1977b; Kobayashi, 1978) and increased mutation frequency in Salmonella typhimurium (Imray and MacPhee, 1975) and in E. coli (Webb et al., 1979; Hass and Webb, 1979).

12.3.3.2. Membrane

Evidence exists for both membrane-bound protein modification and lipid peroxidation with photodynamic damage to membranes. Such membrane damage has been demonstrated with virus [HSV-2, ϕ-6, PM-2 (Snipes et al., 1979)], bacteria [Proteus mirabilis (Jacob and Hammam, 1975), Sarcina lutea (Mathews and Sistrom, 1960; Mathews, 1963; Mathews-Roth and Krinsky, 1970; Penderson and Aust, 1973; Anwar and Prebble, 1977), and E. coli (Wakayama et al., 1980; Wagner et al., 1980)] and yeast [Saccharomyces cerevisiae (Kobayashi and Ito, 1976; Cohn and Tseng, 1977; Ito, 1977, 1978) and Neurospora crassa (Shimizu et al., 1979; Thomas et al., 1981)].

Both lipid peroxidation and polypeptide cross-linking have been found in hemoglobin-free membranes (ghosts) of human red blood cells that have been photooxidized (Girotti, 1975). Although lipid peroxidation is essential for membrane lysis (Deziel and Girotti, 1980a; Lamola and Doleiden, 1980), the membrane can become permeable to cations when membrane-proteins are photooxidized (Deziel and Girotti, 1980b). Lipid peroxidation has also been observed in photooxidized human diploid cell cultures (Pereira et al., 1976).

A number of enzymes associated with the erythrocyte membrane have been shown to be photodynamically inactivated (Na^+, K^+-ATPase; Mg^{2+}-ATPase) (Girotti, 1976; Odell *et al.*, 1972; John, 1975). These same enzymes were found to be inactivated in rat brain microsomes (Duncan and Bowler, 1969). Acetylcholinesterase activity was also affected (Girotti, 1976). Glyceraldehyde-3-phosphate dehydrogenase was reported to be inactivated in both red cell membrane systems (Girotti, 1976) and rabbit muscle (Francis *et al.*, 1973). Flavin dehydrogenase complexes (NADPH-cytochrome P_{450} reductase and cytochrome P_{450}) are preferentially damaged when rat liver microsomes are photooxidized (Augusto and Packer, 1981). Photodynamic membrane damage also results in the inhibition of respiration in isolated mitochondria (Ramadan-Talib and Prebble, 1978) in rat liver microsomes (Aggarwal *et al.*, 1978) and in *Neurospora crassa* (Shimizu-Takahama *et al.*, 1981), as well as inhibition of nucleoside and amino acid transport in L1210 cells (Kessel, 1977). Some cell systems have repair mechanisms capable of reversing membrane damage. Incubation of *Proteus mirabilis* after photooxidation before osmotic shock resulted in reduced lysis (Jacob and Hammam, 1975). Photodynamically treated *E. coli* lost its sensitivity to lysozyme after a period of incubation indicating repair of outer membrane damage (Wagner *et al.*, 1980).

12.3.3.3. Cytoplasm

Evidence for photodynamic damage to RNA and ribosomes comes primarily from cell-free systems. However, *in vivo* studies on the distribution of labeled thiopyronine in yeast cells indicated that most of the accumulated dye was bound to ribosomes, making them sensitive to photodynamic action (Marquardt and Von Laer, 1966). Alteration of ribosomal proteins has also been found (Garvin *et al.*, 1969). Little is known about photooxidative alterations of RNA or ribosomes in cultured mammalian cells; however, based on studies with cell-free systems, similar effects should be seen.

12.3.3.4. Effects on Macromolecular Synthesis

Synthesis of DNA, RNA and protein is inhibited in yeast cells after photodynamic inactivation (Lochmann, 1967). This effect follows directly upon irradiation, thus indicating damage to cell components such as RNA, enzymes and ribosomes, as well as to DNA.

Immediate cessation of cell growth, net protein synthesis and DNA replication was also noted with L-strain fibroblasts when photooxidized with acridine orange [3,6-bis(dimethylamino) acridine hydrochloride] (Hill *et al.*, 1960). Inhibition of ^{3}H-thymidine incorporation into the DNA of several mammalian cell lines due to photodynamic inactivation has been reported (Trosko and Isoun, 1971; Litwin and Reisterer, 1973; Speck *et al.*, 1979). DNA, RNA and protein syntheses are inhibited immediately after proflavine-treated HeLa cells are irradiated (Roberts, 1981a). Again, this suggests damage to other cellular targets in addition to DNA.

12.3.3.5. Cytological Changes

In mammalian cell cultures photodynamic damage to the cell is first manifested by cytoretraction, cytoplasmic blebbing and vacuolation, followed shortly by the development of marked pyknosis, and cytoplasmic plus nuclear granularity (Bolande and Wurz, 1963; Lewis, 1945; Klein and Goodgal, 1959; Hill *et al.*, 1960). In cases where cell injury develops rapidly, the cell may abruptly swell and become granular without cytoretraction (Bolande and Wurz, 1963). In the most advanced stages of cellular injury, the cells become stained with dye and lose the ability to adhere to glass (Bolande and Wurz, 1963). These effects may be noticed within 30 min after treatment.

12.3.4. PHOTODYNAMIC INACTIVATION OF VIRUSES

Viruses were first shown to be photosensitive in the 1930s. Inactivation of staphylococcus bacteriophage by methylene blue was reported by Schultz and Krueger (1930). Later the effect of methylene blue on several bacteriophages was compared by Perdrau and Todd (1933a) and Burnet (1933). Dye alone was not sufficient for viral inactivation; light and oxygen were also required (Clifton, 1931). Thus, a true photodynamic effect (as defined by Spikes, 1968) was the mechanism for viral inactivation by these dyes.

Susceptibility of certain animal viruses to photodynamic inactivation by methylene blue and visible light was reported by Perdrau and Todd (1933b). These results were similar to those reported for bacteriophages and were of interest to researchers involved with viral diseases (Perdrau and Todd, 1933c). This led to a series of investigations involving the action of photosensitizing dyes on a wide range of animal viruses.

Beginning with the report of Perdrau and Todd (1933b) on photodynamic inactivation of vaccinia virus, herpesvirus, and fowl plague virus, the following viruses were added to the list of animal viruses susceptible to photodynamic inactivation: rabiesvirus (Galloway, 1934), poliovirus (Rosenblum et al., 1937; Crowther and Melnick, 1961), poxviruses, adenoviruses and papovaviruses (Hiatt et al., 1960), arboviruses (Tomita and Prince, 1963), enteroviruses (Wallis and Melnick, 1963) and murine leukemia virus (Sinkovics et al., 1965).

12.3.4.1. Isolated Virus Particles

In most early work, cell-free preparations of viruses were incubated in the presence of a photosensitizing dye and then exposed to visible light. Different viruses showed markedly different susceptibilities to such treatment. The T-even bacteriophages were much more sensitive than the T-odd bacteriophages (Yamamoto, 1958). Certain animal viruses (Crowther and Melnick, 1961; Hiatt et al., 1960) appeared to be more resistant to photodynamic action than others (Tomita and Prince, 1963; Hiatt, 1960). Differences in virus permeability to dye were usually cited as the reason for these discrepancies (Hiatt, 1960). Later, poliovirus, previously thought to be resistant, was shown to be photodynamically sensitive when stringent controls were followed (Wallis and Melnick, 1963). Other supposedly resistant 'free' viruses were also reported to be susceptible to photodynamic inactivation (Wallis and Melnick, 1964).

12.3.4.2. Virus-infected Cells

Living bacteria or cells were at first reported to protect bacteriophage or animal viruses from photodynamic inactivation (Perdrau and Todd, 1933a, 1933b). These results led to the belief that only 'free' virus could be rendered inactive by photodynamic treatment. However, it must be remembered that these qualitative experiments were completed before the advent of quantitative methods of cell and tissue culture. Although in early studies by Rosenblum et al. (1937) photodynamic inactivation of poliovirus was reported, in later studies it was claimed that free poliovirus could not be inactivated in this manner (e.g. Hiatt et al., 1960). However, it was shown that proflavine (Schaffer, 1962) or neutral red (Crowther and Melnick, 1961) could be incorporated into poliovirus if present at the time of intracellular viral development. Dye was intercalated into the nucleic acid of the developing virions, encapsulated by the viral protein coat, and remained irreversibly bound to the viral nucleic acid when the virions left the host cell (Melnick and Wallis, 1975). Subsequent irradiation with light rendered these 'free' virus particles inactive. This method produced maximally photosensitive viruses (Jarratt, 1977).

12.3.4.3. Dye Permeability of Viral Capsids, Viral and Cellular Membranes

In order for photodynamic inactivation to occur, the dye molecule must be present in close proximity to the molecule(s) with which it is to react. Initially, most dyes bind to their target molecule(s) by ionic or Van der Waals forces which fall off rapidly with distance (Mayor, 1962). If the viral target molecule is nucleic acid, then for whole virions the dye molecule must penetrate the viral capsid and, if present, the viral membrane. During intracellular viral assembly, only penetration of the cell membrane by dye is required.

The only studies that reported direct evidence of dye permeability of either viral capsids or viral membranes were those of Mayor and Diwan (1961) and Mayor (1962). The permeability of the capsids of eleven different viruses to acridine orange was studied. Dye penetration was measured with a fluorescence microscope. It was found that capsids did not act simply as molecular sieves, since capsomere spacing formed 'holes' that were larger than the dye molecules. Thus, all the viral capsids in this study should have been completely permeable. However, certain viruses (e.g. poliovirus and polyoma virus) were not as permeable as expected. The availability of specific sites for dye attachment on the target molecule was postulated as the 'limiting' factor in determining the amount of dye that penetrates the viral capsid.

All other studies of capsid permeability to dye offered only indirect evidence. Usually the effect of the dye (photodynamic inactivation) was used as the criterion for penetration estimates. Evidence that neutral red, toluidine blue (3-amino-7-dimethylamino-2-methylphenazathionine) and proflavine could penetrate viral capsids was reported by Wallis and Melnick (1963), Wallis and Melnick (1964) and Tomita and Prince (1963).

Dye penetration of viral membranes has not been extensively studied. Most authors offer only secondary evidence for membrane permeability to dye. Studies were published by Wallis and Melnick (1963) on dye penetration into several viruses, especially poliovirus. Uptake of neutral red by 'free' virus was found to be a complicated phenomenon and permeability depended upon high pH, the absence of the organic components present in tissue culture medium, and optimal temperature (37°C) (Wallis and Melnick, 1963, 1964). The buffer of choice for preparing photosensitized poliovirus was phosphate buffered saline (Wallis and Melnick, 1963). Herpesvirus could be photosensitized even in the presence of tissue culture medium (Wallis and Melnick, 1964).

The situation involving dye penetration of cell membranes is simpler. Vital dyes (e.g. proflavine and neutral red) penetrate living cell membranes rapidly. Fluorescein dyes bind to cell membranes first and appear to penetrate into the cytoplasm after the cell is damaged (Blum, 1964). A 1 hr pretreatment of monkey kidney cells with neutral red was necessary to assure that dye molecules were available at the site of viral replication (Wallis *et al.*, 1967). After such pretreatment, cells retained their ability to produce photosensitive virus for 72 hr.

12.3.4.4. Herpes Simplex Virus

The sensitivity of HSV to toluidine blue was first demonstrated by Perdrau and Todd (1933b); the first quantitative *in vitro* studies involving this virus were reported by Wallis and Melnick (1964). Herpesvirus was used as a model virus for determining the optimal conditions for inactivating a variety of 'free' particles of animal viruses (Wallis and Melnick, 1964). For herpesvirus, these conditions included: alkaline pH (9.0), incubation at 37°C, and proper dye concentration (10^{-5} M for toluidine blue). Adherence to these precautions produced irreversibly photosensitized virions. Later it was shown that herpesvirus grown in cells that contained a photosensitive dye was maximally photosensitive (Wallis *et al.*, 1967). The events involved in this method of preparing photosensitive virus are identical to those reported above for poliovirus, except that with recent procedures proflavine is substituted for neutral red, since herpesvirus is more sensitive to the former dye (Wallis and Melnick, 1965; Melnick and Wallis, 1977; Melnick *et al.*, 1977).

A comparative study of the efficiency of seven common photosensitizing agents, their effects on the inactivation of free HSV, and their effects on *in vivo* herpetic keratitis has been reported by Tano *et al.* (1977). In their studies only proflavine hemisulfate worked in the *in vivo* situation, most likely due to its ability to penetrate the nuclear membrane of the host cells. Proflavine was also the most effective compound for inactivating free HSV. Methylene blue and eosin Y were next in effect, followed by toluidine blue and neutral red. Riboflavin was weak in viral inactivation, while fluorescein sodium had no effect even at high concentrations.

The exact mechanism of photodynamic inactivation of HSV is unknown. The following hypothetical mechanism (Felber *et al.*, 1973; Rapp *et al.*, 1973) of photoinactivation of HSV has been proposed on the basis of *in vitro* studies discussed above with several virus-host cell systems: during replication of HSV in cells containing a heterotricyclic dye, the dye molecules are intercalated between the stacked bases of the viral DNA. The dye-DNA complex absorbs light energy, resulting in an oxidation reaction that disrupts the structure of the DNA. This leads to loss of guanine, leaving gaps in the base sequence, and the virus particles are unable to complete the replicative cycle.

Another explanation to account for at least a part of the inactivation of HSV-infected cells by photodynamic treatment has been proposed on the basis of *in vitro* studies with proflavine and light (Lytle and Hester, 1976): if cells in the treated herpetic lesions are themselves photo-inactivated, this could result in decreased capacity of the cells to support HSV growth. A similar conclusion was reached in another *in vitro* study on HSV photoinactivation using neutral red and light (Fife *et al.*, 1976). Both results indicated that the concentrations of neutral red or proflavine used for clinical trials are sufficient to cause antiviral activity by cellular photodynamic toxicity.

Other studies have shown that the photosensitizing drug 8-methoxypsoralen and ultraviolet radiation (UV) in the wavelength region 300–400 nm (PUVA treatment) inactivate either free HSV or HSV in virus-infected cells (Hanson *et al.*, 1978; Oill *et al.*, 1978; Redfield *et al.*, 1981). Psoralen derivatives easily penetrate plasma membranes, nuclear membranes, viral envelopes and viral capsids (Hanson *et al.*, 1978). Once present in the area of viral DNA, irradiation of these compounds with UV radiation causes rapid viral killing without loss of virus antigenicity (Redfield *et al.*, 1981). In addition, PUVA treatment inhibits cellular capacity for HSV production (Coppey *et al.*, 1979) and this inhibition follows an action spectrum response that corresponds to the absorption of the drug in the near UV region (Coohill and James, 1979). A comparison of the relative efficiencies for inactivation of HSV by various psoralen derivatives has been reported by Hanson *et al.* (1978). *In vivo* PUVA treatment of HSV-2 in guinea-pig skin resulted in accelerated healing and a lower rate of vesicular development than in untreated animals (Oill *et al.*, 1978).

12.4. CLINICAL PHOTODYNAMIC THERAPY

In view of the evidence linking HSV with carcinogenesis, clinicians have felt a need for more effective therapy for herpetic infections. A therapeutic procedure based on photodynamic inactivation of HSV was developed in 1973 (Felber *et al.*, 1973) and rapidly gained use by clinicians. Development of the clinical procedure from *in vitro* and animal studies, and representative human clinical trials are described in this section.

12.4.1. DEVELOPMENT OF THE THERAPEUTIC PROCEDURE

The *in vitro* photodynamic inactivation of virus studies described in Section 12.3.4 served as a basis for the clinical therapeutic procedure. It was suggested from these studies that treatment of herpetic lesions by photodynamic inactivation might be clinically feasible. Photodynamic inactivation was first tested as a potential therapeutic procedure for curing vaccinia virus lesions in rabbit corneas (Herzberg *et al.*, 1963) and for treating herpesvirus-induced keratitis in rabbits (Moore *et al.*, 1972).

Following a limited number of animal studies, human clinical photodynamic therapy was developed by Felber *et al.* (1973). The procedure was reported to be effective in resolving HSV infections (types 1 and 2) and in reducing reinfection. The original therapeutic procedure consisted of rupturing early vesicular lesions with a sterile needle, applying a 0.1 per cent aqueous solution of neutral red to the base of the ruptured vesicles and subsequently exposing the infected area to fluorescent (15 W) or incandescent (100 W) light at a distance of 6 in. for 15 min. The lesions were reexposed to light for 15 min from 1 to 6 hr later. In cases where new lesions developed within 24–72 hr after treatment, the procedure was repeated in similar manner.

In later studies it was reported that proflavine (usually proflavine-sulfate; 0.1 per cent aqueous solution) is preferable, because it is a more effective photosensitizer than neutral red (Jarratt and Knox, 1974, 1975). In addition, neutral red can produce allergic dermatitis (Goldenberg and Nelson, 1975). After the initial exposure to light, reexposure is presently recommended at 8 hr and again at 24 hr (Melnick and Wallis, 1977) or 36 hr (Jarratt and Knox, 1974).

Results of representative clinical trials are described below.

12.4.2. CLINICAL TRIALS

A summary of representative clinical trials including successes and failures is given in Table 1. Details are described below.

TABLE 1. *Overview of Clinical Studies on Herpes Simplex Virus Photodynamic Therapy**

Clinical study	Type of dye	Type of HSV infection	Number of patients	Reported efficacy of treatment
Felber *et al.* (1973) (double-blind)	neutral red (or placebo)	types 1 + 2 recurrent	20 (+ 12 controls)	effective
Friedrich (1973)	neutral red	type 2 recurrent	30	effective
Kaufman *et al.* (1973)	proflavine	type 2 primary and recurrent	49	effective
Roome *et al.* (1975) (double-blind)	neutral red (or placebo)	types 1 + 2 primary and recurrent	11 (+ 8 controls)	ineffective.
Taylor and Doherty (1975)	proflavine (or iodoxuridine, or normal saline)	type 2 primary and recurrent	16 (+ 20 controls)	ineffective
Myers *et al.* (1975) (double-blind)	neutral red (or placebo)	types 1 + 2 recurrent	96 (including controls)	ineffective
Kaufman *et al.* (1978) (double-blind)	proflavine (or placebo)	type 2 primary and recurrent	75 (+ 82 controls)	ineffective

*Fluorescent or incandescent visible light exposure used in each study; further details given in Section 12.4.2.

12.4.2.1. Successes

Photodynamic therapy was first tested in a clinical double-blind study (Felber *et al.*, 1973) with a group of patients having recurrent HSV infections. Some of the patients were treated with neutral red dye and light, while others served as controls, who were given placebo dye plus light. The majority (eighteen out of twenty) of patients treated with dye and light noted relief from pain and other symptoms superior to that experienced with other types of therapy. There was, however, a 50 per cent symptomatic improvement in control patients (total of twelve). An improvement in healing time of 50 per cent was noted in all twelve patients, and in follow-up studies a decrease in recurrence rate was observed as compared with control patients.

Photodynamic therapy was used by Friedrich (1973) for herpesvirus infection of the vulva. Neutral red (1.0 per cent aqueous solution) was applied to lesions and 5 min later they were exposed to fluorescent light (22 W at a distance of 6 in.) for a period of 15 min. When necessary, the treatment was repeated. In a group consisting of thirty treated patients, symptomatic improvement was noted, the frequency of recurrence decreased, and tissue healed completely within 7–12 days.

Kaufman *et al.* (1973) treated forty-nine women for herpes genitalis using proflavine (0.1 per cent aqueous solution) applied to herpetic ulcers of the vulva and subsequent exposure to incandescent (150 W) or fluorescent light (wattage unspecified) at a distance of 6–8 in. for a minimum of 10 min. This was followed immediately by a second similar treatment. About 40 per cent of these patients had primary infections, and the remainder had the recurrent type. For patients with primary infection, although symptoms were rapidly relieved, the clinical course did not appear to be altered. For cases with recurrent infection, once symptoms were relieved, the clinical course of the disease was shortened (Kaufman *et al.*, 1973).

Methylene blue has also been used successfully in Brazil, although no clinical trials have been reported (Caldas *et al.*, 1982).

12.4.2.2. Failures

Four clinical studies which question the efficacy of photodynamic treatment of HSV infections have been completed. Roome *et al.* (1975) compared photodynamic treatment of genital herpesvirus infections using neutral red (0.1 per cent aqueous solution) with that of phenol red, a nonphotosensitizing dye. A 15-W fluorescent tube was used as the light source at a distance of 6 in. from the lesions. Exposure was for 15 min and the treatment was repeated once within 4–12 hr. Of nineteen patients, eleven were treated with neutral red and eight with phenol red; no difference in response to therapy was observed using either of the two dyes.

Taylor and Doherty (1975) compared proflavine (0.1 per cent), iodoxuridine ointment (0.5 per cent) and normal saline in a clinical trial which included thirty-six patients with herpes genitalis. These investigators also used a 15-W fluorescent tube for 15 min at a distance of 6 in. Treatment was repeated after 24 and 48 hr. They found that proflavine-light treatment had no greater efficacy than iodoxuridine or saline.

In a clinical double-blind placebo-controlled study (Myers *et al.*, 1975, 1976; Oxman, 1977), ninety-five patients with 170 episodes of recurrent herpes simplex (oral, genital and other sites) were treated with either neutral red (0.1 per cent aqueous solution) or phenolsulfonaphthalein placebo. Patients were exposed to a 100-W white incandescent lamp for 15 min at a distance of 12 in. Exposure to light was repeated after 4–6 hr and again after 24 hr. Photodynamic treatment with neutral red had no measurable benefit in healing recurrent lesions or in reducing the frequency of subsequent recurrences.

Kaufman *et al.* (1978) performed a clinical double-blind study which included 157 women patients with primary or recurrent genital herpes simplex. Of these patients, seventy-five were treated with proflavine (0.1 per cent aqueous solution) and eighty-two with placebo dye, followed by exposure to light (100-W incandescent lamp) for 15 min at a distance of 6–8 in. The light exposure was repeated 12 hr later and again 18–24 hr following the initial treatment. No apparent difference was observed in time of healing of lesions or frequency of recurrent lesions.

Thus, the efficacy of neutral red and proflavine in photodynamic antiviral therapy is questionable.

Weber (1976) has used PUVA therapy to treat HSV eruptions in human patients. In contrast, Morison *et al.* (1978), Segal and Watson (1978) and Mackey (1979) have reported that PUVA therapy can cause herpetic lesions to appear. Mackey (1979) attributes this to the UV component of the treatment, whereas Segal and Watson (1978) conclude that the case they report may be fortuitous. Morison *et al.* (1978) suggest that the physician be vigilant in diagnosing and managing herpes simplex outbreaks during the course of PUVA therapy.

12.5. POTENTIAL ADVERSE EFFECTS

The photodynamic treatment of a herpetic lesion results in damage to virus particles, infected cells, and surrounding uninfected cells (see Section 12.3). While aspects of these events may be necessary for successful therapy, there may also be some deleterious effects, because the photodynamic treatment used clinically to date can damage the genetic material. At present, there is little *in vivo* data on possible long-term risks from the therapeutic procedure. There are arguments, however, based on a number of *in vitro* studies which demonstrate that mechanisms exist for possible long-term adverse effects. Discussion relating the results of *in vitro* studies to potential *in vivo* risk is presented here.

12.5.1. Possible Adverse Effects from Photodynamic Treatment of Virus

12.5.1.1. Unmasking the Oncogenic Potential of Herpesvirus

The genetic material of tumor viruses includes information for different virus functions, including replicative and oncogenic properties. Because DNA and RNA are target molecules, photodynamic action, like UV radiation and x-rays, can differentially inactivate genetically controlled virus functions. For several groups of tumor viruses, UV or x-irradiation has been used to differentially inactivate replicative and oncogenic properties. Typical survival curves of lytic and oncogenic functions of irradiated virus are shown schematically in Fig. 2. These viruses include members of the papovavirus (Latarjet *et al.*, 1967a, 1967b; Benjamin, 1965), adenovirus (Finklestein and McAllister, 1969; Jensen and Defendi, 1968; Casto, 1968), and sarcoma virus (Latarjet *et al.*, 1967a; Toyoshima *et al.*, 1970) groups. It has also been shown that irradiation (by UV or gamma rays) of certain DNA-containing tumor viruses can enhance their oncogenicity (Defendi and Jensen, 1967; Seemayer and Defendi, 1973; Schell *et al.*, 1968).

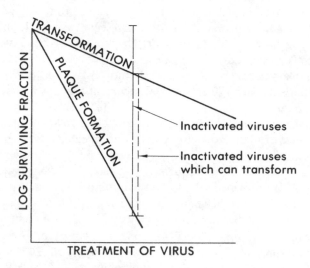

Fig. 2. This generalized diagram applies to any typical DNA-containing tumor virus which possesses genetic information for both lytic and oncogenic functions. In cells which permit untreated virus to replicate and form plaques, the oncogenic potential (transforming ability) of the virus is not readily observable since the cells are lysed, i.e. the oncogenic potential of the virus is masked. The diagram indicates that treatment of the virus, e.g. by irradiation (or photodynamic action), can unmask its transforming ability. For a given quantity of virus treatment (abscissa), a portion of virus particles which are inactivated with respect to plaque-forming (lytic) ability, are still capable of cell transformation.

Using the above rationale, Rapp and colleagues (Duff and Rapp, 1971, 1973; Albrecht and Rapp, 1973; Duff *et al.*, 1972) demonstrated that UV irradiation can separate oncogenic from lytic properties of HSV-1, HSV-2, human cytomegalovirus and SV40 (PARA)-adenovirus 7 hybrid virus. A diagrammatic representation of this rationale is present in Fig. 2. The lytic function of these viruses was inactivated, permitting their suspected oncogenic potential to be unmasked. Detection of the ability of the viruses to oncogenically transform hamster embryo cells *in vitro* then became possible. These studies presented the first evidence that HSV-1, HSV-2 and cytomegalovirus are capable of inducing transformation of normal cells.

Subsequently, Rapp *et al.* (1973) showed that photodynamic inactivation (using neutral red and fluorescent light) of HSV-1 and HSV-2 could likewise unmask the oncogenic potential of these viruses. The viruses were rendered defective with respect to lytic ability; however, they were able to transform hamster embryo cells *in vitro*. (In addition, the treatment allowed retention of the transformation ability of a known oncogenic virus, SV40.) Cell lines were established from clones of these cells. As found with many tumor cells, these cells exhibited decreased contact inhibition. HSV-specific antigens were demonstrated in the cytoplasm of both HSV-1 and HSV-2 transformed cells. From subsequent work (Rapp and Kemeny, 1977) it was shown that these cells caused malignant tumors and metastases when inoculated into hamsters.

Several other cell lines have been transformed with different UV-irradiated herpesviruses. Of particular interest is the evidence with human embryonic lung fibroblasts, where UV-irradiated HSV-2 and cytomegalovirus were the transforming agents (Darai and Munk, 1973; Geder *et al.*, 1976). Furthermore, photodynamically treated (neutral red and visible light) HSV-2 has been used to transform human and rat embryonic fibroblasts (Kucera and Gusdon, 1976; Kucera *et al.*, 1977).Thus, the evidence concerning unmasking oncogenic potential of HSV has been expanded to several viruses and to several cells (including human) with UV and neutral red photodynamic treatment. Treatment with other photodynamic compounds (such as proflavine or methylene blue) which affect the viral DNA would be expected to give similar results.

12.5.1.2. Inducing Endogenous Type C RNA Tumor Virus

A number of mammalian cells have been shown to harbor latent endogenous tumor viruses (Tooze, 1973). It has been hypothesized that all vertebrate cells may contain genetic information for type C RNA-containing tumor viruses (Huebner and Todaro, 1969). Current evidence suggests that such latent viruses may exist in cells much as prophage do in bacteria.

HSV can induce endogenous latent type C viruses in mouse cells, a finding possibly related to the oncogenic potential of HSV. Hampar and colleagues (Hampar *et al.*, 1976; Hampar and Hatanaka, 1977) showed that UV-irradiated HSV-1 and HSV-2 induce endogenous mouse type C virus in normal and Kirsten murine sarcoma virus-transformed Balb/c mouse embryo cells. UV-irradiated HSV-1 also induced endogenous type C virus from Balb/c mouse cells transformed by Gazdar murine sarcoma virus (Gz-MSV) (Brewer and Hellman, 1980b). Reed and Rapp (1976) showed that untreated HSV-1, HSV-2 and human cytomegalovirus can induce endogenous virus information, even in a cell line not readily inducible by conventional means. This reasoning leads to the prediction that photodynamically treated HSV might induce endogenous type C virus. Brewer and Hellman (1980a) have recently found that proflavine photodynamically treated HSV-1 can induce endogenous mouse type C virus from a Balb/c cell line nonproductively transformed by Gz-MSV. Thus, photodynamically treated or UV-irradiated HSV can induce endogenous type C tumor virus.

12.5.1.3. Mutating Herpesvirus

Several photodynamic compounds such as proflavine, toluidine blue and acridine orange have been shown to be mutagenic for microorganisms (Spikes and Livingston, 1969). Recently, the compound first used in clinical photodynamic therapy, neutral red, was shown to be mutagenic in the bacterium *Salmonella typhimurium* (Gutter *et al.*, 1977a). Neutral red caused mutations of the same type as UV radiation in that they are both of the base substitution type.

Methylene blue, also used for photodynamic therapy, produced genetic reversions in two mutant strains of the bacterium *Proteus mirabilis* in the presence of visible light (Bohme and Wacker, 1963). Methylene blue also caused mutations of the base-substitution type (Gutter *et al.*, 1977b). Psoralen compounds are photomutagenic in cells and viruses (Ashwood-Smith *et al.*, 1980; Yarosh *et al.*, 1980). Flavine appears to be a mutagenic agent in human cells (HeLa cells and peripheral lymphocytes) with and without light (Buchinger, 1969). The risk associated with HSV mutation is presently unknown. It is possible that certain mutant herpesviruses might be more virulent or more oncogenic than wild type virus.

12.5.2. POSSIBLE ADVERSE EFFECTS FROM PHOTODYNAMIC TREATMENT OF CELLS

The following adverse effects might result from photodynamic treatment of viral-infected or uninfected cells.

12.5.2.1. Mutating Cells

The evidence indicated above for mutation by photodynamic action suggests that mammalian cells could also be mutated by the dye-light treatment. The exact molecular basis of photodynamic mutation is not known, but possible mechanisms include specific destruction of guanine residues in DNA and/or interaction of free radicals or associated peroxides with the genetic material as mentioned previously (Spikes and Livingston, 1969).

Since mutation can result in changes of cell-growth characteristics or degree of cell differentiation, such endpoints as carcinogenesis might occur.

12.5.2.2 Enhancing Cellular Susceptibility to Transformation by Possible Tumor Viruses

Irradiation of cultured mammalian cells can enhance their susceptibility to oncogenic transformation by certain DNA-containing tumor viruses. For example, x-irradiation of human, mouse (Pollock and Todaro, 1968) and hamster (Stoker, 1963; Coggin, 1969) cells enhanced *in vitro* transformation by papovaviruses and a human adenovirus (Coggin, 1969). A similar enhancement of oncogenesis by a papovavirus can also occur *in vivo* (Harwood and Coggin, 1970).

Ultraviolet radiation has been shown to enhance transformation of mouse and hamster cells by papovaviruses (Lytle *et al.*, 1970) and adenoviruses (Casto, 1973a, 1973b). Certain chemicals, including photosensitizing compounds (Casto, 1973b; Todaro and Green, 1964), also enhance viral transformation. Thus, x-rays, UV radiation and chemicals can increase cellular susceptibility to transformation by several different DNA-containing tumor viruses.

On the basis of the studies described, it would seem reasonable to expect that photodynamic action within cells in or surrounding herpetic lesions might increase their susceptibility to transformation by possible tumor viruses, such as those which might be produced in the HSV population within the photodynamically treated herpetic lesion, or which might enter from elsewhere.

12.5.2.3. Inducing Possible Latent Tumor Viruses

Physical and chemical agents which induce productive expression of prophage from bacteria also induce expression of latent tumor viruses from mammalian and other animal cells. For example, x-irradiation of virus-transformed rat (Fogel and Sachs, 1969; Fogel, 1972) and hamster (Sabin and Koch, 1963; Rothschild and Black, 1970) cells induced production of tumor viruses of the papovavirus group, while irradiation of mouse (Rowe *et al.*, 1971) or avian (Weiss *et al.*, 1971) cells induced endogenous tumor viruses of the leukemia-leukosis type. Similarly, exposure of each of these cells to UV radiation induced latent tumor viruses (Fogel, 1972; Rothschild and Black, 1970; Rowe *et al.*, 1971; Weiss *et al.*, 1971; Fogel and Sachs, 1970; Hellman and Brewer, 1979).

Certain chemicals and photosensitizing compounds induce tumor viruses in cells when used alone (Fogel, 1972; Rothschild and Black, 1970; Lowy *et al.*, 1971; Gerber, 1964) or in conjunction with UV radiation (Fogel, 1972), x-rays (Fogel, 1972; Teich *et al.*, 1973) or visible light (Fogel, 1973). Photosensitizing compounds have also been shown to induce viral genetic information in human tumor (Burkitt's lymphoma) cells (Gerber, 1972; Stewart *et al.*, 1972a, 1972b).

This information, together with the fact that photodynamic treatment has been shown to be capable of inducing prophage in bacteria (Molina *et al.*, 1971; Freifelder, 1966), indicates that photodynamic treatment of mammalian cells could activate latent tumor viruses. Evidence in support of this prediction came from *in vitro* studies (Bockstahler and Adams, 1976) in which it was shown that proflavine-visible light treatment of SV40-transformed hamster cells resulted in induction of this DNA-containing tumor virus. *In vitro* PUVA treatment of these cells also resulted in induction of SV40 (Moore and Coohill, 1981).

12.5.2.4. *Photocarcinogenesis*

Partly as a result of earlier published concerns that photochemotherapy may be carcinogenic, Santamaria *et al.* (1980) have tested proflavine, neutral red and 8-methoxypsoralen as photocarcinogens. Using female Swiss albino mice, these authors demonstrated that each dye-light treatment produced tumors in this experimental animal. The tumors were mammary adenocarcinomas, skin carcinomas, sarcomas, lymphomas and a thyroid adenocarcinoma. Other investigators have also shown psoralens to be photocarcinogens (Stern *et al.*, 1979; Dall'Acqua, 1981; Averbeck, 1981). Thus, the predictions based on basic photochemical and cellular photobiological findings were confirmed in one experimental mammal. No contradictory evidence has been demonstrated.

12.6. CONCLUSIONS AND FUTURE PROSPECTS

As frequently occurs with new therapeutic procedures, a controversy has arisen concerning the continued use of the dye-light therapy for herpetic infections. There are reasons both for and against continued use of the therapy with human patients. Arguments in support of continuation include:

1. Since herpesvirus has been associated with carcinogenesis, it is important that the potentially oncogenic insult be removed as soon as possible following diagnosis. Recurrent infection may be more of an oncogenic risk than curtailed infection (Jarratt and Knox, 1974).
2. Heterotricyclic dyes have been used in the past to treat wounds and burns before the development of antibiotics with no apparent harmful effect (Melnick and Wallis, 1977).
3. Daily administration of a heterotricyclic dye to test animals known to be highly susceptible to carcinogenic agents had no ill effects (Melnick and Wallis, 1977).
4. Although photoinactivated herpesvirus particles may cause transformation of hamster cells in culture, there is no proven association of this to carcinogenesis in humans.

Arguments against continuation (with presently used dyes) include:

1. Photodynamic therapy is photocarcinogenic in mice and, therefore, is potentially hazardous to man, with the possible long-term adverse effect of cancer. Photodynamic treatment might lead to cancer by: (a) unmasking the oncogenic potential of HSV particles; (b) inducing latent tumor virus from treated cells; (c) converting uninfected cells surrounding the lesions into malignant cells by mutagenic or other effects.
2. Since herpesvirus is believed to remain in a latent state in the nerve sheath and sensory ganglia, it may be useless to treat the ends of the nerves in the skin in order to eliminate recurrent herpesvirus (Oxman, 1977).

3. In general, long-term effects of photodynamic therapy on humans are at present unknown. More animal studies are needed before the procedure be further used with human patients.

4. Several medical studies cast doubt on the efficacy of the procedure.

The question arises whether the discrepancy between studies demonstrating no effect and those showing beneficial effects are due to differences in technique. One of the studies (Myers *et al.*, 1975), in which efficacy of therapy could not be demonstrated, has been criticized (Melnick and Wallis, 1977) on the basis of inadequate light-exposure technique, and has been defended (Myers *et al.*, 1976) with regard to adequacy of light exposure. It appears from the light-irradiance measurements reported by Myers *et al.* (1976) that this group probably had exposed patients to as much light energy of appropriate wavelengths as groups who had reported neutral-red light therapy to be effective.

From the standpoint of efficacy, if future clinical trials are carried out, it will be important that investigators take basic principles into consideration. These include aspects of photobiology and photochemistry concerned with photodynamic action, problems of dye penetration in infected and uninfected skin, light-radiation dosimetry in the skin, as well as herpes simplex virology and pathology. The number of significant variables to be considered is large. Examples [see, for example, Jarratt (1977); Melnick *et al.* (1977); Myers *et al.* (1976); Oxman (1977) and Regan and Setlow (1977)] include type of dye, dye concentration, pH of dye solution, temperature, total amount of dye applied to lesions, amount of residual dye remaining on lesion surface, type of light source, light intensity, spectral distribution of light, light exposure time, amount and wavelength of light absorbed by the skin, time of photodynamic treatment after infection, time of and number of light or dye-light treatment reapplications, interval between herpesvirus recurrences, and assessment of the therapeutic response. Relationships between the variables are also important. For example, the wavelengths of light maximally absorbed by a particular DNA-dye complex may not equal those maximally absorbed by skin.

In vitro virus and cell studies can be useful for predicting both potential benefits and adverse effects of photodynamic therapy (see Table 2). Quantitative estimates of the potential adverse effects of photodynamic therapy are not possible at present, since there is little directly pertinent data and because exposure dosimetry in a dye-stained herpetic lesion is extremely difficult. If the dye-light treatment is actually apable of transforming cells in some patients, it may be several years before such cells produce clinically recognisable tumors.

TABLE 2. *Information Obtained from Representative* In Vitro *Studies Suggesting Potential Benefits and Risks of Antiviral Photodynamic Therapy*

Useful for therapy*	Suggesting potential risk†

Virus ('free' and in infected cells) can be inactivated
  Hiatt (1960)
  Wallis and Melnick (1964; 1965)
	Tumorigenicity of virus can be unmasked
	  Rapp *et al.* (1973)
	  Rapp and Kemeny (1977)
	Possible latent tumor virus can be induced from cells by treatment of virus or cells

Cell capacity for virus growth can be inactivated
  Lytle and Hester (1976)
  Fife *et al.* (1976)
	Fogel (1973)
	  Bockstahler and Adams (1976)
	  Brewer and Hellman (1980a)
	Cell suspectibility to transformation by possible tumor virus(es) might be increased
	  Todaro and Green (1964)
	  Lytle *et al.* (1970)
	  Casto (1973b)
	Virus or cells might be mutated
	  Bohme and Wacker (1963)
	  Review by Spikes and Livingston (1969)
	  Gutter *et al.* (1977a, b)
	Carcinogenesis in Mice
	  Santamaria *et al.* (1980)

*Details given in Section 12.3.4.
†Details given in Section 12.5.

Relatively little *in vivo* data is presently available on long-term effects of the procedure. Friedrich *et al.* (1976) obtained biopsies of treated areas from sixteen patients given neutral red plus fluorescent light for genital herpesvirus infections. The study was carried out at intervals ranging from 9 to 52 months, and no histologically identifiable premalignant changes could be found from examination of nearly 4000 tissue sections.

One case report (Berger and Papa, 1977) does, perhaps, provide some evidence of carcinogenic risk. A 21-year-old male patient, who had received neutral red photodynamic therapy for a genital herpesvirus infection, developed Bowen's disease, a rare (particularly in young men) intraepidermal squamous cell carcinoma, on the genital area which had been treated. However, the disease did not occur at the precise site of the herpetic lesion, and the latent period (6 months) between treatment and clinical manifestation of the disease was an unusually short time for cancer development.

Future work may show other dyes to be more effective and less hazardous than those presently used to treat herpetic infections. Caldas (1982) has pointed out that a dye which is selectively taken up by viral-infected cells would be particularly useful; preliminary results show selective uptake of methylene blue by herpesvirus-infected tissue. If antiviral photodynamic therapy is eventually proven both safe and beneficial, the procedure may be applied to the treatment of other viral infections. So far there have been few clinical studies on the treatment of viral infections other than herpesvirus; photodynamic treatment of viral warts in a pilot clinical study has been reported (Morison, 1975).

Independent of whether photodynamic inactivation becomes an accepted antiviral therapy, it is possible it may become useful as an antitumor therapy. Berg and Jungstand (1966) obtained high cure rates by photodynamic treatment of intradermal tumors of white mice with methylene blue.

It may turn out that photodynamic agents which act primarily on viral components other than the DNA will be more efficacious and have fewer potential adverse effects (e.g. mutagenesis). An example is the use of phenothiazine (Snipes *et al.*, 1977), a photodynamic compound which inactivates at the virus membrane level. It is also possible that a further developed alternative therapy for herpetic infections will become the treatment of choice, e.g. the use of chemicals specific for virus growth or the immunological approach through the use of specific antigen therapy.

For the present, the possibility of long-term serious risk indicates that careful consideration of treatment by the dye-light procedure be exercised. The procedure should be used on human patients only in carefully controlled clinical studies. Careful follow-up clinical observation of patients should be undertaken. *In vitro* cellular and viral studies as well as long-term animal studies should be continued for risk evaluation.

It is possible that some of the potential risks from photodynamic therapy discussed in Section 12.5 may also apply to photochemotherapeutic procedures utilizing near UV plus oral intake of psoralen currently used for other dermatological diseases as, for example, psoriasis (Wolff *et al.*, 1976) and atopic eczema (Morison *et al.*, 1976). The rationale for this is that although the molecular photochemical mechanisms of photodynamic therapy and photochemotherapy differ, the treatments do share the same major target (DNA) and some biological effects such as cellular DNA synthesis inhibition, viral and cellular inactivation, and mutagenicity (Scott *et al.*, 1976). Photochemotherapeutic treatment of hairless mice by 365 nm UV radiation plus topical application of 8-methoxypsoralen is known to be carcinogenic (Grube *et al.*, 1977). Further information on photocarcinogenesis associated with PUVA treatment is given in Section 12.5.2.4.

12.7. SUMMARY

The purpose of this review is to summarize available experimental and clinical data concerning benefits and potential risks of photodynamic therapy for oral and genital herpes simplex virus infections. Since such infections are a source of discomfort and pain, and since recent evidence links the virus itself with carcinogenesis, clinicians have felt an increased need for more effective therapy for herpesvirus infections. In 1973 a human clinical therapeutic procedure based on photodynamic inactivation was developed. The treatment consists of applying a photosensitizing dye to herpesvirus lesions and then exposing them to visible light. A number of human clinical trials have been completed; earlier trials seemed to show reduction of herpesvirus infectivity, whereas later, more detailed trials question the efficacy of the procedure. Data from a number of *in vitro* virus-host cell studies suggest the presently used procedures may be potentially carcinogenic and therefore clinically hazardous. Future work may show other photodynamic procedures to be more effective and less hazardous.

This review gives the reader a basis for understanding the basic principles of photo-dynamic inactivation, medical aspects of herpesvirus infections, development of the therapeutic procedure, results of clinical studies, and results of *in vitro* studies which indicate potential long-term adverse effects.

Acknowledgments—The authors are grateful to Dr. David Shugar for the invitation to prepare this review and for valuable advice. We thank Pamela Brewer and Dr. Michael Jarratt for sharing with us results of their studies prior to publication. We are indebted to Drs. Michael Jarratt, Angelo Lamola, Zosia Zarebska, Kendric Smith and colleagues of the Bureau of Radiological Health for their comments and suggestions.

REFERENCES

ADAM, E., KAUFMAN, R. H. and MELNICK, J. L. (1972) Seroepidemiologic studies of herpesvirus type 2 and carcinoma of the cervix. Houston, Texas. *Am. J. Epid.* **96**: 427–442.

AITKEN-SWAN, J. and BAIRD, D. (1966) Cancer of the uterine cervix in Aberdeenshire: epidemiological aspects. *Br. J. Cancer* **20**: 624–641.

AGGARWAL, B. B., QUINTANILLA, A. T., COMMACK, R. and PACKER, L. (1978) Damage to mitochondrial electron transport and energy coupling by visible light. *Biochem. biophys. Acta* **502**: 367–382.

ALBRECHT, T. and RAPP, F. (1973) Malignant transformation of hamster embryo fibroblasts following exposure to ultraviolet-irradiated human cytomegalovirus. *Virology* **55**: 53–61.

ALFORD, C. A. and WHITLEY, R. J. (1976) Treatment of infections due to herpes virus in humans: a critical review of the state of the art. *J. infect. Dis. Suppl. A* **133**: 101–103.

AMAGASA, J. and ITO, T. (1970) Photointeraction of transfer RNA in the presence of acridine orange. *Radiat. Res.* **43**: 45–55.

ANDERSON, S. M. and KRINSKY, N. I. (1973) Protective action of carotenoid pigments against photodynamic damage to liposomes. *Photochem. Photobiol.* **18**: 403–408.

ANDERSON, S. M., KRINSKY, N. I., STONE, M. J. and CLAGETT, D. C. (1974) Effect of singlet oxygen quenchers on oxidative damage to lyposomes initiated by photosensitization or by radiofrequency discharge. *Photochem. Photobiol.* **20**: 65–69.

ANWAR, M. and PREBBLE, J. (1977) The photoinactivation of the respiratory chain in *Sarcina lutea* (micrococcus luteus) and protection by endogenous carotenoid. *Photochem. Photobiol.* **26**: 475–481.

ASHWOOD-SMITH, M. J., POULTON, G. A., BARKER, M. and MILDENBERGER, M. (1980) 5-methoxypsoralen, an ingredient in several suntan preparations, has lethal mutagenic and clastogenic properties. *Nature* **285**: 407–408.

AUGUSTO, O. and PACKER, L. (1981) Selective inactivation of microsomal drug metabolizing proteins by visible light. *Photochem. Photobiol.* **33**: 765–767.

AURELIAN, L., ROYSTON, I. and DARIS, H. J. (1970) Antibody to genital herpes simplex virus: association with cervical atypia and carcinoma *in situ*. *J. natn. Cancer Inst.* **45**: 455–464.

AURELIAN, L., STRNAD, B. C. and SMITH, M. F. (1977) Immunodiagnostic potential of a virus-coded, tumor-associated antigen (AG-4) in cervical cancer. *Cancer* **39**: 1834–1849.

AVERBECK, D. (1981) Photobiology of furocoumarins. In: *Trends in Photobiology*. HELENE, C., CHARLIER, M., MONTENAY-GARESTIER, T. and LAUSTRIAT, G. (eds.). Plenum Press, New York.

BALL, C. A. and ROPER, J. A. (1966) Studies on the inhibition and mutation of *Aspergillus nidulans* by acridines. *Genet. Res.* **7**: 207–221.

BARINGER, J. R. and SWOVELAND, M. A. (1973) Recovery of herpes simplex virus from human trigeminal ganglions. *New Engl. J. Med.* **288**: 648–650.

BASTIAN, F. O., RABSON, A. S., YEE, C. L. and TRALKA, T. S. (1972) Herpesvirus hominis: isolation from human trigeminal ganglion. *Science* **178**: 306–307.

BELLIN, J. S. and GROSSMAN, L. I. (1965) Photodynamic degradation of nucleic acids. *Photochem. Photobiol.* **4**: 45–53.

BELLIN, J. S. and OSTER, G. (1960) Photodynamic action of transforming principle. *Biochim. Biophys. Acta* **42**: 533–535.

BELLIN, J. S. and YANKUS, C. A. (1966) Effects of photodynamic degradation on the viscosity of deoxyribonucleic acid. *Biochim. Biophys. Acta* **112**: 363–371.

BENJAMIN, T. L. (1965) Relative target sizes for the inactivation of the transforming and reproductive abilities of polyoma virus. *Proc. natn. Acad. Sci. USA* **54**: 121–124.

BERG, H. and JUNGSTAND, W. (1966) Photodynamische Wirkung auf das solide Ehrlich-Karzinom. *Naturwissenschaften* **53**: 481–482.

BERG, H., GOLLMICK, F. A., JACOB, H. E. and TRIEBEL, H. (1972) Sensitized photooxidation using methylene blue, thiopyronine and pyronine II. Physiochemical basis of the photodynamic effect of thiopyronine. *Photochem. Photobiol.* **16**: 125–138.

BERGER, R. S. and PAPA, C. M. (1977) Photodye herpes therapy—Cassandra confirmed? *J. Am. Med. Ass.* **238**: 133–134.

BLANK, H. and BRODY, M. W. (1950) Recurrent herpes simplex: a psychiatric and laboratory study. *Psychosom. Med.* **12**: 254–260.

BLANK, H. and RAKE, G. W. (1955) *Viral and Rickettsial Diseases of the Skin, Eye, and Mucous Membranes of Man.* Little, Brown & Co., Boston, Mass.

BLUM, H. F. (1964) *Photodynamic Action and Diseases Caused by Light.* Hafner Pub. Co., New York.

BOCKSTAHLER, L. E. and ADAMS, S. A. (1976) *In vitro* photodynamic induction of a tumor virus. In: *Symposium on Biological Effects and Measurements of Light Sources*, pp. 195–202. HAZZARD, D. G. (ed.). HEW Publ. No. (FDA)77-8002. Bureau of Radiological Health. Rockville, Md., USA 20857.

BOCKSTAHLER, L. E., COOHILL, T. P., HELLMAN, K. B., LYTLE, C. D. and ROBERTS, J. E. (1979) Photodynamic therapy for herpes simplex: a critical review. *Pharmac. Ther.* **4**: 473–499.

BOHME, H. and WACKER, A. (1963) Mutagenic activity of theopyronine and methylene blue in combination with visible light. *Biochem. biophys. Res. Commun.* **12**: 137–139.

BOLANDE, R. P. and WURZ, L. (1963) Photodynamic action. I. Mechanisms of photodynamic cytotoxicity. *Archs Path.* **75**: 115–122.

BOURDON, J. and SCHNURIGER, B. (1967) Photosensitization of organic solids. In: *Physics and Chemistry of the Organic Solid State*, pp. 59–131 (Vol. 3). Wiley & Sons, New York.

BOYE, E. and MOAN, J. (1980) The photodynamic effect of hematoporphyrin on DNA. *Photochem. Photobiol.* **31**: 223–228.

BREWER, P. P. and HELLMAN, K. B. (1980a) Induction of endogenous murine type C virus by photodynamically treated herpes simplex virus. *IRCS Medical Science* **8**: 763.

BREWER, P. P. and HELLMAN, K. B. (1980b) Induction of endogenous murine type C Virus by ultraviolet-irradiated herpes simplex virus: effect of metabolic inhibitors. *J. gen. Virol.* **46**: 267–275.

BUCHINGER, G. (1969) Die Wirkung von Trypaflavin allein und in Kombination mit sichtbarem Licht auf die Chromosomen von Hela-zellen und menschliche Leukocyten. *Hum. Genet.* **7**: 323–336.

BURNET, F. M. (1933) The classification of dysentery-coli bacteriophages. III. A correlation of the serological classification with certain biochemical tests. *J. Path. Bact.* **37**: 179–184.

CALBERG-BACQ, C. M., SIQUET-DECANS, F. and PIETTE, J. (1977) Photodynamic effects of proflavine on bacteriophage φX 174 and its isolated DNA. *Photochem. Photobiol* **26**: 573–579.

CALDAS, L. R. (1982) Photodynamic therapy of infections. In: *Trends in Photobiology*, pp. 349–366. HELENE, C., CHARLIER, M., MONTENAY-GARESTIER, T. and LAUSTRIAT, G. (eds.). Plenum Press, New York.

CALDAS, L. R., MENEZES, S. and TYRRELL, R. M. (1982) Photodynamic therapy of infections. In: *Trends in Photobiology*, pp. 349–366. HELÉNÈ, C., CHARLIER, M. and MONTENAY-GARESTIER, TH. (eds.). Plenum Press, New York.

CARTON, C. A. and KILBOURNE, E. D. (1952) Activation of latent herpes simplex by trigeminal sensory-root section. *New Engl. J. Med.* **246**: 172–176.

CARTON, C. A. (1953) Effect of previous sensory loss on the appearance of herpes simplex: following trigeminal sensory root section. *J. Neurosurg.* **10**: 463–468.

CASTO, B. C. (1968) Effects of ultraviolet irradiation on the transforming and plaque-forming capacities of simian adenovirus SA7. *J. Virol.* **2**: 641–642.

CASTO, B. C. (1973a) Enhancement of adenovirus transformation by treatment of hamster cells with ultraviolet irradiation, DNA base analogs, and dibenz(a,h)anthracene. *Cancer Res.* **33**: 402–407.

CASTO, B. C. (1973b) Biologic parameters of adenovirus transformation. *Prog. exp. Tumor Res.* **18**: 166–198.

CAUZZO, G. G., JORI, G. and SPIKES, J. D. (1977) The effect of chemical structure on the photosensitizing efficiencies of porphyrins. *Photochem. Photobiol.* **25**: 389–395.

CHANDRA, P. and WACKER, A. (1966) Photodynamic effect on template activity of nucleic acids. *Z. Naturf.* **21b**: 663–666.

CHANG, T. W. (1971) Recurrent viral infection (reinfection). *New Engl. J. Med.* **284**: 765–773.

CHRISTENSON, B., and ESPMARK, A. (1977) Long-term follow-up studies on herpes simplex antibodies in the course of cervical cancer: Patterns of neutralizing antibodies. *Am. J. Epid.* **105**: 296–302.

CHURCHILL, A. E. and BIGGS, P. M. (1967) Agent of Marek's disease in tissue culture. *Nature, Lond.* **215**: 528–530.

CLIFTON, C. E. (1931) Photodynamic action of certain dyes on the inactivation of staphylococcus bacteriophage. *Proc. Soc. exp. Biol. Med.* **28**: 745–746.

COGGIN, J. H., Jr. (1969) Enhanced virus transformation of hamster embryo cells *in vitro. J. Virol.* **3**: 458–462.

COHN, G. E. and TSENG, H. Y. (1977) Photodynamic inactivation of yeast sensitized by Eosin Y. *Photochem. Photobiol.* **26**: 465–474.

COOHILL, T. P. and JAMES, L. C. (1979) The wavelength dependence of 8-methoxypsoralen photosensitization of host capacity inactivation in a mammalian cell-virus system. *Photochem. Photobiol.* **30**: 243–246.

COPELAND, E. S., ALVING, C. R. and GRENAN, M. M. (1976) Light induced leakage of spin label marker from liposomes in the presence of phototoxic phenothiazines. *Photochem. Photobiol.* **24**: 41–48.

COPPEY, J., AVERBECK, D. and MORENO, G. (1979) Herpes virus production in monkey kidney and human skin cells treated with angelicin or 8-methoxypsoralen plus 365 nm light. *Photochem. Photobiol.* **29**: 797–801.

CROWTHER, D. and MELNICK, J. (1961) The incorporation of neutral red and acridine orange into developing poliovirus particles making them photosensitive. *Virology* **14**: 11–21.

DALL'ACQUA, F. (1981) Photochemical reactions of furocoumarins. In: *Trends in Photobiology.* HELENE, C., CHARLIER, M., MONTENAY-GARESTIER, T. and LAUSTRIAT, G. (eds.). Plenum Press, New York.

DARAI, G. and MUNK, K. (1973) Human embryonic lung cells abortively infected with herpes virus hominis type 2 show some properties of cell transformation. *Nature New Biol.* **241**: 268–269.

DEFENDI, V. and JENSEN, F. (1967) Oncogenicity by DNA tumor viruses: enhancement after ultraviolet and Cobalt-60 radiations. *Science* **157**: 703–705.

DEZIEL, M. R. and GIROTTI, A. (1980a) Bilirubin – photosensitized lysis of resealed erythrocyte membranes. *Photobiol. Photochem.* **31**: 593–596.

DEZIEL, M. R. and GIROTTI, A. (1980b) Photodynamic action of bilirubin on liposomes and erythrocyte membranes. *J. biol. Chem.* **255**: 8192–8198.

DOUGLAS, R. G., Jr. and COUCH, R. B. (1970) A prospective study of chronic herpes simplex virus infection and recurrent herpes labialis in humans. *J. Immun.* **104**: 289–295.

DOWDLE, W. R., NAHMIAS, A. J. and HARWELL, R. W. (1967) Association of antigenic type of herpesvirus hominis with site of viral recovery. *J. Immun.* **99**: 974–980.

DUFF, R., KNIGHT, P. and RAPP, F. (1972) Variation in oncogenic and transforming potential of PARA (defective SV40)-Adenovirus 7. *Virology* **47**: 849–853.

DUFF, R. and RAPP, F. (1971) Properties of hamster embryo fibroblasts transformed *in vitro* after exposure to ultraviolet irradiated herpes simplex virus type 2. *J. Virol.* **8**: 469–477.

DUFF, R. and RAPP, F. (1973) Oncogenic transformation of hamster embryo cells after exposure to inactivated herpes simplex virus type 1. *J. Virol.* **12**: 209–217.

DUNCAN, C. J. and BOWLER, K. J. (1969) Permeability and photoxidative damage of membrane enzymes. *J. Cell Physiol.* **74**: 259–2.

EPSTEIN, M. A., ACHONG, B. G. and BARR, Y. M. (1964) Virus particles in cultured lymphoblasts from Burkitt's lymphoma. *Lancet* **1**: 702–703.

FELBER, T. D., SMITH, E. B., KNOX, J. M., WALLIS, C. and MELNICK, J. L. (1973) Photodynamic inactivation of herpes simplex. *J. Am. Med. Ass.* **223**: 289–292.

FENNER, F. and WHITE, D. O. (1970) *Medical Virology*. Academic Press, New York.

FIFE, T., CÉSARIO, T. C. and TILLES, J. G. (1976) Effect of neutral red and light on herpes virus hominus type 1 in cell culture. *J. infect. Dis.* **134**: 324–327.

FINKLESTEIN, J. Z. and MCALLISTER, R. M. (1969) Ultraviolet inactivation of the cytocidal and transforming activities of human adenovirus type 1. *J. Virol.* **3**: 353–354.

FOGEL, M. (1972) Induction of virus synthesis in polyoma-transformed cells by DNA antimetabolites and by irradiation after pretreatment with 5-bromodeoxyuridine. *Virology* **49**: 12–22.

FOGEL, M. (1973) Induction of polyoma virus by fluorescent (visible) light in polyoma-transformed cells pretreated with 5-bromodeoxyuridine. *Nature New Biol.* **241**: 182–184.

FOGEL, M. and SACHS, L. (1969) The activation of virus synthesis in polyoma-transformed cells. *Virology* **37**: 327–334.

FOGEL, M. and SACHS, L. (1970) Induction of virus synthesis in polyoma transformed cells by ultraviolet light and mitomycin C. *Virology* **40**: 174–177.

FOOTE, C. S. (1968) Mechanisms of photosensitized oxidation. *Science* **162**: 963–970.

FOWLKS, W. L. (1959) The mechanism of the photodynamic effect. *J. invest. Derm.* **32**: 233–247.

FRANCIS, S. H., MERRIWETHER, B. P. and PARK, J. H. (1973) Effects of photooxidation of histidine-38 on the various catalytic activities of glyceraldehyde-3-phosphate dehydrogenase. *Biochemistry* **12**: 346–355.

FREIFELDER, D. (1966) Acridine orange – and methylene blue-sensitized induction of *Escherichia coli* lysogenic for phage. *Virology* **30**: 567–568.

FREIFELDER, D., DAVISON, P. F. and GERDUSCHEK, E. P. (1961) Damage by visible light to the acridine orange – deoxyribonucleic acid (DNA) complex. *Biophys. J.* **1**: 389–400.

FREIFELDER, D. and URETZ, R. B. (1966) Mechanism of photoinactivation of coliphage T_7 sensitized by acridine orange. *Virology* **30**: 97–103.

FRENKEL, N., ROIZMAN, B., CASSAI, E. and NAHMIAS, A. (1972) A DNA fragment of herpes simplex 2 and its transcription in human cervical cancer tissue. *Proc. natn. Acad. Sci. USA* **69**: 3784–3789.

FRIEDRICH, E. G., Jr. (1973) Relief for herpes vulvitis. *Obstet. Gynec.* **41**: 74–77.

FRIEDRICH, E. G., Jr., KAUFMAN, R. H., LYNCH, P. J. and WOODRUFF, J. D. (1976) Vulvar histology after neutral red photoinactivation of herpes simplex virus. *Obstet. Gynec.* **48**: 564–570.

GALLOWAY, I. A. (1934) The 'fixed' virus of rabies: The antigenic value of the virus inactivated by the photodynamic action of methylene blue and proflavine. *Br. J. exp. Path.* **15**: 92–105.

GARVIN, R. T., JULIAN, G. R. and ROGERS, S. J. (1969) Dye-sensitized photooxidation of the *Escherichia coli* ribosome. *Science* **164**: 583–584.

GEDER, L., LAUSCH, R., O'NEILL, F. and RAPP, F. (1976) Oncogenic transformation of human embryo lung cells by human cytomegalovirus. *Science* **192**: 1135–1137.

GENTRY, G., ASWELL, J., ALLEN, G. and CAMPBELL, P. (1977) Arabinosylthymine: *in vivo* effectiveness in a systemic herpesvirus infection. Abstract, Third International Symposium on Oncogenesis and Herpesviruses, Cambridge, Mass., 25–29 July.

GEORGHIOU, S. (1977) Interaction of acridine drugs with DNA and nucleotides. *Photochem. Photobiol.* **26**: 59–68.

GERBER, P. (1964) Virogenic hamster tumor cells: Induction of virus synthesis. *Science* **145**: 833.

GERBER, P. (1972) Activation of Epstein–Barr virus by 5-bromodeoxyuridine in 'virus-free' human cells. *Proc. natn. Acad. Sci. USA* **69**: 83–85.

GHIRON, C. A. and SPIKES, J. D. (1965a) The flavin-sensitized photoinactivation of trypsin. *Photochem. Photobiol.* **4**: 13–26.

GHIRON, C. A. and SPIKES, J. D. (1965b) The photoinactivation of trypsin as sensitized by methylene blue and eosin Y. *Photochem. Photobiol.* **4**: 901–905.

GIROTTI, A. W. (1975) Photodynamic action of billirubin on human erythrocyte membranes. Modification of polypeptide. *Biochemistry* **14**: 3377–3383.

GIROTTI, A. W. (1976) Billirubin-sensitized photoinactivation of enzymes in the isolated membrane of human erythrocytes. *Photochem. Photobiol.* **24**: 525–532.

GIROTTI, A. W., LYMAN, S. and DEZIEL, M. R. (1979) Methylene blue-sensitized photooxidation of hemoglobin: evidence for cross-link formation. *Photochem. Photobiol.* **29**: 1119–1125.

GOLDENBERG, R. L. and NELSON, K. (1975) Dermatitis from neutral red therapy of herpes genitalis. *Obstet. Gynec.* **46**: 359–360.

GROSSWEINER, L. I. (1969) Molecular mechanisms in photodynamic action. *Photochem. Photobiol.* **10**: 183–191.

GROSSWEINER, L. I. (1976) Photochemical inactivation of enzymes. In: *Current Topics in Radiation Research Quarterly*, Vol. II, 141–199. EBERT, M. and HOWARD, A. (eds.). North Holland, Amsterdam.

GRUBE, D. D., LEY, R. D. and FRY, R. M. M. (1977) Photosensitizing effects of 8-methoxypsoralen on the skin of hairless mice—II. Strain and spectral differences for tumorigenesis. *Photochem. Photobiol.* **25**: 269–276.

GUTTER, B., SPECK, W. T. and ROSENKRANZ, H. S. (1977a) Light-induced mutagenicity of neutral red (3-amino-7-dimethylamino-2-methylphenazine hydrochloride). *Cancer Res.* **37**: 1112–1114.

GUTTER, B., SPECK, W. T. and ROSENKRANZ, H. S. (1977b) A study of the photo-induced mutagenicity of methylene blue. *Mutat. Res.* **44**: 177–182.

GUTTER, B., SPECK, W. T. and ROSENKRANZ, H. S. (1977c) The photodynamic modification of DNA by hematoporphyrin. *Biochim. biophys. Acta* **475**: 307–314.

HAMPAR, B. G., AARONSON, S. A., DERGE, J. G., CHAKRABARTY, H., SHOWALTER, S. D. and DUNN, C. T. (1976) Activation of an endogenous mouse type C virus by ultraviolet- irradiated herpes simplex virus types 1 and 2. *Proc. natn. Acad. Sci. USA* **73**: 646–650.

HAMPAR, B. and HATANAKA, M. (1977) Type C virus activation in 'nontransformed' mouse cells by UV-irradiated herpes simplex virus. *Virology* **76**: 876–881.

HANSON, C. V., RIGGS, J. L. and LENNETTE, E. H. (1978) Photochemical inactivation of DNA and RNA viruses by psoralen derivatives. *J. Gen. Virol.* **40**: 345–348.

HARWOOD, S. E. and COGGIN, J. H., Jr. (1970) Radiation-stimulated SV40 oncogenesis *in vivo*. (Abstracts) 70th Ann. Meet. Amer. Soc. Microbiol., Boston, Mass., April 26–May 1, *Bact. Proc.*, pp. 187–188.

HASS, B. S. and WEBB, R. B. (1979) Photodynamic effects of dyes on bacteria. III. Mutagenesis by acridine orange and 500 nm monochromatic light in strains of *Escherichia coli* that differ in repair capacity. *Mutat. Res.* **60**: 1–11.

HEISE, E. R., KUCERA, L. S., RABEN, M. and HOMESLEY, H. (1979) Serological response patterns to herpesvirus type 2 early and late antigens in cervical carcinoma patients. *Cancer Res.* **39**: 4022–4026.

HELLMAN, K. B. and BREWER, P. B. (1979) Ultraviolet radiation induction of endogenous murine type C virus. *Mutat. Res.* **62**: 205–212.

HERZBERG, K., REUSS, K. and DAHN, R. (1963) Photodynamische Wirkung und Virus Inaktivierung durch Methylenblau und Thiopyronin. *Naturwissenschaften* **50**: 376–377.

HIATT, C. W. (1960) Photodynamic inactivation of viruses. *Trans. N.Y. Acad. Sci.* **23**: 66–78.

HIATT, C. W., KAUFMAN, E., HELPRIN, J. J. and BARON, S. (1960) Inactivation of viruses by the photodynamic action of toluidine blue. *J. Immun.* **84**: 480–484.

HILL, R. B. Jr., BENSCH, K. G. and KING, D. W. (1960) Photosensitization of nucleic acids and proteins. The photodynamic action of acridine orange on living cells. *Expl. Cell Res.* **21**: 106–117.

HSIUNG, G. D. and KAPLOW, L. S. (1969) Herpeslike virus isolated from spontaneously degenerated tissue culture derived from leukaemia-susceptible guinea pigs. *J. Virol.* **3**: 355–357.

HUEBNER, R. J., and TODARO, G. J. (1969) Oncogenes of RNA tumor viruses as determinants of cancer. *Proc. natn. Acad. Sci. USA* **64**: 1087–1094.

IMRAY, F. P. and MACPHEE, D. G. (1975) Induction of base pair substitution and frameshift mutations in wild-type and repair-deficient strains of *Salmonella typhimurium* by the photodynamic action of methylene blue. *Mutat. Res.* **27**: 299–306.

ITO, T. (1977) Toluidine blue: the mode of photodynamic action in yeast cells. *Photochem. Photobiol.* **25**: 47–53.

ITO, T. (1978) Cellular and subcellular mechanisms of photodynamic action: the $^1O_2$ hypothesis as a driving force in recent research. *Photochem. Photobiol.* **28**: 493–508.

ITO, T. (1980) The dependence of photosensitizing efficacy of acridine orange and toluidine blue on the degree of sensitizer-cell interaction. *Photochem. Photobiol.* **31**: 565–570.

ITO, T. and KOBAYASHI, K. (1975) An acridine probe into the physiological state of the cell. *Biochim. biophys. Acta* **378**: 125–132.

ITO, T. and KOBAYASHI, K. (1977a) *In vivo* evidence for the photodynamic membrane damage as a determining step in the inactivation of yeast cells sensitized by toluidine blue. *Photochem. Photobiol.* **25**: 399–401.

ITO, T. and KOBAYASHI, K. (1977b) A survey of *in vivo* photodynamic activity of xanthenes, thiazines and acridines in yeast cells. *Photochem. Photobiol.* **26**: 581–587.

JACOB, H-E. (1971) *In vivo* production of DNA single-stranded breaks by photodynamic action. *Photochem. Photobiol.* **14**: 743–745.

JACOB, H-E. (1974) Photooxidation sensitized by methylene blue, thiopyronine, and pyronine – IV. The behavior of thiopyronine in suspensions of bacteria. *Photochem. Photobiol.* **19**: 133–137.

JACOB, H-E. and HAMMAM, M. (1975) Photodynamic alterations of the cell envelope of proteus mirabilis and their repair. *Photochem. Photobiol.* **22**: 237–241.

JACOB, H-E., SARFERT, E. and TRIEBEL, H. (1973) Physicochemical investigations on DNA isolated from bacteria after photodynamic inactivation. *Z. allg. Microbiol.* **13**: 207–219.

JARRATT, M. (1977) Photodynamic inactivation of herpes simplex virus. *Photochem. Photobiol.* **25**: 339–340.

JARRATT, M. and KNOX, J. M. (1974) Photodynamic action: theory and application. *Prog. Dermat.* **8**: 1–4.

JARRATT, M. and KNOX, J. (1975) Die photodynamische Wirkung bei Herpes simplex: Eine Übersicht. *Hautarzt* **26**: 345–348.

JENSEN, F. and DEFENDI, V. (1968) Transformation of African green monkey kidney cells by irradiated adenovirus 7–simian virus 40 hybrid. *J. Virol.* **2**: 173–177.

JOHN, E. (1975) Complications of phototherapy in neonatal hyperbilirubinaemia. *J. Aust. Pediat.* **11**: 53–55.

JOSEY, W. E., NAHMIAS, W. E. and NAIB, Z. M. (1968) Genital infection with type 2 herpesvirus hominis. *Am. J. Obstet. Gynec.* **101**: 718–729.

KAUFMAN, R. H., ADAM, E., MIRKOVIC, R. R., MELNICK, J. L. and YOUNG, R. L. (1978) Treatment of genital herpes simplex virus infection with photodynamic inactivation. *Am. J. Obstet. Gynecol.* **132**: 861–869.

KAUFMAN, R. H., GARDNER, H. L., BROWN, D., WALLIS, C., RAWLS, W. E. and MELNICK, J. L. (1973) Herpes genitalis treated by photodynamic inactivation of virus. *Am. J. Obstet. Gynec.* **117**: 1144–1146.

KAUTSKY, H. (1937) Reciprocal action between sensitizers and oxygen in light. *Z. Biochem.* **291**: 271–284.

KAWANA, T. and YOSHINO, K. (1980) Estimation of type-specific neutralizing antibody to herpes simplex virus type 2 in uterine cervical cancer patients by a new absorption method. *Microbiol. Immunol.* **24**: 1163–1174.

KESSEL, D. (1977) Effects of photoactivated porphyrins at the cell surface of Leukemia LI 210 cells. *Biochem.* **16**: 3443–3449.

KESSLER, I. I. (1976) Human cervical cancer as a venereal disease. *Cancer Res.* **36**: 783–791.

KESSLER, I. I. (1977) Venereal factors in human cervical cancer: Evidence from marital clusters. *Cancer* (Suppl.) **39**: 1912–1919.

KIBRICK, S. and GOODING, G. W. (1965) Pathogenesis of infection with herpes simplex virus with special reference to nervous tissue. In: NINDB Monograph No. 2: *Slow Latent, and Temperate Virus Infections,* pp. 143–154. GAJDUSEK, D. C., GIBBS, C. J., Jr. and ALPERS, M. (eds.). Government Printing Office, PHS publication No. 1378, Washington, D.C.

KLEIN, S. W. and GOODGAL, S. H. (1959) Photodynamic inactivation of monkey kidney cell monolayers. *Science* **130**: 629.

KOBAYASHI, K. (1978) Effect of sodium azide on photodynamic induction of genetic changes in yeast. *Photochem. Photobiol.* **28**: 535–538.

KOBAYASHI, K. and ITO, T. (1976) Further *in vivo* studies on the participation of singlet oxygen in the photodynamic inactivation and induction of genetic changes in *Saccharomyces cerevisiae. Photochem. Photobiol.* **23**: 21–28.

KOFFLER, H. and MARKERT, I. L. (1951) The effect of photodynamic action on the viscosity of desoxyribonucleic acid. *Proc. Soc. exp. Biol. Med.* **76**: 90–92.

KOPECKY, K. R. and REICH, H. V. (1965) Reactivities in photosensitized olefin oxidations. *Can. J. Chem.* **43**: 2265–2270.

KUCERA, L. S. and GUSDON, J. P. (1976) Transformation of human embryonic fibroblasts by photodynamically inactivated herpes simplex virus, type 2, at supra-optimal temperature. *J. Gen. Virol.* **30**: 257–261.

KUCERA, L. S., GUSDON, J. P., EDWARDS, I. and HERBST, G. (1977) Oncogenic transformation of rat embryo fibroblasts with photoinactivated herpes simplex virus: rapid in vitro cloning of transformed cells. *J. Gen. Virol.* **35**: 473–485.

KURATOMI, K. and KOBAYASHI, Y. (1976) Photodynamic action of lumiflavin on the template DNA of RNA polymerase. *FEBS Letters* **72**: 295–298.

LAMOLA, A. A. and DOLEIDEN, F. H. (1980) Cross-linking of membrane proteins and protoporphyrin-sensitized photohemolysis. *Photochem. Photobiol.* **31**: 597–601.

LAMOLA, A. A., YAMONE, T. and TROZZOLO, A. M. (1973) Cholesterol hydroperoxide formation in red cell membranes and photochemolysis in erythropoetic protoporphyria. *Science* **179**: 1131–1133.

LATARJET, R., CRAMER, R., GOLDE, A. and MONTAGNIER, L. (1967a) Irradiation of oncogenic viruses: dissociation of viral functions. In *Carcinogenesis: A Broad Critique,* pp. 677–695. Proceedings 20th Symposium on Fundamental Cancer Research, Houston, 1966, Williams and Wilkins, Baltimore.

LATARJET, R., CRAMER, R. and MONTAGNIER, L. (1967b) Inactivation, by UV-, X-, and γ-radiations, of the infecting and transforming capacities of polyoma virus. *Virology* **33**: 104–111.

LEDOUX-LEBARD, M. (1902) Action de la lumiere sur la Toxicite de l'eosine et de quelques autres substances pour les paramecies. *Annls. Inst. Pasteur, Paris* **16**: 587–594.

LEIDER, W., MAGOFFIN. R. L., LENNETTE, E. H. and LEONARDS, L. N. R. (1965) Herpes-simplex-virus encephalitis: Its possible association with reactivated latent infection. *New Engl. J. Med.* **273**: 341–347.

LENNETTE, E. H. and MAGOFFIN, R. L. (1973) Virologic and immunologic aspects of major oral ulcerations. *J. Am. dent. Ass.* **87**: 1055–1073.

LERMAN, L. S. (1961) Structural considerations in the interaction of DNA and acridines. *J. molec. Biol.* **3**: 18–30.

LERMAN, L. S. (1964) Amino group reactivity in DNA–amino acridine complexes. *J. molec. Biol.* **10**: 367–380.

LEWIS, M. R. (1945) The injurious effects of light upon dividing cells in tissue culture containing fluorescent substances. *Anat. Rec.* **91**: 199–207.

LITWIN, J. and REISTERER, Z. (1973) The effect of photosensitizing dyes on the H³-thymidine incorporation of cells grown in vitro. *Expl. Cell Res.* **79**: 191–198.

LOBER, G. and KITTLER, L. (1977) Selected topics in photochemistry of nucleic acids. Recent results and perspectives. *Photochem. Photobiol.* **25**: 215–233.

LOCHMANN, E-R. (1967) Über photodynamische Wirkung von Farbstoffen. VII. Hemmung der RNS-synthese bei Saccharomyceszellen verschiedenen Ploidegrades durch Farbstoffe in Gegenwart und in Abwesenheit von sichtbarem Licht. *Z. Naturf.* **22b**: 196–200.

LOCHMANN, E-R. and MICHELER, A. (1973) Binding organic dyes to nucleic acid and the photodynamic effect. In: *Physico-Chemical Properties of Nucleic Acids,* pp. 223–267. DUCHESNE, J. (ed.). (Vol. 1) Academic Press, New York.

LOCHMANN, E-R., STEIN, W. and UNLAUF, C. (1965a) The photodynamic effect of dyes. III. The effect of dyes on Saccharomyces cells of various degrees of ploidy and on their nucleic acids, in the presence and absence of light. *Z. Naturf.* **206**: 778–785.

LOCHMANN, E-R., STEIN, W. and UNLAUF, C. (1965b) The photodynamic action of thiopyronin. *Biophysik* **2**: 271–275.

LOWY, D. R., ROWE, W. P., TEICH, N. and HARTLEY, J. W. (1971) Murine leukemia virus: high frequency activation *in vitro* by 5-iododeoxyuridine and 5-bromodeoxyuridine. *Science* **174**: 155–156.

LYTLE, C. D., HELLMAN, K. B. and TELLES, N. C. (1970) Enhancement of viral transformation by ultraviolet light. *Int. J. Radiat. Biol.* **18**: 297–300.

LYTLE, C. D. and HESTER, L. D. (1976) Photodynamic treatment of herpes simplex virus infection *in vitro. Photochem. Photobiol.* **24**: 443–448.

MACKEY, J. P. (1979) Clinical side-effects of longwave ultraviolet light and oral 8-methoxypsoralen in patients treated for psoriasis. *Irish J. Med. Sci.* **148**: 36–38.

MARQUARDT, H. and VON LAER, U. (1966) Nicht-Mutagenität von Theopyronin in einem Vorwarts-und Rückwartsmutationssystem der Hefe. *Naturwissenschaften* **53**: 185.

MATHESON, I. B. C., ETHERIDGE, R. D., KRATOWICH, N. R. and LEE, J. (1975) The quenching of singlet oxygen by amino acids and proteins. *Photochem. Photobiol.* **21**: 165–171.

MATHESON, I. B. C. and LEE, J. (1979) Chemical reaction rates of amino acids with singlet oxygen. *Photochem. Photobiol.* **29**: 879–881.

MATHEWS, M. M. (1963) Comparative study of lethal photosensitization of *Sarcina lutea* by 8-methoxypsoralen and by toluidine blue. *J. Bact.* **85**: 322–328.

MATHEWS, M. M. and SISTROM, W. R. (1960) The function of the carotenoid pigments of Sarcina lutea. *Arch. Mikrobiol.* **35**: 139–146.

MATHEWS-ROTH, M. M. and KRINSKY, N. I. (1970) Protective function of the carotenoid pigments of *Sarcina lutea. Photochem. Photobiol.* **11**: 419–428.

MAYOR, H. D. (1962) Biophysical studies on viruses using the fluorochrome acridine orange. *Prog. med. Virol.* **4**: 70–86.

MAYOR, H. D. and DIWAN, A. R. (1961) Studies on the acridine orange staining of two purified RNA viruses; poliovirus and tobacco mosaic virus. *Virology* **14**: 74–82.

McDOUGALL, J. K., GALLOWAY, D. A. and FENOGLIO, C. M. (1979) *In situ* cytological hybridization to detect herpes simplex virus RNA in human tissues. In: *Antiviral Mechanisms in the Control of Neoplasis*, pp. 233–240. CHANDRA, P. (ed.). Plenum Press, New York.

McDOUGALL, J. K., GALLOWAY, D. A. and FENOGLIO, C. M. (1980) Cervical carcinoma: detection of herpes simplex virus RNA in cells undergoing neoplastic change. *Int. J. Cancer* **25**: 1–8.

McLAREN, A. D. and SHUGAR, D. (1964) *Photochemistry of Proteins and Nucleic Acids.* Pergamon Press, Oxford.

MELENDEZ, L. V., HUNT, R. D. and DANIEL, M. D. (1968) An apparently new herpesvirus from primary kidney cultures of the squirrel monkey (*Saimiri sclurens*). *Lab. Anim. Care* **18**: 374–381.

MELNICK, J. L. and RAWLS, W. E. (1970) Herpesvirus type 2 and cervical carcinoma. *Ann. N.Y. Acad. Sci.* **174**: 993–998.

MELNICK, J. L. and ADAM, E. (1978) Epidemiological approaches to determining whether herpesvirus is the etiological agent of cervical cancer. *Prog. Exp. Tumor Res.* **21**: 49–69.

MELNICK, J. L. and WALLIS, C. (1975) Photodynamic inactivation of herpesvirus. *Viral Perspectives* **9**: 297–314.

MELNICK, J. L. and WALLIS, C. (1977) Photodynamic inactivation of herpes simplex virus: a status report. *Ann. N.Y. Acad. Sci.* **284**: 171–181.

MELNICK, J. L., KHAN, N. C. and BISWAL, N. (1977) Photodynamic inactivation of herpes simplex virus and its DNA. *Photochem. Photobiol.* **25**: 341–342.

MENKE, J. F. (1935) The hemolytic action of photofluorescein. *Biol. Bull.* **68**: 360–362.

MOAN, J., WAKSWIK, H. and CHRISTENSEN, T. (1980) DNA single-strand breaks and sister chromatid exchanges induced by treatment with hematoporphyrin and light or by X-rays to human NHIK 3025 cells. *Cancer Res.* **40**: 2915–2918.

MOLINA, A., CALENDI, E., MASALA, B. and SANTAMARIA, L. (1971) Evidence of phage induction in *Streptococcus pyogenes* by photodynamic action of 3,4-benzpyrene. *Boll. chim.-farm.* **110**: 377–379.

MOORE, S. P. and COOHILL, T. P. (1981) The wavelength dependence of the effect of 8-methoxypsoralen plus ultraviolet radiation on the induction of latent simian virus 40 from a mammalian cell. *Photochem. Photobiol.* **34**: 609–615.

MOORE, C., WALLIS, C., MELNICK, J. L. and KUNS, M. D. (1972) Photodynamic treatment of herpes keratitis. *Infec. Immunity* **5**: 169–171.

MORISON, W. (1975) Anti-viral treatment of warts. *Br. J. Derm.* **92**: 97–99.

MORISON, W. L., PARRISH, J. A. and FITZPATRICK, T. B. (1976) Oral psoralen photochemotherapy of atopic eczema. *J. invest. Derm.* **67**: 561.

MORISON, W. L., PARRISH, J. A. and FITZPATRICK, T. B. (1978) Oral psoralen photochemotherapy of atopic eczema. *Brit. J. Dermatol.* **98**: 25–30.

MULLER-RUNKEL, R. and GROSSWEINER, L. I. (1981) Dark membrane lysis and photosensitization by 3-carboxypsoralen. *Photochem. Photobiol.* **33**: 399–402.

MYERS, M. G., OXMAN, M. N., CLARK, J. E. and ARNDT, K. A. (1975) Failure of neutral red photodynamic inactivation in recurrent herpes simplex virus infections. *New Engl. J. Med.* **293**: 945–949.

MYERS, M. G., OXMAN, M. N., CLARK, J. E. and ARNDT, K. A. (1976) Photodynamic inactivation in recurrent infections with herpes simplex virus. *J. infect. Dis.* **133**, Suppl. A: 145–150.

NAGATA, C., KODAMA, M., TAGASHIRA, Y. and IMAMURA, A. (1966) Interaction of polynuclear aromatic hydrocarbons, 4-nitro-quinoline l-oxides and various dyes with DNA. *J. Polm. Sci. Part D* **4**: 409–428.

NAHMIAS, A. J., DOWDLE, W. R. and NAIB, Z. M. (1968) Relation of pock size on chorioallantoic membrane to antigenic type of herpesvirus hominis. *Proc. Soc. exp. Biol. Med.* **127**: 1022–1028.

NAHMIAS, A. J., HIRSCH, M. S. and KRAMER, J. H. (1969) Effect of antithymocyte serum on herpesvirus hominis (type 1) infection in adult mice. *Proc. Soc. exp. Biol. Med.* **132**: 696–698.

NAHMIAS, A. J., JOSEY, W. E. and NAIB, Z. M. (1971) Perinatal risk associated with maternal genital herpes simplex virus infection. *Am. J. Obstet. Gynec.* **110**: 825–837.

NAHMIAS, A. J., NAIB, Z. M. and JOSEY, W. E. (1970a) Sarcomas after inoculation of newborn hamsters with herpes virus hominis type 2 strains. *Proc. Soc. exp. Biol. Med.* **134**: 1065–1069.

NAHMIAS, A. J., NAIB, Z. M. and JOSEY, W. E. (1970b) Herpesvirus hominis type 2 infection: association with cervical cancer and perinatal disease. In: *From Molecules to Man—Perspectives in Virology*, pp. 73–89. POLLARD, M. (ed.). (Vol. VII) Academic Press, New York.

NAIB, Z. M., NAHMIAS, A. J. and JOSEY, W. E. (1966) Cytology and histopathology of cervical herpes simplex infection. *Cancer* **19**: 1026–1030.

NASEMANN, T. (1970) Neuere Behandlungsmethoden unterschiedlicher herpes simplex-Infektionen. *Arch. f. klin. u. exp. Derm.* **237**: 234.

NASEMANN, T. and SCHAEG, G. (1973) Herpes simplex-virus, typ 2: mikrobiologische and klinische Erfahrungen mit einer abgetöteten Vakzine. *Der Hautarzt.* **24**(4): 133–139.

NAZERIAN, K., SOLOMON, J. J., WITTER, R. L. and BURMEISTER, B. R. (1968) Studies on the etiology of Marek's disease. II. Finding of a herpesvirus in cell culture. *Proc. Soc. exp. Biol. Med.* **127**: 177–182.

ODELL, G. B., BROWN, R. S. and KOPELMAN, A. E. (1972) The photodynamic action of bilirubin on erythrocytes. *J. Pediat.* **81**: 473–483.

OILL, P. A., GALPIN, J. E., FOX, M. A. and GUZE, L. B. (1978) Treatment of cutaneous herpesvirus hominis type 2 infection with 8-methoxypsoralen and long-wave ultraviolet light in guinea pigs. *J. infect. Dis.* **137**: 715–721.

OSTER, G., BELLIN, J. S., KIMBALL, R. W. and SCHRADER, M. E. (1959) Dye-sensitized photooxidation. *J. Am. chem. Soc.* **81**: 5095–5099.

OXMAN, M. N. (1977) The clinical evaluation of photodynamic inactivation for the therapy of recurrent herpes simplex virus infections. *Photochem. Photobiol.* **25**: 343–344.

PAINE, T. F., Jr. (1964) Latent herpes simplex infection in man. *Bact. Rev.* **28**: 472–479.

PARK, R. K., GOLTZ, R. W. and CAREY, T. B. (1967) Unusual cutaneous infections associated with immunosuppressive therapy. *Archs Derm.* **95**: 345–350.

PEARSON, G. R. and SCOTT, R. E. (1977) Potential for immunization against herpesvirus infections with plasma membrane vesicles. Abstract, Third International Symposium on Oncogenesis and Herpesviruses, Cambridge, Mass., 25–29 July.

PENDERSON, T. C. and AUST, S. D. (1973) The role of superoxide and singlet oxygen in lipid peroxidation promoted by xanthine oxidase. *Biochem. biophys. Res. Commun.* **52**: 1071–1078.

PERDRAU, J. R. and TODD, C. (1933a) The photodynamic action of methylene blue on bacteriophage. *Proc. R. Soc.* (B) **112**: 277–287.

PERDRAU, J. R. and TODD, C. (1933b) Photodynamic action of methylene blue on certain viruses. *Proc. R. Soc.* (B) **112**: 288–298.

PERDRAU, J. R. and TODD, C. (1933c) Canine distemper. The high antigenic value of the virus after photodynamic inactivation by methylene blue. *J. Comp. Path. Ther.* **46**: 78–89.

PEREIRA, O. M., SMITH, J. R. and PACKER, L. (1976) Photosensitization of human diploid cell cultures by intracellular flavins and protection by antioxidants. *Photochem. Photobiol.* **24**: 237–242.

PEREYRA, A. J. (1971) The relationship of sexual activity to cervical cancer. *Obstet. Gynec.* **17**: 154–159.

PIETTE, J., CALBERG-BACQ, C. M. and VAN DE VORST, A. (1978) Photodynamic effect of proflavine on ϕ X 174 bacteriophage, its DNA replicative form and its isolated single-stranded DNA: inactivation, mutagenesis and repair. *Mol. Gen. Genet.* **167**: 95–103.

PIETTE, J., CALBERG-BACQ, C. M. and VAN DE VORST, A. (1979) Production of breaks in single and double stranded forms of bacteriophage ϕ X 174 DNA by proflavine and light treatment. *Photochem. Photobiol.* **30**: 369–378.

PIETTE, J., CALBERG-BACQ, C. M. and VAN DE VORST, A. (1981) Alteration of guanine residues during proflavine mediated photosensitization of DNA. *Photochem. Photobiol.* **33**: 325–333.

POLLOCK, E. J. and TODARO, G. J. (1968) Radiation enhancement of SV40 transformation in 3T3 and human cells. *Nature, Lond.* **219**: 520–521.

PRITCHARD, N. J., BLAKE, A. and PEACOCKE, A. R. (1966) Modified intercalation model for the interaction of amino acridines and DNA. *Nature, Lond.* **212**: 1260–1361.

RAMADAN-TALIB, Z. and PREBBLE, J. (1978) Photosensitivity of respiration in *Neurospora* mitochondria. A protective role for carotenoid. *Biochem. J.* **176**: 767–775.

RAPP, F. and KEMENY, B. A. (1977) Oncogenic potential of herpes simplex virus in mammalian cells following photodynamic inactivation. *Photochem. Photobiol.* **25**: 335–337.

RAPP, F., LI, J. H. and JERKOFSKY, M. (1973) Transformation of mammalian cells by DNA-containing viruses following photodynamic inactivation. *Virology* **55**: 339–346.

RAWLS, W. E., TOMPKINS, W. A. and FIGUEROA, M. E. (1968) Herpesvirus type 2: association with carcinoma of the cervix. *Science* **161**: 1255–1256.

RAWLS, W. E., TOMPKINS, W. A. and MELNICK, J. L. (1969) The association of herpesvirus type 2 and carcinoma of the uterine cervix. *Am. J. Epid.* **89**: 547–554.

RAWLS, H. R. and VAN SANTEN, P. J. (1970) Singlet oxygen and the initiation of fatty acid autoxidation. *J. Am. Oil Chem. Soc.* **47**: 121–125.

RAY, W. J., Jr. and KOSHLAND, D. E., Jr. (1962) Identification of amino acids involved in phospho-glucomutase activity. *J. Biol. Chem.* **237**: 2493–2505.

REDFIELD, D. C., RICHMAN, D. D., OXMAN, M. N. and KRONENBERG, L. H. (1981) Psoralen inactivation of influenza and herpes simplex viruses and of virus-infected cells. *Infect. Immun.* **32**: 1216–1226.

REED, C. L. and RAPP, F. (1976) Induction of murine p30 by superinfecting herpes viruses. *J. Virol.* **19**: 1028–1033.

REGAN, J. D. and SETLOW, R. B. (1977) The effect of proflavin plus visible light on the DNA of human cells. *Photochem. Photobiol.* **5**: 345–346.

RIZZUTO, F. and SPIKES, J. D. (1977) The eosin-sensitized photooxidation of substituted phenylalanines and tyrosines. *Photochem. Photobiol.* **25**: 465–476.

ROBERTS, J. E. (1981a) The effects of photooxidation by proflavine on Hela cells—I. The molecular mechanism. *Photochem. Photobiol.* **33**: 55–59.

ROBERTS, J. E. (1981b) The effects of photooxidation proflavine on Hela cells—II. Damage to DNA. *Photochem. Photobiol.* **33**: 61–64.

ROIZMAN, B., SPEAR, P. G. and KIEFF, E. D. (1972) Herpes simplex viruses I and II: a biochemical definition. In: *Persistent Virus Infections – Perspectives in Virology*, pp. 129–169. POLLARD, M. (ed.). (Vol. VIII) Academic Press, New York.

ROOME, A. P., TINKLER, A. E., HILTON, A. L., MONTEFIORE, D. G. and WALLER, D. (1975) Neutral red with photoinactivation in the treatment of herpes genitalis. *Br. J. Vener. Dis.* **51**: 130–133.

ROSENBLUM, L. A., HOSKWITH, B. and KRAMER, S. D. (1937) Photodynamic action of methylene blue on poliomyelitis virus. *Proc. Soc. Exp. Biol. Med.* **37**: 166–169.

ROTHSCHILD, H. and BLACK, P. H. (1970) Analysis of SV40-induced transformation of hamster kidney tissue *in vitro*. VII. Induction of SV40 virus from transformed hamster cell clones by various agents. *Virology* **42**: 251–256.

ROTKIN, I. P. (1973) A comparison review of key epidemiological studies in cervical cancer related to current searches for transmissable agents. *Cancer Res.* **33**: 1353–1367.

ROWE, W. P., HARTLEY, J. W., LANDER, M. R., PUGH, W. E. and TEICH, N. (1971) Noninfectious AKR mouse embryo cell lines in which each cell has the capacity to be activated to produce infectious murine leukemia virus. *Virology* **46**: 866–876.

ROYSTON, I. and AURELIAN, L. (1970) Immunofluorescent detection of herpesvirus antigens in exfoliated cells from human cervical carcinoma. *Proc. natn. Acad. Sci. USA* **67**: 204–212.

SABIN, A. and KOCH, M. A. (1963) Behavior of noninfectious SV40 viral genome in hamster tumor cells: Induction of synthesis of infectious virus. *Proc. natn. Acad. Sci. USA* **50**: 407–417.

SABIN, A. and TARRO, G. (1973) Herpes simplex and herpes genitalis viruses in etiology of some human cancers. *Proc. natn. Acad. Sci. USA* **70**: 3225–3229.

SANTAMARIA, L., BIANCHI, A., ARNABOLDI, A. and DAFFARA, P. (1980) Photocarcinogenesis by methoxypsoralen, neutral red and proflavine. Possible implications in photochemotherapy. *Medecine Biologie Environnement* **8**: 171–181.

SASTRY, K. S. and GORDON, M. P. (1966) The photosensitized degradation of guanosine by acridine orange. *Biochim. Biophys. Acta* **129**: 42–48.

SCHAFFER, F. L. (1962) Binding of proflavine by and photoinactivation of poliovirus propagated in the presence of the dye. *Virology* **18**: 412–425.

SCHELL, K., MARYAK, J., YOUNG, J. and SCHMIDT, M. (1968) Adenovirus transformation of hamster embryo cells. II. Inoculation conditions. *Arch. ges. Virusforsch.* **24**: 342–351.

SCHENCK, G. O., BECKER, H-D., SCHULTE-ELTE, K-H. and KRAUCH, C. H. (1963) Mit Benzophenon photosensibilisierte Autoxydation von sek. Alkoholen und Äthern. Darstellung von α-Hydroperoxyden. *Chem. Ber.* **96**: 509–516.

SCHNEIDER, J. and ROHDE, B. (1972) Zur Antigentherapie des rezidivierenden herpes simplex mit dem herpes simplex Impfstoff lupidon H and G. *Z. Haut–u. GeschlKrankh.* **47**: (24): 973–980.

SCHULTZ, E. W. and KRUEGER, A. P. (1930) Inactivation of staphylococcus bacteriophage by methylene blue. *Proc. Soc. Exp. Biol. Med.* **26**: 100–101.

SCOTT, B. R., PATHAK, M. A. and MOHN, G. R. (1976) Molecular and genetic basis of furocoumarin reactions. *Mutat. Res.* **39**: 29–74.

SCOTT, T. F. (1957) Epidemiology of herpetic infections. *Am. J. Ophthal.* **43**: 134–147.

SCOTT, T. F. and TOKUMARU, T. (1965) The herpesvirus group. In: *Viral and Rickettsial Infections of Man*, pp. 892–1000. HORSFALL, F. L. and TAMM, I. (eds.). (4th edn.) J. B. Lippincott Co., Philadelphia.

SCRIBA, M. (1977) Protection of guinea pigs against primary and recurrent herpes simplex virus (HSV) infection by live and killed herpes vaccines. Abstract, Third International Symposium on Oncogenesis and Herpesviruses, Cambridge, Mass., 25–29 July.

SEEMAYER, N. H. and DEFENDI, V. (1973) Analysis of minimal functions of simian virus 40. II. Enhancement of oncogenic transformation *in vitro* by UV irradiation. *J. Virol.* **12**: 1265–1271.

SEGAL, R. J. and WATSON, W. (1978) Kaposi's varicelliform eruption in mycosis fungoides. *Arch. Dermatol.* **114**: 1067–1069.

SHIMIZU, M., EGASHIRA, T. and TAKAHAMA, U. (1979) Inactivation of *Neurospora crassa* conidia by singlet molecular oxygen generated by a photosensitized reaction. *J. Bacteriol.* **138**: 293–296.

SHIMIZU-TAKAHAMA, M., EGASHIRA, T. and TAKAHAMA, U. (1981) Inhibition of respiration and loss of membrane integrity by singlet oxygen generated by a photosensitized reaction in *Neurospora crassa* conidia. *Photochem. Photobiol.* **33**: 689–694.

SIMON, M. I. and VANVUNAKIS, H. (1962) The photodynamic reaction of methylene blue with deoxyribonucleic acid. *J. Molec. Biol.* **4**: 488–499.

SIMON, M. I., GROSSMAN, L. and VANVUNAKIS, H. (1965) The photosensitized reaction of polyribonucleotides I. Effects on their susceptibility to enzyme digestion and their ability to act as synthetic messengers. *J. Molec. Biol.* **12**: 50–59.

SINKOVICS, J. G., BERTIN, B. A. and HOWE, C. D. (1965) Some properties of the photodynamically inactivated rauscher mouse leukemia virus. *Cancer Res.* **25**: 624–627.

SMITH, C. C., AURELIAN, L., GUPTA, P. K., FROST, J. K., ROSENSHEIN, N. B., KLACSMANN, K. and GEDDES, S. (1980) An evaluation of herpes simplex virus antigenic markers in the study of established and developing cervical neoplasia. *Anal. Quant. Cytol.* **2**: 131–143.

SMITH, J. W., TORRES, J. and HOLMQUIST, N. (1977) Cellular immunity to HSV-1 and HSV-2 in women with invasive carcinoma of the cervix. Abstract, Third International Symposium on Oncogenesis and Herpesviruses, Cambridge, Mass., 25–29 July.

SMITH, J. W., TORRES, J. E. and HOLMQUIST, N. D. (1979) Association of herpes simplex virus (HSV) with cervical cancer by lymphocyte reactivity with HSV-1 and HSV-2 antigens. *Am. J. Epidemiol.* **110**: 141–147.

SMITH, J. W., TORRES, J. E. and HOLMQUIST, N. D. (1981) Herpes simplex virus type 2 and human cervical cancer: relationship between cellular and immune assays for the detection of previous infection. *J. Natn. Cancer Inst.* **66**: 1031–1036.

SMITH, K. C. (1962) Dose dependent decrease in extractability of DNA from bacteria following irradiation with ultraviolet or with visible light plus dye. *Biochem. Biophys. Res. Commun.* **8**: 157–163.

SMITH, K. C. and HANAWALT, P. C. (1969) *Molecular Photobiology, Inactivation and Recovery*. Academic Press, New York.

SNIPES, W., KELLER, G., WOOG, J., VICKROY, T., DEERING, R. and KEITH, A. (1979) Inactivation of lipids containing viruses by hydrophobic photosensitizers and near-ultraviolet radiation. *Photochem. Photobiol.*, pp. 785–790.

SNIPES, W., VICKROY, T., WOOG, J. and DEERING, R. A. (1977) Inactivation of enveloped viruses by photosensitized membrane damage. Abstract Ei-2, 25th Radiation Research Meeting, San Juan, Puerto Rico, 8–12 May.

SPECK, W. T., CHEN, C. C. and ROSENKRANZ, H. S. (1973) *In vitro* studies of effects of light and riboflavin on DNA and Hela cells. *Pediat. Res.* **9**: 150–153.

SPECK, W. T., SANTELLA, R. M., BREM, S. and ROSENKRANZ, H. S. (1979) Alteration of human cellular DNA by neutral red in the presence of visible light. *Mutat. Res.* **66**: 95–98.

SPIKES, J. D. (1968) Photodynamic action. In: *Photophysiology*, pp. 33–64, Vol. 3. GIESE, A. C. (ed.). Academic Press, New York.

SPIKES, J. D. (1975) Porphyrins and related compounds as photodynamic sensitizers. *Ann. N.Y. Acad. Sci.* **244**: 496–508.

SPIKES, J. D. (1977) Kinetics of the Eosin Y sensitized photooxidation of substituted uracils. *Abstr. Am. Soc. Photobiol.* **5**: 47.

SPIKES, J. D. and GHIRON, C. A. (1964) Photodynamic effects in biological systems. In: *Physical Processes in Radiation Biology*, pp. 309–338, AUGENSTEIN, L. G., MASON, R. and ROSENBERG, B. (eds.). Academic Press, New York.

SPIKES, J. D. and LIVINGSTON, R. (1969) The molecular biology of photodynamic action: sensitized photoautoxidations in biological systems. *Adv. Radiat. Biol.* **3**: 29–121.

SPIKES, J. D. and MACKNIGHT, M. L. (1971) Dye-sensitized photooxidation of proteins. *Ann. N.Y. Acad. Sci.* **171**: 149–161.

SPIKES, J. D. and STRAIGHT, R. (1967) Sensitized photochemical processes in biological systems. *Am. Rev. Phys. Chem.* **18**: 409–435.

SPRECHER-GOLDBERGER, S., THIRY, L. and CATTOOR, J. P. (1970) Herpesvirus type 2 infection and carcinoma of the cervix. *Lancet* **2**: 266.

STERN, R. S., THIBODEAU, L. A., KLEINERMAN, R. A., PARRISH, J. A. and FITZPATRICK, T. B. (1979) Risk of cutaneous carcinoma in patients treated with oral methoxalen photochemotherapy for psoriasis. *N. Engl. J. Med.* **300**: 809–813.

STEWART, S. E., KASNIC, G., DRAYCOTT, C. and BEN, T. (1972a) Activation of viruses in human tumors by 5-iododeoxyuridine and dimethyl sulfoxide. *Science* **175**: 198–199.

STEWART, S. E., KASNIC, G., DRAYCOTT, C., FELLER, W., GOLDEN, A., MITCHELL, E. and BEN, T. (1972b) Activation *in vitro*, by 5-iododeoxyuridine, of a latent virus resembling C-type virus in a human sarcoma cell line. *J. Natn. Cancer Inst.* **48**: 273–277.

STOKER, M. (1963) Effect of x-irradiation on susceptibility of cells to transformation by polyoma virus. *Nature, Lond.* **200**: 756–758.

SUSSENBACH, J. S. and BERNEDS, W. (1965) Photodynamic degradation of guanine. *Biochim. Biophys. Acta* **95**: 184–185.

SYSAK, P. K., FOOTE, C. S. and CHING, T. Y. (1977) Chemistry of singlet Oxygen-XXV. photooxygenation of methionine. *Photochem. Photobiol.* **26**: 19–27.

TANO, Y., KINOSHITA, S., KISHIDA, K., HARA, J., SATO, K. and MANABE, R. (1977) Photodynamic inactivation of herpes simplex virus. *Jpn. J. Ophthalmol.* **21**: 392–398.

TAYLOR, P. K. and DOHERTY, N. R. (1975) Comparison of the treatment of herpes genitalis in men with proflavine photoinactivation, idoxuridine ointment, and normal saline. *Br. J. Vener. Dis.* **51**: 125–129.

TEICH, N., LOWRY, D. R., HARTLEY, J. W. and ROWE, W. P. (1973) Studies of the mechanism of induction of infectious murine leukemia virus from ADR mouse embryo cell lines by 5-iododeoxyuridine and 5-bromodeoxyuridine. *Virology* **51**: 163–173.

TERRIS, M., WILSON, F. and SMITH, H. (1967) Epidemiology of cancer of the cervix. V. The relationship of coitus to carcinoma of the cervix. *Am. J. Publ. Hlth.* **57**: 840–847.

THIRY, L., SPRECHER-GOLDBERGER, S., FASSIN, Y., GOULD, I., GOMPEL, C., PESTIAU, J. and DEHALLEUX, F. (1974) Variations of cytotoxic antibodies to cells with herpes simplex virus antigens in women with progressing or regressing cancerous lesions of the cervix. *Am. J. Epid.* **100**: 251–261.

THOMAS, S. A., SARGENT, M. A. and TUVESON, R. W. (1981) Inactivation of normal and mutant *Neurospora crassa* conidia by visible light and near-UV: role of $^1O_2$, carotenoid composition and sensitizer location. *Photochem. Photobiol.* **33**: 349–354.

THYGESON, P., HOGAN, M. J. and KIMURA, S. J. (1953) Cortisone and hydrocortisone in ocular infections. *Trans. Am. Acad. Ophthal. Oto-lar.* **57**: 64–85.

TODARO, G. J. and GREEN, H. (1964) Enhancement by thymine analogs of susceptibility of cells to transformation by SV40. *Virology* **24**: 393–400.

TOMITA, Y. and PRINCE, A. M. (1963) Photodynamic inactivation of arbor viruses by neutral red and visible light. *Proc. Soc. Exp. Biol. Med.* **112**: 887–890.

TOOZE, J. (1973) *The Molecular Biology of Tumor Viruses*. Cold Spring Harbor Monograph Series, Cold Spring Harbor Lab., pp. 470–495, Cold Spring Harbor, New York.

TOYOSHIMA, K., FRIIS, R. R. and VOGT, P. K. (1970) The reproductive and cell-transforming capacities of avian sarcoma virus B77: inactivation with UV light. *Virology* **42**: 163–170.

TRIEBEL, H., BAR, H., JACOB, H. E., SARFERT, E. and BERG, H. (1978) Sedimentation analysis of DNA photooxidized in the presence of thiopyronine. *Photochem. Photobiol.* **28**: 331–337.

TROSKO, J. E. and ISOUN, M. J. (1971) Photosensitizing effect of tresoralen on DNA synthesis in human cells grown in vitro. *J. Radiat. Biol.* **19**: 87–92.

UEHARA, K., MIZOGUCHI, T. and OKADA, Y. (1964) Photooxidation of adenine and its nucleotides in the presence of riboflavin. *J. Biochem., Tokyo* **55**: 685–687.

WACKER, A., DELLWEG, H., TRAGER, L., KORNHAUSER, A., LODEMANN, E., TURCH, G., SELZER, R., CHANDRA, P. and ISHIMOTO, M. (1964) Organic photochemistry of nucleic acids. *Photochem. Photobiol.* **3**: 369–394.

WAGNER, S., TAYLOR, W. D., KEITH, A. and SNIPES, W. (1980) Effects of acridine plus near ultraviolet light on *Escherichia coli* membranes and DNA *in vivo*. *Photochem. Photobiol.* **32**: 771–779.

WAKAYAMA, Y., TAKAGI, M. and YANO, K. (1980) Photosensitized inactivation of *E. coli* cells in toluidine blue-light system. *Photochem. Photobiol.* **32**: 601–605.

WALLIS, C. and MELNICK, J. L. (1963) Photodynamic inactivation of poliovirus. *Virology* **21**: 332–341.

WALLIS, C. and MELNICK, J. L. (1964) Irreversible photosensitization of viruses. *Virology* **23**: 520–527.

WALLIS, C. and MELNICK, J. L. (1965) Photodynamic inactivation of animal viruses: A review. *Photochem. Photobiol.* **4**: 159–170.

WALLIS, C., SCHEIRIS, C. and MELNICK, J. L. (1967) Photodynamically inactivated vaccines prepared by growing viruses in cells containing neutral red. *J. Immun.* **99**: 1134–1139.

WALZ, M. A., PRICE, R. W., HAYAFHI, K., KATZ, B. J. and NOTKINS, A. L. (1977) Effect of immunization on acute and latent infections of vaginouterine tissue with herpes simplex virus types 1 and 2. *J. Infect. Dis.* **135**: 744–752.

WASKELL, L. A., SASTRY, K. S. and GORDON, M. P. (1966) Studies on the photosensitized breakdown of guanosine by methylene blue. *Biochim. Biophys. Acta* **129**: 49–53.

WEBB, R. B. and KUBITSCHEK, H. E. (1963) Mutagenic and antimutagenic effects of acridine orange in *Escherichia coli. Biochem. Biophys. Res. Commun.* **13**: 90–94.

WEBB, R. B., HASS, B. S. and KUBITSCHEK, H. E. (1979) Photodynamic effects of dyes on bacteria II. Genetic effects of broad-spectrum visible light in the presence of acridine dyes and methylene blue in chemostat cultures of *Escherichia coli. Mutat. Res.* **59**: 1–13.

WEBER, G. (1976) Effects and side-effects of 8-methoxypsoralen-black-light-therapy in more than 1500 patients. *Brit. J. Derm.* **95**: 21.

WEISS, R. A., FRIIS, R. R., KATZ, E. and VOGT, P. K. (1971) Induction of avian tumor viruses in normal cells by physical and chemical carcinogens. *Virology* **46**: 920–938.

WILSON, T. J. (1966) Excited singlet molecular oxygen in photooxidation. *J. Am. Chem. Soc.* **88**: 2898–2902.

WOLFE, L. G., FALK, L. A. and DIENHARDT, F. (1971) Oncogenicity of herpesvirus saimiri in marmoset monkeys. *J. Natn. Cancer Inst.* **47**: 1145–1162.

WOLFF, K., FITZPATRICK, T. B., PARRISH, J. A., GSCHNAIT, F., GILCHREST, B., HONIGSMANN, H., PATHAK, M. A. and TANENBAUM, L. (1976) Photochemotherapy for psoriasis with orally administered methoxalen. *Archs. Derm.* **112**: 943–950.

YAMAGATA, S., TAKAHASHI, K. and EGAMI, F. (1962) The structure and function of ribonuclease T_1. II. The photooxidation of ribonuclease T_1. *J. Biochem., Tokyo* **52**: 261–271.

YAMAMOTO, N. (1958) Photodynamic inactivation of bacteriophage and its inhibition. *J. Bact.* **75**: 443–448.

YAROSH, D. B., JOHNS, V., MUFTI, S., BERNSTEIN, C. and BERNSTEIN, H. (1980) Inhibition of UV and psoralen-plus-light mutagenesis in phage T4 by gene 43 antimutator polymerase alleles. *Photochem. Photobiol.* **31**: 341–350.

ZAMPIERI, A. and GREENBERG, J. (1965) Mutagenesis by acridine orange and proflavine in *Escherichia coli* strain S. *Mutat. Res.* **2**: 552–556.

CHAPTER 13

IMMUNOPOTENTIATING SUBSTANCES WITH ANTIVIRAL ACTIVITY

GEORGES H. WERNER and AURELIO ZERIAL

Département d'Immunologie, Cancérologie et Virologie, Centre Nicolas Grillet,
Rhone-Poulenc Recherches, 94400 Vitry-sur-Seine, France

CONTENTS

13.1. INTRODUCTION

A purposeful struggle against virus diseases of man and domestic animals began almost two centuries ago with Jenner's discovery that inoculation of cowpox to humans made them immune to smallpox. Since that time, through the combined efforts of virologists and immunologists – two scientific disciplines which, until recently, represented a common field of endeavour – effective vaccines have been found against yellow fever, poliomyelitis, influenza, measles, mumps, rubella and rabies while vaccination against hepatitis B, adenovirus, respiratory syncytial virus, cytomegalovirus and varicella virus infections will most likely become a reality before long. In the veterinary field, effective vaccines are used against a number of economically important diseases of cattle, swine and poultry. By comparison with these achievements of specific vaccination, those of antiviral chemotherapy – an area in which intensive work started about 30 years ago – are quite modest indeed, since only a handful of drugs have been shown to exert prophylactic and/or therapeutic activity on poxvirus, herpes virus and influenza virus infections (Table 1). At the present stage, neither vaccines nor antiviral agents show broad spectrum efficacy: in the case of vaccines, their high specificity was to be expected from their very design; it was less obvious for antiviral chemotherapy, although it was reasonable to infer from the diverse mechanisms of viral replication that it would be hard to find inhibitors which might, at the same time, be highly active on many possible viral processes and nontoxic to the host cells at effective antiviral doses. At that point, one may ask whether interferon does not provide an

TABLE 1. *Viral Vaccines versus Antiviral Chemotherapy*

Year first described	Vaccines in present use	Antiviral drugs in present use
1798	Smallpcx (vaccinia)	
1885	Rabies	
1937	Yellow fever	
1940	Influenza	
1954	Poliomyelitis (inactivated)	
1956	Dengue	
1957	Poliomyelitis (live)	
1959	Mumps	
1960	Measles	1960 Methisazone (a)
		1961 Idoxuridine (b)
1966	Rubella	1963 Vidarabine
	Adenoviruses	(ara-A) (b)
1970	Japanese encephalitis	1964 Amantadine (c)
1971	Hepatitis B	1965 Rimantadine (c)
1974	Chickenpox	1972 Ribavirin (d)
1978	Respiratory syncytial virus*	1977 Bromovinyl-deoxyuridine (b)*
1979	Cytomegalovirus*	1977 Acyclovir (b)
		1978 Sodium phosphonoformate (b)*

* Under investigation in man.
(a) Poxvirus infections. (b) Herpesviruses. (c) Influenza A. (d) Relatively broad-spectrum.

example of a broad spectrum antiviral substance and indeed, in spite of uncertainties about the future of its therapeutic applications, this natural inhibitor appears much less limited in its scope than the synthetic antiviral substances. One must recall that the discovery of interferon in 1957 by Isaacs and Lindenmann was the outcome of investigations on the phenomenon of interference between viruses, which is readily demonstrable in experimental systems but also certainly takes place in nature. One may thus wonder whether one could not fruitfully exploit towards nonspecific prophylactic and/or therapeutic applications the various mechanisms which underlie natural resistance to and recovery from virus infections (Lagrange, 1977): such an attempt, which was systematically initiated about a decade ago, is the subject of the present review. It will first be necessary to summarize our present knowledge about immunity in viral infections, especially with respect to the immunological mechanisms of recovery from such infections; we shall then review the available evidence according to which one can experimentally enhance the host's resistance against viral infections in a nonspecific manner through the use of various so-called immunopotentiating or immunomodulating substances and, finally, we shall try to speculate about the possible applications of such manipulations to human or veterinary medicine, with regard to what is known about the immunopathology of virus infections and against the background of what has already been achieved through specific vaccinations.

13.2. IMMUNITY IN VIRAL INFECTIONS

For the purpose of this review, it is important to distinguish between natural and acquired resistance to virus infections and also between resistance to and recovery from such infections: using immunomodulating agents, one may wish to increase the host's relative resistance, by lifting the threshold of infection which is necessary to cause overt disease, but one may also attempt to improve the acquisition of specific resistance by supplementing vaccines with suitable adjuvants; finally, the most important objective may well be to find ways of improving on those nonspecific and specific mechanisms which, under natural circumstances, result finally in the recovery of the host, after a more or less severe and prolonged illness. The mechanisms of natural and acquired resistance and those of spontaneous recovery do have much in common and the drugs capable of exerting such activities may finally turn out to be similar, but the experimental approaches to their discovery and the conditions of their uses will be different.

Natural resistance of animals to a given virus infection, in the absence of any previous experience with this virus or with an antigenically related agent, may be absolute or relative. Immunity has nothing to do with the fact that it is not possible to infect chickens with poliomyelitis viruses or mice with human rhinoviruses and this species resistance manifests itself at the cellular level (except when infectious nucleic acids can be artificially introduced into the cells of the resistant species): beside classes of viruses which are capable of infecting several animal species, there are a number of others which are strictly species-specific in their infectivity, although they may be closely related in other respects, a fact which can be best explained by evolutionary mechanisms (see, for instance, measles virus in humans, canine distemper in dogs and rinderpest in cattle). Mechanical or physical barriers also play an important role: a given species will not be infected by a virus if its physiological body temperature lies well below or above the temperature range at which this virus can replicate. Much more important for our purpose is the relative resistance to viral infection which, within the same animal species or population, varies from one individual or subgroup to another and will manifest itself in significant differences with respect to illness rate or severity. The mechanisms of specific acquired resistance to virus infections will be discussed later; we are dealing here with nonspecific resistance, independent of previous experience with a given virus and, inasmuch as this relative resistance will enable the host to go through a particular virus infection without apparent illness or with minimal symptoms, it is clear that the mechanisms of such resistance may be in many ways similar to those which operate in the spontaneous recovery from a viral disease.

Genetic factors play a role in the resistance to virus infections as do other factors such as age, nutrition, sex, hormonal influences. In man, it is difficult to determine the relative importance of these factors: for instance, the fact that in black Africa measles is a highly lethal disease (mortality up to 5 per cent) may be due to racial factors but also to severe malnutrition (protein deficiency). At any rate, these various factors influencing resistance to viral (and other) infections cannot be dismissed as being entirely nonimmunological in nature: very young animals are more susceptible but this parallels their immunological immaturity, and gross protein deficiency is known to exert a suppressive effect on some immune reactions. But even genetic differences in resistance to virus infections are expressed at the level of cells which are part of the immune system; for instance, genetic susceptibility to mouse hepatitis virus and its phenotypic alteration (induced by drugs and immune responses) respond in a parallel manner in the intact mouse and in *in vitro* cultures of its macrophages, which mirror the susceptibility of the host (Weiser and Bang, 1977): *in vitro*, genetically susceptible macrophages are converted into resistant cells by administration of concanavalin A and, *in vivo*, this lectin can prevent mortality in susceptible mice. Similarly, a strain of avian influenza A virus grows *in vitro* in the peritoneal macrophages of mouse lines which are susceptible *in vivo* to the lethal effect of a human influenza A virus and does not grow in the macrophages of mouse lines which naturally survive the latter infection (Lindenmann *et al.*, 1978). *In vitro* replication of herpes simplex virus (HSV) in murine spleen cells requires simultaneous stimulation with a B cell mitogen like lipopolysaccharide (LPS); spleen cells from C_3H/HeJ mice that do not respond to stimulation by LPS do not either support replication of HSV and, in addition, mice of that line are intrinsically resistant to HSV infection *in vivo* (Kirchner *et al.*, 1978). Mouse lines have been selected according to the intensity of their antibody responses to sheep red blood cells (Biozzi *et al.*, 1975); the low responders possess more 'active' macrophages (in terms of antigen processing) than do high responders. When these two lines were compared with respect to their relative resistance to a number of murine or mouse-adapted human viruses, it was found that the high responders were more resistant than the low responders to murine hepatitis, to herpes simplex and to AO influenza viruses, while the reverse was true with respect to encephalomyocarditis virus (Floc'h and Werner, 1978a): the genetic factors influencing the macrophage directly govern resistance or susceptibility to virus infections.

In strictly immunological terms, resistance against and recovery from virus infections is dependent, in vertebrates, on the three major types of immune response which have probably appeared in the following chronological order, in the course of their evolution: (a) a system based on the cells which mediate largely nonspecific effects of immune reactions, such cells comprising what was previously called the reticulo-endothelial system and is now more adequately designated as the mononuclear phagocyte system and which includes the marrow promonocytes, the blood monocytes and the macrophages (subcutaneous, alveolar, splenic and synovial macrophages, Kupffer cells) and to which should be added granulocytes and mast cells; (b) a system based on specialized sets of T lymphocytes, which, in a more or less broadly specific way, are capable among other functions of lysing virus-infected target cells by direct interaction with the latter; (c) a highly specific and refined system, based on B lymphocytes which produce equally specific antibodies, capable of neutralizing only those viruses against the antigens of which they have been sensitized (either in the course of infection, as a result of past experience or following active immunization). This is of course a grossly simplified picture of the situation, to which should be added, in order to visualize more completely the immunological orchestra which may be called to perform in the course of a virus infection, helper and suppressor T cells, delayed-type hypersensitivity (DTH) reactions, K and NK cells, complement and polymorphonuclear cells.

The role that the cells of the mononuclear phagocyte system, or, more briefly, the macrophages, play in the pathogenesis of virus infections and in protection against them is a very complex one, inasmuch as it is nonspecific. Macrophages are generally considered to be the first line of defense against viruses: they play, indeed, an important role in clearing viruses from the blood stream and preventing the infection of susceptible cells in target organs. Many viruses, however, far from being digested by the macrophages which ingest them, do multiply in these cells and infected monocytes may actually transport viruses around the body. It may be that the ability to grow or simply to reside in macrophages is a vital factor in the virulence of a given virus since, by infecting the macrophages, the virus produces a break in the body's major nonspecific defense mechanism. We were able to show, for example (Zerial and Werner, 1981), that i.p. injection of resident murine peritoneal cells which were infected *in vitro* with HSV-1 could cause lethality in recipient mice, even though the great majority of these cells were not permissive for virus growth. Roughly speaking, the macrophage can be pictured as an advanced fortress but also, at times, as a Trojan horse. The first feature epitomizes what happens in viral infections of the respiratory tract and of the alimentary tract as well as in viral infections of the skin, while obviously the macrophage barrier is at least partly ineffective in the infections usually marked by a viremic phase (such as the generalized infections with rash, those involving the central nervous system and the congenital infections). In fact, within the same species and in the face of the same virus infection, macrophages may be permissive or defensive: herpes simplex virus grows readily in the macrophages of newborn mice and causes their rapid death, while, in adult mice, the same peritoneal macrophages certainly act as barrier, as evidenced by the fact that specific killing of these cells with silica greatly increases the susceptibility of the adult animal to this infection and that transfer of adult macrophages to newborn mice enhances their resistance (Zisman *et al.*, 1970; Hirsch *et al.*, 1970). Indeed, a correlation between the antiviral resistance which develops in the course of the maturation of the host (age-related resistance) and a more restricted virus replication within macrophages from old mice, as compared to young ones, has been found in the case of HSV-1 (Hirsch *et al.*, 1970), HSV-2 (Mogensen, 1978; Mogensen and Anderson, 1978) and mouse hepatitis virus (Taguchi *et al.*, 1979). However, the resistance (or, respectively, the susceptibility) displayed by some strains of mice to a given virus infection (genetic resistance) cannot always be correlated with restriction (or permissivity) of virus growth within macrophages (Brautigan *et al.*, 1979; Lopez and Dumas, 1979; Mogensen, 1979; Taguchi *et al.*, 1981). As in genetic resistance, the mechanism of the antiviral activity of some immunostimulants (e.g. *C. parvum*) does not seem to involve a reduced permissivity of virus growth in macrophages from treated animals (Morse and Morahan, 1981; Zerial and Werner, 1981). Instead, the ability of activated macrophages to restrict virus growth in adjacent infected cells (extrinsic resistance) appears, in the context of immunostimulating agents, to be more important than the intrinsic resistance. Activated macrophages obtained from mice treated with immunostimulants such as pyran copolymer, BCG, *C. parvum* or thioglycollate-elicited peritoneal macrophages were found capable to reduce replication of HSV-2, EMC and vaccinia virus in infected cells (Morahan *et al.*, 1977a, 1980). Extrinsic antiviral resistance, which can be exerted on syngeneic, allogeneic or even xenogeneic cells, requires viable macrophages and does not appear to involve production of interferon (Morse and Morahan, 1981). Its mechanism, which is thought to be different from that of the intrinsic antiviral resistance (Morse and Morahan, 1981), and its role in the pathology of virus infections remain to be determined.

Besides the multifaceted and nonspecific functions of macrophages, it must also be mentioned that these cells can be 'activated' by lymphocytes or 'armed' with specific antibody, although the role of such mechanisms in viral infections is still speculative; finally, the macrophages are among the cells which can produce interferon, as will be discussed later.

It is only recently that the role of cell-mediated immunity (CMI) in the pathogenesis of virus infections (and in resistance against or recovery from them) has been precisely analyzed. That viruses elicit CMI reactions could be inferred from the delayed type hypersensitivity (DTH) reactions which follow intradermal injection of various viral antigens (vaccinia, mumps, for instance) into a previously infected host. T cell-mediated immunity can be abrogated in mice by neonatal thymectomy or treatment with anti-thymocytic globulin: such manipulations aggravate infections of mice with pox- and herpes viruses but show little effect on entero- or togavirus infections and are even possibly beneficial in some cases. In man, some virus infections are particularly severe and frequent in congenital or acquired immunodeficiencies affecting T cells (see Table 2): vaccinia, measles, herpes simplex, varicella-zoster, cytomegalovirus, while congenital or acquired immuno-deficiencies affecting antibody production aggravate infections with poliovirus (attenuated strains, nonvirulent for immunologically normal subjects) or hepatitis B. T cell response to virus infection manifests itself by DTH reactions but also by the appearance of sensitized lymphocytes which are capable of selectively lysing the cells which are bearing the viral antigens on their surface (Blanden, 1974). Available evidence suggests that, at least in the mouse, the class of T cells which is responsible for initiating mechanisms of viral clearance *in vivo* is the same as that which is directly cytotoxic for virus-infected target cells *in vitro*. Furthermore, it was shown that cytotoxic T cells generated in response to lymphocytic choriomeningitis virus (LCM) infection in the mouse can efficiently lyse LCM-infected target cells only when the latter share the H-2 K or H-2 D region determinants (of the murine histocompatibility complex) with the donors of these cytotoxic cells (Doherty *et al.*, 1974; Zinkernagel and Welsh, 1976). One explanation for this important restriction phenomenon would be that cytotoxic T cells express two distinct receptors, one specific for self (H-2) the

TABLE 2. *Viral Diseases Affecting (with Unusual Frequency and/or Severity) Patients Presenting Congenital or Acquired Immunodeficiencies*

| Syndrome or disease | Defect in | | Viral infections |
	HI*	CMI†	
Congenital:			
Severe combined immunodeficiency	+	+	Vaccinia, measles, V–Z,‡ adenovirus
Wiskott-Aldrich	+	+	Measles, V–Z, herpes simplex, cytomegalovirus
Thymic dysplasia	+	+	
(Swiss type)			Vaccinia, measles,
(Di George)	–	+	cytomegalovirus
Hypogammaglobulinemia	+	–	Paralytic poliomyelitis, persistent entero-virus infection
Acquired:			
Leukemia	+	+	Measles, cytomegalovirus, hepatitis B
Hodgkin	–	+	V–Z, herpes simplex, cytomegalovirus
Non-Hodgkin lymphomas	+	+	V–Z, vaccinia
Immunosuppressive chemotherapy	+	+	Measles, V–Z, herpes simplex, cytomegalovirus

* HI: Humoral immunity.
† CMI: Cell-mediated immunity.
‡ V–Z: Varicella-Zoster.

other for nonself (virus) antigen, but it could also be that these cells possess receptors which are specific for the 'altered self' antigen produced by the interaction of virus and H-2 molecules. Cytotoxic T-cell responses have been shown to occur in the following acute viral infections of mice: Sindbis and Semliki Forest alphaviruses, ectromelia and vaccinia (poxviruses), Sendai paramyxovirus, influenza (orthomyxovirus), rabies (rhabdovirus), Coxsackie (enterovirus), adenoviruses, and, of course, LCM (see review by Blanden, 1977); in all these cases, the peak cytotoxic T cell response was observed from 5 to 9 days after infection, i.e. before production of circulating neutralizing antibody and shortly before activation of macrophages by products from sensitized lymphocytes. Mice infected with herpes simplex virus or murine cytomegalovirus develop weak and variable cytotoxic T cell responses. It has been shown, however, that high levels of H_2-restricted virus-specific cytotoxic cells could be induced in cultures of lymph node cells (Pfizenmaier *et al.*, 1977) or spleen cells (Lawman *et al.*, 1980; Rouse and Lawman, 1980; Eberle *et al.*, 1981; Ho, 1981; Schmid *et al.*, 1981) obtained from virus-primed mice, upon secondary stimulation with herpes simplex – or murine cytomegalovirus-infected cells. Transfer of CMV-specific cytotoxic T lymphocytes, as generated *in vitro*, was found capable of reducing virus titers in the spleens of recipient mice, previously (1 day before) infected with CMV.

It is reasonable to assume that the CTL* generated during the 5 to 9 days which follow virus inoculation in a mouse exert a favorable influence on recovery by the fact that they destroy virus-infected cells before infectious virus progeny is actually assembled (Zinkernagel and Althage, 1977), thereby preparing their elimination by macrophages; indeed, peak activity of CTL in the spleen coincides in time with a rapid decline of infectious virus titer in the same organ (Blanden and Gardner, 1976) and this was also shown to occur with respect to respiratory infection of mice with the Sendai strain of paramyxovirus (Anderson *et al.*, 1977). More direct evidence on the role of CTL in natural recovery has been brought recently by the demonstration (Yap *et al.*, 1978) that transfer of specific cytotoxic T lymphocytes protects mice from death following intranasal inoculation of a virulent strain of influenza A virus: there was a striking correlation between the level of cytotoxic activity of injected immune spleen cells and the capacity of the latter to protect the recipient mice from death. Spleen cell suspensions with the highest cytotoxic activity actually gave complete protection. Comparative analysis of the pathology of influenza pneumonia in athymic (nude) and normal mice has revealed that nude mice, as compared to normal ones, experience higher mortality, longer persistence of virus in the lung and no cytotoxic T cell response to influenza virus (Wells *et al.*, 1981a). Recovery of nude mice from influenza infection and ultimate resolution of pneumonia could be obtained by passive i.v. transfer of virus-specific cytotoxic T cells, without concomitant enhancement of the humoral antibody response (Wells *et al.*, 1981b). Indirect evidence also favors an important role of CTL in resistance to and recovery from influenza A virus infection in the mouse: T cells cytotoxic to influenza virus-infected cells occur in the course of a primary immune response to influenza virus and, while exhibiting H-2 restriction, these cells have a broad specificity for viral determinants, since T cells generated against one strain of influenza virus can lyse cells infected with another A strain containing serologically distinct surface antigens (hemagglutinin and neuraminidase) (Effros *et al.*, 1977; Zweerink *et al.*, 1977). It so happens that mice inoculated with live A influenza viruses by a nonlethal route exhibit subsequently a marked resistance against respiratory challenge with a normally lethal dose of another A strain, differing from the first one by both surface antigens and that this state of heterotypic immunity begins 5 days after parenteral inoculation of the first virus, i.e. at the time when it is known that broadly specific CTL appear in the spleen (Floc'h and Werner, 1978b). It must also be stressed that, in this model, delayed type hypersensibility reactions to the whole virions were equally cross-reactive.

It is important to note that after recovery from a virus infection, the cytotoxic T cells which survive, after having disseminated through foci of infection, become part of the small T lymphocyte pool which carries immunological memory; the importance of CTL memory in

---

* CTL: cytotoxic T lymphocytes.

resisting secondary infection is still speculative but it would seem to be a significant factor in all cases where viruses escape neutralization by antibody on route from the portal of entry to target organs (Blanden, 1977).

On the other hand, in several virus infections it is clear that the immune response itself is a major factor in causing some pathological changes. A pertinent example is provided by lymphocytic choriomeningitis (LCM) in adult mice: the cell-mediated response, and particularly the CTL, is both beneficial by clearing virus from lung, liver and spleen and detrimental in causing lethal inflammatory reactions in the brain. CTL can be isolated from the spinal fluid of moribund mice and transfer of such cells can induce lesions in the choroid plexus and meninges. In man, one may suspect that encephalitis caused by arenaviruses results largely from the destruction of infected cells by CTL. On the other hand, it is reasonable to assume that in measles and other exanthematous diseases of childhood, CTL mechanisms are responsible for the recovery from the infection and also for the rash, which is one of the main symptoms of disease. Subjects with congenital or acquired immunodeficiencies at the T cell level may present atypical cases of measles, without rash but with growth of the virus in the lungs.

The CTL response, though probably quite important both in the recovery from and resistance to virus infections and in some aspects of the immunopathology of such infections, is certainly not the only compartment of cell-mediated immunity which comes into play. Sensitized T lymphocytes can liberate various lymphokines and thereby induce migration and specific activation of macrophages: such a mechanism has been clearly demonstrated in infections with nonviral intracellular organisms and deserves further study in the case of virus infections. Delayed-type hypersensitivity reactions have actually been detected following infection with practically all membrane-associated viruses so far studied (poxviruses, myxoviruses, herpesviruses, arenaviruses) and are seldom seen with nonmembrane-associated viruses (i.e. picornaviruses).

Natural killer (NK) cells are mononuclear cells which possess cytotoxic properties against tumor cells and virus-infected cells (see Welsh, 1978, 1981; Herbermann et al., 1979, for review). There is some evidence that, at least in the mouse, NK cells participate in the rejection process of transplanted tumors (Ojo, 1979; Karre et al., 1980; Talmadge et al., 1980; Hanna and Burton, 1981; Reid et al., 1981). Several functional aspects of NK cells suggest that they might be also involved in the resistance to virus infections.

First, endogenous NK cells lyse preferentially virus-infected rather than uninfected cells (Santoli et al., 1978; Ault and Weiner, 1979). Second, NK cell activity can be boosted, in vivo or in vitro, by a variety of substances, which are known to potentiate antiviral mechanisms of the host. These substances include interferon types I and II as well as interferon inducers such as tilorone, statolon, poly I:C, pyran copolymer, C. parvum, BCG, endotoxins and a multitude of infectious DNA and RNA viruses (Welsh, 1978, 1981; Djeu et al., 1979; Ojo, 1979; Tracey, 1979; Senik et al., 1980). Activation of NK cells has also been described, however, with products which apparently do not induce interferon, such as doxorubicin (Santoni et al., 1980), FTS (facteur thymique sérique, thymuline) (Bardos et al., 1979) and mumps glycoproteins (Harfast et al., 1980). Activation of NK cells, which in the case of interferon inducers appears to be mediated by macrophages (Djeu et al., 1979; Tracey, 1979), is, however, accompanied by a loss of specificity: cells, even primary fibroblast cultures, which are rather insensitive to endogenous NK activity, may become targets of activated NK cells (McFarland et al., 1979; Welsh, 1979, 1980). Third, resistance of mice to viruses such as herpes simplex virus type I (Lopez, 1978; Lopez et al., 1980) and mouse hepatitis virus (Levy-Leblond and Dupuy, 1978; Tardieu et al., 1980), similarly to resistance to allogeneic marrow graft (Bennett et al., 1976), can be impaired by ^{89}Sr irradiation, a treatment which markedly depresses NK cell functions (Haller and Wigzell, 1977). Morahan et al. (1981), however, could not increase the sensitivity of mice to herpes simplex virus type II and EMC virus by in vivo irradiation with ^{89}Sr.

Fourth, individuals suffering from severe disseminated HSV-1 infections (Ching and Lopez, 1979) or EB virus infections (Sullivan et al., 1980) present NK activity levels which are lower than those present in healthy individuals. It is interesting to note that deficient NK responses have been also found in patients affected with multiple sclerosis, a disease related perhaps to a chronic measles virus-like infection (Hauser *et al.*, 1981).

The participation of NK cells in viral infections has been evaluated in the murine model (beige mouse) of NK deficiency. The beige homozygous mouse (bg/bg) has, as compared with the heterozygous (bg/+) or the wild type (+/+), a low endogenous NK activity which cannot be boosted by interferon treatment or infection with viruses (McKinnon *et al.*, 1981). Although the beige model has been found suitable in assessing the role of NK cells in the rejection of tumor cells (Karre *et al.*, 1980; Talmadge *et al.*, 1980), it gave conflicting results when tested against virus infections. Welsh and Kiessling (1980) found no difference in LCMV growth in spleens of bg/bg or bg/+mice and Hirsch (1980) found that the recovery of bg/bg mice from Sindbis virus infection was not substantially different from that of bg/+ mice. In the latter model, transfer of NK cells from resistant (35-day-old) mice into susceptible (7-day-old) recipients failed to protect them from the fatal infection, implying that NK cells are not involved in the resistance of adult mice to Sindbis virus infection (Hirsch, 1980).

In contrast, Shellam *et al.* (1981) found that beige mice were more susceptible to lethal infection with murine cytomegalovirus than bg/+ mice. Furthermore, they were able to induce resistance to the virus in bg/bg mice, by passive transfer of marrow cells of bg/+ mice. From these observations, it appears that the role played by NK in viral infections is a very complex one and that it is intimately connected with the type of virus model under study. Clearly, further work is needed to establish the participation of these cells in antiviral immunity.

The last, but certainly not the least important, immune mechanism of defense against virus infections is represented by the production of specific antibodies. These antibodies are capable of neutralizing free virions and, in addition, they can, in association with complement, lyse virus-infected cells; we are therefore in the presence of two distinct processes which play a vital role in limiting viral infections: (a) virus neutralization by serum IgG or by secretory IgA at the mucosal surfaces, (b) immune cytolysis, through the interaction of antibody, complement, K cells, polymorphs and macrophages. The essential role of circulating IgG antibody and of mucosal IgA antibody in resistance to reinfection by a virus, following recovery from a viral infection or vaccination with a killed or attenuated virus, need not be emphasized.

In contrast, the role played by humoral antibodies in the resistance to a primary viral infection has been underestimated. The situation is exemplified by the herpes simplex virus infection in the mouse. The fact that a more severe disease occurs in T cell-deprived mice, as compared to normal mice (Nahmias *et al.*, 1969; Nagafuchi *et al.*, 1979; Oakes, 1975), and that protection in recipient mice can be achieved by passive transfer of immune spleen cells (Oakes, 1975; Rager-Zisman and Allison, 1976; Mogensen and Andersen, 1981) suggests that cell-mediated immunity plays a prominent role in the control of the pathogenesis of herpes simplex virus infection. However, impairment of cell-mediated immunity (e.g. by antithymocyte serum, X-irradiation) exerts marked suppressive effects on the amount of circulating antibodies against the viral antigens (thymus-dependent), which appear quite rapidly following a primary infection (Worthington *et al.*, 1980). Passive transfer of virus-specific antibodies into T cell-deprived (Worthington *et al.*, 1980) or nude mice (Nagafuchi *et al.*, 1979) increased both the survival time and the number of survivors. The best results were obtained in T cell-deprived mice passively transferred with physiological amounts of antibodies before being challenged by the i.p. route with the virus, in which case the level of mortality obtained was comparable with that seen in nonimmunosuppressed controls. The importance of circulating antibodies in preventing infection of the central nervous system accounts for the efficacy of inactivated poliovirus vaccines and of passive administration of gammaglobulins and is exemplified by the fact that patients with B cell deficiencies but intact T cell functions are more prone to paralytic poliomyelitis. Prolonged presence of an enterovirus (echovirus) in the central nervous system of patients with agammaglobulinemia—such a persistence being associated with progressive symptomatic illness—has been recently reported (Wilfert *et al.*, 1977). On the other hand, progressive vaccinia gangrenosa may be observed in patients with T cell deficiencies, even in the presence of adequate circulating antibody levels: depending on the nature of the virus, the limiting effects of antibody on viremia may not suffice to stop the progression of the disease. Similarly, recurrences of herpes simplex skin lesions can occur in patients with high titers of neutralizing antibody in their serum.

Antibody-dependent cell-mediated cytotoxicity (ADCC), effected through K cells, may play a more important role than circulating neutralizing antibody in the actual process of natural recovery from virus infections and immune cytolysis, which occurs later than the production of cytotoxic T lymphocytes, probably concurs with the latter in terminating many viral infections. The importance of antibody-dependent cell-mediated cytotoxicity in the immunity conferred by smallpox vaccination in humans has recently been demonstrated (Perrin *et al.*, 1977; Møller-Larsen and Haahr, 1978).

It is worth mentioning at this point that polymorphonuclear leucocytes (PMNLs) can behave as effectors, although less efficiently than mononuclear cells, of ADCC against antibody-sensitized herpes virus-infected cells (Russell and Essery, 1977; Wardley *et al.*, 1977; Russell and Miller, 1978).

Furthermore, bovine PMNLs have been shown to release an interferon-like mediator when exposed to cells infected with some (herpes viruses) but not all viruses (Rouse *et al.*, 1980). These observations, together with the fact that neutrophils accumulate in great abundance in sites of HSV-1 lesions (Hill *et al.*, 1975), suggest a potential participation of PMNLs in the recovery from herpes virus infections. It is likely, however, that they do not play a major role in acute viral infections. In fact, we have shown that treatment of mice with an irritant known to induce granuloma formation and to increase the number of circulating neutrophils, had no effect with respect to their protection against EMC virus, HSV1 and MHV (Zerial *et al.*, 1980). In contrast such a treatment has been found effective in enhancing resistance against bacterial, fungal and protozoal infections (Fauve, 1978).

As in the case of cell-mediated immunity, antibody production can also exert deleterious effects and contribute to the pathology of some viral infections. A typical example is provided by LCM virus infection in newborn mice: mice infected neonatally exhibit partial immunological tolerance with lifelong persistence of virus in their tissues, but discrete amounts of antibody are produced, which react with virus in the blood to form immune complexes; the latter deposit in the kidney glomeruli, causing glomerulonephritis. Immune complexes certainly play a role in the pathogenesis of persistent viral infections, such as in man chronic hepatitis B, dengue hemorrhagic fever and subacute sclerosing panencephalitis (SSPE). A similar mechanism may account for the severe pattern of disease which was shown to occur in individuals vaccinated with formalin-inactivated measles virus when they were exposed to an outbreak of natural measles or revaccinated with live attenuated measles virus. It may also explain in part the severe bronchiolitis observed in children immunized with inactivated respiratory syncytial virus (RSV) when they were exposed later to wild RSV.

Interferon and interferon inducers are discussed in detail in another review. Although interferon is produced by lymphoid cells and by macrophages, it can also be produced *in vitro* or *in vivo* by almost any type of cell or tissue as a consequence of viral infection and cannot therefore be strictly regarded as an immunological reaction. The role of interferon in host resistance to and recovery from viral infections is mostly based on indirect evidence: (a) there is a temporal association between the presence of virus and interferon in tissues (and, in many cases, the amount of interferon appears to be mainly a reflection of the extent of virus multiplication); (b) in some situations, such as herpes zoster—varicella virus infection in immunosuppressed patients, there is a good association between the appearance of high titers of interferon in the vesicle fluid and the commencement of healing (Stevens *et al.*, 1973); (c) passive administration of large amounts of exogenous interferon has been shown, by many investigators, to confer resistance to or to hasten recovery from viral infections in laboratory animals and, in some cases, in man.

Defective production of α and γ interferon in humans has been recently described. Isaacs *et al.* (1981) have analyzed the production of α and γ interferons *in vitro* by leucocytes (in response to NDV and allogeneic cells respectively) of thirty children affected with recurrent respiratory infections. Four of these children were classified as deficient interferon α producers, since they presented a long-lasting deficit in interferon α production *in vitro* while production of γ-interferon was normal. In addition, interferon α could not be detected in rhinovirus-positive nasopharyngeal secretions of deficient interferon α producers while it was present in 86 per cent of rhinovirus isolates of normal interferon producers. A correlation between deficiency in interferon production and susceptibility to rhinovirus infections could not be clearly established, since the clinical status of deficient and normal interferon α producers was not substantially different. Deficiencies in γ-interferon production and in NK cell functions have been described by Virelizier and Griscelli (1980, 1981) in children affected with severe and repeated bacterial and viral infections, who were otherwise normal for B and T cell responses. Intramuscular administration of exogenous leucocyte interferon was reported beneficial in restoring, at least transiently, NK cell activity, in terminating the infections and in improving the overall clinical status of the patients. These observations, although preliminary, indicate that deficiencies in interferon (e.g. γ type) production, like the 'classical' immunological deficiencies, may have deleterious effects on the resistance to viral and bacterial infections. Furthermore, it seems that these patients can benefit from therapy involving exogenous interferon or possibly interferon inducers.

Following experiments showing increased susceptibility to Semliki Forest virus infection in mice treated with sheep anti-mouse interferon serum (Fauconnier, 1970), recent investigations (Gresser *et al.*, 1976a) have convincingly demonstrated that neutralization of interferon production can markedly aggravate several virus infections in the mouse. For instance, in the case of infection with encephalomyocarditis (EMC) virus, the course of the disease in the mice which were inoculated with a potent sheep anti-mouse interferon globulin was entirely different from that affecting control mice similarly infected but treated with a control globulin preparation: the latter died towards the fourth or fifth day after infection, with signs of central nervous system involvement; by contrast, the anti-interferon-serum-treated mice died within 24–48 hr of an overwhelming systemic infection before virus had multiplied to high titer in the brain. The same authors (Gresser *et al.*, 1976b) also studied the effect of treatment with anti-interferon globulin on the course of the infection of mice with herpes simplex, vesicular stomatitis, influenza A and Moloney sarcoma viruses. With the exception of influenza, such a treatment resulted, in all the other systems, in an accelerated appearance of signs of infection and in a marked aggravation of the disease. It was shown, in addition, that anti-interferon globulin did not block the synthesis of interferon by virus-infected cells but rather neutralized extracellularly its activity. The unavoidable conclusion from these data is that early interferon *in situ* production must play a significant role in limiting viral multiplication and spread and thereby contributing to recovery. On the contrary, interferon has been shown responsible of the severe disease which follows s.c. infection of newborn mice with LCMV. This conclusion could be drawn from two observations. First, production of endogenous interferon in mouse strains correlates with strain sensitivity to LCMV infection (Rivière *et al.*, 1980). Second, administration of antiserum to interferon into LCMV-infected mice exerts a marked protective effect against the development of the fatal disease.

Summarizing this long, still very sketchy, introduction, one may state that vertebrates possess several mechanisms which enable them to survive through virus infections (Table 3): first, a nonspecific and not always very efficient barrier, represented by cells of the mono-nuclear phagocyte system; then, the various functions exerted by specifically sensitized T lymphocytes followed later by humoral events, either narrowly specific (antibodies) or nonspecific (interferon). There are, of course, multiple interactions between these various systems such as the effect on macrophages of the products from sensitized T lymphocytes, the role of T helper cells in antibody production by B cells and the recently demonstrated inhibition by interferon of some T and B cell reactions. Furthermore, as already mentioned several times, some of these immune reactions actually contribute to the pathogenesis of the viral disease.

While specific vaccination with inactivated or live attenuated viruses does nothing more, immunologically speaking, than mimic the natural disease, the mechanisms and possible uses

TABLE 3. *Simplified Representation of Immunological Mechanisms of Resistance to and/or Recovery from Virus Infections*
(arrows indicate: activity on or production by)

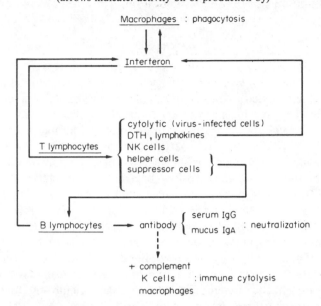

of 'immunopotentiating' drugs – which may be specific with respect to some aspects of the immune response but, by definition, are not specific with respect to the infecting virus – appear extremely complex.

13.3. IMMUNOPOTENTIATING SUBSTANCES OF NATURAL ORIGIN

13.3.1. MISCELLANEOUS MICROBIAL INFECTIONS AND PRODUCTS

Remarkable resistance against challenge with normally lethal doses of the Mengo strain of encephalomyocarditis virus (EMC) was observed in mice which had been infected with the obligate intracellular protozoa *Toxoplasma gondii* and *Besnoitia jellisoni* and with the facultative intracellular bacterium *Listeria monocytogenes* (Remington and Merigan, 1969). In contrast to the prolonged resistance (1 year or more) demonstrable in the animals chronically infected with protozoa, the resistance to viral challenge of listeria-infected mice lasted only 1–3 months and was less striking. Sustained 'activation' of the macrophages in mice chronically infected with protozoa was considered as the most likely explanation for this enhanced resistance to viruses.

Repeated administration to mice of those combined bacterial vaccines which are employed by some physicians for the treatment of bronchial asthma and of recurrent chronic respiratory infections was shown (Degré and Dahl, 1973) to afford protection against intranasal infection with an A2 influenza virus. The combined bacterial vaccine gave some protection when it was administered only once, a few hours before virus inoculation, but the effect was greater when the mice received a first intraperitoneal dose of vaccine 14 days and a second dose 4 hr before virus inoculation. The increased protection produced by this immunizing schedule was paralleled by an increased serum interferon production in the mice upon i.p. inoculation of Newcastle Disease Virus. The importance of eliciting delayed-type-hypersensitivity reactions to the bacterial product before viral challenge in order to obtain optimal nonspecific protection has been clearly demonstrated, – as described in the section devoted to mycobacterial products – in the case of *Mycobacterium tuberculosis* and old tuberculin; similarly, it was shown (Allen and Mudd, 1973) that infection of mice with a nonlethal strain of *Staphylococcus aureus* did not significantly alter their sensitivity to tail vein inoculation with vaccinia virus, but that specific elicitation of the staphylococcus-sensitized animals with a staphylococcal phage lysate a few hours before viral challenge resulted in decreased lesions in the tail.

13.3.2. LIPOPOLYSACCHARIDES (ENDOTOXINS)

The presence of biologically active substances in gram-negative bacteria was recognized during the previous century; it was later found that these were constituents of the cell wall and, because of their toxicity, they were named endotoxins. These endotoxins are lipopolysaccharides (LPS), i.e. heteropolymers containing polysaccharide covalently bound to a phospholipid, termed lipid A. LPS exert a wide variety of biological effects and it is now reasonably clear that lipid A is the active part in most of such effects (Galanos *et al.*, 1977).

Nonspecific effects of LPS upon resistance have been demonstrated in experimental infections by gram-negative and gram-positive bacteria, mycobacteria, fungi, parasites and viruses (Cluff, 1970). Relevant to the enhancement by LPS of the resistance of mice to virus infections, which was first demonstrated in the case of ectromelia (mouse pox) (Gledhill, 1959), is the fact that these substances are highly pyrogenic, at minute doses, and that they cause the release of interferon in the circulation of the animals injected with them. *In vivo* and *in vitro* activation of macrophages by LPS is readily demonstrable by various tests, and it is interesting to note that, while viruses can induce interferon in many types of cells in tissue culture, LPS are only effective in cultures of cells of the reticulo–endothelial system. It is therefore likely that interferon production (or, probably, rather release) as well as hyperthermia are the consequences of a direct effect of LPS on such cells.

The effects of the administration of a purified preparation of LPS on the infection of mice with influenza AO, A2 and B viruses (inoculated intranasally), with EMC virus (s.c. or i.m.), with vesicular stomatitis (i.c.), herpes simplex type 1 (i.p.) and vaccinia (i.p.) viruses have been studied (Rolly *et al.*, 1974). LPS was administered intranasally, i.v., i.m., i.p. or i.c. Although, at appropriate doses and times of administration of the LPS, an enhancing effect on resistance was seen in all these systems, the most striking activity was observed when the substance was given intranasally, at 0.3 to 10 μg per mouse, 24 hr before influenza-virus inoculation by the same route. In this system, protection was still significant when LPS was administered as early as 120 hr and as late as 3 hr before infection, but treatment after infection was ineffective. From the respective kinetics of protection against mortality and of release of circulating interferon by LPS in the mouse, the authors conclude that the latter effect cannot by itself account for the antiviral activity of LPS (which is inactive *in vitro*).

We have studied the effects of LPS preparations from *Salmonella typhimurium* and *Escherichia coli* on infections of mice with EMC, murine hepatitis, influenza, Semliki Forest (arbovirus), herpes simplex type 1 and mouse-adapted foot-and-mouth disease viruses and reached essentially similar conclusions (Floc'h and Werner, unpublished): at minute doses and by various routes, these preparations exerted significant protective effects, and the activity observed when infection was performed at the time of peak interferon levels in the blood (i.e. 2 to 6 hr after LPS injection) was not higher than when it took place after a considerable drop in the titer of circulating interferon (i.e. 24 hr after LPS injection). It is noteworthy that, in these experimental systems, the transient increase of sensitivity to infections by LPS, which is readily demonstrable in many bacterial infections a few hours after the injection of the substance and which precedes enhancement of resistance, was not seen on virus infections. One should also note that the various virus infections tested did not respond equally well to LPS, the least sensitive being herpes simplex.

Even in those systems which respond well to enhancement of resistance by LPS, dose-effect relationships are not linear: curves are often bell-shaped, with peak activity at an intermediary dose, or they may present M, V or W shapes, as was already observed in other circumstances (Bliznakov and Adler, 1972).

The toxicity of LPS makes it somewhat doubtful that such substances could be used in nonspecific protection of man and domestic animals against virus infections; attempts at detoxification of LPS by various chemical procedures have generally resulted in loss of only some of their interesting biological activities, but enhancement of resistance against infections and interferon release were among the effects which were most severely affected by such manipulations, together with the least desirable effects, such as pyrogenicity (Chedid et al., 1975; McIntire et al., 1976). Deleterious effects of LPS in experimental virus infections have also been seen: Newcastle disease virus (an avian virus) produces no signs of infection of the central nervous system in normal mice but causes meningoencephalitis in mice treated with LPS 24 hr previously; this enhancement of infection was ascribed to transudation of the virus resulting from injury to cerebral blood vessels by LPS (Rahman and Lattrell, 1963).

One should finally mention that crude extracts from some gram-positive bacteria have also been shown to enhance resistance of mice against several virus infections: it appears that, in the main, their other biological activities, namely interferon release, macrophage activation and pyrogenicity, are qualitatively similar to those of LPS. For instance, it was recently shown (Nozaki-Renard, 1978) that extraction of *Bacillus subtilis* by methods used to obtain LPS from gram-negative organisms yields substances which cause the release of interferon in mice and exhibit mitogenic as well as pyrogenic activities, while they appear to be of a different chemical nature from that of endotoxins.

13.3.3. Mycobacteria and Mycobacterial Products

It was shown, more than 20 years ago, that inoculation of live bacillus Calmette-Guérin (BCG) induces in the mouse a sustained hyperactivity of the phagocytic cells (Biozzi et al., 1954). BCG-inoculated mice exhibit enhanced resistance to infection with virulent staphylococci (Dubos and Schaedler, 1957) or to challenge with several transplanted tumors (Biozzi et al., 1959). Following the pioneer investigations of Mathé and his group (Mathé et al., 1969), BCG was until recently the most widely used agent in immunotherapy trials against malignant diseases of man.

Enhanced resistance of BCG-infected mice (1 mg/mouse i.v.) to the Mengo strain of encephalomyocarditis virus was reported several years ago (Old et al., 1963). A 1.0 to 2.5 $\log_{10}$ reduction in the virus LD_{50} by the i.v., i.p. or s.c. routes was observed in comparison with control mice, in animals previously infected with BCG; increased resistance was evident by the eighth day following BCG inoculation and persisted for at least 3.5 months; BCG infection did not protect mice against intracerebral virus challenge. Additional interesting observations were made: serum from BCG-inoculated mice did not neutralize Mengo virus nor did it confer passive protection against this challenge; splenectomy of BCG-inoculated mice did not abolish their resistance to the viral challenge (while it is known to inhibit enhanced antibody production against bacterial antigens); *in vitro* the extent of replication of Mengo virus in peritoneal macrophages from BCG-infected mice was not different from that in cells from control mice, but, as the authors rightly stressed, the behavior of the peritoneal cells did not necessarily reflect that of spleen and liver macrophages.

BCG infection by the i.v. route 10 to 7 days prior to intravaginal inoculation of herpes simplex type 2 virus (HSV-2) in adult female mice did not alter the subsequent disease, characterized by vaginitis, posterior paralysis, encephalitis and death (Baker et al., 1974): it even appeared, in some cases, to enhance the severity of the disease, while passive immunization of the mice with specific HSV-2 antiserum 4 hr before virus inoculation provided significant protection. It is interesting to note, however, that the combination of BCG inoculation (7 days before infection) and antiserum treatment (4 hr before) produced the greatest degree of protection.

Different results were obtained when HSV-2 was inoculated i.p. into newborn mice (Starr et al., 1976): in that situation, BCG administered i.p. or intradermally 6 days before virus challenge increased survival rate, while the other immunopotentiating substances studied (levamisole, typhoid or brucella vaccines) were ineffective. Clearly, in the newborn mouse infected i.p., stimulation of the peritoneal macrophages by BCG is sufficient to enhance resistance against HSV-2, while the mechanisms of resistance of adult mice against intravaginal herpes infection must be less simple.

The effect of BCG infection (1 mg/mouse, i.e. about 10^6 live bacilli, intravenously) on the resistance of adult mice to virus infections was investigated using EMC virus (inoculated s.c.), murine hepatitis (i.p.), herpes simplex types 1 and 2 (i.p.), foot-and-mouth disease virus (s.c.), and A0 and A2 influenza viruses (aerosol) (Floc'h and Werner, 1976). In most cases, BCG-inoculated mice exhibited a significantly higher resistance to these lethal infections than control mice: the overall survival rate in the latter was 18 per cent versus 41 per cent in the BCG-inoculated animals. Enhanced resistance following BCG inoculation (which was performed from 31 to 15 days before virus challenge) was especially marked in infections with EMC, HSV-1 and influenza A2 viruses; intercurrent infection of BCG-inoculated mice with nonlethal doses of viruses did not abolish their resistance towards subsequent challenge with lethal doses of an unrelated virus. It is noteworthy that, in the case of A2 influenza-virus infection, the BCG-inoculated mice did not show earlier or higher serum antibody production against the virus than the control mice and that their lung lesions were not markedly diminished: the only difference between the two groups which might explain the higher survival rate of the BCG-inoculated mice was a more rapid virus clearance from their lungs. On the other hand, while BCG-inoculated mice were more resistant than controls to HSV-1, they did not exhibit enhanced resistance to a strain of HSV-2 which required immunosuppression with cyclophosphamide to cause a lethal infection.

Nonspecific protection of mice against A0 influenza virus infection following systemic immunization with BCG was recently confirmed (Spencer et al., 1977); it was found in addition that greater protection was afforded by intranasal BCG than by intraperitoneal BCG immunization against this intranasal virus challenge. This 'compartmentalization' of the response was maximal 4 weeks after BCG inoculation, decreased at 6 weeks and disappeared at 8 weeks, in agreement with what was seen with respect to specific cell-mediated immunity following BCG inoculation to guinea pigs by systemic or intranasal route. The same authors reported that in vitro peritoneal exudate cells from BCG-sensitized guinea pigs showed a more rapid fall in the intracellular titer of influenza virus than did macrophages from unimmunized animals.

BCG has also been reported to modify tumor development in mice following inoculation of oncornaviruses such as Moloney sarcoma virus: mice injected with BCG 28 days before virus inoculation had shorter latent periods for tumor development but longer survivals than control animals; when BCG was mixed with the virus at the time of inoculation, there was a decrease in mortality, tumor incidence and tumor size compared with controls inoculated with the virus alone; inoculation of mice with BCG 28 days before attempted induction of tumors with the BCG-virus mixture completely inhibited tumor development and protected the animals against death (Schwartz et al., 1971).

Thus far, all the experiments reported have been performed in mice, but it has also been shown that BCG immunization of rabbits enhanced their resistance to infection with type 2 herpes simplex virus (Larson et al., 1972). While control rabbits died from encephalitis subsequent to vaginal or corneal inoculation of the virus, animals which had been inoculated i.v. with 4×10^7 viable units of BCG 4 weeks before viral challenge also developed encephalitis but, in most cases, did not die.

On the clinical scene, attempts have been made to treat recurrent herpes genitalis in men and women by nonspecific stimulation of their immunity with BCG. In one study (Anderson et al., 1974), fifteen patients with frequent recurring genital herpes manifestations were injected intradermally with BCG: all of them experienced a decrease in the frequency and severity of their recurrences and the best responses were obtained in those patients who became and remained tuberculin-positive following BCG administration. These encouraging results have not been confirmed in a recent and more extensive study carried out on 100 patients (Corey et al., 1976): patients with previously documented recurrent genital herpes received BCG or placebo (candida antigen) intradermally and were followed at monthly intervals during 6 months. During this study period, there were on the average 2.30 recurrences/100 days in the BCG recipients compared to 2.18 recurrences/100 days in placebo recipients; the mean duration of lesions during recurrences of genital herpes was similar between the BCG and the placebo group, but, among women, the mean duration of pain was shorter (average: 3.5 days) in BCG recipients than in placebo recipients (6.0 days).

One may also mention, in view of the probable viral etiology of this condition, that immunostimulation with BCG failed to affect the clinical course of Burkitt's lymphoma, in a randomized trial carried out on forty patients (twenty-one treated with BCG, nineteen with placebo): no significant differences in the length of remission or the site of relapse were observed that could be attributed to the BCG treatment, in spite of the fact that antibody titers to the membrane antigen associated with Epstein—Barr virus increased greatly in the BCG-injected patients but not in control patients and that BCG treatment increased the rate of recovery from the tumor-induced state of immunosuppression (Magrath and Ziegler, 1976).

An avirulent strain of *Mycobacterium tuberculosis hominis* (H 37 Ra) has also been used to induce resistance of mice against viral challenge, in that case intravenous inoculation of vaccinia virus (Allen and Mudd, 1973): infection with this agent did afford some protection against tail lesions resulting from this challenge but the enhancement of resistance was definitely greater when the H 37 Ra-sensitized mice received an injection of old tuberculin shortly before virus challenge.

All the experiments reported thus far have been performed with live Mycobacteria, but Freund's complete adjuvant (FCA), in which the bacilli are killed, was shown to cause inhibition of multiplication of foot-and-mouth disease virus (FMDV) in adult mice (Gorhe, 1967; Gorhe *et al.*, 1968). Mice received a first intradermal injection of FCA 10 days before intraperitoneal challenge with FMDV and a second one 3 days before that challenge: only 33 per cent of the animals treated in that way showed evidence of viremia, versus 100 per cent in the control mice and the extent of virus multiplication in their pancreas was greatly diminished.

Increased resistance was also shown by the fact that it took about 100 times more virus in FCA-treated mice than in controls to kill 50 per cent of the animals. An important observation was that, in FCA-treated mice, the titer of interferon in the spleen rose rapidly after virus inoculation to a significant level and actually preceded the peak of viral replication while it followed the latter in control animals. A wax D preparation from M. *tuberculosis*, containing lipid, polysaccharide and peptide moieties, exerted essentially the same activities as FCA.

It is important to note that in these positive experiments, the killed bacilli or their wax fraction were injected as an emulsion in mineral oil and that two injections were performed 1 week apart. We found (unpublished observations) that a single treatment of mice with delipidated *Mycobacterium phlei*, in aqueous suspension, shortly (48 hr to 2 hr) before viral challenge did not significantly protect the animals against infection with encephalomyocarditis (EMC), murine hepatitis, herpes simplex or influenza viruses. On the other hand, Lodmell and Ewalt (1978) have reported that i.p. or i.v. injection (but not i.m. or s.c.) of killed M. *tuberculosis* in oil droplet emulsion exerted a marked protection against mortality in mice infected with EMC virus (by the i.p., s.c. or i.m. route), 7—30 days post-treatment.

Relatively little information is available, on the other hand, concerning the activity on virus infections of the various fractions which have recently been isolated from Mycobacteria by several groups. A water soluble fraction consisting of a polysaccharide bound to a peptidoglycan, with a molecular weight of 15 to 30,000, extracted from M. *tuberculosis hominis* was shown to protect mice against EMC virus infection, when it was administered i.v. (at doses ranging from 0.5 to 4.5 mg/kg) 2 hr before viral challenge by the s.c. route (Werner *et al.*, 1975); this same substance was without effect against respiratory infection with influenza virus, when it was administered intranasally 2 to 6 hr before challenge.

Only indirect evidence is available concerning an antiviral activity of the MER (methanol extraction residue) fraction of Mycobacteria, a powerful immunostimulating agent often used in tumor immunotherapy trials in man: mice that had been injected with MER remained free of symptoms during outbreaks of a naturally occurring pneumonitis, of presumed viral origin, which affected animal quarters in which they were housed (Weiss *et al.*, 1964). Similarly there does not seem to exist any information about possible antiviral activities of cord factor (trehalose-6,6'-dimycolate), a glycopeptid produced by mycobacteria, which, in addition to exerting antitumor immunopotentiation, has been shown, together with synthetic other trehalose-6,6'-diesters, to enhance resistance of mice to infection with *Klebsiella pneumoniae* and with *Listeria monocytogenes* when they were administered in oily emulsion 14 days before challenge (Parant *et al.*, 1978).

The minimal structure required for the adjuvant activity of mycobacterial cell walls preparations has been shown to consist of a muramyldipeptide, namely *N*-acetylmuramyl-L-alanyl-D-isoglutamine (MDP), of which various analogs have been synthesized (Adam *et al.*, 1976). While MDP exhibits, in addition to its adjuvant effect on antibody production and delayed-type hypersensitivity, an enhancing effect on resistance of mice to bacterial infections (Chedid *et al.*, 1976), even when administered orally, it does not appear that its activity on viral infections has been investigated. It is known, on the other hand, that MDP, injected together with a vaccine consisting of sub-units of influenza virus, exerts, in the mouse and in the hamster, a definite adjuvant effect on the production of antibodies to the virus hemagglutinin (Audibert *et al.*, 1977; Webster *et al.*, 1977).

In view of the remarkable effects of infection with a live attenuated *Mycobacterium* strain like BCG on nonspecific resistance to virus infections – at least in laboratory models – it is hoped that more information will soon become available on the activity in this area of the mycobacterial products which exhibit many of the immunopotentiating effects of the whole bacilli. Direct stimulation of the mononuclear phagocyte system is the most likely mechanism accounting for the antiviral activity of BCG; in addition, in animals inoculated with this agent, there appear after some time specifically sensitized T lymphocytes which, through interaction with the microbial antigen persisting in their organism, are induced to release factors capable of activating macrophages. Such a phenomenon may be difficult to reproduce with a nonliving fraction, unless the substance can actually persist in the tissues or be administered in a way which will make a similar reaction possible. In other words, BCG takes at least 10 days after inoculation to enhance resistance against viral infections but this state of enhanced resistance is long-lasting, while a mere primary and transient stimulation of the macrophages will only have a short-lived effect on resistance. Repeated administrations of the nonliving immunopotentiating substances may, however, lead to a more prolonged and marked effect. In this connection, one may recall that in the experiments showing a sparing effect of Freund's complete adjuvant on the infection of mice with foot-and-mouth disease virus, this substance, in an oily emulsion, was administered twice, 10 and 3 days before viral challenge.

13.3.4. BRUCELLA AND BORDETELLA

Microorganisms of the genus *Brucella*, which cause disease in man, cattle, sheep, swine and other animal species, and *Bordetella pertussis*, the etiologic agent of whooping cough in man, share with *Mycobacterium tuberculosis* the capacity of surviving and dividing inside phagocytic cells. Their continued presence within macrophages induces the formation of granuloma and, as a result of interaction between macrophages and sensitized lymphocytes, macrophage "activation" and delayed type hypersensitivity reactions take place conspicuously. It is not surprising therefore that *Brucella* and *Bordetella* organisms, as well as products extracted from them, have been intensively studied as 'immunostimulating' agents.

Live *Brucella abortus* was the first bacterium shown to induce the appearance of circulating interferon in mice and chicks following parenteral administration (Stinebring and Youngner, 1964; Youngner *et al.*, 1964). In contrast to the short duration (from 6–12 to 24–48 hr after injection) of this interferon response, protection of mice infected with *B. abortus* against viral infections can last several weeks (Billiau *et al.*, 1970). Studies on the mechanism of enhanced resistance of live *B. abortus*-inoculated mice to i.p. infection with the Mengo strain of encephalomyocarditis virus (Muyembe *et al.*, 1972) have shown that stimulation of the phagocytic and virucidal activity of the peritoneal macrophages and of the blood monocytes was a more valid explanation than serum and tissue interferon induction for this increased resistance. The resistant state lasted for at least 3 weeks; when the bacteria were inoculated by the i.p. route passage of the virus from the peritoneal cavity was inhibited; this was not observed when the bacteria were inoculated intravenously but, in that case, replication of virus in the spleen was decreased.

Heat-killed *B. abortus* was shown to induce in mice, following i.p. inoculation, a 'virus-type' interferon response (with serum peak titers at 6.5 hr) as well as a state of increased resistance against i.p. challenge with the Semliki Forest species of alphavirus (Feingold *et al.*, 1976). Extraction of heat-killed *B. abortus* with a mixture of chloroform-methanol (CM) yielded an insoluble residue (extracted cells) and a soluble extract: neither of those substances induced interferon production or afforded protection against viral challenge. On the other hand, extraction of live *B. abortus* with aqueous ether yielded a nonviable insoluble residue with low toxicity, named BRU-PEL, which induced interferon and protected mice against viral challenge; extraction of BRU-PEL with CM again destroyed these activities (Youngner *et al.*, 1974). Full activities were restored when the CM extracts were recombined with the extracted cells; furthermore, a CM extract of *Escherichia coli* was also capable of restoring activity to the extracted *B. abortus* cells. One may thus conclude that the interferon-inducing and antiviral properties of *B. abortus* reside in a CM-extractable component, which is common to *B. abortus* and *E. coli*, and in an unextractable component which is unique to *B. abortus*. The CM extract from *Brucella* was shown to contain 92 per cent lipids. Since virus challenge, in these experiments, was performed shortly after injection of the preparations, i.e. at the time when interferon was present in the blood, one cannot determine whether these nonviable preparations are as capable as live *B. abortus* to induce a long-lasting state of antiviral resistance.

This was, however, demonstrated to be the case in experiments performed with the BRU-PEL extract mentioned above (Kern *et al.*, 1976). The kinetics of the interferon response to BRU-PEL was similar to that induced by viruses or double-stranded ribonucleotides and, given shortly before intranasal infection with herpes simplex virus type 2 virus (HSV-2) in 3-week old mice or i.p. infection with encephalomyocarditis virus (EMC) in adult mice, the substance markedly protected them against mortality. In adult mice infected i.p. with HSV-2, protection by BRU-PEL was significant when it was administered by the same route 1 day before infection, nonexistent when treatment was performed 4 days before infection but again significant when injection took place 7, 10 or 14 days before viral challenge. Altogether when BRU-PEL was administered as an interferon inducer (i.e. shortly before infection), its antiviral activity was less marked than that of poly I : C, but when it was administered several days before infection, its antiviral activity was comparable to that of live *Brucella*. As in the case of the latter, the conclusion is that this substance (which is insoluble and may therefore persist in macrophages having ingested it) protects against viral infections through a mechanism of stimulation of the phagocytic cells rather than through interferon induction.

Intravenous inoculation of mice with *Bordetella pertussis* vaccine (in which the microorganisms are killed with heat or formaldehyde) causes transient hypertrophy of the spleen and a very striking hyperleucocytosis, in which lymphocytosis predominates (Morse, 1965). The increase in circulating lymphocytes likely results from release of cells from various lymphoid organs; a lymphocytosis-promoting factor (LPF) has recently been isolated from *Bordetella* and shown to exert a mitogen-like activity *in vitro* on murine lymphocytes (Kong and Morse, 1977). Mice inoculated with *B. pertussis* show enhanced humoral immune responses to heterologous antigens (Floersheim, 1965) while cell-mediated immune responses tend to decrease (Finger *et al.*, 1967); furthermore, an 'endotoxin-like' interferon response is induced (Borecky and Lackovič, 1967). In spite of the recognition of these various activities, the only investigation we are aware of on the effect of *B. pertussis* on a murine virus infection was the demonstration (Anderlik *et al.*, 1972) that adult mice infected intracerebrally with 100 LD_{50} of lymphocytic choriomeningitis virus (LCM) and treated intravenously on the same day with *B. pertussis* vaccine had a definitely longer survival time than control mice, similarly inoculated with LCM virus but untreated. Thus, in a particular case where cell-mediated immune (CMI) responses are detrimental to the host by causing encephalitis, an immunopotentiating agent with selective activity (enhancement of humoral immunity, inhibition of CMI) may exert a favorable activity.

13.3.5. CORYNEBACTERIUM PARVUM

The immunostimulating activities of heat – and formaldehyde – killed *Corynebacterium parvum* or *granulosum* microorganisms have aroused considerable interest because of their potential application to nonspecific immunotherapy of cancer, which was demonstrated in several experimental and clinical studies. *C. parvum* is presently used in several oncology centers throughout the world and it is of more than academic interest to know its activity on virus infections. *C. parvum* injected i.p. (12 or 25 mg/kg) to mice 7 and again 2 days before infection by the same route with encephalomyocarditis virus (EMC) greatly enhanced survival of the animals (Cerutti, 1974). It was shown, in addition, that cell-free peritoneal exudate obtained from *C. parvum*-treated mice 2 to 5 days after injection contained a factor capable of inhibiting the replication of EMC and vesicular stomatitis virus in L cell cultures; several characteristics distinguished that factor from interferon. Intraperitoneal injection of *C. parvum* (10 mg/kg) 6 to 8 days before i.p. inoculation of mice with herpes simplex type 1 virus (HSV-1) protected them from encephalitis and death (Kirchner *et al.*, 1977). Mice immunosuppressed with cyclophosphamide and showing enhanced susceptibility to HSV-1 infection were also protected by *C. parvum* treatment; treatments performed shortly before or after virus inoculation were ineffective. Essentially similar results were obtained in another study (Glasgow *et al.*, 1977): mice treated 7 to 10 days before inoculation of virus were protected against lethal infections with HSV-2, EMC, murine cytomegalovirus and Semliki Forest arbovirus. Moreover, i.p. injection of *C. parvum* protected mice against i.p. or intranasal infection with EMC virus, showing that the immunostimulant exerts a systemic, rather than local, effect. Enhanced resistance against HSV-2 could be transferred to recipient mice by peritoneal exudate cells from *C. acnes*-treated animals. The same authors (Morahan *et al.*, 1977b) showed that suppression of macrophage function by *in vivo* treatment with silica increased susceptibility of mice to HSV-2 infection by a 10- to 100-fold factor, but that such a treatment, causing early and sustained viral replication in visceral organs, did not inhibit the antiviral activity of *C. acnes*. It is interesting to note that a similar observation, suggesting that macrophages may not play a major role in the immunostimulating activity of Corynebacteria, was made with respect to the antitumor activities of *C. parvum* (Biozzi *et al.*, 1978).

Unpublished results from our laboratory were generally in agreement with those of the studies summarized above: we found that adult mice were protected against lethal subcutaneous infection with a mouse-adapted C type strain of foot-and-mouth disease virus or against lethal intranasal infection with Semliki Forest virus when they received a single i.p. administration from 11 days to 1 day before infection; very small doses of *C. parvum* (2 mg/kg i.p.) enhanced resistance against murine hepatitis virus, also inoculated i.p., even when treatment preceded infection by only 6 hr. With respect to subcutaneous infection of mice with EMC virus, a single intravenous inoculation of *C. parvum* provided higher enhancement of resistance against lethality when it was performed 6 days rather than 4 days before virus inoculation and, in both cases, there was a clear-cut dose–effect relationship between the amount of *C. parvum* injected and the degree of protection. Intranasal administration of minute doses of *C. parvum* (0.5 or 2 mg/kg), 1 day before exposure to an aerosol of AO influenza virus, significantly enhanced survival of the mice. On the other hand, in the case of i.p. infection with HSV-1, protection of the mice was evident only when treatment with *C. parvum* was performed at least 5 days before virus inoculation; *in vivo* transfer of increased resistance could be made with spleen or peritoneal cells from treated mice.

Enhanced resistance against infection with Junin virus (an arenavirus which is the etiologic agent of Argentine hemorrhagic fever in humans) was reported in newborn mice treated with *C. parvum* (Budzko *et al.*, 1978) and it is noteworthy that the kinetics of optimal activity in this system (in which both *C. parvum* and the virus were injected intraperitoneally) was quite different from that seen in the experiments described above: maximal protection was afforded when *C. parvum* was administered simultaneously with the virus; a small but significant degree of protection was induced by *C. parvum* given 3 or 6 days after infection, while treatment 3 days before infection was ineffective. Furthermore, brain viral titers at various times after infection were comparable in control and *C. parvum*-treated mice. Depression of macrophages by silica injection *in vivo* was shown to actually enhance resistance to Junin virus infection, suggesting that the protective effect of *C. parvum* is unlikely to be due, in this system, to its capacity to stimulate macrophages. Neonatal thymectomy had been shown previously to prevent the onset of the disease caused by Junin virus in newborn mice (Weissenbacher *et al.*, 1969) and it is tempting to speculate that, in this system, *C. parvum* exerts its protective activity by inducing suppression at the level of the thymus. One must also note that, in the case of infection with HSV-2, newborn mice, in contrast to adult mice, were not protected by *C. parvum* injection. As in the case of the infection with Junin virus it was found (Schindler *et al.*, 1981) that protection of mice against MHV3 infection could be achieved when *C. parvum* was administered shortly *after* infection or simultaneously with it.

One must therefore conclude that *C. parvum* may exert its antiviral activities through different sorts of mechanisms, depending on the nature of the host–virus immunological and immunopathological relationship in the experimental systems in which this agent is being tested. What the experiments with Junin virus clearly indicate is that *C. parvum* can exert a protective effect even against an infection in which immunological reactions, rather than viral replication in target organs, play a major role in the pathology.

An insight into one of the possible mechanisms of immunopotentiation by *C. parvum* is provided by a study of its effect on natural killer (NK) cell activity against tumor cells in mice (Ojo *et al.*, 1978): when given intravenously, *C. parvum* caused a dramatic decrease in NK cell activity, whereas, administered intraperitoneally, it caused a sharp increase in rapidly cytolytic effector cells, which were also shown to be NK cells, among the peritoneal exudate cells. One may recall that, in most studies on the antiviral activity of *C. parvum*, this agent was indeed administered by the intraperitoneal route and that NK cells are known to be able to lyse virus-infected cells.

Two recent reports have brought important additional information on the possible mechanism of the antiviral activity of *C. parvum*. On the one hand, it was shown (Hirt *et al.*, 1978) that mouse spleen cells produced considerable amounts of interferon when tested *in vitro* 5 to 20 days after *in vivo* injection of *C. parvum*; the highest levels of interferon were obtained when spleen cells from *C. parvum*-treated mice (10 mg/kg i.p.) were again challenged *in vitro* with *C. parvum* (20 µg/ml). Interferon production in cultures of mouse spleen cells incubated with *C. parvum* has been also described by Evans and Johnson (1981). There is disagreement, however, with respect to the type of interferon produced. While Hirt *et al.* (1978) reported induction of type II interferon, production of both type I and type II interferons has been described by Evans and Johnson (1981).

On the other hand, evidence has been presented that interferon and interferon inducers (Newcastle disease virus, tilorone, statolon) can markedly enhance NK (natural killer) cell activity in mice (Gidlund *et al.*, 1978). The kinetics of induction of NK cell activity after injection of tilorone or statolon was shown to parallel the known kinetics of interferon induction and injection of potent murine interferon preparations also led to a marked increase of NK cell activity *in vivo*. Furthermore, anti-interferon globulin, when injected into mice, inhibited the capacity of tilorone and Newcastle disease virus to enhance NK cell activity *in vivo*; it also inhibited, but to a lesser degree, the NK cell activity of peritoneal exudate cells taken from mice injected with *C. parvum*.

It is therefore possible to conclude that, at least in the experimental systems in which this activity requires injection of *C. parvum* several days before infection, the antiviral activity is due to stimulation of NK cells, probably in part mediated through the production of interferon, rather than stimulation of macrophages. It is also noteworthy that, in the case of infection of mice with HSV-2, two treatments with *C. parvum*, the first one 7 days and the second one 1 day before infection are more effective than a single treatment 7 days before, while a single treatment 1 day before is ineffective (Zerial and Werner, unpublished).

On the other hand, the protective effect of *C. parvum* when given shortly before or after infection, as in the case of the MHV3 infectious model in mice (Schindler *et al.*, 1981), appears to involve local macrophage stimulation rather than interferon induction or activation of NK cells.

Several attempts have been made to isolate from *C. parvum* cell wall material or other constituents and to demonstrate that they could exert the same immunopotentiating activities as the whole organism. With respect to the activities on tumor development, these attempts appear to have been generally unsuccessful, but water-soluble substances extracted from delipidated cells of *C. parvum* – including a fraction of relatively low molecular weight (6000 daltons) of peptidoglycan nature – were shown to exert some of the activities of the whole cells, in particular enhancement of resistance of mice against EMC virus infection (when administered intravenously 2 hr before s.c. inoculation of the virus) and against the plasma variant of Moloney sarcoma virus – as judged by inhibition of splenomegaly 3 weeks after virus inoculation – when administered i.v. 4 days before infection (Migliore-Samour *et al.*, 1974). It would be interesting to test the activity of such fractions in a system like herpes virus infection, which is known to respond to whole *C. parvum* preparations only when they are administered several days before infection. It may well be that in the case of an infection like EMC virus, mere transient stimulation of the macrophages is sufficient to afford increased resistance.

In spite of the impressive experimental evidence in favor of an antiviral activity of *Corynebacterium parvum*, but possibly because of the known complexity of its activity mechanisms and of its side-effects, it does not appear that clinical studies have been performed to demonstrate a beneficial effect of this agent in viral illnesses of humans. The only study we are aware of consisted in injecting *C. parvum* intradermally to asymptomatic chronic carriers of hepatitis B surface antigen (HBsAg), to persons with serum antibodies to HBsAg (anti-HBs) and to control individuals without HBsAg nor anti-HBs (Papaevangelou *et al.*, 1977): *C. parvum* caused a significant increase of anti-HBs titers in persons with preexisting such antibodies, but anti-HBs responses were not induced in carriers and HBsAg was not eliminated, its titer remaining practically unchanged.

It has also been suggested, but not established, that the benefit derived from *C. parvum* treatment in some forms of cancer may to some extent be due to the enhanced resistance of these immunologically compromised patients against viral and other infections.

13.3.6. GLUCANS

Glucan, a water-insoluble β-1,3-glucopyranose polysaccharide with a helical configuration, which is extracted from yeast cell walls, as well as related polyglucoses with a β-1,3 linkage extracted in Japan from some edible mushrooms (lentinan, pachymaran, schizophyllan) potentiate cellular and humoral immunity and nonspecifically enhance host resistance to malignant cells and to bacterial, fungal and protozoan infections. It has been shown (Reynolds *et al.*, 1980) that intravenous pretreatment of mice with glucan enhanced the survival of mice challenged intraperitoneally with Venezuelan equine encephalomyelitis virus (VEE) or subcutaneously with Rift Valley fever virus (RVF). It is interesting to note that optimal pretreatment time was 3 days in the case of VEE challenge and 7 days in the case of RVF challenge. Post-challenge treatments were ineffective. More recently, the same group of investigators (Di Luzio *et al.*, 1982) reported a markedly enhanced resistance of mice pretreated intravenously with glucan to intraperitoneal challenge with a strain of murine hepatitis virus (MHV) and with a strain of human herpes simplex type 2 virus. In the latter case, the animals received relatively large doses of glucan (23 mg/kg) on days 19, 8, 6, 4 and 2 prior to infection: by 16 days post-challenge, 87 per cent survival was noted in the treated group versus 27 per cent in the controls.

In both studies, particulate, water-insoluble glucan was used: this form is known to induce granuloma formation in the liver when injected intravenously: such an effect could explain the enhanced resistance to hepatotropic viruses. In this respect, it is of interest that a soluble form of glucan was also found capable of modifying viral hepatitis in the mouse (80 per cent survival in the soluble glucan-treated animals versus 25 per cent in the controls, with no evidence of granuloma formation in the liver), in another study by Di Luzio and his group (reported by Chirigos and Jacques, 1981).

13.3.7. TRANSFER FACTOR

Strictly speaking, the term transfer factor (TF) refers to a dialysable extract of leukocytes, which can transfer specific cellular immunity from a skin-test-positive donor to a skin-test-negative recipient. Although first considered, according to this definition, as a specific agent, transferring reactivity only to antigens or haptens to which the leukocytes donor is sensitive, TF has gradually come to be regarded as being able to enhance in a less specific manner induction or expression of cell-mediated immunity ('adjuvant' effect).

Several attempts have been made to use TF therapeutically in persistent viral infections and various degrees of success have been reported in progressive vaccinia, herpes zoster, 'giant cell' measles pneumonia, subacute sclerosing panencephalitis, chronic active hepatitis and cytomegalovirus retinitis (see review by Mazaheri et al., 1977). In all such studies, evidence for activity of TF was largely anecdotal, since they were not double-blind controlled trials and since most such diseases go through natural cycles of relapse or remission. A small double-blind trial of TF was performed in eight patients with chronic active hepatitis: all four patients who received TF from donors who had recovered from hepatitis B and A showed biochemical improvement (fall in serum transaminase levels) and some histological improvement, but HBsAg remained present in the serum (Schulman et al., 1976).

In another study (Jain et al., 1977), six patients with HBsAg-positive chronic liver disease were treated with TF prepared from leukocytes of normal blood donors with no history of hepatitis and with TF from subjects recently recovered from B hepatitis. The administration of the latter preparation provoked a hepatic reaction manifested by elevation of serum aspartate transaminase, representing damage or destruction of hepatocytes; TF from nonimmune donors did not provoke this reaction. All patients returned to their previous clinical status after the period of the study and permanent benefit was not achieved.

On the other hand, a double-blind study was undertaken to evaluate TF efficacy in patients with severe recurrent herpes simplex type 1 (six patients) or type 2 (twenty-two patients). TF had been obtained from eight donors who showed evidence of humoral and cellular immunity to HSV-1 and HSV-2 antigens but were free from recurrences. Each patient received TF or saline subcutaneously every 2 months for a total of six doses. Results were entirely negative: TF treatment did not decrease the numbers and severity of recurrences when compared with patients receiving the placebo and, furthermore, TF did not change the in vitro responsiveness of the recipients' lymphocytes to HSV antigens (Oleske et al., 1978). Interestingly enough, subjective improvement was reported by two-thirds of the patients both in the placebo and the TF group.

As described in a recent report (Steele, 1980), transfer factor prepared from leukocytes of adults convalescing from chickenpox, was administered s.c. to fifteen children with acute lymphocytic leukemia, twelve in remission and three in relapse. All children had negative histories of varicella-zoster infection and all presented negative responses in virus-specific immune tests (cytotoxicity against VZ-infected cells; VZ-induced blastogenesis; leukocyte inhibitory factor (LIF) production upon stimulation with VZ-infected cells). Nine out of the twelve patients in remission became positive, 3 weeks after treatment, in the cytotoxicity test; five became positive in the blastogenesis test and seven in the LIF test. None of the patients in relapse, who ultimately died, developed a response in these tests. Although cellular immune reactivity to VZ virus could be transferred with transfer factor, there is no indication that VZ-specific transfer factor can prevent the onset of the disease, or accelerate the recovery of it, in high-risk patients. An encouraging result has been obtained in a child affected by a combined EB virus and cytomegalovirus infection (Jones et al., 1981). The patient was treated orally with xenogeneic transfer factor, obtained from leukocytes from a cow immunized with M. tuberculosis and which presented CMI to infectious bovine tracheitis virus. Treatment with transfer factor coincided with the development of lymphocytes blastogenesis to CMV, disappearance of CMV from urines and clinical resolution of illness.

The use of experimental models could help in clarifying the possible usefulness of TF in the treatment of some viral illnesses; thus marmosets have been protected from fatal HSV-1 infection using dialysable leukocyte extract prepared from a human donor with marked cellular immunity to the virus (Steele *et al.*, 1976).

13.3.8. THYMIC HORMONES (OR FACTORS)

There is little doubt nowadays that the thymus fulfills at least part of its action through the operations of soluble mediators; thymic hormones (or: factors) is the term applied to substances which are produced by the thymus gland and which act within the thymus or at a distance, to induce T cell differentiation (see review by Bach, 1978). Thymic factors comprise polypeptides of various degrees of purity and identification and which are called by the teams investigating them: thymosin (A. L. Goldstein), thymopoietin (G. Goldstein), thymic humoral factor, THF (Trainin) and serum thymic factor, FTS (J. F. Bach).

Considerable progress has been made over the last few years in the knowledge of these various thymic hormones. Available now for clinical studies are fraction 5 of thymosin, TP-1 (which is an extract prepared in a way similar to that of thymosin fraction 5) and THF (prepared from calf thymus by ultracentrifugation and dialysis). Since the amino acid sequence of some of the thymic hormones has been established, synthetic polypeptides are also available for clinical use; they include thymosin alpha-1, TP-5 (a pentapeptide patterned after thymopoietin) and FTS (or: thymuline, a zinc-containing nonapeptide). All these substances are capable of normalizing various functional parameters of T lymphocytes (such as E rosette formation and response to mitogens) in animals and humans with corresponding deficiencies. It has already been mentioned that thymuline (FTS) can stimulate NK cell activity *in vitro* and *in vivo* in the mouse. Thymic hormones could therefore be useful for treating patients with congenital or acquired defects in T-cell-mediated immunity which would make them especially prone to some virus infections. The first report of such an application described THF therapy in four children treated with immunosuppressive cytostatic drugs for lymphoproliferative malignancies, who had come down with varicella (Zaizov *et al.*, 1977). It is known that such patients are at an increased risk of developing severe forms of generalized varicella (mortality close to 7 per cent, vs. 0.1–0.4 per cent in the general population). In this study, the patients received daily intramuscular injections of THF for 5–16 days, starting on the first day of the varicella eruption. All four children recovered uneventfully and therapy was shown to increase the number of peripheral blood lymphocytes and of rosette-forming cells. In a more recent study (Handzel *et al.*, 1981), sixty-three patients suffering from varicella or zoster complicating acute lymphocytic leukemia, acute myeloblastic leukemia, Hodgkin or non-Hodgkin lymphoma, neuroblastoma or rhabdomyosarcoma received daily intramuscular injections of THF; based on clinical and laboratory findings, there was ample evidence for a prompt restoring effect of the treatment on the immunological recovery mechanisms. The same authors quote five cases of severe viral encephalitis which showed a dramatic clinical recovery after short courses of THF therapy (usually within 1 to 3 days after institution of the treatment).

Experimental evidence for the antiviral activity of THF has been provided by Rager-Zisman *et al.* (1980) who treated with this substance (300 μg/mouse i.p. on days 2, 3, 4, 7 and 9 post-infection) mice which had been inoculated intranasally with Sendai virus. While loss of body weight, involution of the thymus and pneumonia were observed in control mice, the THF-treated mice kept on gaining weight, their thymus involution was stopped and they showed less frequent lung lesions.

A number of clinical studies are presently under way with thymuline (FTS) and encouraging results in severe viral infections—such as a case of generalized herpes in a thymectomized patient—have been reported (Bach and Dardenne, 1982). The same authors observed that, in three children with IgA deficiency, treatment with FTS led to the appearance of normal IgA levels in the serum.

It then appears that there is a considerable potential for the use of thymic factors and hormones in immunosuppressed patients exhibiting severe infections with 'thymus-dependent' viruses (herpes, varicella-zoster, cytomegalovirus). They might also be used in the treatment of neonatal rubella, of HBs-positive hepatitis and of recurrent herpes, but it must be kept in mind that such a treatment might stimulate suppressor T lymphocytes, thus possibly counteracting its beneficial effects (Bach and Dardenne, 1982).

13.4. INTERFERON AND INTERFERON INDUCERS

The topic of interferon and interferon inducers as antiviral agents is comprehensively treated in another chapter.

It will suffice to recall here that many of the immunopotentiating substances described in this review are capable of inducing the production or the release of interferon and that, on the other hand, interferon as well as classical interferon inducers are known to exert various immunomodulating effects. Double-stranded interferon-inducing polyribonucleotides, like poly I : C for instance, exert immunostimulating and adjuvant activities that resemble those of endotoxins; a simple synthetic interferon inducer, like tilorone, has been shown to enhance antibody production while depressing cell-mediated immune responses.

Interferon itself has been shown, under some experimental conditions, to inhibit antibody production (Gisler et al., 1974) and to inhibit DNA synthesis induced in lymphocytes by phytohemagglutinin or by allogeneic cells (Lindahl-Magnusson et al., 1972), while also enhancing the specific cytotoxicity of sensitized lymphocytes for allogeneic target tumor cells (Lindahl et al., 1972) and the expression of cell-surface components, such as Fc receptors (Fridman et al., 1980) and histocompatibility antigens (Lindahl et al., 1976; Vignaux and Gresser, 1978; Fellous et al., 1979), which play a major role in antiviral immunity (e.g. T cell cytotoxicity, ADCC). On the other hand, murine interferon can enhance the phagocytic activity (Huang et al., 1971) and the antitumor properties (Schultz and Chirigos, 1979) of mononuclear cells from the mouse peritoneal cavity as well as NK cell activity (see Section 13.2). Recently it has been shown that type I and type II interferons can act synergistically with respect to inhibition of EMC virus multiplication (Fleischmann et al., 1979) and intracellular induction of 'antiviral' enzymes, such as the 2–5 A synthetase and the 67 K protein kinase (Zerial et al., 1982). This suggests that simultaneous production of both types of interferon by immunostimulating agents (Evans and Johnson, 1981) may represent an advantageous mechanism of antiviral defense.

13.5. SYNTHETIC SUBSTANCES

13.5.1. COPOLYMER PYRAN, POLYCARBOXYLATES

Pyran is the name given to a copolymer of divinyl ether and maleic anhydride, to which a high density of negative charges gives a polyanionic nature, as it is the case also with dextran sulfate or with poly I : C. It has been shown to induce interferon in mouse and man, to stimulate or to depress various immune responses, to prevent adjuvant-induced arthritis in the rat and to enhance macrophage functions (particularly cytostatic activity for tumor cells). It is active, by parenteral routes, against many transplanted, viral or carcinogen-induced tumors in the mouse and it underwent clinical trials in cancer patients (Regelson et al., 1978). It appears that toxicity of pyran preparations is, to a large extent, related to their molecular weight, the polymers with the lowest molecular weight (15,000) being the least toxic, while retaining their antitumor activity (Breslow et al., 1973).

A pyran preparation (MW not indicated) was shown to protect both normal mice and mice which had been adult thymectomized, lethally irradiated and bone marrow reconstituted (T × B mice) against mortality following intravenous (i.v.) or intravaginal infection with herpes simplex type 2 virus (HSV-2) (Morahan and McCord, 1975). T × B mice were found to be about 10 times more sensitive to that infection than normal mice. The protective effect required that the compound was administered i.v. or i.p. 24 hr before viral challenge: in pyran-treated mice, virus appeared later and in lower titers in the spinal cord than in the control animals (McCord *et al.*, 1976). While pyran and *Corynebacterium parvum* were both effective in protecting mice against i.v. infection with HSV-2, only pyran showed activity against intravaginal infection; depression of macrophage function by *in vivo* administration of silica, although markedly enhancing the sensitivity of the mice to HSV-2 infection by the i.v. route, did not inhibit the activity of pyran or of *C. parvum* (Morahan *et al.*, 1977b). The possible mechanisms of the protective effect of pyran on intravaginal infection of mice with HSV-2 have been analyzed (Breinig *et al.*, 1978): treatment effectively limited viral replication in the vaginal area and survival of mice was correlated with elimination of the early replication of HSV-2 in this area and thus prevention of its spread to the central nervous system. No evidence was found for increased neutralizing antibody production to HSV-2 in pyran-treated mice; on the contrary, antibody production in these mice was delayed and decreased, as was HSV-2 specific delayed hypersensitivity response. These decreased humoral and cell-mediated immune responses in pyran-treated mice were considered to be a reflection of the early decreased growth of the virus. On the other hand, adherent peritoneal cells stimulated by *in vivo* i.p. treatment with pyran were found to possess antiviral activity *in vitro* and to transfer resistance to suckling mice *in vivo*.

Since it is likely that their mode of action is similar to that of pyran, one may also mention here the antiviral activity *in vivo* of polycarboxylates, such as polyacrylic acid, poly-methacrylic acid and chlorite-oxidized oxyamylose. The general structure of polyacrylic acids is:

$$[-CH_2-CH(COOH)-]_n.$$

Polycarboxylates have been shown to exert many effects on host defense mechanisms, such as interferon induction, pyrogenicity, stimulation of macrophage activities, adjuvant activity on humoral and cell-mediated immune reactions, and consequently they protect animals against viral, bacterial, fungal and protozoal infections and against grafted tumors and leukemias (see review by De Clercq, 1973). The fact that their antiviral activity is not solely mediated through their interferon-inducing properties was shown by the kinetics of this activity: for instance, carbopol, a polymer of acrylic acid cross-linked with allylsucrose, imparts resistance to mice which receive an i.p. injection of the compound 1 to 4 days before intravenous challenge with vaccinia virus or intranasal challenge with herpes simplex virus, whereas a modest peak of interferon activity in the serum occurs 20 to 40 hr after treatment (De Clercq and Luczak, 1976). The ratios between toxic (i.e. causing significant mortality in uninfected mice) and active doses (enhancing resistance to intranasal challenge with herpes virus), by the i.p. route were found to be 5 for carbopol and polyacrylic acid and 25 for chlorite-oxidized oxyamylose. It is noteworthy that, like BCG or *C. parvum*, polyacrylic acids increased the sensitivity of the mice to the lethal effect of endotoxin injection when they were administered 14 to 7 days before the latter (Maral, R., personal communication). Polymethylmethacrylate has also been reported to exert adjuvant activity on immunization of mice and guinea pigs with influenza vaccines consisting of viral subunits (Kreuter *et al.*, 1976).

13.5.2. Levamisole

Tetramisole and its levorotatory isomer, levamisole, have been known for more than a decade for their high effectiveness as anthelmintics in man and domestic animals; they are active against most pathogenic nematodes and levamisole is widely used in man, especially for treating ankylostomiasis and ascariasis. It was later found (Renoux and Renoux, 1971) that mice immunized with an only moderately active anti-*Brucella* vaccine were completely protected against challenge with live *Brucella* bacilli when they had received levamisole or tetramisole together with the vaccine. This observation aroused considerable interest, since it was the first time that a synthetic agent was reported to exert an immunoadjuvant effect and since it was readily possible to undertake clinical trials with a drug which was already in use in humans. To summarize the mass of experimental and clinical data which have been published about the immunomodulating activities of levamisole would be a formidable task and the reader is referred to recently published reviews (Renoux, 1978; Symoens, 1978); we shall borrow from these reviews the following conclusions: 'Levamisole stimulates recruitment and functions of macrophage and T cell under a narrow range of doses and time of administration in normal or immunoimpaired man and animal. Strain, sex, age and antigen modulate the activity of levamisole from enhancement to inhibition; stimulation is mediated through a serum factor able also to promote thymocytes in thymusless mice (Renoux). Studies on isolated phagocytes and lymphocytes show that levamisole influences virtually all cell functions involved in cell mediated immune responses. It seems to be the first member of a new series of simple chemical agents that mimic hormonal regulation of the immune system (Symoens).'

Chemical structure of levamisole, tetramisole

Before reviewing clinical data concerning immunoenhancing activities of levamisole in some viral infections, we shall analyze experimental evidence in favor of such an activity. This can be simply done by stating that, to our knowledge, the only positive result to be reported was that levamisole treatment significantly increased survival rates of suckling rats inoculated intraperitoneally, at 10 days of age, with a strain of herpes simplex type 2 virus (HSV-2) (Fischer et al., 1975; Fischer et al., 1977). Survival, 14 days after infection, was 4 per cent in control rats, 30 per cent in animals receiving levamisole subcutaneously (3 mg/kg, 4 and 24 hr after infection), 20 per cent in animals treated with adenine arabinoside, and 11 per cent in rats receiving combined treatments with both drugs – suggesting antagonism between their activities. Splenectomy studies indicated that levamisole requires an intact spleen if it is to provide protection against encephalitis caused by HSV-2 and it is possible that the drug enhances splenic entrapment of the virus, thus preventing its dissemination.

On the other hand, studies in mice seem to have been uniformly negative at least with respect to protection by levamisole of newborn or adult mice infected intraperitoneally or intravaginally with HSV-2 (Starr et al., 1976; Morahan et al., 1977b). In our own laboratory (unpublished results), using several types of virus infections in adult mice, we failed to observe any significant or consistent activity of levamisole, except for a slight increase in survival time in animals infected with murine hepatitis virus or with influenza A2 virus and receiving levamisole in their drinking water throughout the experiment.

Experiments in larger animals have proven more encouraging. Single intramuscular doses of 1–6 mg/kg levamisole were given to 149 cattle and 26 goats affected with foot-and-mouth disease (type C virus): within 48 hr, there was dramatic improvement of symptomatology in the treated animals as compared with controls (Rojas and Olivari, 1974). Levamisole was also tested for therapeutic activity in Aleutian disease of mink, a persistent infection caused by a parvovirus. The drug was incorporated into the mink ration (1 mg/kg daily for 14 days, followed by 14 days without treatment and again 14 days of treatment): the health status of the treated animals after 3 months was improved, as indicated by an increased body weight, lower incidence of bile duct proliferation and periportal infiltrates and reduced hyper-gammaglobulinemia (Kenyon, 1978).

With respect to clinical evidence on the efficacy of levamisole (always administered orally) in human viral diseases, several studies have been performed in patients afflicted with recurrent herpes labialis or recurrent herpes progenitalis. Most of these studies were uncontrolled, i.e. they did not include placebo-treated subjects: clinical improvement and decreased frequency of recurrences were reported in several cases of facial, labial, corneal and genital herpes (Kint and Verlinden, 1974; Kint et al., 1974; Lods, 1976). Clinical improvement was associated with enhanced in vitro response of lymphocytes to herpes virus antigen in one study (O'Reilly *et al.*, 1977) and with a decreased response in another study (Spitler *et al.*, 1975).

More recently, the results of a double-blind, controlled trial of levamisole in the treatment of recurrent herpes labialis were reported (Russell *et al.*, 1978); it included ninety-nine subjects with recurrent circumoral herpes at least 4 times a year. Forty-eight subjects received the drug (2.5 mg/kg) on 2 consecutive days each week for 6 months and the fifty-one controls were given a placebo. During the 6 months of the study, there were no significant differences between the two groups in the duration or severity of the lesions or in the subjective assessment of drug efficacy by the patients; as far as the last parameter is concerned, it is noteworthy that 60 per cent of subjects on placebo evaluated this treatment as excellent. No difference was found between the levamisole and control groups in their lymphocyte responses to the virus or to PHA. It must be noted that before treatment, the frequency of lesions in the levamisole group was higher than in the control group: when this factor was taken into account, there was a significant difference between the two groups, with the group receiving levamisole demonstrating a greater improvement than controls.

Several other controlled double-blind clinical studies have been performed on the activity of levamisole in recurrent herpes simplex episodes. Mehr and Albano (1977) found no beneficial effect in twenty-eight patients with recurrent herpes labialis and genitalis. The patients had been instructed to initiate a 3-day treatment regimen (with 50, 100 or 150 mg levamisole orally per day) at the onset of each clinical episode. This same regimen was applied, in another study, to forty-two patients with a high frequency of recurrent herpes labialis, who were followed for a mean of 7–8 months (Spruance *et al.*, 1979). Statistical analysis revealed that, as the dosage increased, so did the frequency of recurrences; conversely, the duration of lesions and of lesion pain decreased with increasing dosage. The authors concluded that levamisole was not an appropriate agent for the treatment of recurrent herpes labialis, adding that the paradoxical response to this immunomodulator – i.e. increased frequency and decreased severity – provided evidence that altered host responses may contribute to the pathogenesis of this disease. In still another study (Jose and Minty, 1980), levamisole was tested in thirty-three patients with frequently recurring attacks of herpes labialis or herpes genitalis, all of whom had experienced monthly recurrent episodes for at least 6 months. The patients were randomly allocated to receive 2.5 mg/kg levamisole or placebo orally on 2 consecutive days each week for 26 weeks; the tablets were reversed for a second consecutive 6-month period. The results showed a reduction in frequency, severity and total duration of attacks in six out of twelve patients with herpes labialis and in seventeen out of twenty-one patients with herpes genitalis. Whereas the symptoms of 20 per cent of patients showed improvement while on placebo, the additional benefit from levamisole was reported to be clinically obvious and statistically significant. A notable feature was the considerable delay period (up to 8 weeks) after the start of levamisole administration before any clinical response to the drug could be seen; the drug was not beneficial in treating existing attacks but was useful in the prevention of recurrences—a conclusion which seems to contradict that of the previously described study. The latter was, however, concerned only with herpes labialis and levamisole treatment was not applied in the intervals between recurrences. Side effects, usually mild, were indeed frequently seen in the study involving weekly levamisole treatments.

Reviewing ten placebo-controlled studies on the effect of levamisole in recurrent labial or genital herpes, Symoens *et al.* (1979) note that, overall, 107 out of 172 patients (62 per cent) improved with levamisole versus 86 out of 194 (44 per cent) who received a placebo. These authors add that the differences between placebo and levamisole are usually most pronounced when individual responsiveness is considered rather than group mean differences and conclude that patients with recurrent herpes simplex are highly hetero-geneous groups, comprising subpopulations responding to levamisole, placebo, both or neither.

Clinical studies have concluded to a beneficial effect of levamisole treatment in various other viral diseases: an uncontrolled trial showed rapid regression of warts (due to molluscum contagiosum virus) in nine out of ten children (Helin and Bergh, 1974); a double-blind study on seventy children with frequent respiratory diseases during the winter months – actual viral etiology was not assessed by laboratory tests – showed decreased frequency and severity of these infections in the levamisole-treated group (Van Eygen et al., 1976); a placebo-controlled trial was performed in fifty consecutive patients with acute viral hepatitis: disappearance of antibodies against the core antigen was faster in levamisole- than in placebo-treated patients with type B hepatitis and, by the end of the third month, one only of the twenty-three levamisole-treated patients had not recovered from the acute disease (as judged by transaminases, HBsAg presence and histology) versus eight out of twenty-seven patients in the control group (Par et al., 1977).

More recent open or controlled studies on the possible usefulness of levamisole in hastening recovery from viral infections – such as influenza, hepatitis and measles – have been reviewed by Symoens et al. (1979).

Further to a study summarized above, Van Eygen et al. (1979) tested levamisole in a double-blind manner in 106 children with recurrent upper respiratory tract infections of various etiologies. They received levamisole (2.5 mg/kg orally) or placebo b.i.d. for 2 consecutive days each week for 6 months, a control examination being performed every 2 months only. Improvement, with respect to number of infectious episodes and duration and severity of these episodes, was observed more frequently on the levamisole group than in the placebo group. If an incidence of only one infection every winter is considered to be 'normal', then 70 per cent of the levamisole-treated children, against only 26 per cent of those receiving the placebo, exhibited a normal defense against such infections.

In view of the hypothetical viral etiology of Crohn disease, improvement of this condition by levamisole therapy is worth mentioning (Bertrand et al., 1974).

In conclusion, it appears difficult, at the present time, to get a clear and definite view of the possible usefulness of levamisole in immunomodulating therapy of viral illnesses. The contrast between the rather negative results of experiments in laboratory animals and the often encouraging data from clinical trials may be due in part to the fact that, in the first case, the drug was given prophylactically while it was administered in a therapeutic manner to the patients. In the latter case, levamisole may have exerted its beneficial effect by restoring immune responses which had been impaired by the virus infection; better information on this last point might indeed help in selecting the patients who would be more likely to benefit from treatment with levamisole or other immunomodulating drugs.

At any rate, the potential danger of long-term levamisole therapy—mainly the occurrence of agranulocytosis – must be weighed against the probability of benefit from such a therapy; as seen above this benefit is far from being obvious in most situations.

13.5.3. INOSIPLEX

Together with levamisole, inosiplex (Isoprinosine (R)) differs from the other immuno-potentiating substances described in this review by the fact that it has already been extensively used in man, but, unlike levamisole which began its career as an anthelminthic drug, inosiplex was from the start put on the market, in some countries as an antiviral agent.

Inosiplex is a compound formed from inosine and the para-acetamidobenzoate salt of 1-dimethylamino-2-propanol, with a molar ratio of 1:3.

Early studies, showing that inosiplex could inhibit cytopathic effect of a rhinovirus or of influenza A2 virus in cell cultures, led to consider this compound as an antiviral agent in the usual meaning of the term. Inhibition of cytopathic effect was only moderate, however, even at high concentrations of inosiplex and in spite of daily medium change of the cultures to compensate for degradation of the purine portion (see review by Ginsberg and Glasky, 1977). Evidence for an in vivo antiviral activity of inosiplex in laboratory animals was first contradictory, depending on how the animals were treated with the compound. Negative results were reported when this substance was evaluated in a coordinated study at five different laboratories (Glasgow and Galasso, 1972): no antiviral effect could be demonstrated in mice infected with encephalomyocarditis (EMC), type 2 herpes simplex,

Structural formula of inosiplex

influenza and rabies viruses, in rabbits infected with vaccinia virus, in cats infected with feline rhinotracheitis and panleukopenia viruses, in ferrets infected with distemper virus and in swine infected with influenza and transmissible gastroenteritis viruses. The only antiviral activity observed was suppression of fibroma virus lesions in rabbits receiving large i.p. doses of inosiplex. In mice, therapy at a dose of 300 mg/kg had been initiated at various times before or after virus inoculation (in most cases early after) and was administered once daily either i.p. or orally.

Suspicion that inosiplex did not behave like a classical antiviral agent arose when it was noticed (Muldoon *et al.*, 1972) that treatment initiated 24 hr prior to infection and continued daily thereafter did not increase survival in mice infected intranasally with A2 influenza virus, while treatment started 24 hr *after* infection resulted in significantly increased survival time. Other experiments suggested that optimal activity of inosiplex, administered in a therapeutic manner, i.e. following virus inoculation, required the presence of adequate immune responses in the animal: in mice challenged with a dose of influenza virus causing 60 per cent mortality in untreated controls, inosiplex treatment reduced mortality to 30 per cent while cortisone increased it to 85 per cent, but combined inosiplex and cortisone treatments led to a 100 per cent mortality; similar results were obtained when mice were immunosuppressed with anti-lymphocyte serum (Ginsberg and Glasky, 1977). Direct evidence for an interaction of inosiplex with the immune system was provided by experiments in which mice were immunized with sheep erythrocytes and their spleen cells assayed 4 days thereafter for production of hemolytic plaques in an erythrocyte–agar overlay in the presence of various concentrations of the drug: in this *in vitro* situation, concentrations of 100, 300 and 500 μg/ml of inosiplex significantly increased the number of plaques (Ginsberg and Glasky, 1977). It was also shown (Hadden *et al.*, 1976) that, in *in vitro* cultures of human peripheral blood lymphocytes, inosiplex, over a concentration range from 0.2 to 250 μg/ml, slightly but significantly augmented proliferation induced by phytohemagglutinin (PHA); in the absence of PHA the drug had no effect on lymphocyte proliferation.

Inosiplex has shown some protective effect on experimental virus infections of laboratory animals when care was taken to administer this drug following a therapeutic schedule (i.e. in beginning treatment *after* the animals had been infected) and at appropriate dosage (in most cases, in the drinking water, at a 1 per cent concentration). For instance, A/J mice which are highly susceptible to the lethal effect of an i.p. inoculation of herpes simplex virus type 1 were converted to moderate susceptibility, similar to that of BALB/c mice, when inosiplex was added to their drinking water starting 24 hr after infection (Hadden *et al.*, 1977). In our own studies (Floc'h and Werner, unpublished), in which inosiplex was administered in the same manner, increased survival as a result of treatment was seen in mice inoculated i.p. with murine hepatitis virus or with two strains of herpes simplex type 1 virus but not in mice infected s.c. with EMC virus or through an aerosol of influenza A2 virus. Enhancement of the partial protective effect of a suboptimal dose of tilorone (given 24 hr before infection) was seen in EMC-virus-infected mice receiving inosiplex in their drinking water from the first day after infection. There was some difficulty in confirming these various encouraging results in repeat experiments, the actual degree of efficacy of inosiplex being variable from one test to another.

An attempt at integrating the antiviral and immunoenhancing effects of inosiplex has been presented recently (Simon et al., 1978). Using a hemadsorption assay, it was shown that at two distinct concentration ranges (from 0.005 to 1.0 μg/ml and from 10 to 150 μg/ml) inosiplex inhibited infection of HeLa cells with the AO/PR8 strain of influenza virus and also decreased intracellular levels of the virus. This inhibition was moderate, however, and rarely exceeded 50 per cent (which, with the hemagglutination technique used to measure virus levels, means a two-fold dilution difference). At about the same two concentration ranges, inosiplex increased the proliferating effect of concanavalin A and of A2 influenza virus on murine spleen cells cultured in vitro: again, this stimulation was slight, thymidine incorporation being around 1.5 times higher in cultures containing appropriate amounts of the drug than in cultures stimulated by Con A or by virus alone. When inosiplex' effect on influenza virus replication was compared, by linear regression analysis, with its potentiation of virus-induced splenocyte proliferation, the correlation coefficients obtained at the two concentration ranges suggested that both of these effects must have a common biological basis. Furthermore, the authors showed that intraperitoneal inoculation of mice with live influenza AO/PR8 virus caused, 7 days later, a slight decrease below normal levels of in vitro response of their spleen cells to Con A; treatment with inosiplex, initiated after inoculation of the virus, normalized this response and, in addition, considerably increased the degree of spleen cell proliferation induced in vitro by the viral antigen. Mice which had received a high dilution of the virus by the i.p. route showed only partial immunity (30 per cent survival) when they were challenged intranasally 20 days later with a lethal dose of virus; their immunity was much stronger (100 per cent survival) when they had been treated with inosiplex from the time of the immunization.

It has also been shown that inosiplex was able to greatly enhance the antiviral protection afforded by a single dose of murine interferon against lethal infection with EMC virus (Chany and Cerutti, 1977). In these experiments, mice were infected i.p. with 100 LD_{50} of virus; the administration of 20,000 units of interferon 1 hr after infection only slightly delayed death; inosiplex alone exerted no effect, but when the animals received 1000 mg/kg i.p. of inosiplex 24 hr before and interferon 1 hr after infection, 80 per cent of the animals survived and were resistant to subsequent reinfection. In contrast with what was seen in other experimental systems, therapeutic administration of inosiplex (7 hr after the virus, 1 hr after interferon) had no protective effect whatsoever in this system. It appears possible that inosiplex enhances the response of cells to interferon by interacting with their membranes, in a way similar to its enhancing effect on the response of lymphocytes to some mitogens.

As inosiplex is a nontoxic substance, there have been many studies on its antiviral activity in man following oral administration. We shall first review trials performed in volunteers who were artificially infected.

Inosiplex was given orally to twenty-two volunteers who, along with twenty-three other volunteers receiving a placebo, were inoculated intranasally with two strains of human rhinovirus (RV-9 and RV-31); treatment had been started 48 hr before infection, daily treatments consisted of 4 times 1.5 g of inosiplex daily. Results of this trial were entirely negative: inosiplex treatment exerted no effect on the average clinical score of the colds induced and on laboratory evidence of infection with either or both viruses (reisolation of virus, seroconversion) (Soto et al., 1973). In another study, fifteen volunteers treated with inosiplex (2.5 g twice daily for 10 days, beginning 48 hr before infection) and fifteen placebo-treated volunteers were inoculated intranasally with A/Hong Kong/8/68 (H3N2) influenza virus: treatment with inosiplex did not result in any appreciable modification of the clinical course of the illness and the only demonstrable beneficial effect of the drug was that the total number of virus isolates was slightly but significantly lower in the volunteers receiving it (decrease in virus shedding); acquisition of neutralizing antibodies was similar in both groups (Longley et al., 1973). Prophylactic efficacy of inosiplex was again evaluated in a double-blind study in which volunteers were challenged intranasally with rhinovirus type 32 or type 44 (Pachuta *et al.*, 1974); the drug was given orally, at a daily dosage of 6 g, for 2 days prior to intranasal challenge with either virus and for 7 post-challenge days. Results were unimpressive: in both trials (each including nine volunteers on inosiplex and nine others on placebo), the occurrence and severity of the colds were greater in the placebo group but the difference with the drug-treated group was not considered significant; the average numbers of rhinovirus isolations during the post-challenge days were similar in the placebo- and in the drug-treated group; post-challenge antibody titers in serum and nasal secretions were not significantly different between the two groups.

In view of the experimental evidence that inosiplex behaves as an immunomodulating agent and is more effective when treatment is initiated after than before viral challenge, a double-blind study was performed more recently on the therapeutic efficacy of the drug in rhinovirus infection of volunteers (Waldman and Ganguly, 1977). Thirty-nine volunteers were randomly assigned to inosiplex or placebo groups; drug or placebo was started either at the time of, or 48 hr *after*, nasal challenge with rhinovirus type 21. Illness was assessed in terms of typical common cold symptoms (sneezing, sore throat, nasal stuffiness, nasal discharge, cough) and infection was determined by virus isolation from nasal washings and serum antibody rises. Evaluation of individual symptoms revealed a fairly uniform decrease in mean scores for all symptoms in volunteers taking inosiplex as compared to controls (statistically significant for nasal stuffiness and nasal discharge). The illness rate was reduced in the volunteers receiving inosiplex: eleven volunteers among the twenty on placebo were judged to be ill, versus only three out of ten in volunteers receiving inosiplex since the day of challenge and two out of nine in those who started taking the drug 2 days after challenge. The number of volunteers from whom virus was isolated was nearly the same in the placebo and inosiplex groups, but the mean duration of virus isolation was reduced in the treated group and fewer in the latter had serological evidence of infection as determined by antibody rise: these differences were not statistically significant, however. Interestingly, peripheral blood lymphocytes of volunteers treated with placebo showed 4, 8 and even 21 days after infection a decreased *in vitro* response to PHA, by comparison with pre-infection values, whereas in individuals receiving inosiplex, PHA response after infection was actually increased.

As part of a double-blind study of the therapeutic activity of inosiplex on herpes labialis (type 1) and herpes genitalis (type 2), the cell-mediated immune responses of patients were investigated prior to and after initiation of therapy, using as parameters the PHA response of peripheral blood lymphocytes and their ability to produce lymphotoxin following stimulation by PHA (Bradshaw and Sumner, 1977). After a week of treatment, thirteen patients on inosiplex and nine patients on placebo showed an increased response to PHA (and this increase was greater in the drug-treated group), while seven patients on inosiplex and twelve patients on placebo showed a decreased response to PHA (this decrease being more marked in the placebo group than in the drug group). With respect to changes in lymphotoxin titers, nine patients on inosiplex showed a marked increase versus four placebo-treated individuals, whose increase was small, whereas ten placebo-receiving patients and five inosiplex-receiving patients showed a decrease in such titers. Interpretation of such data is difficult but they suggest that inosiplex acts as an immunomodulating agent in humans and, furthermore, that actual response to this treatment may well vary from one individual to another.

In another double-blind placebo-controlled study (Corey *et al.*, 1979), the immunomodulatory and therapeutic effects of inosiplex were evaluated in patients affected by genital herpes. In such a study, thirty-nine patients were enrolled within 7 days since the beginning of the lesions: nineteen were treated orally with 4 g daily of inosiplex and twenty received placebo. Analysis of lymphocyte transformation responses to lectins (Con A, PWM, PHA) did not reveal differences among the two groups of patients. However, blood lymphocytes from inosiplex-treated patients displayed, as compared to those of the placebo group, a higher response to herpes simplex virus antigens, which was statistically significant, particularly when patients affected by a primary infection were considered. The clinical course of the primary infection was also positively affected by inosiplex: drug-treated patients experienced, as compared to the placebo group, a shorter duration of itching, a shorter duration of viral shedding from genital lesions as well a shorter time to heal them.

Beneficial effects of inosiplex against a variety of herpetic infections have been claimed in clinical studies, recently carried out. These include open studies in the case of herpes keratitis (Di Tizio *et al.*, 1979), zoster (Torregrossa, 1978; Carcó *et al.*, 1979), herpetic encephalitis (Lesourd *et al.*, 1980), a double-blind placebo-controlled study on recurrent mucocutaneous herpes (Bouffaut and Saurat, 1980) and a placebo-controlled study on recurrent genital herpes (Lassus and Salo, personal communication).

Therapeutic and prophylactic–therapeutic efficacy of inosiplex against influenza A (H3N2) challenge infection in human volunteers has been recently reassessed (Waldman *et al.*, 1978). This double-blind study was performed on forty-one adult volunteers who were inoculated intranasally with the A/Dunedin/73 strain. Inosiplex, at a daily dose of 4 g (in six administrations of either 1 or 0.5 g) was started either 2 days prior to challenge or 2 days following it and treatment was continued in both groups for a total of 9 days. When the number of volunteers with clinical illness suggestive of influenza was considered in each group, a lower illness rate was seen in each of the two treatment groups compared with placebo; although the infection rate, determined by an increase in serum antibody titer, was not different in the three groups, both frequency and severity of illness was lower in each of the treatment groups compared to placebo. A marked increase in the *in vitro* response to PHA of peripheral blood lymphocytes was seen 2, 4 and 21 days following virus inoculation in volunteers receiving inosiplex in a therapeutic manner, this increase was more modest in individuals receiving the drug according to a prophylactic–therapeutic schedule and even more discrete (although still significant) in placebo-treated patients.

In another double-blind placebo-controlled study (Schiff *et al.*, 1978) inosiplex was administered orally at 4 g daily to sixteen young volunteers, for 6 days beginning 24 hr after intranasal challenge with influenza virus A (Dunedin/73, H_3N_2). Fourteen subjects received placebo. Surprisingly, there was no serological evidence of influenza infection in two recipients of inosiplex and in five recipients of placebo. Evaluation was therefore carried out in only fourteen volunteers treated with the drug and in nine placebo. The average total symptom score was reported as being statistically lower for the treated group than for the placebo one and such a difference was more apparent 3 days after challenge. With respect to the individual symptoms, the score difference was maintained statistically for chills, headache, nasal and post-nasal discharge, sore throat, malaise and hoarse voice. The score for fever, nasal obstruction, myalgia as well as other parameters (virus shedding, antibody response, PHA lymphocyte stimulation) did not differ significantly between the drug and the placebo-treated groups.

In a similar study carried out by Betts *et al.* (1978), eighteen volunteers received the drug (4 g daily for 6 days) and fifteen placebo, 24 hr after challenge with A/Victoria 3/74 (H_3N_2) influenza virus. As in the previous study (Schiff *et al.*, 1978), the mean symptom score for the two groups was essentially the same during the first 3 days post-infection but, the fourth and fifth day, there was a lower score for the inosiplex-treated group. At days 5, 6 and 7 (but not for the first 4 days) there was furthermore a statistically lower percentage of individuals shedding virus in the recipients of inosiplex. Twelve subjects, from each group, underwent lymphocyte studies (PHA and influenza antigen stimulation on day 3, and cytotoxicity against influenza virus-infected cells on day 6, the three responses being compared with those obtained on day 0). The number of individuals responding in the PHA stimulation test and in the cytotoxicity test was higher for the inosiplex group (8 and 7 out of 12) than for the placebo (2/12). In contrast, no difference was noted for the response to influenza antigen.

In addition to studies performed in volunteers, clinical trials of inosiplex have been conducted in several areas. According to a recent clinical overview (Glasky *et al.*, 1978), 165 such studies have now been performed, involving a total of 4259 patients with viral illnesses as diverse as influenza, hepatitis A, recurrent herpes simplex, herpes zoster, varicella, mumps and measles. The majority of these trials consisted of open studies but a number of controlled double-blind studies have been described (hepatitis A, measles, mumps and varicella); the general conclusion to be derived from the accumulated data is that inosiplex, described as both an antiviral and a 'pro-host' drug, with a virtual absence of side effects, exerted a significantly favorable influence on the intensity and duration of symptoms and accelerated recovery.

Recent studies on the evaluation of inosiplex on SSPE* patients have suggested that long-term treatment with the drug might be favorable to the clinical course of the disease. Haddad and Risk (1980) did not observe, on the basis of historical controls, a clinical improvement in eighteen patients treated for short periods (2–27 weeks) with inosiplex. Dyken and Swift (1982) reported that, out of fifteen SPEE patients treated with inosiplex (100 mg/kg), four did not respond to therapy and died. Eleven patients, however, were still alive 2 years after the onset of the disease (73 per cent survival versus 38 per cent expected). Clinical improvements (decrease of the disability index) have been noted in nine patients, although they differed from case to case and fluctuated considerably throughout the therapy.

A higher long-term survival, in SSPE patients treated with inosiplex as compared to historical controls, has been also claimed by Jones *et al.* (personal communication). They obtained 78 per cent survival at 2 years (versus 38 per cent), 69 per cent at 4 years (versus 20 per cent) and 65 per cent at 8 years (versus 14 per cent).

Jabbour *et al.* (1980) reported the percentage of survival for forty-five drug-treated patients and for twenty-nine control (untreated) patients, the difference being highly encouraging for the inosiplex treatment (97.6 per cent versus 74 per cent at 2 years, 92 per cent versus 58.5 per cent at 3 years, 81.1 per cent versus 42.90 per cent at 5 years and 81.1 per cent versus 19 per cent at 13 years). In the latter analysis, patients (treated or untreated) who died within 6 months since the onset of the disease were not included. Evaluation of compounds against SSPE is not a simple task and rigorous controlled trials are difficult to set up. The results presented above suggest, but cannot presently prove, the efficacy of inosiplex in the treatment of such a disease.

13.5.4. MISCELLANEOUS IMMUNOMODULATING AGENTS

Over the last few years, a number of synthetic substances endowed with immunomodulating activities have been described, some of which have already reached the stage of clinical evaluation.

BM 12,531 or: azimexon, 1-[1-(2-cyano-1 aziridinyl-1-methylethyl]-2 aziridinecarboxamide, increases the resistance of normal mice to *Candida albicans* and that of cyclophosphamide-immunosuppressed mice to *Ps. aeruginosa* and *C. albicans* (Bicker *et al.*, 1979). It also exerts in mice and rats anti-tumor effects mediated through immunostimulation. Phase I studies are under way in cancer patients. To our knowledge, the only report about the activity of this drugs on virus infections concerns the infection of baby mice with vesicular stomatitis virus and suggests some protection when azimexon is administered i.p. 1 day before infection (Bicker, personal communication).

Bestatin, a streptomyces metabolite of known chemical structure [(2S, 3R)-3-amino-2-hydroxy-4-phenylbutanoyl-L-leucine], is an inhibitor of aminopeptidases associated with outer membranes of lymphoid cells. It potentiates humoral and cell-mediated immunity in the mouse and, under conditions of prolonged treatment, restores some of the impaired immune functions of aged mice (Umezawa, 1981). Bestatin is undergoing clinical investigation in cancer patients, with a suggestion of enhancement of NK cell activity. As far as we know, there has been no report on the activity of bestatin in experimental or clinical virus infections. The same applies to another interesting substance with modulating activities on T lymphocytes, sodium diethyldithiocarbamate (Renoux and Renoux, 1979).

On the other hand, one must mention observations according to which therafectin, a synthetic substance [1,2-*O*-isopropylidene-3-*O*-3'-(*N'*,*N'*-dimethylamino-n-propyl)-D-glucofuranose], protected normal and cyclophosphamide-immunosuppressed mice from influenza A and vaccinia virus infections and protected hamsters from lethal herpes virus encephalitis (Gordon, personal communication).

---

* Subacute sclerosing panencephalitis.

NPT 15392 is a novel synthetic immunomodulating substance [erythro-9-(2-hydroxy-3-nonyl) hypoxanthine] for which various *in vitro* and *in vivo* activities on immune functions have been reported. These activities are said to be similar to those of inosiplex in many respects but different in others (Hadden and Wybran, 1981). The main features of *in vitro* actions involve: (a) induction of T cell receptor display and enhancement of the display of pre-existing receptors; (b) stimulation or inhibition (according to the concentration) of mitogen-induced proliferation of lymphocytes; (c) induction of T suppressor cells and modulation of lymphocyte-induced suppression; (d) enhancement of helper and of cytolytic T cells. *In vivo*, administration of NPT 15392 to young adult mice (at a dose of 100 μg/kg by the i.p. route) stimulated natural killer (NK) activity in the spleen and in the peritoneal cell populations, with two peaks of stimulation, one 3 days and the other one 14 days after treatment (Florentin *et al.*, 1981). Clearly NPT 15392 appears as a valid candidate for immunomodulation studies in virus infections and further information concerning this specific application is awaited with interest.

13.6. POSSIBLE MECHANISMS OF THE ANTIVIRAL ACTIVITY OF IMMUNOPOTENTIATING SUBSTANCES

It is useful to make an inquiry about the mechanisms through which immunopotentiating substances enhance resistance to virus infections: such knowledge may help in defining what could be the practical applications of such substances as well as their limitations and also in designing more active and better tolerated agents. We have seen in the introduction that the immunological mechanisms which are part of the natural defenses of the host against virus infections are diverse and complex, that they may vary from one virus infection to another and that they are closely interrelated; furthermore, some immune reactions do contribute to the pathogenesis of some viral infections. The purpose one has in mind when using immunopotentiating substances for combating viral illnesses is to enhance those reactions which play a favorable role in the outcome of the infection without stimulating the detrimental ones.

One must admit, however, that for most of the immunopotentiating substances which have shown antiviral activity, the precise immunological mechanisms through which they act are not known. Lipopolysaccharides, for instance, cause a variety of reactions, usually 'toxic' in nature, such as stimulation of lysosomal enzymes in macrophages, production of fever, release of interferon from phagocytic cells, thus temporarily creating a situation which is not favorable to viral multiplication and spread in the treated organism. This state of enhanced resistance to viral infection is rather short-lived and requires administration of the LPS a few hours or, at most, a few days before virus inoculation. Whole microorganisms, whether live like BCG or killed like *Corynebacterium parvum*, cause the formation of granuloma from which, through the interaction with the microorganism of specifically sensitized lymphocytes, substances are released which nonspecifically activate cells of the mononuclear phagocyte system: as a result, these cells, in which virus replication normally takes place, oppose a barrier to virus multiplication and spread. This state of enhanced resistance may be long-lived since the mechanism of macrophage activation is self-perpetuating as long as the injected microorganism, or its products, persist in the tissues. In this situation again, injection of the microorganism and sensitization to it must precede virus inoculation, at least by a few days in that case, for effective protection against infection. Interferon inducers may protect against virus infections through local and systemic stimulation of interferon production, but, like lipopolysaccharides, some of them, such as the double-stranded polyribonucleotides, also stimulate macrophage functions and cause hyperthermia, thus creating a temporarily unfavorable environment for the infecting virus. Tilorone, a simple synthetic interferon inducer, has been shown, in addition to causing greatly enhanced levels of circulating interferon within 24 hr after its administration, to stimulate B lymphocytes and antibody production, to stimulate macrophages but also to inhibit production of delayed-type hypersensitivity reactions by T lymphocytes: do all these mechanisms come into play in the antiviral activity of tilorone? It is interesting to note that tilorone as well as pyran copolymer, another interferon inducer and immunopotentiating agent, cause the appearance, as early as 48 hr after i.p. injection in the mouse, of cytoplasmic granules in monocytes and polymorphonuclear leukocytes of the peripheral blood and that these granules persist for long periods, although the antiviral state is not as long-lived as in the case of a persisting microbial infection such as BCG.

With microorganisms like BCG, with endotoxins or some interferon inducers, the antiviral state appears to be essentially a nonspecific expression of a more or less prolonged general solicitation of the immune system, an indirect benefit from a situation which may be described as temporarily pathological, an increased ability of coping with viral intruders in a host which has been put in a state of alarm. It is, of course, more difficult to explain in similar terms the much more discrete antiviral effects of immunomodulating substances such as levamisole or inosiplex, which are also more difficult to demonstrate in laboratory animals. In the case of inosiplex, for instance, it is known that in most cases, it is more active when administered shortly after viral inoculation than before, in contrast with other immunopotentiating substances which, at least in experimental infections, are completely inactive when administered to an animal already infected. It may be therefore that inosiplex enhances defense mechanisms which have been already triggered by the viral infection itself: it would be fruitful, with this and other immunomodulating drugs showing antiviral activity, to analyse their effects on the responses of T and B lymphocytes to the viral infection, i.e. cytotoxic T cells, NK cells, delayed-type hypersensitivity and antibody production.

Delayed-type hypersensitivity (DTH) reactions with an antigen unrelated to the infecting virus is another mechanism of local or systemic enhancement of resistance and, as already mentioned, it may at least partly explain the effect of microbial agents or products (BCG, C. parvum) which are able to sensitize and to persist in the sensitized host. For instance, it has been shown that in rabbits immunized with Freund's complete adjuvant, induction of a DTH reaction by tuberculin purified protein derivative (PPD) at the site of dermal vaccinia virus infection accelerated elimination of the virus and led to clinical recovery (Lodmell et al., 1976). Low concentrations of acid-labile 'immunological' (type II, or γ) interferon were found in the skin of uninfected tuberculin-sensitized animals challenged with PPD; high concentrations of acid-stable ('viral') interferon were found in the skin of tuberculin-sensitized rabbits infected with vaccinia virus and challenged with PPD or saline, but the time of appearance of acid-stable interferon was greatly accelerated in the animals challenged with PPD instead of saline. Increased resistance to the lethal effect of a subcutaneous (s.c.) inoculation of encephalomyocarditis virus (EMC) was observed in mice which had been sensitized to sheep red blood cells (SRBC) by s.c. inoculation and challenged by the same route 6 days later with SRBC, 1 day before virus inoculation (Floc'h and Werner, unpublished).

It would be erroneous to believe that only those substances which stimulate, i.e. increase or elicit immune reactions in a broad sense, are capable of enhancing resistance to virus infections. Selective depression of some of these immune reactions can also be beneficial, in keeping with the notion that not all the immune reactions to the infecting virus are favorable to the host's survival. For instance, repeated injections of rabbit anti-mouse thymocyte globulin were found to increase the survival rates of mice infected with low doses of influenza A2 virus (Suzuki et al., 1974) and nude mice, which are deficient in T lymphocytes, die later than normal mice following respiratory infection with A0 influenza virus (Sullivan et al., 1976). Such nude mice show also minimal antibody response to the virus and, interestingly, those which do not die do not eliminate the virus, which persists 2 to 3 weeks in their lungs and spleen. On the other hand, a drug which inhibits B lymphocytes, cyclophosphamide, was shown to lower the mortality of mice infected with a virulent influenza A0 virus (Singer et al., 1972), while administration of the same drug converted a relatively harmless infection with an avirulent strain into a fatal pneumonic illness (Hurd and Heath, 1975). Thus, depending on the nature of the host–virus relationship (of which virulence is one aspect), T and B cell responses may be considered as beneficial or harmful to the final outcome of the infection and stimulation or depression of these responses may have widely different results.

A better insight into the mechanisms of the antiviral activities of immunomodulating substances (i.e. stimulating, restoring or depressing, according to the case) will be gained through experiments in which such substances will be administered, before or after virus infection, to animals in which defined compartments of the immune system are selectively suppressed, for instance through treatment with immunosuppressive drugs, as a consequence of a genetic defect, following surgical ablation of thymus or spleen or killing of macrophages with silica. Very important also will be *in vivo–in vitro* experiments in which, following *in vivo* administration of the immunomodulating agent to an animal subsequently or simultaneously infected with a virus, lymphocytes and cells of the monocyte-macrophage system will be studied *in vitro* with respect to a number of functions known to play a role in natural resistance to and recovery from that infection: phagocytic activity, toxicity for virus-infected cells, hypersensitivity to the viral antigen (i.e. *in vitro* proliferation in the presence of this agent), antibody production. Antiviral activity of normal, stimulated or activated mouse peritoneal cells can, for instance, be measured *in vitro*, by absorbing them to mouse embryo fibroblast infected with herpes simplex virus, removing nonadherent cells by washing and measuring later the virus yields in the cultures' supernatant fluids (Morahan and Kaplan, 1978); using this technique, it was found that stimulation of the peritoneal cells by i.p. injection of glycogen exerted a weak effect on their antiviral activity while activation with *Corynebacterium parvum* or pyran copolymer strongly enhanced it.

13.7. POSSIBLE THERAPEUTIC APPLICATIONS OF IMMUNOPOTENTIATING DRUGS WITH ANTIVIRAL ACTIVITY

Thus far, with relatively few exceptions, experimental studies on the antiviral activity of immunopotentiating substances have mostly consisted in treating animals with these substances and demonstrating that they were more resistant than untreated controls to a *subsequent* virus infection. If we try to deduce directly from the results of such studies the kinds of application to human or veterinary medicine immunopotentiating substances could have in the field of viral illnessess, we are forced to consider these substances as being nothing more than 'nonspecific vaccines', with the added restriction that specific viral vaccines generally induce long-lasting immunity, while the enhanced resistance against viral infections afforded by nonspecific immunostimulators is of relatively short duration (except in the case of a living infectious agent like BCG). Practically, it appears difficult to envisage frequent and repeated administrations of such substances to healthy subjects in order to maintain constantly their resistance at a high level, inasmuch as many of the immunopotentiating agents presently available are not devoid of often serious side effects (see review by Werner *et al.*, 1977). There may be some exceptions to that rule, however, such as the possibility of frequent stimulation, by intranasal administration of nonirritating and nonallergenic drugs, of the local immune defense mechanisms against infection with respiratory viruses. Nontoxic drugs which would exert their immunopotentiating activity following oral administration could also be used to raise the level of resistance of susceptible subjects, young children, for instance, against virus infections; with regard to the controversial participation of vitamin C (ascorbic acid) in protection against some virus infections, it is noteworthy that inclusion of this vitamin in the drinking water of mice, while exerting no effect on their humoral antibody response, increased T lymphocyte response to concanavalin A and enhanced response to interferon induction (Siegel and Morton, 1977). Other possibilities for short-term prophylactic use of immunostimulating substances exist in the veterinary field, as a means of protecting young animals (especially cattle and swine) against the virus illnesses of complex and multiple etiology which commonly affect them and cause severe losses; most such illnesses occur, however, in animals which are immunologically immature and it should be demonstrated that immunopotentiating agents can exert their activities in such animals.

On the basis of available experimental data, one can only speculate as to the possible therapeutic uses, *stricto sensu*, of immuno-potentiating drugs endowed with antiviral activities. As stated previously, the great majority of experiments have been performed in systems in which, because of the rapidly lethal character of the infection, administration of the drug after inoculation of the virus would be ineffective. Although the mechanisms of recovery from a virus infection are not essentially different from those underlying resistance to that infection, one cannot be sure that substances increasing nonspecifically that resistance would facilitate recovery if they were administered to the host after it has been infected. Clinically, BCG and levamisole may have shown some activity in cases of recurrent herpes simplex, when administered during the periods free of overt disease and, to our knowledge, inosiplex is the only immunopotentiating drug which has been claimed to show efficacy when administered in a truly therapeutic way, that is after infection with the virus and even after appearance of symptoms.

Many virus infections cause at least transient disturbances in the immune system of the infected host and this fact must be kept in mind when attempting to visualize the value of treating viral illnesses with immunopotentiating drugs.

Immunologic dysfunction induced by virus infection in man and animals include suppression or inhibition of cell-mediated immunity (temporary depression of delayed-type hypersensitivity, enhanced allograft survival, inhibition of in vitro reactivities of lymphocytes), abnormalities in antibody response (suppression or enhancement of antibody production, changes in serum immunoglobulin levels, suppression of tolerance induction) and there are many possible ways through which viruses can cause these dysfunctions: alteration of macrophage functions by viruses replicating within them, destruction of B and T lymphocytes, inhibition of T cell activation (through cell destruction, receptor blockade, or arrest of macro-molecular synthesis), alteration of lymphocyte traffic or stimulation of suppressor cells. All these situations are well documented with several examples (see review by Woodruff and Woodruff, 1975). For instance, in man, measles has been known for a long time to cause temporary loss of tuberculin skin reactivity and, following immunization with live measles vaccine, this anergic state may last several weeks; similarly, rubella infection or vaccination with live virus suppress for several days the in vitro response of peripheral blood lymphocytes to phytohemagglutinin (McMorrow et al., 1974); during acute influenza illness, lymphopenia is observed, which can last up to 4 weeks, and blastogenic responses of lymphocytes to phytohemagglutinin (PHA) and concanavalin A are depressed and remain so for 4 weeks after infection (Dolin et al., 1977). In patients with hepatitis A or hepatitis B, PHA-responsiveness of peripheral blood lymphocytes was impaired during the first week after the onset of jaundice and there was less marked but prolonged impairment for a further period of 6 to 10 weeks; serum from patients with hepatitis A or B was found to contain an inhibitor of lymphocyte response to PHA (Newble et al., 1975). Among the many investigations performed in animals in order to analyse immunological disturbances caused by virus infection, we shall only quote two studies, because of the light they throw on possible mechanisms and pathological consequences. In the mouse, infection with murine hepatitis virus (MHV-3) modified the humoral immune response to sheep red blood cells (SRBC): infecting mice before antigen administration caused immunodepression, simultaneous injection of virus and SRBC resulted in immunostimulation; on the other hand, persistent MHV-3 infections (which may be induced in some mouse lines, like C3H or A2G) were associated with a chronic state of immunodepression. Moreover, the presence of circulating interferon (the immunomodulating properties of which are well documented) was well correlated with these modifications: interferon peaking before antigen administration was associated with immunodepression, interferon production after antigen administration was associated with immunostimulation, whereas low and permanent levels of circulating interferon were associated with chronic immunodepression (Virelizier et al., 1976). On the other hand, mice lethally infected with street rabies virus failed to develop cytotoxic T lymphocytes specific for rabies virus-infected target cells, while high-level cytotoxicity was generated after nonfatal infection with attenuated rabies virus strains; furthermore, concurrent infection with street rabies virus suppressed development of a cell-mediated cytotoxic response specific for influenza-virus-infected cells (Wiktor et al., 1977): it thus appears that street rabies virus (which is not known to replicate in cells of the immune system) induces a general defect in cell-mediated cytotoxic response and development of fatal rabies may reflect the operation of this selective immunosuppressive mechanism.

What could be the benefit to be gained from treating virus-infected patients with immunopotentiating drugs, on the basis of the knowledge summarized above about virus-induced disturbances of the immune system? Theoretically, there should be wide possibilities in this area: virus-induced immunodepression is likely to play a role in the severity of the disease itself and it may, in addition, increase the susceptibility of the host to other viral illnesses, to bacterial, fungal or parasitic infections and possibly to malignancies. Compensating through immunomodulating drugs the immunological dysfunctions occurring in many viral infections should therefore have interesting therapeutic applications, but it remains to be proven that this is indeed feasible. There is clearly a need for testing immunopotentiating substances in experimental systems in which such effects would be demonstrable.

This brings us naturally to another possible field of application for antiviral immunopotentiating drugs: enhancing resistance to virus infections in immunologically compromised patients or animals. In such situations, these drugs could conceivably be administered in a prophylactic manner. The increased severity of several viral illnesses – notably measles, varicella-zoster, cytomegalovirus infection, herpes simplex – in immunologically deficient patients has already been stressed in the introduction, as indirect evidence for the importance of an intact immune system in resistance to viral infections. In the realm of congenital immunodeficiencies, such as thymic dysplasia or severe combined immunodeficiency, immunopotentiating drugs may have little to offer, except for those agents, like thymic hormones or transfer factor which, in principle, should substitute for missing immunological functions in such patients. The situation appears quite different, however, with respect to acquired immunodeficiencies, be they due to malignant conditions (leukemia and lymphomas) or to immunosuppressive therapy with cytostatic drugs. For instance, herpes zoster is a frequent complication of lymphoreticular malignancy and increased susceptibility to clinical infection with varicella-zoster virus (VZV) correlates with deficiencies in *in vitro* lymphocyte responses to VZV antigen (Arvin *et al.*, 1978). Severe forms of cytomegalovirus infection have been shown to occur in patients receiving immunosuppressive therapy for rheumatological disorders or before kidney or bone-marrow transplantation and it appears that most such patients are at risk from endogenous infection (Anonymous, 1977). Deficiencies in cell-mediated immunity to cytomegalovirus, in the presence of normal antibody levels, have been observed in cardiac transplant patients; such deficiencies took up to 3 years after transplant to resolve and were associated with a syndrome of unexplained fever, hepatitis, pneumonitis and leukopenia (Pollard *et al.*, 1978). Whether enhancement of cytomegalovirus infection was due to immunosuppressive therapy or to graft-versus-host reactions (GVHR) is not established, but it has been shown in mice that GVHR alone can enhance murine cytomegalovirus infection in a chronically infected host (Dowling *et al.*, 1977). With respect to deficiencies in humoral immunity, it is noteworthy that patients with lepromatous leprosy have an impaired immune response that diminishes their efficiency in terminating hepatitis B virus infection with the production of circulating antibodies (Serjeantson and Woodfield, 1978).

In all such acquired immunodeficiencies, selective stimulation of the impaired immune response through administration of an appropriate immunopotentiating drug should help in preventing the occurrence of or in decreasing the severity of virus infections. It seems possible that part of the benefit derived from nonspecific immunotherapy by cancer patients is due to an enhancement of their resistance to viral infections, to which treatment with cytostatic drugs makes them prone. In other situations associated with immunodeficiency, usefulness of immunopotentiating drugs for decreasing susceptibility to virus infections can also be suggested, with the proviso that these drugs should not antagonize the beneficial effects expected from immunosuppressive treatment, i.e. stimulate graft rejection, for instance.

It is probable also that, beside obvious and severe cases of acquired immunodeficiencies, there occur in the life of any individual short or prolonged periods of discrete immunodeficiency, due to many possible reasons, which predispose him to clinically overt virus infections. This may be the case, for instance, in those young children who exhibit excessively frequent infections of the respiratory tract and finally improve as they grow older. Interesting applications of immunopotentiating drugs are provided by such situations, but it will first be necessary to find reliable and sensitive laboratory techniques to detect these discrete and transient states of immunodeficiency. Veterinary studies could be useful to test the possibility of combating through immunopotentiation the susceptibility to virus infections of immunologically deficient animals: immunodeficiency disorders in young horses have been shown to correlate with a high prevalence of adenovirus infections (McGuire et al., 1977) and the outcome of canine distemper virus inoculation in gnotobiotic dogs was shown to be correlated with their cell-mediated immunity level, assessed by skin tests with phytohemagglutinin (Krakowka et al., 1977).

The possibility of using immunopotentiating substances for the management of persistent (also called chronic) viral infections is a highly speculative topic, since relatively little is known presently about the various mechanisms of such persistence. These mechanisms may include unique properties of the virus (such as the nonimmunogenicity of viroids implicated in the subacute spongiform encephalopathies) as well as a inadequate host defenses. Agents causing latent infections, such as herpes simplex and varicella-zoster viruses, escape immune elimination by remaining in nerve cells during the intervals between disease episodes and, on the other hand, in several chronic infections, the viruses seem to grow mainly in lymphoid tissue, particularly in macrophages (this was shown to be the case with LCM and lactic dehydrogenase viruses in the mouse, aleutian disease virus in minks and equine infectious anemia virus in horses). Under such circumstances, one does not see clearly how immunopotentiation could be beneficial, but there are reasons for believing that persistent viral infections may, in some cases, be associated with hyporesponsiveness of humoral (hepatitis B) or cellular immune mechanisms. Burkitt lymphoma, associated with Epstein–Barr virus (EBV) infection, has been attributed to a state of immunodepression perhaps caused by endemic malaria. It remains for the future to explore the clinical value of immunomodulating treatments in persistent viral infections of humans, such as hepatitis B, the rubella syndrome, cytomegalovirus and EBV infections, subacute sclerosing pan-encephalitis (SSPE) and progressive multifocal leukoencephalopathy (PML). Immunological disturbances are evident in some of these conditions; enhanced susceptibility of immunosuppressed patients to hepatitis B and cytomegalovirus has already been mentioned; antibody levels to measles virus are abnormally high in SSPE and PML occurs only in subjects whose immunological responsiveness has been severely lowered by malignant disease and/or immunosuppressive drugs. There are also other poorly understood chronic diseases which may be due to persistent virus infections, such as multiple sclerosis and amyotrophic lateral sclerosis. Several animal models of persistent viral infections are available and it should be feasible, albeit not without technical difficulties, to study the effects of immunopotentiating drugs on such diseases. For instance, mouse hepatitis virus (MHV-3) exerts different effects on different strains of mice: strain A mice are completely resistant, most strains die of acute hepatitis and, thirdly, in certain strains (such as C3H and A2G) the virus produces a state of persistent virus infection which leads to neuropathological manifestations (Virelizier et al., 1975). It was later shown (Virelizier and Allison, 1976) that MHV-3 replicates freely, with giant cell formation, in macrophages from susceptible mice, that it does not replicate in macrophages from resistant A mice and, finally, that macrophage cultures from C3H or A2G mice showed intermediate susceptibility. It would be highly interesting to see whether treatment of the latter strains of mice with immunopotentiating substances, after they have been infected with the virus, would help them getting rid of the infection.

Many, if not most, persistent viral infections, in a wide variety of hosts, are associated with the production of virus-induced immune complexes which are present in the circulation or may deposit in the tissues, thereby causing disease. Glomeruli in the kidney, blood vessels and choroid plexus are the main sites where circulating immune complexes deposit. Immune complexes less often deposit in the joints, heart, lungs and liver. Circulating immune complexes likely represent a quite common phenomenon that occurs whenever the host mounts an antibody response against the infecting virus. In acute viral infections, symptoms like myalgia or joint pain may result from immune complex deposits which locally activate various possible mediators of inflammation; in chronic infections, in which ongoing viral replication coexists with a continuous host immune response, immune complexes commonly cause nephritis and arteritis (see review by Oldstone and Dixon, 1975). As in the case of persistent viral infections, the immunopathology of which is largely dependent on deposition of immune complexes in the tissues, it would be premature to speculate about the possible uses of immunopotentiation for the therapy of immune complex diseases: one may imagine that further stimulation of antibody production might help in dissolving the circulating complexes before they deposit in critical tissues or that stimulated macrophages might have an increased capacity to clear such complexes. There are several models of immune complex diseases in the mouse (infections with lactic dehydrogenase virus, with lymphocytic choriomeningitis virus, with various oncornaviruses) and the possible impact of immunopotentiating substances on such diseases is amenable to experimental analysis.

The provisional conclusion one may reach concerning the possible uses in human and veterinary medicine of immunopotentiating substances endowed with antiviral activity is that the situation may be, for exactly opposite reasons, just as difficult and complicated as in the case of antiviral chemotherapy. In the latter field, nontoxic agents which can effectively inhibit viral replication are usually very narrowly specific, which severely limits their usefulness; on the other hand, while there are many different mechanisms through which viruses are known to replicate, the mechanisms through which the infected host's immune responses cope with virus invasion are equally diverse and they do not always interact harmoniously in order to preserve the host's integrity. Therefore, just as it is difficult to visualize a single broad-spectrum 'antiviral' drug, it appears illusory to envisage an immunopotentiating substance which could be used to stimulate resistance to and hasten recovery from all possible virus infections.

The contradiction between *antiviral chemotherapy* and *antiviral immunotherapy* is only apparent and both approaches could conceivably be used concurrently. It is known, for instance, that effective antiviral substances like *amantadine* or *methisazone*, when applied *in vivo*, do not block totally virus replication in target tissues (such as lungs and brain): they only reduce it to a level which, owing to the intervention of the host's immune response, is compatible with his survival.

Combined treatments of virus infections with a selective antiviral drug (when precise diagnosis can be done on time) and with an appropriate immunopotentiating substance could be of definite therapeutic advantage. A great deal of experimental work, based on models of virus infections which should be more relevant than many of those which are presently in use, is still necessary. 'Good applied science in medicine requires a high degree of certainty about the basic facts at hand, and especially about their meaning, and we have not yet reached this point. . . .' (Lewis Thomas, *The Medusa and the Snail*, 1980, p. 143.)

Acknowledgement—The authors are indebted to Mrs. Françoise Chaselas for her valuable help in organizing and typing the manuscript.

REFERENCES

ADAM, A., DEVYS, M., SOUVANNAVONG, V., LEFRANCIER, P., CHOAY, J. and LEDERER, E. (1976) Correlation of structure and adjuvant activity of *N*-acetyl muramyl-L-alanyl-D-isoglutamine (MDP) and analogues. *Biochem. Biophys. Res. Comm.* **72**: 339–346.

ALLEN, E. G. and MUDD, S. (1973) Protection of mice against vaccinia virus by bacterial infection and sustained stimulation with specific bacterial antigens. *Infect. Immun.* **7**: 62–67.

ANDERLIK, P., SZERI, I., BANOS, Zs., FÖLDES, I. and RADNAI, B. (1972) Interaction of *Bordetella pertussis* vaccine treatment and lymphocytic choriomeningitis virus infection in mice. *Experientia* **28**: 985–986.

ANDERSON, F. D., USHIJIMA, R. N. and LARSON, C. L. (1974) Recurrent herpes genitalis: treatment with attenuated *Mycobacterium bovis* (BCG). *Obstetr. Gynecol.* **43**: 797–805.

ANDERSON, M. J., BAINBRIDGE, D. R., PATTISON, J. R. and HEATH, R. B. (1977) Cell-mediated immunity to Sendai virus infection in mice. *Infect. Immun.* **15**: 239–244.

ANONYMOUS (Editorial) (1977) Cytomegalovirus in immune conpromised hosts. *Br. Med. J.* **1**: 1048–1049.

ARVIN, A. M., POLLARD, R. B., RASMUSSEN, L. E. and MERIGAN, T. C. (1978) Selective impairment of lymphocyte reactivity to varicella-zoster virus antigen among untreated patients with lymphoma. *J. infect. Dis.* **137**: 531–540.

AUDIBERT, F., CHEDID, L. and HANNOUN, C. (1977) Augmentation de la réponse immune au vaccin grippal par administration d'un glycopeptide synthétique (*N*-acétyl-muramyl-L-alanyl-D-isoglutamine) doué d'activité adjuvante. *C.R. Acad. Sci.* (Paris) **285**: 467–470.

AULT, K. and WEINER, H. L. (1979) Natural killing of measles-infected cells by human lymphocytes. *J. Immun.* **122**: 2611–2617.

BACH, J. F. (1978) Thymic hormones. In: *Pharmacology of Immunoregulation*, pp. 165–170. WERNER, G. H. and FLOC'H, F. (eds.). Academic Press, New York, London, publ.

BACH, J. F. and DARDENNE, M. (1982) L'utilisation clinique des hormones thymiques. In: *Actualités de Chimie Thérapeutique*, 9ème série, pp. 91–100. Technique et Documentation – Lavoisier, Paris.

BAKER, M. B., LARSON, C. L., USHIJIMA, R. N. and ANDERSON, F. D. (1974) Resistance of female mice to vaginal infection induced by *herpesvirus hominis* type 2: effects of immunization with *Mycobacterium bovis*, intravenous injection of specific herpesvirus hominis type 2 antiserum and a combination of these procedures. *Infect. Immun.* **10**: 1230–1234.

BARDOS, P., CARNAUD, C. and BACH, J. F. (1979) Augmentation de l'activité des cellules naturelles tueuses (cellules NK) par le facteur thymique sérique. *C.R. hebd. Séanc. Acad. Sci., Paris*, D **289**: 1251–1254.

BENNETT, M., BAKER, E. E., EASTCOTT, J. W., KUMAR, V. and YONKOSKY, D. (1976) Selective elimination of marrow precursors with the bone-seeking isotopes Sr⁸⁹: implications for hemopoiesis, lymphopoiesis, viral leukemogenesis and infections. *J. Reticuloendothel. Soc.* **20**: 71–87.

BERTRAND, J., RENOUX, G., RENOUX, M. and PALAT, A. (1974) Maladie de Crohn et lévamisole. *Nouv. Presse méd.* **3**: 2265.

BETTS, R. F., DOUGLAS, Jr., R. G., GEORGE, S. D. and RINEHART, C. J. (1978) Isoprinosine in experimental influenza in volunteers. 78th Annual Meeting of American Society for Microbiology, Las Vegas, Nevada. May 14–19, 1978.

BICKER, U., ZIEGLER, A. E. and HEBOLD, G. (1979) Investigations in mice on the potentiation of resistance to infections by a new immunostimulant compound. *J. inf. Dis.* **139**: 389–395.

BILLIAU, A., SCHONNE, E., EYSKMANS, L. and DE SOMER, P. (1970) Interferon induction and resistance to virus infection in mice infected with *Brucella abortus*. *Infect. Immun.* **2**: 698–704.

BIOZZI, G., BENACERRAF, B., GRUMBACH, F., HALPERN, B. N., LEVADITI, J. C. and RIST, N. (1954) Etude de l'activité granulopexique du système réticulo-endothélial au cours de l'infection tuberculeuse expérimentale de la souris. *Ann. Inst. Pasteur* **87**: 291–300.

BIOZZI, G., STIFFEL, C., HALPERN, B. N. and MOUTON, D. (1959) Effet de l'inoculation du bacille de Calmette-Guérin sur le développement de la tumeur ascitique d'Ehrlich chez la souris. *C.R. Soc. Biol. (Paris)* **153**: 987–989.

BIOZZI, G., STIFFEL, C. and MAZUREK, C. (1978) Studies on the mechanisms of antitumor protection by *Corynebacterium parvum*. In: *Pharmacology of Immunomodulation*, pp. 353–366. WERNER, G. H. and FLOC'H, F. (eds.). Academic Press, London, New York, publ.

BIOZZI, G., STIFFEL, C., MOUTON, D. and BOUTHILLIER, Y. (1975) Selection of lines of mice with high and low antibody responses to complex immunogens. In: *Immunogenetics and Immunodeficiency*, pp. 180–227. BENACERRAF, B. (ed.). MTP Publisher, Lancaster, England.

BLANDEN, R. V. (1974) T cell response to viral and bacterial infection. *Transplant. Rev.* **19**: 56–88.

BLANDEN, R. V. (1977) Cell-mediated immune response to acute viral infection. In: *Progress in Immunology III*, pp. 463–471. MANDEL, T. E. (ed.). Proc. 3rd Intl. Congress Immunol., Australian Academy of Science, Canberra, publ.

BLANDEN, R. V. and GARDNER, I. D. (1976) The cell-mediated immune response to ectromelia virus infection. *Cell. Immun.* **22**: 271–279.

BLIZNAKOV, E. V. and ADLER, A. D. (1972) Nonlinear response of the reticulo-endothelial system upon stimulation. *Path. Microbiol.* **38**: 393–410.

BORECKY, L. and LACKOVIČ, V. (1967) The cellular background of interferon production *in vivo*. Comparison of interferon induction by Newcastle disease virus and *B. pertussis*. *Acta virol.* **11**: 150–156.

BOUFFAUT, P. and SAURAT, J. H. (1980) Isoprinosine as a therapeutic agent in recurrent mucocutaneous infections due to herpes virus. *J. Immunopharm.* **2**: 193 (abstract).

BRADSHAW, L. J. and SUMNER, H. L. (1977) *In vitro* studies on cell-mediated immunity in patients treated with inosiplex for herpes virus infection. *Ann. N.Y. Acad. Sci.* **284**: 190–196.

BRAUTIGAN, A. R., DUTKO, F. J., OLDING, L. B. and OLDSTONE, M. B. (1979) Pathogenesis of murine cytomegalovirus infection: the macrophage as a permissive cell for cytomegalovirus infection, replication and latency. *J. gen. Virol.* **44**: 349–359.

BREINIG, M. C., WRIGHT, L. L., McGEORGE, M. B. and MORAHAN, P. S. (1978) Resistance to vaginal or systemic infection with herpes simplex virus type 2. *Arch. Virol.* **57**: 25–34.

BRESLOW, D. S., EDWARDS, E. I. and NEWBURG, N. R. (1973) Divinyl ether-maleic anhydride (Pyran) copolymer used to demonstrate the effect of molecular weight on biological activity. *Nature* **246**: 160–162.

BUDZKO, D. B., CASALS, J. and WAKSMAN, B. H. (1978) Enhanced resistance against Junin virus infection induced by *Corynebacterium parvum*. *Infect. Immun.* **19**: 893–897.

BURNS, W. H. (1977) Immune responses to herpesvirus infections. In: *Progress in Immunology III*, pp. 472–479. MANDEL, T. E. (ed.). Proc. 3rd Intl. Congress Immunol., Australian Academy of Science, Canberra, publ.

CARCÓ, F. P., FRUTTALDO, L. and SALIVA, G. (1979) Studio preliminare sulla valutazione clinica dell'efficacia terapeutica dell'Isoprinosina nelle infezioni acute da herpes-virus. *Archivio di Medicina Intern.* **21** (6): 589–603.

CERUTTI, I. (1974) Propriétés antivirales du *C. parvum*. *C.R. Acad. Sci. (Paris)* D **279**: 963–966.

CHANY, C. and CERUTTI, I. (1977) Effet stimulant de l'isoprinosine sur l'action antivirale de l'interféron. *C.R. Acad. Sci. (Paris)* D **284**: 499–501.

CHEDID, L., AUDIBERT, F., BONA, C., DAMAIS, C., PARANT, F. and PARANT, M. (1975) Biological activities of endotoxins detoxified by alkylation. *Infect. Immun.* **12**: 714–721.

CHEDID, L., AUDIBERT, F., LEFRANCIER, P., CHOAY, J. and LEDERER, E. (1976) Modulation of the immune response by a synthetic adjuvant and analogs. *Proc. natn. Acad. Sci. USA* **73**: 2472–2475.

CHING, C. and LOPEZ, C. (1979) Natural killing of herpes simplex virus type 1 – infected target cells: normal human responses and influence of antiviral antibody. *Infect. Immun.* **26**: 49–56.

CHIRIGOS, M. A. and JACQUES, P. (1981) Polysaccharides and related substances. In: *Advances in Immuno-pharmacology*, p. 487. HADDEN, J., CHEDID, L., MULLEN, P. and SPREAFICO, F. (eds.). Pergamon Press, Oxford, New York.

CLUFF, L. E. (1970) Effects of endotoxins on susceptibility to infections. *J. inf. Dis.* **122**: 205–215.

COREY, L., REEVES, W. C., VONTVER, L. A., ALEXANDER, E. R. and HOLMES, K. K. (1976) Trial of BCG vaccine for the prevention of recurrent genital herpes. Abstract No. 403, 16th Interscience Conference on Antimicrobial Agents and Chemotherapy, Chicago, Ill.

COREY, L., CHIANG, W. T., REEVES, W. C., STAMM, W. E., BREWER, L. and HOLMES, K. K. (1979) Effect of isoprinosine on the cellular immune response in initial genital herpes virus infection. *Clin. Res.* **27**: 41A.

DE CLERCQ, E. (1973) Nonpolynucleotide interferon inducers. In: *Selective Inhibitors of Viral Functions*, pp. 177–198. CARTER, W. A. (ed.). Chemical Rubber Company Press, Cleveland, Ohio, publ.

DE CLERCQ, E. and LUCZAK, M. (1976) Antiviral activity of carbopol, a cross-linked polycarboxylate. *Arch. Virol.* **52**: 151–158.

DEGRÉ, M. and DAHL, H. (1973) Enhanced effect of repeated administration of bacterial vaccine against viral respiratory infection. *Infect. Immun.* **7**: 771–776.

DI LUZIO, N. R., WILLIAMS, D. L. and BROWDER, W. (1982) Immunopharmacology of glucan: the modification of infectious diseases. In: *Advances in Pharmacology and Therapeutics*, II, pp. 101–112. YOSHIDA, H., HAGIHARA, Y. and EBASHI, S. (eds.). Pergamon Press, Oxford, New York.

DI TIZIO, A., MUTOLO, A., GLORIALANZA, G., CATONE, E. and ROMANI, G. P. (1979) Methisoprinol, valutazione clinica della sua efficacia terapeutica nella cheratite da herpes virus hominis. Studio preliminare. *Annali Ottalmologia Clinica Oculistica.* **105**: 341–350.

DJEU, J. Y., HEINBAUGH, J. A., HOLDEN, H. T. and HERBERMAN, R. B. (1979) Augmentation of mouse natural killer cell activity by interferon and interferon inducers. *J. Immun.* **122**: 175–181.

DOHERTY, P. C., ZINKERNAGEL, R. M. and RAMSHAW, I. A. (1974) Specificity and development of cytotoxic thymus-derived lymphocytes in lymphocytic choriomeningitis. *J. Immun.* **112**: 1548–1559.

DOLIN, R., RICHMAN, D. D., MURPHY, B. R. and FAUCI, A. S. (1977) Cell-mediated immune responses in humans after induced infections with influenza A virus. *J. infect. Dis.* **135**: 714–719.

DOWLING, J. N., WU, B. C., ARMSTRONG, J. A. and HO, M. (1977) Enhancement of murine cytomegalovirus infection during graft-vs.-host reaction. *J. infect. Dis.* **135**: 990–996.

DUBOS, R. J. and SCHAEDLER, R. W. (1957) Effects of cellular constituents of Mycobacteria on the resistance of mice to heterologous infections. I. Protective effects. *J. exp. Med.* **106**: 703–717.

DYKEN, P. and SWIFT, A. (1982) Long term follow-up of subacute sclerosing panencephalitis (SSPE). Patients treated with inosiplex (Isoprinosine). *Ann. Neurol.* (in press).

EBERLE, R., RUSSELL, R. G. and ROUSE, B. T. (1981) Cell immunity to herpes simplex virus. Recognition of type-specific and type-common surface antigens by cytotoxic T cell population. *Infect. Immun.* **34**: 795–803.

EFFROS, R. B., DOHERTY, P. C., GERHARD, W. and BENNINK, J. (1977) Generation of both cross-reactive and virus-specific T-cell populations after immunization with serologically distinct influenza A viruses. *J. exp. Med.* **145**: 557–568.

EVANS, S. R. and JOHNSON, H. M. (1981) The induction of at least 2 distinct types of interferon in mouse spleen cell cultures by *Corynebacterium parvum. Cell. Immun.* **64**: 64–72.

FAUCONNIER, B. (1970) Augmentation de la pathogénicité virale par l'emploi de sérum anti-interféron *in vivo. C.R. Acad. Sci. (Paris)* D **271**: 1464–1466.

FAUVE, R. M. (1978) Inflammation and host resistance against pathogens. In: *Pharmacology of Immunoregulation*, pp. 319–333. WERNER, G. H. and FLOC'H, F. (eds.). Academic Press, London, New York, publ.

FEINGOLD, D. S., KELETI, G. and YOUNGNER, J. S. (1976) Antiviral activity of *Brucella abortus* preparations: separation of active components. *Infect. Immun.* **13**: 763–767.

FELLOUS, M., KAMOUN, M., GRESSER, I. and BONO, R. (1979) Enhanced expression of HA antigens and β_2-microglobulin on interferon-treated human lymphoid cells. *Eur. J. Immun.* **9**: 446–449.

FINGER, H., EMMERLING, P. and SCHMIDT, J. (1967) Accelerated and prolonged multiplication of antibody-forming spleen cells by *Bordetella pertussis* in mice immunized with sheep red blood cells. *Experientia* **23**: 591–592.

FISCHER, G. W., PODGORE, J. K., BASS, J. W., KELLEY, J. L. and KOBAYASHI, G. Y. (1975) Enhanced host defense mechanisms with levamisole in suckling rats. *J. infect. Dis.* **132**: 578–581.

FISCHER, G. W., BALK, M. W., CRUMRINE, M. H. and BASS, J. W. (1976) Immunopotentiation and antiviral chemotherapy in a suckling rat model of herpesvirus encephalitis. *J. infect. Dis* **133** (A): 217–220.

FLEISCHMANN, W. R. Jr., GEORGIADES, J. A., OSBORNE, L. C. and JOHNSON, H. M. (1979) Potentiation of interferon activity by mixed preparations of fibroblast and immune interferon. *Infect. Immun.* **26**: 248–253.

FLOC'H, F. and WERNER, G. H. (1976) Increased resistance to virus infections of mice inoculated with BCG (Bacillus Calmette-Guérin). *Ann. Immunol. (Inst. Pasteur)* **127** C: 173–186.

FLOC'H, F. and WERNER, G. H. (1978a) Comparative studies on susceptibility to some virus infections of mice with respect to their antibody responsiveness to an unrelated antigen. In: *Pharmacology of Immunoregulation*, pp. 153–161. WERNER, G. H. and FLOC'H, F. (eds.). Academic Press, New York, London.

FLOC'H, F. and WERNER, G. H. (1978b) Heterotypic protective immune reactions in mice infected with distinct serotypes of human influenza virus. *Ann. Microbiol. (Inst. Pasteur)* **129** A: 509–524.

FLOERSHEIM, G. L. (1965) Effect of pertussis vaccine on the tuberculin reaction. *Int. Arch. Allergy* **26**: 340–344.

FLORENTIN, I., BRULEY-ROSSET, M., SCHULZ, J., DAVIGNY, M., KIGER, N. and MATHÉ, G. (1981) Attempts at functional classification of chemically defined immunomodulators. In: *Advances in Immunopharmacology*, pp. 311–325. HADDEN, J., CHEDID, L., MULLEN, P. and SPREAFICO, F. (eds.). Pergamon Press, Oxford, New York.

FRIDMAN, W. H., GRESSER, I., BANDU, M. T., AGUET, M. and NEAUPORT-SAUTES, C. (1980) Interferon enhances the expression of Fcγ receptors. *J. Immun.* **124**: 2436–2441.

GALANOS, C., FREUDENBERG, M., HASE, S., JAY, F. and RUSCHMANN, E. (1977) Biologic activities and immunological properties of lipid A. In: *Microbiology 1977*, pp. 269–276. SCHLESSINGER, D. (ed.). American Society for Microbiology, Washington, D.C. publ.

GIDLUND, M., ÖRN, A., WIGZELL, H., SENIK, A. and GRESSER, I. (1978) Enhanced NK cell activity in mice injected with interferon and interferon inducers. *Nature* **273**: 759–761.

GINSBERG, T. and GLASKY, A. J. (1977) Inosiplex: an immunomodulation model for the treatment of viral disease. *Ann. N.Y. Acad. Sci.* **284**: 128–138.

GISLER, R. H., LINDHAL, P. and GRESSER, I. (1974) Effects of interferon on antibody synthesis *in vitro*. *J. Immun.* **113**: 438–444.

GLASGOW, L. A. and GALASSO, G. J. (1972) Isoprinosine: lack of antiviral activity in experimental model infections. *J. infect. Dis.* **126**: 162–169.

GLASGOW, L. A., FISCHBACH, J., BRYANT, S. M. and KERN, E. R. (1977) Immunomodulation of host resistance to experimental virus infections in mice: effects of *Corynebacterium acnes*, *Corynebacterium parvum* and Bacille Calmette-Guérin. *J. infect. Dis.* **135**: 763–770.

GLASKY, A. J., KESTELYN, J. and ROMERO, M. (1978) Isoprinosine Ⓡ: a clinical overview of an antiviral/immunomodulating agent. Presented at the 7th International Congress of Pharmacology, Paris, July 1978. Abstract No. 2267.

GLEDHILL, A. W. (1959) The effect of bacterial endotoxin on resistance of mice to ectromelia. *Br. J. exp. Pathol.* **40**: 195–202.

GORHE, D. S. (1967) Inhibition of multiplication of foot and mouth disease virus in adult mice pretreated with Freund's complete adjuvant. *Nature* **216**: 1242–1244.

GORHE, D., ASSO, J. and PARAF, A. (1968) Effet du traitement préalable par les adjuvants de l'immunité sur la multiplication du virus de la fièvre aphteuse chez la souris adulte. *Ann. Inst. Pasteur* **115**: 446–464.

GRESSER, I., TOVEY, M. G., BANDU, M. T., MAURY, C. and BROUTY-BOYE, D. (1976a). Role of interferon in the pathogenesis of virus diseases of mice as demonstrated by the use of anti-interferon serum. I. Rapid evolution of encephalomyocarditis virus infection. *J. exp. Med.* **144**: 1305–1315.

GRESSER, I., TOVEY, M. G., MAURY, C. and BANDU, M. T. (1976b) Role of interferon in the pathogenesis of virus diseases in mice as demonstrated by the use of anti-interferon serum II. Studies with herpes simplex, Moloney sarcoma, vesicular stomatitis, Newcastle disease and influenza viruses. *J. exp. Med.* **144**: 1316–1323.

HADDAD, F. S. and RISK, W. S. (1980) Isoprinosine treatment in 18 patients with subacute sclerosing panencephalitis: a controlled study. *Ann. Neurol.* **7**: 185–188.

HADDEN, J. W., HADDEN, E. M. and COFFEY, R. G. (1976) Isoprinosine augmentation of phytohemagglutinin-induced lymphocyte proliferation. *Infect. Immun.* **13**: 382–388.

HADDEN, J. W., LOPEZ, C., O'REILLY, R. J. and HADDEN, E. M. (1977) Levamisole and inosiplex: antiviral agents with immunopotentiating action. *Ann. N.Y. Acad. Sci.* **284**: 139–152.

HADDEN, J. W. and WYBRAN, J. (1981) Isoprinosine, NPT 15392 and Azimexone; Modulators of lymphocyte and macrophage development and function. In: *Advances in Immunopharmacology*, pp. 327–340. HADDEN, J., CHEDID, L., MULLEN, P. and SPREAFICO, F. (eds.). Pergamon Press, Oxford, New York.

HALLER, O. and WIGZELL, H. (1977) Suppression of natural killer cell activity with radioactive strontium: effector cells are marrow-dependent. *J. Immun.* **118**: 1503–1505.

HANDZEL, Z. T., ZAIZOV, R., VARSANO, I., LEVIN, S., PECHT, M. and TRAININ, N. (1981) The influence of thymic humoral factor on immunoproliferative disorders and viral infections in humans. In: *Advances in Immunopharmacology*, pp. 83–88. HADDEN, J. W. (ed.). Pergamon Press, Oxford, New York.

HANNA, N. and BURTON, R. C. (1981) Definitive evidence that natural killer (NK) cells inhibit experimental tumor metastasis *in vivo*. *J. Immun.* **127**: 1754–1758.

HARFAST, B., ÖRVELL, C., ALSHEIKHLY, A., ANDERSSON, T., PERLMAN, P. and NORRBY (1980) The role of viral glycoproteins in mumpsvirus dependent lymphocyte-mediated cytotoxicity in vitro. *Scand. J. Immun.* **11**: 391–400.

HAUSER, S. L., AULT, K. A., LEVIN, M. J., GAROVOY, M. R. and WEINER, H. L. (1981) Natural killer cell activity in multiple sclerosis. *J. Immun.* **127**: 1114–1117.

HELIN, P. and BERGH, M. (1974) Levamisole for warts. *New Engl. J. Med.* **291**: 1311.

HERBERMANN, R. B., DJEU, J. Y., KAY, H. D., ORTALDO, J. R., RICCARDI, C., BONNARD, G. D., HOLDEN, H. T., FAGNANI, R., SANTONI, A. and PUCCETTI, P. (1979) Natural killer cells: characteristics and regulation of activity. *Immunol. Rev.* **44**: 43–70.

HILL, T. J., FIELD, H. J. and BLYTH, W. A. (1975) Acute and recurrent infection with herpes simplex virus in the mouse: a model for studying latency and recurrent disease. *J. gen. Virol.* **28**: 341–353.

HIRSCH, M. S., ZISMAN, B. and ALLISON, A. C. (1970) Macrophages and age-dependent resistance to herpes simplex virus in mice. *J. Immun.* **104**: 1160–1165.

HIRSCH, R. L. (1980) Natural killer cells appear to play no role in the recovery of mice from Sindbis virus infection. *Immunology* **43**: 81–89.

HIRT, H. M., BECKER, H. and KIRCHNER, H. (1978) Induction of interferon production in mouse spleen cell cultures by *Corynebacterium parvum*. *Cell. Immun.* **38**: 168–175.

HO, M. (1981) Role of specific cytotoxic lymphocytes in cellular immunity against murine cytomegalovirus. *Infect. Immun.* **27**: 767–776.

HUANG, K. Y., DONAHOE, R. M., GORDON, F. B. and DRESSLER, H. R. (1971) Enhancement of phagocytosis by interferon-containing preparations. *Infect. Immun.* **4**: 581–588.

HURD, J. and HEATH, R. B. (1975) Effect of cyclophosphamide on infections in mice caused by virulent and avirulent strains of influenza virus. *Infect. Immun.* **11**: 886–889.

ISAACS, A. and LINDENMANN, J. (1957) Virus interference. I. Interferon. *Proc. R. Soc.* B **157**: 258–267.

ISAACS, D., TYRRELL, D. A. J., CLARKE, J. R., WEBSTER, A. D. B. and WALMAN, H. B. (1981) Deficient production of leucocyte interferon (interferon α) *in vitro* and *in vivo* in children with recurrent respiratory tract infections. *Lancet* **2**: 950–952.

JABBOUR, J. T., VAN DER ZWAAG, R., BALDRIDGE, G., KESTELYN, J. and MAXWELL, K. (1980) A comparative analysis of the therapeutic effect of isoprinosine in the course of SSPE. Abstract 18. 6b. 10. 4th Int. Congr. Immunol., Paris, July 1980.

JAIN, S., THOMAS, H. C. and SHERLOCK, S. (1977) Transfer factor in the attempted treatment of patients with HBsAg-positive chronic liver disease. *Clin. exp. Immun.* **30**: 10–15.

JONES, J. F., JETER, W. S., FULGINITI, V. A., MINNICH, L. L., PRITCHETT, R. F. and WEDGWOOD, R. J. (1981) Treatment of childhood combined Epstein–Barr virus/cytomegalovirus infection with oral bovine transfer factor. *Lancet* **2**: 122–124.

JOSE, D. G. and MINTY, C. C. J. (1980) Levamisole in patients with recurrent herpes infection. *Med. J. Austral.* **2**: 390–394.

KARRE, K., KLEIN, G. O., KIESSLING, R., KLEIN, G. and RODER, J. (1980) Low natural *in vivo* resistance to syngeneic leukemias in natural killer-deficient mice. *Nature* **284**: 624–626.

KENYON, A. J. (1978) Treatment of Aleutian mink disease with levamisole. In: *Current Chemotherapy*, vol. 1, pp. 357–358. SIEGENTHALER, W. and LÜTHY, R. (eds.). American Society for Microbiology, Washington, D.C., publ.

KERN, E. R., GLASGOW, L. A. and OVERALL, J. C., Jr. (1976) Antiviral activity of an extract of *Brucella abortus*: induction of interferon and immunopotentiation of host resistance. *Proc. Soc. exp. Biol. Med.* **152**: 372–376.

KINT, A. and VERLINDEN, L. (1974) Levamisole for recurrent herpes labialis. *New Engl. J. Med.* **291**: 308.

KINT, A., COUCKE, C. and VERLINDEN, L. (1974) The treatment of recurrent-herpes infections with levamisole. *Arch. Belges Dermatol.* **30**: 167–171.

KIRCHNER, H., HIRT, H. M. and MUNK, K. (1977) Protection against herpes simplex virus infection in mice by *Corynebacterium parvum*. *Infect. Immun.* **16**: 9–11.

KIRCHNER, H., HIRT, H. M., ROSENSTREICH, D. L. and MERGENHAGEN, S. E. (1978) Resistance of C3H/HeJ mice to lethal challenge with herpes simplex virus. *Proc. Soc. exp. Biol. Med.* **157**: 29–32.

KONG, A. S. and MORSE, S. I. (1977) The *in vitro* effects of *Bordetella pertussis* lymphocytosis promoting factor on murine lymphocytes. 1. Proliferative response. *J. exp. Med.* **145**: 151–158.

KRAKOWKA, S., COCKERELL, G. and KOESTNER, A. (1977) Intradermal mitogen response in dogs: correlation with outcome of infection by canine distemper virus. *Am. J. Vet. Res.* **38**: 1539–1542.

KREUTER, J., MAULER, R., GRUSCHKAU, H. and SPEISER, P. P. (1976) The use of new polymethacrylate adjuvants for split influenza vaccines. *Expl. Cell Biol.* **44**: 12–19.

LAGRANGE, P. H. (1977) Non-specific resistance to virus infection induced by immunostimulation. *Bull. Inst. Pasteur* **75**: 291–307.

LARSON, C. L., USHIJIMA, R. N., KARIM, R., BAKER, M. B. and BAKER, R. E. (1972) Herpesvirus hominis type 2 infection in rabbits: effect of prior immunization with attenuated *M. bovis* (BCG) cells. *Infect. Immun.* **6**: 465–468.

LAWMAN, M. C., ROUSE, B. T., COURTNEY, R. J. and WALKER, R. D. (1980) Cell mediated immunity against herpes simplex. Induction of cytotoxic T lymphocytes. *Infect. Immun.* **127**: 133–139.

LESOURD, B., RANCOUREL, G., HURAUX, J. M., POMPIDOU, A., JACQUE, C., DENVIL, D., BUGE, A. and MOULIAS, R. (1980) Immunological restoration *in vivo* and *in vitro*, isoprinosine therapy and prognosis of acute encephalitis. *Int. J. Immunopharm.* **2**: 195 (abstract).

LÉVY-LEBLOND, E. and DUPUY, J. M. (1978) Neonatal susceptibility to MHV_3 infection in mice. I. Transfer of resistance. *J. Immunol.* **118**: 1219–1222.

LINDAHL, P., LEARY, P. and GRESSER, I. (1972) Enhancement by interferon of the specific cytotoxicity of sensitized lymphocytes. *Proc. natn. Acad. Sci. USA* **69**: 721–725.

LINDAHL, P., GRESSER, I., LEARY, P. and TOVEY, M. (1976) Interferon treatment of mice: enhanced expression of histocompatibility antigens on lymphoid cells. *Proc. natn. Acad. Sci. USA* **73**: 1284–1287.

LINDAHL-MAGNUSSON, P., LEARY, P. and GRESSER, I. (1972) Interferon inhibits DNA synthesis induced in mouse lymphocyte suspensions by phytohemagglutinin or by allogeneic cells. *Nature New Biol.* **237**: 120–121.

LINDENMANN, J., DEUEL, E., FANCONI, S. and HALLER, O. (1978) Inborn resistance of mice to Myxoviruses: macrophages express phenotype *in vitro*. *J. exp. Med.* **147**: 531–540.

LODMELL, D. L. and EWALT, L. C. (1978) Enhanced resistance against encephalomyocarditis virus infection in mice, induced by a nonviable *Mycobacterium tuberculosis* oil-droplet vaccine. *Infect. Immun.* **19**: 225–230.

LODMELL, D. L., EWALT, L. C. and NOTKINS, A. L. (1976) Inhibition of vaccinia virus replication in skin of tuberculin-sensitized animals challenged with PPD. *J. Immunol.* **117**: 1757–1763.

LODS, F. (1976) Traitement de l'herpes cornéen récidivant et des zonas ophtalmiques par le lévamisole. *Nouv. Presse Méd.* **5**: 148.

LONGLEY, S., DUNNING, R. L. and WALDMAN, R. H. (1973) Effect of isoprinosine against challenge with A (H3N2)/Hong Kong influenza virus in volunteers. *Antimicrob. Agents Chemother.* **3**: 506–509.

LOPEZ, C. (1978) Immunological nature of genetic resistance of mice to herpes simplex-type 1 infection. In: *Oncogenesis and Herpes Virus*, III. pp. 775–778. DE THE, G., HENLE, W. and RAPP, F. (eds.). International Agency for Research on Cancer, Lyon, France.

LOPEZ, C. and DUMAS, G. (1979) Replication of herpes simplex virus type 1 in macrophages from resistant and susceptible mice. *Infect. Immun.* **23**: 432–437.

LOPEZ, C., RYSHKE, R. and BENNETT, M. (1980) Marrow-dependent cells depleted by Sr^{89} mediate genetic resistance to herpes simplex virus type 1 infection in mice. *Infect. Immun.* **28**: 1028–1032.

McCORD, R. S., BREINIG, M. K. and MORAHAN, P. S. (1976) Antiviral effect of Pyran against systemic infection of mice with herpes simplex virus type 2. *Antimicrob. Agents Chemother.* **10**: 28–33.

McFARLAND, R. I., CEREDIG, R. and WHITE, D. O. (1979) Comparison of natural killer cells induced by Kunjin virus and *Corynebacterium parvum* with those occurring naturally in nude mice. *Infect. Immun.* **26**: 832–836.

McGUIRE, T. C., BANKS, K. L. and PERRYMAN, L. E. (1977) Immunodeficiency disorder in young horses. In:

Progress in Immunology, III, pp. 658–661. MANDEL, T. E. (ed.). Proc. Intl. Congress Immunol., Australian Academy of Sciences, Canberra, publ.

McINTIRE, F. C., HARGIE, M. P., SCHENCK, J. R., FINLEY, R. A., SIEVERT, H. W., RIETSCHEL, E. T. and ROSENSTREICH, D. L. (1976) Biologic properties of nontoxic derivatives of a lipopolysaccharide from *Escherichia coli* K 235. *J. Immunol.* **117**: 674–678.

McKINNON, K. P., HALE, A. H. and RUEBUSH, M. J. (1981) Elicitation of natural killer cells in beige mice by infection with vesicular stomatitis virus. *Infect. Immun.* **32**: 204–210.

McMORROW, L. E., VESIKARI, T., WOLMAN, S. R., GILES, J. P. and COOPER, L. Z. (1974) Suppression of the response of lymphocytes to phytohemagglutinin in rubella. *J. infect. Dis.* **130**: 464–469.

MAGRATH, I. T. and ZIEGLER, J. L. (1976) Failure of BCG immunostimulation to affect the clinical course of Burkitt's lymphoma. *Br. Med. J.* **1**: 615–618.

MATHÉ, G., AMIEL, J. L., SCHWARZENBERG, L., SCHNEIDER, M., CATTAN, A., SCHLUMBERGER, J. R., HAYAT, M. and DE VASSAL, F. (1969) Active immunotherapy for acute lymphoid leukemia. *Lancet* **1**: 697–699.

MAZAHERI, M. R., HAMBLIN, A. S. and ZUCKERMAN, A. J. (1977) Immunotherapy of viral infections with transfer factor. *J. Med. Virol.* **1**: 209–217.

MEHR, K. A. and ALBANO, L. (1977) Failure of levamisole in herpes simplex. *Lancet* **ii**: 773–774.

MIGLIORE-SAMOUR, D., KORONTZIS, M., JOLLÈS, P., MARAL, R., FLOC'H, F. and WERNER, G. H. (1974) Hydrosoluble immunopotentiating substances extracted from *Corynebacterium parvum*. *Immunol. Commun.* **3**: 593–603.

MOGENSEN, S. C. (1978) Macrophages and age-dependent resistance to hepatitis induced by herpes simplex virus type 2 in mice. *Infect. Immun.* **19**: 46–50.

MOGENSEN, S. C. (1979) Role of macrophages in natural resistance to virus infections. *Microbiol. Rev.* **1**: 26.

MOGENSEN, S. C. and ANDERSEN, K. H. (1978) Role of activated macrophages in resistance of congenitally athymic nude mice to hepatitis induced by herpes simplex virus type 2. *Infect. Immun.* **19**: 792–798.

MOGENSEN, S. C. and ANDERSEN, K. H. (1981) Recovery of mice from herpes simplex virus type 2 hepatitis: adoptive transfer of recovery with immune spleen cells. *Infect. Immun.* **33**: 743–747.

MØLLER-LARSEN, A. and HAAHR, S. (1978) Humoral and cell-mediated immune responses in humans before and after revaccination with vaccinia virus. *Infect. Immun.* **19**: 34–39.

MORAHAN, P. S. and KAPLAN, A. M. (1978) Antiviral and antitumor functions of activated macrophages. In: *Immune Modulation and Control of Neoplasia by Adjuvant Therapy*, pp. 447–457. CHIRIGOS, M. A. (ed.). Raven Press, New York, publ.

MORAHAN, P. S. and McCORD, R. S. (1975) Resistance to herpes simplex type 2 virus induced by an immunopotentiator (Pyran) in immunosuppressed mice. *J. Immun.* **115**: 311–313.

MORAHAN, P. S., GLASGOW, L. A., CRANE, J. L., Jr. and KERN, E. R. (1977a) Comparison of antiviral and antitumor activity of activated macrophages. *Cell. Immun.* **28**: 404–415.

MORAHAN, P. S., KERN, E. R. and GLASGOW, L. A. (1977b) Immunomodulator-induced resistance against herpes simplex virus. *Proc. Soc. exp. Biol. Med.* **154**: 615–620.

MORAHAN, P. S., MORSE, S. S. and McGEORGE, M. B. (1980) Macrophage extrinsic antiviral activity during herpes simplex virus infection. *J. gen. Virol.* **46**: 291–300.

MORAHAN, P. S., COLEMAN, P. H., MORSE, S. S. and WALKMAN, A. (1981) Resistance factors in beige (Chediak-Higashi) mice and Sr89-treated mice. *Abstracts of the 5th Intl. Congr. Virol. (Strasbourg)*, p. 152.

MORSE, S. I. (1965) Studies on the lymphocytosis induced in mice by *Bordetella pertussis*. *J. exp. Med.* **121**: 49–68.

MORSE, S. S. and MORAHAN, P. S. (1981) Activated macrophages mediate interferon-independent inhibition of herpes simplex virus. *Cell. Immun.* **58**: 72–84.

MULDOON, R. L., MEZNY, L. and JACKSON, G. G. (1972) Effects of isoprinosine against influenza and some other viruses causing respiratory diseases. *Antimicrob. Ag. Chemother.* **2**: 224–228.

MUYEMBE, J. J., BILLIAU, A. and DE SOMER, P. (1972) Mechanism of resistance to virus challenge in mice infected with *Brucella abortus*. *Arch. gesamte Virusforsch.* **38**: 290–296.

NAGAFUCHI, S., ODA, H., MORI, R. and TANIGUCHI, T. (1979) Mechanism of acquired resistance to herpes simplex virus infection as studied in nude mice. *J. gen. Virol.* **44**: 715–723.

NAHMIAS, A., HIRSCH, M. S., KRAMER, J. H. and MURPHY, F. A. (1969) Effect of antithymocyte serum on herpes virus hominis (type 1) infection in adult mice. *Proc. Soc. exp. Biol. Med.* **132**: 696–698.

NEWBLE, D. I., HOLMES, K. T., WANGEL, A. G. and FORBES, I. J. (1975) Immune reactions in acute viral hepatitis. *Clin. exp. Immunol.* **20**: 17–28.

NOZAKI-RENARD, J. (1978) Induction d'interféron par *Bacillus subtilis*. *Ann. Microbiol. (Inst. Pasteur)* **129A**: 525–543.

OAKES, J. E. (1975) Role for cell-mediated immunity in the resistance of mice to subcutaneous herpes simplex virus infection. *Infect. Immun.* **12**: 166–172.

OJO, E. (1979) Positive correlation between the levels of natural killer cells and *in vivo* resistance to syngeneic tumor transplants as influenced by various routes of administration of *Corynebacterium parvum* bacteria. *Cell Immun.* **45**: 182–187.

OJO, E., HALLER, O., KIMURA, A. and WIGZELL, H. (1978) An analysis of conditions allowing *Corynebacterium parvum* to cause either augmentation or inhibition of natural killer cell activity against tumor cells in mice. *Int. J. Cancer* **21**: 444–452.

OLD, L. J., BENACERRAF, B. and STOCKERT, E. (1963) Increased resistance to Mengo virus following infection with bacillus Calmette-Guérin. In: *Rôle du Système Réticulo-Endothélial dans l'Immunité Antibactérienne et Antitumorale*, pp. 319–336. HALPERN, B. N. (ed.). C.N.R.S. Symposium No. 115, Paris.

OLDSTONE, M. B. A. and DIXON, F. J. (1975) Immune complex disease associated with viral infections. In: *Viral Immunology and Immunopathology*, pp. 341–356. NOTKINS, A. L. (ed.). Academic Press, New York, London, publ.

OLESKE, J. M., STARR, S., KOHL, S., SHABAN, S. and NAHMIAS, A. (1978) Clinical evaluation of transfer factor in patients with recurrent herpes simplex virus infections. In: *Current Chemotherapy*, vol. I, pp. 359–360. SIEGENTHALER, W. and LÜTHY, R. (ed.). American Society for Microbiology, Washington, D.C., publ.

O'REILLY, R. J., CHIBBARO, A., WILMOT, R. and LOPEZ, C. (1977) Correlation of clinical and virus-specific immune responses following levamisole therapy of recurrent herpes progenitalis. *Ann. N.Y. Acad. Sci.* **284**: 161–170.

PACHUTA, D. M., TOGO, Y., HORNICK, R. B., SCHWARTZ, A. R. and TOMINAGA, S. (1974) Evaluation of isoprinosine in experimental human rhinovirus infection. *Antimicrob. Ag. Chemother.* **5**: 403–408.

PAPAEVANGELOU, G., SPARROS, L., VISSOULIS, CH., KYRIAKIDOU, A., GIOKAS, G., HADZIMANOLIS, J. and TRICHOPOULOS, D. (1977) The effect of intradermal administration of *Corynebacterium parvum* on the immune response to hepatitis Bs antigen. *J. Med. Virol.* **1**: 15–19.

PAR, A., BARNA, K., HOLLOS, I., KOVACS, M., MISZLAI, ZS., PATAKFALVI, A. and JAVOR, T. (1977) Levamisole in viral hepatitis. *Lancet* **1**: 702.

PARANT, M., AUDIBERT, F., PARANT, F., CHEDID, L., SOLER, E., POLONSKY, J. and LEDERER, E. (1978) Nonspecific immunostimulant activities of synthetic trehalose-6,6′ diesters (lower homologs of cord factor). *Infect. Immun.* **20**: 12–19.

PERRIN, L. H., ZINKERNAGEL, R. M. and OLDSTONE, M. B. A. (1977) Immune response in humans after vaccination with vaccinia virus: generation of a virus-specific cytotoxic activity by human peripheral lymphocytes. *J. exp. Med.* **146**: 949–968.

PFIZENMAIER, K., JUNG, H., STARZINSKI-POWITZ, A., RÖLLINGHOFF, M. and WAGNER, H. (1977) The role of T cells in antiherpes simplex virus immunity. I. Induction of antigen-specific cytotoxic T lymphocytes. *J. Immunol.* **119**: 939–945.

POLLARD, R. B., RAND, K. H., ARVIN, A. M. and MERIGAN, T. C. (1978) Cell-mediated immunity to cytomegalovirus infection in normal subjects and cardiac transplant patients. *J. infect. Dis.* **137**: 541–547.

RAGER-ZISMAN, B. and ALLISON, A. C. (1976) Mechanism of immunologic resistance to herpes simplex virus 1 (HSV-1) infection. *J. Immunol.* **116**: 35–40.

RAGER-ZISMAN, B., HARISH, Z., ROTTER, V., YAKIR, Y. and TRAININ, N. (1980) Treatment of mice infected with Sendai virus with THF, a thymic hormone. In: *Advances in Allergology and Immunology*, pp. 25–31. OEHLING, A. (ed.). Pergamon Press, Oxford, New York.

RAHMAN, A. N. and LUTTRELL, C. N. (1963) Pathogenesis of viral meningoencephalitides: enhancement of viral penetrance into the brain. *Bull. Johns Hopkins Hosp.* **112**: 1–14.

REGELSON, W., SHNIDER, B. I., COLSKY, J., OLSON, K. B., HOLLAND, J. F., JOHNSTON, C. L., Jr. and DENNIS, L. H. (1978) Clinical study of the synthetic polyanion pyran copolymer (NSC 46015, Diveema) and its role in future clinical trials. In: *Immune Modulation and Control of Neoplasia by Adjuvant Therapy*, pp. 469–490. CHIRIGOS, M. A. (ed.). Raven Press, New York, publ.

REID, L. M., MINATO, N., GRESSER, I., HOLLAND, J., KADISH, A. and BLOOM, B. (1981) Influence of anti-mouse interferon serum on the growth and metastasis of tumor cells persistently infected with virus and of human prostatic tumors in athymic nude mice. *Proc. natn. Acad. Sci. USA* **78**: 1171–1175.

REMINGTON, J. S. and MERIGAN, T. C. (1969) Resistance to virus challenge in mice infected with protozoa or bacteria. *Proc. Soc. exp. Biol. Med.* **131**: 1184–1188.

RENOUX, G. (1978) Modulation of immunity by levamisole. *J. Pharmacol. and Therapeutics* **2**: 397–423.

RENOUX, G. and RENOUX, M. (1971) Effet immunostimulant d'un imidazothiazole dans l'immunisation des souris contre l'infection par *Brucella abortus*. *C.R. Acad. Sci. (Paris)* **D 272**: 349–350.

RENOUX, G. and RENOUX, M. (1979) Immunopotentiation and anabolism induced by sodium diethyldithiocarbamate. *J. Immunopharmacol.* **1**: 247–253.

REYNOLDS, J. A., KASTELLO, M. D., HARRINGTON, D. G., CRABBS, C. L., PETERS, C. J., JEMSKI, J. V., SCOTT, G. H. and DI LUZIO, N. R. (1980) Glucan-induced enhancement of host resistance to selected infectious diseases. *Infect. Immun.* **30**: 51–57.

RIVIÈRE, Y., GRESSER, I., GUILLON, J. C. and TOVEY, M. G. (1977) Inhibition by anti-interferon serum of lymphocytic choriomeningitis virus disease in suckling mice. *Proc. natn. Acad. Sci. USA* **74**: 2135–2139.

RIVIÈRE, Y., GRESSER, I., GUILLON, J. C., BANDU, M. T., RONCO, P., MOREL-MAROGER, L. and VERROUST, D. (1980) Severity of LCM virus disease in deficient strains of suckling mice correlates with increasing amounts of endogenous interferon. *J. exp. Med.* **152**: 632–640.

ROJAS, A. and OLIVARI, A. J. (1974) Levamisole: effect in foot and mouth disease. Preliminary note. *Rev. Med. Vet. Argentina*, **55**: 263–265.

ROLLY, H., VERTESY, L. and NEUFARTH, A. (1974) Studies on the chemotherapeutic actions of antiviral lipopolysaccharides. In: *Progress in Chemotherapy*, vol. 2, pp. 1013–1018. DAIKOS, G. K. (ed.). Hellenic Society of Chemotherapy, Athens, publ.

ROUSE, B. T. and LAWMAN, M. J. D. (1980) Induction of cytotoxic T lymphocytes against herpes simplex type 1: role of accessory cells and amplifying factor. *J. Immun.* **124**: 2340–2341.

ROUSE, B. T., BABIUK, L. A. and HENSON, P. M. (1980) Neutrophils in antiviral immunity: inhibition of virus replication by a mediator produced by bovine neutrophils. *J. Infect. Dis.* **141**: 223–232.

RUSSELL, A. S. and ESSERY, G. (1977) Cellular immunity to herpes simplex virus in man. VII. K-cell activity to HSV-1-infected target in disease. *Cancer.* **40**: 42–48.

RUSSELL, A. S. and MILLER, C. (1978) A possible role for polymorphonuclear leucocytes in the defense against recrudescent herpes simplex virus infection in man. *Immunology.* **34**: 371–378.

RUSSELL, A. S., BRISSON, E. and GRACE, M. (1978) A double-blind controlled trial of levamisole in the treatment of recurrent herpes labialis. *J. infect. Dis.* **137**: 597–600.

SANTOLI, D., TRINCHIERI, G. and LIEF, F. S. (1978) Cell mediated cytotoxicity against virus-infected target cells in humans. *J. Immun.* **121**: 526–531.

SANTONI, A., RICCARDI, C., SORCI, V. and HERBERMAN, R. B. (1980) Effects of adriamycin on the activity of mouse natural killer cells. *J. Immun.* **124**: 2329–2335.

SCHIFF, G. M., ROSELLE, G., YOUNG, B., MAY, D., ROTTE, T. and GLASKY, A. J. (1978) Clinical evaluation of isoprinosine in artificially-induced influenza in humans. 78th Annual Meeting of American Society for Microbiology, Las Vegas, Nevada, May 14–19, 1978.

SCHINDLER, L., STREISSLE, G. and KIRCHNER, H. (1981) Protection of mice against mouse hepatitis virus by *Corynebacterium parvum*. *Infect. Immun.* **32**: 1128–1131.

SCHMID, D. S., LARSEN, H. S. and ROUSE, B. T. (1981) The role of accessory cells and T cell growth factor in induction of cytotoxic T-lymphocytes against herpes simplex virus antigens. *Immunology* **44**: 755–763.

SCHULMAN, S. T., HUTTO, J. H., SCOTT, B., AYOUB, E. M. and McGUIGAN, J. E. (1976) Transfer factor therapy of chronic aggressive hepatitis. In: *Transfer Factor, Basic Properties and Clinical Applications*, pp. 439–447. ASCHER, M. S., GOTTLIEB, A. A. and KIRKPATRICK, C. H. (ed.). Academic Press, New York, London, Publ.

SCHULTZ, R. M. and CHIRIGOS, M. A. (1979) Selective neutralisation by antiinterferon globulin of macrophage activation by L-cell interféron, *Brucella abortus* ether extract, *Salmonella typhimurium* lipopolysaccharide and polyanions. *Cell Immun.* **48**: 52–58.

SCHWARTZ, D. B., ZBAR, B., GIBSON, W. T. and CHIRIGOS, M. A. (1971) Inhibition of murine sarcoma virus oncogenesis with living BCG. *Int. J. Cancer* **8**: 320–325.

SENIK, A., STEFANOS, S., KOLB, J. P., LUCERO, M. and FALCOFF, E. (1980) Enhancement of mouse natural killer cell activity by type II interferon. *Ann. Immun. (Inst. Pasteur)* **131** C: 349–361.

SERJEANTSON, S. and WOODFIELD, D. G. (1978) Immune response of leprosy patients to hepatitis B virus. *Am. J. Epidemiol.* **107**: 321–328.

SHELLAM, G. R., ALLAN, J. E., PAPADIMITRIOU, J. M. and BRANCOFT, G. J. (1981) Increased susceptibility to cytomegalovirus infection in beige mutant mice. *Proc. natn. Acad. Sci. USA* **78**: 5104–5108.

SIEGEL, B. V. and MORTON, J. I. (1977) Vitamin C and the immune response. *Experientia* **33**: 393–395.

SIMON, L. N., SETTINERI, R., COATS, H. and GLASKY, A. J. (1978) Isoprinosine: integration of the antiviral and immunoproliferative effects. In: *Current Chemotherapy*, vol. 1, pp. 366–368. SIEGENTHALER, W. and LÜTHY, R. (eds.). American Society for Microbiology, Washington, D.C. publ.

SINGER, S. H., NOGUCHI, P. and KIRSCHSTEIN, R. L. (1972) Respiratory disease in cyclophosphamide-treated mice. II. Decreased virulence of PR8 influenza virus. *Infect. Immun.* **5**: 957–960.

SOTO, A. J., HALL, T. S. and REED, S. E. (1973) Trial of the antiviral action of isoprinosine against rhinovirus infection of volunteers. *Antimicrob. Ag. Chemother.* **3**: 332–334.

SPENCER, J. C., GANGULY, R. and WALDMAN, R. H. (1977) Nonspecific protection of mice against influenza virus infection by local or systemic immunization with bacille Calmette-Guérin. *J. inf. Dis.* **136**: 171–175.

SPITLER, L. E., GLOGAU, R. G., NELMS, D. C., BASCH, C. M., OLSON, J. A., SILVERMAN, S. and ENGLEMAN, E. P. (1975) Levamisole and lymphocyte response in herpes simplex virus infections. In: *Symposium on Antivirals with Clinical Potential, Stanford, Calif.*

SPRUANCE, S. L., KRUEGER, G. G., MacCALMAN, J., OVERALL, J. C., Jr. and KLAUBER, M. R. (1979) Treatment of recurrent herpes simplex labialis with levamisole. *Antimicrob. Ag. Chemother.* **15**: 662–665.

STARR, S. E., VISINTINE, A. M., TOMEH, M. O. and NAHMIAS, A. J. (1976) Effects of immunostimulants on resistance of newborn mice to herpes simplex type 2 infection. *Proc. Soc. exp. Biol. Med.* **152**: 57–60.

STEELE, R. W. (1980) Transfer factor reactivity to varicella-zoster antigen in childhood leukemia. *Cell. Immun.* **50**: 282–289.

STEELE, R. W., HEBERLING, R. L., EICHBERG, J. W., ELLER, J. J., KALTER, S. S. and KNIKER, W. T. (1976) Prevention of herpes simplex virus type 1 fatal dissemination in primates with human transfer factor. In: *Transfer Factor, Basic Properties and Clinical Applications*, pp. 381–386. Academic Press, New York, London, publ.

STEVENS, D. A., JORDAN, G. W., WADDELL, T. F. and MERIGAN, T. C. (1973) Adverse effects of cytosine arabinoside on disseminated zoster in a controlled trial. *New Engl. J. Med.* **289**: 873–878.

STINEBRING, W. R. and YOUNGNER, J. S. (1964) Patterns of interferon appearance in mice injected with bacteria or bacterial endotoxin. *Nature* **204**: 712–713.

SULLIVAN, J. L., MAYNER, R. E., BARRY, D. W. and ENNIS, F. A. (1976) Influenza virus infection in nude mice. *J. inf. Dis.* **133**: 91–94.

SULLIVAN, J. L., BYRON, K. S., BREWSTER, F. E. and PURTILLO, D. T. (1980) Deficient natural killer cell activity in X-linked lymphoproliferative syndrome. *Science.* **210**: 543–545.

SUZUKI, F., OHYA, J. and ISHIDA, N. (1974) Effect of antilymphocyte serum on influenza virus infection in mice. *Proc. Soc. exp. Biol. Med.* **146**: 78–84.

SYMOENS, J. (1978) Treatment of the compromised host with levamisole, a synthetic immunotherapeutic agent. In: *Immune Modulation and Control of Neoplasia by Adjuvant Therapy*, pp. 1–9. CHIRIGOS, M. A. (ed.). Raven Press, New York, publ.

SYMOENS, J., DECREE, J., VAN BEVER, W. F. M. and JANSSEN, P. A. J. (1979) Levamisole. In: *Pharmacological and Biochemical Properties of Drug Substances*, pp. 407–464. GOLDBERG, M. E. (ed.). American Pharmaceutical Association, Washington, D.C.

TAGUCHI, F., YAMADA, A. and FUJIWARA, K. (1979) Factors involved in the age-dependent resistance of mice infected with low-virulence mouse hepatitis virus. *Arch. Virol.* **62**: 333–340.

TAGUCHI, F., YAMAGUCHI, R., MAKINO, S. and FUJIWARA, K. (1981) Correlation between growth potential of mouse hepatitis viruses in macrophages and their virulence for mice. *Infect. Immun.* **34**: 1059–1061.

TALMADGE, J. E., MEYERS, K. M., PRIEUR, D. J. and STARKEY, J. R. (1980) Role of NK cells in tumour growth and metastasis in beige mice. *Nature* **284**: 622–624.

TARDIEU, M., HÉRY, C. and DUPUIS, J. M. (1980) Neonatal susceptibility to MHV$_3$ infection in mice. II. Role of natural effector marrow cells in transfer of resistance. *J. Immun.* **124**: 418–423.

THOMAS, L. (1980) *The Medusa and the Snail. More Notes of a Biology Watcher*. Bantam Books, New York.

TORREGROSSA, F. (1978) Risultati terapeutici preliminari nel trattamento dell'herpes zoster con un nuovo agente antivirale, il Methisoprinol. *Acta Gerontol.* **28**: 105–112.

TRACEY (1979) The requirement for macrophages in the augmentation of natural killer cell activity by B.C.G. *J. Immun.* **123**: 840–845.

UMEZAWA, H. (1981) *Small Molecular Immunomodifiers of Microbial Origin. Fundamental and Clinical Studies of Bestatin.* Pergamon Press, Oxford, New York.

VAN EYGEN, M., ZNAMENSKY, P. Y., HECK, E. and RAYMAEKERS, I. (1976) Levamisole in prevention of recurrent upper respiratory tract infections in children. *Lancet* **1**: 382–385.

VAN EYGEN, M., DILS, F., GILLEROT, J. and VERSCHUEREN, E. (1979) A double-blind pediatric evaluation of levamisole in the prevention of recurrent upper respiratory tract infections. *Eur. J. Pediatr.* **131**: 147–153.

VIGNAUX, F. and GRESSER, I. (1978) Enhanced expression of histocompatibility antigens on interferon-treated mouse embryonic fibroblasts. *Proc. Soc. exp. Biol. Med.* **157**: 456–460.

VIRELIZIER, J. L. and ALLISON, A. C. (1976) Correlation of persistent mouse hepatitis virus (MHV-3) infection with its effect on mouse macrophage cultures. *Arch. Virol.* **50**: 279–285.

VIRELIZIER, J. L. and GRISCELLI, C. (1980) Interferon administration as an immunomodulatory and anti-microbial treatment in children with defective interferon secretions. In: *Primary Immunodeficiencies.* INSERM Symp. No. 16, pp. 473–484. SELIGMANN, M. and HITZIG, W. H. (ed.). Elsevier/North Holland Biomedical Press.

VIRELIZIER, J. L. and GRISCELLI, C. (1981) Défaut sélectif de sécrétion d'interféron associé à un déficit d'activité cytotoxique naturelle. *Arch. Fr. Pediat.* **38**: 77–81.

VIRELIZIER, J. L., DAYAN, A. D. and ALLISON, A. C. (1975) Neuropathological effects of persistent infection of mice by mouse hepatitis virus. *Infect. Immun.* **12**: 1127–1140.

VIRELIZIER, J. L., VIRELIZIER, A. M. and ALLISON, A. C. (1976) The role of circulating interferon in the modifications of immune responsiveness by mouse hepatitis virus (MHV-3). *J. Immun.* **117**: 748–753.

WALDMAN, R. H. and GANGULY, R. (1977) Therapeutic efficacy of inosiplex (Isoprinosine Ⓡ) in rhinovirus infection. *Ann. N.Y. Acad. Sci.* **284**: 153–160.

WALDMAN, R. H., KHAKOO, R. A. and WATSON, G. (1978) Isoprinosine: efficacy against influenza challenge infection in humans. In: *Current Chemotherapy*, vol. 1, pp. 368–370. SIEGENTHALER, W. and LÜTHY, R. (eds.). American Society for Microbiology, Washington D.C., publ.

WARDLEY, R. C., ROUSE, B. T. and BABIUK, L. A. (1977) Antibody dependent cytotoxicity mediated by neutrophils: a possible mechanism of antiviral defense. *J. Reticuloendothel. Soc.* **19**: 29–36.

WEBSTER, R. G., GLEZEN, W. P., HANNOUN, C. and LAVER, W. G. (1977) Potentiation of the immune response to influenza virus subunit vaccines. *J. Immun.* **119**: 2073–2077.

WELLS, A. M., ALBRECHT, P. and ENNIS, F. D. (1981a) Recovery from a viral respiration infection. I. Influenza pneumonia in normal and T-deficient mice. *J. Immun.* **126**: 1036–1041.

WELLS, A. M., ENNIS, F. A. and ALBRECHT, P. (1981b) Recovery from a viral respiration infection. II. Passive transfer of immune spleen cells to mice with influenza pneumonia. *J. Immun.* **126**: 1042–1046.

WEISER, W. Y. and BANG, F. B. (1977) Blocking of *in vitro* and *in vivo* susceptibility to mouse hepatitis virus. *J. exp. Med.* **146**: 1467–1472.

WEISS, D. W., BONHAG, R. S. and PARKS, J. A. (1964) Studies on the heterologous immunogenicity of a methanol-insoluble fraction of attenuated tubercle bacilli (BCG). 1. Antimicrobial protection. *J. exp. Med.* **119**: 53–70.

WEISSENBACHER, M., SCHMUNIS, L. and PARODI, A. S. (1969) Junin virus multiplication in thymectomized mice. Effect of thymus and immunocompetent cell grafting. *Arch. gesamte Virusforsch.* **26**: 63–66.

WELSH, R. M. (1978) Mouse natural killer cells: induction, specificity and function. *J. Immun.* **121**: 1631–1635.

WELSH, R. M. (1981) Do natural killer cells play a role in virus infections? *Antivir. Res.* **1**: 5–12.

WELSH, R. M. and KIESSLING, R. W. (1980) Natural killer cell response to lymphocytic choriomeningitis virus in beige mice. *Scand. J. Immun.* **11**: 363–368.

WELSH, R. M., ZINKERNAGEL, R. M. and HALLENBECK, L. A. (1979) Cytotoxic cells induced during lymphocytic choriomeningitis virus infection of mice. II. Specificities of natural killer cells. *J. Immun.* **122**: 475–481.

WERNER, G. H., MARAL, R., FLOC'H, F., MIGLIORE-SAMOUR, D. and JOLLÈS, P. (1975) Adjuvant and immunostimulating activities of water-soluble substances extracted from *Mycobacterium tuberculosis* (var. *hominis*). *Biomedicine* **23**: 440–452.

WERNER, G. H., MARAL, R., FLOC'H, F. and JOUANNE, M. (1977) Toxicological aspects of immunopotentiation by adjuvants and immunostimulating substances. *Bull. Inst. Pasteur* **75**: 5–84.

WHITE, D. O. (1977) Antiviral immunity. In: *Progress in Immunology* III, pp. 459–462. MANDEL, T. E. (ed.). Proc. 3rd Intl. Congress Immunol., Australian Academy of Science, Canberra, publ.

WIKTOR, T. J., DOHERTY, P. C. and KOPROWSKI, H. (1977) Suppression of cell-mediated immunity by street rabies virus. *J. exp. Med.* **145**: 1617–1622.

WILFERT, C. M., BUCKLEY, R., ROSEN, F. S., WHISNANT, J., OXMAN, M. N., GRIFFITH, J. F., KATZ, S. L. and MOORE, M. (1977). Persistent enterovirus infections in agammaglobulinemia. In: *Microbiology 1977*, pp. 488–493. SCHLESSINGER, D. (ed.). American Society for Microbiology, Washington, D.C. publ.

WOODRUFF, J. F. and WOODRUFF, J. J. (1975) The effect of viral infections on the function of the immune system. In: *Viral Immunology and Immunopathology*, pp. 393–418. NOTKINS, A. L. (ed.). Academic Press, New York, publ.

WORTHINGTON, M., CONLIFFE, M. A. and BARON, S. (1980) Mechanism of recovery from systemic herpes simplex virus infection. I. Comparative effectiveness of antibody and reconstitution of immune spleen cells in immunosuppressed mice. *J. infect. Dis.* **142**: 163–174.

YAP, K. L., ADA, G. L. and McKENZIE, I. F. C. (1978) Transfer of specific cytotoxic lymphocytes protects mice inoculated with influenza virus. *Nature* **273**: 238–239.

YOUNGNER, J. S. and STINEBRING, W. R. (1964) Interferon production in chickens injected with *Brucella abortus*. *Science* **144**: 1022–1023.

YOUNGNER, J. S., KELETI, G. and FEINGOLD, D. S. (1974) Antiviral activity of an ether-extracted nonviable preparation of *Brucella abortus*. *Infect. Immun.* **10**: 1202–1206.

ZAIZOV, R., VOGEL, R., COHEN, I., VARSANO, I., SHOHAT, B., ROTTER, V. and TRAININ, N. (1977) Thymic hormone (THF) therapy in immunosuppressed children with lymphoproliferative neoplasia and generalized varicella. *Biomedicine* **27**: 105–108.

ZERIAL, A. and WERNER, G. H. (1981) Effect of immunomodulating agents on viral infections. *Acta Microb. Acad. Sci. Hung.* **28**: 325–337.

ZERIAL, A., FLOC'H, F. and WERNER, G. H. (1980) Comparative effects of an inflammatory reaction on the resistance of mice to bacterial and viral infections. *Ann. Immunol. (Institut Pasteur)* **131** C, 177–184.

ZERIAL, A., HOVANESSIAN, A. G., STEFANOS, S., HUYGEN, K., WERNER, G. H. and FALCOFF, E. (1982) Synergistic activities of type I (α, β) and type II (γ) murine interferons. *Antiv. Res.* **2**: 227–239.

ZINKERNAGEL, R. M. and ALTHAGE, A. (1977) Antiviral protection by virus immune cytotoxic T cells: infected target cells are lysed before infectious virus progeny is assembled. *J. exp. Med.* **145**: 644–651.

ZINKERNAGEL, R. M. and WELSH, R. M. (1976) H-2 compatibility requirement for virus-specific T-cell mediated effector functions *in vivo*. I. Specificity of T cells conferring antiviral protection against lymphocytic choriomeningitis virus is associated with H-2K and H-2D. *J. Immun.* **17**: 1495–1503.

ZISMAN, B., HIRSCH, M. S. and ALLISON, A. C. (1970) Selective effects of antimacrophage serum, silica and anti-lymphocyte serum on pathogenesis of herpes virus infection of young adult mice. *J. Immun.* **104**: 1155–1159.

ZWEERINK, H. J., ASKONAS, B. A., MILLICAN, D., COURTNEIDGE, S. A. and SKEHEL, J. J. (1977) Cytotoxic T cells to type A influenza virus; viral hemagglutinin induces A-strain specificity while infected cells confer cross-reactive cytotoxicity. *Eur. J. Immunol.* **7**: 630–635.

INDEX